PROCEDURES

KINN'S

THE CLINICAL MEDICAL ASSISTANT

AN APPLIED LEARNING APPROACH

14th **EDITION**

Brigitte Niedzwiecki, MSN, RN, RMA
Medical Assistant Program Director & Instructor
Chippewa Valley Technical College
Eau Claire, Wisconsin

Julie Pepper, BS, CMA (AAMA)
Medical Assistant Instructor
Health Navigator Program Director
Chippewa Valley Technical College
Eau Claire, Wisconsin

P. Ann Weaver, MSEd, MT (ASCP)
Medical Assistant Instructor
Chippewa Valley Technical College
Eau Claire, Wisconsin

ELSEVIER

Elsevier
3251 Riverport Lane
St. Louis, Missouri 63043

KINN'S THE CLINICAL MEDICAL ASSISTANT: AN APPLIED LEARNING APPROACH, FOURTEENTH EDITION

ISBN: 978-0-323-61357-6

Notices

Practitioners and researchers must always rely on their own experience and knowledge in evaluating and using any information, methods, compounds or experiments described herein. Because of rapid advances in the medical sciences, in particular, independent verification of diagnoses and drug dosages should be made. To the fullest extent of the law, no responsibility is assumed by Elsevier, authors, editors or contributors for any injury and/or damage to persons or property as a matter of products liability, negligence or otherwise, or from any use or operation of any methods, products, instructions, or ideas contained in the material herein.

International Standard Book Number: 978-0-323-61357-6

Publishing Director: Kristin Wilhelm
Content Development Manager: Ellen Wurm-Cutter
Senior Content Development Specialist: Becky Leenhouts
Publishing Services Manager: Julie Eddy
Senior Project Manager: Richard Barber
Design Direction: Ryan Cook

Printed in the United States of America

Last digit is the print number: 9   8   7   6   5   4   3

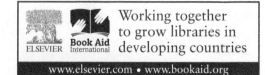

REVIEWERS

Kristi Bertrand, MPH, CMA (AAMA)
Owner/Founder, Chief Academic Officer
Medical Career & Technical College
Richmond, Kentucky

Michelle Buchman, MA, BSN
Michel Assisting Chair and Assistant Professor
Medical Assisting
Cox College
Springfield, Missouri

Candace S. Dailey, MSN, RN, CMA (AAMA)
Dean Health Occupations
Medical Assistant Program Director
Health Occupations
Nicolet College
Rhinelander, Wisconsin

Amy Eady, MT (ASCP), MS, RMA
Medical Assistant Program Director
Dean of Occupations & Program Assessment
Montcalm Community College
Sidney, Michigan

Michael Freeman, CMA
Roseville, Ohio

Tracie Fuqua, BS, CMA (AAMA)
Program Director
Medical Assistant Program
Wallace State Community College
Hanceville, Alabama

Pamela Harvey, RN, MSNED, CPR
Medical Assistant Instructor
North Florida Technical College
Santa Fe College
Gainesville, Florida
Starke, Florida

Angela Kortemeier, MS, RHIA, CHTS-TR, CCMA
Instructor
Business – Medical Coding and Billing
Gogebic Community College
Ironwood, Michigan

Brandi Lippincott, BS, MOS Master
Director
Merit Training Institute
Mount Laurel, New Jersey

LaToya N. Mason, CMA (AAMA), MBA, MHA
Director, Health Sciences
Health Sciences
Lake Michigan College
Benton Harbor, Michigan

Penny Mints, MSB, CCMA, RDMS (AB,OB/GYN), MT (ASCP)
Faculty
Allied Health Department
Northern Maine Community College
Presque Isle, Maine

Norma Moore, BS, MSHA, MT (ASCP), CCMA
Medical Assistant Program Director
Health Sciences Division
Laredo Community College
Laredo, Texas

Robert W. Mun
Program Coordinator of the General Sciences
Department of Education
Hawaii Medical College
Honolulu, Hawaii

PREFACE

Medical assisting as a profession has changed dramatically since *The Office Assistant in Medical and Dental Practice,* by Portia Frederick and Carol Towner, was first published in 1956. Each subsequent edition of this textbook has reflected the age in which it was published. Now, *Kinn's The Medical Assistant: An Applied Learning Approach,* fourteenth edition, continues to represent a long-standing commitment to high-quality medical assisting education with its engaging, straightforward writing style and demonstrated positive outcomes. Hundreds of instructors in classrooms across the country have used this text to teach thousands of students over the years. Many of these students have gone on to teach students of their own with this very same trusted resource. To continue the use and growth of this text and its features, the fourteenth edition continues to offer the most comprehensive, up-to-date, and innovative approach to teaching this subject today.

This textbook has endured throughout the years because it has been able to keep pace with an ever-changing profession while producing students who are well trained and qualified to enter medical practices across the country. This dependability is the reason the market continues to rely on this text, edition after edition. Underlying this dependability is a foundation of pedagogic features that has stood the test of time and that has been expanded and improved upon yet again in this latest edition. Such features include the following:

- An easy-to-read, highly interactive writing style that engages students through practical applications of medical assistant competencies
- An emphasis on skill development, with procedural steps outlining each skill, supported by rationales that provide meaning to each step
- A pedagogic framework based on the use of learning objectives, vocabulary terms, and supportive student supplements
- A package of supportive materials to accommodate a wide variety of student learning types and instructor teaching styles

NEW TO THIS EDITION

- **New chapter** on medical terminology, anatomy, and pathology
- **Reorganized and expanded content** on medical office accounts, law and ethics, math skills, behavioral health, and disease processes
- **New artwork** focused on the workings of a modern medical office, with updated illustrations and photographs of office procedures and medical records
- **Streamlined presentation** with combined chapters and an easier-to-read format
- **New Patient Coaching** section addresses providing information to patients in a supportive environment that allows them to grow, change, or improve their situation
- **More certification practice** with expanded and updated sample exams

EVOLVE

The Evolve site features a variety of student resources, including Chapter Review Quizzes, new Procedure Videos, Medical Terminology Audio Glossary, practice certification exams, and much more! The instructors' Evolve Resources site consists of TEACH Instructor Resources, including Lesson Plans, PowerPoint Presentations, Answer Keys for Chapter Review Quizzes, and a retooled Test Bank with more than 5000 questions.

STUDY GUIDE AND PROCEDURE CHECKLIST MANUAL

The Study Guide provides students with the opportunity to review and build on information they have learned in the text through vocabulary reviews, case studies, workplace applications, and more. The updated Procedure Checklists include CAAHEP and ABHES competencies that can be traced to the online correlation grid.

FEATURES

A Scenario is presented at the beginning of each chapter so the student can envision a real-world situation when reading the chapter content.

Scenario questions provide a way for students to apply the concepts they are learning and think about decisions they would make in real situations.

Learning Objectives emphasize the cognitive and performance objectives presented in the chapter.

Each chapter contains a vocabulary list with definitions so students can first familiarize themselves with the important terms associated with each chapter.

---

10 HEALTH RECORDS

SCENARIO

Susan Beezler has just begun her career in the medical assisting profession. In the morning, she is attending medical assisting school, and in the afternoon, she works part-time for the Walden-Martin Family Medical Clinic (WMFM) as a records assistant. Susan is eager to learn about healthcare and looks forward to taking on more responsibility at the office.

Dr. David Kahn is a new provider who has recently joined WMFM. Dr. Kahn has enjoyed working with Susan and feels that her energy will be just what his patients need. He has taken a professional interest in Susan and often lets her assist him with patients when her other duties allow.

Susan knows that although she is a beginner in the office, she will gain trust from her supervisors and patients as long as she projects a teachable attitude. The office has recently converted to an electronic records system but is also still using paper records. Susan uses the information she learned in school about both types of health records. She cheerfully performs filing and even does some transcription for Dr. Kahn. The other staff members are pleased with her willingness to perform the most mundane tasks.

Susan enjoys sharing her experiences with her classmates. She is the only student currently working in the medical field, and the ... has lots of questions about the "real world" of medical assisting ... ... to breach patient confidentiality, she discusses situation... ... never mentioning any patients' names.

Susan feels a great sense of pride that she is ... healthcare team and able to contribute to the live...

While studying this chapter, think about the following questions:
- What is the definition and application of subjective information?
- What is the definition and application of objective information?
- How does the HITECH act impact health records?
- How can you maintain a connection with the patient when using an EHR?
- What are the different ways to back up...
- How do you correctly destroy health re...
- How do you document in health rec...
- What equipment and supplies are...
- What are the indexing rules for al...

LEARNING OBJECTIVES

1. Discuss the two types of patient records.
2. State several reasons that accurate health records are important.
3. Differentiate between subjective and objective information in creating a patient's health record.
4. Explain who owns the health record.
5. Distinguish between an electronic health record (EHR) and an electronic medical record (EMR).
6. Do the following related to healthcare legislation and EHRs:
   - Define meaningful use and relate it to the healthcare industry.
   - List the three main components of meaningful use legislation.
7. Discuss the importance of nonverbal communication with patients when an EHR system is used.
8. Discuss backup systems for the EHR, in addition to the transfer, destruction, and retention of health records as related to the EHR.
9. Discuss retention and destruction of medical records as related to paper records.
10. Describe how and when to... discuss health information...
11. Identify and discuss the... medical record.
12. Discuss how to docu... record, and how to...
13. Discuss dictation a...
14. Identify the filing... store, and main...
15. Describe index... health record...
16. Discuss the... patient he...
17. Discuss...

VOCABULARY

age of majority The age at which the law recognizes a person to be an adult; it varies by state.

alphabetic filing Any system that arranges names or topics according to the sequence of the letters in the alphabet.

alphanumeric Describes systems made up of combinations of letters and numbers.

anthropometric (an thruh po ME trik) Pertaining to the measurement of the size and proportions of the human body.

caption A heading, title, or subtitle under which records are filed.

compliance (kuhm PLIE uhns) Meeting the standards and regulations of the practice's established policies and procedures. Can also mean cooperation.

computerized provider/physician order entry (CPOE) The process of entering medication orders or other provider instructions into the EHR.

concise (kuhn SICE) Using as few words as possible to express a message.

continuity of care The smooth continuation of care from one provider to another. This allows the patient to receive the most benefit with no interruption or duplication of care.

dictation (dik TEY shuhn) To say something aloud for another person to write down.

direct filing system A filing system in which materials can be located without consulting another source of reference.

electronic health record (EHR) An electronic record that conforms to nationally recognized standards and contains health-related information about a specific patient. It can be created, managed, and consulted by authorized clinicians and staff from more than one healthcare organization.

e-prescribing The use of electronic software to communicate with pharmacies and send prescribing information. It takes the place of writing a prescription by hand and giving it to a patient; most new or refill prescriptions can be submitted electronically, cutting down on fraud and errors.

hereditary (huh RED i ter ee) Passed from parents to offspring through the genes.

incidence (IN si duhns) How often something happens or occurs.

interface An interconnection between systems.

interoperability (in ter op er uh BIL i tee) The ability to work with other systems.

numeric filing The filing of records, correspondence, or cards by number.

objective information Data obtained through physical examination, laboratory and diagnostic testing, and by measurable information.

obliteration (ub lit uh REY shun) To remove or destroy all traces of; do away with; destroy completely.

out guides Sturdy cardboard or plastic file-sized cards used to replace a folder temporarily removed from the filing space.

parameters (puh RAM i ters) Rules that control how something should be done; guidelines or boundaries.

patient portal A secure online website that gives patients 24-hour access to personal health information using a username and password.

prognosis (prog NOH sis) The likely outcome of a disease, including the chance of recovery.

provisional diagnosis (die ug NOH sis) A temporary diagnosis made before all test results have been received.

quality control A process to ensure the reliability of test results, often using manufactured samples with known values.

retention schedule A method or plan for retaining or keeping health records and for their movement from active to inactive to closed.

reverse chronologic order The most recent item is on top, and the oldest item is last.

subjective information Data or information obtained from the patient, including the patient's feelings, perceptions, and concerns; this information is obtained through interviews or written questions.

subsequent (SUHB si kwuhnt) Occurring later or after.

tickler file A chronologic file used as a reminder that something must be dealt with on a certain date.

transcription (tran SKRIP shuhn) A typed or written copy of dictated material.

vested Granted or endowed with a particular authority, right, or property; to have a special interest in.

Health records can be found in two different formats, electronic and paper. Most healthcare facilities have switched to electronic health records (EHRs). Some of the benefits of EHRs include:
- Easy storage of patient information
- Availability to multiple users at the same time
- More efficient claim submission process

The federal government has also offered financial incentives for providers to implement EHRs. Although most providers are using EHRs, there are still some who are using paper records and others who are using a combination of electronic and paper records. When a provider is making a switch to an EHR, he or she may decide to keep the patient's previous records in the paper format and just use the electronic format moving forward. Some providers may decide to scan in the last 3 to 5 years of the paper record into the electronic record. Whatever the scenario the healthcare facility has chosen, it is important for the medical assistant to understand both systems and to be able to perform well with either one.

TYPES OF RECORDS

Paper health records have been shown to be much less efficient than an EHR. In most cases, only one person at a time can use the paper record. It is fairly common for information to be filed in the incorrect record. The entire record also can be misfiled. Gathering data for research and quality control is more challenging. Data are difficult to share in facilities with multiple departments or locations. The paper-based record is good for documentation of patient care, but it is not nearly as useful in other capacities.

UNIT FIVE FUNDAMENTALS OF CLINICAL MEDICAL ASSISTING

416

CRITICAL THINKING APPLICATION 19.4

Rosa is caring for an injured 3-year-old child with an open wound on his right knee. She puts on disposable gloves to clean the wound, and the mother demands to know why. How can she explain her actions?

FIGURE 19.5 Personal Protective Equipment.

shoe covers, laboratory coats, masks and respirators, protective eyewear, and face shields (Fig. 19.5).

Gloves are the most commonly used PPE in a healthcare facility. Gloves must be worn if the medical assistant is at all likely to be involved in any of the following activities (see Procedure 19.1, p. 425):

- Touching a patient's blood, body fluids, mucous membranes, or skin that is not intact.
- Handling items and surfaces contaminated with blood and body fluids.
- Performing venipuncture, fingerstick/capillary puncture, injections, and other vascular procedures.
- Assisting with any surgical procedure. If a glove is torn during the procedure, the glove should be removed, the hands washed carefully, and new gloves put on as soon as possible.
- Handling, processing, and disposing of all blood and body fluid specimens.
- Cleaning and decontaminating spills of blood or other body fluids.

The same pair of gloves cannot be worn for the care of more than one patient; new disposable gloves must be used for each individual patient.

Safety Alert

Protective equipment contaminated with body fluids of any kind must be removed and placed in a designated area or biohazard waste container. The hands or any other exposed areas must be washed or flushed as soon as possible. Face shields that cover the mouth, nose, and eyes must be worn whenever splashes, sprays, or droplets are possible. Utility gloves may be reused if they are intact (i.e., have no cracks, tears, or punctures). All PPE must be removed before the medical assistant leaves the medical facility (Fig. 19.6).

Environmental Protection

Environmental protection refers to minimizing the risk of injury by isolating or removing any physical or mechanical health hazard in the workplace. Every medical assistant must adhere to these safety rules:

- Read warning labels on biohazard waste containers and equipment.
- Minimize splashing or spraying of OPIM. Blood that splatters onto exposed areas of the skin or mucous membranes is a proven mode of HBV transmission.
- Bandage any breaks or lesions on your hands before gloving.
- If any body surface is exposed to potentially infectious material, scrub the area with soap and warm, running water as soon as possible after the exposure.
- If your eyes come in contact with body fluids, continuously flush them with water as soon as possible for a minimum of 15 minutes using an eye wash unit. A stationary unit connected to warm, running water is the best method for properly flushing potentially infectious material out of the eyes.
- Contaminated needles and other sharps should never be recapped, bent, broken, or resheathed; needle units must have protective safety device to cover the contaminated needle after injection.
- Contaminated sharp instruments, such as operating scissors, should not be processed in a way that requires employees to reach into containers to grasp them.
- Immediately after use, dispose of syringes and needles, scalpel blades, and other disposable sharp items in a labeled, leakproof, puncture-resistant biohazard container. The container must be located as close as possible to the area where the item is used.
- All specimens must be placed in a container that prevents leakage during collection, handling, processing, storage, transport, and shipping. Avoid contaminating the outside of the container or the label with the specimen substance. The container must have a biohazard label to alert others that it holds potentially infectious material. Gloves should be worn throughout this procedure.
- Equipment requiring repair that has been contaminated with blood or body fluids should be decontaminated before being repaired in the office or transported for repair. There is no documented evidence of HIV transmission from contaminated environmental surfaces, but surface contamination is a proven mode of transmission of HBV.
- Smoking, eating, drinking, applying cosmetics or lip balm, and handling contact lenses are prohibited in work areas where there is a reasonable likelihood of contamination by pathogens.
- Food and beverages cannot be kept in refrigerators, freezers, or cabinets or on countertops where infectious materials could be present.

Safety Alert boxes alert students to important safety information and reinforce the importance of safety in the profession.

Critical Thinking Application boxes prompt students to apply what they have learned as they read and study the chapter.

452   **UNIT FIVE** FUNDAMENTALS OF CLINICAL MEDICAL ASSISTING

PROCEDURE 20.4 Obtain a Temperature Using a Tympanic Thermometer

Task: Accurately determine and record a patient's temperature using a tympanic thermometer.

EQUIPMENT and SUPPLIES

- Patient's record
- Tympanic thermometer
- Disposable probe covers
- Alcohol wipes
- Waste container

PROCEDURAL STEPS

1. Wash hands or use hand sanitizer.
   <u>PURPOSE</u>: To ensure infection control.
2. Gather the necessary equipment and supplies.
3. Greet the patient. Identify yourself. Verify the patient's identity with full name and date of birth. Explain the procedure to be performed in a manner that the patient understands. Answer any questions the patient may have about the procedure.
   <u>PURPOSE</u>: Identification of the patient prevents errors, and explanations are a means of gaining implied consent and patient cooperation.
4. Clean the probe with an alcohol wipe if indicated. Place a disposable cover on the probe (see the following figure).
   <u>PURPOSE</u>: To ensure a clean surface and prevent cross-contamination.

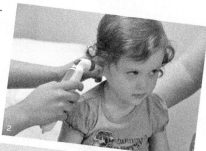

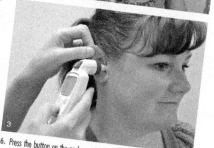

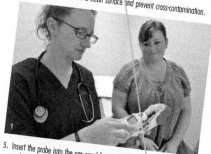

5. Insert the probe into the ear canal far enough to seal the opening. Do not apply pressure. For children younger than age 3, gently pull the earlobe down and back (see the first of the following figures); for patients older than age 3, gently pull the top of the ear (pinna) up and back (see the second of the following figures).
   <u>PURPOSE</u>: The external ear must be pulled gently to open the external auditory canal and expose the tympanic membrane for an accurate reading.

6. Press the button on the probe as directed. The temperature will appear on the display screen in 1 to 2 seconds.
7. Remove the probe, note the reading, and discard the probe cover into a waste container without touching it.
   <u>PURPOSE</u>: The probe cover is contaminated and must be discarded in a waste container.
8. Wash hands or use hand sanitizer and disinfect the equipment if indicated. See the manufacturer's manual for cleaning the equipment. Many recommend cleaning the probe lens with alcohol wipes.
   <u>PURPOSE</u>: To ensure infection control.
9. Document the reading in the patient's medical record (e.g., T: 98.6°F [T]).
   <u>PURPOSE</u>: Procedures that are not recorded are considered not done.

7/11/20xx 2:20 p.m. T: 101.2°F (T) --
-------------------------------------- C. Ricci, CMA (AAMA)

Step-by-step Procedure boxes demonstrate how to perform and document procedures encountered in the healthcare setting.

the anger or become argumentative. Medical assistants must use good listening skills with angry people and must be empathetic. Notify the facility's administrator of all difficult patients or ask for help from co-workers.

There should be a policy in place for dealing with potentially dangerous individuals. Policies can include:

- Making sure that you can reach the exit if you take the patient to another room
- Having another employee close by
- Knowing under what circumstances you should contact the police or building security for assistance

Patient Checkout

When patients return to the front office for checkout, greet them with a friendly smile and call the individual by name. Form the habit of asking patients if they have any questions. Check the health record to determine when the provider wants the patient to return. Most providers note this information on the encounter form. Make the return appointment. Remember to give the patient an appointment reminder card. If the time and day. Give the patient an appointment reminder card. If the copayment was not collected prior to the visit it may be collected during checkout.

The medical assistant can convey a sense of caring by terminating the visit cordially. Thank the patient for coming. If the patient will return for another visit, the assistant can say something such as, "We'll see you next week." If the patient will not be returning soon, a pleasant "I hope you'll be feeling better soon" is appropriate. In addition, tell patients to call the facility if they have any questions or if they need additional care. Whatever words of goodbye are chosen, all patients should leave the facility feeling that they have received top-quality care and were treated with friendliness, respect, and courtesy.

CLOSING COMMENTS

Patient Coaching

Providing patients with an information booklet about the healthcare facility can familiarize them with policies and procedures. Many providers compile an extensive booklet that even provides tips as to when the provider should be called immediately, listing symptoms and signs of emergencies.

Educating the patient about the healthcare facility's policies helps the facility run smoothly from day to day. All patients should be familiar with the policies about appointments. This leads to fewer misunderstandings and conflicts over bills that might include a charge for a missed appointment.

If the facility offers internet-based appointment scheduling or forms completion, patients must be taught how to use the system. A printed pamphlet or information sheet is helpful for providing instructions to the patient. A wise option is to have a special phone number that patients can call if they have problems with the system. For best results, choose a program that is simple to use, easy to understand, and does not breach patient confidentiality.

Legal and Ethical Issues

As mentioned earlier, the appointment schedule may be used as a legal record and could be brought by subpoena into a court of law.

Make sure all handwriting in the book is completely legible and that information is routinely collected in a consistent manner for each entry. Do not fail to note a no-show both in the patient's health record and the appointment schedule. This often is helpful when a provider must prove that the patient did not follow medical advice or that the patient contributed to his or her poor condition by missing appointments. Old appointment schedules should be kept for a time equal to that of the statute of limitations in the state where the practice is located.

A medical assistant must never offer medical advice to a patient. The patient sees the medical assistant as an extension of the provider and tends to weigh advice and comments by the medical assistant with the same validity as if they came from the provider. Provide only information the provider has approved or that is included in the healthcare facility's policies and procedures manual.

When a patient complains, listen carefully and try to resolve the problem or assure the patient that the issue will be discussed with the appropriate staff member to find a solution. If someone other than the patient asks for information about the patient, refrain from discussion unless the patient or provider has authorized the release of information.

Patient-Centered Care

Going to a healthcare facility can be intimidating and uncomfortable for many patients. It is important that the medical assistant try to put everyone at ease. Cultivate the habit of greeting each patient immediately in a friendly, self-assured manner. Establish eye contact and smile while introducing yourself to the patient.

Small talk can help put a patient at ease. Talking about the weather or an uncontroversial topic may make the patient more comfortable. Asking personalized questions can also help. Providers and staff members sometimes make brief notes in the health record about the current events in the patient's life. On the next visit, the staff or provider can use this information to start a conversation with the patient. For instance, the patient may state she is going to Florida for a vacation. During the next visit, the provider may start off the visit by asking how her Florida trip was. Asking personalized questions will solidify the personal connection with patients. They may feel important, less intimidated, and more comfortable. It is a great way to provide excellent customer service.

Professional Behaviors

When working in scheduling and helping patients move through the healthcare facility, medical assistants have many opportunities to demonstrate professionalism. It is important to remember that we are often seeing patients when they are not at their best, so we must learn not to take all of the responses personally. When an angry patient approaches the reception desk, you should smile politely, ask how you can help the person, and respond in a soothing tone of voice. When a patient calls for an appointment and demands a day and time when the provider is not available, you should remain calm and explain why that day and time are not an option. As a medical assistant in the front office, you have the opportunity to make an amazing first impression on patients. Remember to always behave professionally.

Patient Coaching sections address how the MA can provide information to patients in a supportive environment that allows them to grow, change, or improve their situation.

NEW! Professional Behaviors boxes provide tips on professional behavior that are specific to each chapter's content.

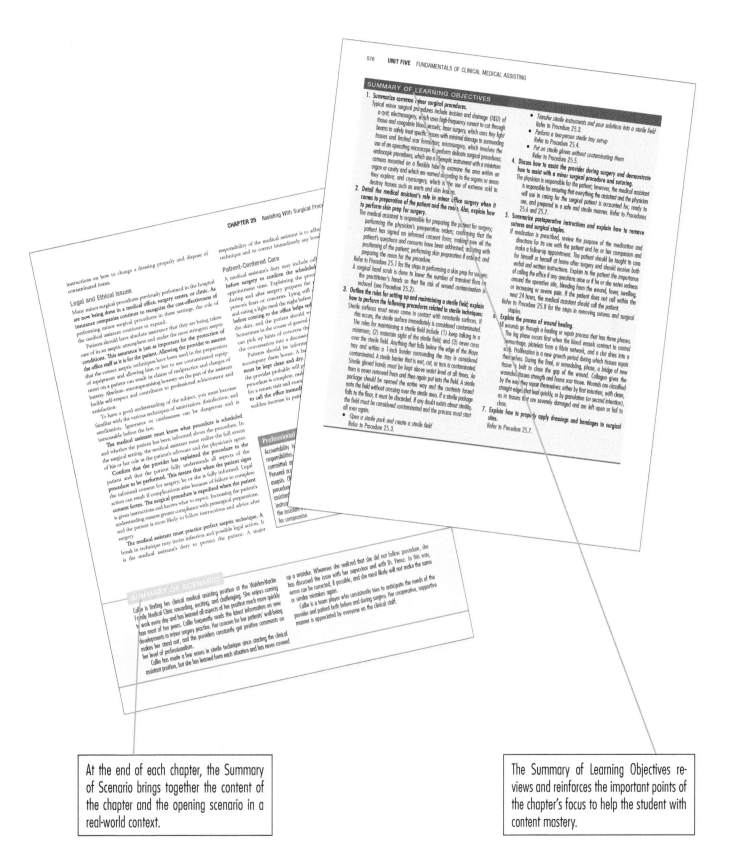

At the end of each chapter, the Summary of Scenario brings together the content of the chapter and the opening scenario in a real-world context.

The Summary of Learning Objectives reviews and reinforces the important points of the chapter's focus to help the student with content mastery.

CONTENTS

THE PROFESSIONAL MEDICAL ASSISTANT AND THE HEALTHCARE TEAM

1

SCENARIO

Carmen Angelos is a new student in a medical assisting program accredited by the Commission on Accreditation of Allied Health Education Programs (CAAHEP) at Butler County Community College. Carmen is returning to school after working at a local pharmacy for 5 years, where she became very interested in pursuing a career in medical assisting. She has been out of high school for a few years but is very excited about her new career choice.

While studying this chapter, think about the following questions:
- Why is professionalism an important attribute in the field of medical assisting?
- What is a typical job description for an entry-level medical assistant?
- How will scope of practice and standards of care determine your role as a medical assistant?
- Why is it important to learn about professional medical assisting organizations?
- Studying may be a challenge for Carmen. What skills can she use to help her learn new material and prepare for examinations?

- Why is it important for medical assisting students to learn about the various healthcare facilities and medical specialties?
- How can Carmen show professional behavior toward all patients in the healthcare setting?
- How can time management strategies help Carmen prioritize her responsibilities as a member of the healthcare team?

LEARNING OBJECTIVES

1. Discuss the typical responsibilities of a medical assistant and describe the role of the medical assistant as a patient navigator.
2. Discuss the attributes of a professional medical assistant, project a professional image in the ambulatory care setting, and describe how to show respect for individual diversity.
3. Differentiate between scope of practice and standards of care for medical assistants.
4. List and discuss professional medical assisting organizations.
5. Examine your learning preferences and interpret how your learning style affects your success as a student.
6. Integrate effective study skills into your daily activities, design test-taking strategies that help you take charge of your success, and incorporate critical thinking skills and reflection to help you make mental connections as you learn material.

7. Summarize the history of medicine and its significance to the medical assisting profession.
8. Summarize the various types of medical professionals, allied health professionals, and healthcare facilities.
9. Define a patient-centered medical home (PCMH) and discuss its five core functions and attributes.
10. Explain the reasons professionalism is important in the medical field, describe work ethics, and stress the importance of cooperation.
11. Apply time management strategies to prioritize the medical assistant's responsibilities as a member of the healthcare team.
12. Respond to criticism, problem-solve, identify obstacles to professional behaviors, and define the principles of self-boundaries.

VOCABULARY

allopathic (al uh PATH ik) A system of medical practice that treats disease by the use of remedies, such as medications and surgery, to produce effects different from those caused by the disease under treatment; medical doctors (MDs) and osteopaths (DOs) practice allopathic medicine; also called conventional medicine.

complementary and alternative medicine (CAM) A group of diverse medical and healthcare systems, practices, and products that are not generally considered part of conventional medicine. Complementary medicine is used in combination with conventional medicine (allopathic or osteopathic); alternative medicine is used instead of conventional medicine.

conscientious (kon shee EN shuhs) Meticulous, careful.

contamination (kun tam i NAY shun) The process by which something becomes harmful or unusable through contact with something unclean.

critical thinking The constant practice of considering all aspects of a situation when deciding what to believe or what to do.

demeanor (dih MEE ner) Behavior toward others; outward manner.

detrimental (de truh MEN tl) Harmful.

holistic (hoh LIS tik) A form of healing that considers the whole person (i.e., body, mind, spirit, and emotions) in individual treatment plans.

hospice (HOS pis) A concept of care that involves health professionals and volunteers who provide medical, psychological, and spiritual support to terminally ill patients and their loved ones.

indicator (IN di kay ter) An important point or group of statistical values that, when evaluated, indicates the quality of care provided in a healthcare facility.

initiative (i NISH eh tive) The ability to determine what needs to be done and to take action on your own.

integrity (in TEG ri tee) Adhering to ethical standards or right conduct standards.

learning style The way an individual perceives and processes information to learn new material.

mnemonic (ni MON ik) A learning device (e.g., an image, a rhyme, or a figure of speech) that a person uses to help him or her remember information.

morale (muh RAL) Emotional or mental condition with respect to cheerfulness or confidence.

negligence (NEG li jens) Failure to act as a reasonably prudent person would under similar circumstances; such conduct falls below the standards of behavior established by law for the protection of others against unreasonable risk of harm.

overlearn To learn or memorize beyond the point of proficiency or immediate recall.

patient navigator A person who identifies patients' needs and barriers; then assists by coordinating care and identifying community and healthcare resources to meet the needs. May also be called *care coordinator*.

perceiving (per SEEV ing) How an individual looks at information and sees it as real.

processing (prah CES ing) How an individual internalizes new information and makes it his or her own.

reflection (ree FLEK shun) The process of thinking about new information so as to create new ways of learning.

reliable (ree LIE ah bul) Dependable, able to be trusted.

triage (tree AHZH) The process of sorting patients to determine medical need and the priority of care.

What an exciting and challenging career you have chosen! Medical assistants are multiskilled healthcare workers who function under the direction of a licensed provider and are primarily employed in outpatient or ambulatory care facilities, such as medical offices and clinics. According to the U.S. Bureau of Labor Statistics, medical assisting is one of the nation's fastest growing careers, and employment opportunities are projected to grow 29% through 2026.

This growth in job opportunities for medical assistants is due to multiple factors, including a steady increase in the aging population as baby boomers spur demand for preventive health services from physician offices and ambulatory care centers. Since medical assistants are trained in both administrative and clinical skills, they are the perfect employees to meet the needs of this increasing population. In addition, the switch to electronic health records (EHRs) in ambulatory care centers will also open up employment opportunities for medical assistants who are trained in EHR computer software.

RESPONSIBILITIES OF THE MEDICAL ASSISTANT

Medical assistants are the only allied health professionals specifically trained to work in ambulatory care settings, such as physicians' offices, clinics, and group practices. That training includes both clinical and administrative skills, covering a multitude of medical practice needs. The skills performed by an entry-level medical assistant depend on his or her place of employment, but all graduates of accredited programs are taught a similar skill set.

Clinical skills include:

- Assisting during physical examinations
- Performing patient screening procedures
- Assisting with minor surgical procedures, including sterilization procedures
- Performing electrocardiograms (ECGs)
- Obtaining and recording vital signs and medical histories
- Performing phlebotomy
- Performing tests permitted by the Clinical Laboratory Improvement Amendments (i.e., CLIA-waived tests)
- Collecting and managing laboratory specimens
- Following Occupational Safety and Health Administration (OSHA) regulations on infection control
- Administering vaccinations and medications as ordered by the provider
- Performing patient education and coaching initiatives within the scope of practice
- Documenting accurately in a paper record or an EHR
- Performing first aid procedures as needed
- Performing infection control procedures
- Applying therapeutic communication techniques
- Adapting to the special needs of a patient based on his or her developmental life stage, cultural diversity, and individual communication barriers

- Acting as a patient advocate or navigator, including referring patients to community resources
- Acting within legal and ethical boundaries

Administrative skills include:
- Answering telephones
- Managing patient scheduling
- Creating and maintaining patient health records
- Documenting accurately in a paper record and an EHR
- Performing routine maintenance of facility equipment
- Performing basic practice finance procedures
- Coordinating third-party reimbursement
- Performing procedural and diagnostic coding
- Communicating professionally with patients, family members, practitioners, peers, and the public
- Managing facility correspondence
- Performing patient education and coaching initiatives within the scope of practice
- Following legal and ethical principles
- Complying with facility safety practices

These lengthy lists of capabilities that make up the basic skill set are not all that is expected of entry-level medical assistants; they also play a significant role as the patient's advocate. Current research describes this role as being a **patient navigator** (Fig. 1.1). If you have ever had a loved one who was very ill and required medical attention from a number of different practitioners and allied health specialty groups, you understand what a complex and overwhelming task it can be to make decisions and coordinate a loved one's care. Care coordination originated from the patient navigator program. This program was established at the Harlem Hospital Center in 1990. The goal was to assist cancer patients in accessing quality healthcare. Many patient navigator positions were funded with the assistance of the Patient Navigator, Outreach and Chronic Disease Prevention Act of 2005. Today, patient navigator positions are commonly called *care coordinators*. These positions can be found in ambulatory care settings and hospitals. In hospitals, the care coordinators help manage the acute care services and also help patients transition home or to other healthcare settings.

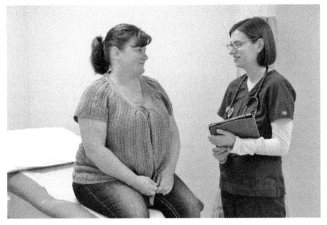

FIGURE 1.1 The medical assistant as a patient navigator.

Customer Service

Another aspect of being a medical assistant is providing excellent customer service. Customer service closely relates to professional behaviors. One must be professional to provide exceptional customer service. In healthcare today, many of our patients have the ability to choose where they go to seek care. The ambulatory care facility needs to attract and retain patients to remain open and for you to have a job. Two of the quickest ways to lose patients are to treat them poorly and to act in an unprofessional manner. Happy patients will tend to tell others about their experiences. Great customer service leads to a successful healthcare facility and allows growth.

To understand customer service, we first need to know who our customers are. A *customer* is one who purchases goods or services. A customer can also be a person whom you deal with in the work environment. By that definition, we can see that patients are our customers. They choose our ambulatory care facility to seek healthcare services. They (or their insurance company) pay for the services provided. Patients are considered *external customers,* or people we do business with who are "outside" (i.e., not employed by) the healthcare facility. Other external customers include medical equipment and supply vendors and pharmaceutical representatives.

The second part of the customer definition relates to *internal customers,* or people whom you deal with in the work environment. These are individuals we interact with inside the facility. They include our co-workers, employees in other departments, and the administrative staff. Both internal and external customers are important for the success of the healthcare facility.

Customer service is whatever we do for our customers to improve their experience at our healthcare facility. People may have different ideas about how they should be treated during their interactions. Our goal is to provide *customer satisfaction,* or a sense of contentment with the interaction. Typically, the more we get to know the customer, the better we can provide customer service. This might not always be possible. For instance, a new patient comes for an appointment.

If you are at the reception desk, you do not have a lot of time to get to know the patient. The most important things for you to do are:

- Be considerate and treat the patient as you would want to be treated
- Look and act professional

CRITICAL THINKING APPLICATION   1.2

During Carmen's orientation, she learned about customer service and customer satisfaction. In your own words, how would you define both of these phrases?

CHARACTERISTICS OF PROFESSIONAL MEDICAL ASSISTANTS

Medical assistants must have professional *characteristics*, or distinguishing traits. You will start developing these traits while in school. You will put them into practice during practicum. They will follow you into your first job. If a student is unprofessional during practicum, it will be difficult to get a job. That behavior may be **detrimental** to the medical assistant's professional career.

Professionalism

As a healthcare professional, medical assistants represent the healthcare facility. They are viewed as an extension of the provider and the facility. A healthcare professional:

- has high ethical standards.
- displays **integrity**.
- completes work accurately and in a timely fashion.

It is important for successful professionals to show *professionalism*; that is, having courteous, **conscientious**, and respectful behaviors. This approach is used during all interactions and situations in the workplace. Our patients and co-workers expect professional behavior. Patients base much of their trust and confidence in those who show professionalism. How health professionals act is a direct reflection on the facility and provider. If a medical assistant is rude to a patient, the patient may think that the provider is rude. The perceived quality of care will be negative. Medical assistants must always display professionalism. This includes their attitude, appearance, and behavior. Regardless of the situation, they must always act professionally.

Courtesy and Respect

Courtesy, respect, and dignity often come together when discussing professionalism. *Courtesy* is having good manners or being polite. Courteous behavior is polite, open, and welcoming. *Respect* means to show consideration or appreciation for another person. *Dignity* is the state or quality of being worthy of respect.

We show our patients dignity by treating all patients the way we would want to be treated. It does not matter if the patient has bad body odor or is dressed in tattered clothes. The patient is a person worthy of respect. Patients expect to be treated as individuals who matter. They want to be respected and not to be treated as an annoyance or a medical condition. How can the medical assistant treat others with courtesy and respect?

- Make patients feel welcome and respected. A pleasant greeting and eye contact should be the first things patients experience. Thanking patients at the end of the visit is also important.
- Display positive nonverbal behaviors. Use a calm tone of voice, eye contact when appropriate, and provide privacy for patients. Maintain patient confidentiality.

- Learn about other cultures in your area. When working with patients from those cultures, make sure to avoid gestures, words, and behaviors that could be perceived as disrespectful.
- Always use proper grammar, without slang words. Explain medical treatments and conditions in simple lay language. If you need to use a medical term, explain it to the patient.

Empathy and Compassion

It is important that professional medical assistants demonstrate empathy and compassion to their patients. Empathy, sympathy, and compassion can easily be confused. *Empathy* is the ability to understand another's perspective, experiences, or motivations. We can share another's emotional state. Empathy differs from sympathy. *Sympathy* is feeling sorrow, concern or pity for what the other person has gone through. *Compassion* means we have a deep awareness of the suffering of another and wish to ease it. These characteristics will help to build our positive relationship with our patients.

Tact and Diplomacy

Tact and diplomacy are extremely valuable traits in healthcare professionals. Being *tactful* means being acutely sensitive to what is proper and appropriate when interacting with others. A tactful person has the ability to speak or act without offending others. Being *diplomatic* means using tact and sensitivity when interacting with others. The medical assistant must be sensitive to the needs of others. How can a medical assistant use these traits when communicating with others?

- Consistently be polite and honest during your communication. Show sensitivity to others through your communication and behaviors.
- Recognize the needs and rights of others. Attempt to reach a mutually beneficial resolution to the problem.
- Assess your personal response to the situation. Your personal beliefs and biases should not prevent you from interacting diplomatically and tactfully with others.

CRITICAL THINKING APPLICATION   1.3

During Carmen's orientation, she learned about the importance of courtesy, respect, empathy, compassion, tact, and diplomacy. Select three of these words and share with a peer examples of how a medical assistant could display these traits.

Respect for Individual Diversity

Medical assistants work with diverse populations. Your patients will come from different backgrounds. *Diversity* describes the differences and similarities in identity, perspective, and points of view among people. When talking about diversity people usually think of things such as nationality or race, but diversity can also include things such as age and economic status.

It is important to be open and nonjudgmental when working with patients and workers who are different than ourselves. Be aware and accepting of other cultural differences. Be aware of your own cultural values. What preconceived ideas do you have of other diverse groups? How might your biases affect the care you provide to those in different groups?

It is important to educate yourself about other groups. Get to know their customs and practices. Culture can affect healthcare. It can influence how people describe their symptoms, when healthcare is sought, and how treatment plans are followed. For instance, people in some cultures eat traditional foods high in sodium. This could be an issue if a person has high blood pressure or kidney disease. Understanding and accepting the differences represented by your patients will help you provide the best care possible for them.

Honesty, Dependability, and Responsibility

Honest means to be sincere and upright. *Dependable* is the same as trustworthy. *Responsible* is defined as being trusted or depended upon. These are three traits that employers value in their employees. Professional medical assistants should be honest, dependable, and responsible. When given a task, they should complete it accurately, on time, and to the best of their ability. If they make an error, they should be upfront about it. Patient safety is the number one priority. Any mistake in patient care needs to be reported immediately to the provider and to the supervisor. Dependability and honesty are critical components in earning the trust and respect of others. How can medical assistants perform their duties using these three characteristics?

- Be honest and straightforward when interacting with others.
- Accept responsibility for your mistakes. Determine how to prevent them in the future.
- Follow through on your promises.
- Complete your work to the best of your abilities. Complete it on time.
- Be self-motivated. Don't wait to be asked to complete a task.
- Embrace change.

Professional Appearance

Most ambulatory healthcare facilities have dress codes for employees. Medical assistants are usually required to wear scrubs, along with the facility's nametag (and a photo) clearly visible (Fig. 1.2). Table 1.1 provides a typical dress code. Dress codes will vary by facility. Some communities are more conservative, and thus the dress codes reflect this.

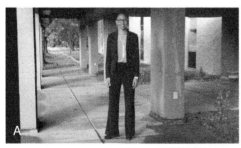

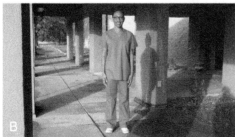

FIGURE 1.2 A professional appearance is important for a medical assistant. **(A)** Business attire. **(B)** Scrubs.

Typically, healthcare facilities include terms such as "modest" and "business attire" in describing their dress codes. The rule of thumb is to make sure the employee does not expose too much at the neckline, the abdomen, and below the waist when bending and raising the arms. Business attire is not casual clothing. Casual clothes include jeans, T-shirts, shorts, exercise/sports clothing, and so on. Business attire is considered dressier, more professional, than casual clothes. Dress pants and a dress shirt would be considered business attire for men. Dress pants, a dress shirt, modest dresses, and modest skirts and blouses would be considered business attire for women.

CRITICAL THINKING APPLICATION   **1.4**

Rosie, a business office employee at Walden-Martin Family Medical Clinic, is allowed to dress in business attire. She interacts with patients who have questions about their bill. Describe how Rosie should dress.

SCOPE OF PRACTICE AND STANDARDS OF CARE FOR MEDICAL ASSISTANTS

Scope of practice is defined as the range of responsibilities and practice guidelines that determine the boundaries within which a healthcare worker practices. What is the scope of practice of a medical assistant? There is no single definition of the scope of practice for medical assistants throughout the United States, but some states have enacted scope of practice laws covering medical assistant practice. These states include Alaska, Arizona, California, Florida, Georgia, Illinois, Maine, Maryland, Montana, Nevada, New Jersey, New York, Ohio, South Dakota, Virginia, Washington, and West Virginia. Medical assistants working in those states must refer to the identified roles specified in the law. However, for those employed in states without scope of practice laws, medical assistant practice is guided by the norms of that particular location, facility policies and procedures, and individual physician-employers. In some states, medical assistants are overseen by the board of nursing, whereas in others, the board of medicine oversees medical assistants. Make sure you are aware of your state's rules governing medical assistant scope of practice.

One fact is absolutely true about all practicing medical assistants – they are not independent practitioners. Whether certified or not, regardless of length of training or experience, every medical assistant must practice under the direct supervision of a physician or other licensed provider (e.g., nurse practitioner or physician assistant).

Earlier in this chapter we discussed the typical tasks performed by a medical assistant, so you already know generally what duties medical assistants perform in ambulatory care centers; however, some specific tasks are beyond the scope of practice of medical assistants, including the following:

- Performing telephone or in-person **triage**; medical assistants are not legally authorized to assess or diagnose symptoms
- Prescribing medications or making recommendations about over-the-counter drugs and remedies
- Giving out drug samples without provider permission
- Automatically submitting refill prescription requests without provider orders
- Administering intravenous (IV) medications and starting, flushing, or removing IV lines unless permitted by state law
- Analyzing or interpreting test results

TABLE 1.1   Typical Dress Code for Medical Assistants

DRESS CODE	PROFESSIONAL	UNPROFESSIONAL	COMMENTS
Uniform: scrubs and white shoes	• Scrubs must be clean, pressed (ironed), and fit properly. • Scrub pants must be hemmed to the appropriate length. • Closed-toed shoes must be white and clean.	• Dirty, wrinkled, ripped scrubs • Scrub pants dragging on the floor • Scruffy, dirty shoes • Open shoes (sandals), fabric shoes	• Shoes need to protect your feet. Cloth and open-toed shoes provide very little protection. • Pants dragging on floors pick up and transfer bacteria.
Hair	• Natural colors; clean and styled • Long hair must be tied back	• Unnatural colors; dirty, messy hair • Hair in face or hanging down	• Hair hanging in front can interfere with patient care, spread bacteria, and get caught in equipment.
Fingernails	• Cut short, unpolished	• Long, polished, artificial nails	• Bacteria can multiply and grow under long, artificial, and/or polished nails.
Cosmetics and body odors	• Professional makeup • No odors on the body	• Overuse of makeup • Wearing perfume, cologne, etc. • Using scented lotions • Smelling like a cigarette • Body odor (from not bathing)	• Too much makeup can look unprofessional. • Smells like perfumes, colognes, or cigarettes can trigger allergies in others. • Offensive body odor is unprofessional because we are in patients' intimate/personal space.
Jewelry	• Wedding band (no stones) • One pair of earrings (studs) • Watch	• Rings with stones • Multiple earrings on each ear • Necklaces, bracelets • Lanyards	• Bacteria can accumulate in rings and bracelets. • Necklaces and lanyards can be choking hazards if grabbed by a patient.
Tattoos and body piercings	• Tattoos and body piercings must follow the healthcare facility's policy	• Not following the healthcare facility's policy	• In conservative communities, body piercings and tattoos may be perceived as unprofessional.
Professional dress (street clothes) for special events	• Blouse, top, or sweater • Dress pants • Dress or skirt (to the top of the knee) • Dress shoes	• Low-cut tops; sheer tops • Jeans, ripped pants, exercise clothes • Flip-flops, tennis shoes • Mini skirts	• Clothes should look professional; should not be ripped or casual in appearance.

• Operating laser equipment
• Performing laboratory tests that are not CLIA-waived
• Ordering diagnostic or radiographic tests/procedures

What is the difference between scope of practice and standards of care? The scope of practice for a medical assistant is what has been established by law in some states or by practice norms, institutions, or physician-employers in states without scope of practice laws. *Standards of care,* however, is a legal term that refers to whether the level and quality of patient service provided is the same as what another healthcare worker with similar training and experience in a similar situation would provide. Standards of care set minimum guidelines for job performance. They define what the expected quality of care is and provide specific guidelines on whether the care standard has been met. Medical assistants not meeting the expected standard of care may be charged with professional **negligence** (discussed in greater detail in Chapter 3).

The following are examples of breaks in the standards of care in medical assisting.

• A patient calls reporting a persistent headache for 3 days. You tell the patient to get some rest and take ibuprofen, without referring the call to a provider. What standard of care has been broken?
• A patient asks you to explain his lab report. You do your best to explain what his blood count levels mean. What is the problem here?
• An elderly patient tells you she cannot afford to get her prescriptions filled. The provider is busy, but you know there are samples of the prescribed drug in the medication cupboard, so you give her several packets. Does this follow standard of care?
• A patient tells you her son fell on the playground yesterday, and he is complaining that his arm hurts. You tell the mother

it is probably just a strain and suggest she wrap the arm with an elastic bandage. Why is this a problem?

- You overhear a patient calling one of the other medical assistants "nurse." Should your co-worker correct the patient? Why?

Hopefully you are beginning to see that the practice of medical assisting is limited not only by individual state laws or norms, but also by the standards and scope of practice established by the supervising providers where the medical assistant is employed. Remember, the scope of practice and expected standards of care for licensed medical professionals are quite different from those for medical assisting practice. The medical assistant must refer to the provider for orders and guidance on what behaviors are expected for medical assistants in that facility. The medical assistant can *never* independently diagnose, prescribe, or treat patients. She or he must *always* have the written order of a provider or follow established policies and procedures when performing clinical skills.

PROFESSIONAL MEDICAL ASSISTING ORGANIZATIONS, CREDENTIALS, AND CONTINUING EDUCATION

Becoming a member of a professional organization, obtaining credentials, and participating in continuing education are all part of being a professional medical assistant. In this next section you will find information about professional organizations, how to obtain a medical assistant credential, and continuing education.

Professional Organizations for Medical Assistants

Most healthcare occupations have a professional organization that sets high standards for quality and performance. A code of ethics is also developed by the organization to help guide the actions of those in that particular profession. Professional organizations provide many benefits to their members, including opportunities for continuing education, national and regional conventions, and networking opportunities. Medical assisting is no different. Becoming a member of a professional organization will also show your employer that you are committed to being the best possible medical assistant. The following sections provide descriptions of three of the professional medical assisting organizations available.

American Association of Medical Assistants

The American Association of Medical Assistants (AAMA) was created in 1956 and remains the only association devoted exclusively to the medical assisting profession. According to the AAMA's website (*www.aama-ntl.org*), becoming a member includes the following benefits:

- AAMA legal counsel represents medical assistants across the United States to fight for the rights of medical assistant practice; in addition, the counsel stays abreast of federal and state laws regarding medical assisting.
- Members receive a complimentary subscription to *CMA Today*, an informative magazine devoted entirely to the medical assistant profession; each issue (six per year) offers continuing education unit (CEU) articles, medical assisting news, and healthcare information.

More information about the AAMA is available on the organization's website: *www.aama-ntl.org*.

American Medical Technologists (AMT)

The American Medical Technologists (AMT) was founded in 1939 as a nationally recognized certification agency for multiple allied health professionals, including Medical Assistant (RMA), Medical Laboratory Technician (MLT), Phlebotomy Technician (RPT), Medical Administrative Specialist (CMAS), and Dental Assistant (RDA).

According to the AMT's website (*www.americanmedtech.org*), becoming a member includes the following benefits:

- Professional publications
- Annual convention
- State society meeting and seminars
- Continuing education
- Career services
- Awards and scholarships

Additional information on the AMT is available on the organization's website: *www.americanmedtech.org.*

The National Healthcareer Association (NHA)

The National Healthcareer Association (NHA) was established in 1990 to offer certification examinations in a number of allied health programs; for example, certification is granted for pharmacy, phlebotomy, and electrocardiography (ECG) technicians. The NHA also offers two different medical assisting certifications: Certified Clinical Medical Assistant (CCMA) and Certified Medical Administrative Assistant (CMAA). The NHA is not involved in program curriculum standards or program accreditation. It simply offers certification if the applicant can successfully pass the NHA examination developed for each particular medical discipline. You can find out more about the certifications offered through the NHA at the association's website: *www.nhanow.com/.*

Achieving a Credential

Medical assistants have several options if they choose to become credentialed. Being a credentialed medical assistant has certain benefits:

- Credentialed medical assistants have had to pass a national standardized exam. Passing the exam indicates that they have the knowledge to perform the medical assistant's duties.
- Some employers require the credential prior to hiring or within a few months after hiring.
- Some employers will pay more if a person has achieved a medical assistant credential.

There are several national agencies that will provide credentials to medical assistants upon successful completion of their exam. Table 1.2 presents some of the more common medical assistant credentials. It is important for graduating medical assistants to research whether credentials are preferred or required by local employers. It is also important to identify which credential is most wanted by local employers. Your instructors are also excellent resources if you have additional questions on credentials for medical assistants.

Continuing Education

For a professional medical assistant, it is important to stay current (up-to-date) with the newest medications, treatments, and diagnostic tests. Education beyond your medical assistant degree is considered continuing education. Most healthcare professionals need to do continuing education to renew their certification or license. There are many opportunities for continuing education. These include:

TABLE 1.2 Credentialing Agencies for Medical Assistants		
AGENCY/WEBSITE	**CREDENTIAL**	**RECERTIFICATION METHODS**
American Association of Medical Assistants (AAMA) http://www.aama-ntl.org	Certified Medical Assistant (CMA [AAMA])	Recertify every 5 years either by exam or by earning 60 continuing education points. Specific points must be achieved in the three content areas. At least 30 points must be from AAMA-approved continuing education units (CEUs).
American Medical Technologists (AMT) https://www.americanmedtech.org	Registered Medical Assistant (RMA)	Recertify every 3 years either by exam or by completing specific activities.
National Healthcareer Association (NHA) https://www.nhanow.com	Clinical Medical Assistant (CCMA) Medical Administrative Assistant (CMAA)	Recertify every 2 years either by exam or by earning 10 continuing education credits.
National Center for Competency Testing (NCCT) https://www.ncctinc.com	Medical Assistant (NCMA)	Recertify every year either by exam or by completing 14 contact hours of continuing education.

- Reading professional journals and reputable health websites
- On-the-job educational conferences
- Local, state, and national medical assistant conferences

Typically, additional continuing education opportunities exist if a medical assistant is a member of an organization.

HOW TO SUCCEED AS A MEDICAL ASSISTANT STUDENT

Who You Are as a Learner: How Do You Learn Best?

You have taken the first step toward becoming a successful student by choosing your profession and field of study. Becoming a medical assistant opens the doors to a wide variety of opportunities in both administrative and clinical practice at ambulatory or institutional healthcare facilities. To become a successful medical assistant, you first must become a successful student. This section will help you discover the way you learn best, and it provides multiple strategies to assist you in your journey toward success.

Think about what you do when you are faced with something new to learn. How do you go about understanding and learning the new material? Over time you have developed a method for **perceiving** and **processing** information. This pattern of behavior is called your **learning style**. Learning styles can be examined in many different ways, but most professionals agree that a student's success depends more on whether the person can "make sense" of the information than on whether the individual is "smart." Determining your individual learning style and understanding how it applies to your ability to learn new material are the first steps toward becoming a successful student.

Learning Style Inventory

For you to learn new material, two things must happen. First, you must perceive the information. This is the method you have developed over time that helps you examine new information and recognize it as real. Once you have developed a method for learning about the new material, you must process the information. Processing the information is how you internalize it and make it your own. Researchers believe that each of us has a preferred method for learning new material. By investigating your learning style, you can figure out how to combine different approaches to perceiving and processing information that will lead to greater success as a student.

The first step in learning new material is determining how you perceive it, or as some experts explain, what methods you use to learn the new material. Some learners opt to watch, observe, and use **reflection** to think about and learn the new material. These students are *abstract perceivers,* who learn by analyzing new material, building theories about it, and using a step-by-step approach to learning. Other students need to perform some activity, such as rewriting notes from class, making flash cards, and outlining chapters, to learn new information. Students who learn by "doing" are called *concrete perceivers.* Concrete learners prefer to learn things that have a personal meaning or that they believe are relevant to their lives. So, which type of perceiver do you think you are? Before you actually learn new material, do you need time to think about it, or do you prefer to "do" something to help you learn the material?

The second step in learning new material is information processing, which is the way learners internalize the new information and make it their own. New material can be processed by two methods. *Active processors* prefer to jump in and start doing things immediately. They make sense of the new material by using it *now.* They look for practical ways to apply the new material and learn best with practice and hands-on activities. *Reflective processors* have to think about the information before they can internalize it. They prefer to observe and consider what is going on. The only way they can make sense of new material is to spend time thinking and learning a great deal about it before acting. Which type of information processor do you think you are? Do you prefer to jump in and start doing things to help you learn, or do you need to analyze and consider the material before you can actually learn it?

Using Your Learning Profile to Be a Successful Student: Where Do I Go From Here?

No one falls completely into one or the other of the categories just discussed. However, by being aware of how we generally prefer first to perceive information and then to process it, we can be more sensitive to our learning style and can approach new learning situations with a plan for learning the material in a way that best suits our learning preferences.

Your preferred perceiving and processing learning profile will fall into one of the following four stages of the Learning Style Inventory, which was created by David Kolb of Case Western Reserve University.

- *Stage 1* learners have a *concrete reflective* style. These students want to know the purpose of the information and have a personal connection to the content. They like to consider a situation from many points of view, observe others, and plan before taking action. They feel most comfortable watching rather than doing, and their strengths include sensitivity toward others, brainstorming, and recognizing and creatively solving problems. If you fall into this stage, you enjoy small-group activities and learn well in study groups.
- *Stage 2* learners have an *abstract reflective* style. These students are eager to learn just for the sheer pleasure of learning, rather than because the material relates to their personal lives. They like to learn lots of facts and arrange new material in a clear, logical manner. Stage 2 learners plan studying and like to create ways of thinking about the material, but they do not always make the connection with its practical application. If you are a stage 2 learner, you prefer organized, logical presentations of material and therefore enjoy lectures and readings and generally dislike group work. You also need time to process and think about new material before applying it.
- *Stage 3* learners have an *abstract active* style. Learners with this combination learning style want to experiment and test the information they are learning. If you are a stage 3 learner, you want to know how techniques or ideas work, and you also want to practice what you are learning. Your strengths are in problem solving and decision making, but you may lack focus and may be hasty in making decisions. You learn best with hands-on practice by doing experiments, projects, and laboratory activities. You enjoy working alone or in small groups.

CRITICAL THINKING APPLICATION   1.5

- Consider the two ways to perceive new material. Are you a concrete perceiver, who ties the information to a personal experience, or are you an abstract perceiver, who likes to analyze or reflect on the meaning of the material? Choose the type you think most accurately describes your method of learning.
- Now, think about the way you process learning. Are you an active processor, who always looks for the practical applications of what you learn, or are you a reflective processor, who has to think about new material before internalizing it?
- After completing this activity, write down the combination of your perceiving and processing learning styles and share it with your instructor.

- *Stage 4* learners are *concrete active* learners. These students are concerned about how they can use what they learn to make a difference in their lives. If you fall into this stage, you like to relate new material to other areas of your life. You have leadership capabilities, can create on your feet, and usually are vocal in a group, but you may have difficulty completing your work on time. Stage 4 learners enjoy teaching others and working in groups and learn best when they can apply new information to real-world problems.

To get the most out of knowing your learning profile, you need to apply this knowledge to how you approach learning. Each of the learning stages has pluses and minuses. When faced with a learning situation that does not match your learning preference, see how you can adapt your individual learning profile to make the best of the information. For example, if you are bored by lectures, look for an opportunity to apply the information being presented to a real problem you are facing in the classroom or at home. If you are an abstract perceiver, take time outside of class to think about new information so that you are ready to process it into your learning system. If you benefit from learning in a group, make the effort to organize review sessions and study groups. If you learn best by teaching others, offer to assist your peers with their learning. By taking the time now to investigate your preferred method of learning, you will perceive and process information more effectively throughout your school career.

CRITICAL THINKING APPLICATION   1.6

Take a few minutes to reflect on a time when you really enjoyed learning about something new. How was the material presented, and what did you do to "make it your own"? What do you need to do to become a more effective learner?

Study Skills: Tricks for Becoming a Successful Student

Let's investigate some ideas that are useful for learning new material. These study skills include memory techniques, active learning, brain tricks, reading methods, and note-taking strategies.

Several techniques can help you store and remember information. The first of these involves organizing information into recognizable groups so that the brain can find it easily. You can organize information by getting the big picture first before trying to learn the details. One way to implement this strategy is to skim a reading assignment before actually reading and taking notes on the material, thus getting a general impression of what you need to learn before tackling the details. Depending on your learning style, it may also help to find a way of making the new information meaningful. Think about your educational goals and how the new material will help you achieve those goals.

Another way of remembering material is to create an association with something you already know. If new material is grouped with already stored material, the brain remembers it much more easily. For example, maybe you took a biology class in high school and learned the basics about human anatomy and physiology. Try to create a link between what you previously learned and the details of the new information you are expected to learn now. Or maybe you have a family member who suffers from a particular disease. Think about that individual's signs and symptoms while learning more details about the disease so that you can apply your learning to his or her situation.

A useful study skill for some learners is to be physically active while learning. Some students learn best if they walk or talk out loud while studying. Besides encouraging learning, moving and talking while studying relieve boredom and keep you awake. Another way to be actively involved in learning is to use pictures or diagrams to represent the material you are studying. Some people are visual learners, and creating pictures of the material is the easiest method for them to retain the information. Other students find that rewriting notes, making lists of information, creating flash cards, color-coding notes, or highlighting important material in a textbook helps them retain the material. Writing also helps students who need to "do" something to learn.

Studying goes much more smoothly if you work with your brain rather than against it. If you tend to get anxious and worried while studying, you may be acting as your own worst enemy. One way of dealing with a topic you are anxious about is to **overlearn** it. If material is overlearned, you are much less likely to experience test anxiety. Another method for remembering material is to review it quickly after class. This mini-review helps the new information become part of your long-term memory system.

Many students find creating songs, dances, or word associations an effective way to learn and remember new material. Putting details into a familiar song and moving to it can help trick the brain into remembering the information. This is especially helpful when trying to learn anatomy and physiology. For example, think about one of your favorite songs and "dance" your way through the blood flow through the heart. Or, if you are finding the organization of the body especially tricky to remember, such as the movement of food through the gastrointestinal (GI) system, create a **mnemonic** that helps you remember the information. The most common one suggested for the parts of the intestines is: **D**ow **J**ones **I**ndustrial **C**limbing **A**verage **C**losing **S**tock **R**eport. The first letter of each word stands for an anatomic part of the intestines – *d*uodenum, *j*ejunum, *i*leum, *c*ecum, *a*ppendix, *c*olon, *s*igmoid, and *r*ectum. You can make up your own mnemonics or memory tricks to help you learn complicated material.

Another excellent way of learning information is to actually teach it to someone else. Teaching requires you to have a good understanding of the material and the ability to describe it for others. It can be an effective reinforcement of complicated material.

A great deal of the learning process is expected to take place from assigned readings. You can use several methods to make reading assignments more meaningful. If you find a reading assignment challenging or difficult to understand, the first step is to take the time to read it again. Sometimes the first time through the material is not enough to gain understanding. As you read, highlight important words or thoughts and stop periodically to summarize the material. Some students find outlining new material helpful. This is another way to use active learning to help you make the information "your own."

If you get bored while reading, use your body; walk or talk your way through the assignment. Take the time to look up words or terms you do not understand or ask your instructor or tutor for help. The best way to determine whether you have learned anything from your reading is to try to explain the material to someone else. For example, you can meet with other students and explain to them what you learned. If you can do that effectively, you know you have acquired the knowledge needed from the reading assignment.

Many students find effective note taking a challenge. The big question is, "How much of what the instructor says do I actually need to write down?" The first step in effective note taking is to come to class prepared. The more familiar you are with the material, the easier it will be to determine the important parts of the instructor's lecture. Pay attention to the instructor and look for clues to what he or she thinks is important. Ask questions about the material if you do not understand it, rather than writing down information that makes no sense to you. Think critically about what you hear before you write it down, so you can start to build relationships among the things you want or need to know.

If your instructor uses PowerPoint presentations to teach a lesson, request copies of the slides before the lecture so you have an opportunity to review them as you are doing your reading. Many courses have an online website where PowerPoints or other lecture materials are available for review. Take advantage of these added materials to be prepared for each class so that you can ask questions about anything you don't understand. In addition, this textbook has an extensive online site that you can access for learning resources. Investigate the site and see whether something there can help you reach your learning goals.

When it comes to actual note taking, some strategies can make the process of recording notes an active learning tool. Organize the information as much as possible while you are writing or typing, either in an outline or a paragraph format. If you take notes on a laptop or tablet, make sure your keyboarding skills are good enough for you to keep up with the flow of information and that you review your notes shortly after class to fill in any missing details. If you take notes on paper, use only one side of the page (for easier reading) and leave blank spaces where needed to fill in details later. Use key words to help you remember the material and create pictures or diagrams to help visualize it. If permitted, record the lecture and make sure you have copies of any handouts or notes distributed by your instructor that cover material written on the board or provided in a PowerPoint presentation. If your instructor refers the class to a YouTube video or other website, transcribe the site address correctly to refer to it at a later time. Another helpful tool is to develop your own system of abbreviations to help simplify the note-taking process.

The most effective way to use your notes is to review them shortly after class and then find a time to review them every day. This is the time to add details, clarify information, or make notes about asking the instructor for explanations during the next class. You could even exchange notes with students you trust to compare information. Some students find it beneficial to create an electronic copy of their notes (if they wrote them out on paper) or to rewrite them. This gives you an opportunity to learn the material as you transcribe it. As you are reviewing your notes, you also can draw mind maps of the information or diagram outlines to help you better understand and remember the material.

Creating mind maps is a way of representing the main idea of a topic and supporting important details with a figure or picture. Healthcare textbooks present complicated concepts with multiple main ideas, each with its own important details. Mind maps are a way of combining complex details and organizing them into a format that is easier to remember. The *spider map* (Fig. 1.3) presents a method for including several main ideas with details in one study guide. The *fishbone map* (Fig. 1.4) can be used to learn complicated causes of disease. The *chain-of-events map* (Fig. 1.5) displays the cause and effect of events, such as infection control or the history of medicine. The *cycle map* (Fig. 1.6) shows the connection between factors, such

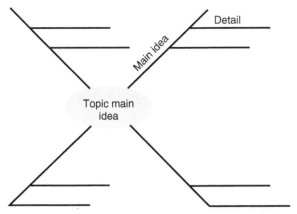

FIGURE 1.3 Spider map showing multiple main ideas with supporting details.

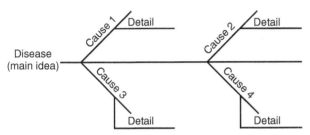

FIGURE 1.4 Fishbone map used to describe cause of disease.

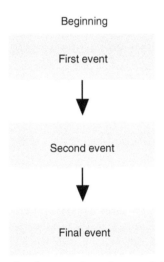

FIGURE 1.5 Chain-of-events map showing the cause and effect of events.

as in the chain of infection. Creating your own mind maps is a way of making the information more meaningful and easier for you to understand and remember.

Although many techniques can help you study, perhaps the most important one is your attitude toward learning. Some students fall into the "I can't possibly learn this material" trap. That type of attitude only leads to self-defeat. The way to overcome barriers is first to recognize that they exist. Once you know your weak spots, use the suggested study skills to improve in those areas. Do not be afraid to ask questions or to ask for help if you do not understand the material. Use as many different strategies as necessary to become a successful student.

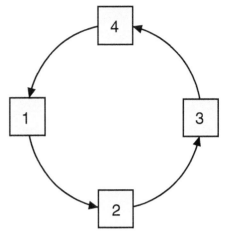

FIGURE 1.6 Cycle map illustrating the way one action leads to another.

CRITICAL THINKING APPLICATION   **1.7**
Write down at least two barriers to learning that you face. Review the study skills suggestions and choose four to try out. Use them over the next week to help you learn new material. Reflect on whether the chosen study skills helped you learn the material better.

Test-Taking Strategies: Taking Charge of Your Success

What happens when you do not know the answer to the first question on a test? What if you do not know the next one? Are you able to go on without panicking? Many people find taking tests the most challenging part of being a successful student. Multiple approaches are available that you can use to take charge of your success and improve your ability to take tests. These include such strategies as adequate preparation, controlling negative thoughts during test time, and understanding ways to manage various types of questions.

The first step is to go into a test adequately prepared. Use the time management skills discussed later in this chapter to prepare for the big day. Recognize and use your preferred learning style to overlearn the material and increase your confidence. Use memory tools (e.g., flash cards, checklists, and mind maps) to help you visualize the material. Form a study group if you are the type of learner who benefits from studying in groups. Schedule and plan study time and reward yourself for your hard work. It also is important to go into the test rested and relaxed; therefore, you should eat, exercise to relieve stress, and sleep before the test so that you are as alert as possible.

Before you start the test, make sure you read the directions carefully. If possible, begin with the easiest or shortest questions to build your confidence. Be aware of the amount of time allotted for the examination, and pace yourself accordingly. As you go through the test, look for clues to answers in other questions. During test time, remember to use positive self-talk at the first indication of panic. Repeatedly remind yourself that you are well prepared; relax and think about the material before you get worried. You need to stop negative thoughts as soon as they arise and instead visualize yourself being successful. Use slow, deep breathing to relax and, if helpful, close your eyes for a minute and visualize a relaxing place before you go on with the test.

Certain strategies are useful for answering different types of questions. With multiple choice questions, try to identify key words or clues in each question. Read the question carefully and answer it in your head before you review the provided answers. If you are not absolutely sure of the answer, make an educated guess or follow your instincts in choosing an answer. If there are answers that you know are not correct, that can eliminate the "all of the above" answer choice. By eliminating the answers that you know are incorrect, you can focus on the other answer choices.

"True or false" questions give you a 50/50 chance of being correct. Remember that if any part of the question is not true, then the statement is false. Again, check the statements for key words that help indicate the direction of the answer. Look for qualifying terms (e.g., *always, never, sometimes*) that are the key to understanding the meaning of the true or false statement.

CRITICAL THINKING APPLICATION   1.8
Think about a time you experienced test anxiety. Write down the details of the situation and how you felt. Choose four test-taking strategies you think would be beneficial for handling similar situations in the future.

Becoming a Critical Thinker: Making Mental Connections

The ability to process information and arrive at reasonable conclusions is crucial to all healthcare workers. The process of **critical thinking** involves (1) sorting out conflicting information, (2) weighing your knowledge about that information, (3) ignoring or letting go of personal biases, and (4) deciding on a reasonable belief or action. Critical thinking is actually an active search for the truth.

Critical thinking could be described as thorough thinking because it requires learners to keep an open mind to all possibilities. Successful students are thorough thinkers because they must determine the facts about a topic and come to logical conclusions about the material. Critical thinkers also are inquisitive learners; they constantly analyze and sort out conflicting information to reach conclusions.

A crucial step in critical thinking is evaluating the results of your learning. Reflection is the key to critical thinking. "How did I learn what I learned?" and "What does it mean in my life?" are questions that must be asked consistently to continue to learn. Becoming a successful student, and ultimately a successful member of the allied health team, requires critical thinking skills.

Using these tools to become the best possible medical assistant student will also help you become the best possible professional medical assistant.

THE HISTORY OF MEDICINE

Although religious and mythologic beliefs were the basis for care for the sick in ancient times, evidence suggests that drugs, surgery, and other treatments based on theories about the body were used as early as 5000 BC. Moses presented rules of health to the Hebrews in approximately 1205 BC. He was the first advocate of preventive medicine and is considered the first public health officer. Moses knew that some animal diseases could be passed to humans and that **contamination** existed; therefore, a religious law was developed forbidding humans to eat or drink from dirty dishes. The people of

that era believed that doing so would defile their bodies, and they would lose their souls.

Hippocrates, known as the Father of Medicine, is the most famous of the ancient Greek physicians. He was born in 450 BC on the island of Cos in Greece. He is best remembered for the Hippocratic Oath, which has been administered to physicians for more than 2000 years. To this day, most graduating medical school students swear to some form of the oath (Fig. 1.7).

Hippocrates is credited with taking mysticism out of medicine and giving it a scientific basis. During this period of history, most believed that illness was caused by demonic possession; to cure the illness, the demon had to be removed from the body. Hippocrates' clinical descriptions of diseases and his volumes on epidemics, fevers, epilepsy, fractures, and instruments were studied for centuries. He believed that the body had the capacity to heal itself and that the physician's role was to help nature. It is also interesting to see that Hippocrates addressed confidentiality and understood that it was important to maintain patient privacy.

Medical knowledge developed slowly, and distribution of such knowledge was poor. In the 17th century, European academies or societies were established, consisting of small groups of men who met to discuss subjects of mutual interest. One of the earliest academies was the Royal Society of London, formed in 1662. In the United States, medical education was greatly influenced by the Johns Hopkins University School of Medicine in Baltimore, Maryland, established in the early 1890s. The school admitted only college graduates with at least one year's training in the natural sciences. The clinical education at Johns Hopkins was superior because the school partnered with Johns Hopkins Hospital, which had been created expressly for teaching and research by members of the medical faculty. Table 1.3 presents selected medical pioneers and their achievements.

The History of Medical Assisting

As physicians made the switch from going to patients' homes for treatment to having the patient come to their office, some physicians hired nurses to help in their practices. Gradually, the administrative part of running a practice became increasingly complicated and time-consuming, and physicians realized that they needed an assistant with both administrative and clinical training. Nurses were likely to have training only in clinical skills; therefore, many physicians began training individuals – medical assistants – to assist with all the office duties.

The first medical assistants started working in individual physicians' offices with on-the-job training to help out when an extra pair of hands was needed. Today medical assisting is one of the most respected allied health fields in the industry, and training is readily available through community colleges, junior colleges, and private educational institutions throughout the United States.

CRITICAL THINKING APPLICATION   1.9
- In Table 1.3, review the list of individuals who have made significant contributions to medicine. Which one do you believe had the greatest impact on modern healthcare?
- Consider how the medical assisting profession began. How do you think advances in medicine throughout history have affected the current practice of medical assisting?

I swear to fulfill, to the best of my ability and judgment, this covenant:

I will respect the hard-won scientific gains of those physicians in whose steps I walk, and gladly share such knowledge as is mine with those who are to follow.

I will apply, for the benefit of the sick, all measures [that] are required, avoiding those twin traps of overtreatment and therapeutic nihilism.

I will remember that there is art to medicine as well as science, and that warmth, sympathy, and understanding may outweigh the surgeon's knife or the chemist's drug.

I will not be ashamed to say "I know not," nor will I fail to call in my colleagues when the skills of another are needed for a patient's recovery.

I will respect the privacy of my patients, for their problems are not disclosed to me that the world may know. Most especially must I tread with care in matters of life and death. If it is given me to save a life, all thanks. But it may also be within my power to take a life; this awesome responsibility must be faced with great humbleness and awareness of my own frailty. Above all, I must not play at God.

I will remember that I do not treat a fever chart, a cancerous growth, but a sick human being, whose illness may affect the person's family and economic stability. My responsibility includes these related problems, if I am to care adequately for the sick.

I will prevent disease whenever I can, for prevention is preferable to cure.

I will remember that I remain a member of society, with special obligations to all my fellow human beings, those sound of mind and body as well as the infirm.

If I do not violate this oath, may I enjoy life and art, respected while I live and remembered with affection thereafter. May I always act so as to preserve the finest traditions of my calling and may I long experience the joy of healing those who seek my help.

Written in 1964 by Louis Lasagna, Academic Dean of the School of Medicine at Tufts University, and used in many medical schools today.

FIGURE 1.7 Modern version of the Hippocratic Oath.

MEDICAL PROFESSIONALS

Now that you have an understanding of the medical assistant profession, let's take a look at other areas in healthcare. Physicians and providers (e.g., nurse practitioners and physician assistants) are portals of entry or first contacts for patients seeking medical care. *Primary care providers* (PCPs) are healthcare practitioners who monitor a patient's overall health. Family medicine, internal medicine, and pediatrics are generally considered primary care specialties. After the initial assessment or with the diagnosis of a more complex health issue, patients may be referred to a medical specialist for further examination and treatment.

Doctors of Medicine

Medical doctors (Doctor of Medicine [MD]) are considered **allopathic** physicians. They are the most widely recognized type of physician. They diagnose illness and disease and prescribe treatment for their patients. MDs have a wide variety of rights, including writing prescriptions, performing surgery, offering wellness advice, and performing preventive medicine procedures. Becoming an MD requires 4 years of undergraduate university training (premed) and 4 years of medical school. Regardless of where premed students attend college, a national standard of course work is required to apply to medical school. They must take entry and advanced levels of biology, physics, organic and inorganic chemistry, mathematics, English, humanities, and social sciences. The United States has approximately 125 allopathic medical schools. After medical school, the student faces 3 to 8 years of residency

programs, depending on the medical specialty he or she pursues. After completion of a residency program, a physician can obtain board certification in one or more of 37 different specialty areas recognized by the American Board of Medical Specialties (Table 1.4). An MD must have a state license to practice, and continuing education is required to maintain the license. Graduates of foreign medical schools usually can obtain a license in the United States after passing an examination and completing a residency program in this country.

Doctors of Osteopathy

Osteopathic physicians (Doctor of Osteopathy [DO]) complete requirements similar to those of MDs to graduate and practice medicine. Osteopaths use medicine and surgery, in addition to osteopathic manipulative therapy (OMT), in treating their patients. Andrew Taylor Still is considered the father of osteopathic medicine, which he established in 1874. He believed in a more **holistic** approach to medicine, and although he was an MD, he founded the American School of Osteopathy in Kirksville, Missouri. The school originally was chartered to offer an MD degree but later focused more on the osteopathic approach. DOs stress preventive medicine and holistic patient care, in addition to a special focus on the musculoskeletal system and OMT. Premed students moving toward osteopathic medicine complete the same undergraduate course work as allopathic candidates and 4 years of medical studies at a school for osteopathic medicine. Over the years there have become fewer differences between allopathic and osteopathic programs, with many DO physicians earning residency programs in the same institutions as MDs.

TABLE 1.3   Medical Pioneers and Their Achievements

NAME	ACHIEVEMENT	NAME	ACHIEVEMENT
Andreas Vesalius (1514–1564)	Father of modern anatomy; wrote first anatomy book	Robert Koch (1843–1910)	Developed Koch's postulates, a theory of causative agents for disease; discovered the cause of cholera
William Harvey (1578–1657)	Discovered the circulatory system	William Roentgen (1845–1923)	Discovered the x-ray
Anton van Leeuwenhoek (1632–1723)	First to observe microbes through a lens; developed the first microscope	Walter Reed (1851–1902)	Proved that yellow fever was transmitted by mosquito bites while in the U.S. Army serving in Cuba
John Hunter (1728–1793)	Founder of scientific surgery	Paul Ehrlich (1854–1915)	Injected chemicals for the first time to treat disease (syphilis)
Edward Jenner (1749–1823)	Developed smallpox vaccine	Marie Curie (1867–1934)	Discovered radium and polonium
Ignaz Semmelweis (1818–1865)	First physician to recommend hand washing to prevent puerperal fever; believed there was a connection between performing autopsies and then delivering babies that caused puerperal fever in new mothers	Alexander Fleming (1881–1955)	Discovered penicillin
		Albert Sabin (1906–1993)	Developed the oral live-virus vaccine for polio 10 years after Salk developed the first injected vaccine
Florence Nightingale (1820–1910)	Founder of nursing	Virginia Apgar (1909–1974)	Founded neonatology; developed the Apgar score, which assesses the status of newborns
Clara Barton (1821–1912)	Established the American Red Cross	Jonas Salk (1914–1955)	Developed the first safe and effective injectable vaccine for polio
Elizabeth Blackwell (1821–1910)	First woman in the United States to earn a Doctor of Medicine degree	Christiaan Barnard (1922–2001)	Performed the first human heart transplant
Louis Pasteur (1822–1895)	Father of bacteriology and preventive medicine; developed pasteurization and established the connection between germs and disease	Edwin Carl Wood (1929–2011)	Pioneered the technique of in vitro fertilization (IVF)
Joseph Lister (1827–1912)	Father of sterile surgery; developed antiseptic methods for surgery	David Ho (1952–)	Research pioneer in acquired immunodeficiency syndrome (AIDS)

TABLE 1.4   Examples of Medical Specialties

SPECIALTY	PRACTITIONER'S TITLE	DESCRIPTION
Allergy and immunology	Allergist/ immunologist	Allergists/immunologists are trained to evaluate disorders and diseases of the immune system. This includes conditions such as adverse reactions to drugs and food, anaphylaxis, and problems related to autoimmune diseases, asthma, and insect stings.
Anesthesiology	Anesthesiologist	Anesthesiologists provide pain relief and pain management during surgical procedures and also for patients with long-standing conditions accompanied by pain.
Colon and rectal surgery	Colorectal surgeon	Colorectal surgeons diagnose and treat conditions affecting the intestines, rectum, and anal area, in addition to organs affected by intestinal disease.
Dermatology	Dermatologist	Dermatologists work with adult and pediatric patients in treating disorders and diseases of the skin, hair, nails, and related tissues. Dermatologists are specially trained to manage conditions such as skin cancers, cosmetic disorders of the skin, scars, allergies, and other disorders, both malignant and benign.

TABLE 1.4   Examples of Medical Specialties—*continued*

SPECIALTY	PRACTITIONER'S TITLE	DESCRIPTION
Emergency medicine	Emergency physician	Emergency physicians are experts in assessing and treating a patient to prevent death or serious disability. They provide immediate care to stabilize the patient's condition, and then refer the patient to the appropriate professional for further care.
Family medicine	Primary care provider (PCP)	PCPs offer care to the whole family, from newborns to elderly adults. They are familiar with a wide range of disorders and diseases, and preventive care is their primary concern.
General surgery	Surgeon	General surgeons correct deformities and defects and treat diseases or injured parts of the body by means of operative treatment.
Genetics	Medical geneticist	Geneticists are physicians trained to diagnose and treat patients with conditions related to genetically linked diseases. They provide genetic counseling when indicated.
Internal medicine	Internist	Internists are concerned with comprehensive care, often diagnosing and treating those with chronic, long-term conditions. They must have a broad understanding of the body and its ailments.
Neurologic surgery	Neurosurgeon	Neurosurgeons provide surgical care for patients with conditions of the central, autonomic, and peripheral nervous systems.
Neurology/psychiatry	Neurologist/psychiatrist	Neurologists diagnose and treat disorders of the nervous system. Psychiatrists are physicians who specialize in the diagnosis and treatment of people with mental, emotional, or behavioral disorders. A psychiatrist is qualified to conduct psychotherapy and to prescribe medications.
Nuclear medicine	Nuclear medicine specialist	These specialists use radioactive substances to diagnose, treat, and detect disease.
Obstetrics and gynecology	Obstetrician/gynecologist	Obstetricians provide care to women of childbearing age and monitor the progress of the developing child. Gynecologists are concerned with the diagnosis and treatment of the female reproductive system.
Ophthalmology	Ophthalmologist	Ophthalmologists diagnose, treat, and provide comprehensive care for the eye and its supporting structures. These physicians also offer vision services, including corrective lenses.
Otolaryngology	Otolaryngologist	Otolaryngologists treat diseases and conditions that affect the ear, nose, and throat and structures related to the head and neck. Problems that affect the voice and hearing are also referred to this specialist.
Pathology	Pathologist	Pathologists study the causes of diseases. They study tissues and cells, body fluids, and organs themselves to aid in the process of diagnosis.
Pediatrics	Pediatrician	Pediatricians promote preventive medicine and treat diseases that affect children and adolescents. They monitor the child's growth and development and provide a wide range of health services.
Physical medicine and rehabilitation	Physiatrist	Physiatrists assist patients who have physical disabilities. This may include rehabilitation, patients with musculoskeletal disorders, and patients suffering from pain as a result of injury or trauma.
Plastic surgery	Plastic surgeon	Plastic surgeons work with patients who have a physical defect as a result of some type of injury or condition. They perform reconstructive cosmetic enhancements and elective procedures.
Preventive medicine	Preventive medicine specialist	Preventive medicine specialists are concerned with preventing mental and physical illness and disability. They also analyze current health services and plan for future medical needs.
Radiology	Radiologist	Radiology is a specialty in which x-rays are used to diagnose and treat disease. A diagnostic radiologist specializes in using x-rays, ultrasound, nuclear medicine, computed tomography, and magnetic resonance imaging to detect abnormalities throughout the body.
Thoracic surgery	Thoracic surgeon	Thoracic surgeons are concerned with the operative treatment of the chest and chest wall, lungs, heart, heart valves, and respiratory passages.
Urology	Urologist	Urologists are concerned with the treatment of diseases and disorders of the urinary tract. They diagnose and manage problems with the genitourinary system and practice endoscopic procedures related to these structures.

Doctors of Chiropractic

Chiropractors (Doctor of Chiropractic [DC]) focus on the relationship between the spine and the function of the body. The goal is to correct alignment problems and thereby alleviate pain, improve function, and support the body's natural ability to heal itself. Spinal manipulation has been shown to be beneficial for low back pain, headaches, neck pain, whiplash-associated disorders, and upper and lower extremity joint conditions. Chiropractic care is one of the most common fields of **complementary and alternative medicine (CAM)**. Examples of complementary and alternative medicine can be found in the following box.

Complementary and Alternative Medicine Therapies

- Chiropractic
- Massage therapy
- Acupuncture
- Biofeedback
- Meditation
- Guided imagery
- Healing touch
- Natural products
- Yoga, Tai Chi, or Qi Gong
- Homeopathy
- Naturopathy
- Progressive relaxation
- Hypnotherapy
- Ayurvedic medicine

Chiropractic doctors have at least 4 years of additional training beyond a bachelor's degree. The training includes both classroom and direct patient care. The doctors must pass the national licensing exam. State law regulates their practice, and many state boards require continuing education to maintain the license.

Hospitalists

Hospitalists are physicians whose primary professional focus is the general medical care of hospitalized patients. Most hospitalists are employed by the healthcare facility instead of having individual freestanding offices in which patients are seen and treated. Perhaps the most attractive benefit of becoming a hospitalist is the quality of life for the physician and his or her family. Hospitalists work a specific, set number of hours each week and receive a set salary from their employers. In addition, most institutions that employ hospitalists cover these physicians with blanket malpractice insurance, saving the practitioner the expense of costly premiums. Although the hospitalist is in charge of the patient while the person is in the hospital, if the patient has a PCP, he or she may still visit the patient. The hospitalist would still refer the patient to medical specialists as needed for more advanced care.

Nurse Practitioners

Nurse practitioners (NPs) provide basic patient care services, including diagnosing and prescribing medications for common illnesses, or they may have additional training and expertise in a specialty area of medicine. These professionals must have advanced academic training beyond the registered nurse (RN) degree and also vast clinical experience. An NP is licensed by individual states and can practice independently or as part of a team of healthcare professionals.

Physician Assistants

A physician assistant (PA) is a certified healthcare professional who provides diagnostic, therapeutic, and preventive healthcare services under the supervision of a medical doctor. Physician assistants must be licensed, which requires completion of a physician assistant program that is typically at the master's degree level. Physician assistants must pass the Physician Assistant National Certifying Examination to practice in any state. They may also complete advanced training to focus on a particular specialty practice.

ALLIED HEALTH PROFESSIONALS

In addition to doctors, nurse practitioners, and physician assistants the healthcare team includes allied health professionals. The definition of an allied health professional can vary, but it loosely refers to those who can act only under the authority of a licensed medical practitioner (e.g., MD, DO, optometrist, dentist, pharmacist, podiatrist, or chiropractor). Allied health professionals include respiratory therapists, radiation therapists, occupational therapists, physical therapists, technologists of various types, dental hygienists, medical assistants, phlebotomists, pharmacy technicians, and other professionals who do not independently diagnose and prescribe treatment, but perform diagnostic procedures, therapeutic services, and provide care.

The allied health professions fall into two broad categories: technicians (assistants) and therapists. Technicians are trained to perform procedures, and their education lasts 2 years or less. They are required to work under the supervision of medical providers or licensed therapists. This part of the allied health field includes, among others, physical therapy assistants, medical laboratory technicians, radiology technicians, occupational therapy assistants, recreational therapy assistants, respiratory therapy technicians, and medical assistants (Table 1.5).

The educational process for nurses and therapists is more intensive. These professions require a state-issued license and an advanced degree, showing that the individual is trained to evaluate patients, diagnose conditions, develop treatment plans, and understand the rationale behind various treatments (Table 1.6).

Allied health professionals typically work as part of a healthcare team, which is what you will do as a professional medical assistant.

As a new medical assistant, you will enter the ranks of an ever-growing group of allied health professionals who provide services for patients in a variety of settings in today's healthcare system. Allied health professionals comprise nearly 60% of the healthcare workforce. The term "allied health" is used to identify a cluster of health professions, encompassing as many as 200 careers. In the United States, about 5 million allied health professionals work in more than 80 different professions; they represent approximately 60% of all healthcare providers.

TYPES OF HEALTHCARE FACILITIES

Hospitals

Hospitals are classified according to the type of care and services they provide to patients and by the type of ownership. There are three different levels of hospitalized care, which are interconnected.

TABLE 1.5	Allied Health Occupations Recognized by the American Medical Association	
TITLE	CREDENTIAL	JOB DESCRIPTION
Anesthesiology assistant	AA	Functions as a specialty physician assistant under the direction of a licensed and qualified anesthesiologist; assists in developing and implementing the anesthesia care plan.
Art therapist	ATR	Uses drawings and other art and media forms to assess, treat, and rehabilitate patients with mental, emotional, physical, and/or developmental disorders.
Athletic trainer	ATC	Provides a variety of services, including injury prevention, assessment, immediate care, treatment, and rehabilitation after physical injury or trauma.
Audiologist	CCC-A	Identifies individuals with symptoms of hearing loss and other auditory, balance, and related neural problems; assesses the nature of those problems and helps individuals manage them.
Blood bank technology specialist	SBB	Performs routine and specialized tests in blood center and transfusion services, using methods that conform to the accepted standards in the blood bank industry.
Diagnostic cardiovascular sonographer/ technologist	RDCS, RVT	Using invasive or noninvasive techniques (or both), performs diagnostic examinations and therapeutic interventions for the heart and blood vessels at the request of a physician.
Clinical laboratory science/medical technologist	MT, MLT	In conjunction with pathologists, performs tests to diagnose the causes and nature of disease; also develops data on blood, tissues, and fluids of the human body using a variety of methodologies.
Counseling-related professional	LPC, LMHC	Deals with human development through support, therapeutic approaches, consultation, evaluation, teaching, and research; practices the art of helping people to grow.
Cytotechnologist	CT	Works with pathologists to evaluate cellular material from all body sites, primarily through use of the microscope; examines specimens for normal and abnormal cytologic changes, including malignancies.
Dance therapist	DTR, ADTR	Uses the psychotherapeutic properties of movement as a process that furthers the emotional, cognitive, social, and physical integration of the patient as a tool for healing.
Dental assistant, dental hygienist, dental laboratory technician	CDA, RDH, CDT	Performs a wide range of tasks, from assisting the dentist to teaching patients how to prevent oral disease and maintain oral health.
Diagnostic medical sonographer	RDMS	Uses medical ultrasound to gather sonographic data, which can aid the diagnosis of a variety of conditions and diseases; also monitors fetal development.
Dietitian, dietetic technician	DTR	Integrates and applies the principles of food science, nutrition, biochemistry, physiology, food management, and behavior to achieve and maintain good health.
Electroneurodiagnostic technologist	REEG-T	Records and studies the electrical activity of the brain and nervous system; obtains interpretable recordings of patients' nervous system function.
Genetics counselor	IGC	Provides genetic services to individuals and families seeking information about the occurrence or risk of a genetic condition or birth defect.
Health information management professional	RHIA, RHIT	Provides expert assistance in the systems and processes for health information management, including planning, engineering, administration, application, and policy making.
Kinesiotherapist	RKT	Provides rehabilitation exercise and education designed to reverse or minimize debilitation and enhance the functional capacity of medically stable patients.
Massage therapist	MT	Applies manual techniques, and may apply adjunctive techniques, with the intention of positively affecting the health and well-being of a patient or client.

Continued

TABLE 1.5   Allied Health Occupations Recognized by the American Medical Association—*continued*

TITLE	CREDENTIAL	JOB DESCRIPTION
Medical assistant	CMA, RMA, CCMA, CMAA	Functions as a member of the healthcare delivery team and performs both administrative and clinical procedures and duties; a multiskilled health professional.
Medical illustrator	MI	Specializes in the visual display and communication of scientific information; creates visuals and designs communication tools for teaching both medical professionals and the public.
Music therapist	MT-BC	Uses music in a therapeutic relationship to address the physical, emotional, cognitive, and social needs of individuals of all ages; assesses the strengths and needs of clients and patients.
Nuclear medicine technologist	RT	Uses the nuclear properties of radioactive and stable nuclides to make diagnostic evaluations of anatomic or physiologic conditions of the body; also provides therapy with unsealed radioactive sources.
Ophthalmic laboratory technician, medical technician/technologist	COT, COMT	Collects data and performs clinical evaluations; performs tests and protocols required by ophthalmologists; assists in the treatment of patients.
Orthoptist	CO	Performs a series of diagnostic tests and measurements on patients with visual disorders; helps design a treatment plan to correct disorders of vision, eye movements, and alignment.
Orthotist/prosthetist	RTO, RTP, RTPO	Designs and fits devices (orthoses) to patients who have disabling conditions of the limbs and spine and/or partial or total absence of a limb.
Perfusionist	CCP	Operates extracorporeal circulation and autotransfusion equipment during any medical situation in which the patient's respiratory or circulatory function must be supported or temporarily replaced.
Pharmacy technician	CPhT	Assists pharmacists with duties that do not require the expertise or judgment of a licensed pharmacist.
Radiation therapist, radiographer	RRTD	Delivers prescribed dosages of radiation to patients for therapeutic purposes; provides appropriate patient care and maintains accurate records of the treatment provided.
Rehabilitation counselor	CRC	Determines and coordinates services to assist people with disabilities in moving from psychological and economic dependence to independence.
Respiratory therapist, respiratory therapy technician	RRT, CRT, RPFT, CPFT	Evaluates, treats, and manages patients of all ages with respiratory illnesses and other cardiopulmonary disorders. Advanced respiratory therapists exercise considerable independent judgment.
Surgical assistant	CSA	Assists in exposure, hemostasis, closure, and other intraoperative technical functions that help surgeons carry out a safe operation with optimal results for the patient.
Surgical technologist	ST, CST	Helps prepare patients for surgery and maintain the sterile field in the surgical suite, making sure all members of the surgical team follow sterile technique.
Therapeutic recreation specialist	CTRS	Uses treatment, education, and recreation services to help people with illnesses, disabilities, and other conditions develop and use their leisure in ways that enhance their health.

- Primary level of care
  - Smaller city or community hospitals
  - Usually serve as the first level of contact between the community members and the hospital setting
- Secondary level of care
  - Both PCPs and specialists provide care
  - Larger municipal or district hospitals that provide a wider variety of specialty care and departments

- Tertiary level of care
  - Referral system for primary or secondary care facilities
  - Provide care for complicated cases and trauma
  - Medical centers, regional and specialty hospitals

Private hospitals are run by a corporation or other organization and usually are designed to produce a profit for the owners or stockholders. *Nonprofit* hospitals exist to serve the community in which they are located and are normally run by a board of directors.

TABLE 1.6   Licensed Healthcare Professions

TITLE	CREDENTIAL	JOB DESCRIPTION
Certified nurse midwife	CNM	Registered nurse (RN) with additional training and certification; performs physical exams; prescribes medications, including contraceptive methods; orders laboratory tests as needed; provides prenatal care, gynecologic care, labor and birth care, and health education and counseling to women of all ages.
Diagnostic cardiac sonographer or vascular technologist	DCS or DVT	Assists in the diagnosis and treatment of cardiac and vascular diseases and disorders; performs noninvasive tests, including echocardiographs and electrocardiographs.
Emergency medical technician	EMT	Progresses through several levels of training, each providing more advanced skills. EMTs' medical education encompasses managing respiratory, cardiac, and trauma cases and often emergency childbirth. Some states also recognize specialties in the EMT field, such as EMT-Cardiac, which includes training in cardiac arrhythmias, and EMT-Shock Trauma, which includes starting intravenous fluids and administering specific medications.
Licensed practical or vocational nurse	LPN or LVN	Provides bedside care, assisting with the day-to-day personal care of inpatients; assesses patients, documents their progress, and administers medications and intravenous fluids when allowed by law; often works in hospitals or skilled nursing facilities and in physicians' offices.
Medical technologist	MT	Performs diagnostic testing on blood, body fluids, and other types of specimens to assist the provider in arriving at a diagnosis.
Nurse anesthetist	NA	RN who administers anesthetics to patients during care provided by surgeons, physicians, dentists, or other qualified health professionals.
Nurse practitioner	NP	Provides basic patient care services, including diagnosing and prescribing medications for common illnesses; must have advanced academic training, beyond the registered nurse (RN) degree, and also must have extensive clinical experience.
Occupational therapist	OT	Assists in helping patients compensate for loss of function.
Paramedic	Paramedic	Specially trained in advanced emergency skills to aid patients in life-threatening situations.
Physical therapist	PT	Assists patients in regaining their mobility and improving their strength and range of motion. Devises treatment plans in conjunction with the patient's physician.
Physician assistant	PA	Provides direct patient care services under the supervision of a licensed physician; trained to diagnose and treat patients as directed by the physician. In most states is allowed to write prescriptions; take patient histories, order and interpret tests, perform physical examinations, and make diagnostic decisions.
Radiology technician	RT	Uses various machines to help the provider diagnose and treat certain diseases; machines may include x-ray equipment, ultrasonographic machines, and magnetic resonance imaging (MRI) scanners.
Registered dietitian	RD	Thoroughly trained in nutrition and the different types of diets patients require to improve or maintain their condition. Designs healthy diets for patients during hospital stays and can help plan menus for home use. Also teaches patients about their recommended diet.
Registered nurse	RN	Provides direct patient care, assesses patients, and determines care plans; has many career options.
Respiratory therapist	RT	Commonly uses oxygen therapy to assist with breathing; also performs diagnostic tests that measure lung capacity. Most work in hospitals. All types of patients receive respiratory care, including newborns and geriatric patients.

The term *nonprofit* sometimes is misleading, because "profit" is different from "making money." A nonprofit hospital or organization may make money in a campaign or fundraiser, but all of the money is returned to the organization. Nonprofit hospitals and organizations must follow strict guidelines in the area of finance and must account to the government for the money brought in and the purposes for which it is used.

A *hospital system* is a group of facilities that are affiliated and work toward a common goal. Hospital systems may include a hospital and a cancer center in a small community or may consist of a group of separate hospitals in a specific geographic region. Many hospital systems are designed as integrated delivery systems. An integrated delivery system (IDS) is a network of healthcare providers and organizations that provides or arranges to provide a coordinated continuum of services to a defined population and is willing to be held clinically and fiscally accountable for the clinical outcomes and health status of the population served. An IDS may own or could be closely aligned with an insurance product, such as a type of insurance policy. Services provided by an IDS can include a fully equipped community and/or tertiary hospital, home healthcare and **hospice** services, primary and specialty outpatient care and surgery, social services, rehabilitation, preventive care, health education and financing, and community provider offices. An IDS can also be a training location for health professional students, including physicians, nurses, and allied health professionals.

Accreditation is considered the highest form of recognition for the quality of care a facility or an organization provides. Not only does it indicate to the public that the facility is concerned with providing high-quality care, it also provides professional liability insurance benefits and plays a role in regulatory agency relicensure and certification efforts. Hospitals and other healthcare facilities are accredited by The Joint Commission, an organization that promotes and evaluates the quality of care in healthcare facilities. Standards or **indicators** have been developed that help determine when patients are receiving high-quality care. The term "quality" refers to much more than whether the patient liked the food served or had to wait to have a procedure or test performed. Categories of compliance include:

- Assessment and care of patients
- Use of medication
- Plant, technology, and safety management
- Orientation, education, and training of staff
- Medical staff qualifications
- Patients' rights

Accreditation by The Joint Commission is required to obtain reimbursement from Medicare, managed care organizations, and insurance companies. Besides accrediting healthcare facilities, The Joint Commission carefully evaluates patient safety. It has established the National Patient Safety Goals, which must be addressed by member facilities. The 2018 safety goals for ambulatory organizations took effect January 1, 2018. They included:

- Identifying patients correctly
- Using medicines safely
- Preventing infection
- Preventing mistakes in safety

All these safety factors are addressed in future chapters.

Ambulatory Care

Ambulatory care centers include a wide range of facilities that offer healthcare services to patients who seek outpatient health services. Physicians' offices, group practices, and multispecialty group practices are common types of ambulatory care facilities, and medical assistants can be employed in all of these practices. Group practices may involve a single specialty, such as pediatrics, or may be a multispecialty. A multispecialty practice might consist of an internal medicine physician, an oncologist, a cardiologist, and an endocrinologist.

Usually the providers in the practice refer patients to each other when indicated. This is not only more convenient for the patients, but also more profitable for the members in the practice. A patient seeing a provider for the first time is considered a *new* patient, whereas a patient who has seen the provider on previous occasions is called an *established* patient. Most providers charge new patients more than established patients because the levels of decision making, the extent of the physical examination, and the complexity of the medical history require that more time be directed toward the new patient.

Occupational health centers are concerned with helping patients return to work and productive activity. Often, physical therapy is used in conjunction with rehabilitation services to assist the patient in regaining as much of his or her previous level of ability as possible. Also, freestanding rehabilitation centers can assist patients with a wide range of services. Pain management centers help patients deal with discomfort associated with their condition. Sleep centers diagnose and treat people with sleep problems. Freestanding urgent or emergency care centers provide patients with an alternative to hospital emergency departments (EDs) and are typically open when traditional provider offices are closed.

Surgery has become more convenient because of the number of ambulatory surgical centers that exist today. Many insurance companies now prefer day surgery because it is more cost-effective. A wide variety of outpatient surgical facilities is available, offering procedures in ophthalmology, plastic surgery, and gastrointestinal concerns, including colonoscopies.

Dialysis centers offer services to patients with severe kidney disorders, and many of the larger cities across the country have cancer centers for patients who need treatment by oncologists. Among the many other types of ambulatory care facilities are centers that provide magnetic resonance imaging (MRI), student health clinics, dental clinics, community health centers, and women's health centers.

Other Healthcare Facilities

Several other types of healthcare facilities deserve attention in the broad overview of the healthcare industry. Diagnostic laboratories offer testing services for patients referred by their providers. The enactment of CLIA in 1967 and its amendment in 1988 established that the only laboratory tests that can be performed in a physician's office lab are those designated as *CLIA-waived*. You will learn how to perform many CLIA-waived tests in your medical assistant program. Larger ambulatory care centers may contain an on-site advanced diagnostic laboratory where all studies can be completed. Smaller or independent practices typically have to send non-CLIA-waived tests to an outside diagnostic facility.

Home health agencies or hospital-affiliated home healthcare organizations provide crucial services to patients who require medical

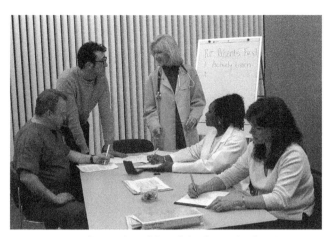

FIGURE 1.8 Teamwork is a vital part of the medical profession. All staff members must work together to care for the patient and perform required duties in the healthcare facility.

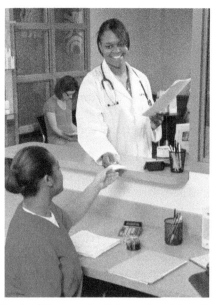

FIGURE 1.9 Knowing which employee to call when help is needed promotes goodwill among employees and often gets a task done more efficiently.

follow-up but are not in a hospital setting. Home healthcare includes therapy services, administration of and assistance with medications, wound care, and other services so that the patient can remain at home, yet still obtain consistent medical attention. Hospice care is a type of home health service that provides medical care and support for patients facing end-of-life issues and their families. The goal of hospice is to provide peace, comfort, and dignity while controlling pain and promoting the best possible quality of life for the patient. Some communities have inpatient hospice services available either in a special unit in a hospital or in an independent hospice center.

THE HEALTHCARE TEAM

To deliver comprehensive quality care, everyone who interacts with patients, from the time they enter the facility to the time they leave, must work as a cooperative member of the healthcare team. If managers were asked to name the most important attributes for medical professionals, teamwork would be high on the list (Fig. 1.8). Staff members must work together for the good of the patients. They must be willing to perform duties outside a formal job description if they are needed in other areas of the office. Many supervisors frown on employees who state, "That's not in my job description." A professional medical assistant should perform the duty and later discuss with the supervisor any valid reasons that the task should have been assigned to someone else. However, if the task is illegal, unethical, or places the patient or anyone else in danger, it should not be done. If you are ever concerned about patient safety, you should discuss the situation with your supervisor before performing the task.

Although we all would enjoy working in an office where everyone gets along and likes every other employee, this does not always happen. Personal feelings must be set aside at work, and all employees must cooperate with others to get the job done efficiently. If a medical assistant has an issue with another employee, the first move would be to discuss it privately with the other person. If the situation does not improve, perhaps a supervisor (office or practice manager) should be involved for further discussions. Do not bring the provider into the discussion unless there is no choice because the facility manager is expected to deal with personnel issues (Fig. 1.9).

Patient-Centered Medical Home

The Patient Centered Medical Home (PCMH) is a model of patient care. In this model, patient care is looked at from a holistic approach. The healthcare team wants to be able to assist that patient with any issues that come up about his or her care. This means having multiple team members available. The provider and the medical assistant would provide the primary care. There would also be a nurse who coordinates all of the care for the patient, including issues about home healthcare, financial issues, transportation issues, and so on. Many models include a clinical pharmacist who is available to discuss medication questions and concerns with the patient.

Research indicates that PCMHs are saving money by reducing hospital and ED visits while at the same time improving patient outcomes. The Agency for Healthcare Research and Quality (AHRQ), which is part of the Department of Health and Human Services (HHS), believes that improving our primary care system is the key to achieving high-quality, accessible, efficient healthcare for all Americans. The agency recognizes that health information technology (IT) plays a central role in the successful implementation of the key features of the primary care medical home. According to the AHRQ, the PCMH has five core functions and attributes:

1. *Comprehensive care:* The primary care practice has the potential to provide physical and mental healthcare, prevention and wellness, acute care, and chronic care to all patients in the practice. However, comprehensive care cannot be provided by only the practicing physician. It requires a team of care providers. The healthcare team for a PCMH includes physicians, nurse practitioners, physician assistants, nurses, pharmacists, nutritionists, social workers, educators, and medical assistants. If these specialty individuals are not readily available to smaller physician practices, virtual teams can be created online to link providers and patients to services in their communities.
2. *Patient-centered care:* The PCMH provides primary healthcare that is holistic and relationship based, always considering the

individual patient and all facets of his or her life. However, establishing a partnership with patients and their families requires understanding and respect of each patient's unique needs, culture, values, and preferences. Medical assistants are trained to provide respectful patient care regardless of individual patient factors. The goal of the PCMH is to encourage and support patients in learning how to manage and organize their own care. Patients and families are recognized as core members of the care team.

3. *Coordinated care:* The PCMH coordinates care across all parts of the healthcare system, including specialty care, hospitals, home healthcare, and community services. Coordination is especially important when patients are transitioning from one site of care to another, such as from hospital to home. The PCMH works at creating and maintaining open communication among patients and families, the medical home, and members of the broader healthcare team.

4. *Accessible services:* The PCMH is designed to deliver accessible care. This is achieved by establishing policies that create shorter wait times for urgent needs, expanded office hours, around-the-clock telephone or electronic access to a member of the care team, and alternative methods of communication, such as email and telephone care.

5. *Quality and safety:* The PCMH is committed to delivering quality healthcare by providing evidence-based medicine and shared decision making with patients and families; assessing practice performance and working on improvements; collecting safety data; and measuring and responding to patients' experiences and satisfaction. All of this information is made public to allow an open assessment of the practice and suggestions for possible methods of improvement.

The goal of the PCMH is to improve patient outcomes and reduce costs. There are accreditation processes that must be completed for a healthcare facility to be recognized as a PCMH. For further information about the PCMH model, refer to the Patient Centered Medical Home Resource Center, Department of Health and Human Services: http://pcmh.ahrq.gov.

PRACTICING PROFESSIONALISM AS A TEAM MEMBER

A *team* is a group of people organized for work or a specific purpose. In the healthcare setting, usually the team consists of the employees working in the same department. A broader definition could include all the employees at the facility. A *team member* is loyal to the group and works well with the other people in the group. As a member, the medical assistant must help the team function. To do this, it is important to know the roles of the different team members. Tables 1.5 and 1.6 describe various healthcare professionals found in ambulatory care facilities.

To be a valuable team member, it is important to have several qualities. Work ethic, punctuality, cooperation, and the willingness to help are important traits in a team member. It takes all members working together to make an effective and productive team. When a member "drops the ball," others must step in and do extra work.

Exceptional Customer Service

To provide exceptional customer service, medical assistants need to:
- Remember that patients, family members, and co-workers are all customers.
- Be professional in behavior and appearance.
- Consider cultural differences when using nonverbal communication.
- Prepare clear, concise verbal communication (written and oral).
- Use therapeutic communication, including active listening.

To help promote professionalism when you first meet a patient, it is important to GIVE:
- **G**reet the patient.
- **I**dentify yourself.
- **V**erify the patient's identity by asking for the person's full name and date of birth.
- **E**xplain the procedure to be performed in a manner that is understood by the patient.

The Meaning of Professionalism

Professionalism is defined as having a courteous, conscientious, and respectful approach to all interactions and situations in the workplace. It is characterized by or conforms to the recognized standard of care for the profession. Conducting themselves in a professional manner is essential for successful medical assistants. The attitude of those in the medical profession generally is more conservative than that seen in other career fields. Patients expect professional behavior and base much of their trust and confidence in those who show this type of **demeanor** in the healthcare facility (Fig. 1.10).

Work Ethic and Punctuality

A *work ethic* is composed of sets of values based on hard work and diligence. The medical assistant should always display **initiative** and be **reliable**. People with a good work ethic arrive on time, are rarely absent, and always perform to the best of their ability. Co-workers become frustrated if another employee consistently arrives late or is absent. This forces others to take on additional duties, and it may prevent them from completing their own work. One missing employee

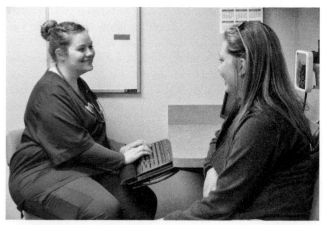

FIGURE 1.10 The professional medical assistant is an asset to the healthcare facility.

can disrupt the entire day. Phones may not be answered promptly. Patients may have to wait longer for appointments. Lunch breaks may be shortened to allow all the work to be done. All employees should know and follow the attendance policies of the facility as outlined in the policies and procedures manual.

Most new hires have a probationary period that may last 30 to 90 days. Excessive absences or *tardiness* (being late) will negatively affect the employee. It may be grounds for *termination* (job loss). If the medical assistant must be absent or tardy, the supervisor must be notified prior to the start time. Make sure to follow the office policy. All employees must be *punctual* (on time) every day. Providers and patients alike expect this reliability.

CRITICAL THINKING APPLICATION   **1.10**

Carmen tends to arrive at the clinic with about 1 minute to spare. She realizes that she needs to change her habits and arrive about 10 minutes before her start time. This would give her a little "cushion" if traffic is slow. If you were Carmen, what strategies could you use to make sure to get to the healthcare facility 10 minutes before the start time?

Cooperation and Willingness to Help

Each team member must be willing to cooperate and help others on the team. It is not uncommon that one team member might be very busy or handling an emergency. Other team members must be willing to step up and lend a helping hand. For instance, a medical assistant may be tied up caring for a very sick patient. Other patients who have appointments are waiting to be seen. One of the other team members needs to help room the patients (e.g., take their vital signs and histories for the provider). This is how the department can provide exceptional customer service. Team members watch out for each other. If someone is getting behind, others help out.

Through cooperation, the team is more productive. Team members have greater job satisfaction. When members cooperate and work together, there is a great sense of communication and understanding in a team. Most importantly, the patients are cared for, and great customer service is provided.

Prioritizing and Time Management Skills

Prioritizing duties and using time management skills are critical for the success of medical assistants. *Prioritizing* means to arrange and complete duties in the order of most importance. *Time management strategies* are methods that maximize personal efficiencies and prioritize tasks. This means that we are to use our time efficiently and concentrate on the most important duties first. To do this, we must first prioritize our duties. We must arrange our schedules to ensure that these duties can be performed. The first way to improve time management is to plan the tasks that need to be done that day. Take 10 minutes to write down the tasks for the day. This helps ensure the tasks get done. Make sure to reference the list throughout the day to keep on track. Don't schedule too much to do each day, so that it is impossible to get everything done. Keep the list manageable. You need to build in some extra time in case of emergencies or urgent issues that come up. The key to managing time is prioritizing.

Time Management Strategies

- Organize and review your daily "to do" list. If you honestly believe you can't possibly get everything that is a priority done, ask for help. It is better to admit you can't do it all than to ignore a task that is important.
- Brainstorm with your peers about ways to achieve all the tasks facing everyone each day. Maybe someone can come up with a unique way to solve a problem; but if not, at least all of you will be on the same page.
- Make a master list of important tasks so nothing is forgotten.
- Try to accomplish like tasks in the same block of time. If you have phone calls to return or insurance referrals to complete, do both at the same time to be more efficient.
- At the end of each day, create a new "to do" list for the next day so that nothing important is forgotten.

When prioritizing your tasks, use a code system to indicate when they need to be done. For instance:
- Use an "M" for tasks that *must* be done that day.
- Use an "S" for tasks that *should* be done that day.
- Use a "C" for tasks that *could* be done if time permits.

Once the tasks have been divided into these categories, they can be further classified in each section. For instance, if category *M* has six tasks, they can be numbered in the order they should be performed. The same process is completed with the tasks in categories *S* and *C*. As the tasks are completed, they are checked off. At the end of each day, create a new "to do" list for the next day so that nothing important is forgotten.

CRITICAL THINKING APPLICATION   **1.11**

Carmen needs to practice her time management skills. Using the system described, make your "to do" list. Use M, S, and C to categorize your activities.

Responding to Criticism

As we work, we are evaluated by others. It may be informal or formal for a job evaluation. We learn from others' feedback on our performance. This criticism can be hard to take. It threatens our confidence and self-esteem. We need to realize the value of the feedback. It will help us improve our skills and refine our professional skills. When a person gives us feedback or criticism, it is important to take it as a professional. Becoming defensive or blaming others is not professional. This type of behavior will be a negative reflection on you.

Problem Solving and Chain of Command

When you are working as part of a team, it is important to understand how to solve differences with other members. Typically, it is best to talk with the person with whom you are having an issue. Try not to use statements that accuse the other person. Refrain from using sentences that start with "You are…" Try to remove the emotion from the situation if you can. Use more "I feel…" statements. If your attempt to resolve the situation is unsuccessful, then it is usually recommended that you talk with the supervisor.

If the issue is related to theft, confidentiality, or harassment, you may need to follow the chain of command in the healthcare facility. Usually, you need to start with your supervisor or the person you report to. Then the next step is the supervisor of your supervisor, and so on. Most employee handbooks discuss the facility's chain of command.

Barriers to Professionalism

At times it is not easy to be a professional. Sometimes patients and co-workers try our patience. It can be difficult to maintain a professional attitude in these cases. Some of the obstructions to professional behavior are discussed in this section.

Attitude

Having a negative attitude can bring down the **morale** of the whole team. Patients can sense when the staff is unhappy, and this makes them wonder why. It is not the patient's responsibility to cheer up the medical assistants. The patients will also be less likely to share personal information with someone who has a negative attitude. Try to find the positive in any given situation.

Complaining can be considered having a negative attitude. If you have a problem you should discuss it, constructively, with someone who can help resolve the situation. Sitting in the break room and complaining to another medical assistant about your schedule will not help to resolve the situation. Talking with your supervisor would be a better solution.

Procrastination

Delaying or putting off tasks can be detrimental to patient care and your relationship with your co-workers. If there is a task that you dread doing, do it quickly and efficiently and you will not have to think about it until the next time. When you are working in healthcare, waiting to do something can put a patient at risk or require that your co-workers do it for you. Either situation can put your job at risk.

Personal Problems and "Baggage"

We all have a personal life. Sometimes things happen in our lives before we go to work. It is important that we push these issues aside and focus on our job. If we carry this "baggage" to work, it can interfere with our ability to do our job. We may be tempted to make personal calls, check emails, and so on. This takes time away from our job, and our focus is not on our job. If the "baggage" is so important and concerning, the medical assistant needs to speak with the supervisor. It might not be appropriate to be working if one cannot concentrate on the job at hand. The patient must be the prime concern of all the employees in the healthcare facility.

Gossip

Gossip is casual or idle chat (rumors) about other people and their business. Many times, the "discussion" is based on someone's opinion and not fact. Most people enjoy working in an environment in which employees cooperate and get along with each other. Rumors and gossip can cause problems with employee morale. They can affect how a team functions. A medical assistant should refuse to participate in the rumor mill (Fig. 1.11). Attempting to be cordial and friendly

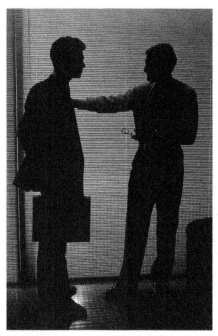

FIGURE 1.11 Gossip and rumors have no place in the medical profession. Avoid employees who participate in this type of activity.

to everyone at work is important. Supervisors regard those who gossip or spread rumors as unprofessional and untrustworthy. You should always avoid passing along work-related rumors to patients and family members.

Personal Communication

The medical assistant should not take unnecessary phone calls from friends and family at the office. The office phone is a business line and must be used as such, except in emergencies. Using personal cell phones during working hours is not acceptable. Use breaks and lunch hours to take care of business on the phone. Never take a personal call or respond to text messages on a cell phone while working with a patient. Many healthcare facilities require cell phones to be silenced and out of sight during the workday. Because most phones have cameras, facility administrators are concerned about unlawful pictures being taken. Many healthcare computer networks block certain nonhealthcare websites (e.g., social media sites). Table 1.7 describes acceptable and unacceptable activities for digital communication devices and online activities.

CRITICAL THINKING APPLICATION   **1.12**

Carmen loves her phone. But she learned very quickly that her phone was to be turned off and put away during work hours. Explain why having cell phones out and turned on can create issues in the healthcare facility.

Visitors should not frequent the office, especially the area where the medical assistant is working. If someone must come to the office, always offer the reception area as a waiting room. Visitors should never be allowed to enter patient areas.

Checking personal email also should be avoided in the workplace. Any type of personal business, such as studying, looking up information on the internet for personal use, internet shopping, or using social

TABLE 1.7　Using Digital Communication Devices and Online Activities in Healthcare Facilities		
DEVICE/ACTIVITY	**ACCEPTABLE, PROFESSIONAL**	**UNACCEPTABLE, UNPROFESSIONAL**
Phone calls/text messages	• Emergency calls only • Turn off or silence ringer • Make personal calls only on break time	• Frequent checking for calls received • Making personal calls • Have phone out and visible when working with patients • Taking pictures
Personal emails and social media	• Do not open, read, or post	• Sending and reading personal emails • Viewing social media postings
Online activities	• Work-related web-related activity	• Shopping, gaming, nonwork websites

media, should be done at home and not in the office. All of these actions distract the medical assistant from the job at hand; the focus should be on serving the patients in the office at all times. Many employees are fired each year for surfing or shopping on the internet for personal reasons or for checking personal email. Make sure all personal business is handled outside of business hours.

Dating Co-Workers

Given the amount of time that we spend with our co-workers, it is not surprising that personal relationships can develop. Dating someone you work with can present professionalism issues. Maintaining a professional demeanor while at work becomes that much harder, especially if you are both on the same team. Other co-workers might think that there is favoritism, especially if one person is the supervisor of another. There can also be issues if the relationship ends badly and both must continue to work together.

Self-Boundaries

When you are working in healthcare, it is important to develop a solid professional relationship with your patients. By establishing realistic self-boundaries, you can protect that relationship.

CLOSING COMMENTS

Medical assisting has developed over the years into a profession that makes considerable contributions to quality patient care in ambulatory care centers. Medical assistants are uniquely trained to manage both the administrative and clinical needs of patients in physicians' offices, clinics, and outpatient facilities. One of the crucial roles of medical assistants is to act as the patient's navigator; that is, to help patients understand and comply with complex care issues. The medical assistant joins a wide range of allied health professionals as part of a healthcare team in which all members work together to best meet the needs of patients. Medical assistants can work in a variety of healthcare facilities and alongside medical specialists to care for patients. They also can act as core members of the PCMH and, along with a variety of community resources, can help provide holistic care to patients in the healthcare system. However, the medical assisting practice must align with the state and regional scope of practice laws and must meet expected standards of care. Medical assistants must always act

under the direction of a physician or provider; they cannot diagnose, prescribe, or treat patients independently.

Patients expect and deserve professional behavior from those who work in medical facilities. Display courtesy and respect toward patients, families, and peers. A diplomatic and tactful person always attempts to interact honestly without giving offense. By displaying these attributes, the medical assistant earns the respect of co-workers and becomes indispensable to his or her employer. Behaving in a professional manner in the medical office helps the medical assistant gain the patient's trust. Trust is one of the most important factors in preventing cases of medical liability. Treating patients with care and not subjecting them to negative behaviors keeps the patient-provider relationship strong and conducive to the health and recovery of the patient. Performing as a cooperative team member goes a long way in promoting a positive healthcare environment for the patient. Incorporating time management strategies into each day not only helps you perform tasks more efficiently, but also ensures that no important tasks are left uncompleted. The entry-level medical assistant can promote professional behavior by joining one of the professional medical assistant organizations and seeking national credentialing.

Patient Coaching

Some patients have very little knowledge about the healthcare industry and may need instruction and explanations about details important to their healthcare. They often call the healthcare facility with questions; therefore, medical assistants must understand the wide variety of healthcare facilities and medical resources available in the community. Become familiar with community resources to make provider-approved referrals for patients who need help from various sources. If a patient seems to have a need, speak with him or her privately and determine whether any agency or organization might help with the issues at hand. The PCMH model relies on all healthcare workers to participate in the care of patients.

Legal and Ethical Issues

Medical assistants are responsible for understanding and following the scope of practice in their communities and for always meeting the expected standards of care. Not meeting these responsibilities can result in serious liability for themselves and their employers.

Remember, the medical assistant must act under the direct supervision of a physician or licensed provider. You must know the limitations placed on your practice by the state in which you live or by the facility or provider who employs you. There is nothing more important than patient safety, so always act within the guidelines of the law and according to the policies and procedures of the facility where you work. Medical assistants are multiskilled healthcare workers who can have a lasting positive effect on patient outcomes. However, never forget that you do not have the authority or education to diagnose, prescribe, or treat patients' clinical problems. Professional credentialing is becoming more important each year.

The workday should be centered around patient care, so never allow personal business to intrude on time that should be spent assisting patients and the provider. Otherwise, the patient may be left with the impression that the medical assistant, or the entire staff, is unprofessional, and this often leads to trust issues with the individuals employed at the facility.

Patient-Centered Care

Patient-centered care involves taking care of the whole patient, not just the physical problems. As a professional medical assistant, you can be instrumental in helping the patient with coordination and integration of care, providing information and education as directed by the provider, involving the family with the patient's care, and above all, respecting the patient's preferences.

Professional Behaviors

Much of this chapter has focused on an introduction to what it means to be a medical assistant and what you will need to learn so you can perform all the skills expected of an entry-level medical assistant. However, working with patients and providing quality care go beyond being able to perform administrative and clinical skills. Each patient must be viewed holistically. This means considering the following patient factors:

- What is the patient's physical condition, and how is it affecting his or her life?
- What is the patient's psychological state; is it preventing the person from following treatment regimens?
- Are any communication barriers preventing the patient from understanding the diagnosis or suggested treatment?
- Is the patient's culture, age, or lifestyle preventing him or her from following the provider's orders?
- Are insurance issues or financial problems preventing the patient from following through with treatment plans?

These are just a few of the factors that can affect patient outcomes. Again, because you will be trained in both administrative and clinical duties, you will be in a unique position to understand all the factors that might affect patient care. It is your responsibility to treat all patients with respect and empathy and to do whatever you can to support them throughout the healthcare experience.

SUMMARY OF SCENARIO

Carmen is a bit overwhelmed but very excited about what she has learned about the role of medical assistants in ambulatory care. She finds it hard to believe that she will become competent in all aspects of the typical medical assistant's job description, but she anticipates learning both administrative and clinical skills. She is looking forward to joining the local AAMA chapter so that she can take advantage of professional development opportunities and networking with other medical assistant professionals and students in her community. Carmen now appreciates the significance of scope of practice and of meeting standards of care, and she is researching the laws affecting medical assistant practice in her state. She can't wait until she is actually able to work with the healthcare team to meet the holistic needs of patients in the practice where she will be employed.

SUMMARY OF LEARNING OBJECTIVES

1. **Discuss the typical responsibilities of a medical assistant and describe the role of the medical assistant as a patient navigator.**
   Medical assistants are trained in both clinical and administrative skills that are applicable to ambulatory care settings, such as providers' offices, clinics, and group practices. Graduates of accredited programs are all taught a similar skill set that prepares students for an entry-level position. The actual duties will depend on the place of employment.

   Medical assistants have long been encouraged to act as patient advocates in the ambulatory care setting. That role is now described as acting as a patient navigator or care coordinator to help patients manage the complexities of their care. Given their multilevel training, medical assistants can help patients navigate through a wide variety of confusing issues.

2. **Discuss the attributes of a professional medical assistant, project a professional image in the ambulatory care setting, and describe how to show respect for individual diversity.**
   Professional medical assistants display courteous, respectful behaviors and communicate with tact and diplomacy. They demonstrate responsible and honest behaviors and always act with integrity. Professional medical assistants view constructive criticism as a way of improving their skill level. Important assumptions are made within seconds of meeting someone based only on how the person looks. Most medical facilities require that medical assistants wear a uniform or scrubs or professional clothing that is not too tight and projects a professional, businesslike appearance. In addition, name badges should be visible; hair should be clean, and longer hair should be tied back; shoes should be clean; nails should be short

and without nail polish (no artificial nails); and no jewelry should be worn.

It is important to recognize that diversity is more than just nationality or race. It can include age, economic status, disabilities, and so on. As professional medical assistants we should learn as much about our patient population as possible, learning about its customs and practices. Being informed will help us to better serve our patients.

3. **Differentiate between scope of practice and standards of care for medical assistants.**

Scope of practice determines the range of responsibilities and practice guidelines for healthcare workers. The scope of practice for a medical assistant is what has been established by law in some states or by practice norms, institutions, or physician-employers in states without scope of practice laws. The standard of care (a legal term) sets the minimum guidelines for job performance. It defines the level and quality of patient service that should be provided by healthcare workers with similar training and experience in a similar situation.

Licensed healthcare professionals have a different scope of practice and expected standard of care than medical assistants. Medical assistants can never diagnose, prescribe, or treat patients. The medical assistant's actions are always done under the supervision of a provider such as a physician, nurse practitioner, or physician assistant. The medical assistant should follow the written order or follow established policies and procedures.

4. **List and discuss professional medical assisting organizations.**

Three professional medical assisting organizations were discussed in this chapter. The American Association of Medical Assistants (AAMA), American Medical Technologists (AMT), and the National Healthcareer Association (NHA). All three organizations offer certification and continuing education.

5. **Examine your learning preferences and interpret how your learning style affects your success as a student.**

Learning preferences are the ways you like to learn and that have proven successful in the past. Your learning style is determined by your individual method of perceiving or examining new material and the way you process it or make it your own. People are either concrete or abstract perceivers and either active or reflective processors.

6. **Integrate effective study skills into your daily activities, design test-taking strategies that help you take charge of your success, and incorporate critical thinking skills and reflection to help you make mental connections as you learn material.**

Study skills, such as memory techniques, active learning, brain tricks, effective reading methods, note-taking strategies, and mind maps, all help students to be more successful.

Test-taking strategies include preparing adequately for the examination, controlling negative thoughts during the examination, and understanding how to deal with different types of questions.

Critical thinking can be defined as thorough thinking because it considers all sides of the information without bias.

Reflection is the process of thinking about or reviewing information before acting.

7. **Summarize the history of medicine and its significance to the medical assisting profession.**

The history of medicine can be traced to ancient practices as far back as 5000 BC. In 1205 BC Moses presented rules of health to the Hebrews, thus becoming the first advocate of preventive medicine. Hippocrates, known as the Father of Medicine, is the most famous of the ancient Greek physicians and is best remembered for the Hippocratic Oath, which has been administered to physicians for more than 2000 years. The medical assisting profession relies on previous medical discoveries to provide patients with safe care in today's healthcare environment. Table 1.3 summarizes medical pioneers and their achievements.

8. **Summarize the various types of medical professionals, allied health professionals, and healthcare facilities.**

Physicians and other providers (e.g., nurse practitioners and physician assistants) are portals of entry or first contacts for patients seeking medical care. Medical professionals include physicians (MDs, DOs), dentists, chiropractors, optometrists, podiatrists, pharmacists, nurse practitioners, and physician assistants. Table 1.4 presents a list of medical specialties.

The definition of an allied health professional can vary, but it loosely refers to those who can act only under the authority of a licensed medical practitioner. Allied health professions fall into two broad categories: technicians (assistants) and therapists. Allied health professionals, including professional medical assistants, typically work as part of a healthcare team. Table 1.5 presents a list of allied health occupations, and Table 1.6 shows a list of licensed healthcare professions.

Healthcare facilities include different levels of hospitals, ambulatory care facilities, and a variety of other institutions that provide specialty care for patients.

9. **Define the Patient-Centered Medical Home (PCMH) and discuss its five core functions and attributes.**

The PCMH is a concept that is transforming the organization and delivery of primary care. The healthcare team looks at patient care from a holistic approach. Improving our primary care system is the key to achieving high-quality, accessible, efficient healthcare for all Americans. The PCMH has five core functions and attributes: (1) comprehensive care, (2) patient-centered care, (3) coordinated care, (4) accessible services, and (5) evidence-based, high-quality, safe care.

10. **Explain the reasons professionalism is important in the medical field, describe work ethics, and stress the importance of cooperation.**

Professionalism is the characteristic of conforming to the technical or ethical standards of a profession. Professionalism is vital in the medical profession because patients expect and deserve to be treated in a professional way. When the medical assistant acts in a professional way, he or she establishes trust with the patient. Patients notice professional behavior, even when it is not directed at them specifically. They notice how others are treated in the reception room and in other areas of the office. Always act in a professional manner while at work.

Continued

SUMMARY OF LEARNING OBJECTIVES—*continued*

Work ethics are sets of values based on the moral virtues of hard work and diligence, involving a whole range of activities, from individual acts to the philosophy of the entire facility.

Each team member must be willing to cooperate and help others on the team. Through cooperation, the team is more productive.

11. **Apply time management strategies to prioritize the medical assistant's responsibilities as a member of the healthcare team.**

Medical assistants need to use time efficiently, prioritize duties, and arrange schedules to ensure that duties can be performed in a timely manner. This can be done by planning tasks that need to be done that day. Most tasks can be prioritized into three general categories: those that must be done that day, those that should be done that day, and those that could be done if time permits.

12. **Respond to criticism, problem-solve, identify obstacles to professional behaviors, and define principles of self-boundaries.**

Criticism can be hard to take, but we need to realize the value of feedback. When you are working as a part of a team, it is important to understand how to resolve differences with other members. If there is an issue related to theft, confidentiality, or harassment, you may need to follow the chain of command in the healthcare facility. Everyone has a life outside the workplace, and sometimes we face challenges and difficult times that are hard to put aside. The professional medical assistant never transfers personal problems or baggage to anyone at the medical facility. The medical assistant should refuse to participate in the office rumor mill and should be cordial and friendly to everyone at work. Avoid personal phone calls and visits unless it is an absolute emergency.

Awareness of personal boundaries helps us determine the actions and behaviors that we find unacceptable. Healthy self-boundaries make it possible to respect our strengths, abilities, and individuality and those of others.

HEALTH RECORDS

2

SCENARIO

Susan Beezler has just begun her career in the medical assisting profession. In the morning, she is attending medical assisting school, and in the afternoon, she works part-time for the Walden-Martin Family Medical Clinic (WMFM) as a records assistant. Susan is eager to learn about healthcare and looks forward to taking on more responsibility at the office.

Dr. David Kahn is a new provider who has recently joined WMFM. Dr. Kahn has enjoyed working with Susan and feels that her energy will be just what his patients need. He has taken a professional interest in Susan and often lets her assist him with patients when her other duties allow.

Susan knows that although she is a beginner in the office, she will gain trust from her supervisors and patients as long as she projects a teachable attitude. The office has recently converted to an electronic records system but is also still using paper records. Susan uses the information she learned in school about both types of health records. She cheerfully performs filing and even does some transcription for Dr. Kahn. The other staff members are pleased with her willingness to perform the most mundane tasks.

Susan enjoys sharing her experiences with her classmates. She is the only student currently working in the medical field, and the others ask her lots of questions about the "real world" of medical assisting. She is very careful not to breach patient confidentiality; she discusses situations only in general terms, never mentioning any patients' names.

Susan feels a great sense of pride that she is already a member of the healthcare team and able to contribute to the lives of her patients.

While studying this chapter, think about the following questions:

- What is the definition and application of subjective information?
- What is the definition and application of objective information?
- How does the HITECH act impact health records?
- How can you maintain a connection with the patient when using an EHR?
- What are the different ways to back up an EHR?
- How do you correctly destroy health records?
- How do you document in health records?
- What equipment and supplies are needed for a paper records system?
- What are the indexing rules for alphabetic and numeric filing systems?

LEARNING OBJECTIVES

1. Discuss the two types of patient records.
2. State several reasons that accurate health records are important.
3. Differentiate between subjective and objective information in creating a patient's health record.
4. Explain who owns the health record.
5. Distinguish between an electronic health record (EHR) and an electronic medical record (EMR).
6. Do the following related to healthcare legislation and EHRs:
   - Define meaningful use and relate it to the healthcare industry.
   - List the three main components of meaningful use legislation.
7. Discuss the importance of nonverbal communication with patients when an EHR system is used.
8. Discuss backup systems for the EHR, in addition to the transfer, destruction, and retention of health records as related to the EHR.
9. Discuss retention and destruction of medical records as related to paper records.
10. Describe how and when to release health record information; also, discuss health information exchanges (HIEs).
11. Identify and discuss the two methods of organizing a patient's paper medical record.
12. Discuss how to document information in an EHR and a paper health record, and how to make corrections/alterations to health records.
13. Discuss dictation and transcription.
14. Identify the filing equipment and filing supplies needed to create, store, and maintain paper health records.
15. Describe indexing rules, and how to create and organize a patient's health record.
16. Discuss the pros and cons of various filing methods and how to file patient health records.
17. Discuss the organization of files and of health-related correspondence.

age of majority The age at which the law recognizes a person to be an adult; it varies by state.

alphabetic filing Any system that arranges names or topics according to the sequence of the letters in the alphabet.

alphanumeric Describes systems made up of combinations of letters and numbers.

anthropometric (an thruh po ME trik) Pertaining to the measurement of the size and proportions of the human body.

caption A heading, title, or subtitle under which records are filed.

compliance (kuhm PLIE uhns) Meeting the standards and regulations of the practice's established policies and procedures. Can also mean cooperation.

computerized provider/physician order entry (CPOE) The process of entering medication orders or other provider instructions into the EHR.

concise (kuhn SICE) Using as few words as possible to express a message.

continuity of care The smooth continuation of care from one provider to another. This allows the patient to receive the most benefit with no interruption or duplication of care.

dictation (dik TEY shuhn) To say something aloud for another person to write down.

direct filing system A filing system in which materials can be located without consulting another source of reference.

electronic health record (EHR) An electronic record that conforms to nationally recognized standards and contains health-related information about a specific patient. It can be created, managed, and consulted by authorized clinicians and staff from more than one healthcare organization.

e-prescribing The use of electronic software to communicate with pharmacies and send prescribing information. It takes the place of writing a prescription by hand and giving it to a patient; most new or refill prescriptions can be submitted electronically, cutting down on fraud and errors.

hereditary (huh RED i ter ee) Passed from parents to offspring through the genes.

incidence (IN si duhns) How often something happens or occurs.

interface An interconnection between systems.

interoperability (in ter op er uh BIL i tee) The ability to work with other systems.

numeric filing The filing of records, correspondence, or cards by number.

objective information Data obtained through physical examination, laboratory and diagnostic testing, and by measurable information.

obliteration (ub lit uh REY shun) To remove or destroy all traces of; do away with; destroy completely.

out guides Sturdy cardboard or plastic file-sized cards used to replace a folder temporarily removed from the filing space.

parameters (puh RAM i ters) Rules that control how something should be done; guidelines or boundaries.

patient portal A secure online website that gives patients 24-hour access to personal health information using a username and password.

prognosis (prog NOH sis) The likely outcome of a disease, including the chance of recovery.

provisional diagnosis (die ug NOH sis) A temporary diagnosis made before all test results have been received.

quality control A process to ensure the reliability of test results, often using manufactured samples with known values.

retention schedule A method or plan for retaining or keeping health records and for their movement from active to inactive to closed.

reverse chronologic order The most recent item is on top, and the oldest item is last.

subjective information Data or information obtained from the patient, including the patient's feelings, perceptions, and concerns; this information is obtained through interviews or written questions.

subsequent (SUHB si kwuhnt) Occurring later or after.

tickler file A chronologic file used as a reminder that something must be dealt with on a certain date.

transcription (tran SKRIP shuhn) A typed or written copy of dictated material.

vested Granted or endowed with a particular authority, right, or property; to have a special interest in.

Health records can be found in two different formats, electronic and paper. Most healthcare facilities have switched to **electronic health records (EHRs)**. Some of the benefits of EHRs include:

- Easy storage of patient information
- Availability to multiple users at the same time
- More efficient claim submission process

The federal government has also offered financial incentives for providers to implement EHRs. Although most providers are using EHRs, there are still some who are using paper records and others who are using a combination of electronic and paper formats. When a provider is making a switch to an EHR, he or she may decide to keep the patient's previous records in the paper format and just use the electronic format moving forward. Some providers may decide to scan in the last 3 to 5 years of the paper record into the electronic record. Whatever the scenario the healthcare facility has chosen, it is important for the medical assistant to understand both systems and to be able to perform well with either one.

TYPES OF RECORDS

Paper health records have been shown to be much less efficient than an EHR. In most cases, only one person at a time can use the paper record. It is fairly common for information to be filed in the incorrect record. The entire record also can be misfiled. Gathering data for research and **quality control** is more challenging. Data are difficult to share in facilities with multiple departments or locations. The paper-based record is good for documentation of patient care, but it is not nearly as useful in other capacities.

With an EHR, multiple users can access the record at the same time. There are fewer errors because handwritten notes do not have to be interpreted. Most EHRs link the clinical information needed for billing purposes. An EHR also includes practice management capabilities that allow for patient scheduling and generation of reports needed for research and quality control.

It is important for the medical assistant to be aware of the differences between the practice management software and the EHR. You may use both during your day as a medical assistant. The EHR contains a record of patient interactions and health history. The practice management software allows the facility to operate the business side by maintaining schedules and financial information for revenue cycle management for reimbursement.

CRITICAL THINKING APPLICATION 2.1

Some of Dr. Kahn's patients are concerned that computer-based health records may not be completely private. They are worried that unauthorized individuals could access their information on the computer and do them harm. Should patients be allowed to decide whether their records are kept on computer or on paper? Why or why not?

IMPORTANCE OF ACCURATE HEALTH RECORDS

Health records are kept for five basic reasons:

- *To provide the best possible medical care for the patient.* The provider examines the patient and enters the findings in the patient's health record. These findings are clues to the diagnosis. The provider may order many types of tests to confirm the clinical findings. As the reports of these tests come in, the findings fall into place, much like the pieces of a jigsaw puzzle. With these data, the provider can prescribe treatment and form an opinion about the patient's **prognosis.** The health record provides a complete history of all the care given to the patient.
- *To provide critical information for others.* By reading through the record and discovering the methods used to treat the patient, healthcare professionals can provide **continuity of care.** Each provider knows what services have been provided and can continue the care, even from one facility to another.
  - For example, when a patient is transferred from a hospital to a skilled nursing facility, the information from the patient's hospital record helps the nursing facility staff to better care for the patient. When patients move from place to place or caregivers change, copies of the pertinent information should move with the patient to provide this continuity of care.
- *To provide legal protection for those who provided care to the patient.* A well-documented health record is excellent proof that certain procedures were performed or that medical advice was given. An accurate record is the foundation for a legal defense in cases of medical professional liability. This is one reason that writing legibly in the paper record to document exactly what happened to the patient and the provider's response are critical. Remember: If it is not documented, it did not happen.
- *To provide statistical information that is helpful to researchers.* The patient's record provides information about medications taken and the reactions to them. Health records may be used to evaluate the effectiveness of certain kinds of treatment or to determine the

incidence of a given disease. Providers often take part in drug studies that track adverse reactions and side effects. The effects of various treatments and procedures also can be tracked, and statistics gathered from patients' records. When statistical information is tracked, the patient-specific data are removed. This information may result in a new outlook on some phases of medicine and can lead to revised techniques and treatments. The statistical data from health records also are valuable in the preparation of scientific papers, books, and lectures.
- *To provide support for claims reimbursement.* This is required by most insurance companies.

CONTENTS OF THE HEALTH RECORD

The patient's health record is the most important record in a healthcare facility. For completeness, each patient's record should contain **subjective information** provided by the patient and **objective information** obtained by the provider and staff of the healthcare facility. If all entries are complete, the health record will stand the test of time. No branch of medicine is exempt from the need to keep patient health records.

Subjective Information
Personal Demographics
The patient's health record begins with routine personal data, which the patient usually supplies on the first visit when the health record is established. Most patients are required to complete a patient information form (Fig. 2.1; see Procedure 2.1, p. 54). The basic facts are:

- Patient's full name, spelled correctly
- Names of parents/guardians if the patient is a child or legally incompetent
- Patient's gender
- Date of birth (DOB)
- Marital status
- Name of spouse if married
- Home address, telephone number, and email address
- Occupation
- Name of employer
- Business address and telephone number
- Employment information for spouse
- Healthcare insurance information
- Source of referral
- Social Security number

Past Health, Family, and Social History
The past health, family, and social histories are often obtained by having the patient complete a questionnaire. The medical assistant may review the form for completeness, and he or she may need to clarify any questions or missing information with the patient before the patient is seen by the provider. The provider will also add information provided during the patient interview. The responses provide information about:

- Any past illnesses (including injuries and/or physical defects, whether congenital or acquired)
- Hospitalizations, or surgeries the patient has had (Fig. 2.2).
- Patient's daily health habits

Welcome

Thank you for selecting our health care team! To help us meet all your health care needs, please fill out this form completely in ink. If you have any questions or need assistance, please ask us - we will be happy to help.

Patient # _____

Soc. Sec. # _____

Patient Information (CONFIDENTIAL)

Date _____

Name _____ Birth date _____ Home phone _____

Address _____ City _____ State _____ Zip _____

Check appropriate box: ☐ Minor ☐ Single ☐ Married ☐ Divorced ☐ Widowed ☐ Separated

If student, name of school/college _____ City _____ State _____ ☐ Full time ☐ Part time

Patient's or parent's employer _____ Work phone _____

Business address _____ City _____ State _____ Zip _____

Spouse or parent's name _____ Employer _____ Work phone _____

Whom may we thank for referring you? _____

Person to contact in case of emergency _____ Phone _____

Responsible Party

Name of person responsible for this account _____ Relationship to patient _____

Address _____ Home phone _____

Driver's license # _____ Birth date _____ Financial institution _____

Employer _____ Work phone _____ SSN# _____

Is this person currently a patient in our office? ☐ Yes ☐ No

Insurance Information

Name of insured _____ Relationship to patient _____

Birth date _____ Social Security # _____ Date employed _____

Name of employer _____ Union or local # _____ Work phone _____

Address of employer _____ City _____ State _____ Zip _____

Insurance company _____ Group # _____ Policy/ID # _____

Ins. co. address _____ City _____ State _____ Zip _____

How much is your deductible? _____ How much have you used? _____ Max. annual benefit _____

DO YOU HAVE ANY ADDITIONAL INSURANCE? ☐ Yes ☐ No   IF YES, COMPLETE THE FOLLOWING:

Name of insured _____ Relationship to patient _____

Birth date _____ Social Security # _____ Date employed _____

Name of employer _____ Union or local # _____ Work phone _____

Address of employer _____ City _____ State _____ Zip _____

Insurance company _____ Group # _____ Policy/ID # _____

Ins. co. address _____ City _____ State _____ Zip _____

How much is your deductible? _____ How much have you used? _____ Max. annual benefit _____

I authorize release of any information concerning my (or my child's) health care, advice and treatment provided for the purpose of evaluating and administering claims for insurance benefits. I also hereby authorize payment of insurance benefits otherwise payable to me directly to the doctor.

X _____

Signature of patient or parent if minor _____ Date _____

FIGURE 2.1 The patient information form provides all of the information that the medical assistant needs to construct the patient's record.

Stickers can be used on the front of paper health records to indicate allergies, advance directives, and other information (Fig. 2.3). In an EHR, there will be alerts that may appear as a pop-up window when the record is accessed that will indicate that the patient has allergies, that immunizations are due, or that there is no advance directive on file. The alerts are helpful for the health professional because they keep important facts about the patient in the forefront of the professional's mind while he or she is treating the individual.

Past Health History. The past health history will include information about:

- previous illnesses/injuries (including childhood illnesses, such as chickenpox or measles)

- previous hospitalizations
- previous surgeries

The dates that these occurred will need to be documented, along with any complications that occurred. The provider needs to be aware of this information because it could affect the patient's current condition.

Family History. The family history includes:

- The physical condition of the various members of the patient's family
- Any illnesses or diseases individual members may have had
- Causes of death

This information is important because certain diseases may have a **hereditary** pattern. Most providers are interested in the immediate family: parents, grandparents, siblings, and children.

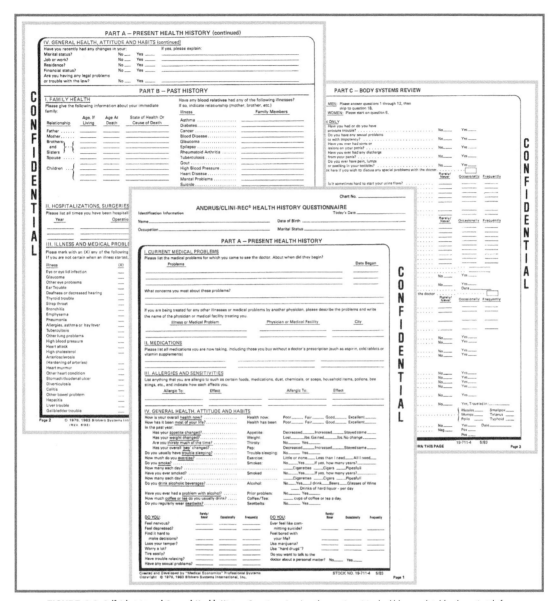

FIGURE 2.2 Self-Administered General Health History Questionnaire. Lengthy questionnaires should be completed by the patient before the individual is seen by the provider. Either mail the questionnaire to the patient in advance or ask the patient to come in early to complete the paperwork. (Courtesy Bibbero Systems, An InHealth Company, Petaluma, CA. *www.bibbero.com.*)

Social History. The social history includes information about the patient's lifestyle, such as:

- Living situation
- Marital status
- Employment
- Tobacco use
- Alcohol and drug use
- Exercise
- Nutrition

All of these factors can have an impact on a patient's overall health; they also can help highlight risk factors.

CRITICAL THINKING APPLICATION 2.2

While taking a patient's medical history, Susan asks about his social history. She asks whether he drinks alcohol. The patient immediately becomes defensive and accuses Susan of getting too personal about his affairs.

- How might Susan explain her reasons for asking these questions? What options are available if the patient refuses to discuss his social history with Susan?
- Could this opposition to questions about the social history raise suspicion in Susan's mind? What might she suspect?

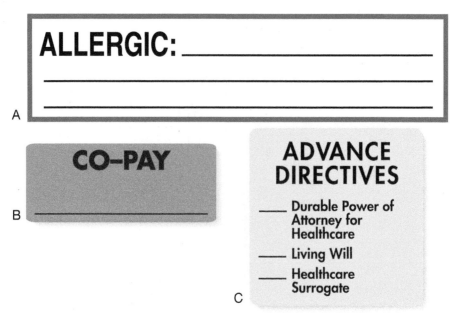

FIGURE 2.3 Record Stickers. Information on stickers on the outside of the record allows the provider and medical staff to see important information about the patient quickly. (Courtesy Bibbero Systems, An InHealth Company, Petaluma, CA. *www.bibbero.com.*)

Chief Complaint. The patient's chief complaint is a **concise** account of the patient's symptoms, explained in the patient's own words. It should include:

- The nature, location, frequency, and duration of pain, if any
- When the patient first noticed the symptoms
- Treatments the patient may have tried before seeing the provider and whether they have helped with the symptoms or not; when the last dose was taken
- Whether the patient has had the same or a similar condition in the past
- Other medical treatment received for the same condition in the past

Most healthcare facilities use a pain scale to determine the severity of the patient's discomfort. The medical assistant might ask, "How bad is your pain on a scale of 0 to 10, with 0 being almost no pain, and 10 being the worst pain you've ever experienced?" The pain scale or wording used in individual facilities should be documented in the office policies and procedures manual and followed by the medical assistant.

Objective Information

Objective findings, sometimes referred to as *signs,* are findings that can be observed and measured. They can include vital signs, measurements, observations made by the medical assistant, and findings from the provider's examination of the patient.

Vital Signs and Anthropometric Measurements

The medical assistant's responsibilities include:

- Taking the patient's vital signs (i.e., temperature, pulse, respirations, blood pressure, and pulse oximetry reading)
- Obtaining the person's **anthropometric** measurements (i.e., height and weight)

These measurements are documented in the patient's health record and are used by the provider in his or her assessment. If the medical assistant observes other signs, such as a rash, this would also be documented in the patient's health record and brought to the provider's attention.

Findings, Laboratory and Radiology Reports

After the provider has examined the patient, the physical findings are documented in the health record. The results of other tests or requests for these tests are then documented. If the tests were done elsewhere, the report is attached to the paper record. When an EHR is used, the separate sheet may be scanned so that it is in an electronic format and can be added to the patient's EHR.

Diagnosis

Based on all the evidence provided in the patient's past history, the provider's examination, and any supplementary tests, the provider notes his or her diagnosis of the patient's condition in the health record. If some doubt remains, this may be labeled a **provisional diagnosis**. A *differential diagnosis* is the process of weighing the probability of one disease causing the patient's illness against the probability that other diseases are causative. For example, the differential diagnosis of rhinitis, or a runny nose, could indicate allergic rhinitis (i.e., hay fever), the common cold, or even abuse of drugs or nasal decongestants.

Treatment Prescribed and Progress Notes

The provider's suggested treatment is listed after the diagnosis. Generally, instructions to the patient to return for follow-up treatment within a specific period also are noted here. If surgery or other treatment is going to be performed during the current visit, the patient must sign a consent form.

On each **subsequent** visit, when a paper record is used, the date must be entered on the record; information about the patient's condition and the results of treatment, based on the provider's observations, must be added to the health record. Notations of all medications prescribed, or instructions given, in addition to the patient's own report of how he or she is doing, should be documented in the health record. If the patient is hospitalized, the name of the hospital, the reason for admission, and the dates of admission and discharge are documented. Much of this information can be obtained from the hospital discharge summary.

The Medical Assistant's Role

It is important to ensure patient privacy when documenting in the health record. If you are interviewing the patient to obtain history information, do it where the patient's answers cannot be heard by others. If privacy is not possible, the patient should be given a form to fill out. The information can be transferred to the permanent record later. When privacy is available, the medical assistant may ask the patient questions and document the answers directly into the health record. This allows you to become better acquainted with the patient while completing the necessary records. It can also ensure that the patient understands the meaning of all of the questions.

If new patients must complete a lengthy form, there are several options:

- It can be mailed to the patient. The accompanying letter can request that it be completed and returned to the provider before the appointment.
- If the record is electronic, the patient may access his or her record through a patient portal. Using this method, the information is documented directly into the EHR system. It would then be reviewed by the medical assistant and provider during the office visit.
- Another option with an EHR is for the patient to complete a paper form, and the medical assistant enters the information into the EHR while reviewing the form with the patient.

The medical assistant may document the patient's chief complaint. The provider will question the patient in more detail. Many providers write their own entries in the record in longhand if a paper record is used. Some may document the findings directly into the computer if an electronic record is used. Others may dictate the material directly into the EHR. Another option is for a medical assistant or scribe to document the provider's findings. A final option is for the provider to use a recording device. If the material is dictated and transcribed, the provider should verify each entry. The entry must be initialed by the provider before it is entered into the patient's record. For a record to be admissible as evidence in court, the person dictating or writing the entries must be able to verify that they were true and correct at the time they were written. The best indication of this is the provider's signature or initials on the typed entry. In an EHR, the provider's electronic signature is proof of the accuracy of the entries.

Use of a Medical Scribe

A medical scribe should have an understanding of medical terminology, excellent computer skills, and a strong attention to detail. It is important that medical scribes understand that they are not obtaining the information from the patient. Their role is to document the information obtained by the provider and enter it into the EHR, per the provider's instructions.

Those healthcare facilities that have hired scribes have found that both the patients and providers are more satisfied with patient encounters. Providers are establishing a better relationship with patients because they are able to spend their time with face-to-face interaction rather than interacting with a computer.

OWNERSHIP OF THE HEALTH RECORD

Who owns the health record? Patients often assume that because the information in the health record is about them, ownership of the record is rightfully theirs. However, the owner of the physical health record is the provider or medical facility, often called the "maker," that initiated and developed the record. The patient has the right of access to the information within the record but does not own the physical record or other documents pertaining to the record. The patient has a **vested** interest and therefore has the right to demand confidentiality of all information placed in the record.

The actual paper health record should never leave the medical facility where it originated. Even the provider should refrain from taking the record from the office to the hospital or nursing facility. If information from the record is needed, copies can be made, and progress notes can be written on site and placed into the original record later. This is not an issue with an EHR because the record can be accessed by multiple users at the same time. Patients' paper records should be kept in a locked room or locked filing cabinets when the office is closed. EHRs must be protected from unauthorized access. Regulations established by the Health Insurance Portability and Accountability Act (HIPAA) state that each user must have a unique user name and password; individual access is determined by the system administrator.

Written health records must be legible. Each record should be written as if the provider and staff expect it to eventually be involved in a lawsuit; therefore, every word must be legible to an average reader years after it is written. The record can help the provider prove that he or she treated a patient in a competent manner. It can also prove that the patient was not given competent care. Every person on staff at the provider's office is responsible for writing legibly in every health record.

EHRs eliminate the issue of legibility in the record, but it is just as important to be sure that all patient care is documented in the electronic record. If care is not documented, this will leave the healthcare facility open to potential lawsuits and can affect patient care. In addition, if services are not documented, they cannot be billed to the patient or the patient's insurance company.

CRITICAL THINKING APPLICATION 2.3

On Susan's third day at work, a man comes into the office and demands to see his mother's health record. Susan accesses the record and sees that the mother has not granted permission for information to be given to her son. What should Susan do in this situation? Are there any viable reasons the son should have access to his mother's medical information?

TECHNOLOGIC TERMS IN HEALTH INFORMATION

There is some confusion regarding the acronyms *EHR* and *EMR*. These acronyms have been used interchangeably for many years. The Office of the National Coordinator for Health Information Technology (ONC) has established definitions for EHR and EMR that are easy to understand. Table 2.1 shows the definitions of EHR and EMR.

EMR is being used less and less as the federal regulations regarding electronic records have been established. There is a significant push toward having all electronic records meet the definition of an EHR. There are many advantages to having an electronic record system

TABLE 2.1   Electronic Health Record (EHR) versus Electronic Medical Record (EMR)

ELECTRONIC HEALTH RECORD (EHR)	ELECTRONIC MEDICAL RECORD (EMR)
• Electronic record of health-related information about a patient • Conforms to nationally recognized interoperability standards • Can be created, managed, and consulted by authorized clinicians and staff from more than one healthcare organization	• An electronic record of health-related information about an individual • An electronic version of a paper record • Can be created, gathered, managed, and consulted by authorized clinicians and staff within a single healthcare organization

that can be accessed from more than one healthcare organization. The continuity of patient care is much more easily established when all providers have access to the same records regardless of what organization they are working for. There should be less running of duplicate tests and procedures, which will help reduce the cost of providing healthcare.

A *personal health record* (PHR) is defined by the ONC as an electronic record of health-related information about an individual that conforms to nationally recognized **interoperability** standards and that can be drawn from multiple sources, but that is managed, shared, and controlled by the individual. There are several ways that a PHR can be created. Some health insurance companies offer PHRs for those they insure; some employers offer it as a service for their employees; and some healthcare facilities offer it to their patients. It is important to remember that the patient maintains a PHR. The information from an EHR does not automatically transfer to a PHR.

Another way for patients to access their healthcare information is through a **patient portal**. Patient portals allow patients to access their actual EHRs. At any time, a patient can view progress notes, laboratory results, medications, or immunizations. Many patient portal systems also allow:

• Communication between the patient and provider
• Completion of forms online
• Requests to be made for prescription refills
• Scheduling of appointments

By establishing effective patient portals, healthcare facilities can meet some of the meaningful use requirements.

HIPAA uses the term *protected health information* (PHI), which is any information about health status, the provision of healthcare, or payment for healthcare that can be linked to an individual patient. HIPAA requires that all PHI be safeguarded. This applies to:

• EHRs
• EMRs
• PHRs
• Patient portals

THE HEALTH INFORMATION TECHNOLOGY FOR ECONOMIC AND CLINICAL HEALTH ACT (HITECH) AND MEANINGFUL USE

The HITECH Act provides financial incentives for the meaningful use of certified EHR technology to achieve health and efficiency goals. It was part of the American Recovery and Reinvestment Act to promote the adoption and meaningful use of health information technology. Remember, HIPAA was created in large part to simplify administrative processes using electronic devices. *Meaningful use* means that providers must show that they are using EHR technology in ways that can be measured significantly in quality and quantity. If providers meet the meaningful use requirements, they will qualify for incentive payments. Three main components of meaningful use can be identified:

• Use of certified EHR technology in a meaningful manner, such as **e-prescribing**
• Use of certified EHR technology for electronic exchange of health information to improve the quality of healthcare
• Use of certified EHR technology to submit clinical quality reports, procedure and diagnosis codes, surveys, and other measures

Providers can expect reductions in the amounts they are paid from Medicare and Medicaid if they are not in **compliance**. Remember, the computer system in the medical office must be more than a tool for data recall to be considered an EHR system; the provider must use the system for tasks, at a minimum, such as e-prescribing and **computerized provider/physician order entry (CPOE)**.

CRITICAL THINKING APPLICATION   **2.4**

Some of the patients who visit Dr. Kahn and Dr. Martin have expressed concern that electronic health records (EHRs) may not be private enough and that their health information will be "floating around on the internet." They are worried that unauthorized individuals could somehow access their information on the computer and do them harm.

• How might Susan alleviate the patients' fears about their records being available on the internet?
• What disadvantages with regard to confidentiality are associated with the EHR?

CAPABILITIES OF ELECTRONIC HEALTH RECORD SYSTEMS

The EHR system can perform a multitude of tasks, saving time and money in the provider's office (Fig. 2.4). The following are some of the features of a typical EHR system.

• **Specialty software.** Patient data are captured and processed into a system that is specialty-specific. The terminology and patient care treatments are compatible with the provider's specialty. However, additional features can allow the provider to include terminology from other specialties.
• **Appointment scheduler.** The appointment scheduler (Fig. 2.5) allows the staff to:
  • Track and schedule appointments
  • Create the schedule matrix

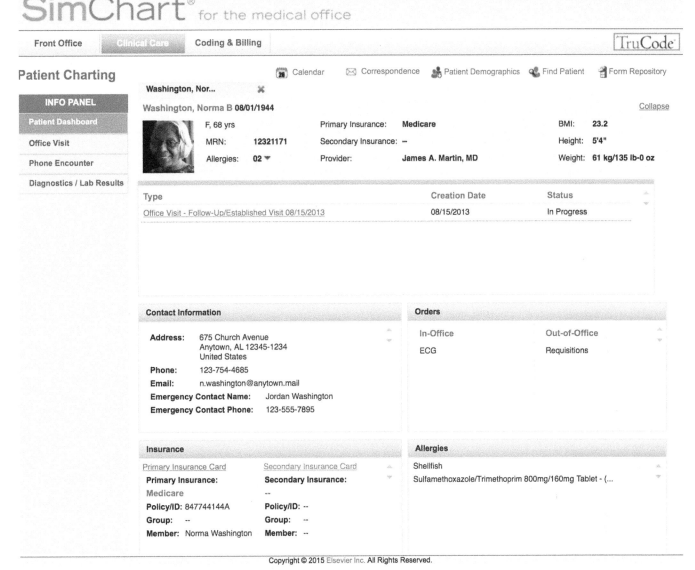

FIGURE 2.4 The electronic health record (EHR) can perform numerous tasks, in addition to displaying personal information about the patient. This allows the provider and medical assistants to interact with patients and provide better service.

- Account for recurring time blocks
  The appointments can be merged into specific types with default times so that lengthy procedures are not scheduled in short appointment blocks. The scheduler features also allow various search **parameters**; if a patient calls because he or she cannot remember the appointment time, a search can be initiated using:
- Date
- Provider's name
- Patient's name
- Keywords
- **Appointment reminder and confirmation.** The system can be programmed to automatically remind patients with a confirmation call. The staff can record the message to be sent, and patients are prompted to choose options, such as "Press one" to confirm or reschedule appointments.
- **Prescription writer.** The EHR system can produce electronic prescriptions, which can be printed and given to patients or

automatically submitted to a pharmacy. Lists can be created with the provider's most common drug choices and dosages. An allergy function can be linked to the patient's list of allergies and alert the provider of an issue. The system can also generate a patient information sheet on new prescriptions.
- **Medical billing system.** Also known as a *practice management system*. The EHR billing system can manage all of the practice's billing and accounting systems. The system also can **interface** with clearinghouses for electronic claims submission and tracking. Reports can be generated that provide accurate details of the financial state of the practice at certain intervals or whenever requested.
- **Charge capture.** The charge capture functions can store lists of billing codes, such as:
  - International Classification of Diseases (ICD)
  - Current Procedural Terminology (CPT)
  - Charges for procedures, supplies, and laboratory tests

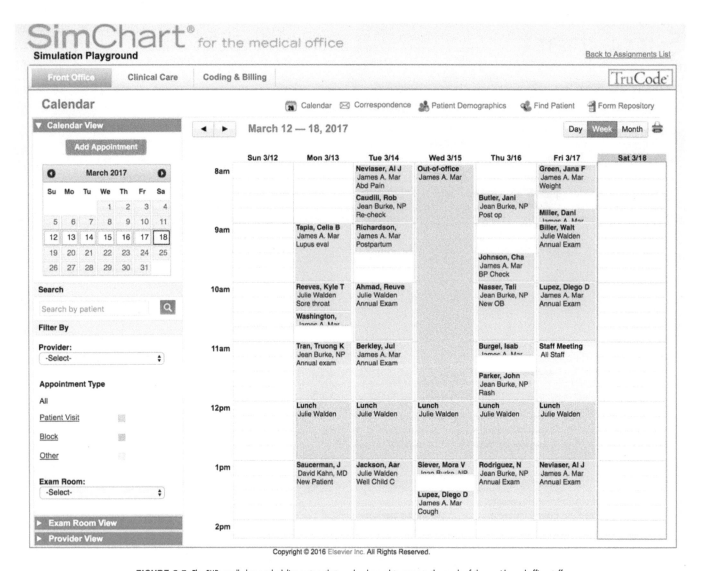

FIGURE 2.5 The EHR usually has a scheduling system that can be changed to manage the needs of the provider and office staff.

Alerts can let the user know when a certain charge does not match a diagnosis code; for instance, a blood glucose test done for a sore throat. In such cases, the software alerts the user and helps prevent errors that can lead to denial of insurance claims.

- **Eligibility verification.** EHR billing systems can perform online verification of insurance eligibility and can capture demographic data.
- **Referral management.** In the case of a referral or consultation, sharing information with another provider can be done electronically. The patient does not have to obtain copies of the record and then bring them to the new provider. This also eliminates the cost of making copies and is faster and more efficient than copying and mailing patients' records.
- **Laboratory order integration.** The laboratory order integration feature allows the user to interact with outside laboratories. The EHR can receive and post laboratory results to patients' records. Tests can be ordered from the provider's laptop, tablet, or smart phone. Results can be transmitted by fax, scan, or email and uploaded directly into the patient's record (see Procedure 2.2, p. 55).

CRITICAL THINKING APPLICATION   2.5

Jennifer, the office manager, has noticed that Susan seems overwhelmed in the training classes for the EHR system used by the clinic. During a break, Jennifer asks Susan whether she is having any specific problems with the training classes. She also asks for Susan's input on the system. Susan says that she just prefers clinical work and that her typing skills are a little "rusty." She is determined to do her best to learn the system and asks if she could have extra practice time.

- How might Jennifer respond to Susan's comments?
- What can Susan do to overcome her issues with the EHR system?

MAINTAINING A CONNECTION WITH THE PATIENT WHEN USING THE ELECTRONIC HEALTH RECORD

Many patients are required to choose a primary care provider (PCP) to be referred to a specialist. They also have the option of changing the PCP or specialist. The patient may decide to change providers

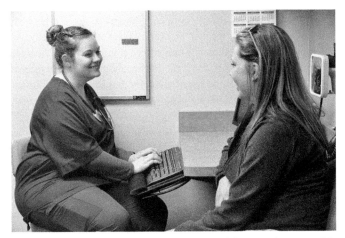

FIGURE 2.6 The medical assistant must make eye contact with the patient when using an EHR.

simply because he or she does not feel comfortable with that particular provider.

Because the change process is relatively easy, the healthcare facility should strive to provide excellent care and service to its patients. If the care begins to seem impersonal, patients may feel a strong desire to change providers. Patients are consumers of healthcare services, and they expect quality healthcare and service.

When using the EHR, the medical assistant must make sure that his or her nonverbal communication sends the right message to the patient. Eye contact is essential (Fig. 2.6). If the medical assistant constantly looks at the electronic device, the patient feels left out of the process. Make eye contact with the patient while asking questions and look at the screen only when needed to enter information. Do not shield the device from the patient's view when entering information. This can give the impression you are hiding something from the patient. Although patients may not understand anything they see on the screen, they will feel more at ease if their information is not hidden from them. Also, modify your position so that the patient feels like a part of the information process. Just as sitting in a chair across from a supervisor's desk can be intimidating, the patient may feel the same emotions sitting across from a medical assistant entering information into the EHR. Sit next to or at an angle to the patient to support the impression that those in the healthcare facility and the patient are partners in the healthcare plan.

Because patients have the right to make decisions in most aspects of their healthcare plans, offer choices wherever possible. Never expect patients to make quick decisions about their care. They may want to consult family members or give some thought to important medical decisions. The medical assistant needs to allow the patient time to think unless the patient is faced with a critical, time-sensitive decision. Providers often assume that patients will automatically follow their instructions or orders; however, some patients prefer some time to consider their options. Always follow up and make note of any wait time the patient requests, notify the provider, and enter that information into the EHR. Make sure timely communication is accomplished with the patient and that any additional orders that need to be put in place are completed. The many features of the EHR allow the medical assistant to be efficient and highly competent if he or she is willing to make an extra effort to master the EHR system.

Also, make sure patients understand all instructions given to them regarding test procedures or preparation for procedures. Most EHRs can print an instruction sheet, which the medical assistant can review with the patient. The customer service aspect of patient care is even more important when the facility uses an EHR system (see Procedure 2.3, p. 55).

CRITICAL THINKING APPLICATION   2.6

Jennifer walks behind Susan's desk and notices that she is looking at the progress notes on a patient who was recently arrested and indicted for child abuse. The case has been in the newspaper and on television consistently for several weeks. Jennifer asks Susan why she has accessed that record. Susan hesitates and then says she must have entered the wrong patient ID number. Does Susan's explanation sound convincing? Why is Jennifer concerned about Susan looking at the patient's record? Just because the individual is a patient at the clinic, does that mean any employee has the right to look at the patient's EHR?

BACKUP SYSTEMS FOR THE ELECTRONIC HEALTH RECORD

Even the best or most expensive EHR system cannot function without power. If a natural disaster occurs and the provider's office is without electricity for several days or weeks, the provider must have a backup system to protect the information contained in the EHR. HIPAA requires that the facility adopt a backup and recovery plan that includes daily offsite software backup for the EHR system. Three options are available for data preservation and backup.

- *External hard drive.* An external hard drive connects to the main computer, and with fairly simple programming it can copy the information in the EHR daily. Seven electronic folders, one for each day of the week, can hold the information from the previous day; these folders are replaced with new, updated information at designated periods. CDs and DVDs can hold daily data, and some thumb drives have enough capacity to perform this task. Once a habit of a daily backup to the external hard drive has been established, the method is relatively simple and reliable.
- *Full server backup.* The provider may want to back up the EHR system on a dedicated server, which is a large-capacity computer set aside specifically for the EHR system. With these servers, a full backup should be performed monthly. Many large medical facilities and hospitals have one or more dedicated servers for the EHR system.
- *Online backup system.* An online backup system can be used, usually for a subscription fee. Although the cost may be higher than for some other methods, online systems are easy to use because there is no external drive to carry and no CD or thumb drive to put through the process of downloading data. However, time investment is involved, because the process of contacting the company that offers the service and then downloading all the data takes several hours. Also, the initial download can take quite a while. Even so, an online system is stable and reliable.

All of these backup methods require an alternative power source in case of a disaster that interrupts electrical service. Remember that backup systems are not effective if the data are stored at the medical facility and the disaster happens at or affects that physical address. Information technology professionals usually recommend using two of the three methods for the best protection. The system must be protected from theft and unauthorized use, just like the onsite system.

Medical assistants should keep their paper health records skills sharp in case the EHR system is down for an extended period. Always have a supply of the most commonly used forms in a paper format available for use in such instances. When the EHR system comes back up, these paper forms can be scanned into the patients' EHRs.

RETENTION AND DESTRUCTION OF HEALTH RECORDS

In most medical offices, records are classified in three ways:
- *Active:* Records of patients currently receiving treatment
- *Inactive:* Records of patients whom the provider has not seen for 6 months or longer
- *Closed:* Records of patients who have died, moved away, or otherwise terminated their relationship with the provider

The process of moving a file from active to inactive status is called *purging.* An EHR system can be set up to automatically move the inactive records to another server so that processing time will not be slowed down, but the records are still readily accessible if the patient returns to the healthcare facility. Closed EHRs are also separated from the active records and are typically stored elsewhere. They may be placed on CDs or computer hard drives or maintained in inactive cloud space by the EHR vendor.

As with EHRs, paper health records are classified as active, inactive, and closed. A paper record system must have a system established for regular transfer of files from active to inactive status or possibly destruction. The expansion of records and the file space available can influence the transfer period. Records for patients currently hospitalized may be kept in a special section for quick reference and then placed in the regular active file when the patient is discharged from the hospital. In a surgical practice, the record frequently includes the specific date on which the patient is discharged from the provider's care, and the notation is made on the record, "Return prn" (from the Latin *pro re nata,* "as the occasion arises" or "when needed"). This record may safely be placed in the inactive file.

Most medical facilities use a year sticker on the file folder that indicates the last year the patient visited the clinic. If the file has a sticker showing that the patient's last visit was in 2018, and he or she presents to the clinic on January 5, 2020, a 2020 sticker should be placed over the one that indicates 2018. These stickers often are included with color-coded filing systems. The medical assistant can easily look at a group of files and see which ones need to be changed to inactive or closed status.

According to the American Medical Association (AMA) Council on Ethical and Judicial Affairs, providers have an obligation to retain patient records whether they are paper or electronic. Currently, no nationwide standard rule exists for establishing a records **retention schedule.**

Medical considerations are the primary basis for deciding how long to retain health records. For example, operative notes and chemotherapy records should always be part of the patient's health record. The laws regarding the retention of health records vary from state to state, and many governmental programs have their own guidelines for specific records retention. When no rules specify the retention of health records, the best course is to keep the records for 10 years. However, for minors, the facility should keep the records until the minor reaches the **age of majority** plus the statute of limitations. It is best to know the state requirements related to health records retention and follow those guidelines. The office policies and procedures manual should address records retention pertaining to the state where the practice exists.

The records of any patient covered by Medicare or Medicaid must be kept at least 10 years. The HIPAA Privacy Rule does not include requirements for the retention of health records. However, the rule does require that appropriate administrative, technical, and physical safeguards be applied so that the privacy of health records is maintained.

Some providers refuse to destroy or discard old records. Storage is less of an issue with EHRs because they take up much less physical space. Always refer to state laws when discarding health records.

Before old records are destroyed, patients should be given an opportunity to claim a copy of the records or have them sent to another provider. The medical facility should keep a master list of all records that have been destroyed. To legally destroy an EHR, the record, including the backup record, has to be overwritten using utility software.

RELEASING HEALTH RECORD INFORMATION

The healthcare facility must be extremely careful when releasing any type of medical information. The patient must sign a release for information to be given to any third party.

Requests for medical information should be made in writing (Fig. 2.7). HIPAA has designated that specific information must be included on the release of information form:
- Who is releasing the information
- To whom the information is being released
- What specific information is to be released
- An expiration date for the release

Accepting a faxed request for medical information or a faxed release of information from a patient is unwise. Even requests from the patient's attorney or insurance companies must be cleared by the patient for them to obtain information.

If a provider is involved in a liability suit, there will be a required exchange of information. As both parties to a lawsuit begin to prepare their cases, they enter the discovery process. Each side must disclose the pertinent facts of the case that may influence the final outcome of that case. On each occasion that information is needed from the provider, a separate request must be sent. Because the patient signs this request form, it serves as a release.

Most offices charge a fee to print or copy health records, whether it is a per-page charge or a per-record fee. If the records are sent electronically, no fee is charged. Follow the steps in the policies and procedures manual for the release of records. Some providers designate the office manager to handle requests for records releases.

Pay particular attention to records release requests involving a minor. In most cases, the parent or legal guardian is entitled to read through the patient's health records; however, according to the US Department of Health and Human Services (HHS), there are three

Central Texas Dermatology Clinic   •   102 Westlake Drive   •   Austin, Texas 78746

AUTHORIZATION TO DISCLOSE HEALTH INFORMATION

I hereby authorize the use or disclosure of information from the medical record of:

Patient Name: _____   Date of Birth: _____

Social Security# _____   Daytime Phone: _____

I authorize the following individual or organization to disclose the above named individual's health information:

_____   Address: _____

This information may be disclosed TO and used by the following individual or organization:

_____   Address: _____

Please release the following:

____ Progress Notes   ____ Pathology Reports   ____ Lab Reports   ____ Any and all Records

____ Other Diagnostic reports (specify _____

____ Other (specify) _____

Including Information (if applicable) pertaining to:

____ Mental Health   ____ Drug/Alcohol   ____ HIV/AIDS   ____ Communicable Treatment

Purpose or Need for Disclosure:

____ **Continued Patient Care**   ____ Personal Use

____ **Attorney/Legal**   ____ Insurance Claim/Application

____ Disability Determination   ____ Other(specify) _____

I understand that the information in my health record may include information relating to sexually transmitted disease, acquired immunodeficiency syndrome (AIDS), or human immunodeficiency virus (HIV). It may also include information about behavioral or mental health services, and treatment for alcohol and drug abuse.

I understand that the information released is for the specific purpose stated above. Any other use of this information without the written consent of the patient is prohibited.

I understand that I have the right to revoke this authorization at any time. I understand that if I revoke this authorization I must do so in writing and present my written revocation to the individual or organization releasing information. I understand that the revocation will not apply to information already released in response to this authorization. I understand that the revocation will not apply to my insurance company when the law provides my insurer the right to contest a claim under my policy. Unless otherwise revoked, this authorization will expire on following date, event or condition: _____

_____

If I fail to specify an expiration date, event or condition, this authorization will expire in six months.

I understand that authorizing the disclosure of this health information is voluntary. I can refuse to sign the authorization. I need not sign this form in order to ensure treatment. I understand that I may inspect or copy the information to be used or disclosed, as provided in CFR 164.524. I understand that any disclosure of information carries with it the potential for an unauthorized re-disclosure and the information may not be protected by federal confidentiality rules. If I have questions about disclosure of my health information, I can contact Theresa Farren at 512-327-7779.

_____   _____
Signature of Patient or Legal Representative   Date

_____   _____
Relationship to Patient (If Legal Representative)   Witness

> **COMPLETE ONLY IF INFORMATION IS TO BE RELEASED DIRECTLY TO PATIENT:**
> I understand that my medical record may contain reports, test results, and notes that only a physician can interpret. I understand and have been advised that I should contact my physician regarding the entries made in my medical record to prevent my misunderstanding of the information contained in these entries. I will not hold Central Texas Dermatology liable for any misinterpretation of the information in my medical record as a result of not contacting my physician for the correct interpretation.
>
> _____   _____
> Signature of Patient or Legal Representative   Date
>
> _____   _____
> Relationship to Patient (If Legal Representative)   Witness

Dr. review/signature/date _____

Date request completed _____   # of pages copied _____

Staff Signature _____

PHI Log completed _____

FIGURE 2.7 Authorization to Release Health Records. All requests for health records should be in writing, and the request should be kept in the patient's health record.

situations in which the parent may not be legally entitled to review the records of his or her minor child:

- When the minor is the one who consents to care, and the parent is not required to also consent to care under state law
- When the minor obtains medical care at the direction of a court or a person authorized by the court
- When the minor, parent, and provider all agree that the doctor and minor patient can have a private, confidential relationship

If the provider believes that the minor might be in an abusive situation or that the parent or legal guardian may be harming the patient, the provider is required, both legally and ethically, to report the abuse.

Sometimes patients want to look at their own records. They certainly have a right to see this information, but some patients may not understand the terminology used in the record. A staff member should always remain with a patient who is looking at his or her health record. Remember, the original health record should never leave the medical facility. Always follow office policy when releasing health records.

When a release is presented to the office, provide only the records requested in the release. Do not provide information that is not requested. The patient must specify that substance abuse, mental health, or human immunodeficiency virus (HIV) records are to be released. Remember that the patient ultimately decides whether a record can be released. If any question arises about what is to be released, consult the office manager or the provider.

Health Information Exchanges

The demand for electronic health information exchange (HIE) between one healthcare facility and another, together with nationwide efforts to improve the efficiency and quality of healthcare, is creating a demand for HIEs. As more and more providers move to EHRs, it only makes sense to have a system in place that will facilitate the exchange of that information electronically to improve the timeliness of that exchange. Patient care can be improved because all providers will have access to the information needed to treat the patient.

The ONC states, There are currently three forms of HIE:

- *Directed Exchange* – The ability to send and receive secure information electronically between care providers to support coordinated care
- *Query-Based Exchange* – The ability of providers to find and/ or request information on a patient from other providers, often used for unplanned care
- *Consumer-Mediated Exchange* – The ability of patients to aggregate and control the use of their health information among providers

The implementation of HIE varies from state to state. Some of the federal funding for the implementation of HIE is administered by the ONC.

ORGANIZATION OF THE HEALTH RECORD

Source-Oriented Records

The traditional patient record is a source-oriented record (SOR). Observations and data are cataloged according to their source:

- Provider (progress notes)
- Laboratory
- Radiology
- Hospital
- Consultations

Forms and progress notes are filed in **reverse chronologic order** and in separate sections of the record according to the type of form or service rendered (e.g., all laboratory reports together, all x-ray reports together, and so on). Reverse chronologic order is used so that the provider and staff members do not have to search to the bottom of the record to find a recent laboratory report or a test.

Problem-Oriented Records

The problem-oriented medical record (POR) is a departure from the traditional system of keeping patient records. The POR is a method of recording data in a problem-solving system. This system is divided into four components:

- The *database* includes the chief complaint, present illness, patient profile, review of systems, physical examination, and laboratory reports.
- The *problem list* is a numbered, titled list of every problem the patient has that requires management or workup. This may include social and demographic troubles in addition to strictly medical or surgical ones.
- The *treatment plan* includes management, additional workups needed, and therapy. Each plan is titled and numbered with respect to the problem.
- The *progress notes* include structured notes that are numbered to correspond with each problem number.

Several companies have developed file folders for organizing patient data according to the POR. The problem list (Fig. 2.8) is placed at the front of the record. Special sections are provided for current major and chronic diagnoses/health problems and for inactive major or chronic diagnoses/health problems. Progress notes usually follow the SOAP approach. SOAP is an acronym for the following:

- **S**ubjective impressions or patient reports
- **O**bjective clinical evidence or observations
- **A**ssessment or diagnosis
- **P**lans for further studies, treatment, or management

Some medical offices also use an *E* in the record to represent *evaluation*; others include *E* for *education* and *R* for *response*. The education notation shows that the patient was educated about his or her condition or given a patient information sheet. The response section is used to record an assessment of the patient's understanding of and possible compliance with the treatment plan.

The POR has the advantage of creating order and organization in the information added to a patient's health record. The records are more easily reviewed, and the likelihood of overlooking a problem is greatly reduced. The SOAP method forces a rational approach to the patient's problems and assists in forming a logical, orderly plan of patient care (Fig. 2.9). The POR is especially helpful in clinics, group practices, and hospitals, where more than one person must be able to find essential information in the record.

MASTER PROBLEM LIST
For use of this form, see AR 40-66; the proponent agency is the Office of The Surgeon General

MAJOR PROBLEMS

PROBLEM NUMBER	DATE ONSET	DATE ENTERED	PROBLEM	DATE RESOLVED
1.				
2.				
3.				
4.				
5.				
6.				
7.				
8.				
9.				
10.				
11.				
12.				

TEMPORARY (MINOR) PROBLEMS

PROBLEM LETTER	PROBLEM	DATES OF OCCURRENCES					
A.							
B.							
C.							
D.							
E.							
F.							
G.							
H.							

PATIENT'S IDENTIFICATION (Use mechanical imprint if available; for typed or written entries give: Name, SSN, Unit, Sex, Birthdate, and Duty Phone)

SUMMARY OF PROBLEMS, ALLERGIES, MEDICATIONS, SURGERIES AND TRAUMAS:

NOTE: DO NOT DISCARD FROM CHART

FIGURE 2.8 A problem list designed for a problem-oriented record (POR).

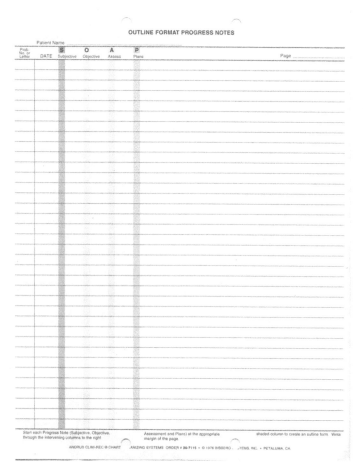

OUTLINE FORMAT PROGRESS NOTES

FIGURE 2.9 SOAP Progress Notes. The SOAP method keeps information organized and in a logical sequence. An actual progress note would include the provider's or medical assistant's signature or initials after each entry. (Courtesy Bibbero Systems, An InHealth Company, Petaluma, CA. *www. bibbero.com.*)

CRITICAL THINKING APPLICATION   **2.7**

Susan learned about SOAP documentation in school and is eager to use it in her new job. Dr. Kahn is seeing a patient who reports to Susan that she has had nausea and vomiting for the past 3 days. Susan obtains a weight of 132.5 pounds, temperature (T) 101.2° F tympanically, pulse (P) 94 beats/min, respiration (R) 14 breaths/min, and blood pressure (BP) 122/84 mm Hg in the right arm. What information would be documented in the Subjective field? What information would be documented in the Objective field? Who would document information in the Assessment field?

DOCUMENTING IN AN ELECTRONIC HEALTH RECORD

Documentation in an EHR involves using radio buttons, drop-down menus, and free-text boxes. The radio buttons and drop-down menus allow for standardization of the content in the EHR, and the free-text boxes allow for the documentation of the unique circumstance found with each patient (Fig. 2.10). It is important to carefully review the choices made with the radio buttons and drop-down menus. Information documented using the free-text boxes should be proofread before submitting.

DOCUMENTING IN A PAPER HEALTH RECORD

When you are documenting in a paper health record, the entry will always start with the date in the MM/DD/YYYY format. The date will be followed by the time. This may be written in standard or military time. If standard time is used, it must be followed by a.m. or p.m. (e.g., 2:00 p.m.). If military time is used, it is in a four-digit format without a colon (e.g., 1400). All entries must be written in black or blue ink, following the format designated by the healthcare facility. Documentation should be in the order in which the steps were completed. If a temperature, pulse, and respiration (TPR) measurement is done, it would be documented in the "O" or Objective section of the SOAP note starting with temperature, then pulse, and, lastly, respirations.

MAKING CORRECTIONS AND ALTERATIONS TO HEALTH RECORDS

Sometimes corrections must be made to health records. The first step is to verify the proper procedure for making corrections in the facility's policy and procedures manual. Some providers prefer a specific method for correcting errors in the health record. Erasing, using correction fluid, or any other type of **obliteration** is never acceptable. To correct a handwritten entry:

1. Draw a line through the error.
2. Insert the correction above or immediately after the error in a spot where it can be read clearly.
3. If indicated by the policies and procedures manual, write "Error" or "Err." in the margin.
4. The person making the correction should write his or her initials or signature and the date below the correction. Follow the format indicated in the policy and procedures manual (Fig. 2.11).

Errors made while using the computer are corrected in the usual way. However, an error discovered in an entry at a later date is corrected in the same manner as for a handwritten entry. This is sometimes called an *addendum*. Never attempt to alter health records without using this specific correction procedure, because this alteration of records may indicate a fraudulent attempt to cover up a mistake made by a staff member or the provider. Do not hide errors. If the error could, in any way, affect the patient's health and well-being, it must be brought to the provider's attention immediately. An EHR system will track the changes made within the record.

DICTATION AND TRANSCRIPTION

With the increased use of EHRs and voice recognition software, there is decreased need for **transcription**. If **dictation** is still done in the healthcare facility, the administrative medical assistant may find that transcribing the dictation is a job she or he will sometimes perform. Transcription can be done from handwritten notes or, more likely, from machine dictation. Smooth operation of the facility may depend on the timely, accurate performance of assigned responsibilities, such as record documentation and the preparation of special reports. Accuracy and speed are the primary requirements, along with a strong grasp of medical terminology and anatomy and physiology.

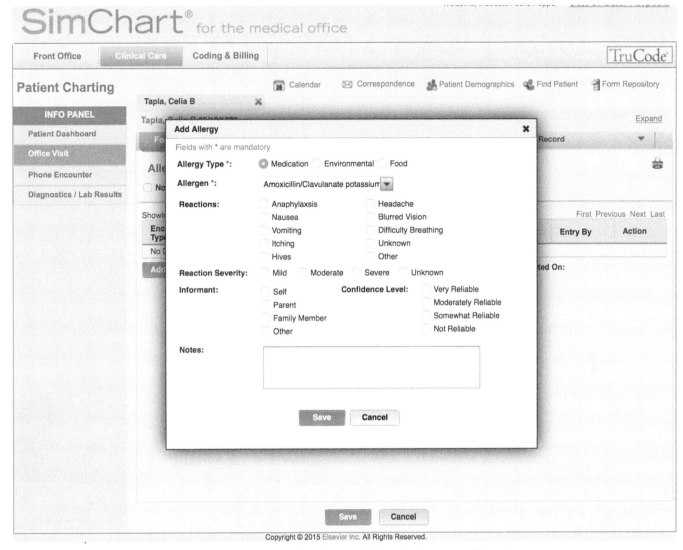

FIGURE 2.10 Documentation in an EHR is done using radio buttons, drop-down menus, and free-text boxes.

Dictation may be done using a machine transcription unit or a portable transcription unit. Many healthcare facilities now use a system that is accessed by telephone; the provider calls the system, using passwords or access codes, and records the information for the health record while speaking into the telephone. Later, employees transcribe the information into the health record. The provider must acknowledge and initial all transcripts before they are placed in the health record.

Voice Recognition Software

Some healthcare facilities use voice recognition software for transcription. When first installed, the software requires the user to say several sentences into the unit so that it "learns" to recognize the user's voice. The system can be used to dictate the following:

- Progress notes
- Letters
- Emails
- Any document in the healthcare facility that needs to be created

The provider will need to approve these documents before they are permanently attached to the patient's record. Some systems have

an authentication component that allows a type of electronic signature, such as those needed for hospital record dictation.

CREATING AN EFFICIENT PAPER HEALTH RECORDS MANAGEMENT SYSTEM

The paper health records management system should provide an easy method of retrieving information. The files should be organized in an orderly fashion. The information must be documented accurately, and corrections should be made and documented properly. The wording in the record should be easily understood and grammatically correct. An efficient method of adding documents to the record must be established so that the provider always has the most up-to-date information. Above all, the health records management system must work for the individual facility.

Filing Equipment

For years, the traditional filing system involved a vertical, four-drawer steel filing cabinet, used with manila folders with the patient's name

10/31/20XX	1:30pm T: 98.4 (TA), P̶6̶2̶ ⁷²ᵉʳʳᵒʳ ˢ· ᴮᵉᵉᶻˡᵉʳ ᶜᴹᴬ ⁽ᴬᴬᴹᴬ⁾ reg, strong
	R: 14 reg, deep, BP: 116/72 Ⓡ arm sitting
	——————————————— Susan Beezler, CMA (AAMA)

10/15/20XX	9:30am Mantoux test: ∅ ¹⁰ ᵉʳʳᵒʳ ˢ· ᴮᵉᵉᶻˡᵉʳ ᶜᴹᴬ ⁽ᴬᴬᴹᴬ⁾ mm induration
	——————————————— Susan Beezler, CMA (AAMA)

FIGURE 2.11 Corrections to health records must be done in a legible manner and must be clearly understood. Always initial and date corrections to health records.

on the tab. The most popular system today is color coding on open horizontal shelves. Rotary, lateral, compactable, and automated files also are available. Some records are kept in card or tray files. Several factors should be considered when selecting filing equipment:

- Office space availability
- Structural considerations
- Cost of space and equipment
- Size, type, and volume of records
- Confidentiality requirements
- Retrieval speed
- Fire protection
- Cost

Drawer Files

Drawer files should be full suspension; they should roll easily, close securely, and be equipped with a locking device. The best cabinets have a center trough at the bottom of each drawer with a rod for holding divider guides. A drawback of the vertical four-drawer files is that only one person can use a file cabinet at a time. Also, filing is slower, because the drawer must be opened and closed each time a file is pulled or filed.

File cabinets are heavy and can tip over, causing serious damage or injury unless reasonable care is taken. Open only one file drawer at a time and close it when the filing has been completed. A drawer left even slightly open can injure a passerby.

Horizontal Shelf Files

Shelf files should have doors that lock to protect the contents. A popular type of shelf file has doors that slide back into the cabinet; the door from a lower shelf may be pulled out and used for workspace. Open shelf units hold files sideways and can go higher on the wall because no drawers need to be pulled out (Fig. 2.12). File retrieval is faster, because several individuals can work simultaneously.

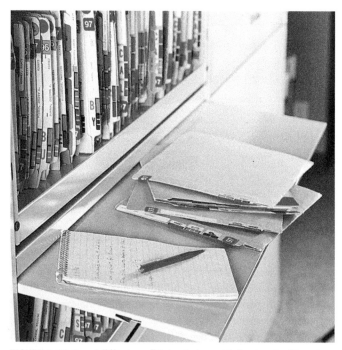

FIGURE 2.12 Open shelf filing is an efficient method, especially for color-coding filing systems. The shelf doors often can be used as workspace.

Rotary Circular Files

Rotary circular files can hold a large volume of records. They save space and clerical motion. The files revolve easily; some have push-button controls. Several people can work at one rotary file and use records at the same time. One disadvantage is that they afford less privacy and protection than files that can be closed and locked.

Compactible Files

An office with little space and a great volume of records might use compactible files, which are a variation of open shelf files. The files are mounted on tracks in the floor, and the units slide along the tracks so that access is gained to the needed records. One drawback is that not all records are available at the same time.

Automated Files

Automated files are initially very expensive, and they also require more maintenance than other types of filing equipment. They are likely to be found only in large facilities, such as clinics or hospitals. These files bring the record to the operator instead of the operator going to the record. When the operator presses a button indicating the appropriate shelf, the shelf automatically moves into position in front of the operator for record retrieval. The automated or power file is fast and can store large numbers of records in a small amount of space. However, only one person can use the unit at a time.

Card Files

Almost every office has some occasion to use a card file. This may be for patient ledgers, a patient index, a library index, an index of surgical tray setups, telephone numbers, or numerous other records. A good-quality steel box or tray is a sound investment.

Filing Supplies
Divider Guides

Each file drawer or shelf should be equipped with plenty of dividers or guides. Some authorities recommend one guide for approximately each 1½ inch of material, or every eight to 10 folders. Guides should be of good-quality heavy cardstock or strong plastic. Less-well-constructed guides soon become bent and frayed and have to be replaced. Divider guides have a protruding tab, which may be an integral part of the card or may be made of metal or plastic. The guides reduce the area of search and serve as supports for the folders. They are available in single, third, or fifth cut (i.e., one, three, or five different positions).

Out Guides

Out guides are made of heavyweight cardboard or plastic and are used to replace a folder that has been temporarily removed (Fig. 2.13). They may also have a large pocket to hold any filing that may come in while the folder is out. They should be of a distinctive color for quick detection. This makes refiling simpler and alerts the file clerk that a file is missing. Several colors may be used, each color designating the temporary location of the file. The out guide may have lines for recording information, or it may have a plastic pocket for inserting an information card.

File Folders

Most records to be filed are placed in covers or tabbed folders. The most commonly used is a general purpose, third-cut manila folder that may be expanded to ¾ of an inch. These are available with a double-thickness, reinforced tab, which greatly extends the life of the folder. Folders kept in drawers have tabs at the top; those kept on shelves have tabs at the side. Many folder styles are available for special purposes.

Hanging, or suspension, folders are made of heavy stock and hang on metal rods from side to side in a drawer. They can be used only with file cabinets equipped with suspension equipment.

Binder folders have fasteners that are used to bind papers in the folder. These offer some security for the papers, but filing the materials is time-consuming.

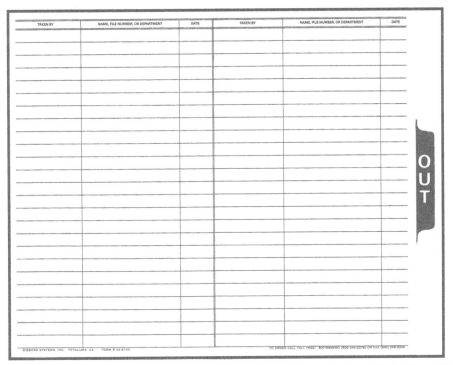

FIGURE 2.13 Out guides allow tracking of a file not in its proper location by providing information on the location of the file. (Courtesy Bibbero Systems, An InHealth Company, Petaluma, CA. *www.bibbero.com*.)

The number of papers that will fit in one folder depends on the thickness of the papers and the capacity of the folder. Near the bottom edge of most folders are one or more score marks, which should be used as the contents of the folders expand. Papers should never protrude from the folder edges, and they should always be inserted with their tops to the left. When papers start to ride up in any folder, the folder is overloaded.

Labels

The label is a necessary filing and finding device. Use labels to identify each shelf, drawer, divider guide, and folder. A label on the drawer or shelf identifies the nature of its contents. It should also indicate the range (i.e., alphabetic, numeric, or chronologic) of the material filed in that space.

The label on the divider guide identifies the range of folder headings following that divider guide up to the next divider (e.g., Ba-Bo). The label on the folder identifies the contents of that folder only, such as the following:

- Name of the patient
- Subject matter of correspondence
- Business topic

Label a folder when a new patient is seen, existing folders are full, or materials need to be transferred within the filing system.

Labels are available in almost any size, shape, or color to meet the individual needs of any facility. Visit an office supply website and review the catalogs to find the best product to meet the needs of the facility.

A narrow label applied to the front of the folder tab is the easiest to use and is satisfactory for folders kept in a drawer file. Labels for shelf filing should be identifiable from both front and back. Always type the label before separating it from the roll or protective sheet. Type the **caption** on the label in indexing order (see Procedure 2.4, p. 56).

INDEXING RULES

Indexing rules (Table 2.2) are standardized and based on current business practices. The Association of Records Managers and Administrators takes an active part in updating these rules. Some establishments adopt variations of these basic rules to accommodate their needs. In any case, the practices need to be consistent within the system:

TABLE 2.2	Applying Indexing Rules				
INDEXING RULE	NAME	UNIT 1	UNIT 2	UNIT 3	
1	Robert F. Grinch	Grinch	Robert	F.	
	R. Frank Grumman	Grumman	R.	Frank	
2	J. Orville Smith	Smith	J.	Orville	
	Jason O. Smith	Smith	Jason	O.	
3	M. L. Saint-Vickery	Saint-Vickery	M.	L.	
	Marie-Louise Taylor	Taylor	Marielouise		
4	Charles S. Anderson	Anderson	Charles	S.	
	Anderson's Surgical Supply	Andersons	Surgical	Supply	
5	Ah Hop Akee	Akee	Ah	Hop	
6	Alice Delaney	Delaney	Alice		
	Chester K. DeLong	Delong	Chester	K.	
7	Michael St. John	Stjohn	Michael		
8	Helen M. Maag	Maag	Helen	M.	
	Frederick Mabry	Mabry	Frederick		
	James E. MacDonald	Macdonald	James	E.	
9	Mrs. John L. Doe (Mary Jones)	Doe	Mary	Jones (Mrs. John L.)	
10	Prof. John J. Breck	Breck	John	J. (Prof.)	
	Madame Sylvia	Madame	Sylvia		
	Sister Mary Catherine	Sister	Mary	Catherine	
	Theodore Wilson, MD	Wilson	Theodore (MD)		
11	Lawrence W. Jones, Jr.	Jones	Lawrence	W. (Jr.)	
	Lawrence W. Jones, Sr.	Jones	Lawrence	W. (Sr.)	
12	The Moore Clinic	Moore	Clinic (The)		

1. Last names are considered first in filing; then the given name (first name), second; and the middle name or initial, third. Compare the names beginning with the first letter of the name. When a letter is different in the two names, that letter determines the order of filing.
2. Initials precede a name beginning with the same letter. This illustrates the librarian's rule, "Nothing comes before something."
3. With hyphenated personal names, the hyphenated elements, whether first name, middle name, or surname, are considered to be one unit.
4. The apostrophe is disregarded in filing.
5. When you are indexing a foreign name in which you cannot distinguish between the first and last names, index each part of the name in the order in which it is written. If you can make the distinction, use the last name as the first indexing unit.
6. Names with prefixes are filed in the usual alphabetic order, with the prefix considered part of the name.
7. Abbreviated parts of a name are indexed as written if that person generally uses that form.
8. Mac and Mc are filed in their regular place in the alphabet. If the files have a great many names beginning with Mac or Mc, some offices file them as a separate letter of the alphabet for convenience.
9. The name of a married woman who has taken her husband's last name is indexed by her legal name (her husband's surname, her given name, and her middle name or maiden surname). There should be a cross-reference, such as an out guide placed where her maiden name falls directing you to her new name.
10. When followed by a complete name, titles may be used as the last filing unit if needed to distinguish the name from another, identical name. Titles without complete names are considered the first indexing unit.
11. Terms of seniority or professional or academic degrees are used only to distinguish the name from an identical name.
12. Articles (e.g., the, a) are disregarded in indexing.

FILING METHODS

The three basic filing methods used in healthcare facilities are:
- Alphabetic by name
- Numeric
- Subject

Patients' records are filed either alphabetically by name or by one of several numeric methods. Subject filing is used for business records, correspondence, and topical materials.

Alphabetic Filing

Alphabetic filing by name is the oldest, simplest, and most commonly used system. It is the system of choice for filing patients' records in most small providers' offices.

The alphabetic system of filing is traditional and simple to set up, requiring only a file cabinet or shelf, folders, and some divider guides (see Procedure 2.5, p. 57). It is a **direct filing system** in that the person filing needs to know only the name to find the desired file. Alphabetic filing does have some drawbacks:

- The correct spelling of the name must be known.
- As the number of files increases, more space is needed for each section of the alphabet. This results in periodic shifting of folders to allow for expansion.
- As the files expand, more time is required for filing or retrieving each folder because of the greater number of folders involved in the search. The time can be greatly reduced by color coding.

Numeric Filing

Practically every large clinic or hospital uses some form of **numeric filing**, combined with color and shelf filing. Management consultants differ in their recommendations; some recommend numeric filing only if more than 5000 to 10,000 records are involved. Others recommend nothing but numeric filing. Numeric filing is an *indirect filing system*, or one that requires use of an alphabetic cross-reference to find a given file. Some object to this added step and overlook the advantages of numeric filing:

- It allows unlimited expansion without periodic shifting of folders, and shelves are usually evenly filled.
- It provides additional confidentiality to the record.
- It saves time in retrieving and filing records quickly. One knows immediately that the number 978 falls between 977 and 979. By contrast, an alphabetic system, even with color coding, requires a longer search to locate the exact spot.

Several types of numeric filing systems can be used:

- In a straight, or consecutive, numeric system, patients are given consecutive numbers as they first start using the practice. This is the simplest numeric system and works well for files of up to 10,000 records. It is time-consuming, and the chance for error is greater when documents with five or more digits are filed. Filing activity is greatest at the end of the numeric series.
- In a terminal digit system, patients also are assigned consecutive numbers, but the digits in the number usually are separated into groups of twos or threes and are read in groups from right to left instead of from left to right. The records are filed backward in groups. For example, all files ending in 00 are grouped together first, then those ending in 01, and so on. Next the files are grouped by their middle digits so that the 00 22s come before the 01 22s. Finally, the files are arranged by their first digits, so that 01 00 22 precedes 02 00 22.
- Middle-digit filing begins with the middle digits, followed by the first digits, and finally by the terminal digits. Numeric filing requires more training, but once the system has been mastered, fewer errors occur than with alphabetic filing.

CRITICAL THINKING APPLICATION 2.8

Susan is unsure whether alphabetic or numeric filing is best in the healthcare facility. What are some advantages and disadvantages of each method?

Subject Filing

Subject filing can be either alphabetic or **alphanumeric** (e.g., A 1-3, B 1-1, B 1-2, and so on) and is used for general correspondence. The main difficulty with subject filing is indexing, or classifying; that is, deciding where to file a document. Many papers require *cross-referencing*. An example would be if you had a subject folder for

Laboratory Supplies and the same organization provides you with your General Medical Supplies; there should be a notation in the Laboratory Supplies folder stating, "See Also General Medical Supplies," and vice versa. All correspondence dealing with a particular subject is filed together. The papers in the folders are filed chronologically with the most recent on top. The subject headings are placed on the tabs of the folders and filed alphabetically.

Color-Coding

When a color-coding system is used, both filing and finding files is easier, and misfiling of folders is kept to a minimum. The use of color visually restricts the area of search for a specific record. A misfiled record is easily spotted even from a distance of several feet. In color coding, a specific color is selected to identify each letter of the alphabet. Any selection of colors may be used, and the division of the alphabet is determined by one's own needs. However, studies have shown that the frequency with which different letters occur varies widely.

Alphabetic Color-Coding

As medicine continues to consolidate into larger facilities with more patients in one system, the filing of patients' records becomes more complicated, and color coding becomes more useful. Several color-coding systems use two sets of 13 colors: one set for letters A to M, and a second set of the same colors on a different background for letters N to Z.

Many ready-made systems are available for use. Self-adhesive, colored letter blocks with either two or three letters in the specific colors are supplied in rolls. The color blocks with the appropriate letter are placed on the index tab of the folder, along with the patient's full name. The letters are in pairs so that they can be seen from either side of the record. Strong, easily differentiated colors are used, creating a band of color in the files that makes spotting out-of-place folders easy (Fig. 2.14).

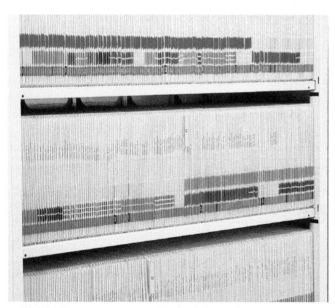

FIGURE 2.14 With color-coding of patients' records, a misplaced file is easily spotted. (Courtesy Bibbero Systems, An InHealth Company, Petaluma, CA. *www.bibbero.com*.)

Numeric Color-Coding

Color coding is also used in numeric filing. Numbers 0 through 9 are each assigned a different color. In a terminal digit filing system, the colors for the last two numbers are affixed to the tab. If the number 1 is red and 5 is yellow, all files with numbers ending in 15 have a red and yellow band. Usually a predetermined section of the number is color coded.

Other Color-Coding Applications

Color can work in many other ways for the efficient healthcare facility. Small tabs in a variety of colors can be used to identify certain types of insured patients and other specific information. For example, a red tab over the edge of the folder may identify a patient on Medicare; a blue tab may identify a Medicaid patient; a green tab may identify a workers' compensation patient; matching tabs may be attached to the insured's ledger card; research cases may be identified by a special color tab; and brightly colored labels on the outside of a patient's record can indicate certain health conditions, such as drug allergies. In a partnership practice, a different color folder or label may identify each provider's patients. Color also can be used to differentiate dates: one color for each month or year.

The use of color in filing is limited only by the imagination. One word of caution: Every person in the facility who uses the files must know the key to the coding, and the key should also be written in the facility's policy and procedures manual.

ORGANIZATION OF FILES

Providers find studying a disorganized patient record very difficult. Some systematic method must be followed in placing items in the patient folder. From the filing standpoint, it should be emphasized that when a patient record is not in actual use, it should be in only one place – the filing cabinet or on the shelf. Many precious hours can be wasted searching for misplaced or lost records that were carelessly left unfiled.

The patient's full name, in indexing order, should be typed on a label and the label attached to the folder tab. A strip of transparent tape can be placed on the label to prevent smudging. The patient's full name should also be typed on each sheet in the folder. Some types of records common to the healthcare setting, other than patient records, are health-related correspondence, general correspondence, practice management files, miscellaneous files, and tickler or follow-up files.

Health-Related Correspondence

Correspondence pertaining to patients' health should be filed in the patient's health record. Other medical correspondence should be filed in a subject file.

General Correspondence

The provider's office operates as both a business and a professional service. Correspondence of a general nature pertaining to the operation of the office is part of the business side of the practice. Usually, a special drawer or shelf is set aside for the general correspondence.

The correspondence is indexed according to subject matter or the names of the correspondents. The guides in a subject file may appear in one, two, or three positions, depending on the number of headings, subheadings, and subdivisions.

Practice Management Files

Of course, the most active financial record is the patient ledger. In facilities that still use a manual system, this is a card or vertical tray file, and the accounts are arranged alphabetically by name. At least two divisions are used: active accounts and paid accounts.

Miscellaneous Files

Papers that do not warrant an individual folder are placed in a miscellaneous folder. In that folder, all papers relating to one subject or with one correspondent are kept together in chronologic order, with the most recent on top, and then filed alphabetically with other miscellaneous material. Related materials may be stapled together. Never use paper clips for this purpose. When as many as five papers accumulate with one correspondent or subject, a separate folder should be prepared. Other business files include records of income and expenses, financial statements, income and payroll tax records, canceled checks, and insurance policies. These papers may be filed chronologically.

Tickler or Follow-Up Files

The most frequently used follow-up method is a **tickler file**, so called because it tickles the memory that something needs to be done or followed up on a particular date. The tickler file is always in a chronologic arrangement. In its simplest form, it consists of notations on the daily calendar. If information, such as an x-ray report or a laboratory report, is expected about a patient with an appointment to come in, the medical assistant might make a note on the calendar or tickler file a day ahead to check on whether the report has arrived.

The tickler file can be a part of a computerized health record system or could be as simple as an email sent to oneself. Many people put reminders on their cell phones using an application (app) specially designed for memos and reminders. The tickler file could also be a card file: 12 guides, one for each month, are placed at the front of the cabinet, container, or other object used to hold the folders. Notations of actions to be taken are placed behind the guides for specific days of the current month. Notations for future months are placed behind the guide for that month. To be effective, the tickler file must be checked first thing each day.

The tickler file can be used in many ways. It is a useful reminder of recurring events, such as payments, meetings, and so forth. On the last day of each month, all the notations from behind the next month's guide are distributed among the daily numbered guides, and the guide for the month just completed is placed at the back of the file.

CRITICAL THINKING APPLICATION   2.9

Susan is responsible for checking the tickler file daily. What types of documents and duties might she find inside these files?

Transitory or Temporary File

Many papers are kept longer than necessary because no arrangement is made for separating those with a limited usefulness. This situation can be prevented by having a transitory or temporary file. For example, if a medical assistant writes a letter requesting a reprint of the new patient brochure, the file copy is placed in the transitory folder until the reprint is received. When the reprint is received, the file copy is destroyed. The transitory file is used for materials with no permanent value. The paper may be marked with a "T" and then destroyed when the action is completed.

CLOSING COMMENTS

Just as in every aspect of the medical profession, advances in health records management are occurring rapidly, allowing providers and other caregivers to perform their duties more efficiently and accurately. A medical assistant must constantly be willing to learn and to adapt to changes arising from legislation and technologic advances. Computers have become generally accepted as a means of recording health information.

A primary goal of all healthcare facilities is to provide efficient, high-quality patient care. The EHR system can help the staff reach that goal. In the future, every provider's office, hospital, pharmacy, and healthcare facility may be able to access information in minutes, which will improve patient care and save lives. Stay abreast of news and articles related to EHR systems. The healthcare industry is one of constant growth and learning, and today's information technology provides the medical assistant with endless opportunities to make that growth rewarding and applicable to her or his current position.

Legal and Ethical Issues

The authority to release information from the health record lies solely with the patient unless such a release is required by law through a subpoena duces tecum. Ownership of the record often is a subject of controversy. The record belongs to the provider; the information belongs to the patient.

Remember that the EHR system contains information that is confidential at all times. The patient must authorize the release of health information in electronic form, just as if it were a piece of paper. EHR systems must:
- Maintain the security and confidentiality of data
- Be easily retrievable
- Have safeguards against the loss of information
- Protect patients' rights to confidentiality and privacy
- Require identification and authentication for access

By supporting these requirements, the medical facility remains in compliance with applicable laws and gains the trust of patients, who are reassured that their health information is secure and safe.

Patient-Centered Care

Patients worry about the security of their information, particularly about who can access it. Lawsuits are often filed when patients discover that an unauthorized person has accessed their protected health information. The medical assistant should listen to a patient's concerns and explain the safety procedures that apply to the EHR in language the patient can understand. Some facilities prepare a brochure to explain the conversion process to the patient and the advantages of the EHR system.

The medical assistant should expect hesitation and even reluctance from patients who are concerned about the privacy of their health information. Patients are concerned about lack of control over who views their records. Be prepared to answer their questions about the safety of their records as related to the EHR. The medical assistant must know how the EHR is protected and what security measures are in place to be able to reassure the patients that their records are protected at all times.

Professional Behaviors

Once the medical assistant has been trained on the EHR system and has had the opportunity to use it for a time, daily use should become second nature. In fact, it may be difficult to imagine a workday without the system! By being open to change and willing to learn, the medical assistant can set a good example for all employees and will be more receptive to the process of change. Be encouraging to other staff members while training on the system, and if technology comes easily to you, share your knowledge with others and assist wherever possible. Do not expect to master the system in a week; instead, realize that a new system has a learning curve and be patient with and receptive to the educational process. Keep technical support phone numbers handy and feel free to use them whenever a new or complicated issue arises. Work as a team, and if possible, help others who might find learning the system more of a struggle. Above all, while getting used to the new technology, make sure your attitude is one of enthusiasm, interest, and curiosity.

SUMMARY OF SCENARIO

Susan looks forward to attending her medical assisting classes each day and works diligently to perform to the best of her ability in the classroom. She strives to do well on each procedure check-off and each examination she completes. Her instructors provide excellent feedback and appreciate her contributions to the class.

Susan has the attitude that everything she is allowed to do in the healthcare facility is a learning tool. She regularly asks for additional responsibilities and is always ready to assist a co-worker. Dr. Kahn has recognized that she has the desire to learn, and he gives her many opportunities to glean more knowledge through the everyday activities in the office.

Although she is new to the medical profession, Susan learns quickly and thinks logically. She knows the rules and regulations on patient confidentiality and is always careful about the information she provides to those who request it. She is never hesitant about asking her office manager for guidance if she is unsure about any aspect of her duties. Susan is understanding and respectful when patients are concerned about their privacy. Her confidence and warm personality play a role in the trust she earns from the patients at the clinic.

Susan is willing to admit when she has made an error and has sought advice from Dr. Kahn and her office manager when an error needed correction. Although filing is not one of her favorite duties, she can be counted on to do her best while completing this important task. She realizes that filing is critical because the documents in the patient's health record direct the care provided to the patient. An abnormal laboratory report that is missing can make a crucial difference in the patient's care. She takes pride in her work, and she is efficient and accurate where health records are concerned. When she is faced with a new task, she considers it a learning experience and asks for help if she is not completely sure about the way to handle a situation.

Susan's co-workers are supportive and always willing to help her as she learns to be the best medical assistant she can be. Her future as a professional medical assistant certainly holds opportunity and chances for advancement. Just as important, patients trust her. She has alleviated patients' concerns about EHRs by taking the time to explain privacy policies and exactly what information will be accessible to third parties. This trust also gives patients the confidence to reveal personal information and to know that it will be held in the strictest confidence, not just by Susan, but by each employee in the provider's office.

SUMMARY OF LEARNING OBJECTIVES

1. **Discuss the two types of patient records.**

   The two major types of patient records are the paper health record and the electronic health record (EHR). The EHR is much more efficient than the paper record, and most healthcare facilities have switched to EHRs for a number of reasons.

2. **State several reasons that accurate health records are important.**

   Health records must be accurate primarily so that the correct care can be given to the patient. The record also helps ensure continuity of care between providers so that no lapse in treatment occurs. The

   record serves as indication and proof in court that certain treatments and procedures were performed on the patient; therefore, it can be excellent legal support if it is well maintained and accurate. Health records also aid researchers with statistical information.

3. **Differentiate between subjective and objective information in creating a patient's health record.**

   Subjective information is provided by the patient, whereas objective information is provided by the provider. Examples of subjective information include the patient's address, Social Security number, insurance information, and description of what he or she is experiencing. Objective information is obtained through the provider's questions and observations made during the examination.

Refer to Procedure 2.1 to see how to create a patient's health record and register a new patient in practice management software.

4. **Explain who owns the health record.**

    The provider owns the physical health record, but the patient controls the information contained in it.

5. **Distinguish between an electronic health record (EHR) and an electronic medical record (EMR).**

    The EHR is an electronic record of health-related information about an individual that conforms to nationally recognized interoperability standards and that can be created, managed, and consulted by authorized clinicians and staff from more than one healthcare organization. The EMR is an electronic record of health-related information about an individual that can be created, gathered, managed, and consulted by authorized clinicians and staff within one healthcare organization.

6. **Do the following related to healthcare legislation and EHRs:**

    - *Define meaningful use and relate it to the healthcare industry.*
      Meaningful use, defined simply, means that providers must show that they are using EHR technology in ways that can be measured significantly in quality and quantity. If providers meet the meaningful use requirements, they will qualify for incentive payments.

    - *List the three main components of meaningful use legislation.*
      The three main components of meaningful use are (1) use of certified EHR in a meaningful manner, such as e-prescribing; (2) use of certified EHR technology for electronic exchange of health information to improve the quality of health care; and (3) use of certified EHR technology to submit clinical quality reports, procedure and diagnosis codes, surveys, and other measures.

7. **Discuss the importance of nonverbal communication with patients when an EHR system is used.**

    Eye contact is critical when an EHR system is used with patients. Body language must indicate that the medical assistant is open to and listening to the patient's concerns, not just concentrating on data entry. Providers and medical assistants alike may have to relearn how to interact with patients in a natural way while using the laptop or tablet in the examination room. Realize that during the implementation period, processing and serving patients may take longer because the staff is using new technology. Most patients are understanding about this if the medical assistant explains that a new system is in place and asks for patience. Because patients are not always technologically savvy, most will be supportive and interested in the EHR system.

8. **Discuss backup systems for the EHR, in addition to the transfer, destruction, and retention of health records as related to the EHR.**

    The provider must have a backup system for the EHR in case a medical office is without power for a significant amount of time. The EHR systems can be set to automatically back up the information at specified times during the day. This means that a minimum amount of data would be lost if the power went out. Options include external hard drive, full server backup, and online backup systems. In most medical offices, records are classified in three ways: active, inactive, and closed. The process of moving a file from active to inactive is called *purging*. Providers have an obligation to retain patient records. The records of any patient covered by Medicare or Medicaid must be kept at least 10 years.

9. **Discuss retention and destruction of medical records as related to paper records.**

    As with EHRs, paper health records are classified as active, inactive, or closed. Large healthcare facilities may find it advisable to convert their paper health records to microfilm.

10. **Describe how and when to release health record information; also, discuss health information exchanges (HIEs).**

    The healthcare facility must be extremely careful when releasing any type of medical information; the patient must sign a release for information to be given to any third party. Requests for medical information should be made in writing. Pay particular attention to records release requests involving a minor.

    There are currently three kinds of HIE — directed exchange, query-based exchange, and consumer-mediated exchange — and the implementation of HIE varies from state to state.

11. **Identify and discuss the two methods of organizing a patient's paper medical record.**

    The source-oriented medical record (SOMR) categorizes the content by its source, such as provider, laboratory, radiology, hospital, and consultation. Within each source category the content is arranged in reverse chronologic order so that the most recent content is viewed first.

    The problem-oriented medical record (POMR) categorizes each of the patient's problems and elaborates on the findings and treatment plans for all concerns. Detailed progress notes are kept for each individual problem. This method addresses each of the patient's concerns separately, whereas a source-oriented record may address all problems and concerns at one time, usually covering one to three patient concerns per office visit. The POMR helps ensure that individual problems are all addressed.

12. **Discuss how to document information in an EHR and a paper health record, and how to make corrections/alterations to health records.**

    Documenting information in an EHR involves using radio buttons, drop-down menus, and free-text boxes. When you are documenting in a paper health record, the entry will always start with the date in the MM/DD/YYYY format. All entries must be written in black or blue ink and follow the format designated by the healthcare facility.

    To create a handwritten correction to a health record, a line should be drawn through the error, the correction inserted above or immediately after, and the person making the correction should write his or her initials or signature and the date below the correction. Errors made while using an EHR are corrected in the usual way; however, an error discovered in an entry at a later date is corrected in the same manner as for a handwritten entry.

Continued

13. **Discuss dictation and transcription.**

    With the increased use of EHRs and voice recognition software, there is decreased need for transcription. Transcription can be done from handwritten notes, or more likely from machine dictation. Accuracy and speed are important. Some healthcare offices use voice recognition software for transcription.

14. **Identify the filing equipment and filing supplies needed to create, store, and maintain paper health records.**

    Several types of equipment and supplies are needed to manage patients' records. Office space availability; structural considerations; cost of space and equipment; size, type, and volume of medical records; confidentiality requirements; retrieval speed; fire protection; and cost should all be considered when choosing filing equipment. Filing equipment includes drawer files, horizontal shelf files, rotary circular files, compactible files, automated files, and card files. Filing supplies include divider guides, out guides, file folders, and labels.

15. **Describe indexing rules, and how to create and organize a patient's health record.**

    Five basic steps are involved in document filing: (1) The papers are conditioned, which is the preparatory stage for filing. (2) The documents are released, which means they are ready to be filed because they have been reviewed or read and some type of mark has been placed on the document to indicate this. (3) The documents are indexed, which involves deciding where each document should be filed and coding it with some type of mark on the paper indicating

    that decision. (4) Sorting involves placing the files in filing sequence. (5) The actual filing and storing of the documents are the last step. Refer to Table 2.2 for indexing rules. Refer to Procedure 2.4 for information on creating and organizing a paper health record.

16. **Discuss the pros and cons of various filing methods and how to file patient health records.**

    Both the alphabetic and numeric filing systems have advantages and disadvantages. Perhaps most important is the staff's preference. Some find it easier to retrieve files that are in standard alphabetic order, whereas others prefer a numeric system. The numeric system is more confidential than an alphabetic system. Some staff members prefer a combination of the two, called the alphanumeric system. Both effectively keep health records in good order and allow the medical assistant to spot a misfiled record quickly.

    Refer to Procedure 2.5 to see how to file patient health records.

17. **Discuss the organization of files and of health-related correspondence.**

    When a patient record is not in actual use, it should only be in the filing cabinet or on the shelf. Health-related correspondence, including general correspondence, should be filed appropriately. Practice management files are usually divided into active and paid accounts. Papers that do not warrant an individual folder are placed in the miscellaneous folder. Follow-up files are frequently called "tickler files." Transitory (i.e., temporary) files can be helpful for material with no permanent value.

PROCEDURE 2.1   Register a New Patient in the Practice Management Software

Task: Register a new patient in the practice management software, prepare a Notice of Privacy Practices (NPP) form and a Disclosure Authorization form for the new patient, and document this in the electronic health record (EHR).

Scenario: The patient received both documents and signed the Disclosure Authorization form.

EQUIPMENT and SUPPLIES

- Computer with SimChart for the Medical Office or practice management and EHR software
- Completed patient registration form
- Scanner

PROCEDURAL STEPS

1. Obtain the new patient's completed registration form. Log into the practice management software.
   PURPOSE: The registration form will provide the information needed to create the new record in the practice management system.

2. Using the patient's last and first names and date of birth, search the database for the patient.
   PURPOSE: To help ensure the integrity of the practice management and EHR systems, a search for the new patient's name must always be done before registering that person. This prevents a double record from

being created if the patient had been entered into the database at an earlier time.

3. If the database does not contain the patient's name, add a new patient and enter the patient's demographics from the completed registration form.
   PURPOSE: This will create the patient's record in the practice management system.

4. Verify that the information entered is correct and that all fields are completed before saving the data.
   PURPOSE: Errors during the registration process can affect the communication with the patient (e.g., if a wrong address or email is entered) or can affect billing (e.g., if the incorrect insurance information is added). Accuracy is extremely important when entering the patient's information.
   Note: The software will generate a health record number for the patient.

5. Using the EHR software, prepare and print a copy of the NPP and a Disclosure Authorization form for the new patient. The Disclosure Authorization form should indicate the disclosure will be to the patient's insurance company.

PROCEDURE 2.1   **Register a New Patient in the Practice Management Software—***continued*

PURPOSE: Before the medical office can release patient information to the insurance company, the patient has to give consent in writing.

6. Using the EHR, document that the patient received a copy of the NPP and signed the Disclosure Authorization form. Scan the Disclosure Authorization form and upload it into the EHR.

PURPOSE: Documentation in the health record provides a legal record of what was done or communicated to the patient.

7. Log out of the software upon completion of the procedure.
PURPOSE: Logging into and out of the software helps to protect the integrity of the data saved in the software and prevents unauthorized people from viewing the information.

PROCEDURE 2.2   **Upload Documents to the Electronic Health Record**

Task: Scan paper records and upload digital files to the EHR.

Scenario: A new patient brings in a laboratory report and a radiology report that he would like to have added to his EHR. You need to scan in the original documents and upload them to the EHR.

EQUIPMENT and SUPPLIES

- Scanner
- Computer with SimChart for the Medical Office or EHR software
- Patient's laboratory and radiology reports

PROCEDURAL STEPS

1. Obtain the patient's name and date of birth if not on the reports.
   PURPOSE: You will need the patient's name and date of birth to find the patient's EHR.
2. Using a scanner that is connected to the computer, scan each document, creating an individual digital image for each.
   PURPOSE: The reports should be scanned separately and not combined to create one file. Each type of report must be uploaded separately to the correct location in the EHR.
3. Locate the file of the two scanned images in the computer drive. Open the files to ensure the images are clear.

PURPOSE: When you are scanning and uploading documents to the EHR, it is crucial that the image of the document is clear and can be easily read by the provider. If the image is blurred, rescan the document.

4. In the EHR, search for the patient, using the patient's last and first names. Verify the patient's date of birth.
   PURPOSE: Before you begin uploading to or documenting in the EHR, it is critical to verify that the correct record is opened.
5. Locate the window to upload diagnostic/laboratory results and add a new result. Enter the date of the test. Select the correct type of result. Browse for the image file of the laboratory file and attach it. Save the information. Select the option to add a new result and repeat the steps to upload the second report. Verify that both documents were uploaded correctly.
   PURPOSE: Errors during the upload may affect the ability to see the files. Verifying at the time of the upload will help you ensure that providers can see the results in the future.

PROCEDURE 2.3   **Protect the Integrity of the Medical Record**

Task: Protect the integrity of the medical record.

Scenario: You are mentoring a medical assistant student, who is in practicum. You notice the student routinely does not sign out of the electronic health record before leaving the desk. The facility's policy is to sign out or lock the computer before leaving it.

Directions: Role-play the scenario with a peer, who plays the student. You, the medical assistant, must explain to the "student" the facility's policy. Also address the hazards of not protecting the medical record. If the student does not change this behavior, you will need to address the situation with the department supervisor.

PROCEDURAL STEPS

1. Professionally and respectfully discuss the situation with the student.
2. Inform the student about the facility's policy and the hazards of not protecting the electronic health record.
   PURPOSE: It is important that the student be knowledgeable about the policies and the hazards of not protecting the EHR.
3. Provide the student with strategies to protect the electronic health record.
4. Inform the student what will occur if he or she does not protect the electronic record.

PROCEDURE 2.4   Create and Organize a Patient's Paper Health Record

Task: Create a paper health record for a new patient. Organize health record documents in a paper health record.

EQUIPMENT and SUPPLIES

- End tab file folder
- Completed patient registration form
- Divider sheets with different color labels (4)
- Progress note sheet (1)
- Name label
- Color-coding labels (first two letters of last name and first letter of first name)
- Year label
- Allergy label
- Black pen or computer with word processing software to process labels
- Health record documents (i.e., prior records, laboratory reports)
- Hole puncher

PROCEDURAL STEPS

1. Obtain the patient's first and last names.
   PURPOSE: To customize the record for the patient, the first and last names will be required.
2. Neatly write or word-process the patient's name on the name label. Left justify the last name, followed by a comma, the first name, middle initial, and a period (e.g., Smith, Mary J.).
   PURPOSE: The label should be easy to read. The last name always comes before the first name.
3. Adhere the name label to the bottom left side of the record tab. When you hold the record by the main fold in your left hand, the writing should be easy to read. (For directional purposes, assume the record main fold is on the left and the tab is at the bottom.)
   PURPOSE: Placing the labels in correct position will make it easier to find the information needed.
4. Put the color-coding labels on the bottom right edge of the folder. Start by placing the first letter of the last name at the farthest right edge. Working left, place the second letter of the last name, then the first letter of the first name, and lastly the year label. The year label should be close to the name label.
   PURPOSE: When the folders are in the file cabinet, they are sorted by the colored labels, starting with the top label (first letter of the last name), followed by the second and remaining labels.

5. Place the allergy label on the front of the record. If allergies are known, clearly write the allergy on the label in red ink.
   PURPOSE: Allergies need to be clearly identified on medical records.
6. Place the divider labels on the record divider sheets if they come separately. Ensure the labels on the divider sheets are staggered so they do not overlap. Print the name of the section on the front and back of the label. The print should be easy to read when the record is held by the main fold. (Suggested names for dividers: Progress Notes, Laboratory, Correspondence, and Miscellaneous.)
   PURPOSE: Placing divider labels on the divider sheets in a staggered pattern allows the provider to easily see all sections of the health record.
7. Using the prongs on the left-hand side of the record, secure the registration form.
   PURPOSE: The registration form should be in an easy-to-find location in the record.
8. Using the prongs on the right-hand side of the record, secure the index dividers with a progress note sheet under the progress note tab.
   PURPOSE: The provider will need the progress note sheet to document data regarding the visit.

Scenario: The patient authorized his or her prior provider to send health records to your agency. You need to organize these records within the paper health record.

9. Verify the name and the date of birth on the health record, and ensure they match the information on the health record.
   PURPOSE: Before you organize and file documents in a patient's health record, it is critical to ensure the health record is for the correct patient.
10. Open the prongs on the right side of the record, and carefully remove the record to the point at which the documents need to be inserted. For the documents being inserted, punch holes in the proper location. Insert the papers into the record, and then reassemble the remaining part of the record. Continue to do this until all the documents are filed within the health record.
    PURPOSE: Documents need to be placed in the correct location in the record so the provider can easily find information.

PROCEDURE 2.5	File Patient Health Records

Task: File patient health records using two different filing systems: the alphabetic system and the numeric system.

Scenario: The agency uses the alphabetic system. You need to file health records in the correct location.

EQUIPMENT and SUPPLIES

- Paper health records using the alphabetic filing system
- Paper health records using the numeric filing system
- File boxes or file cabinet

PROCEDURAL STEPS

1. Using alphabetic guidelines, place the records to be filed in alphabetic order.
   PURPOSE: Placing the records in alphabetic order before filing in the box or cabinet will make the filing process more efficient.
2. Using the file box or file cabinet, locate the correct spot for the first file.
   PURPOSE: It is important that you place the record in the correct spot so that others can locate the record.
3. Place the health record in the correct location. Continue these filing steps until all the health records are filed.
4. Using numeric guidelines, place the records to be filed in numeric order.
   PURPOSE: Placing the records in numeric order before filing in the box or cabinet will make the filing process more efficient.
5. Using the file box or file cabinet, locate the correct spot for the first file.
   PURPOSE: It is important that you place the record in the correct spot so that others can locate the record.
6. Place the health record in the correct location. Continue these filing steps until all the health records are filed.

3

INTRODUCTION TO ANATOMY AND MEDICAL TERMINOLOGY

SCENARIO

Daniela Garcia has just been hired as a part-time float receptionist at Walden-Martin Family Medical Clinic (WMFM). She also has just started the medical assistant program at the local community college. She is currently taking a medical terminology course and a human body and disease course. She understands that learning medical terminology is very much like learning a foreign language. She also understands that by learning the meanings of different word parts, she can easily figure out the meaning of a new medical term.

Daniela was excited to accept this position. She feels that this job would give her a foot in the door for a possible medical assistant position in the future.

It will also allow her to learn more about healthcare. Having just graduated from high school in May, she does not have a lot of previous work experience.

During her first week on the job, Daniela realizes there is a lot to learn. As a float she will be assisting in the specialty clinic, where providers from other agencies hold outreach clinics. During outreach, these providers see patients and provide specialty services not offered by WMFM providers. From patients to providers, everyone seems to use medical terminology, body-related terms, and language describing disease states. Daniela is happy to know a bit from her course, but she realizes she has a lot more terminology to learn.

While studying this chapter, think about the following questions:
- How do you decode medical terms using the CARD method?
- How do you identify combining forms, suffixes, and prefixes used in medical terminology?
- How do you apply spelling rules to medical terminology?
- How do you recognize and use terms related to the basic anatomy and pathology concepts?
- How do you describe the organization of the body?
- How do you describe body systems?
- How do you recognize and use surface anatomy, directional, and positional terms?
- How do you describe body cavities and abdominopelvic quadrants?
- What are common predisposing factors and causes of disease?

LEARNING OBJECTIVES

1. Review the origins of medical terminology and discuss the difference between decodable and nondecodable terms.
2. Describe how to decode terms using the check, assign, reverse, and define (CARD) method.
3. Use the rules given to build and spell healthcare terms.
4. Describe the structural organization of the human body.
5. Properly use surface anatomy, positional, and directional terminology.
6. Describe body cavities, abdominopelvic quadrants, and body planes.
7. Discuss the acid-base balance in the human body.
8. Discuss pathology basics, including pathology terminology, protection mechanisms, predisposing factors, and the causes of disease.

VOCABULARY

anaplastic (an uh PLAS tic) A rapidly dividing cancer cell that has little to no similarity to normal cells.

antibodies Protein substances, produced in the blood or tissues in response to a specific antigen, that destroy or weaken the antigen. Part of the immune system.

antigens Substances that stimulate the production of an antibody when introduced into the body. Antigens include toxins, bacteria, viruses, and other foreign substances.

biopsy (BIE op see) Process of viewing living tissue that has been removed for the purpose of diagnosis or treatment.

chromosomes (KROH muh sohms) Rod-shaped structures found in the cell's nucleus; they contain genetic information.

combining forms The "subjects" of most terms. They consist of the word root with its respective combining vowel.

diaphragm A broad, dome-shaped muscle used for breathing that separates the thoracic and abdominopelvic cavities.

differentiated (dif uh REN shee ayt ed) Describes the degree to which malignant tissue looks like the normal tissue it came from – poorly differentiated means it does not look like the normal tissue; well differentiated means it looks like the normal tissue.

endoscopy (en DOS kuh pee) An examination using a scope with a camera attached to the long, thin tube that can be inserted into the body.

homeostasis (hoh mee uh STAY sis) The internal environment of the body that is compatible with life. A steady state that is created by all the body systems working together to provide a consistent and unvarying internal environment.

intercellular Located between cells.

mitosis (mie TOH sis) A cell division process by which two daughter cells are formed from one parent cell; each daughter has a complete copy of the parent's chromosomes.

nondecodable terms Words used in healthcare whose definitions must be memorized without the benefit of word parts.

oncologist A specially trained doctor who diagnoses and treats cancer.

organelle Structures inside of the cell that have specific functions to maintain the cell.

pathogen A disease-causing organism.

pathologist A physician specially trained in the nature and cause of disease.

pathology The study of disease.

peristalsis (per uh STAL sis) Wavelike motion.

prefixes Word parts that appear at the beginning of terms.

suffixes Word parts that appear at the end of terms.

toxins (TOK sins) Substances created by microorganisms, plants, or animals that are poisonous to humans.

vasoconstriction Contraction of the muscles, causing narrowing of the inside tube of the vessel.

Medical terminology is a specialized vocabulary that has its roots in Greek and Latin word components. Professionals in healthcare use this terminology to communicate with each other. By applying the process of "decoding," or recognizing the word components and their meanings, you will be able to interpret literally thousands of medical terms. By using **combining forms**, **suffixes**, and **prefixes** you can break down medical terms and easily learn their meaning. This chapter presents a review of medical terminology to help you fully communicate as a healthcare professional.

This chapter also will review general anatomy, directional terms, and **pathology** terms and testing. This will help you before you start the specialty chapters of the book. Review is key to remembering and using information that has been presented in your education. Having a mastery of medical terminology, basic anatomy terms and concepts, and disease terminology and testing will give you the tools to understand the language and procedures presented in each medical specialty.

TYPES OF MEDICAL TERMS

Decodable Terms

Decodable terms are those that can be broken into their Greek and Latin word parts and given a working definition based on the meanings of those word parts. Most medical terms are decodable, so learning word parts is important. The word parts are as follows:

Combining form: Word root with its respective combining vowel.
Word root: Foundation of the medical term.
Combining vowel: A letter sometimes used to join word parts. Usually an "o" but occasionally an "a," "e," "i," or "u."
Suffix: Word part that appears at the end of a term. Suffixes are used to modify the meaning of the combining form.
Prefix: Word part that sometimes appears at the beginning of a term. Prefixes also modify the meaning of the combining form. They usually are used to further define the absence, location, number, quantity, or state of the term.

For our first examples, we will use ophthalm- (Greek) and ocul- (Latin). These combing forms both mean "eye." Both of the word

roots use an "o" as their combining vowel. Therefore ophthalmo/o and ocul/o are the combining forms related to "eye." Figs. 3.1 and 3.2 demonstrate the decoding of the terms *ophthalmology* and *extraocular*. Throughout the text, we will be using combining forms so that you will learn the appropriate combining vowel for that particular term.

Nondecodable Terms

Not all terms are composed of word parts that can be used to determine the definition. These terms are known as **nondecodable terms**. For these types of terms, the meaning must be memorized. A medical dictionary is an excellent tool to help with finding the definition of nondecodable terms. Examples of nondecodable terms include the following:

Cataract: From the Greek term meaning "waterfall." In healthcare language, this means the condition in which the lens becomes progressively opaque (loss of transparency).

Asthma: From the Greek term meaning "panting." Although this word origin is understandable, the definition is a respiratory disorder characterized by recurring episodes of paroxysmal dyspnea (difficulty breathing).

Diagnosis: The disease or condition that is determined after a healthcare provider evaluates a patient's signs, symptoms, and history. Although the term is built from word parts (dia-, meaning "through," "complete," and -gnosis, meaning "state of knowledge"), using these word parts to form the definition of diagnosis, which is "a state of complete knowledge," is not very helpful.

Prognosis: Similar to *diagnosis*, the term *prognosis* can be broken down into its word parts (pro-, meaning "before" or "in front of," and -gnosis, meaning "state of knowledge"), but this does not give the true definition of the term, which is "a prediction of the probable outcome of a disease or disorder."

Sequela: A condition that follows and is the result of an injury or disease.

Acute: A term that describes a sudden, severe onset (acu- means "sharp") of a disease.

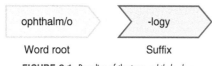

FIGURE 3.1 *Decoding of the term* ophthalmology.

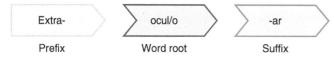

FIGURE 3.2 *Decoding of the term* extraocular.

Chronic: Developing slowly and lasting for 6 months or longer (chron/o means "time"). Diagnoses may be additionally described as being either acute or chronic.

Sign: An objective finding of a disease state (e.g., fever, high blood pressure, rash).

Symptom: A subjective report of a disease (pain, itching).

Other types of terms that are not built from word parts include the following:

Eponyms: Terms that are named after a person or place associated with the term. Examples include the following:

Alzheimer disease, which is named after Alois Alzheimer, a German neurologist. The disease is a progressive mental deterioration.

Achilles tendon, which is a body part named after a figure in Greek mythology whose one weak spot was this area of his anatomy. Tendons are bands of tissue that attach muscles to bone. The Achilles tendon is the particular tendon that attaches the calf muscle to the heel bone. Unlike some eponyms, this one does have a medical equivalent, the calcaneal tendon.

This text presents eponyms without the possessive. This practice is in accordance with the American Medical Association (AMA) and the American Association for Medical Transcription (AAMT).

Abbreviations and Symbols

Abbreviations are terms that have been shortened to letters or numbers for the sake of convenience, such as AAMA for the American Association of Medical Assistants. Symbols are graphic representations of a term, such as @ for *at*. Abbreviations and symbols are common in written and spoken medical terminology but can pose problems for healthcare workers. The Institute of Safe Medical Practice has provided an extensive list. Each healthcare organization should have an official list, which includes the single meaning allowed for each abbreviation or symbol. Examples of acceptable abbreviations and symbols include the following:

Simple abbreviations: A combination of letters (often, but not always the first letter of significant word parts) and sometimes numbers; for example:
IM: Abbreviation for *intramuscular* (pertaining to within the muscles)
C2: Second cervical vertebra (second bone in neck)

Acronyms: Abbreviations that are also pronounceable; for example:
CABG: Coronary artery bypass graft (a detour around a blockage in an artery of the heart)

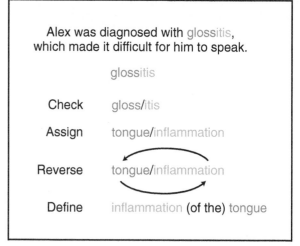

FIGURE 3.3 How to decode a medical term using the check, assign, reverse, and define (CARD) method. (From Shiland B: *Mastering healthcare terminology,* ed 5, St Louis, 2016, Elsevier.)

TURP: Transurethral resection of the prostate (a surgical procedure that removes the prostate through the urethra)

Symbols: Graphic representations of terms
♂ stands for male
♀ stands for female
↑ stands for increased
↓ stands for decreased
+ stands for present
− stands for absent

DECODING TERMS

Check, Assign, Reverse, and Define (CARD) Method

Using Greek and Latin word components to break down the meanings of medical terms requires a simple four-step process – the check, assign, reverse, and define (CARD) method. You need to do the following:

- *Check* for the word parts in a term.
- *Assign* meanings to the word parts.
- *Reverse* the meaning of the suffix to the front of your definition.
- *Define* the term.

Using Fig. 3.3, see how this process is applied to a medical term.

In the tables that follow, the term is in the first column and a definition is in the second column. Table 3.1 introduces six common combining forms and six common suffixes. (The use of prefixes will be introduced later.) Table 3.2 introduces six medical terms that use six different combining forms and suffixes. Success in decoding these terms depends on how well you remember the word parts presented in Table 3.1. Once you have mastered these 12 word parts, you will be able to recognize and define many other medical terms that use these same word parts.

BUILDING TERMS

Now that you've seen how terms are decoded, we will talk about how they are built. First, here are a few rules on how to spell medical terms correctly.

TABLE 3.1 Common Combining Forms and Suffixes

COMBINING FORMS	SUFFIXES
ot/o = ear	**-algia** = pain
cardi/o = heart	**-tomy** = incision
ophthalm/o = eye	**-scope** = instrument to view
nephr/o = kidney	**-logy** = study of
neur/o = nerve	**-plasty** = surgical repair
hepat/o = liver	**-itis** = inflammation

TABLE 3.2 Samples of Decodable Terms

TERM	DEFINITION
otalgia	Pain in the ear, or earache
cardiotomy	Incision of the heart
ophthalmoscope	Instrument used to view the eye
nephrology	Study of the kidney
neuroplasty	Surgical repair of a nerve
hepatitis	Inflammation of the liver

TABLE 3.3 Noun-Ending Suffixes

SUFFIX	MEANING
-icle	small, tiny
-is	structure, thing
-ole	small, tiny
-ule	small, tiny
-um	structure, thing, membrane
-y	process of, condition

Spelling Rules

With a few exceptions, decodable medical terms follow five simple rules.

1. If the suffix starts with a vowel, a combining vowel is *not* needed to join the parts. For example, it is simple to combine the combining form **hepat/o** and suffix **-itis** to build the term **hepatitis**, which means "an inflammation of the liver." The combining vowel "**o**" is not needed because the suffix starts with the vowel "**i.**"
2. If the suffix starts with a consonant, a combining vowel *is* needed to join the two word parts. For example, to build a term using **neur/o** and **-plasty**, the combining vowel is used and the resulting term is spelled **neuroplasty**, which refers to a surgical repair of a nerve.
3. If a combining form ends with the same vowel that begins a suffix, one of the vowels is dropped. The term that means "inflammation of the inside of the heart" is built from the suffix **-itis** (inflammation), the prefix **endo-** (inside), and the combining form **cardi/o**. **Endo-** + **cardi/o** + **-itis** would result in *endocardiitis*. Instead, one of the "i"s is dropped, and the term is spelled **endocarditis**.
4. If two or more combining forms are used in a term, the combining vowel is retained between the two, regardless of whether the second combining form begins with a vowel or a consonant. For example, joining **gastr/o** and **enter/o** (small intestine) with the suffix **-itis**,

results in the term **gastroenteritis**. Notice that the combining vowel is *kept* between the two combining forms (even though **enter/o** begins with the vowel "e"), and the combining vowel is *dropped* before the suffix **-itis**.
5. Sometimes when two or more combining forms are used to make a medical term, special notice must be paid to the order in which the combining forms are joined. For example, joining **esophag/o** (which means esophagus), **gastr/o** (which means stomach), and **duoden/o** (which means duodenum, the first part of the small intestines) with the suffix **-scopy** (process of viewing), produces the term *esophagogastroduodenoscopy*. An esophagogastroduodenoscopy (EGD) is a visual examination of the esophagus, stomach, and duodenum. In this procedure, the examination takes place in a specific sequence (that is, esophagus first, stomach second, and then the duodenum). Thus the term reflects the direction from which the scope travels through the body (Fig. 3.4).

Suffixes

The body system chapters in this text include many combining forms that are used to build terms specific to each system. These combining forms will not be seen in other places, except as a sign or symptom of a particular disorder. Suffixes, however, are used over and over again throughout the text. Suffixes usually can be grouped according to their purposes. Tables 3.3 through 3.8 cover the major suffix categories.

Noun-Ending Suffixes

Noun endings are used most often to describe anatomic terms. Noun endings such as -icle, -ole, and -ule describe a small or tiny structure. See Table 3.3.

Adjective Suffixes

Adjective suffixes usually mean "pertaining to." For example, when the suffix **-ac** is added to the combining form **cardi/o**, the term *cardiac* is formed, which means "pertaining to the heart." Remember that when you see an adjective term, you need to see what it is describing. For example, cardiac pain is pain of the heart, and cardiac surgery is surgery done on the heart. An adjective tells only half of the story. Common adjective suffixes include the following: -ac, -al, -ar, -ary, -eal, -ic, -ous and mean pertaining to.

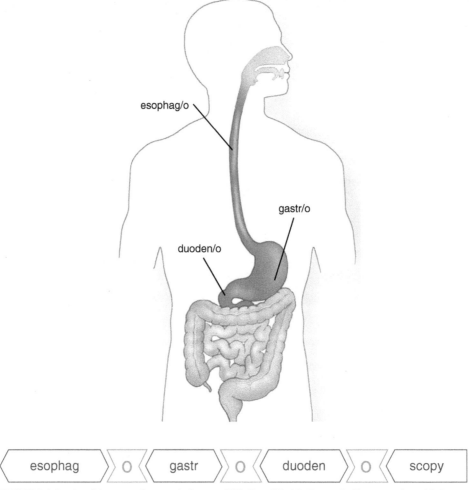

esophag/o

gastr/o

duoden/o

| esophag | O | gastr | O | duoden | O | scopy |

FIGURE 3.4 Decoding of the term *esophagogastroduodenoscopy* (EGD). (From Shiland B: *Mastering healthcare terminology*, ed 5, St Louis, 2016, Elsevier.)

Pathology Suffixes

Pathology suffixes describe a disease process or a sign or symptom. The meanings vary according to the conditions that they describe. See Table 3.4.

Diagnostic Procedure Suffixes

Diagnostic procedure suffixes point to a procedure that helps to determine the diagnosis. Although a few diagnostic procedures also can help to treat a disease, most are used to establish which particular disease or disorder is occurring. See Table 3.5.

Therapeutic Intervention Suffixes

Therapeutic intervention suffixes indicate types of treatment. Treatments may be medical or surgical in nature. See Table 3.6.

Instrument Suffixes

Instruments are indicated by yet another set of suffixes. Note the obvious similarities to their diagnostic and therapeutic cousins. For example, electrocardiography is a diagnostic procedure that is done to measure the electrical activity in the heart; an electrocar-diograph is the instrument used to perform electrocardiography. See Table 3.7.

Specialty and Specialist Suffixes

Specialties and specialists require yet another category of suffixes. Someone who specializes in the study of the heart would be called a *cardiologist*. **Cardi/o** means "heart," and **-logist** means "one who specializes in the study of." See Table 3.8.

CRITICAL THINKING APPLICATION   **3.1**

Daniela understands that by breaking a medical term into word parts (combining forms, suffixes, and prefixes) it will be easier to figure out the meaning of the term. She decides to spend some time reviewing suffixes. She quickly learns that -ia means condition and -itis means inflammation, because they are parts of terms she has heard before. However, she has never heard terms that use these suffixes: -sclerosis, -malacia, -ptosis, -rraphy, and -trite. Find the meaning of each of those suffixes.

TABLE 3.4	Pathology Suffixes
SUFFIX	MEANING
-algia	pain
-cele	herniation
-dynia	pain
-emia	blood condition
-ia	condition
-itis	inflammation
-malacia	softening
-megaly	enlargement
-oma	tumor, mass
-osis	abnormal condition
-pathy	disease process
-ptosis	prolapse, drooping, sagging
-rrhage, -rrhagia	bursting forth
-rrhea	discharge, flow
-rrhexis	rupture
-sclerosis	abnormal condition of hardening
-stenosis	abnormal condition of narrowing

TABLE 3.5	Diagnostic Procedure Suffixes
SUFFIX	MEANING
-graphy	process of recording
-metry	process of measuring
-opsy	process of viewing
-scopy	process of viewing

Prefixes

Prefixes modify a medical term by indicating a structure's or a condition's

- Absence
- Location
- Number or quantity
- State

Sometimes, as with other word parts, a prefix can have more than one meaning. For example, the prefix **hypo-** can mean "below" or "deficient." To spell a term with the use of a prefix, simply add the prefix directly to the beginning of the term. No combining vowels are needed (Table 3.9).

TABLE 3.6	Therapeutic Intervention Suffixes
SUFFIX	MEANING
-ectomy	removal, resection, excision
-plasty	surgical repair
-rrhaphy	suture, repair
-stomy	new opening
-tomy	incision, cutting
-tripsy	crushing

TABLE 3.7	Instrument Suffixes
SUFFIX	MEANING
-graph	instrument to record
-meter	instrument to measure
-scope	instrument to view
-tome	instrument to cut
-tripter	machine to crush
-trite	instrument to crush

TABLE 3.8	Specialty and Specialist Suffixes
SUFFIX	MEANING
-er	one who
-iatrician	one who specializes in treatment
-iatrics	treatment
-iatrist	one who specializes in treatment
-iatry	process of treatment
-ist	one who specializes
-logist	one who specializes in the study of
-logy	study of

CRITICAL THINKING APPLICATION   **3.2**

Daniela has mastered suffixes and is ready to move on to prefixes. She concentrates most on prefixes that are similar to one another in spelling or meaning. Can you explain the difference between inter- and intra-? Para- and peri-? Ante- and anti-?

TABLE 3.9	Prefixes
PREFIX	**MEANING**
a-	no, not, without
an-	no, not, without
ante-	forward, in front of, before
anti-	against
dys-	abnormal, difficult, bad, painful
endo-, end-	within
epi-	above, upon
hyper-	excessive, above
hypo-	below, deficient
inter-	between
intra-	within
neo-	new
par-	near, beside
para-	near, beside, abnormal
per-	through
peri-	surrounding, around
poly-	many, much, excessive, frequent
post-	after, behind
pre-	before, in front of
sub-	under, below
trans-	through, across

SINGULAR/PLURAL RULES

Most medical terms end with Greek or Latin suffixes. Making a medical term singular or plural is not always done the same way as it is in English. Listed below are the most common singular/plural endings and the rules for using them.

- When a singular form of a word ends with -a, keep the -a and add an -e.
  - Example: singular – axilla   plural – axillae
- When a singular form of the word ends with -ax, drop the -x and add -ces.
  - Example: singular – thorax   plural – thoraces
- When a singular form of the word ends with -ex or -ix, drop the -ex or -ix and add -ices.
  - Example: singular – apex   plural – apices
  - Example: singular – cervix   plural – cervices
- When a singular form of the word ends with -is, drop the -is and add -es.
  - Example: singular – diagnosis   plural – diagnoses
- When a singular form of the word ends with -us, drop the -us and add -i.
  - Example: singular – embolus   plural – emboli
- When the singular form of the word ends with -um, drop the -um and add -a.
  - Example: singular – ovum   plural – ova
- When the singular form of the word ends with -y, drop the -y and add -ies.
  - Example: singular – biopsy   plural – biopsies
- When a singular form of the word ends with -x, drop the -x and add -ges.
  - Example: singular – larynx   plural – larynges

COMMON COMBINING FORMS

Table 3.10 lists the common combining forms in medical terminology. This is not a complete list of combining forms, but it covers the most

TABLE 3.10	Common Combining Forms		
COMBINING FORM	**MEANING**	**COMBINING FORM**	**MEANING**
aden/o	gland	cholecyst/o	gallbladder
arteri/o	artery	chondr/o	cartilage
arthr/o	joint	col/o	large intestine, colon
aur/i	ear, hearing	coron/o	crown, heart
bacteri/o	bacteria	cut/o	skin
bi/o	living, life	cutane/o	skin
cardi/o	heart	cyst/o	bladder, sac
carp/o	wrist	dent/i	tooth
cephal/o	head	derm/o	skin
cervic/o	neck, cervix	duoden/o	duodenum

TABLE 3.10   Common Combining Forms—*continued*

COMBINING FORM	MEANING	COMBINING FORM	MEANING
electr/o	electricity	path/o	disease
enter/o	small intestine	ped/o	child
esophag/o	esophagus	pharyng/o	throat
gastr/o	stomach	phleb/o	vein
gingiv/o	gums	phil/o	attraction
gloss/o	tongue	pne/o	breathing
glyc/o	glucose, sugar	pneum/o	lungs
hem/o, hemat/o	blood	psych/o	mind
hepat/o	liver	pulm/o, pulmon/o	lungs
hyster/o	uterus	rhin/o	nose
lingu/o	tongue	somn/o	sleep
lipid/o	lipid, fat	spir/o	breathing
lith/o	stone	splen/o	spleen
mamm/o	breast	therm/o	heat, temperature
muscul/o	muscle	tonsill/o	tonsil
my/o	muscle	trache/o	trachea, windpipe
nat/o	birth, born	troph/o	nourishment
nephr/o	kidney	ur/o, urin/o	urine, urinary system
neur/o	nerve	urethr/o	urethra
ophthalm/o	eye	valvul/o	valve
oste/o	bone	ven/o	vein
ot/o	ear	vertebr/o	backbone, vertebra

commonly used forms. Until you are comfortable with medical terminology, keep a list of common combining forms, prefixes, and suffixes nearby so that you can refer to it as needed.

ANATOMY REVIEW

Structural Organization of the Body

The human body is a collection of many body systems. Examples include the digestive, cardiovascular, musculoskeletal, and respiratory systems. Each system is composed of different organs. For instance, the stomach and intestines are digestive system organs. Each organ is made up of combinations of tissues, and these tissues are composed of cells. So when studying the organization of the body, it is easier to start at the level of cells and work up to the organism (human body) level.

Cells

The basic unit of life is the *cell*. Cells determine the functional and structural characteristics of the entire body. Cells are microscopic in size. They have a variety of shapes and perform a vast array of functions. A cell is covered by a plasma membrane. The cell contains cytoplasm and **organelles**. See Table 3.11 and Fig. 3.5 for the parts of the cells.

Most human cells reproduce by **mitosis**. Mitosis is a process in which one cell splits into two identical daughter cells. The two cells are genetically identical to the parent cell. Prior to the mitosis process, the cell enters the interphase stage. During this stage, the genetic information (i.e., **chromosomes**) replicate. Each sister pair of chromosomes (called *chromatids*) are joined together until they are pulled apart later in the mitosis process. The point where the two chromatids are joined is called the *centromere*. The centromere is also the attachment point for spindle fibers, which will be involved in the mitosis process. The mitosis process consists of four phases; prophase, metaphase, anaphase, and telophase.

Tissues

Tissue is a group of similar cells from the same source that together carry out a specific function. The study of body tissues is known as

TABLE 3.11   Cell Parts

CELL PARTS	DESCRIPTION
Plasma membrane	Outer covering of the cell that allows certain substances to enter the cell and blocks the entrance of other substances. Can also be called the *cell membrane*.
Cytoplasm	Gel that surrounds the nucleus and fills the cells. Organelles are suspended in the cytoplasm.
Ribosome	Organelle that makes enzymes and proteins. Contains ribonucleic acid (RNA).
Rough endoplasmic reticulum (ER)	Organelle that is a network of membranes; connects to the nucleus. The rough appearance is due to the attachment of ribosome to the ER.
Smooth endoplasmic reticulum (ER)	Tube-like organelle; function changes depending on the cell type. Functions may include calcium storage, steroid production, and lipid production.
Golgi apparatus	Processes and packages proteins and lipids produced by the cell. The cell's "processing plant."
Lysosomes	Contain enzymes which digest nutrients and other substances in the cell.
Mitochondrion	Produces energy for the cell. The cell's power plant.
Nucleus	Control center of the cell; contains chromosomes made up of deoxyribonucleic acid (DNA); carries genetic information.
Nucleolus	A small organelle inside of the nucleus; produces ribosomes.
Centrioles	Tube-like structures that help with cell division.
Cilia	Fine, hair-like extensions on the surface of the cell.
Microvilli	Small projections on the surface of the cell; increases the surface area and increases cellular absorption.
Flagellum	Single, long, whip-like extension on the surface of the cell. Used to move the cell.

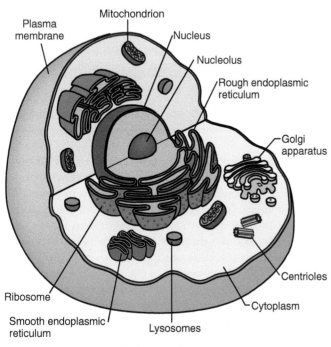

FIGURE 3.5 Cell structures.

histology. All body tissues are grouped into four types. The four types of tissue include the following:

- *Epithelial tissue*: Acts as an internal or external covering for organs. Examples of epithelial tissue include the outer layer of the skin, glands, and linings of body cavities and organs. Epithelial tissue

CRITICAL THINKING APPLICATION   3.3

Daniela was learning about the cell structures in school. While on break one night, she talked to Bella. Bella is a new CMA (AAMA) who just graduated. Daniela mentioned she was learning about cell parts. Bella encouraged Daniela to associate the cell parts to the things she might see in a city. For instance, she stated, "The plasma membrane could be the walls around the city." What other associations could be made between the cell structures and a city?

has the cells packed so closely together that there is little to no **intercellular** material. *Simple epithelium* is a single layer of the same-shaped cells. *Stratified epithelium* contains multiple layers of cells.

- *Connective tissue*: Supports and binds other body tissues. Examples of connective tissue include bone; blood; adipose, fibrous, and areolar tissues; and cartilage. Connective tissue is the most frequently occurring tissue in the body.
- *Muscle tissue*: Produces movement. Table 3.12 shows the classification, characteristics, and roles of the types of muscle tissue.
- *Nervous tissue*: Includes cells that provide transmission of information to control a variety of functions. Nervous tissue controls the body's functions to maintain **homeostasis**. Nervous tissue is made up of neurons (nerve cells) and supportive structures called *neuroglial cells*.

Organs

An *organ* is a structure composed of two or more types of tissue. An organ may have one or more functions. Organs are grouped within

TABLE 3.12	Classification of Muscle Tissue	
CLASSIFICATION	**CHARACTERISTICS**	**ROLE**
Skeletal	Striated, voluntary	Attached to bones and produces voluntary body movements when contracted
Cardiac	Striated, involuntary	Forms the heart muscle wall
Smooth	Nonstriated, involuntary	Lines the blood vessel walls and hollow organs; allows **peristalsis** and **vasoconstriction**

body systems. An organ may be part of one or more systems. Organs can be divided into parts.

Body Systems

A *body system* is composed of several organs and their related structures. These structures work together to perform a specific function in the body. Table 3.13 summarizes the body systems, including their structures and functions.

Organism

The *organism* of the body is made up of many body systems. These work together to maintain a steady environment in the body, called *homeostasis*. If the balance is off or if the environment moves out of the normal range, diseases can occur.

To summarize the structural organization of the body, from simple to complex:

- *Cells:* The most basic unit
- *Tissues:* Groups of similar cells from the same source that carry out a specific function
- *Organ:* A structure made up of two or more types of tissues

TABLE 3.13	Summary of Body Systems	
BODY SYSTEM	**CELLS, STRUCTURES, AND ORGANS**	**FUNCTIONS**
Blood	Arteries, arterioles, veins, venules, white blood cells, red blood cells, platelets, plasma	Transports materials (e.g., oxygen, nutrients) and collects wastes throughout the body; involved with fighting infection and forming clots
Cardiovascular	Heart, valves, arteries, arterioles, veins, venules	Transports materials in the blood throughout the body
Endocrine	Pituitary, pineal gland, hypothalamus, thyroid, pancreas, adrenal cortex and medulla, parathyroid, thymus, ovaries, testes	Produces hormones that circulate in the blood to target tissue that stimulates a particular action. Helps maintain homeostasis.
Gastrointestinal	Mouth, tongue, teeth, pharynx, esophagus, stomach, small intestine, large intestine, liver, gallbladder, pancreas, appendix	Breakdown, digestion, and absorption of nutrients
Integumentary	Skin, subcutaneous tissue, sweat and sebaceous glands, hair, nails, sense receptors	Protection, temperature regulation, senses organ activity
Lymphatic and immune	Lymph, lymph vessels, lymph nodes, thymus, tonsils, spleen, lymphocytes, antibodies	Maintains fluid balance; protects internal environment; provides immunity to many diseases
Musculoskeletal	Bones, joints, muscles, tendons, ligaments, cartilage	Movement, heat production, support, protection
Nervous	Brain, spinal cord, neurons, neuroglial cells, peripheral nerves, autonomic nerves	Controls body structures to maintain homeostasis; receives and processes information
Reproductive	*Female:* estrogen and progesterone, ovum, ovaries, fallopian tubes, uterus, vagina, vulva, mammary glands *Male:* testosterone, sperm, epididymis, vas deferens, prostate gland, testes, scrotum, penis, urethra	Produces hormones; reproduction
Respiratory	Nose, sinuses, pharynx, larynx, trachea, bronchi, lungs, bronchioles, alveoli	Delivers oxygen to cells and removes carbon dioxide
Sensory	Eyes, ears, taste buds, olfactory receptors, sensory receptors	Gathers information through vision, hearing, balance, taste, and smell
Urinary	Nephron unit, kidneys, ureters, bladder, urethra	Eliminates nitrogenous waste; maintains electrolyte, water, and acid-base balances

- *Body system:* Made up of several organs and their related structures
- *Organism:* Made up of many body systems that work together to maintain homeostasis in the body

---

CRITICAL THINKING APPLICATION   3.4

Bella's tip really helped Daniela with the cell structures. Now Daniela needs to remember the organization of the body, in order, from the simplest to the most complex. Bella encourages Daniela to create a phrase or word that would help her remember cells, tissues, organs, body system, and organism. What might be a way to remember these five items in order?

SURFACE ANATOMY TERMINOLOGY

In healthcare we use surface anatomy terminology to describe locations on the body. For instance, when you take a blood pressure reading, you need to place the stethoscope over the brachial artery in the antecubital space. The radial artery is used when you take a radial pulse. Knowing the surface anatomy terminology will help you understand what is being asked of you and will allow you to communicate professionally with others.

Anatomical position is a standard frame of reference. This means the body stands erect with the face forward, arms at the sides, palms forward, and toes pointed forward. Fig. 3.6A shows the body in anatomical position, in addition to the ventral surface anatomy. (Fig.

3.6B shows the dorsal surface anatomy.) Tables 3.14 through 3.17 provide additional information on front (ventral) and back (dorsal) surface anatomy terminology.

CRITICAL THINKING APPLICATION   3.5

As Daniela was learning about surface anatomy terminology, she tried to relate it to things she knew or had learned about in her receptionist position. For instance, *palmar* sounds like *palm* and refers to the palm of the hand. From Tables 3.14 through 3.17, which words have you heard before? How might you remember these surface anatomy terms?

POSITIONAL AND DIRECTIONAL TERMINOLOGY

Positional and directional terms are used to describe up/down, middle/side, and front/back. Many times patients will be in different positions, depending on the situation. Having a standard method to communicate directions and positions allows for clear communication between healthcare professionals. These terms are used commonly in healthcare. For example, x-rays may be taken from the front of the body to the back – an anteroposterior (AP) view, or from the back to the front – a posteroanterior (PA) view.

The *midline* of the body is an imaginary line drawn from the crown of the head down between the eyes, through the chest, and separating the legs. Several of the directional terms use the midline as a reference. See Table 3.18.

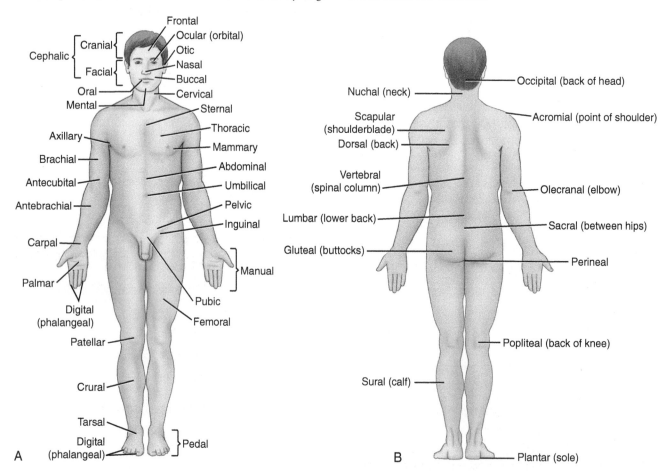

FIGURE 3.6 (A) Ventral surface anatomy. (B) Dorsal surface anatomy. (From Shiland B: *Mastering healthcare terminology*, ed 5, St Louis, 2016, Elsevier.)

TABLE 3.14 Ventral Surface Anatomy: Terms for the Head

TERM	DEFINITION
buccal	Pertaining to the cheek
cephalic	Pertaining to the head
cervical	Pertaining to the neck
cranial	Pertaining to the skull
facial	Pertaining to the face
frontal	Pertaining to the front, the forehead
mental	Pertaining to the chin, or to the mind
nasal	Pertaining to the nose
ocular	Pertaining to the eye
oral	Pertaining to the mouth
otic	Pertaining to the ear; also called *auricular*

TABLE 3.16 Ventral Surface Anatomy: Terms for Arms and Legs

TERM	DEFINITION
antecubital	Pertaining to the front of the elbow
brachial	Pertaining to the arm
carpal	Pertaining to the wrist
crural	Pertaining to the leg
digital	Pertaining to the finger/toe
femoral	Pertaining to the thigh
manual	Pertaining to the hand
palmar	Pertaining to the palm; also termed *volar*
patellar	Pertaining to the kneecap
pedal	Pertaining to the foot
tarsal	Pertaining to the ankle

TABLE 3.15 Ventral Surface Anatomy: Terms for the Trunk

TERM	DEFINITION
abdominal	Pertaining to the abdomen
axillary	Pertaining to the armpit
coxal	Pertaining to the hip
deltoid	The triangular muscle covering the shoulder joint
inguinal	Pertaining to the groin
mammary	Pertaining to the breast
pelvic	Pertaining to the pelvis
pubic	Pertaining to the pubis
sternal	Pertaining to the breastbone
thoracic	Pertaining to the chest; also called *pectoral*
umbilical	Pertaining to the umbilicus

TABLE 3.17 Dorsal Surface Anatomy Terms

TERM	DEFINITION
acromial	Pertaining to the acromion (highest point of shoulder)
dorsal	Pertaining to the back
gluteal	Pertaining to the buttocks
lumbar	Pertaining to the lower back
nuchal	Pertaining to the neck, especially the back of the neck
olecranal	Pertaining to the elbow
perineal	Pertaining to the perineum; the perineum is the space between the external genitalia and the anus
plantar	Pertaining to the sole of the foot
popliteal	Pertaining to the back of the knee
sacral	Pertaining to the sacrum
scapular	Pertaining to the scapula
sural	Pertaining to the calf
ventral	Pertaining to the belly side
vertebral	Pertaining to the spine

CRITICAL THINKING APPLICATION   3.6

Bella continues to help Daniela on breaks during work. Today, Daniela is learning directional terms. Bella encourages Daniela to repeat the term and definition as she points to that part of her body. How else might Daniela learn the directional terms and the opposite pairs?

TABLE 3.18   Positional and Directional Terms

TERM	DEFINITION
anterior	Pertaining to the front
ventral	Pertaining to the belly side
posterior	Pertaining to the back
dorsal	Pertaining to the back of the body
superior	Toward the head
cephalad	Toward the head
inferior	Toward the tail
caudad	Toward the tail
medial	Pertaining to the middle (midline)
lateral	Pertaining to the side
ipsilateral	Pertaining to the same side
contralateral	Pertaining to the opposite side
unilateral	Pertaining to one side
bilateral	Pertaining to two sides
superficial (external)	On the surface of the body
deep (internal)	Away from the surface of the body
proximal	Pertaining to near the origin
distal	Pertaining to far from the origin
dextrad	Toward the right
sinistrad	Toward the left
afferent	Pertaining to carrying toward a structure
efferent	Pertaining to carrying away from a structure
supine	Lying on one's back
prone	Lying on one's belly

BODY CAVITIES

The body contains cavities, or hollowed areas, that are filled with organs. The body is separated into the dorsal (posterior) and ventral (anterior) body cavities. The *dorsal body cavity* protects nervous system organs. It contains the cranial cavity and the spinal cavity. The *ventral body cavity* is divided into the thoracic and abdominopelvic cavities. The **diaphragm** creates a physical separation between the thoracic and the abdominopelvic cavities. Table 3.19 summarizes the structures found in each body cavity.

Abdominopelvic Quadrants and Regions

The abdominopelvic cavity is extensive. To help describe a location in the abdominopelvic area, either the four quadrants or the nine regions can be used. Descriptions that focus on the quadrants are

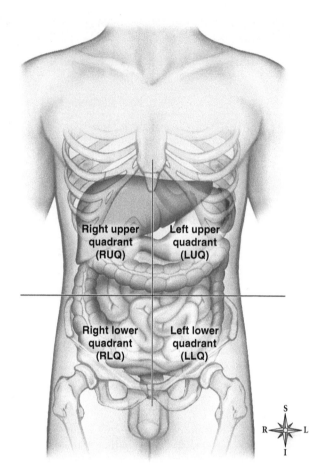

FIGURE 3.7 Abdominopelvic quadrants. (Patton KT, Thibodeau GA: *The human body in health and disease*, ed 7, St Louis, 2018, Elsevier.)

simpler to understand and may be used with patients. The regions are more specific and are typically used by healthcare providers.

With the abdominopelvic quadrants, an imaginary line is drawn down the midline of the body. A horizontal line is drawn across the abdominopelvic cavity, intersecting at the naval (Fig. 3.7). These quadrants are referred to as either right or left and upper or lower. Typically, the abbreviations are used when documenting information about the patient. The four quadrants, and their contents, are as follows:

- *Right upper quadrant* (RUQ): Right lobe of the liver, gallbladder, right kidney, small intestine (duodenum), large intestine (ascending and transverse colon), and head of the pancreas
- *Left upper quadrant* (LUQ): Stomach, spleen, left lobe of the liver, pancreas, left kidney, and large intestine (transverse and descending colon)
- *Right lower quadrant* (RLQ): Appendix, cecum, right ovary, right ureter, right spermatic cord, large intestine (ascending colon), and right kidney
- *Left lower quadrant* (LLQ): Small intestine, large intestine (descending and sigmoid colon), left ovary, left ureter, left spermatic cord, and left kidney

The nine abdominopelvic regions lie over the abdominopelvic cavity. They provide a more specific location than the quadrants. Refer to Fig. 3.8 and Table 3.20 for the nine regions and the related organs.

TABLE 3.19   Body Cavities

MAIN BODY CAVITIES	SUBCATEGORIES	DESCRIPTION
Dorsal body cavity	Cranial cavity	Contains the brain; surrounded and protected by the cranium (skull)
	Spinal cavity	Contains the spinal cord; surrounded and protected by the vertebrae (bones of the spine)
Ventral body cavity	Thoracic cavity	Contains the heart, lungs, esophagus and trachea (windpipe); protected by the ribs, the sternum (breastbone), and the vertebrae (backbones)
	Abdominopelvic cavity	Can be divided as follows: Abdominal cavity – contains the abdominal organs (e.g., stomach, liver, gallbladder, intestines). Pelvic cavity – contains the urinary bladder and the reproductive organs Nothing separates the abdominal and pelvic cavities.

TABLE 3.20   Abdominopelvic Regions With the Underlying Organs

Right Hypochondriac Region	Epigastric Region	Left Hypochondriac Region
Liver, gallbladder, right kidney	Kidneys, pancreas, liver, stomach	Stomach, liver, left kidney, spleen
Right Lumbar Region	**Umbilical Region**	**Left Lumbar Region**
Small intestine, large intestine (ascending colon), liver, right kidney	Small intestine, large intestine (transverse colon), pancreas, stomach	Small intestine, large intestine (descending colon), left kidney
Right Iliac Region	**Hypogastric Region**	**Left Iliac Region**
Appendix, small intestine, large intestine (cecum and ascending colon)	Small intestine, large intestine (sigmoid colon), bladder	Small intestine, large intestine (descending and sigmoid colon)

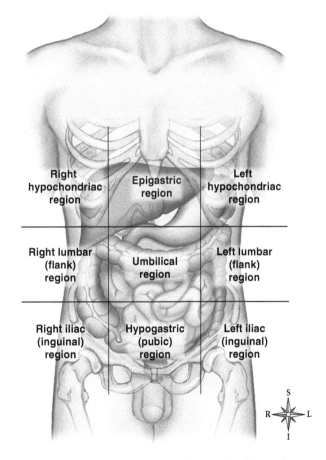

FIGURE 3.8 Abdominopelvic regions. (Patton KT, Thibodeau GA: *The human body in health and disease*, ed 7, St Louis, 2018, Elsevier.)

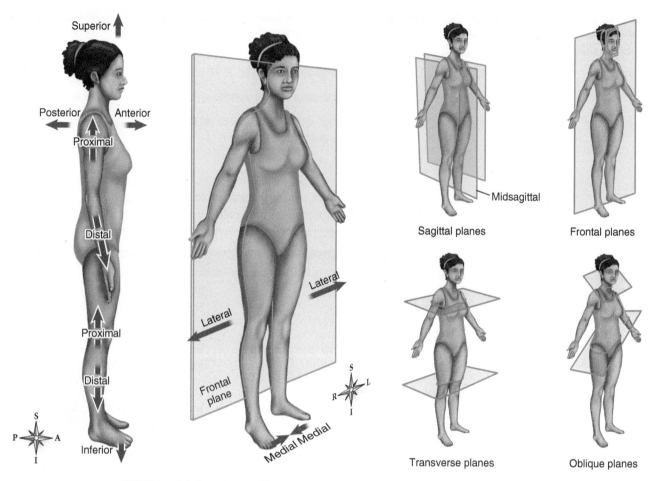

FIGURE 3.9 Body planes. (Patton KT, Thibodeau GA: *The human body in health and disease,* ed 7, St. Louis, 2018, Elsevier.)

CRITICAL THINKING APPLICATION   3.7

Tonight Bella is helping Daniela practice positional and directional terms with the regions. Bella asks Daniela the following questions:
- What regions are lateral to the umbilical region?
- What regions are superior to the lumbar regions?
- What region is medial to the hypochondriac regions and superior to the umbilical region?
- What region is inferior to the umbilical region?
- What regions are lateral to the sides of the hypogastric region?

What should Daniela's answers be to these questions?

BODY PLANES

Another way of describing the body is by dividing it into planes. *Planes* are imaginary cuts or sections through the body. The use of plane terminology is common when diagnostic imaging of the body is discussed (e.g., computed tomography [CT] or computerized axial tomography [CAT] scan). Diagnostic imaging will be discussed in more detail later in the chapter.

A *midsagittal plane,* or *median plane,* separates the body into equal right and left halves. The *coronal plane,* or *frontal*

plane, divides the body into front and back portions. The *transverse plane,* or *horizontal plane,* divides the body horizontally into an upper part and a lower part. An *oblique plane* uses a diagonal cut through the body. See Fig. 3.9 for illustrations of the body planes.

ACID-BASE BALANCE

The *pH* is important to review because it affects body homeostasis. pH refers to the acid-base level of a solution on a scale of 1 to 14. A neutral pH is 7. An acidic solution has a pH less than 7 and contains more hydrogen ions. A base, or alkaline solution, has a pH greater than 7 and contains fewer hydrogen ions. To maintain homeostasis, the body attempts to keep the pH between 7.35 and 7.45. To maintain the acid-base range in the body, the concentration of hydrogen ions must remain constant. If the pH moves outside of this range, serious illness or even death can occur.

The pH of our bodies can change based on the food we eat, the air we breathe, and the urine we excrete. To help maintain the pH range, the urinary system, the respiratory system, and chemical buffers must all work together. *Buffers* (e.g., bicarbonate) work to prevent changes in the pH. If there are more hydrogen ions, lowering the pH, buffers will absorb some of the hydrogen ions. This will raise the pH. If the pH is too high, the buffers will "donate" hydrogen ions, bringing the pH down to the normal range.

The respiratory system regulates the carbon dioxide (CO_2) in our blood. CO_2 in the blood can combine with water to form the buffer bicarbonate. If a person *hyperventilates* (breathes rapidly), the CO_2 levels in the blood decrease, which also causes a decrease in the bicarbonate levels in the blood. This causes the pH of the body to rise.

The urinary system also has a role in acid-base levels. The kidneys can absorb more base or more acid, depending on what the body needs for homeostasis. The kidneys can also produce bicarbonate if needed.

PATHOLOGY BASICS

Pathology is the study of diseases. In the ambulatory care setting, many patients' visits relate to the diagnosis or treatment of one or more disease processes. As a person ages, it is common to have more than one chronic illness. Having an understanding of common diseases is important for medical assistants. The body system chapters that follow will cover the most common diseases impacting the system discussed. This chapter provides you with the basics to help you understand the concepts discussed in future chapters. Common pathology terminology, protective mechanisms in the body, predisposing factors for disease, and causes of disease will be discussed.

Pathology Terminology

As you learn more about diseases, you will notice different terms used. Here is a list of terms commonly used when discussing pathology:

- *Disease*: A specific illness with a recognizable group of signs and symptoms and a clear cause (e.g., infection, environment).
- *Syndrome*: A group of signs and symptoms that occur together and are associated with a condition.
- *Disorder*: A disruption of the function or structure of the body. Many times the words *disorder* and *disease* are used interchangeably in healthcare.
- *Prevalence*: How often the disease occurs.
- *Incidence*: Reflects the number of newly diagnosed people with the disease.
- *Morbidity*: Illness.
- *Mortality*: Death.
- *Acute*: A severe, sudden onset of a disease.
- *Chronic*: A disease, disorder, or syndrome that lasts longer than 6 months.

The upcoming chapters will discuss common diseases in each body system. For most of the diseases, the following sections will be discussed. It is important for the medical assistant to be familiar with the terminology used:

- *Etiology*: The cause of the disorder or disease.
- *Sign*: An indicator that is measured or observed by others; also called *objective data*. Examples of signs include redness, swelling (edema), blood pressure, and pulse.
- *Symptom*: An indicator that is only perceived by the patient; also called *subjective data*. Examples include pain, headache, dizziness, and nausea. Many times *signs* and *symptoms*

are used interchangeably, but there is a difference in their definitions.

- *Diagnostic procedures*: Tests and procedures that are used to help diagnose or monitor a condition. See Table 3.21 and Figs. 3.10 and 3.11 for common diagnostic procedures.
- *Treatments*: Management of a disease or disorder; they can include follow-up care and home treatments (e.g., medications, special diets, testing).

CRITICAL THINKING APPLICATION   **3.8**

Daniela is struggling to remember the difference between signs and symptoms. What might be ways to remember these two terms? What are some examples of signs and symptoms?

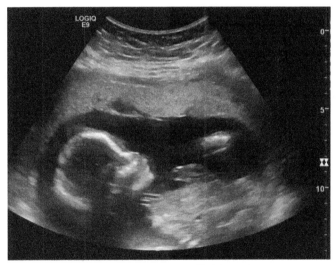

FIGURE 3.10 Two-dimensional fetal ultrasound.

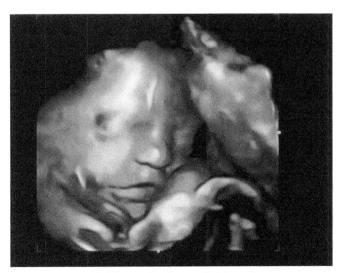

FIGURE 3.11 Three-dimensional fetal ultrasound.

TABLE 3.21	Common Diagnostic Procedures and Tests in Ambulatory Healthcare	
PERFORMED BY/TYPE OF TEST	**PROCEDURE**	**DESCRIPTION**
Medical Laboratory Blood Tests	Blood glucose	Used to detect high or low blood sugar (glucose)
	C-reactive protein (CRP)	Detects inflammation
	Complete blood count (CBC)	Measures red blood cells (RBCs) and white blood cells (WBCs), hemoglobin (Hgb), hematocrit (HCT), and platelets; CBC with differential test provides a breakdown of the number of each type of white blood cell
	Comprehensive metabolic panel (CMP)	Includes different tests that evaluate, for instance, liver function, kidney function, glucose, and electrolytes
	Electrolyte panel (Lytes)	Used to check for electrolyte (e.g., sodium, potassium, chloride) imbalances
	Erythrocyte sedimentation rate (ESR)	Used to measure the degree of inflammation in the body
	Follicle-stimulating hormone (FSH)	Measures the follicle-stimulating hormone, a reproductive hormone
	Glycated hemoglobin test or hemoglobin glycosylated test (HbA1C or A1C)	Measures the average blood glucose (sugar) over 2 to 3 months
	Lipid profile	Used to check cholesterol and triglycerides
	Liver function panel	Measures specific proteins and enzymes to provide information on the liver's functioning; also called the *hepatic function test*
	Partial thromboplastin time (PTT), prothrombin time (PT), and international normalized ratio (INR)	Measures blood clotting time
	Thyroid-stimulating hormone (TSH) test	Measures the amount of thyroid-stimulating hormone in the blood; also part of the thyroid panel, which includes additional tests
Medical Laboratory Tests	Culture and sensitivity (C&S)	Culture detects organism in body fluid (e.g., blood, sputum, urine) and sensitivity testing to determine antibiotics that would inhibit organism growth
	Fecal immunochemical test (FIT)	Uses antibodies to detect human hemoglobin protein
	Guaiac fecal occult blood test (gFOBT)	Used to detect blood in stool
	Stool parasitic examination (O&P)	Used to detect ova and parasites in the stool
	Urinalysis (UA)	Detects abnormalities in the urine that can be used to diagnose many conditions
Endoscopy	Arthroscopy	An arthroscope is inserted through a small incision to view a joint
	Bronchoscopy	A bronchoscope is inserted through the mouth to visualize the trachea and bronchi
	Capsule endoscopy	A camera in a capsule is swallowed and provides pictures of the gastrointestinal tract
	Colonoscopy and sigmoidoscopy	An endoscope is inserted through the anus and used to visualize the large intestine and colon
	Colposcopy	A colposcope is inserted into the vagina to visualize the cervix and vagina
	Cystoscopy and ureteroscopy	An endoscope is inserted into the urethra to look at the urinary system
	Endoscopic retrograde cholangiopancreatography (ERCP)	An endoscope is inserted into the mouth and passed to the duodenum; a thin tube, called a *catheter*, is passed through the endoscope and is used to inject dye into the ducts that lead to the pancreas and gallbladder, then x-rays are used to detect narrowing of structures
	Esophagogastroduodenoscopy (EGD)	An endoscope is inserted through the mouth to visualize the lining of the esophagus, stomach, and duodenum (small intestine)

TABLE 3.21	Common Diagnostic Procedures and Tests in Ambulatory Healthcare—*continued*	
PERFORMED BY/TYPE OF TEST	**PROCEDURE**	**DESCRIPTION**
Imaging Procedures	Computed tomography (CT, CAT) scan	A computerized x-ray imaging modality that provides axial and three-dimensional scans; the patient lies on a table that slides into the circular device that takes the x-rays
	Fluoroscopy	Direct observation of an x-ray image in motion
	Magnetic resonance imaging (MRI)	An imaging modality that uses a magnetic field and radiofrequency pulses to create computer images of both bones and soft tissues in multiple planes
	Nuclear scans	A radioactive substance is injected or ingested and then is detected by a special camera as it moves through a body structure
	Positron emission tomography (PET) scan	Imaging test that uses a radioactive drug (tracer) to show the activity of tissues and organs

	Ultrasound (US) (also called *sonography*)	A transducer is moved over the body and sends out high-frequency sound waves; waves bounce off tissues and the transducer captures the waves:
		  2D US: creates a flat, two-dimensional picture
		  3D US: creates a three-dimensional (3D) picture
		  4D US: creates a 3D picture with sound and motion
		  Doppler US: assesses blood flow through blood vessels

	X-ray (also called *radiograph*)	Uses electromagnetic waves to take pictures of the inside structures of the body; creates black-and-white images based on the amount of radiation that is absorbed:
		  White areas: absorb more radiation (e.g., bones)
		  Gray areas: absorb less (e.g., soft tissue and fat)
		  Black: absorbs none (e.g., air)
		Different views can be ordered:
		  PA (posteroanterior) films: x-ray passes from the back to the front of the person
		  AP (anteroposterior) films: x-ray passes from the front to the back of the person

	Contrast media	Can be used with x-rays, CT, MRI, and US to improve the clarity of the soft tissue picture; ingested, administered by enema, or by injection (via blood vessels) and eliminated via the urine or stool; common contrast media include:
		  X-rays and CT scans: barium and iodine
		  MRIs: gadolinium
		  US: saline (salt water) and air

Predisposing Factors

Predisposing factors are risk factors for disease. These factors make it more likely or increase the risk that the person may develop the disease or condition. Some predisposing factors can be changed to reduce the risk of developing a disease, whereas others cannot be changed. Predisposing factors include the following:

- *Hereditary or genetic factors*: Certain diseases can be inherited, or members of a family can have a higher-than-normal risk for getting a specific disease.

- *Age*: Certain diseases occur in childhood, whereas others occur more often in older adults. Some diseases occur due to changes in the body structures with age. For instance, the ear structures are different in an infant compared with an older person. Degenerative diseases occur in older generations due to the wear and tear on the structures.

- *Gender*: Certain diseases occur specifically, or more often, in one gender than the other. For instance, testicular cancer impacts males. whereas uterine cancer affects females. Sometimes both genders may get a disease, but one gender has a higher risk factor. Women are at higher risk for breast cancer than men.

- *Environmental factors*: Certain diseases are more common when a person has been exposed to pollutants in the air, land, or water. Though pesticides can reduce the risk of disease (e.g., West Nile viral infection and rabies), exposure to certain pesticides has been found to increase the risk of cancer.
- *Lifestyle*: Stress, poor diet, infrequent exercise, or abusing nicotine, alcohol, or drugs can increase the risk for disease.

CRITICAL THINKING APPLICATION   3.9

While on break at work, Daniela works on an assignment. She needs to determine which predisposing factors could be changed and how they could be changed. What could be her answers?

Causes of Disease

Disease can result from a change in homeostasis or can be the result of the body's response to a perceived threat. There are several common causes of disease, including genetics, infectious **pathogens**, inflammatory processes, immunity, nutritional imbalance, trauma and environmental agents, and neoplasms. The following sections describe these causes.

Genetics

Each person is made up of 46 chromosomes, which carry genetic information (genes). We get 23 chromosomes from each of our parents. *Genes* are the basic units of heredity, or the instructions on how our bodies should develop and function. Genes provide the differences among us and the similarities in families. From genes we get our physical appearance and our susceptibility to disease.

Recall that chromosomes are found in the cell's nucleus. During the process of conception and the cell division that follows, an extra chromosome or a change in the chromosome structure may occur. A genetic disease may result from a chromosomal error or from the patient inheriting a defective gene from either parent. Types of genetic disease include the following:

- *Monogenic disorders*: A defective gene is inherited from one or both parents. See Table 3.22 for information on genetic diseases and how a child could develop a disease.
- *Chromosomal disorders*: An abnormal number of chromosomes or a change in the chromosomal structure causes a disease such as Klinefelter syndrome or Turner syndrome.

Infectious Pathogens

Many microorganisms are *nonpathogenic*, which means they do not cause disease. They can be found in our body, maintaining the homeostasis. Other microorganisms are *pathogenic*, which means disease causing (Table 3.23). These pathogens enter our bodies through direct contact, indirect contact, or by vectors (Table 3.24).

When a pathogen enters our body and starts to multiply, we have an infection. Changes occur in our body, yet we do not feel any different. This is the *incubation period*. It starts at the time of exposure

TABLE 3.22   Genetic Diseases

NEEDED FOR DEVELOPMENT OF DISEASE OR TRAIT	EXAMPLES OF GENETIC DISEASES
One copy of the defective dominant gene	Huntington disease
Two copies (one from each parent) of the defective recessive gene	Cystic fibrosis Tay-Sachs disease Sickle cell anemia Phenylketonuria (PKU)

and ends when the signs and symptoms appear. The incubation period is different for each disease. For instance, strep throat has an incubation period of 2 to 5 days, whereas varicella (chickenpox) has an incubation period of 14 to 16 days. As our body tissues become damaged from the infection, we start to see the signs and symptoms. This is when disease occurs.

Some diseases are *noncommunicable*. They cannot be transmitted from one person to another. For instance, a person with tetanus cannot spread the disease to another person. Other diseases are *communicable*. These diseases are transmitted from one person to another. If a communicable disease is known to be easily transmitted, it is called a *contagious disease*. Strep throat and influenza are examples of contagious diseases. For instance, people with strep throat are contagious from the start of the fever until they have been on the appropriate antibiotics for 24 hours. The period during which a disease can spread to another is called the *contagious period*. It is important for people in healthcare to understand the ways diseases are spread. Taking required precautions will minimize your risk of "catching something" from your patients.

CRITICAL THINKING APPLICATION   3.10

At school, Daniela learned about the transmission of pathogens. As a receptionist, she sees a lot of sick people stopping at her desk. She encourages those who cough to wear a mask. Hand sanitizer and tissue are also available. Thinking about disease transmission, why are these three items important in the prevention of disease?

Inflammatory Response

The inflammatory response is the body's efficient way of protecting itself. Inflammation occurs when the tissues are injured. The five key signs of inflammation are redness (erythema), swelling (edema), pain, warmth, and loss of function. The injury could be the result of bacteria, trauma, heat, toxins, or other causes. The cells damaged release chemicals called *histamine*, *prostaglandins*, and *bradykinin*. These chemicals cause the following responses:

- Blood vessels at the site dilate. This causes more local blood flow. With the increase in blood flow, redness and warmth occur in that area.

TABLE 3.23	Common Pathogens	
PATHOGEN	DESCRIPTION	RELATED DISEASES
Fungi	Yeast and molds; only a few cause fungal disease or mycoses	Tinea corporis (ringworm) Tinea pedis (athlete's foot) Thrush
Protozoa	One-celled organisms	Trichomoniasis Malaria Amebic dysentery
Viruses	Smallest microorganism; requires a host cell to multiply	Common cold Measles, mumps Chickenpox, influenza
Bacteria	Single-celled organisms; classified by shape: bacilli (rod shaped), spirilla (spiral shaped), cocci (dot shaped) Many disease-causing bacteria produce **toxins** that create the illness	Bacilli: tuberculosis, whooping cough, *Escherichia coli*, salmonella Spirilla: cholera, syphilis, Lyme disease Cocci: gonorrhea, meningitis, strep throat
Helminths	A group of larger parasites that enter the body and live off the food you eat	Pinworms, tapeworms, flukes
Ectoparasites	A parasite that lives on the outside of the body	Lice, scabies

TABLE 3.24	Modes of Transmission for Pathogens	
MODES OF TRANSMISSION	DEFINITION	EXAMPLES OF DISEASES
Direct contact	Susceptible person comes in contact with an infected person; spread occurs via contact with blood, body fluids, and excretions (e.g., stool, urine, and saliva). Methods of direct contact include: • Person to person (sneezing, touching, coughs) • Animal to person (being bitten or scratched or handling animal waste) • Mother to unborn child	Influenza Pertussis Chickenpox Rabies Gonorrhea Tuberculosis
Indirect contact	Spread occurs through contact with a contaminated object (e.g., water, food, drinking glass, airborne transmission).	*Escherichia coli* Botulism
Vectors (insects)	Most blood-sucking insects consume the disease-causing microorganism from one host and transmit it during a "meal" to another host.	Mosquitoes: yellow fever, malaria, West Nile fever, Zika Ticks: Lyme disease, tick-borne encephalitis, rickettsial diseases Fleas: plague, rickettsiosis

• Blood vessel walls allow more white blood cells and plasma to move out of the vessel into the surrounding tissues. The white blood cells work to protect the cells and clean up the dead tissue. The extra fluid from the blood causes swelling, pain, and loss of movement. For instance, if an injury occurs in your finger joint area, the swelling may be so great that it prevents you from moving your finger.

Even though the inflammatory process can be efficient, it can also be the cause of disease. *Autoinflammatory diseases* (e.g., familial Mediterranean fever) differ from autoimmune diseases, which will be described later in the chapter. Autoinflammatory diseases result from a genetic mutation that causes the inflammatory process to activate without a reason. The person may experience recurring brief attacks of pain and fever, and blood work indicates systemic inflammation.

Immunity Disorders

Our immune system protects our bodies against potentially harmful substances. Our immune system "remembers" the **antigens** from diseases and responds with specific **antibodies**. The antibodies destroy or attempt to destroy the harmful substances. Similar to autoinflammatory conditions, at times the immune response can work against us. These malfunctions are classified as follows:

- *Allergies*: Reactions occur if a person is exposed to a food (e.g., milk, tree nuts, peanuts, eggs, soy, and wheat), pollen, dust mites, mold, pet dander, inhalants, or other substances.
- *Autoimmunity*: The immune system does not recognize the body's own antigens and starts attacking itself. Rheumatoid arthritis, lupus, and psoriasis are examples of autoimmune disorders.
- *Immunodeficiency*: This is caused by a deficiency in one or more of the immune system's key players, such as white blood cells (e.g., B cells and T cells). A person with immunodeficiency has impaired resistance to infections.

Nutritional Imbalances

Nutritional imbalances include too little or too much of a nutrient. Nutritional imbalances can impact growth and disease and can result in death. The following are causes of nutritional imbalances:

- *Vitamin and mineral deficiencies:* Some of these deficiencies can be caused by alcoholism, disease, dietary deficiencies (and poverty), weight loss surgery, and metabolic disorders.
- *Vitamin and mineral excesses:* Vitamin excesses can occur when a person takes too much of a vitamin. The water-soluble vitamins (vitamins B and C) pass through the body fairly quickly. The fat-soluble vitamins (vitamins A, D, E, and K) can accumulate in the body. This can lead to toxic conditions. Mineral excess can be caused by diet, medication, or a metabolic error.
- *Obesity:* Causes include the following:
  - Eating too many calories
  - Getting too little exercise
  - Having an endocrine or a metabolic condition
    Obesity can increase a person's risk for other diseases, including heart disease, diabetes, hypertension (high blood pressure), and stroke.
- *Starvation:* Eating too little food can result from disease or poverty.
- *Trauma and environmental agents:* Trauma from auto accidents, violence, falls, and other events can cause disease. Common traumatic injuries include fractures, lacerated and ruptured organs, bleeding, neck and spinal injuries, and head injuries. Psychological trauma can also cause disorders.

Environmental changes, such as severe heat or cold and extremes of atmospheric pressures, can impact health. Poisonings, insect and animal bites, burns, electric shocks, and near drownings can also cause diseases.

NEOPLASMS

When cells grow quicker than normal or do not die as fast as they should, an abnormal mass is created. This mass is called a *neoplasm,* or *tumor.* Tumors can be *benign* (noncancerous) or *malignant* (cancerous). Table 3.25 shows the difference between benign and malignant tumors.

There are more than 100 different types of cancer. Cancers are classified based on the type of tissue from which they originate. See Table 3.26 for the classifications of cancer. (See also Figs. 3.12 and 3.13.)

As the malignant cells grow, they can break through the *basement membrane.* This delicate membrane separates the epithelial cells from connective tissues. Once this occurs, the cancerous cells can invade blood and lymph vessels. The circulating fluid (blood, lymph fluid) can then carry the cancerous cells to another location in the body. Thus cancerous cells from the primary (or original) tumor can

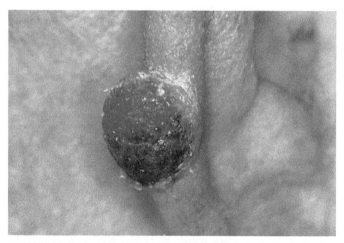

FIGURE 3.12 Squamous cell carcinoma on the ear. (From McCance KL, Huether SE: *Pathophysiology: the biologic basis for disease in adults and children,* ed 6, St. Louis, 2010, Mosby.)

TABLE 3.25	Differences Between Benign and Malignant Tumors	
CHARACTERISTIC	**BENIGN TUMOR**	**MALIGNANT TUMOR**
Cellular structure	Same as surrounding tissue	**Anaplastic** changes and poorly differentiated
Type of growth	Grows within a "shell" (encapsulated)	Infiltrates and *metastasizes;* spreads to distant site(s) in the body via the bloodstream or lymph system
Rate of growth	Usually slow; rarely fatal	May be slow, rapid, or very rapid; almost always fatal if left untreated
Destruction of localized tissue	None	Common; invades and takes over the surrounding tissue

TABLE 3.26	Classification of Cancer	
CLASSIFICATION	**DESCRIPTION**	**DISEASE EXAMPLES**
Carcinoma Types:	Impact skin, lungs, breast, colon, prostate	
Squamous cell carcinoma	Derived from squamous epithelium	Squamous cell carcinoma of the lung
Adenocarcinoma	Derived from an organ or a gland	Gastric adenocarcinoma
Sarcomas	Impact connective tissue (bones, muscle, cartilage, blood vessels, and fat)	Osteosarcoma, chondrosarcoma, hemangiosarcoma, mesothelioma, and glioma
Lymphomas Types:	Impact lymphatic tissue (vessels, nodes, and organs, including the spleen, tonsils, and thymus gland)	
Hodgkin lymphoma	Diagnosed by the detection of Reed-Sternberg cell, a cell specific only to this disease	
Non-Hodgkin lymphoma	All other lymphomas with the exception of Hodgkin lymphoma	
Leukemia	Impacts the bone marrow, causing lots of abnormal blood cells to be created	Acute myelocytic leukemia
Myeloma	Impacts the plasma cells (a type of white blood cell) in the bone marrow	Multiple myeloma
Mixed tumors	Combination of cells from within one classification or between two cancer classifications	Teratocarcinoma, carcinosarcoma

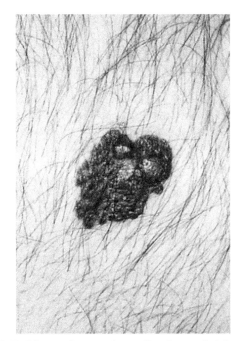

FIGURE 3.13 Malignant melanoma on the arm. (From Damjanov I: *Anderson's pathology*, ed 10, St. Louis, 2000, Mosby.)

metastasize to another location in the body, creating a secondary tumor.

If a provider suspects a patient may have cancer, a number of blood tests and imaging tests will be ordered. A **biopsy** may be performed. The surgeon may also take a biopsy of nearby lymph nodes so the tissue can be checked for malignant cells. Based on the diagnostic results, the **oncologist** or **pathologist** will grade and stage the cancer.

Grade refers to how abnormal the malignant cells look. If the malignant cells and tissues closely resemble normal cells and tissue, the tumor is called "well **differentiated**." These are more slow-growing tumors. If the malignant cells and tissues do not look like normal cells and tissue, they are called "undifferentiated" or "poorly differentiated." The microscopic look of the cell is graded using 1, 2, 3, or 4 to indicate the appearance. Grade 1 means well-differentiated, or the cells and organization of the malignant tissue look close to those of normal tissue. Grade 2 means moderately differentiated, or the tissue does not look like normal tissue; the cells are growing at a faster rate than normal. Grades 3 and 4 do not look like normal tissue and tend to spread quicker.

Stage refers to the extent of the cancer, including the size and if it has spread. A cancer is staged in this manner. Several staging systems are used, and various factors must be taken into consideration with staging systems:

- Location of the tumor
- Type of cell
- Size of the tumor
- If it has spread to nearby lymph nodes

TABLE 3.27	Stages of Cancer: 0 to IV System
STAGE	DESCRIPTION
Stage 0	Abnormal cells are present; no spreading has occurred.
Stages I, II, and III	Malignancy is present. The number is greater for larger tumors and tumors that have spread to nearby tissues.
Stage IV	Cancer has metastasized.

TABLE 3.28	Stages of Cancer: Defined by Terms
STAGE	DEFINITION
In situ	Abnormal cells are present; no spreading has occurred.
Localized	Cancer cells are present; no spreading has occurred.
Regional	Cancer has spread to nearby lymph nodes, organs, or tissues.
Distant	Cancer has metastasized.
Unknown	Not enough information is available.

- If it has spread to other locations in the body
- Tumor grade, or how abnormal the cells look compared with normal cells and how quickly the tumor grows and spreads

The TNM staging system is widely used. The letters T, N, and M will be followed by a number or letter. For instance, a patient may have T1N0M0. It is important to have an understanding of what this means:

T: Refers to the size and extent of the primary tumor
  - TX: Primary tumor cannot be measured
  - T0: Primary tumor cannot be found
  - T1, T2, T3, and T4: Refer to the size and extent of the primary tumor; the higher the number, the larger or more extensive the tumor

N: Refers to the number of nearby lymph nodes impacted by the malignant cells
  - NX: Nearby lymph node cancer cannot be measured
  - N0: No cancer in the nearby lymph nodes
  - N1, N2, and N4: Refers to the location and quantity of nearby lymph nodes that have cancer; the higher the number, the more nodes are impacted

M: Refers to whether the tumor has metastasized
  - MX: Metastasis cannot be measured
  - M0: No metastasis has occurred
  - M1: Metastasis has occurred

Other systems can be used in healthcare to stage cancer. Tables 3.27 and 3.28 provide two additional methods. This information will help you understand references to cancer.

CLOSING COMMENTS

Patient Coaching

Putting medical terminology into understandable language is important for every patient. Many patients will benefit from having medical terms put into simpler, everyday language. Choose your words carefully. Describe body parts, systems, and procedures in language that is clear and understandable to your patient. Ask your patients to repeat instructions back to you so that you know that they are clear on all instructions. Listen to your patient and be open and willing to answer any questions that are within a medical assistant's scope of practice. Have written instructions available whenever possible.

Legal and Ethical Issues

Communication is key to providing the best possible patient care and serving the patient in an ethical manner. Using proper terminology, spelling, and pronunciation will help you inform your patients in a useful way. Being certain that your patients are clear on all instructions is vital. If patients don't receive clear instructions, they may make mistakes in preparing for diagnostic procedures, taking medication, or following treatment or therapy regimens. Clear communication is essential.

Patient-Centered Care

Understanding medical terminology, basic anatomy, and basic pathology allows the medical assistant to help his or her patients in very real ways. The medical assistant can "translate" medical terms into day-to-day language. Medical assistants who can describe procedures in everyday terms help their patients understand what will happen during a procedure and may put a patient's mind at ease. Knowing what to expect helps relieve fear of the unknown.

Professional Behaviors

Having a good understanding of the structural organization of the body will help as you learn about each body system. Knowing how medical terminology relates to body organization, cavities, quadrants, regions, and planes is important for accurate communication. As a medical assistant, you will be communicating with providers and peers. Using correct medical terminology and having a strong understanding of the body systems will help you communicate effectively in the ambulatory care setting.

SUMMARY OF SCENARIO

Daniela continues in her position as a float receptionist. She is gaining a lot of experience in the Walden-Martin Family Medical Clinic. She is excited to be able to understand so many medical terms. When she comes across a new term, she is now able to decode it by breaking it down into word parts. With her knowledge of the most common prefixes and suffixes, she can get a general idea of what the term means even if she does not know the meaning of all the word parts. She can already see how she will be able to use her knowledge of medical terminology in other classes in her medical assistant program.

Bella continues to help Daniela study for her medical terminology and human body courses. Daniela really appreciates the study tips and reviewing assistance that Bella gives her. Some of her favorite ways to study these courses include the following:

- Making flashcards with the term or word part on one side and the definition on the other. Bella warned her to keep the definition short and simple.

For nonmedical terminology, she learned more when she wrote her own definition. She realized the tests did not always use the exact words used in the textbook.

- Daniela realized that she learned better when she listened to the content. So she recorded herself going through her flashcards and review sheets. She found that if she stated the term or question and then paused, when she listened she could fill in the blank before hearing the answer.
- Lastly, Daniela learned that she sometimes felt she knew the content but was not always sure until it came to the test. So she decided to test herself on the content during her study times to see what she really knew.

Daniela is very excited that she will soon complete her human body and disease course and medical terminology course. She is also excited to apply the study practices she is learning to her future medical assistant courses.

SUMMARY OF LEARNING OBJECTIVES

1. **Review the origins of medical terminology and discuss the difference between decodable and nondecodable terms.**

   Medical terminology is a specialized vocabulary that has its root in Greek and Latin word components. Decodable terms are those that can be broken into their Greek and Latin word parts and given a working definition based on the meanings of those word parts. Most medical terms are decodable, so learning word parts is important. The word parts are as follows: **Combining form:** Word root with its respective combining vowel. **Word root:** Foundation of the medical term. **Combining vowel:** A letter sometimes used to join word parts. Usually an "o" but occasionally an "a," "e," "i," or "u." **Suffix:** Word part that appears at the end of a term. Suffixes are used to modify the meaning of the combining form. **Prefix:** Word part that sometimes appears at the beginning of a term. Not all terms are composed of word parts that can be used to determine the definition. These terms are known as **nondecodable terms**. For these types of terms, the meaning must be memorized.

2. **Describe how to decode terms using the check, assign, reverse, and define (CARD) method.**

   Using Greek and Latin word components to break down the meanings of medical terms requires a simple four-step process — the check, assign, reverse, and define (CARD) method. You need to do the following:
   - *Check* for the word parts in a term.
   - *Assign* meanings to the word parts.
   - *Reverse* the meaning of the suffix to the front of your definition.
   - *Define* the term.

   Fig. 3.3 shows how this process is applied to a medical term.

3. **Use the rules given to build and spell healthcare terms.**

   With a few exceptions, decodable medical terms follow five simple rules:
   1. If the suffix starts with a vowel, a combining vowel is not needed to join the parts.

   2. If the suffix starts with a consonant, a combining vowel is needed to join the two word parts.
   3. If a combining form ends with the same vowel that begins a suffix, one of the vowels is dropped.
   4. If two or more combining forms are used in a term, the combining vowel is retained between the two, regardless of whether the second combining form begins with a vowel or a consonant.
   5. Sometimes when two or more combining forms are used to make a medical term, special notice must be paid to the order in which the combining forms are joined.

   Prefixes and suffixes are also used to build medical terms. See Tables 3.1 through 3.10 for an overview of prefixes, suffixes, and root words used in medical terminology.

4. **Describe the structural organization of the human body.**

   The human body is a collection of many body systems. In studying the organization of the body, you will see that it follows this order, from most simple to most complicated: cells make up tissues, tissues make up organs, organs make up systems, systems work together to make up the human body.

5. **Properly use surface anatomy, positional, and directional terminology.**

   In healthcare we use surface anatomy terminology to describe locations on the body. Anatomical position is a standard frame of reference. This means the body stands erect with the face forward, arms at the sides, palms forward, and toes pointed forward. Fig. 3.6A shows the body in anatomical position. Tables 3.14 through 3.17 provide additional information on front (ventral) and back (dorsal) surface anatomy terminology.

   Positional and directional terms are used to describe up/down, middle/side, and front/back. The *midline* of the body is an imaginary line drawn from the crown of the head down between the eyes, through the chest, and separating the legs. Several of the directional terms

Continued

use the midline as a reference. See Table 3.18 for more information on positional and directional terms.

6. **Describe body cavities, abdominopelvic quadrants, and body planes.**

   The body is separated into the dorsal (posterior) and ventral (anterior) body cavities. The *dorsal body cavity* protects nervous system organs. It contains the cranial cavity and the spinal cavity. The *ventral body cavity* is divided into the thoracic and abdominopelvic cavities. The diaphragm creates a physical separation between the thoracic and the abdominopelvic cavities. Table 3.19 summarizes the structures found in each body cavity.

   With the abdominopelvic quadrants, an imaginary line is drawn down the midline of the body. A horizontal line is drawn across the abdominopelvic cavity, intersecting at the naval (Fig. 3.7). These quadrants are referred to as either right or left and upper or lower. The four quadrants are as follows: *Right upper quadrant* (RUQ), *Left upper quadrant* (LUQ), *Right lower quadrant* (RLQ), *Left lower quadrant* (LLQ).

   The nine abdominopelvic regions lie over the abdominopelvic cavity. They provide a more specific location than the quadrants. Refer to Fig. 3.8 and Table 3.20 for the nine regions and the related organs.

   Another way of describing the body is by dividing it into planes. *Planes* are imaginary cuts or sections through the body. The use of plane terminology is common when discussing diagnostic imaging. A *midsagittal plane,* or *median plane,* separates the body into equal right and left halves. The *coronal plane,* or *frontal plane,* divides the body into front and back portions. The *transverse plane,* or *horizontal plane,* divides the body horizontally into an upper part and a lower part. An *oblique plane* uses a diagonal cut through the body. See Fig. 3.9 for illustrations of the body planes.

7. **Discuss the acid-base balance in the human body.**

   pH refers to the acid-base level of a solution on a scale of 1 to 14. A neutral pH is 7. An acidic solution has a pH less than 7 and contains more hydrogen ions. A base or alkaline solution has a pH greater than 7 and contains fewer hydrogen ions. To maintain homeostasis, the body attempts to keep the pH between 7.35 and 7.45. To maintain the acid-base range in the body, the concentration of hydrogen ions must remain constant. If the pH moves outside of this range, serious illness or even death can occur. To help maintain the pH range, the urinary system, the respiratory system, and chemical buffers must all work together. *Buffers* (like bicarbonate) work to prevent changes in the pH.

8. **Discuss pathology basics, including pathology terminology, protection mechanisms, predisposing factors, and the causes of disease.**

   Pathology is the study of diseases. Pathology terminology includes the following terms:

   - Disease, syndrome, disorder, prevalence, incidence, morbidity, mortality, acute, chronic, etiology, sign, symptom, diagnostic procedures, and treatments.

   Protection mechanisms are ways that the body guards itself from disease and death.

   - Mechanisms include the inflammatory response and immunity.

   Predisposing factors are risk factors for disease. Some predisposing factors include:

   - Hereditary or genetic factors, age, gender, environmental factors, and lifestyle

   Disease can result from a change in homeostasis or can be the result of the body's response to a perceived threat. There are several common causes of diseases, including genetics, infectious pathogens, inflammatory processes, compromised immunity, nutritional imbalance, trauma and environmental agents, and neoplasms. See Tables 3.22 through 3.28 for additional information.

INFECTION CONTROL

SCENARIO

Rosa Lucia is a certified medical assistant working for Walden-Martin Family Medical Clinic (WMFM). She is quite concerned about contracting an infectious disease while caring for her patients. Rosa learned about Standard Precautions while enrolled in her medical assisting program and now must implement that knowledge in the workplace. Two important factors in preventing the spread of infection are (1) understanding how to break the chain of infection and (2) recognizing the importance of correct and frequent hand washing.

While studying this chapter, think about the following questions:

- How can Rosa use her understanding of infection control to prevent the spread of infection?
- What is the significance of an Exposure Control Plan in Rosa's pediatric office?
- What are the important details of the office's compliance with the guidelines established by the Occupational Safety and Health Administration (OSHA)?
- How can Rosa implement required infection control procedures at Walden-Martin Family Medical Clinic?

LEARNING OBJECTIVES

1. Describe the characteristics of pathogenic microorganisms.
2. Do the following related to the chain of infection:
   - Apply the chain of infection process to the healthcare practice.
   - Compare viral and bacterial cell invasion.
   - Differentiate between humoral and cell-mediated immunity.
3. Summarize the impact of the inflammatory response on the body's ability to defend itself against infection.
4. Analyze the differences among acute, chronic, latent, and opportunistic infections.
5. Do the following related to the Occupational Safety and Health Administration (OSHA) standards for the healthcare setting:
   - Specify potentially infectious body fluids.
   - Integrate OSHA's requirement for a site-based exposure control plan into facility management procedures.
   - Explain the major areas included in the OSHA Compliance Guidelines.
- Discuss protocols for disposal of biologic chemical materials.
- Remove contaminated gloves while following the principles of Standard Precautions.
- Summarize the management of post-exposure evaluation and follow-up and participate in bloodborne pathogen training and a mock exposure event.
6. Apply the concepts of medical and surgical asepsis to the healthcare setting.
7. Discuss proper hand washing and demonstrate the proper hand washing technique for medical asepsis.
8. Differentiate among sanitization, disinfection, and sterilization procedures, and select barrier/personal protective equipment while demonstrating the correct procedure for sanitizing contaminated instruments.
9. Discuss the role of the medical assistant in asepsis.

VOCABULARY

antibodies Protein substances produced in the blood or tissues, in response to a specific antigen, that destroy or weaken the antigen; part of the immune system.

antiseptics (an ti SEP tiks) Substances that inhibit the growth of microorganisms on living tissue (e.g., alcohol and povidone-iodine solution [Betadine]); they are used to cleanse the skin, wounds, and so on.

autoimmune A disease in which the body produces antibodies that attack its own tissues and cells, leading to the deterioration of structure and/or function.

candidiasis (kan di DIE i sis) An infection caused by a yeast, *Candida albicans,* that typically affects the vaginal mucosa and skin.

communicable (kuh MYOO ni kuh buhl) Diseases spread from person to person either by direct contact or nondirect contact (i.e., insects, examination tables)

defecation (def i KAY shun) The act of voiding waste from the bowels through the anus; the act of having a bowel movement.

degenerative (dih JEN er uh tiv) An illness resulting from the deterioration of tissues and organs.

disinfectant (dis in FEK tant) Any chemical agent used on nonliving objects to destroy or inhibit the growth of harmful organisms; not effective against bacterial spores.

fatigue (fuh TEEG) Extreme tiredness.

germicides (JUR muh sides) Agents that destroy pathogenic organisms.

hereditary (huh RED i ter ee) Passed from parents to offspring through the genes.

impervious (im PUR vee uhs) Not permitting penetration.

inanimate Not animate; lifeless.

inhalation (in huh LAY shuhn) The act of breathing in.

ingested Taken, as food, into the body.

interferon (in ter FEER on) A protein formed when a cell is exposed to a virus; the protein blocks viral action on the cell and protects against viral invasion.

malaise (ma LAYZ) A condition of general bodily weakness or discomfort.

noninvasive procedures Procedures that do not penetrate human tissue.

nosocomial (nos uh KOH mee uhl) **infections** Infections acquired in a healthcare setting.

parenteral (pa REN ter uhl) Taken into the body by any route other than the digestive tract (e.g., subcutaneous, intravenous, or intramuscular administration).

pathogenic Capable of producing disease.

pyemia (pie EE mee uh) The presence of pus-forming organisms in the blood.

relapse The recurrence of the symptoms of a disease after apparent recovery.

remission The partial or complete disappearance of the clinical and subjective characteristics of a chronic or malignant disease.

spore A thick-walled, dormant form of bacteria that is very resistant to disinfection measures.

Standard Precautions A set of infection control practices used to prevent the transmission of diseases that can be acquired by contact with blood, body fluids, nonintact skin, and mucous membranes.

sterile (STER il) Free of all microorganisms, pathogenic and nonpathogenic.

tinea (TIN ee uh) Any fungal skin disease that results in scaling, itching, and inflammation; examples include ringworm and athlete's foot.

transmission The passage or spread of disease.

vectors Animals or insects (e.g., ticks, rodents, mosquitos) that transmit a pathogen.

To gain an understanding of the importance of infection control, you must comprehend the concepts of disease transmission and the body's response to infection. One of the easiest ways to prevent the spread of disease is to wash your hands or use alcohol-based hand sanitizers. Every procedure must begin and end with hand hygiene practices. Making sure that **sterile** technique is used is another huge component of infection control. The fundamental concepts of this chapter should be used whenever you are faced with an infection control issue. The guidelines established by the Occupational Safety and Health Administration (OSHA) also have stated this. The guidelines in this chapter are basic to all clinical skills, and following them can reduce the transmission of disease organisms and lessen the severity of disease. These guidelines also may save a patient's or co-worker's life, or even your own.

DISEASE

Disease is defined as a specific illness with a recognizable group of signs and symptoms and a clear cause (e.g., infection, environment). We recognize and categorize many types of diseases: **hereditary** (genetic), drug-induced, **autoimmune**, **degenerative**, **communicable**, and infectious, to name only a few. Sometimes a specific disease may fit two or more categories.

Any disease caused by the growth of **pathogenic** microorganisms in the body falls into the category of *infectious diseases.* The entrance of a living microbe into the body is not a disease until the infected cell or individual shows harmful changes in structure, function, or biochemistry. In fact, a pathogen may be **ingested**, injected, or inhaled and never cause disease. However, an unaffected person can still transmit the infection to another person. In this case we call the unaffected person a *carrier.*

Microorganisms are almost everywhere. We carry them on our skin, in our bodies, and on our clothing. They can be in ice, boiling water, the soil, and the air. The only places free of microorganisms are certain internal body organs and tissues and sterilized medical equipment and supplies. In the normal state, organs and tissues that do not connect with the outside by means of mucus-lined membranes are free of all living microorganisms.

CHAIN OF INFECTION

Certain factors are required for an infectious disease to spread. These factors, or links, make up the chain of infection. Break the chain and you break the infection process (Fig. 4.1).

The chain of infection starts with the infectious agent. There are five types of potentially pathogenic agents or microorganisms: viruses,

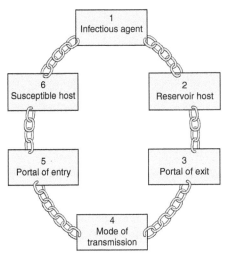

FIGURE 4.1 The chain of infection.

of viral replication. Interferon and the antiviral agents may be prescribed, depending on the specific viral agent. Viral diseases include the following:

- Common cold
- Influenza A and B
- Herpes
- Infectious hepatitis (e.g., hepatitis B and C)
- Acquired immunodeficiency syndrome (AIDS), which is caused by the human immunodeficiency virus (HIV)

Antiviral Agents

- Acyclovir (Zovirax)
- Adefovir dipivoxil (Hepsera)
- Famciclovir (Famvir)
- Oseltamivir (Tamiflu)
- Penciclovir (Denavir)
- Valacyclovir hydrochloride (Valtrex)

bacteria, fungi, protozoa, and helminths. Infection cannot occur without the presence of an infectious microorganism. The best way for healthcare workers to prevent the spread of disease is to use infection control procedures, such as the following:

- Consistent hand washing
- Proper use of **antiseptics**
- Effective disinfection and sterilization methods

Viruses, the smallest of all pathogens, lead the list of important disease-causing agents. Viral particles insert their own deoxyribonucleic acid (DNA) or ribonucleic acid (RNA) into a host cell and then use the host cell to help reproduce more viral particles. Viral invasion may not cause immediate symptoms because host cells infected with viruses can produce a substance called **interferon**. This protects nearby cells. Interferon leaves the infected cell and acts somewhat like Paul Revere, warning neighboring cells that "a virus is coming!" The neighboring cells then produce antiviral proteins, which prevent the virus from replicating inside the cells, slowing or halting the infection.

Antibiotics are unable to destroy viral invaders. The only way to destroy a viral invader is to destroy the host cell. Therefore, the treatment for viral infections typically focuses on relieving symptoms, or *palliative treatment*, and antiviral medications that slow the rate

Bacteria are tiny, simple cells that produce disease in a variety of ways. Pathogenic bacteria can secrete toxic substances that do the following:

- Damage human tissues
- Act as parasites inside human cells
- Grow on body surfaces, disrupting normal functions

Bacteria are classified according to their shape, or *morphology*. Some bacteria can produce resistant internal structures, called **spores**, that make treatment difficult. When bacteria invade the body, the patient can be treated in a number of ways. The most common approach is to use antibiotics to destroy the invader or inhibit its growth. We all have nonpathogenic bacteria that reside in various body systems. For example, a harmless form of *Escherichia coli (E. coli)* lives in the large intestine. These bacteria protect against disease by competing for nutrients, taking up space, and excreting waste. All of these actions discourage pathogens. Common diseases caused by bacteria include the following:

- Tuberculosis
- Urinary tract infections
- Pneumonia
- Strep throat

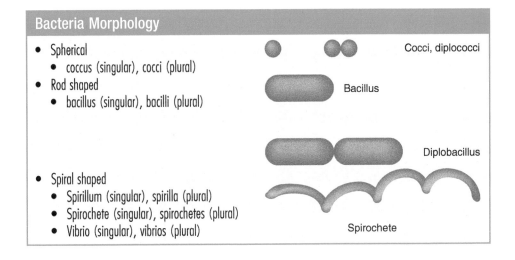

Bacteria Morphology

- Spherical
  - coccus (singular), cocci (plural)
- Rod shaped
  - bacillus (singular), bacilli (plural)

- Spiral shaped
  - Spirillum (singular), spirilla (plural)
  - Spirochete (singular), spirochetes (plural)
  - Vibrio (singular), vibrios (plural)

Cocci, diplococci

Bacillus

Diplobacillus

Spirochete

Antibiotic Resistance

Antibiotic resistance is one of the world's most significant public health problems. Infectious microorganisms that once were easily treated with antibiotics are growing increasingly resistant to the actions of these drugs. The Centers for Disease Control and Prevention (CDC) reported that at least 2 million people in the United States become infected with antibiotic-resistant bacteria, and at least 23,000 people die each year as a direct result of these infections. Resistance occurs when an antibiotic is used inappropriately to treat an infection. This allows the pathologic organism to change or mutate in some way, which reduces or eliminates the effectiveness of the drug. The mutation can occur in the following situations:

- An antibiotic is prescribed when it is not needed (e.g., for a viral infection).
- The antibiotic is prescribed inaccurately (e.g., lower dosage, fewer days than recommended).
- The antibiotic is not taken as prescribed.

Although mutations are rare, overuse of antibiotics provides more opportunity for them to occur. Antibiotics should be used to treat bacterial infections; however, they are not effective against viral infections, such as the common cold, most sore throats, and the flu. Cautious use of antibiotics is the key to preventing the spread of resistance. The CDC makes the following recommendations for providers:

- Prescribe antibiotic therapy only when it will benefit the patient.
- Treat the patient with an antibiotic that is specific to the infecting pathogen.
- Prescribe the recommended dose and treatment duration of the medication.

CRITICAL THINKING APPLICATION   4.1

Susie Chen, a 3-year-old patient, is being seen today. She has been complaining of a cough and nasal congestion. Susie's father does not understand why the pediatrician did not order an antibiotic for his daughter's viral infection. Rosa needs to reinforce the doctor's decision. How can she help the father understand the proper use of antibiotics?

Fungi may be unicellular or multicellular; they include such organisms as mushrooms, molds, and yeasts. Many forms are pathogenic and can cause disease, such as **candidiasis** and **tinea** infections. Fungi grow best in warm, moist environments. Treatment with antifungal agents includes the application of topical preparations (e.g., clotrimazole [Lotrimin]) for tinea infections; vaginal suppositories (e.g., miconazole [Monistat]) for candidiasis; and oral medications (e.g., fluconazole [Diflucan], ketoconazole [Nizoral], and terbinafine [Lamisil]). Fungal infections also are called *mycotic* infections.

Protozoa are unicellular parasites that can replicate and multiply rapidly once inside the host. Examples of diseases caused by protozoa include giardiasis, which is typically caused by the ingestion of water contaminated by feces, and malaria, in which *Plasmodium* organisms invade the blood system. Protozoal infections frequently are seen in tropical climates, which have large insect populations. These insects serve as **vectors** for many protozoal diseases. For example, the mosquito transmits the organisms that cause malaria. Protozoa and helminths (worms) are usually grouped together as parasites.

Helminths are multicellular and include tapeworms, roundworms, and flatworms (flukes). Tapeworms live in the intestines of some animals and can be transferred to humans who eat undercooked meat from infected animals. Most parasitic roundworm eggs are found in the soil and enter the human body when a person picks them up on the hands and then transfers them to the mouth. Roundworms eventually migrate to human intestines and cause infection and disease. Hookworms are intestinal parasites that are spread if the infected person defecates outside in nature or if the feces is used as fertilizer. The eggs are deposited in the soil and mature into larvae. The larvae can penetrate the skin of humans who walk barefoot or ingest contaminated soil (e.g., dirt on fingers or food.) Flatworms with an external sucker are referred to as *flukes*. Flukes are found in raw or improperly cooked fish.

The second link in the chain of infection is the reservoir. The most common reservoirs are people, insects, animals, water, food, and contaminated instruments and equipment. Most pathogens must gain entrance into a host or else they die. The reservoir host supplies all of the conditions needed for microbial growth, allowing the microbes to multiply. The pathogen either causes infection in the host or, in the case of vector-borne diseases, exits the host in great enough numbers to cause disease in another host.

The chain of infection continues with the means, or *portal*, of exit – that is, how the pathogen escapes the reservoir host through the mouth, eyes, intestines, reproductive tract, nose, ears, urinary tract or open wounds. The use of Standard Precautions (e.g., gloves, masks, proper wound care, correct disposal of contaminated products, and hand washing) helps control the ability of infectious material to spread from one host to another.

After exiting the reservoir host, the organism needs to be a mode of **transmission**. Transmission is either direct or indirect. *Direct transmission* occurs from contact with an infected person, with discharges from an infected person (e.g., feces or urine), or with infected soil. Direct transmission includes droplet transmission. This refers to the droplets that come from sneezing, coughing, or even talking. Those droplets land on the next potential host. *Indirect transmission* refers to the transfer of microorganisms by suspended particles in the air, **inanimate** objects, or animals and insects. When microorganisms are suspended particles, this is considered airborne transmission. Transmission occurs through **inhalation** of the microorganisms. *Vectors* are animals or insects that harbor pathogens and can transmit them. Transmission can also occur through contaminated food or drink or through contact with contaminated objects (called *fomites*). Proper sanitation of water and food; the use of sanitization, disinfection, and sterilization procedures; and the use of **germicides** (e.g., Wavicide and Cidex) all help control the transmission of pathogens.

The next link in the chain of infection is the means, or portal, of entry. This is how the transmitted pathogen enters a new host through the mouth, eyes, intestines, reproductive tract, nose, ears, urinary tract, or open wounds. The first line of defense against pathogenic invasion is made up of the body's physical and chemical barriers. An intact *integumentary system*, or skin, serves as a physical barrier to infection. Other anatomic defense mechanisms include the following:

- Tears
- Cilia
- Mucous membranes
- pH of body fluids
- **Defecation** and vomiting

The body's second line of defense is nonspecific chemical and cellular responses. *Phagocytic* cells engulf and destroy the microbes. Inflammation occurs, bringing white blood cells to the area. The inflammatory response produces swelling, redness, heat, and pain.

The third line of defense involves specific immunity. The immune system responds by producing **antibodies** specifically designed to combat the presence of a foreign substance, or *antigen*. This process is called *humoral immunity* and is the responsibility of the body's B cells. Another immune system response involves T cells. This is called *cell-mediated immunity* and causes the destruction of pathogenic cells at the site of invasion or infection.

How Humoral Immunity Is Acquired

There are two ways that antibodies can be acquired: actively or passively. These groups can be further categorized as artificial or natural.

With actively acquired immunity, the body actively makes antibodies after exposure to the disease-causing organism. This could result from having the actual disease or from a vaccination.

With passively acquired immunity, the body is given the antibodies without having to work for them. This could be the result of placental transfer, breastfeeding, or an injection of immunoglobulins.

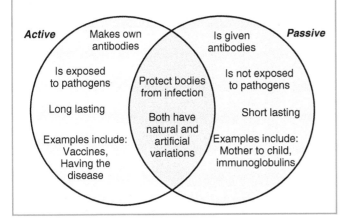

The final link in the chain of infection is exposure of the pathogen to a susceptible host. If the host is *susceptible* (i.e., capable of supporting the growth of the infecting organism), the organism multiplies. Various factors contribute to a host's susceptibility:

- Genetic factors
- Quantity of organisms
- State of the individual's physical health
  - Stress
  - Poor health
  - Poor nutrition
  - Poor hygiene or crowded living conditions

If conditions are right, the organism reaches infectious levels, and the susceptible host can start the chain of infection all over again.

CRITICAL THINKING APPLICATION   4.2

Tommy Anderson, a 5-year-old patient, is in the office because of an outbreak of impetigo. Rosa must apply the concepts of the chain of infection and infection control methods to teach Tommy and his mother how to prevent the spread of the infection to other members of the family. What procedures should she follow after Tommy's visit to prevent the spread of the infection to other patients, other staff members, and herself?

Immunizations trigger the development of antibodies. These antibodies mean that an individual is not susceptible to that disease even if she or he is exposed to the pathogen. However, some people do not develop immunity to diseases even after following immunization guidelines. The Centers for Disease Control and Prevention (CDC) has estimated that, depending on the vaccine, individuals do not develop immunity 1% to 5% of the time. The provider can check for immunity by ordering an antibody titer. A *titer* is a laboratory test that measures the level of antibodies in a blood sample. If a vaccine stimulated a person's immune system to create antibodies to a disease, the antibodies will be present in adequate amounts in the titer. If not, the provider decides whether another dose of the vaccine should be given to try to boost the person's immune response.

The Body's Natural Protective Mechanisms

The body has many levels of protection against the invasion of pathogenic microorganisms.

- Intact skin serves as a natural barrier to disease.
- Mucous membranes lining the openings of the body help protect underlying tissues and trap foreign substances.
- Tiny, hairlike projections, called *cilia,* line the respiratory tract and move in a coordinated upward motion to expel trapped foreign substances.
- Trapped substances can be expelled with sneezing and coughing before the organisms invade underlying tissue.
- Some body secretions, such as tears, have antimicrobial properties that help destroy invading pathogens.
- The natural pH of many of the body's organs discourages the growth of microbes. The acidic pH of urine, the vaginal mucosa, and the stomach helps prevent pathogenic invasion. The body's resident microbes create and maintain this environment.

INFLAMMATORY RESPONSE

The *inflammatory response* (Fig. 4.2) starts when the body experiences trauma or is exposed to pathogens. To defend itself, the body starts certain responses to destroy and remove pathogenic organisms and their byproducts. If this is not possible, it will limit the damage caused by the invading pathogen. This process results in the four classic symptoms of inflammation:

- *Erythema* (redness)
- *Edema* (swelling)
- Pain
- Heat

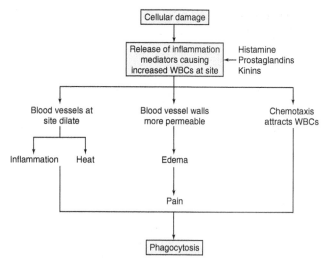

FIGURE 4.2 The inflammatory response. *WBC*, White blood cell.

When the body is exposed to an infectious agent or a foreign substance, cellular damage occurs at the site. Inflammation mediators (i.e., *histamine*, *prostaglandins*, and *kinins*) are released, causing three different responses at the cellular level. All three actions are designed to increase the number of white blood cells (WBCs) at the injury site.

First, blood vessels at the site dilate, causing an increase in local blood flow, which results in redness (inflammation) and heat. Blood vessel walls become more *permeable*, which allows for the movement of WBCs through the vessel wall to the site. The WBCs begin to form a fibrous capsule around the site to protect surrounding cells from damage or infection. Blood plasma also filters out of the more permeable vessel walls, resulting in edema (swelling), which puts pressure on the nerves and causes pain. Finally, *chemotaxis*, or the release of chemical agents, occurs, attracting even more WBCs to the site. The increased number of WBCs at the site results in phagocytosis. Destroyed pathogens, cells, and WBCs collect in the area and form a thick, white substance called *pus*. If the pathogenic invasion is too great for localized control, the infection may collect in the body's lymph nodes, where more WBCs are present to help fight the battle. This causes swollen glands, or *lymphadenopathy*. If the body is too weak or the number of pathogens is too great, the infection may spread to the bloodstream. A systemic infection, called *septicemia* or *blood poisoning*, may occur, which ultimately could affect the entire body. Another term for septicemia is **pyemia**. Without appropriate medical intervention, death can occur from a systemic infection.

TYPES OF INFECTION

Acute Infection

An *acute infection* has a rapid onset of symptoms but lasts a relatively short time. This type of infection will go through the following stages:

- *Incubation:* The period of time between exposure to the pathogen and the appearance of the first symptoms. It can be from a few days to a few months. The incubation period for mononucleosis is 4 to 6 weeks.
- *Prodromal:* The short period of time when the first symptoms appear. With mononucleosis the patient may have 1 to 2 weeks of **fatigue**, **malaise**, *myalgia*, and a low-grade fever.
- *Acute:* The disease is at its peak and symptoms are fully developed. With mononucleosis, *pharyngitis*, *tonsillitis*, and *lymphadenopathy* are common symptoms.
- *Declining:* The symptoms of the disease start to subside. If patients have been prescribed antibiotics, this is when they may decide to stop taking them. It is important to stress to patients that they must take all of the medication. With mononucleosis, the declining stage can take several weeks or even months.
- *Convalescent:* In this stage, patients will regain their strength and return to a state of good health.

The prodromal stage of an acute infection is that time when the patient first shows vague, nonspecific symptoms of disease. For example, the person is not vomiting, nor does he or she have a fever, but the individual just does not feel well. In an acute viral infection, the host cell typically dies within hours or days. In most acute infections, such as the common cold, the body's defense mechanisms eliminate the virus within 2 to 3 weeks.

Chronic Infection

A *chronic infection* is one that persists for a long period of time, sometimes for life. In the case of chronic hepatitis B infection, patients are *asymptomatic,* or without symptoms. The virus is still detectable with blood tests and remains transmissible throughout the person's life. Hepatitis B infection is transmitted by blood or blood products and by all body fluids. It is a serious health hazard to those who work in healthcare. All individuals employed in a healthcare setting should be immunized against hepatitis B. OSHA requires all employers to offer hepatitis B vaccination to their employees.

Latent Infection

A *latent infection* is a persistent infection in which the symptoms cycle through periods of **relapse** and **remission**. Cold sores and genital herpes are latent viral infections caused by the herpes simplex virus (HSV) types 1 and 2, respectively. The virus enters the body and causes the original lesion. It then lies dormant, in nerve cells away from the surface, until a certain trigger (illness with fever, sunburn, or stress) causes it to leave the nerve cell and seek the surface again. Once the virus reaches the superficial tissues, it becomes detectable for a short time and causes a new outbreak at the site. Another herpes virus, varicella-zoster virus, causes chickenpox (varicella). This virus may lie dormant along a nerve pathway for years and later erupt as the painful disease shingles (herpes zoster).

Opportunistic Infections

Opportunistic infections are caused by organisms that are not typically pathogenic but cause disease under certain circumstances. A host with an impaired immune system response, such as individuals infected with HIV, is susceptible to opportunistic infections. Over time, the person's immune system becomes weakened, and diseases result that are not typically seen in patients with a healthy immune system, such as *Pneumocystis jiroveci* pneumonia and oral candidiasis. People without a compromised immune system can have an opportunistic infection.

OCCUPATIONAL SAFETY AND HEALTH ADMINISTRATION STANDARDS FOR THE HEALTHCARE SETTING

In 1987, in response to concern about the increasing prevalence of HIV and hepatitis B virus (HBV), the CDC recommended a new approach to potentially infectious materials, called *Universal Precautions.* The underlying concept of Universal Precautions is that because healthcare workers do not know whether a patient has an infectious organism, all blood and certain body fluids must be treated as if they contain infectious bloodborne pathogens. Therefore, precautions must be implemented for all patients, regardless of the information available about the person's individual health history. In turn, Universal Precautions protect patients from any bloodborne infection the healthcare worker may carry.

In 2001 OSHA developed the Bloodborne Pathogens Standard (**Standard Precautions**), which includes Universal Precautions. The goal of the Bloodborne Pathogens Standard is to safeguard all healthcare employees and their patients who are at risk of exposure from blood and other potentially infectious materials (OPIM). Items contaminated with any of the following potentially infectious materials require special handling:

- Body fluids
  - Semen
  - Vaginal secretions
  - Cerebrospinal fluid (CSF)
  - Synovial fluid
  - Pleural fluid
  - Pericardial fluid
  - Peritoneal fluid
  - Amniotic fluid
  - Saliva in dental procedures
  - Any body fluid that is visibly contaminated with blood
  - All body fluids in situations in which it is difficult or impossible to differentiate between body fluids
- Any unfixed tissue
- Any pathogenic microorganism

Bloodborne Pathogens Standard

In 2000 Congress passed the Needlestick Safety and Prevention Act. This was in response to the CDC's concern about employees' risk when working with sharps. Employers are required to keep a sharps injury log that describes the device involved in the incident and the details of how and where the incident occurred. Employers must also make available to employees effective sharps management devices, such as these:

- Syringes with self-sheathing needles
- Needles that retract after use
- Needleless intravenous (IV) systems

Parenteral exposure includes accidental needlesticks, occupation-related human bites, and exposure of nonintact skin (e.g., cuts and abrasions on the employee's hands) to OPIM. An employer who fails to comply with OSHA's Bloodborne Pathogens Standard could face a maximum penalty of $7,000 for the first violation and up to $70,000 for repeated violations.

The Bloodborne Pathogens Standard also clarifies the use of washing or flushing of any exposed body area or mucous membrane immediately, or as soon as possible, after exposure to OPIM. This includes hand washing after the removal of gloves or other personal protective equipment.

Hands should be washed with soap and warm, running water when available. When running water is not available, alcohol-based hand sanitizers can be used. Studies have shown that correct use of alcohol-based hand sanitizers significantly reduces the number of microorganisms on the skin. It also takes less time than traditional hand washing and causes less irritation to the skin (Fig. 4.3).

The CDC's recommendations for adequate hand hygiene are as follows:

- Visibly soiled hands should be washed for a minimum of 15 seconds with soap and warm, running water (see Procedure 4.2).
- Alcohol-based hand sanitizers that contain at least 60% alcohol should be used before and after contact with each patient, and also after removing gloves, to prevent cross-contamination among patients and healthcare workers (see Procedure 4.2).
- Use an alcohol-based hand sanitizer properly, applying the label-recommended amount to the palm of one hand and rubbing the hands together, covering all surfaces until the hands are dry.
- Artificial nails should not be worn; studies show that even after careful hand hygiene, healthcare workers with artificial nails have more pathogenic microbes under their nails and on their fingertips than workers with natural nails. Artificial nails also cause nail changes that contribute to the transmission of microbes.
- Natural nail tips should be no longer than one-fourth of an inch to prevent microbial growth under the nail.

The best way to reduce the risk of infection is to follow the Bloodborne Pathogens Standard. Healthcare workers must take

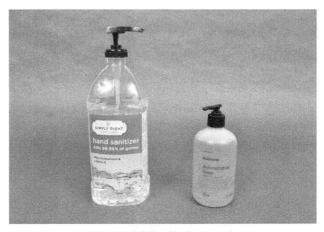

FIGURE 4.3 Alcohol-based hand sanitizer and soap.

Requirements of Employers: OSHA Bloodborne Pathogens Standard

---

EXPOSURE CONTROL PLAN

Each medical office must develop a written exposure control plan (ECP). The purpose of an ECP is to identify tasks where there is the potential for exposure to blood and other potentially infectious materials.

- A timetable must be published indicating when and how communication of potential hazards will occur.
- The employer must offer employees the hepatitis B vaccine within 10 working days of employment (at no cost to the employee). If employees sign a form to refuse the vaccine, they can change their mind at no cost to the employee.
- The employer must document the steps that should be taken in case of an exposure incident, including a postexposure evaluation and follow-up, strict record keeping, implementation of engineering controls, provision for personal protective equipment, and general housekeeping standards.This plan must be posted in the medical office.
- There must also be written procedures for evaluating the circumstances of an exposure incident.
- Training records must be kept for 3 years.

ENGINEERING CONTROLS AND WORK PRACTICES

The employer must provide engineering controls, or equipment and facilities that minimize the possibility of exposure. Examples of engineering controls include the following:

- Providing puncture-resistant containers for used sharps.
- Providing handwashing facilities that are readily accessible.
- Equipment for sanitizing, decontaminating, and sterilizing.

The employer must also enforce work practice controls. Work practice controls also minimize the possibility of exposure by making sure employees are using the proper techniques while working. Examples include the following:

- Enforcing proper handwashing or sanitizing procedures.
- Enforcing proper technique for using and handling needles to prevent needlesticks.
- Enforcing proper techniques to minimize the splashing of blood.

PERSONAL PROTECTIVE EQUIPMENT

Employers must provide, and employees must use, personal protective equipment (PPE) when the possibility exists of exposure to blood or contaminated body fluids. This equipment must not allow blood or potentially infectious material to pass through to the employee's clothes, skin, eyes, or mouth. Examples of PPE include the following:

- Gowns
- Face shields
- Goggles
- Gloves

If an employee has an allergy to powder or latex, the employer must provide hypoallergenic or powderless gloves. The employee cannot be charged for PPEs.

EXPOSURE INCIDENT MANAGEMENT

An exposure incident is contact with blood or biohazard infectious material that occurs when doing one's job. When an exposure incident is reported, the employer must arrange for an immediate and confidential medical evaluation. The information and actions required are as follows:

- Documenting how the exposure occurred.
- Identifying and testing the "source" individual, if possible.
- Testing the employee's blood, if consent is granted.
- Providing counseling.
- Evaluating, treating, and following up on any reported illness.

Medical records must be kept for each employee with occupational exposure for the duration of employment plus 30 years.

COMMUNICATION OF POTENTIAL HAZARDS TO EMPLOYEES

A medical assistant will be exposed to hazardous chemicals on the job. Most chemicals handled by assistants are not any more dangerous than those used in the home. In the workplace, however, exposure is likely to be greater, concentrations higher, and exposure time longer.

The "right to-know" law, OSHA's hazard communication standard, states that each employee has a right to know what chemicals he or she is working with in the workplace. The right-to-know law is intended to make the workplace safer by making certain that all information regarding chemical hazards is known to the employee. This information is supplied in the material safety data sheet (MSDS), a fact sheet about a chemical that includes the following information:

- Identification of the chemical
- Listing of the physical and health hazards
- Precautions for handling
- Identification of the chemical as a carcinogen
- First-aid procedures
- Name, address, and telephone number of manufacturer

Many SDS information sheets can be obtained in repositories on the Internet. An SDS should be updated at least every 3 years. Employers must ensure that all products have an up-to-date SDS when they enter the workplace.

Potential hazards are also communicated with labels and color. Any containers with biohazard waste must be orange (or reddish orange) and must display the biohazard symbol. These labels and colors alert employees to the risk of possible exposure.

FIGURE 4.4 Requirements of Employers: OSHA Bloodborne Pathogens Standard. (Occupational Safety and Health Administration. *https://www.osha.gov.* Accessed September 14, 2018.)

---

adequate and consistent precautions to protect themselves and their patients. Fig. 4.4 summarizes the Bloodborne Pathogens Standard. Healthcare facilities must establish specific policies and procedures for the management of an exposure incident (e.g., accidental needlestick) and the exposed employee.

Compliance Guidelines

The Bloodborne Pathogens Standard is for anyone working in the healthcare field. Only some of the regulations apply to the ambulatory care setting. Safety and infection control go beyond hand washing

and knowledge of the disease cycle. The information presented here applies to the medical assisting profession.

Barrier Protection

Barrier protection, or *personal protective equipment* (PPE), should be used when contact with blood or OPIM is expected. PPE includes specialized clothing or equipment that prevents the healthcare worker from coming in contact with blood or OPIM. This prevents or minimizes the entry of infectious material into the body. Types of PPE used in the healthcare setting include gloves, gowns/aprons,

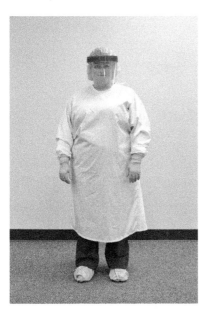

FIGURE 4.5 Personal Protective Equipment.

Environmental Protection

Environmental protection refers to minimizing the risk of injury by isolating or removing any physical or mechanical health hazard in the workplace. Every medical assistant must adhere to these safety rules:

- Read warning labels on biohazard waste containers and equipment.
- Minimize splashing or spraying of OPIM. Blood that splatters onto exposed areas of the skin or mucous membranes is a proven mode of HBV transmission.
- Bandage any breaks or lesions on your hands before gloving.
- If any body surface is exposed to potentially infectious material, scrub the area with soap and warm, running water as soon as possible after the exposure.
- If your eyes come in contact with body fluids, continuously flush them with water as soon as possible for a minimum of 15 minutes using an eye wash unit. A stationary unit connected to warm, running water is the best method for properly flushing potentially infectious material out of the eyes.
- Contaminated needles and other sharps should never be recapped, bent, broken, or resheathed; needle units must have protective safety devices to cover the contaminated needle after injection.
- Contaminated sharp instruments, such as operating scissors, should not be processed in a way that requires employees to reach into containers to grasp them.
- Immediately after use, dispose of syringes and needles, scalpel blades, and other disposable sharp items in a labeled, leakproof, puncture-resistant biohazard container. The container must be located as close as possible to the area where the item is used.
- All specimens must be placed in a container that prevents leakage during collection, handling, processing, storage, transport, and shipping. Avoid contaminating the outside of the container or the label with the specimen substance. The container must have a biohazard label to alert others that it holds potentially infectious material. Gloves should be worn throughout this procedure.
- Equipment requiring repair that has been contaminated with blood or body fluids should be decontaminated before being repaired in the office or transported for repair. There is no documented evidence of HIV transmission from contaminated environmental surfaces, but surface contamination is a proven mode of transmission of HBV.
- Smoking, eating, drinking, applying cosmetics or lip balm, and handling contact lenses are prohibited in work areas where there is a reasonable likelihood of contamination by pathogens.
- Food and beverages cannot be kept in refrigerators, freezers, or cabinets or on countertops where infectious materials could be present.

shoe covers, laboratory coats, masks and respirators, protective eyewear, and face shields (Fig. 4.5).

Gloves are the most commonly used PPE in a healthcare facility. Gloves must be worn if the medical assistant is at all likely to be involved in any of the following activities (see Procedure 4.1, p. 100):

- Touching a patient's blood, body fluids, mucous membranes, or skin that is not intact.
- Handling items and surfaces contaminated with blood and body fluids.
- Performing venipuncture, fingerstick/capillary puncture, injections, and other vascular procedures.
- Assisting with any surgical procedure. If a glove is torn during the procedure, the glove should be removed, the hands washed carefully, and new gloves put on as soon as possible.
- Handling, processing, and disposing of all blood and body fluid specimens.
- Cleaning and decontaminating spills of blood or other body fluids.

The same pair of gloves cannot be worn for the care of more than one patient; new disposable gloves must be used for each individual patient.

Safety Alert

Protective equipment contaminated with body fluids of any kind must be removed and placed in a designated area or biohazard waste container. The hands or any other exposed areas must be washed or flushed as soon as possible. Face shields that cover the mouth, nose, and eyes must be worn whenever splashes, sprays, or droplets are possible. Utility gloves may be reused if they are intact (i.e., have no cracks, tears, or punctures). All PPE must be removed before the medical assistant leaves the medical facility (Fig. 4.6).

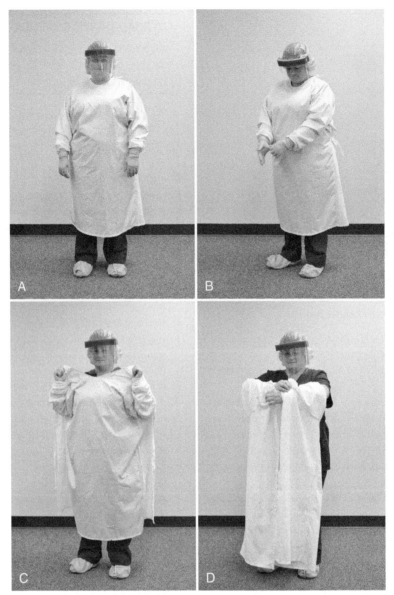

FIGURE 4.6 Removing a contaminated gown.

Housekeeping Controls

The Bloodborne Pathogens Standard requires certain housekeeping measures to ensure a sanitary work area. A schedule must be posted for the cleaning and decontaminating of each work area where exposures could occur. Documentation of these procedures must include information about the surface cleaned, the type of waste encountered, and procedures performed in the designated area.

- After accidental spills of blood or body fluids, at the end of each procedure, and at the end of each shift, work surfaces must be immediately cleaned and then disinfected with a **disinfectant** registered with the Environmental Protection Agency (EPA).
- All reusable containers must be disinfected and decontaminated on a routine basis.
- Sharps containers must be kept as close as possible to the work area. Never attempt to reach inside a sharps container, and do not overfill them. Replace containers on a routine basis, and be

certain that the lid is closed securely before preparing them for biohazard waste disposal.
- Never pick up spilled material or broken glassware with the hands. Brooms, brushes, dustpans, and pickup tongs or forceps should be used. The material should be placed immediately into an **impervious** biohazard waste container at the spill site (Fig. 4.7). Use an absorbent, professional biohazard spill preparation as directed to decontaminate the site.
- Handle soiled linen as little as possible and always wear gloves or other protective equipment during disposal. Linens soiled with blood or body fluids should be double-bagged and transported in labeled, leakproof biohazard bags.
- Contaminated materials and/or infectious waste must be handled with extreme caution to prevent exposure. Biohazard waste must be collected in impermeable, red polyethylene or polypropylene biohazard-labeled bags or containers and sealed (Fig. 4.8). This

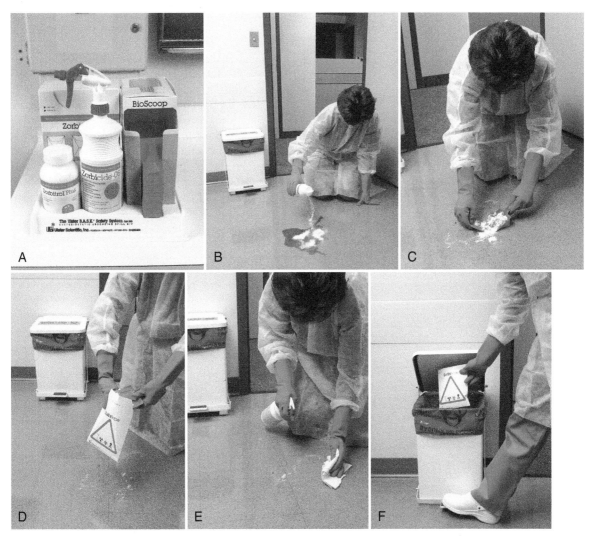

FIGURE 4.7 Cleaning Up Spilled Material. (A) Clean-up kit with printed instructions. (B) Sprinkle congealing powder over the spill. (C) Scoop up the spill. (D) Place the contents in a biohazard bag. (E) Wipe the area thoroughly with a germicide. (F) Place all contaminated material in a biohazard bag or container.

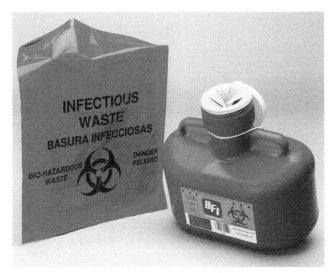

FIGURE 4.8 Biohazard bag and biohazard sharps container.

waste must be disposed of in accordance with all federal, state, and local regulations. Disposal methods include treatment by heat, incineration, steam sterilization, chemical treatment, or other equivalent methods that will render the waste inactive before it is placed in a landfill.

Protocols for Disposal of Biologic Chemical Materials

The Medical Waste Tracking Act set the standards for governmental regulation of medical waste; however, that law expired in 1991. The states were then given responsibility for regulating the disposal of medical waste. Each state varies in its degree of regulation, ranging from no regulation to strict rules. The following are some examples of regulations covering the disposal of hazardous materials:

- Biomedical waste should be collected in containers that are leakproof and strong enough to prevent breakage during handling; the containers must be labeled with the biohazard symbol.

- Workers who handle biomedical waste should observe Standard Precautions.
- Biologic waste containers and boxes should not be held in the healthcare facility for longer than 30 days.
- Sharps are instruments intended to cut or penetrate the skin; they include lancets, scalpel blades, needles, and syringe/needle combinations. Sharps must be placed in red, hard plastic sharps boxes after use; sharps boxes should be closed when three-fourths full.
- Boxes for disposal of chemicals should be labeled with the chemicals' names and any other pertinent data; they must be adequately sealed to prevent breakage or leakage.
- Each healthcare facility must hire a biomedical waste disposal service whose employees are trained to collect and haul away biomedical waste in special containers (usually cardboard boxes or reusable plastic bins) for treatment at a facility designed to handle biomedical waste.

  The cost to the healthcare facility for biomedical waste disposal is typically based on the weight of the contaminated items collected (i.e., the weight of filled sharps containers, biohazard boxes, and bags).

Hepatitis B Vaccine Declination

I understand that due to my occupational exposure to blood or other potentially infectious materials I may be at risk of acquiring hepatitis B virus (HBV) infection. I have been given the opportunity to be vaccinated with hepatitis B vaccine, at no charge to myself. However, I decline hepatitis B vaccination at this time. I understand that by declining this vaccine, I continue to be at risk of acquiring hepatitis B, a serious disease. If in the future I continue to have occupational exposure to blood or other potentially infectious materials and I want to be vaccinated with hepatitis B vaccine, I can receive the vaccination series at no charge to me.

Name: _____   Date: _____

FIGURE 4.9 Sample hepatitis B declination form. (Occupational Safety and Health Administration. https://www.osha.gov/SLTC/etools/hospital/hazards/bbp/declination.html. Accessed September 14, 2018.)

CRITICAL THINKING APPLICATION   4.5
Your office manager asks you to prepare a fact sheet for your co-workers that summarizes the details of OSHA's Bloodborne Pathogens Standard. What should you include?

Hepatitis B Vaccination

HBV vaccination must be available free of charge to all employees at risk for occupational exposure to bloodborne pathogens, within 10 days of starting employment. The vaccine is given by intramuscular injection in three doses. The second injection is given 4 weeks after the first, and the third injection 6 months after the first. Boosters for the hepatitis B immunization are not currently recommended. However, if they are recommended in the future, boosters must be made available to eligible employees without cost.

After three doses of hepatitis B vaccine, more than 90% of healthy adults and more than 95% of infants, children, and adolescents develop adequate antibody responses. Despite this, healthcare workers with a high risk of exposure should have a titer drawn after completing the series to determine whether they have antibodies against the disease. Antibody testing should be done 1 to 2 months after completion of the vaccine series. If the employee did not respond to the first series, or if the series was not completed, revaccination with a second three-dose series is recommended. If antibodies still do not develop, no further vaccination is given.

Employees have the right to decline hepatitis B immunization, but they are required to sign a declination form (Fig. 4.9) that is kept on file as a record of their refusal. The statement can be signed only after the employee has received training about the following:
- Hepatitis B and the hepatitis B vaccination
- Safety, route of administration, and benefits of vaccination

In addition, the employee must be informed that the vaccine will be administered free of charge. Employees who change their mind may receive the vaccine at a future date free of charge.

Post-Exposure Follow-up

If an employee is exposed through an accidental needlestick, a human bite, exposure to broken skin, or from a splash or splatter onto mucous membranes, such as the eyes, certain procedures must be followed. The following specific steps should be taken after exposure to contaminated waste:
- Immediately, or as soon as possible after exposure, the worker should wash or flush the exposed area.
- The exposure incident must be immediately reported to the supervisor.
- The employee must immediately receive a confidential medical evaluation. The provider caring for the exposed employee must receive written details of the exposure incident, including the route and circumstances surrounding the incident. All documentation related to the exposure must do the following:
  - Remain confidential.
  - Not be disclosed to any individual without the employee's express written permission.
  - Be kept for at least the duration of the worker's employment plus 30 years.
- An incident report must be filed that documents the details surrounding the exposure incident, the route or type of exposure, and the identity, if known, of the source individual. The source individual is the person, living or dead, whose blood or potentially infectious material was the source of the occupational exposure.
- The source individual is screened for HBV, hepatitis C virus (HCV), and HIV. Depending on state regulations, consent may or may not be required from the source individual to perform the screening. If consent is required but not given, the employer must document that consent was not received from the source individual. If screening is done, OSHA requires that the employee be informed of the results of the source individual's tests.
- The exposed employee is tested for HBV, HCV, and HIV if consent is given to determine whether the employee already has one of

these infectious diseases. If the employee refuses the tests but blood is drawn, the sample must be stored 90 days for the worker to decide whether screening is wanted.

- If the employee has not been vaccinated against HBV, vaccination is offered.
- The injured employee must receive a copy of the healthcare provider's written opinion within 15 days of completion of the evaluation.
- The exposed employee must receive health counseling about the risk of illness or other adverse outcomes of exposure and the potential for and consequences of transmission of the disease to family, patients, and others.

Healthcare students are at risk for bloodborne pathogen exposure and should follow all OSHA guidelines designed to protect individuals from exposure. A complete, unabridged copy of OSHA's Bloodborne Pathogens Standard may be obtained at the OSHA website (*https://www.osha.gov*).

The CDC has developed a checklist that ambulatory care facilities can use to systematically assess employee adherence to infection prevention and to ensure that the facility has policies and procedures in place and has adequate supplies available to prevent infections at the site. If the answer to any of the questions is no, the facility must do all it can to correct the problems with either staff or supplies (Table 4.1).

Risk of Infection After an Occupational Exposure

Hepatitis B Virus (HBV)

Healthcare workers who have received the hepatitis B vaccine and have developed immunity to the virus are at virtually no risk for infection. For an unvaccinated person, the risk from a single needlestick or a cut exposure to HBV-infected blood ranges from 6% to 30%.

Hepatitis C Virus (HCV)

The estimated risk for infection after a needlestick or cut exposure to HCV-infected blood is approximately 1.8%. The risk after a blood splash is unknown but is believed to be very small.

Human Immunodeficiency Virus (HIV)

The average risk for HIV infection after a needlestick or cut exposure to HIV-infected blood is about 0.23%; the risk after exposure of the eye, nose, or mouth is near zero; the risk after exposure of the skin to HIV-infected blood is estimated to be less than 0.1%.

From the Occupational Safety and Health Administration. *https://www.cdc.gov/hiv/workplace/healthcareworkers.html.*

CRITICAL THINKING APPLICATION   4.6

Rosa's office has been especially busy today. While administering an injection to a frightened 6-year-old child, a co-worker accidentally sticks herself with the needle. She tells Rosa about the incident, but she does not know what to do next. What steps should be taken to manage the situation?

ASEPTIC TECHNIQUES: PREVENTING DISEASE TRANSMISSION

Asepsis means free from infection or infectious material. *Medical asepsis* is defined as the destruction of disease-causing organisms. By using principles of medical asepsis, we can prevent the spread of disease. The goal is to eliminate or minimize pathogens by following OSHA's Bloodborne Pathogens Standard and disinfecting objects as soon as possible after contamination. This creates a healthcare environment as free of pathogens as possible.

Surgical asepsis is the destruction of all organisms. This technique is used for any procedure that enters the body's skin or tissues, such as surgery or injections. Anytime the skin or a mucous membrane is punctured, pierced, or incised, surgical aseptic techniques are practiced. Everything that comes in contact with the patient should be sterile:

- Gowns
- Drapes
- Instruments
- Gloves

Minor surgery, urinary catheterization, injections, and some specimen collections, such as blood collection and biopsies, are performed using surgical aseptic technique.

Because skin cannot be sterilized, the goal of hand hygiene is to reduce the number of microorganisms. Hand washing uses mechanical friction, soap, and warm, running water. Alcohol-based hand sanitizers are also effective in reducing the number of microorganisms. The alcohol kills the microorganisms. If the hands are visibly soiled, hand washing should be done.

Normally, two types of microorganisms are found on the skin: normal *resident flora* and *transient flora*. Normal resident flora lives harmlessly on the skin. Transient flora includes bacteria, viruses, and other organisms picked up on the hands. Resident flora is firmly attached to the skin, whereas transient flora is not. This means that transient flora is easily removed by thorough hand hygiene, preventing the transfer to patients.

The most effective barrier against infection is intact skin. If the skin and mucous membranes are intact, medical asepsis can be used for most **noninvasive procedures**, such as pelvic and proctologic examinations. Instruments and objects used in medical aseptic procedures must be sanitized and disinfected or sterilized before being used on another patient. Medical aseptic procedures may include the use of gowns and masks, but these are not sterile and are worn to protect the healthcare worker more than the patient. Many healthcare facilities are providing masks for patients to use if they present with productive cough, fever, and other influenza-like symptoms. In addition to masks hand sanitizer stations are provided. Both of these measures can help prevent the spread of disease.

Another practical application of medical aseptic technique is to set up work areas in the medical office's laboratory. One side of the laboratory is the "clean" side, where only noninfectious procedures are performed. The other side is the "dirty" side, where potentially infectious materials are processed or cleaned.

Hand Hygiene

Hand hygiene can be accomplished in two different ways. If the hands are visibly soiled, they must be washed using a medical aseptic

TABLE 4.1   Modified CDC Infection Prevention Checklist[a]

FACILITY POLICIES	PRACTICE PERFORMED		IF ANSWER IS NO, DOCUMENT PLAN FOR REMEDIATION
1. Administrative Policies and Facility Practices			
a. Written infection prevention policies and procedures are available, current, and based on evidence-based guidelines, regulations, or standards.	Yes	No	
b. Infection prevention policies and procedures are reassessed at least annually or according to state or federal requirements, and updated if appropriate.	Yes	No	
c. At least one individual trained in infection prevention is employed by or regularly available to the facility.	Yes	No	
d. Supplies necessary for adherence to Standard Precautions are readily available.	Yes	No	
e. Healthcare personnel for whom contact with blood or other potentially infectious material is anticipated are trained in the OSHA Bloodborne Pathogens Standard upon hire and at least annually.	Yes	No	
f. The facility maintains a log of needlesticks, sharps injuries, and other employee exposure events.	Yes	No	
g. Following an exposure event, postexposure evaluation and follow-up, including prophylaxis as appropriate, are available at no cost to the employee.	Yes	No	
h. Hepatitis B vaccination is available at no cost to all employees at risk of occupational exposure.	Yes	No	
i. Postvaccination screening for hepatitis B surface antibodies is conducted.	Yes	No	
j. All personnel are offered annual influenza vaccination at no cost.	Yes	No	
k. All personnel with potential exposure to tuberculosis (TB) are screened for TB upon hire and annually (if negative).	Yes	No	
2. Surveillance and Disease Reporting			
a. Updated list of reportable diseases is readily available to all personnel.	Yes	No	
3. Hand Hygiene			
a. Facility provides training and supplies necessary for adherence to hand hygiene.	Yes	No	
4. Personal Protective Equipment (PPE)			
a. Facility provides training and supplies for appropriate PPE.	Yes	No	
b. Impermeable gowns are worn during procedures in which contact with blood or body fluids is anticipated.	Yes	No	
c. PPE is removed and discarded prior to leaving the exam room.	Yes	No	
d. Hand hygiene is performed immediately after removal of PPE.	Yes	No	
5. Environmental Cleaning			
a. Policies and procedures exist for routine cleaning and disinfection of environmental surfaces.	Yes	No	
b. Cleaning procedures are periodically monitored and assessed to ensure that they are consistently and correctly performed.	Yes	No	
c. The facility has a policy/procedure for decontamination of spills of blood or other body fluids.	Yes	No	

[a]The complete checklist is available at the CDC website for Infection Prevention in Outpatient Settings.
Modified from the Occupational Safety and Health Administration.
www.cdc.gov/HAI/settings/outpatient/checklist/outpatient-care-checklist.html.

technique. If the hands are not visibly soiled, alcohol-based hand sanitizer can be used. Hand hygiene, using the correct technique, must be done before and after each patient is examined or treated, and also when stipulated by the Bloodborne Pathogens Standard.

When you wash your hands for the first time in the morning, spend at least 1 minute on the scrub. For subsequent hand washing, the CDC recommends 15 seconds. Each office sink should be equipped with a liquid soap dispenser. A water-soluble lotion may be rubbed into the hands after they have been washed and dried. Dry, cracked, chapped skin is no longer intact and can provide a means of entry for microorganisms.

Proper hand washing depends on two factors: running water and friction. The water should be warm. Water that is too hot or too cold causes the skin to become chapped. Friction is the firm rubbing of all surfaces of the hands and wrists. Remember that your fingers have four sides, and fingernails have two sides. For medical aseptic hand washing, all jewelry except a plain wedding band is removed. A wristwatch may be left on if it can be moved up on the forearm away from the wrist area. The hands are washed under running water with the fingertips pointing downward. Soap and friction are applied to the hands and wrists. The water is allowed to wash debris away from the wrists and down toward the fingertips (see Procedure 4.2, p. 102).

When you use an alcohol-based hand sanitizer, it should take 20 to 30 seconds to rub all of it into the skin. Be sure to cover all surfaces and continue rubbing it in until your hands are dry (see Procedure 4.2, p. 102). Evidence suggests that hand hygiene with an alcohol-based hand sanitizer is more effective at reducing **nosocomial infections** than plain hand washing. Antimicrobial-impregnated wipes (e.g., towelettes) are not a substitute for an alcohol-based hand sanitizer or soap.

Remember, the goal of hand hygiene is to protect yourself from infection and to prevent cross-contamination from one patient to another.

When to Use Hand Hygiene

Medical aseptic hand washing or alcohol-based hand sanitizer should be used in the following situations:
- After you finish with one patient and before you attend to another patient
- After you finish handling one specimen and before you handle another specimen
- After you use toilet facilities
- Whenever you touch something that causes your hands to become contaminated
- When you arrive at work and before you leave the facility
- After removing gloves
- Before and after eating

According to the CDC, proper hand hygiene must be performed in the following instances, even if disposable gloves are worn:
- Before and after contact with the patient or his or her immediate care environment
- Before performing an aseptic task (e.g., giving an injection, drawing blood)
- After contact with blood, body fluids, or contaminated surfaces
- When hands move from a contaminated body site to a clean body site during patient care

Sanitization

You must carefully clean instruments and other items used in the healthcare facility before proceeding with disinfection or sterilization. *Sanitization* is the cleaning process that reduces the number of microorganisms to a safe level. This cleansing process removes debris such as blood and other body fluids from instruments or equipment. This debris can protect the microorganisms from disinfection or sterilization (see Procedure 4.3, p. 103).

The medical assistant should always wear gloves while performing sanitization. Thick utility gloves will help protect your hands when you work with instruments that have sharp or pointed edges. Gloves prevent possible personal contamination with OPIM that may be present on the articles being cleaned. The procedure should be completed immediately after use of the instruments. A separate workroom, or the "dirty" side of the utility room, is used to prevent cross-contamination of clean instruments and equipment. If sanitization cannot be done immediately, rinse the used items under cold water immediately after the procedure and place them in a detergent solution. Never allow blood or other substances to dry on an instrument.

When you are ready to sanitize instruments, rinse each instrument in cold running water. Sharp instruments should be kept separate from the other instruments. Metal instruments may damage the cutting edges, and sharp instruments may damage other instruments or injure you. Clean all sharp instruments at the same time, when you can concentrate on preventing injury. Open all hinges, and scrub serrations and ratchets with a small scrub brush or toothbrush. Rinse the instruments in hot water, and then check carefully that they are in proper working order before they are disinfected or sterilized. The items should be hand dried with a towel to prevent spotting and allowed to air dry before further processing.

Sanitization is a very important step, and it cannot be overlooked or done carelessly. The use of disposable instruments minimizes the need for sanitization, disinfection, and sterilization.

Ultrasonic Sanitization

Sound waves can be used to sanitize instruments. The instruments are placed in an ultrasonic bath of cleaner and water. Sound waves cause the solution to vibrate, which loosens the materials attached to the instruments. Ultrasonic cleaners are beneficial because they do not damage even the most delicate instruments, and workers do not run the risk of an accidental sharps injury.

Disinfection

Disinfection is the process of killing pathogenic organisms or of rendering them inactive. It is not always effective against spores, tuberculosis bacilli, and certain viruses. Some disinfectant chemicals can kill microbes within a short time, but they are usually hard on instruments. Some chemicals, such as Cidex, are effective enough to kill all organisms, but the usual immersion time for these sterilants is 10 hours or longer. For exam tables and countertop surfaces, there are two common disinfectants: hydrogen peroxide and bleach. Both are low cost and effective.

Many other types of disinfecting agents are available for instruments and equipment. It is important to follow the manufacturer's guidelines on the following factors:
- How to use each product properly
- Advantages and disadvantages
- Possible sources of error

Levels of Disinfectants

The CDC defines three levels of disinfectants:
- Low-level disinfectants can kill most vegetative bacteria, some fungi, and some viruses. Used for exam tables and countertops. Example: hydrogen peroxide.
- Intermediate-level disinfectants can kill mycobacteria, vegetative bacteria, most viruses, and most fungi, but they do not kill spores. Used for noncritical items, such as stethoscopes and percussion hammers. Example: isopropyl alcohol.
- High-level disinfectants will kill all microorganisms except large numbers of bacterial spores. Used for semicritical items, such as a flexible fiberoptic *sigmoidoscope*. Example: Cidex OPA.

Here are common errors that can cause chemicals to lose their effectiveness:
- Instruments are not thoroughly sanitized. Attached organic matter inhibits or prevents the action of the disinfectant. No chemical can kill unless it reaches all instrument surfaces; therefore, complete sanitization is absolutely necessary.
- The disinfectant solution is left in an open container, and evaporation changes its concentration.
- Solutions are not changed after the recommended period for use has expired.
- Solutions are not prepared properly or are not mixed properly before use.
- The manufacturer's recommended temperature for use and storage is not maintained.

Chemical disinfectants cannot be used on skin or tissues because they can damage them. Therefore antiseptics, such as alcohol, are used on the skin to reduce the number of pathogens. Alcohol is the most widely used antiseptic, but studies indicate that it is not as effective as other products in inhibiting the growth and reproduction of microorganisms on the skin's surface. Other antiseptic chemicals, such as povidone-iodine solution (Betadine), are effective antimicrobial agents that are safe to use on a patient's skin.

Sterilization

Sterilization is essential for surgical asepsis. Sterilization can be achieved with moist heat, dry heat, ultraviolet light, ionizing radiation, gas, or chemicals. Medical facilities typically use the autoclave method, which uses moist heat. Steam under pressure in the autoclave offers an excellent method of sterilization because it kills all pathogens and spores. You will learn more about surgical asepsis and the sterilization process in Chapter 9.

> **CRITICAL THINKING APPLICATION**   4.7
> Rosa is responsible for the orientation of the new medical assistant in the office's sanitization and disinfection procedures. Outline the important concepts and methods of each one.

ROLE OF THE MEDICAL ASSISTANT IN ASEPSIS

Asepsis is one of the few procedures that will directly affect the health of the patient, the provider, and the staff. The spread of pathogens in the ambulatory care setting can be controlled only through the effective, consistent application of the Bloodborne Pathogens Standard and by proper sanitization, disinfection, and sterilization of supplies, equipment, and work surfaces.

The medical assistant must develop the skills needed for performing aseptic procedures properly. It is important that these techniques be done on such a routine basis that they become an unbreakable habit. The use of disposable items is highly recommended for infection control purposes. However, when disposable equipment is used, the assistant must follow recommended disposal guidelines to ensure infection control.

CLOSING COMMENTS

Patient Coaching

The medical assistant should take every opportunity to educate patients about the infection process and ways to prevent the transmission of disease. The best time to instruct a patient in aseptic techniques that can be used at home is while performing the aseptic procedure. Consider these examples:
- While washing your hands, explain to the patient that this routine is particularly important for patients who are very young or old or who get sick frequently. Instruct the patient that the hands should be washed before and after meals; after sneezing, coughing, or blowing the nose; after using the restroom; before and after changing a dressing; and after changing an infant's diaper.
- Advise the patient to carry an alcohol-based hand sanitizer and to use it as indicated throughout the day.
- Explain to the patient that coughing or sneezing into a bent elbow is an effective method for preventing the spread of disease.
- Instruct the patient in the differences between sterile and clean dressings and bandages. Demonstrate each step in changing a dressing properly and explain how to dispose of contaminated items.

A medical assistant can help patients live healthier lives in many ways. For example, here are a few more suggestions for teaching the patient about asepsis and infection control:
- Set up an information table in the waiting room with take-home pamphlets and literature.
- Mail, email, or post on the healthcare facility's website a periodic newsletter to patients about infection control, especially during flu season.
- Demonstrate and explain aseptic procedures to patients and family members, inviting them to participate.

Legal and Ethical Issues

Medical asepsis and infection control in ambulatory care practices give rise to numerous legal and ethical concerns. Personal discipline is the primary concern in medical asepsis. Typically, the medical assistant is alone when performing an aseptic procedure; therefore, if contamination occurs, he or she is the only one who knows. If contamination should occur, the medical assistant must start over again with clean supplies.

A primary reason for performing aseptic procedures completely and effectively is to prevent the development of nosocomial infections in susceptible patients. These infections, which are acquired in the healthcare environment, can be especially dangerous for elderly or debilitated patients. Ignorance of the various aseptic techniques or carelessness can be dangerous and is inexcusable before the law.

Professional Behaviors

One of the medical assistant's main responsibilities is to perform sanitization, disinfection, and sterilization procedures with precision and total effectiveness. There is no room for compromise. These procedures have a huge impact on infection control. Patients should have absolute confidence that they are being treated in an aseptic atmosphere and under aseptic conditions. This assurance is just as important for the protection of the provider and staff as it is for the patient. Allowing the provider to assume, incorrectly, that the required aseptic techniques were used to prepare for a procedure, and allowing him or her to use contaminated equipment on a patient, may result in a malpractice lawsuit. Honesty on the part of the medical assistant builds self-respect and contributes to professional achievement.

SUMMARY OF SCENARIO

Implementing Standard Precautions throughout daily practice is crucial to the welfare and protection of both the patient and the healthcare worker. Rosa must be sure to wash her hands routinely or to use an alcohol-based hand sanitizer. She also must familiarize herself with the office's exposure control plan, follow OSHA's Bloodborne Pathogens Standard, use PPE when needed, follow environmental protection guidelines, use appropriate procedures for cleaning up contaminated spills and other housekeeping controls, and understand post-exposure follow-up if an accidental exposure occurs. In addition, Rosa must follow guidelines for sanitization, disinfection, and sterilization of appropriate instruments and equipment.

SUMMARY OF LEARNING OBJECTIVES

1. **Describe the characteristics of pathogenic microorganisms.**

   Pathogenic microorganisms include viruses, bacteria, protozoa, fungi, and helminths. Viruses, the smallest of all pathogens, lead the list of important disease-causing agents. Viral particles insert their own deoxyribonucleic acid (DNA) or ribonucleic acid (RNA) into a host cell and then use the host cell to help reproduce more viral particles. Bacteria are tiny, simple cells that produce disease by secreting toxins, act as parasites inside human cells, or grow on body surfaces, disrupting normal human functions. Bacteria are classified according to their shape. Protozoa are unicellular parasites that can replicate and multiply rapidly once inside the host. They are frequently carried by insects that serve as vectors for the disease. Fungi may be unicellular or multicellular; they include molds and yeasts and cause tinea infections. Helminths are multicellular and include tapeworms, roundworms, and flatworms (flukes).

2. **Do the following related to the chain of infection:**

   - *Apply the chain of infection process to the healthcare practice.*
     The chain of infection is the way infectious disease is spread. It begins with the infectious agent and moves to the host, the means or portal of exit from the host, the mode of transmission, and the means or portal of entry into a new host. It ends with the presence of the infection in a susceptible host. At least one of these links must be broken to stop the spread of infection.
   - *Compare viral and bacterial cell invasion.*
     Bacterial infections can be treated with antibiotics, but viral infections, which involve viral takeover of cellular DNA or RNA material, cannot be treated with antibiotics because viruses are not cells, but parasites within a cell.

   - *Differentiate between humoral and cell-mediated immunity.*
     Humoral immunity creates specific antibodies to combat antigens through the action of B cells. The immune system also reacts at the cellular level with T-cell activity in cell-mediated immunity by causing the destruction of pathogenic cells at the site of invasion.

3. **Summarize the impact of the inflammatory response on the body's ability to defend itself against infection.**

   The inflammatory response is one aspect of the body's ability to defend itself against infection. It involves the body's reaction to the introduction of a foreign substance or an antigen, an increase in blood flow to the site, and the release of inflammatory mediators that attract white blood cells to the site. WBCs isolate and destroy the source of inflammation.

4. **Analyze the differences among acute, chronic, latent, and opportunistic infections.**

   Acute diseases have a rapid onset and short duration. Chronic diseases are present over a long period, perhaps a lifetime. Latent diseases cycle through relapse and remission phases. Opportunistic infections are caused by organisms that are not typically pathogenic but that occur in hosts with an impaired or weakened immune system response, such as individuals with HIV.

5. **Do the following related to the Occupational Safety and Health Administration (OSHA) standards for the healthcare setting:**

Continued

SUMMARY OF LEARNING OBJECTIVES—*continued*

- *Specify potentially infectious body fluids.*
  Potentially infectious body fluids include CSF; mucus; synovial, pleural, pericardial, peritoneal, and amniotic fluids; blood; vaginal and seminal secretions; saliva; and human tissue.

- *Integrate OSHA's requirement for a site-based exposure control plan into facility management procedures.*
  OSHA requires incorporation of a site-based Exposure Control Plan into facility management procedures. The plan must be revised annually and must be available for employees to review. It must reflect current safety technology, identify employees at risk for exposure, and contain specifics about protection from bloodborne pathogens, including PPE, training, hepatitis B immunization, exposure, follow-up, record keeping, and the labeling and disposal of all biohazard waste.

- *Explain the major areas included in the OSHA Compliance Guidelines.*
  The OSHA Compliance Guidelines include barrier protection devices, environmental protection, housekeeping controls, hepatitis B immunization, and post-exposure follow-up.

- *Discuss protocols for disposal of biologic chemical materials.*
  Biologic chemicals must be disposed of in accordance with all federal, state, and local regulations.

- *Remove contaminated gloves while following the principles of Standard Precautions.*
  Refer to Procedure 4.1, p. 100.

- *Summarize the management of post-exposure evaluation and follow-up and participate in bloodborne pathogen training and a mock exposure event.*
  Post-exposure evaluation and follow-up are as follows: The site is cleaned, and the exposed individual reports to his or her supervisor immediately. Medical assessment is performed immediately. Testing of the source individual's and the worker's blood is performed if possible and if consent is given. Health counseling is provided. Strict confidentiality of all medical records is maintained.

6. **Apply the concepts of medical and surgical asepsis to the healthcare setting.**
   Medical asepsis is the removal or destruction of pathogens. Medical aseptic techniques are used to reduce the number of microorganisms as much as possible. Surgical asepsis is destruction of all microorganisms. Surgical asepsis is used when the patient's skin or mucous membranes are disrupted.

7. **Discuss proper hand washing and demonstrate the proper hand washing technique for medical asepsis.**
   Refer to Procedure 4.2, p. 102.

8. **Differentiate among sanitization, disinfection, and sterilization procedures, and select barrier/personal protective equipment while demonstrating the correct procedure for sanitizing contaminated instruments.**
   Sanitization is cleaning of contaminated articles or surfaces to reduce the number of microorganisms (refer to Procedure 4.3, p. 103). Disinfection involves the use of physical or chemical means to destroy pathogens or their components on inanimate surfaces or objects. Sterilization removes all living microorganisms.

9. **Discuss the role of the medical assistant in asepsis.**
   Asepsis is important the health of the patient, the provider, and the staff. The medical assistant must develop the necessary skills, in addition to a firm grasp of the principles involved, for performing aseptic procedures properly.

PROCEDURE 4.1   Remove Contaminated Gloves and Discard Biohazard Material

Task: To minimize exposure to pathogens by aseptically removing and discarding contaminated gloves.

EQUIPMENT and SUPPLIES

- Disposable gloves
- Biohazard waste container with labeled red biohazard bag

PROCEDURAL STEPS

1. With the dominant hand, grasp the glove of the opposite hand near the palm and begin removing the first glove (see the following figure). The arms should be held away from the body with the hands pointed down.
   <u>PURPOSE:</u> Holding the hands down and away from the body helps prevent possible contamination.

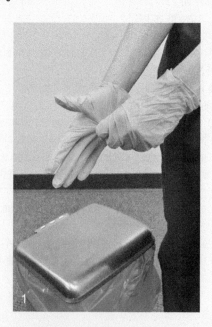

| PROCEDURE 4.1 | Remove Contaminated Gloves and Discard Biohazard Material—*continued* |

2. Pull the glove inside out (see the following figure). After removal, ball it into the palm of the remaining gloved hand.
   PURPOSE: Taking off the glove inside out prevents transmission of pathogens to another surface.

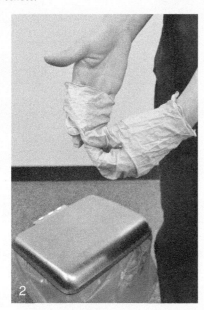

3. Insert two fingers of the ungloved hand between the edge of the cuff of the other contaminated glove and the hand (see the following figure).

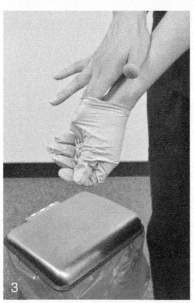

4. Push the glove down the hand, inside out, over the contaminated glove being held, leaving the contaminated side of both gloves on the inside.
   PURPOSE: This technique protects the wearer from the contaminated surfaces of both gloves.

5. Properly dispose of the inside-out, contaminated gloves in a biohazard waste container (see the following figure).
   PURPOSE: To prevent the spread of infection.

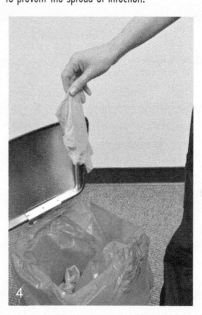

6. Perform a medical aseptic hand wash as described in Procedure 4.2, or sanitize the hands with an alcohol-based sanitizer.
   PURPOSE: To minimize the number of pathogens on the hands, thereby reducing the number of transient flora and the risk of transmission of pathogens.

PROCEDURE 4.2 | Perform Hand Hygiene

Task: To minimize the number of pathogens on the hands, thus reducing the risk of transmission of pathogens.

EQUIPMENT and SUPPLIES

- Sink with warm running water
- Liquid soap in a dispenser (bar soap is not acceptable)
- Disposable nail brush or orange stick
- Paper towels in a dispenser
- Water-based lotion
- Covered waste container with foot pedal
- Alcohol-based hand sanitizer

PROCEDURAL STEPS

Medical Aseptic Hand Washing

1. Remove all jewelry except your wristwatch, if it can be pulled up above your wrist, and a plain wedding ring.
   <u>PURPOSE</u>: Jewelry can harbor microorganisms.
2. Turn on the faucet and regulate the water temperature to lukewarm.
   <u>PURPOSE</u>: Water that is too hot can cause the skin to become dry and chapped.
3. Wet your hands, apply soap, and lather using a circular motion with friction while holding your fingertips downward (see the following figure). Rub well between your fingers. If this is the first hand wash of the day, use a nail brush or an orange stick and clean under every fingernail. Inspect your nails thoroughly.
   <u>PURPOSE</u>: Friction removes soil and contaminants from the hands and wrists.

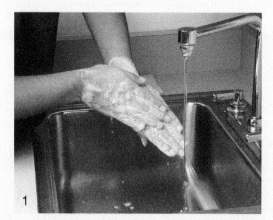

4. Rinse well, holding your hands so that the water flows from your wrists downward to your fingertips (see the following figure).
   <u>PURPOSE</u>: Soil and contaminants will wash off the skin and down the drain.

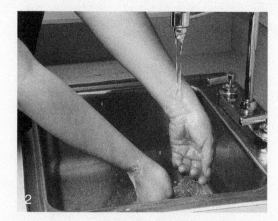

5. If this is the first hand wash of the day or if your hands are obviously contaminated, wet your hands again and repeat the scrubbing procedure using a vigorous, circular motion over the wrists and hands for at least 1 to 2 minutes.
   <u>PURPOSE</u>: Time is required for friction and motion to eliminate all possible soil and contaminants.
6. Rinse your hands a second time, keeping the fingers lower than your wrists.
   <u>PURPOSE</u>: To ensure removal of all transient flora.
7. Dry your hands with paper towels. Do not touch the paper towel dispenser as you are obtaining towels (see the following figure).
   <u>PURPOSE</u>: Touching the dispenser contaminates your hands, and you will need to start over.

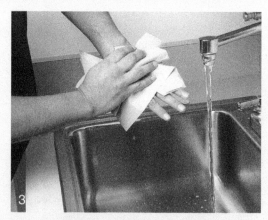

8. If the faucets are not foot operated, turn them off with a dry paper towel (see the following figure).
   <u>PURPOSE</u>: The faucet is dirty and will contaminate your clean hands.

PROCEDURE 4.2	**Perform Hand Hygiene**—*continued*

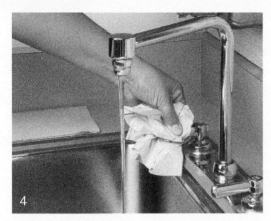

9. After you finish drying your hands and turning off the faucets, discard used towels in a covered waste container.
   <u>PURPOSE</u>: Always discard contaminated waste in a covered waste container immediately to eliminate the source of infection.
10. If needed, apply a water-based antibacterial hand lotion to prevent chapped or dry skin.
   <u>PURPOSE</u>: Chapped skin eliminates the first line of defense against infectious organisms.

11. Repeat the procedure as indicated throughout the day.
   <u>PURPOSE</u>: To eliminate contaminants and prevent the transmission of pathogens to yourself and others.

Applying an Alcohol-Based Hand Sanitizer
1. Inspect your hands to ensure they are not visibly soiled.
   <u>PURPOSE</u>: If the hands are visibly soiled, then the medical aseptic hand wash should be performed.
2. Remove your watch or push it up on your arm; remove rings.
   <u>PURPOSE</u>: Watches and rings can harbor microorganisms
3. Apply alcohol-based hand sanitizer to the palm of one hand: gel or lotion – dime-sized; foam – walnut-sized.
   <u>PURPOSE</u>: Using too much alcohol-based hand sanitizer can be drying to the skin. Dry skin cracks and chaps, creating portals of entry for microorganisms.
4. Thoroughly spread sanitizer over all surfaces of both hands, including around and under the fingernails.
   <u>PURPOSE</u>: All surfaces need to be exposed to the alcohol-based hand sanitizer to effectively kill all microorganisms.
5. Rub your hands until dry (20 to 30 seconds).

PROCEDURE 4.3	**Sanitize Soiled Instruments**

Task: To remove all contaminated matter from instruments in preparation for disinfection or sterilization while following Standard Precautions and wearing appropriate personal protective equipment (PPE).

EQUIPMENT and SUPPLIES

- Sink with cold and hot running water
- Sanitizing agent or low-sudsing soap with enzymatic action
- Decontaminated utility gloves that show no signs of deterioration
- Chin-length face shield or goggles and face mask if contamination with bloodborne pathogens is possible
- Impermeable gown
- Disposable brush
- Disposable paper towels
- Utility gloves

- Disinfectant cleaner prepared according to manufacturer's directions
- Covered waste container with foot pedal
- Biohazard waste container with labeled red biohazard bag

PROCEDURAL STEPS

1. Put on an impermeable gown and face shield or goggles and mask if the potential for splashing of infectious material exists (see the following figure).
   <u>PURPOSE</u>: To provide personal protection against potentially infectious matter.

Continued

PROCEDURE 4.3   **Sanitize Soiled Instruments**—*continued*

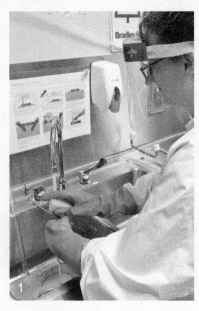

2. Put on utility gloves.
   <u>PURPOSE</u>: To provide personal protection against potentially infectious matter and sharp instruments.
3. Separate the sharp instruments from other instruments to be sanitized.
   <u>PURPOSE</u>: To prevent possible self-injury and exposure to infectious matter.
4. Rinse the instruments under cold running water.
   <u>PURPOSE</u>: To help remove debris and body fluids.
5. Open hinged instruments and scrub all grooves, crevices, and serrations with a disposable brush (see the following figure).
   <u>PURPOSE</u>: Microorganisms can hide under contaminants and may not be destroyed by the disinfection process.

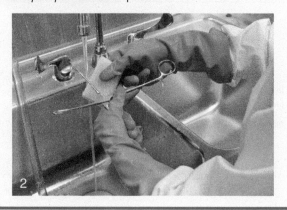

6. Rinse well with hot water.
   <u>PURPOSE</u>: Hot water removes all soap and contaminant residue.
7. Towel-dry all instruments thoroughly and dispose of contaminated towels and disposable brush in a biohazard waste container. Do not touch the paper towel dispenser as you are obtaining towels.
   <u>PURPOSE</u>: All contaminated material must be discarded in a labeled biohazard container and/or a labeled red biohazard bag. Touching the dispenser with the utility gloves contaminates the dispenser. Wet instruments can rust or become dull.
8. Remove the utility gloves and wash your hands according to Procedure 4.2.
   <u>PURPOSE</u>: To remove any contaminants.
9. Towel-dry your hands and put on gloves. Decontaminate the utility gloves and work surfaces using disinfectant cleaner.
   <u>PURPOSE</u>: To prevent personal exposure to contaminants. All equipment and working surfaces should be cleaned and decontaminated with a disinfectant to prevent transmission of infectious organisms.
10. Dispose of the contaminated towels in a covered waste container.
    <u>PURPOSE</u>: All contaminated material must be disposed of in a labeled biohazard container and/or a labeled red biohazard bag.
11. Place sanitized instruments in a designated area for disinfection or sterilization.
    <u>PURPOSE</u>: Sanitized instruments must be removed from the cleaning area to prevent possible cross-contamination.
12. Remove the gloves according to Procedure 4.1. Dispose of the gloves in a biohazard waste container. Sanitize the hands.
    <u>PURPOSE</u>: To prevent the spread of infectious organisms and to remove any possible contaminants.

5

VITAL SIGNS

SCENARIO

Carlos Ricci, CMA (AAMA), is a certified medical assistant who works at Walden-Martin Family Medical (WMFM) Clinic. Carlos graduated from a medical assistant program 3 years ago and enjoys the variety of patients and the patient contact involved in working on the clinical side of WMFM. One of Carlos' primary responsibilities is to accurately measure and record each patient's vital signs before the patient is seen. Over the past 3 years, he has come to understand the importance of taking accurate vital sign measurements and of accurately documenting those results.

While studying this chapter, think about the following questions:

- What factors might alter a patient's vital signs?
- What methods could be used to gather and record a patient's temperature, pulse, respirations, blood pressure, height, weight, and body mass index (BMI)?
- What are the current guidelines for diagnosing and treating hypertension?

LEARNING OBJECTIVES

1. Do the following related to temperature:
   - Cite the average body temperature for various age groups.
   - Describe emotional and physical factors that can cause body temperature to rise and fall.
   - Convert temperature readings between the Fahrenheit and Celsius scales.
   - Obtain and record an accurate patient temperature using three different types of thermometers.
2. Do the following related to pulse:
   - Cite the average pulse rate for various age groups.
   - Describe pulse rate, volume, and rhythm.
   - Locate and record pulse at multiple sites.
3. Do the following related to respiration:
   - Cite the average respiratory rate for various age groups.
   - Demonstrate the best way to obtain an accurate respiratory count.

4. Do the following related to blood pressure:
   - Cite the approximate blood pressure range for various age groups.
   - Specify physiologic factors that affect blood pressure.
   - Differentiate between essential and secondary hypertension.
   - Interpret current hypertension guidelines and treatment.
   - Describe how to determine the correct cuff size for individual patients.
   - Identify the different Korotkoff phases.
   - Accurately measure and document blood pressure.
5. Discuss and perform pulse oximetry.
6. Accurately measure and document height and weight, use the body mass index scale, and convert kilograms to pounds and pounds to kilograms.

VOCABULARY

apnea (AP nee ah) Abnormal, periodic cessation of breathing.

arteriosclerosis (ar teer ee oh sklah ROH sis) Thickening, decreased elasticity, and calcification of arterial walls.

auscultated (AW skuhl tay ted) Listened to with a stethoscope.

bounding Describes a pulse that feels full because of the increased power of cardiac contraction or as a result of increased blood volume.

bradycardia (brad ee KAHR dee uh) A slow heartbeat; a pulse below 60 beats per minute.

bradypnea (brad IP nee ah) Abnormally slow breathing.

calibrated (KAL uh bray ted) Determined by or checked against a standard (as in readings).

cerumen (si ROO muhn) A waxy secretion in the ear canal; commonly called ear wax.

Cheyne-Stokes respiration Deep, rapid breathing followed by a period of apnea.

chronic obstructive pulmonary disease (COPD) A progressive, irreversible lung condition that results in diminished lung capacity.

diurnal (die UR nl) variation Fluctuations that occur during each day.

dyspnea (DISP nee ah) Difficult or painful breathing.

essential hypertension Elevated blood pressure of unknown cause that develops for no apparent reason; sometimes called primary hypertension.

febrile (FEB ruhl) Pertaining to an elevated body temperature.

fluctuate (FLUHK choo ayt) To shift back and forth.

homeostasis (hoh mee oh STAY sis) The internal environment of the body that is compatible with life. A steady state that is created by all the body systems working together to provide a consistent and unvarying internal environment.

hyperpnea (hie PURP nee ah) Excessively deep breathing.

hyperventilation (hie pur ven ti LAY shun) Abnormally increased breathing.

hypotension Blood pressure that is below normal (systolic pressure below 90 mm Hg and diastolic pressure below 50 mm Hg).

idiopathic (id ee uh PATH ik) Of unknown cause.

intermittent pulse A pulse in which beats occasionally are skipped.

larynx (LAR inks) The voice box.

lymphedema (lim fuh DEE mah) A condition in which extra lymph fluid builds up in tissues and causes swelling. It may occur in an arm or leg if lymph vessels are blocked, damaged, or removed by surgery.

malaise (ma LAYZ) A condition of general bodily weakness or discomfort, often marking the onset of a disease.

myocardium (mie oh KAR dee um) The middle layer, and thickest layer, of the heart; composed of cardiac muscles.

occlude To close, shut, or stop up.

orthopnea (or THOP nee ah) A condition of difficult breathing unless in an upright position.

orthostatic (postural) hypotension A temporary fall in blood pressure when a person rapidly changes from a recumbent position to a standing position.

otitis externa Inflammation or infection of the external auditory canal; commonly called swimmer's ear.

peripheral (puh RIF er uhl) Refers to an area outside of or away from an organ or structure.

pulse deficit A condition in which the radial pulse is less than the apical pulse; it may indicate a peripheral vascular abnormality.

pulse pressure The difference between the systolic and diastolic blood pressures (30 to 50 mm Hg is considered normal).

pyrexia (pie REK see ah) A febrile condition or fever.

rales (rayls) An abnormal lung sound heard on auscultation, characterized by discontinuous bubbling noises.

rhonchi (RON kie) An abnormal rumbling sound heard on auscultation, caused by airways blocked by secretions or muscle contractions.

sinus arrhythmia An irregular heartbeat that originates in the sinoatrial node (pacemaker).

stertorous (STUR ter uhs) Heavy, as related to snoring.

syncope (SING kuh pee) Fainting; a brief lapse in consciousness.

tachycardia (tak i KAHR dee ah) A rapid but regular heart rate; one that exceeds 100 beats per minute.

tachypnea (tack ip NEE ah) Rapid, shallow breathing.

thready Describes a pulse that is thin and feeble.

vertigo (VUR tih goh) Dizziness; an abnormal sensation of movement when there is none.

wheezing (WHEE zing) Whistling sound made during breathing.

Almost every patient who visits the healthcare facility will have some vital signs measured. These signs are the body's indicators of internal **homeostasis** and the patient's general state of health. Medical assistants are often responsible for obtaining these measurements. It is crucial that they have confidence in the theory and practical applications of vital sign measurements. A medical assistant who understands the principles of and the reasons for these measurements is a valuable asset to any healthcare facility.

Accuracy is essential. A change in one or more of the patient's vital signs may indicate a change in general health. Variations may suggest the presence or disappearance of a disease process. This may lead to changes in the treatment plan. Taking vital signs is a task that requires consistent attention to accuracy and detail. These findings are necessary to come up with a correct diagnosis. Vital signs should never be measured in an indifferent or a casual manner. In addition to performing measurements accurately, you must take care when documenting the findings in the patient's health record.

The *vital signs* are the patient's temperature, pulse, respiration, and blood pressure. These four signs are abbreviated *TPR* and *BP* and may be referred to as *cardinal signs*. Many organizations consider pulse oximetry, SpO_2, a vital sign also. The medical assistant must understand the significance of the vital signs and must measure and record them accurately. *Anthropometric measurements* are not considered vital signs but are usually obtained at the same time as vital signs. These measurements include height, weight, body mass index (BMI), and other body measurements, such as fat composition.

FACTORS THAT MAY INFLUENCE VITAL SIGNS

Vital signs are influenced by many factors, both physical and emotional. A patient may have had a hot or cold beverage just before the examination or may be anxious or fearful about what the provider may find. For example, consider that a patient has been asked to return for a repeat Papanicolaou (Pap) test because the first one showed the presence of suspicious cells. The medical assistant measures the patient's blood pressure and finds it significantly elevated compared with previous readings. The patient may be anxious and concerned about the test results. The elevated blood pressure readings likely reflect her anxiety.

What impact would it have on a temperature reading if a patient could not find a parking place and had to walk four blocks to the office, knowing he would be late for his appointment? If you said it would be elevated, you are right. Certainly, this patient's metabolism would increase because of the physical exercise. As a result, his temperature would be elevated, along with his pulse, respirations, and blood pressure. The medical assistant should give the patient some time to recover from his sprint to the office before taking any vital sign measurements.

Vital signs are often altered if the patient is in pain. Pay attention to nonverbal signs that might indicate discomfort or pain, especially if the patient's blood pressure, pulse, and respirations are elevated. In addition, many patients are uneasy about being seen by the provider. This may alter vital signs. The medical assistant must help the patient relax before taking any readings. Measurements sometimes must be obtained a second time, after the patient is more calm or comfortable. For a better picture of the patient's vital signs, the medical assistant may be asked to take the vital signs twice: at the beginning of the visit and just before the patient leaves the examination room.

TEMPERATURE

Body temperature is defined as the balance between heat lost and heat produced by the body. It is measured in degrees Fahrenheit (F) or degrees Celsius (C). The process of chemical and physical change in the body that produces heat is called *metabolism*. Body temperature is a result of this process. The core body temperature is maintained within a normal range by the *hypothalamus*. The average body temperature varies from person to person and is different in each person at different times throughout the day. In a healthy adult, this **diurnal variation** ranges from 97.7° to 99.5°F (36.5° to 37.5°C); the average daily temperature is 98.6°F (37°C). Body temperature is lowest in the morning and highest in the late afternoon. Factors that may affect body temperature include the following:

- *Age:* The body temperature of infants and young children fluctuates more rapidly in response to external environmental temperatures. Aging adults lose the insulation of subcutaneous fat and thermoregulatory control.
- *Stress and physical activity:* Both exercise and emotional stress can increase the metabolic rate, causing an elevation in temperature.
- *Gender:* Hormone secretions result in fluctuations of the core body temperature in women throughout the menstrual cycle.
- *External factors:* Smoking, drinking hot fluids, and chewing gum can temporarily elevate an oral temperature. Environmental factors also can change body temperature. Cold weather tends to reduce body temperature, and hot weather tends to increase it.

In illness, an individual's metabolic activity increases. This causes an increase in internal heat production, which in turn raises the body temperature. The increase in body temperature is thought to be the body's defensive reaction, because heat inhibits the growth of some bacteria and viruses.

When a fever is present, superficial blood vessels (those near the surface of the skin) constrict. The small papillary muscles at the base of hair follicles also constrict, creating "goose bumps." Chills and shivering may follow, producing internal heat. As this process repeats itself, more heat is produced, and the body temperature rises above the normal range. When more heat is lost than is produced, the opposite effect occurs, and body temperature drops below the normal range.

Fever

Infection, either bacterial or viral, is the most common cause of fever in both children and adults.

Infants do not usually develop **febrile** illnesses during the first 3 months of life; if one is present, it usually is very serious. However, fever, or **pyrexia**, is very common in young children and accounts for an estimated 30% of office visits. Fevers are classified according to the 24-hour pattern they follow. The three most common patterns are as follows (Fig. 5.1):

- *Continuous fever,* which rises and falls only slightly during a 24-hour period. The temperature consistently remains above the patient's average normal temperature range and **fluctuates** less than 3 degrees.
- *Intermittent fever,* which comes and goes, alternating between elevated and normal levels.

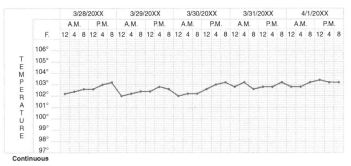

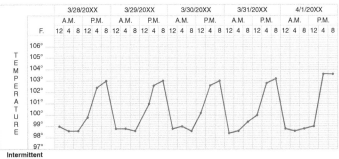

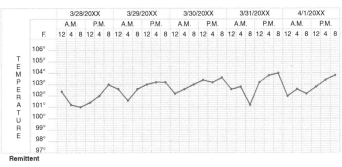

FIGURE 5.1 Fever Patterns.

- *Remittent fever,* which fluctuates considerably (i.e., by more than 3 degrees) and never returns to the normal range.

Variation from the patient's average body temperature range may be the first warning of an illness or a change in the patient's current condition. Patients with fever usually have the following indicators:

- Loss of appetite (*anorexia*)
- Headache
- Thirst
- Flushed face
- Hot skin
- General **malaise**

Some patients experience an acute onset of chills and shivering, followed by an increase in body temperature. A serious possible complication in young children with high fevers is a febrile seizure. Medication to reduce the fever, or *antipyretic* drugs (e.g., acetaminophen or ibuprofen), should be taken as instructed to prevent dangerous spikes in temperature. A rectal, temporal, or aural (ear) temperature over 100.4°F (38°C); an oral temperature over 100°F (37.8°C); and an axillary temperature over 99°F (37.2°C) are all considered a fever.

Sites

Several types of thermometers and various sites can be used to take temperature readings. A digital thermometer is placed under the tongue, in the armpit, or in the rectum; a tympanic thermometer is inserted into the ear; and a temporal artery thermometer is moved across the forehead. Temperatures can be read in either Fahrenheit or Celsius. Most thermometers will convert from one scale to the other. Average temperature values for adults are shown in Table 5.1.

Converting Temperatures

There are many options for converting temperatures between the Fahrenheit and Celsius scales. Most EHRs will do the conversion when the temperature is entered. There also are online options. If you need to do the conversion manually, the following formulas will help you out.

Fahrenheit to Celsius

$°C = (°F − 32) ÷ 1.8$
Example: 101°F
$°C = (101−32) ÷ 1.8$
$°C = 69 ÷ 1.8$
$°C = 38.3$

Celsius to Fahrenheit

$°F = (°C × 1.8) + 32$
Example: 39°C
$°F = (39 × 1.8) + 32$
$°F = 70.2 + 32$
$°F = 102.2$

TABLE 5.1 Average Adult Temperatures

SITE	FAHRENHEIT	CELSIUS
Axillary	97.6°	36.4°
Oral	98.6°	37°
Tympanic	99.6°	37.6°
Rectal	99.6°	37.6°
Temporal artery	99.6°	37.6°

CRITICAL THINKING APPLICATION 5.1

Using the correct formula, convert the following temperatures from one system to the other:

1. 99°F = _____ °C
2. 102°F = _____ °C
3. 38°C = _____ °F
4. 39.5°C = _____ °F

There are a number of factors to consider when determining which site should be used.

Age	Birth–3 months: rectal or temporal artery
	3 months–4 years: rectal, axillary, temporal artery; after the age of 6 months a tympanic thermometer may be used
	4 years or older: oral, axillary, tympanic, temporal artery, rectal
Condition	Mouth breathing – oral is not an option
	Ear infection or occlusion – tympanic is not an option
	Diarrhea – rectal is not an option
	Open wound or rash on forehead – temporal artery is not an option
State of consciousness	If unconscious – oral not an option
Thermometers available in the facility	May only have one or two types of thermometers available
Healthcare facility procedures	Based on patient's condition or provider's preference

When an oral temperature is obtained, you do not have to indicate the site when documenting the reading in the patient's health record. If you use an alternate site, you should document the following identifiers after recording the temperature:

- (T) for tympanic
- (A) for axillary
- (R) for rectal
- (TA) for temporal artery

For example, T: 99.4°F (T) clarifies that an alternate site, tympanic, was used.

Axillary temperatures (A) are approximately 1°F (0.6°C) lower than oral readings because axillary readings are not taken in an enclosed body cavity. Tympanic, rectal, and temporal artery temperatures are approximately 1°F (0.6°C) higher than oral readings. The actual reading from the thermometer should be documented with the correct abbreviation for the site.

The oral site is not typically used with young children. This site requires the patient to hold the thermometer under the tongue and keep the mouth closed, a task that can be difficult for children under the age of 3. A rectal temperature is most often used for infants. It is important to use the proper technique to avoid damaging the rectal tissue (see Procedure 5.3, p. 126). However, most pediatricians prefer that infants' temperatures be taken with a temporal artery thermometer (see Procedure 5.5, p. 128) because it is more comfortable for the baby, less invasive, and eliminates the possible complication of a perforated rectum.

When taken correctly, the tympanic (ear/aural) temperature (T) is an accurate measure because it records the temperature of the blood closest to the hypothalamus. However, research on the temporal artery (TA) thermometer indicates that this method is more accurate than tympanic measurement for identifying elevated temperatures in infants. Pediatricians therefore may prefer TA temperatures in infants suspected of having a fever. The TA thermometer also records accurate temperature readings in all age groups. The tympanic method is still considered a fast, accurate, and noninvasive way of recording temperatures for older children and adults.

For patients younger than 3 years and for those unable to hold a thermometer properly in their mouth during the procedure, a tympanic or temporal artery thermometer can be used; if not, a less accurate axillary temperature can be obtained.

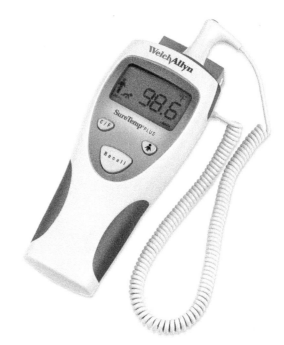

FIGURE 5.2 **Digital Thermometer.** (Courtesy Welch Allyn.)

CRITICAL THINKING APPLICATION   5.2

The mother of a 3-year-old calls the office to report that her child had an axillary temperature of 101°F at 9 o'clock this morning. The schedule is full today, so Carlos has to decide whether the child should be seen today or first thing tomorrow. When should Carlos schedule the appointment? What is the significance of the axillary temperature reading?

TYPES OF THERMOMETERS AND THEIR USES

Digital Thermometer

Digital thermometers are battery operated. Disposable covers fit snugly over the probes and are easily and quickly removed by pushing in the colored end of the probe. The instrument sounds a beep when the process is complete (in 10 to 60 seconds), and the reading appears on a screen on the face of the instrument. Because the only part of the instrument that comes in contact with the patient is the probe, which is covered, the risk of cross-infection is greatly reduced (Fig. 5.2).

When using a digital thermometer to take an oral temperature (see Procedure 5.1, p. 124), it is important to ask if the patient has recently had anything to eat, drink, or smoke. These factors may artificially alter the patient's temperature. Wait 10 to 15 minutes before taking an oral temperature if those factors have occurred. In addition, the patient must be able to hold the thermometer under the tongue with the lips tightly sealed around the probe if an accurate oral reading is to be obtained. Be sure to use the blue probe for an oral temperature.

A digital thermometer with a blue probe can also be used for an axillary temperature (see Procedure 5.2, p. 125). It is important to make sure that there is a tight seal around the probe. This can be done by having the patient hold his or her arm snugly across the chest. Remember, this site is considered the least accurate.

A digital thermometer with a red probe is used for rectal temperatures (see Procedure 5.3, p. 126). This site is used most often for infants. To take an infant's temperature rectally, lubricate the probe tip (most facilities use a lubricating product, such as K-Y Jelly), hold the baby securely with the legs elevated, and insert the probe

approximately 1 inch; hold the probe carefully and continue to secure the infant's legs throughout the procedure to prevent rectal damage.

The digital unit or individual digital thermometers should be routinely cleaned with disinfectant. When ejecting the probe cover, be careful not to contaminate the probe or the processing unit. The probe cover should be deposited directly into a waste container. If a chance exists that a patient's body fluids touched the unit, wipe it with disinfectant before returning it to the storage area.

Tympanic Thermometer

The tympanic membrane of the ear can be used for quick, accurate, and safe assessment of a patient's temperature. It shares the blood supply with the hypothalamus, which is the brain's temperature regulator. The ear canal is a protected cavity. This means factors such as an open mouth, hot or cold drinks, or even a stuffy nose do not affect aural temperature.

The tympanic thermometer system consists of a handheld unit equipped with a tympanic probe, which is covered with a disposable probe cover (Fig. 5.3). When the probe is placed into the ear canal, it gently seals the external opening of the canal, and the sensor detects the infrared energy produced by the tympanic membrane. This signal is digitized by the thermometer and shown on the display screen. Accurate readings are obtained in less than 2 seconds (see Procedure 5.4, p. 127). The tympanic thermometer is popular due to the speed of obtaining the temperature and the comfort it affords the patient. This site should not be used if the patient is complaining of pain in both ears when the ear is touched. He or she may have bilateral **otitis externa**, making the procedure uncomfortable for the patient. In addition, if the patient has a history of or has impacted **cerumen** in both ears, do not use a tympanic thermometer because the reading may be inaccurate.

Insert the probe into the ear canal far enough to seal the opening without applying pressure. To expose the tympanic membrane in

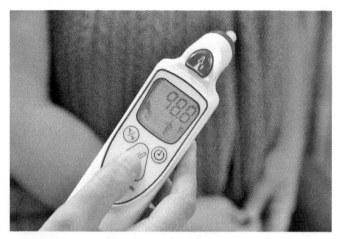

FIGURE 5.3 Tympanic Thermometer.

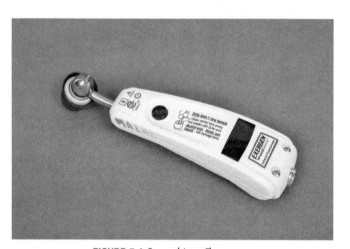

FIGURE 5.4 Temporal Artery Thermometer.

children younger than age 3, gently pull the earlobe down and back; for patients older than age 3, gently pull the pinna (top of the ear) up and back.

Temporal Artery Thermometer

The temporal artery thermometer uses an infrared beam to assess the temperature of the blood flowing through the temporal artery of the forehead, where the artery lies about 1 mm below the skin (Fig. 5.4). Because the artery is so close to the skin, it provides good surface heat conduction, allowing the thermometer to obtain a fast, accurate, and noninvasive measurement of body temperature. To perform the procedure, place the probe in the center of the forehead, halfway between the eyebrows and the hairline. Bangs should be pushed back off the forehead (this method cannot be used if bandages cover the area). Depress the button on the scanner and gently stroke the probe across the forehead toward the hairline (at the temples), keeping the probe flat on the patient's skin. As the scanner moves across the forehead, repeated temperature measurements are taken and the highest measurement is recorded; keeping the button depressed, lift the scanner from the temporal area and lightly place the probe behind the earlobe. Release the button and remove the probe. Recording an accurate temperature takes about 3 seconds (see Procedure 5.5, p. 128). Depending on the facility's infection control procedures, disposable

covers can be used on the scanner, or it can be cleaned between patients with an alcohol wipe.

CRITICAL THINKING APPLICATION   **5.3**

How should the medical assistant adapt temperature-taking techniques in the following scenarios?
- Patient who talks continuously with the thermometer in his mouth
- 7-year-old patient with bilateral otitis externa
- 3-month-old patient when a temporal artery thermometer is available
- 46-year-old patient with a severe asthma attack
- 72-year-old patient with bilateral impacted cerumen
- 28-year-old patient who has just smoked a cigarette

PULSE

A patient's pulse rate reflects the palpable beat of the arteries throughout the body as they expand in response to contraction of the heart. With every beat, the heart pumps an amount of blood, known as the *stroke volume,* into the aorta. Arteries branch off the aorta as it travels down through the center of the abdomen, transferring the pulse beat throughout the body. To measure the pulse, an artery is used that is close to the body surface and can be pushed against a bone. Palpating a **peripheral** pulse gives the rate, rhythm, and volume of the heartbeat and local information about the condition of the artery used.

Pulse Sites

A pulse rate may be counted anyplace an artery is near the surface of the body and the vessel can be pressed against a bone. The most common pulse sites are the temporal, carotid, brachial, radial, femoral, popliteal, and dorsalis pedis arteries (Fig. 5.5). The apical pulse is taken by listening with a stethoscope.

The *temporal* pulse is located in the temple area of the skull, parallel and lateral to the eyes (Fig. 5.6). It is seldom used as a pulse site but may be used as a pressure point to help control bleeding from a head injury.

The *carotid* artery is located between the **larynx** and the *sternocleidomastoid* muscle in the front and to the side of the neck (Fig. 5.7). It most frequently is used in emergencies and to check the pulse during cardiopulmonary resuscitation (CPR). It can be felt by pushing the muscle to the side and pressing against the larynx.

The *brachial* pulse is felt at the inner (*antecubital*) aspect of the elbow. This is the artery that is felt and listened to when blood pressure is measured (Fig. 5.8). It also can be felt in the groove between the biceps and triceps muscles on the inner surface of the middle upper arm. This is the pulse that is checked on infants and young children receiving CPR.

The *radial* artery is the most commonly used site for counting the pulse rate. It is found on the thumb side of the wrist, 1 inch below the base of the thumb (Fig. 5.9).

The *femoral* pulse is located at the site where the femoral artery passes through the groin (see Fig. 5.5). The examiner must press deeply below the *inguinal* ligament to palpate this pulse.

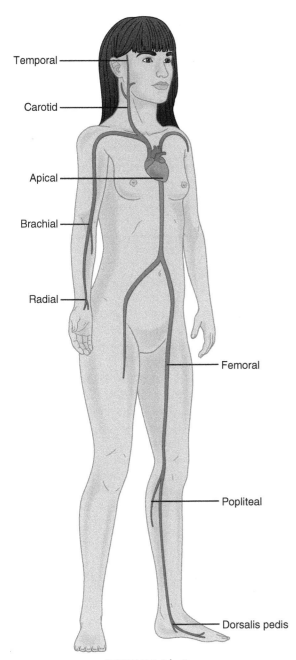

FIGURE 5.5 Pulse Sites.

Labels: Temporal, Carotid, Apical, Brachial, Radial, Femoral, Popliteal, Dorsalis pedis

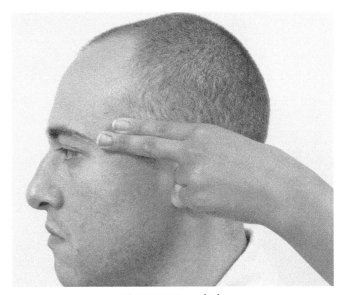

FIGURE 5.6 Temporal Pulse.

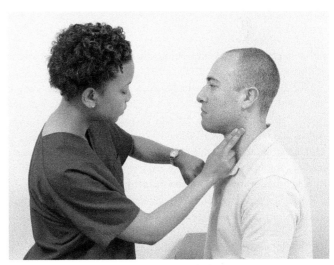

FIGURE 5.7 Carotid Pulse.

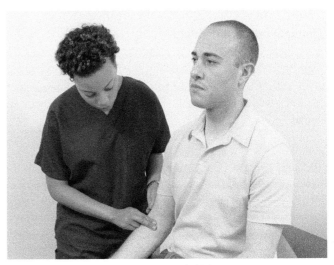

FIGURE 5.8 Brachial Pulse.

The *popliteal* pulse is found at the back of the leg behind the knee (see Fig. 5.5). Palpation of this pulse requires the patient to be in a recumbent position with the knee slightly flexed. The popliteal artery is deep and difficult to feel. It is palpated and also monitored with a stethoscope when a leg blood pressure reading is necessary. The provider checks blood flow through the popliteal artery if a circulatory system problem, such as a blood clot, is suspected in the lower leg.

The *dorsalis pedis* (pedal) artery is felt across the arch of the foot, just slightly lateral to the midline, beside the extensor tendon of the great toe. This pulse may be congenitally absent in some patients. Because a good pulse rate at this site is an indicator of normal lower limb circulation and arterial sufficiency, the provider checks the pedal

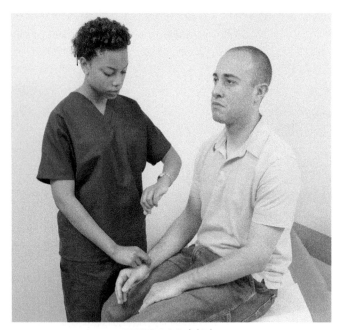

FIGURE 5.9 Radial Pulse.

TABLE 5.2 Approximate Age-Related Pulse Rates		
AGE	RANGE (beats/min)	AVERAGE
Newborn	120–160	140
1–2 years	80–140	120
3–6 years	75–120	100
7–11 years	75–110	95
Adolescence to adulthood	60–100	80

pulses in patients with peripheral vascular problems, such as patients with diabetes mellitus.

The *apical* heart rate, or the heartbeat at the apex of the heart, is heard with a stethoscope. It is used for infants and young children because the radial pulse is difficult to palpate in young patients. Apical rates are also recorded on adult patients who have irregular or difficult-to-feel radial pulses so as to ensure an accurate heart rate reading. An apical count may be requested if the patient is taking cardiac drugs or has **bradycardia** or **tachycardia**. To determine the presence of a **pulse deficit**, the provider may listen to the apical beat while the medical assistant counts the pulse at another site (usually the radial pulse). The stethoscope is placed at the apex of the heart, which is located in the left fifth intercostal space on the midclavicular line – that is, between the fifth and sixth ribs on a line with the midpoint of the left clavicle. The pulse should be counted for 1 full minute and should be documented with (AP) beside the recorded count (see Procedure 5.6, p. 129).

Characteristics of a Pulse

Rate, rhythm, and volume are the factors assessed when taking a pulse. These characteristics vary with the size and elasticity of the artery and the strength and regularity of the heart's contractions. A patient's pulse can reveal valuable information about the cardiovascular system.

Rate

The pulse rate is a measure of the number of beats felt from the movement of blood through an artery. When the heart contracts, blood is pumped into the arteries. The pressure throughout the arteries increases, and the arteries expand. When the heart relaxes, little blood is moving through the arteries, and arterial pressure decreases. Each contraction and relaxation of the heart muscle is a beat. The resulting expansion and relaxation of the arteries creates a pulsation. This is the pulse rate. Normally, the beat (rate) and the pulse rate are the same. The rate of the pulse is the number of beats (pulsations) that occur in 1 minute.

Age, body size, gender, and health status can affect the pulse rate. The rate is also affected by an individual's activities and psychological state and by certain medications. Children tend to have more rapid pulse rates than adults. The rate usually is faster in women (70 to 80 beats per minute) than in men (60 to 70 beats per minute). The rate is more rapid when a person is sitting than when he or she is lying down, and it increases when an individual stands, walks, or runs. During sleep or rest, the pulse rate may drop to as low as 45 to 50 beats per minute. Well-conditioned athletes tend to have pulse rates of 50 to 60 beats per minute because consistent aerobic exercise strengthens the *heart muscle* (the myocardium) so that each heart contraction ejects an increased volume of blood into the arterial system. Table 5.2 lists the normal pulse ranges for various age groups of patients.

Rhythm

The pulse rhythm is the time between pulse beats. A normal rhythm pattern has an even tempo, which indicates that the intervals between the beats are of equal duration. An abnormal rhythm, or arrhythmia, is described according to the rhythm pattern detected. An **intermittent pulse** may occur in healthy individuals during exercise or after drinking a beverage containing caffeine. A common irregularity found in children and young adults is a **sinus arrhythmia**. The heart rate varies with the respiratory cycle, speeding up with inspiration and slowing to normal with expiration. If beats are frequently skipped or if the beats are markedly irregular, the provider should be advised, because this may indicate heart disease. If an irregular rhythm is detected, the pulse should be counted for a full minute to ensure accuracy. A note also should be made that the patient's pulse was irregular – for example, "P: 86 irregular."

Volume

The volume (*pulse amplitude*) reflects the strength of the heart when it contracts. Volume can be assessed by feeling the strength of the pulse as blood flows through the vessel. The force of each pulse beat is described as **bounding**, or full; strong, or normal; or **thready**, or weak. The force of the heartbeat and the condition of the arterial wall (whether hard or soft) influence the volume of the pulse beat. The pulse may vary only in intensity, and otherwise may be perfectly regular. This condition also can indicate heart disease. The pulse volume is recorded using a three-point scale.

Three-Point Scale for Measuring Pulse Volume

3+	Full, bounding pulse	Pulsation is very strong and does not disappear with moderate pressure.
2+	Normal pulse	Pulsation is easily felt but disappears with moderate pressure.
1+	Weak, thready pulse	Pulsation is not easily felt and disappears with slight pressure.

Determining the Pulse Rate
Radial and Apical Pulse Rates

To record an accurate radial pulse, you must have the patient in a comfortable position with the artery to be used at the same level as or lower than the heart (see Procedure 5.7, p. 130). The limb should be well supported and relaxed. The patient may be lying down or sitting. As with all palpated pulse readings, the pads of the first two or three fingers are placed over the artery. Never use your thumb to determine the pulse rate. The thumb has its own pulse, and you may confuse your pulse rate with the patient's rate. Push the radial artery against the bone until the strongest pulsation is felt. Both you and the patient should be in a relaxed position. Too much pressure **occludes** the artery, and too little pressure prevents detection of irregularities or of all the beats. The pulse should be counted for 1 full minute. A 30-second interval may be used once you become proficient at performing the skill. In either case you should document the number of beats in 1 minute.

While counting the rate, you must also be aware of the rhythm and volume. Variations from normal should be noted, such as an arrhythmia or a pulse that is thready or bounding. Some pulses are more difficult to feel than others, and finding the correct pressure to be used for each patient and site requires repeated practice and experience.

For an apical pulse, the patient can be sitting or lying down. Place the stethoscope at the junction of the fifth intercostal space and the midclavicular line on the left side of the patient's chest. You will hear a lubb-dubb sound. Each lubb-dubb sound is one heartbeat. The apical pulse should always be **auscultated** for a full minute to detect any irregularities in rate and rhythm. Remember, one reason you would decide to take an apical pulse on an adult patient is that you noted irregularities in the heart rate when palpating the radial pulse. Therefore, you should listen to an apical pulse for a full minute to make sure you are accurately counting the number of beats per minute. If the pulse rate is counted at any site other than the radial artery, the rate should be documented along with a notation of the site used.

CRITICAL THINKING APPLICATION   5.4

Mrs. Arnez has a documented thready pulse. What site should Carlos use to measure the pulse? Why should he take the pulse for a full minute?

Femoral, Popliteal, and Pedal Pulses

Pulses in the lower extremities may be difficult to find and equally difficult to hear. A Doppler unit, an ultrasound unit that magnifies the pulsation, may be used to locate and count these pulses accurately (Fig. 5.10). A Doppler unit is battery operated and can be attached to a stethoscope so that only the provider can hear the beat, or it can be set so that both the provider and the patient can hear the pulsations.

RESPIRATION

Respiration allows for the exchange of oxygen and carbon dioxide with the atmosphere, the blood, and the body cells. Oxygen is taken into the body to be used for life-sustaining body processes, and carbon dioxide is released as a waste product.

One complete *inhalation* and *exhalation* is called a *respiration*. During the inhalation phase, the diaphragm contracts and drops down. The *intercostal* muscles pull the ribs up and outward; this causes the lungs to expand and fill with air. During the exhalation phase, the diaphragm returns to its normal elevated position and the intercostal muscles relax; this causes the lungs to expel the waste air out of the body.

Both internal and external respirations occur. *External respiration* is the exchange of oxygen and carbon dioxide in the lungs. *Internal respiration* occurs at the cellular level. Oxygen in the bloodstream is transferred into the cells and used with sugars and fatty acids to produce energy. Carbon dioxide is released as a waste product and transported back to the lungs for exhalation.

The respiratory center in the medulla oblongata is sensitive to changes in blood oxygen and carbon dioxide levels. When carbon dioxide levels rise, the respiratory control center sends a message that triggers breathing. Respiration is controlled by the involuntary nervous system. This means that we breathe automatically. Because respiration can be controlled to a certain extent, it also is a voluntary function. However, breathing ultimately is under the control of the medulla oblongata. This is why we can hold our breath only for a short period of time. Once cells become oxygen starved, a stimulus is sent to the

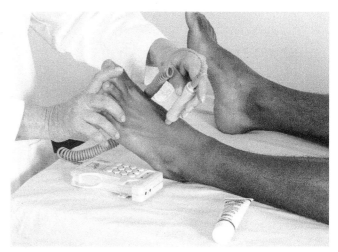

FIGURE 5.10 Doppler ultrasound unit measuring the pedal pulse. (From Jarvis C: *Physical examination and health assessment,* ed 7, St Louis, 2016, Saunders.)

respiratory muscles (the diaphragm and intercostal muscles) and breathing begins involuntarily.

Characteristics of Respirations

Normally, a person's breathing is relaxed, automatic, and silent. However, respiratory disease or chronic conditions can influence the characteristics of an individual's respirations. **Dyspnea** occurs in patients with pneumonia, asthma, or **chronic obstructive pulmonary disease (COPD)**. It also occurs after physical exertion or at very high altitudes. Other alterations in breathing are **bradypnea**, **apnea**, **tachypnea**, and **hyperpnea**. Hyperpnea usually is accompanied by **hyperventilation** and often occurs when the patient is extremely anxious or in pain. **Orthopnea** frequently occurs in patients with congestive heart failure (CHF) or COPD. **Wheezing** signals difficulty breathing in patients with asthma.

When assessing a patient's respirations, you must note three important characteristics: rate, rhythm, and depth:

- *Rate:* The rate of respiration is the number of respirations per minute. Fig. 5.11 shows sample breathing patterns. A ratio of four pulse beats to one respiration is typical. As a rule, both the pulse and respiratory rates respond to exercise or emotional upset. Table 5.3 lists normal respiratory ranges for patients in various age groups.
- *Rhythm:* Refers to the breathing pattern, the space between each breath. A regular breathing pattern is normal in adults; however, the breathing pattern for infants varies. Automatic interruptions, such as sighing, are also considered normal. The terms *regular* or *irregular* are used to document rhythm.
- *Depth:* The depth of respiration is the amount of air inhaled and exhaled. When a patient is at rest, normal respirations have a consistent depth, which can be noted as you watch the rise and fall of the chest. Rapid, shallow breathing at rest occurs with some diseases, such as asthma and emphysema. An alteration in the depth and sometimes the rate of breathing is

also seen in **Cheyne-Stokes respirations**. The terms *normal, deep, shallow,* and *gasping* should be used to document depth.

Normally, no noticeable breath sounds occur during the breathing process, except during snoring. Noticeable breath sounds are a sign of certain diseases, such as pneumonia, asthma, and pulmonary edema. After listening to breath sounds with a stethoscope, the provider can describe the characteristics of breath sounds by using specific terminology (e.g., **rales**, **rhonchi**, or **stertorous** breathing).

When an individual cannot breathe in enough oxygen to supply all body cells with oxygenated blood, normal skin coloring, particularly around the mouth and the nail beds, changes to a bluish, dusky color. This coloration, which indicates an increased level of carbon dioxide in the blood, is called *cyanosis*. The patient also may have other signs and symptoms, such as **vertigo**, chest pain (*angina*), and numbness in the fingers and toes.

Counting Respirations

Because most people can control their breathing to a certain extent, do not mention that you will be counting the person's respirations (see Procedure 5.7, p. 130). Patients may self-consciously alter their breathing rate when they know they are being watched. Count the respirations while appearing to count the radial pulse. Keep your eyes alternately on the patient's chest and your watch while you count the pulse rate; then, without removing your fingers from the pulse site, determine the respiratory rate (Fig. 5.12). If the patient is lying down, the arm on which you are taking the radial pulse may be crossed over the chest so that respirations can be felt with the rise and fall of the chest. Another way of observing respirations is to watch the movement of the patient's shoulders with each inspiration. Count the respirations for 30 seconds and multiply the number by 2. Do not use the 15-second interval because this count can vary by a factor of ±4, which is significant when dealing with such a small number. Note any variation or irregularity in the rhythm or depth. Record the respirations in the health record.

CRITICAL THINKING APPLICATION   **5.5**

Tina Anderson, a 36-year-old patient who is obese, is wearing a heavy knit sweater, and Carlos needs to obtain a respiratory count. What could he do to obtain an accurate measurement of Tina's respiratory rate?

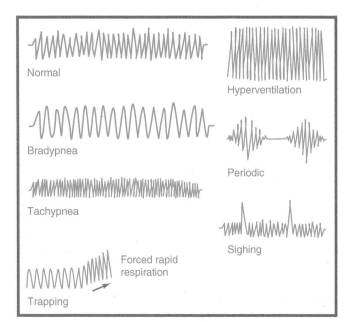

FIGURE 5.11 Breathing Patterns.

TABLE 5.3	Approximate Age-Related Respiration Ranges	
AGE	**RANGE (breaths/min)**	**AVERAGE**
Newborn	30–50	40
1–3 years	20–30	25
4–6 years	18–26	22
7–11 years	16–22	19
Adolescence to adulthood	12–20	16

TABLE 5.4 Approximate Age-Related Blood Pressure Ranges

| AGE | RANGE | |
	SYSTOLIC	DIASTOLIC
Newborn	60–96	30–62
1–3 years	78–112	48–78
4–6 years	78–112	50–79
7–11 years	85–114	52–79
Adolescent	94–119	58–79
Adult	100–119	60–79

TABLE 5.5 Stages of Hypertension

Normal	Less than 120–80 mm Hg
Elevated	Systolic between 120–129 *and* diastolic less than 80 mm Hg
Stage 1	Systolic between 130–139 *or* diastolic between 80–89 mm Hg
Stage 2	Systolic at least 140 *or* diastolic at least 90 mm Hg
Hypertensive crisis	Systolic over 180 *and/or* diastolic over 120

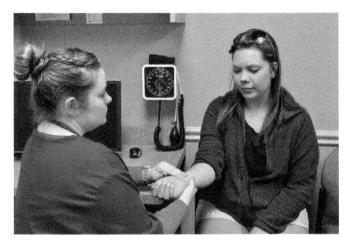

FIGURE 5.12 Hand position when counting respirations. The hands should be left in place as if still counting the patient's pulse.

BLOOD PRESSURE

A BP reading reflects the pressure of the blood against the walls of the arteries. Each time the ventricles contract, blood is pushed out of the heart and into the aorta, exerting pressure on the walls of the arteries. There are actually two BP readings:

- The *systolic* pressure is the highest pressure level that occurs when the heart is contracting and is the first sound heard.
- The *diastolic* pressure is the lowest pressure level when the heart is relaxed and is the last sound heard.

Systole (heart contraction) and diastole (heart relaxation) together make up the cardiac cycle. The difference between systolic and diastolic pressures is the **pulse pressure**.

Blood pressure is read in millimeters of mercury, abbreviated *mm Hg*. However, you need not include the abbreviation when documenting the reading in the patient's health record. BP is recorded as a fraction, with the systolic reading serving as the numerator (top) and the diastolic reading serving as the denominator (bottom) (e.g., 130/80). Table 5.4 lists normal BP ranges for patients of various age groups.

Factors Affecting Blood Pressure

Factors that determine blood pressure include the following:

- Blood volume
- Peripheral resistance created by blood *viscosity* (the thickness of the blood)
- Vessel elasticity
- Condition of the heart muscle and arterial walls

Volume is the amount of blood in the arteries. An increased blood volume raises BP, and a decreased blood volume lowers BP. With extensive bleeding, or hemorrhage, the blood volume drops, and so does the BP.

The *peripheral resistance* of blood vessels refers to the lumen (the diameter of the vessel) and the amount of blood flowing through it. The smaller the lumen, the greater the resistance to blood flow. BP is higher with a small or reduced-size lumen and lower with a large lumen. Vessels affected by fatty cholesterol deposits (*atherosclerotic plaque*) become narrower over time. This results in smaller vessel lumens and therefore higher blood pressure.

Vessel elasticity is the ability of an artery to expand and contract to supply the body with a steady flow of blood. With advancing age, certain lifestyle factors, or the presence of **arteriosclerosis**, vessel elasticity may decrease. This causes the arterial walls to become firm and resistant, increasing the BP.

The condition of the **myocardium** is a primary determinant of the volume of blood flowing through the body. A strong, forceful contraction empties the heart and tends to keep the BP within normal limits. If the myocardium becomes weak, pressure in the vessels begins to increase in an attempt to maintain an adequate level of circulating blood to meet the oxygen and nutrient needs of the body.

Evaluating the Blood Pressure

The American Heart Association (AHA) guidelines for the diagnosis and management of hypertension include five categories for diagnostic and treatment purposes (Table 5.5). The goal of the AHA recommendations is to reduce the number of people who die each year from hypertension-related illnesses, such as coronary artery disease, heart attack, heart failure, kidney disease, and stroke.

Hypertension can occur in children or adults, but individuals of African-American descent, middle-aged and older adults, patients with diabetes mellitus, and those with kidney disease are at greatest risk. Hypertension has been called the silent killer because it frequently has no symptoms. Individuals may go for long periods without knowing they have a problem. Hypertension often is discovered during treatment for another problem.

Signs and Symptoms of Hypertension	
• Blurred vision	• Angina
• Vertigo	• Dyspnea
• Fatigue	• Headache
• Flushing	• Nosebleeds (epistaxis)

Essential hypertension is the most common type of hypertension. It is **idiopathic** but is associated with obesity, a high blood level of sodium, elevated cholesterol levels, family history, and race (African Americans, Native Americans, Mexican Americans, Native Hawaiians, some Asian Americans.

When there is a concern about a patient's BP, the individual is often asked to track it. These readings should be taken at about the same time of day and by the same person using the same-size cuff and the same arm. *Secondary hypertension* is caused by another underlying pathologic condition, such as renal disease, complications of pregnancy, endocrine imbalance, or brain injury.

Temporary hypertension may occur with stress, pain, exercise, and exhaustion. Many patients experience "white coat syndrome"; their BP becomes elevated in the medical environment but is normal when they are away from the healthcare facility.

If a patient's BP is persistently in the prehypertension range at two or more office visits over time, essential hypertension is diagnosed. If the patient's BP is elevated initially, it should be checked again after the patient has been allowed to sit comfortably for at least 2 minutes. Check the BP in both arms with a cuff that is the proper size. If the readings are different, the provider uses the higher value for diagnostic purposes. All of the readings must be documented in the patient's record.

Metabolic Syndrome
Metabolic syndrome occurs when a patient has at least three of the five following conditions: • Abdominal obesity • Elevated blood pressure • Elevated fasting plasma glucose • High serum triglycerides • Low high-density lipoprotein (LDL) levels Metabolic syndrome is associated with an increased risk of developing cardiovascular disease and type 2 diabetes. It is estimated that one-quarter of adults in the United States have metabolic syndrome.

Treatment guidelines for hypertension have four basic aspects:
1. Individuals with prehypertension should be diagnosed and encouraged to make lifestyle changes before they require treatment or move into the hypertensive category. The AHA recommends limiting one's intake of salt and eating a diet rich in potassium, calcium, magnesium, and protein while reducing total fat intake,

especially saturated fat. Individuals with prehypertension also should restrict their alcohol intake, engage in regular physical activity, and lose weight if necessary to maintain a healthy BMI range. Many times, just losing 10% of a person's weight lowers the blood pressure.
2. In people older than 50 years of age, the systolic reading is more important than the diastolic reading. Individuals over 50 should be treated if they have a systolic pressure of 140 mm Hg or higher, regardless of their diastolic blood pressure. Medical treatment at this age can reduce the development of cardiac and kidney disease later in life.
3. Most patients with hypertension require two or more medications to achieve desired blood pressure levels. The goal of treatment is to maintain blood pressure below 140/90 mm Hg, or below 130/80 mm Hg in patients with diabetes or kidney disease. Patients should be treated with both a diuretic, to help the body excrete excess amounts of fluid and sodium, and an antihypertensive medication.
4. A patient-centered treatment approach should be implemented to motivate patients and to maintain compliance with hypertension management. The medical assistant can play an active role in establishing a therapeutic relationship with the patient by providing ongoing education and support to ensure compliance with provider-recommended treatment. Using community resources, such as local dietitian referrals, may also help patients comply with treatment.

Hypotension is an abnormally low blood pressure, which may be caused by emotional or traumatic shock, hemorrhage, central nervous system (CNS) disorders, and chronic wasting diseases. Persistent readings of 90/60 mm Hg or lower usually are considered hypotensive. **Orthostatic (postural) hypotension** can cause patients to experience vertigo or **syncope**. Some medications can cause orthostatic hypotension.

CRITICAL THINKING APPLICATION   5.6

Mr. Samuel Long, a 43-year-old patient, recently was diagnosed with essential hypertension. What should Carlos discuss with Mr. Long to emphasize the dangers of his disease and to teach him about possible lifestyle modifications that he must make to improve his health? Are any community resources available that might help Mr. Long and his family effectively manage his disease?

Measuring Blood Pressure

The instrument used to measure blood pressure is called a *sphygmomanometer,* or blood pressure cuff. It consists of an inflatable cuff, an inflation bulb with a control valve, and a pressure gauge. The blood pressure mechanism consists of an aneroid dial attached to an inflatable cuff (Fig. 5.13A); the device may be handheld, wall mounted, or a floor model (Fig. 5.13B). Some systems have a trigger-style air release valve; these can be pumped up and then the air slowly released simply by pushing the trigger (Fig. 5.14). With the more traditional sphygmomanometers, the valve must be unscrewed.

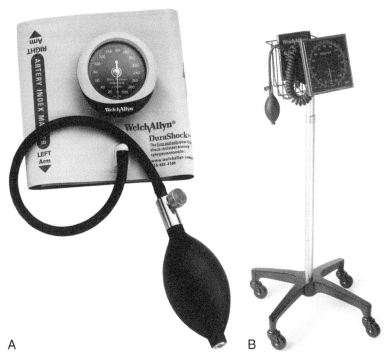

A   B

FIGURE 5.13 (A) Aneroid dial system with an inflatable cuff. (B) Aneroid floor model with a large slanted face.

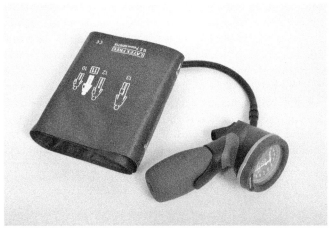

FIGURE 5.14 Trigger-release aneroid blood pressure valve.

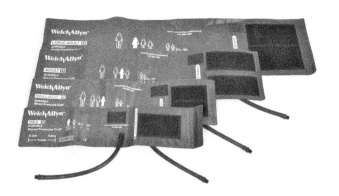

FIGURE 5.15 Variety of blood pressure cuff sizes.

Sphygmomanometers are delicately **calibrated** instruments that must be handled carefully. They should be recalibrated regularly and checked for accuracy by the medical assisstant or by a medical supply dealer. The needle on the aneroid dial sphygmomanometer should rest within the small square or circle at the bottom of the dial. If the sphygmomanometer is not correctly calibrated, the patient's blood pressure reading will be inaccurate.

The sphygmomanometer must be used with a stethoscope. The goal of the procedure is to use the inflatable cuff to stop the circulation through an artery. The stethoscope is placed over the artery just below the cuff. As the cuff is slowly deflated to allow the blood to flow again, cardiac cycle sounds are heard through the stethoscope, and readings are taken when the first (systolic) and last (diastolic) sounds are heard (see Procedure 5.8, p. 131).

To obtain a correct blood pressure reading, the cuff used must be the proper size. The systolic and diastolic blood pressures can be lowered by as much as 5 mm Hg if the cuff is one size larger than appropriate; the blood pressure can be elevated by up to 6 mm Hg if the cuff is one size smaller. The inflatable part (the bladder) of a cuff of the correct size should cover about 80% of the circumference of the upper arm. To help with this, most blood pressure cuffs have predetermined markings on the internal side (the side placed on the patient's arm); as long as the cuff is secured within these lines, it should be the accurate size (Fig. 5.15). Table 5.6 presents the various sizes of blood pressure cuffs available.

When placed on the patient's arm, the cuff should cover two-thirds of the distance from the elbow to the shoulder. The lower edge of the cuff should be 2 to 3 cm (about 2 finger widths, or 1 inch) above the elbow or antecubital space to allow plenty of room to place the stethoscope without touching the cuff. If the stethoscope touches the cuff during the blood pressure reading, the sound of the deflating cuff may interfere with your ability to hear the correct reading. The patient's sleeve must be above the antecubital space; if the sleeve is tight, ask the patient to remove the arm from the sleeve. This is done for two reasons: tight clothing can restrict normal blood flow in the brachial artery, altering the blood pressure, and placing the stethoscope over clothing makes it difficult to hear blood pressure sounds. Provide a patient gown if needed to maintain the patient's privacy.

Blood pressure cuffs and stethoscopes are available in drug and retail stores for patients to use to measure their own blood pressure at home. These units can be aneroid, electronic, or computerized sphygmomanometers (Fig. 5.16). If you have patients who are monitoring their pressure at home, be sure they understand the mechanics of obtaining an accurate reading. It is best to have the patient bring his or her equipment to the office and demonstrate its use. While the patient is showing you the home equipment, you will have an ideal opportunity to check technique and calibration and to answer any questions the patient may have about use of the equipment. This is also a good opportunity to reinforce treatment plans, such as medication, diet, and exercise. It is helpful for a patient who is monitoring blood pressure readings at home to keep a log and review it with the provider during visits to help detect blood pressure variations during normal daily activities.

Some providers will want the BP taken on the leg when a patient has undergone a bilateral mastectomy with lymph node removal or has an arteriovenous shunt (used for dialysis). This is to reduce the risk of **lymphedema.** If a patient has had a mastectomy on one side, the opposite side can be used for BP. When using the leg the BP can be taken at either the thigh or ankle. When using the thigh, a cuff designed for the thigh should be used and the popliteal artery would be auscultated. For the ankle a regular cuff could be used and the posterior tibial artery would be auscultated. It can be difficult to hear Korotkoff sounds at the posterior tibial artery, and a Doppler may need to be used. For either location the patient should be supine (lying down) so that the leg is at the same level as the heart. The cuff should encompass 80% of the circumference of either the thigh or the ankle.

Effects of Body Position on Blood Pressure Measurement

Blood pressure is usually taken with the patient in either the sitting or the supine position. However, the diastolic pressure can be as much as 5 mm Hg higher when patients are sitting than when they are supine. In addition, if the patient's back is not supported and there is some muscle tension in the body (as occurs when the patient is seated on an examination table rather than in a chair), the diastolic pressure may be increased by 6 mm Hg. If patients cross their legs during the reading, the systolic pressure may be raised by 2 to 8 mm Hg. The position of the patient's arm can also have a major influence when the blood pressure is measured. If the upper arm is below the level of the right atrium (e.g., dangling at the patient's side), the reading is artificially elevated; if the arm is above the heart level, the reading is lowered. Or if the patient holds up the arm, muscular

TABLE 5.6	Blood Pressure Cuff Sizes	
	ARM CIRCUMFERENCE	
CUFF	CENTIMETERS	INCHES
Small adult	22–26	9
Adult	27–34	Up to 13
Large adult	35–44	14–17
Adult thigh	45–52	18–20

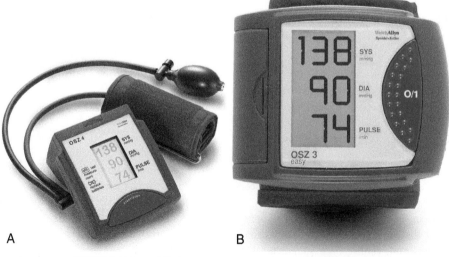

A   B

FIGURE 5.16 Personal blood pressure systems. (A) Digital arm cuff. (B) Digital wrist cuff.

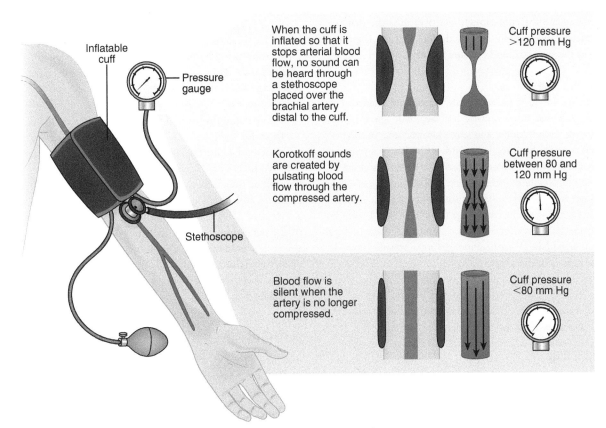

Inflatable cuff

Pressure gauge

Stethoscope

When the cuff is inflated so that it stops arterial blood flow, no sound can be heard through a stethoscope placed over the brachial artery distal to the cuff.

Cuff pressure >120 mm Hg

Korotkoff sounds are created by pulsating blood flow through the compressed artery.

Cuff pressure between 80 and 120 mm Hg

Blood flow is silent when the artery is no longer compressed.

Cuff pressure <80 mm Hg

FIGURE 5.17 The science of taking a blood pressure.

tension will raise the pressure. The arm should be placed at the level of the heart on a table next to an exam room chair or resting on the arm of the chair to avoid these issues (Fig. 5.17).

Common Causes of Errors in Blood Pressure Readings

- The limb used for measurement is above the level of the heart.
- The bladder in the cuff is not completely deflated before a reading is started or retaken.
- The pressure in the cuff is released too rapidly.
- The patient is nervous, uncomfortable, or anxious (may cause a reading to be higher than the patient's actual blood pressure).
- The patient drank coffee or smoked cigarettes within 30 minutes of the blood pressure measurement.
- The cuff was applied improperly.
- The cuff is too large, too small, too loose, or too tight.
- The cuff was not placed around the arm smoothly.
- The bladder is not centered over the artery, or the bladder bulges out from the cover.
- There was a failure to wait 1 to 2 minutes between measurements.
- Instruments are defective:
  - Air leaks in the valve
  - Air leaks in the bladder
  - Aneroid needle not calibrated to zero

Korotkoff Sounds

Korotkoff sounds are the sounds heard during auscultation of blood pressure. Vibrations of the arterial wall produce these sounds when the blood surges back into the vessel after it has been compressed by the blood pressure cuff. The sounds were first discovered and classified into five distinct phases by Russian neurologist Nikolai Korotkoff.

Phase I

Phase I is the first sound heard as the cuff deflates. The blood is resurging into the patient's artery and can be heard clearly as a sharp, tapping sound. Note the gauge reading when this first sound is heard. Record this as the systolic blood pressure.

Phase II

As the cuff deflates, even more blood flows through the artery. The movement of the blood makes a swishing sound. If you did not follow proper procedure in inflating the cuff, you may not hear these sounds because of their soft quality. Occasionally blood pressure sounds completely disappear during this phase. Loss of the sounds, followed by their reappearance later, is called the *auscultatory gap*. The silence may continue as the needle falls another 30 mm Hg. Auscultatory gaps occur particularly in hypertension and certain types of heart disease, so if you notice such a gap, make sure to report it to the provider.

Phase III

In phase III, a great deal of blood is moving down into the artery. The distinct, sharp tapping sounds return and continue rhythmically.

If you do not inflate the cuff enough, you will miss the first two phases completely and you will incorrectly interpret the beginning of phase III as the systolic blood pressure (phase I).

Phase IV

At this point, the blood is flowing easily. The sound changes to a soft tapping, which becomes muffled and begins to grow fainter. Occasionally these sounds continue to zero. This may occur in children, in patients of any age after exercise or with a fever, or in a pregnant patient with anemia. The AHA recommends that the beginning of phase IV be recorded as the diastolic reading for a child. Some providers call the change at phase IV the fading sound and want it recorded between systolic and diastolic recordings (e.g., 120/84/70, with 84 representing the gauge reading when the sounds of phase III have ended and those of phase IV are beginning). Other providers consider phase IV the true diastolic pressure.

Phase V

All sounds disappear in this phase. Note the gauge reading when the last sound is heard. Record this as the diastolic pressure.

Palpatory Method

The systolic pressure may be checked by feeling the radial pulse rather than hearing it with the stethoscope. Place the cuff in the usual position and palpate the radial pulse, noting rate and rhythm. Inflate the cuff until the pulse disappears, then add 30 mm Hg more of inflation to get above the systolic pressure. Do not remove your fingers from the pulse or change the pressure of your fingers. Carefully watch the gauge while slowly releasing the pressure in the cuff and wait until you feel the first pulse beat. Note the reading on the gauge and document the first pulse felt as the systolic pressure. For example, if you first felt the radial pulse return at 102 mm Hg, the palpated blood pressure is recorded as 102/P, with P indicating that the systolic reading was palpated. The diastolic and Korotkoff phases cannot be determined by this method. This method can be very useful in times of a medical emergency, such as shock, when the patient's blood pressure cannot be auscultated. The palpatory method can be used to determine how far you need to pump the cuff to hear that first beat. This is useful for a new patient.

CRITICAL THINKING APPLICATION   **5.7**

Vital signs are documented in a paper record in this order: temperature (T), pulse (P), and respirations (R). Blood pressure is recorded after TPR. Depending on the EHR system, they may be ordered differently. Correctly document the following vital signs:

1. Oral temperature 101.2°F; apical pulse 90, regular rhythm; respirations 22 regular rhythm, shallow volume; and orthostatic blood pressure in the right arm is 138/88 supine in the right arm and 110/70 standing in the right arm

2. Tympanic temperature 36.8°F; radial pulse 66, irregular rhythm, normal volume; respirations 18, regular rhythm, normal volume; and bilateral blood pressure 128/76 in the left arm, sitting and 132/80 in the right arm, sitting

3. Temporal artery temperature 102.4°F; apical pulse 102, irregular rhythm; respirations 27, regular rhythm, normal volume

---

PULSE OXIMETRY

Pulse oximetry is a noninvasive method of evaluating both the pulse rate and the oxygen saturation of the blood. It may also be referred to as saturation of peripheral oxygen (SpO_2). Many ambulatory settings use pulse oximeters to assess a patient's oxygenation status in disorders such as pneumonia, bronchitis, emphysema, or asthma.

To perform the procedure, the medical assistant clips a probe on the patient's earlobe or finger (Fig. 5.18). Fingernail polish must be removed before the clip is applied. If the patient has artificial nails, the earlobe should be used. A beam of infrared light passes through the tissue, and the amount of light absorbed by oxygenated hemoglobin is measured. This is displayed on the digital screen as a percentage. At the same time, the light measures the patient's pulse rate, which also is shown on the screen. A normal pulse oximetry reading is 95% or higher. Treatment, such as oxygen or bronchodilator therapies, usually is started when readings are 90% to 92% or lower (see Procedure 5.9, p. 133).

ANTHROPOMETRIC MEASUREMENTS

Anthropometry is the science that deals with measurement of the size, weight, and proportions of the human body. These measurements often are included in the initial recording of vital signs and before the provider performs a physical examination or a well-baby check. Because they are indicators of the patient's state of health and well-being, height and weight measurements and the associated body mass index are discussed as aspects of the vital signs.

Measuring Weight and Height

A patient's weight and height can be helpful in diagnosis, and the medical assistant must obtain these readings with accuracy and empathy (see Procedure 5.10, p. 133). In many healthcare facilities, weight and height are measured routinely as the patient is taken to the examination room. To safeguard patient confidentiality, the scale

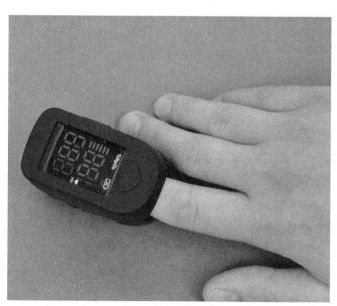

FIGURE 5.18 Pulse Oximeter.

should be located in a private area where other people cannot see the patient's weight. Safeguard the patient's confidentiality by not repeating the measurement out loud. Others nearby might hear this private patient information. If this is the patient's first visit, anthropometric measurements are recorded in the history database and are used as reference information during future visits as needed.

Many providers use the BMI to determine the risk for certain diseases, so the medical assistant may have to use the accurately measured height and weight to determine and record the patient's BMI. This is typically done using a BMI chart that converts the patient's height and weight ratio into a BMI number, or with a wheeled device that calibrates the BMI when the height and weight intersect. BMI numbers also can be determined using an online conversion calculator. Electronic health record (EHR) systems automatically calculate and document the patient's BMI after the height and weight measurements are entered.

Body Mass Index (BMI)

To determine how healthy an adult patient's weight level is, the provider may ask the medical assistant to calculate the patient's BMI. The BMI is the relationship of weight to height that mathematically correlates the patient's measurements with health risks. It is a more accurate predictor of weight-related diseases than traditional height-weight charts because it provides a good estimate of the degree of body fat.

A patient's BMI can be calculated by dividing the weight in kilograms by the square of the height in meters: $BMI = Weight (kg) \div Height (m^2)$. However, to determine the BMI, clinics can use a wheel device that compares the patient's height to weight, an online BMI calculator, or a BMI chart. This is not necessary with EHR systems because the program automatically calculates the BMI after the patient's height and weight have been documented.

Individuals with a BMI of 19 to 22 are thought to live the longest. Death rates are significantly higher for people with a BMI of 25 or above. If the BMI indicates that the patient is overweight or obese, dietary modifications may be needed. The provider makes this decision after evaluating all of the patient's data.

Certain medical specialties and specific medical problems may require continuous monitoring of weight. Hormone disorders (e.g., diabetes), growth patterns (seen in children), and eating disorders (e.g., obesity, bulimia) require accurate weight checks as part of every medical visit. In addition, pregnant patients must have their weight monitored to make sure they are gaining weight, but also as a precaution against too much weight gain, which may indicate fluid retention. Patients with cardiovascular disorders who tend to retain fluid should have their weight checked each time they are seen in the office. Many healthcare facilities document weight in kilograms, but most Americans understand the pound measurements better. When weight must be converted from one to the other, use formulas or an online conversion calculator. EHR systems do the conversion automatically.

Weight Conversion Formulas

Convert Kilograms to Pounds

1 kg = 2.2 lb

Multiply the number of kilograms by 2.2.

Example: A patient weighs 68 kg: 68 × 2.2 = 149.6 lb

Convert Pounds to Kilograms

1 lb = 0.45 kg

Multiply the number of pounds by 0.45 or divide the number of pounds by 2.2 kg.

Example: A patient weighs 120 lb: 120 × 0.45 = 54 kg, or 120 ÷ 2.2 = 54.5 kg.

Accurate height or length measurements are particularly important for children (see Chapter 28). The provider also may request routine height screening for patients diagnosed with osteoporosis because these patients may lose height over time.

CRITICAL THINKING APPLICATION   **5.8**
- A patient weighs 87 kg. How many pounds does he weigh?
- A patient weighs 148 lb. How many kilograms does she weigh?

Weight

Weight can be a sensitive issue for many patients. Maintain a professional attitude when obtaining a patient's weight. Make sure heavy items are removed from pockets and that the patient is not holding a purse. Shoes should also be removed. If patients have difficulty with balance or stability, assist them onto the scale and help them balance themselves. A scale with built-in handrails is ideal for patients who are unable to maintain their balance. If the facility does not have this type of scale, a walker can be placed over the scale for the patient to use as hand support when getting on or off, or to maintain balance while on the scale (Fig. 5.19).

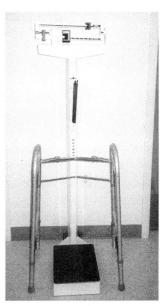

FIGURE 5.19 A walker is placed over the scale to aid the patient's balance.

If the provider prescribes weight measurement at home, make sure the patient understands the importance of getting weighed at the same time each day in clothing of similar weight. Body weight may vary considerably from early morning to late afternoon, so it is usually best if the patient is weighed in the morning. If it is important that the patient be weighed each day, make sure you remind the patient to document each weight and notify the clinic as directed if there are major shifts.

Height

Height can be measured in inches or centimeters. Measurement is easily accomplished by moving the parallel bar attached to a wall ruler or on the scale. Height is usually measured annually for adult patients and documented in feet and inches. If an adult patient has certain medical conditions, such as osteoporosis, height may be measured at each visit. Length measurements used in pediatrics and pediatric BMIs are discussed in Chapter 28.

CRITICAL THINKING APPLICATION   5.9

Mrs. Johnson is being seen at WMFM for the first time. In what order should Carlos take her vital signs and her anthropometric measurements? Should blood pressure be measured in both arms, with the patient both sitting and standing? If so, what is the rationale?

CLOSING COMMENTS

We started this chapter with a discussion of TPR and then moved on to BP and SpO$_2$. We ended with a discussion of weight and height.

A medical assistant should be familiar with the different sites for taking a temperature and the different thermometers used. Using the correct site and thermometer will ensure that a proper temperature is obtained.

Pulse and respiration are often measured at the same time. This way patients are unaware that you are watching them breathe. Until you are proficient at taking a radial pulse, it should be counted for a full minute. An apical pulse is done using a stethoscope. You will hear two sounds, lubb-dubb. Each lubb-dubb is one beat.

When you take a blood pressure, it is important to use the correct size cuff and have it positioned correctly over the brachial artery. By taking a palpated systolic blood pressure first, you can be certain that you do not miss the first Korotkoff sounds.

Pulse oximetry is often done when there is a question about a patient's ability to transport enough oxygen. A finger or earlobe can be used for this procedure. If a finger is used, it should be free of fingernail polish.

Weight and height are anthropometric measurements that are typically taken at a healthcare facility. Weight is usually taken at every visit. Height is usually measured annually for adults, unless the patient has a specific medical condition. These measurements should be taken in a private location for the comfort of the patient. Accurate weight and height measurements are crucial for an accurate BMI calculation. Many providers use the BMI to counsel patients about lifestyle changes.

Patient-Centered Care

Measuring and documenting vital signs are a crucial part of the medical assistant's responsibilities. We must keep in mind that the results can cause the patient anxiety and concern. For example, if you have a patient who is struggling to maintain a healthy blood pressure, it is important that you are sensitive to his or her concerns. If you have a patient who is having difficulty maintaining or losing weight, he or she can be quite apprehensive, embarrassed, or even depressed about weight results. Being aware of the patient's concerns about vital signs and showing sensitivity to his or her needs are part of being a medical assistant.

Professional Behaviors

Taking accurate vital signs and anthropometric measurements is an important aspect of a medical assistant's responsibilities. These measurements give the provider a strong indication of the patient's overall health. Being confident in the process of obtaining these measurements is crucial. Taking vital signs will become second nature over time, but a medical assistant must always take care to be as accurate as possible. It is also important to remember that patients may be concerned about those measurements. Practicing empathy and good listening skills are also part of being a good medical assistant.

SUMMARY OF SCENARIO

Carlos recognizes the significance of measuring and documenting each patient's vital signs and anthropometric measurements. The providers at WMFM rely on Carlos to provide this information accurately. Carlos has never let these procedures become routine. He is always focused on the task, because vital signs are an important reflection of a person's health status.

Carlos knows that a number of factors can alter a patient's vital signs, including the external environment, smoking, drinking hot beverages, exercise, and anxiety and pain. Carlos evaluates patient factors such as age, gender, level of compliance, and the presence of disease to determine the best method of accurately measuring vital signs. In addition, Carlos is sensitive to the need

for safeguarding the patient's privacy. When he was first hired by WMFM, he was concerned about privacy and confidentiality when he discovered that the patient scale was in the hall next to the waiting room. After he discussed this with the office manager, the scale was moved to an examination room so that patients could be weighed in privacy.

Carlos attended a workshop last year on the AHA guidelines for the diagnosis and treatment of hypertension, and he is prepared to explain those recommendations to patients. He recognizes his role in motivating patients diagnosed with prehypertension to stick with recommended lifestyle changes and follow the provider's treatment protocol.

SUMMARY OF LEARNING OBJECTIVES

1. **Do the following related to temperature:**
   - *Cite the average body temperature for various age groups.*
     The average body temperature varies from person to person; in a healthy adult, it is typically between 97.6° and 99°F (36.4° and 37.2°C). (See Table 5.1.)
   - *Describe emotional and physical factors that can cause body temperature to rise and fall.*
     Multiple factors can affect body temperature, including the external environment, age, stress, physical exercise, gender, and illness.
   - *Convert temperature readings between the Fahrenheit and Celsius scales.*
     Using the formulas presented in this chapter, perform correct calculations to convert temperatures between Fahrenheit and Celsius scales.
   - *Obtain and record an accurate patient temperature using three different types of thermometers.*
     The patient's temperature can be measured orally and in the axillary region with a digital thermometer, in the ear using an aural thermometer, and at the temporal artery using a temporal artery scanner. The axillary temperature is approximately 1°F (0.6°C) lower than an accurate oral reading because the reading is not taken in an enclosed body cavity. The tympanic temperature is accurate because it records the temperature of the blood closest to the hypothalamus. The temporal artery scanner is considered most accurate for infants.
     After the temperature reading is documented, (T) is recorded for a tympanic reading; (A) for an axillary reading; and (TA) for a temporal artery reading, to clarify the site. Procedures 5.1 thru 5.5 explain how to take and record patient temperatures using a variety of thermometers.

2. **Do the following related to pulse:**
   - *Cite the average pulse rate for various age groups.*
     Infants and children typically have a faster pulse than adults; as aging progresses, the pulse rate declines. As a rule, both the pulse and respiratory rates respond to exercise or emotional upset. (See Table 5.2 for approximate age-related pulse ranges.)
   - *Describe pulse rate, volume, and rhythm.*
     The pulse *rate* reflects the number of times the heart contracts in 1 minute. The pulse *volume* is the amount of force placed on the arterial walls when the heart beats; the *rhythm* of the pulse is the length of time between beats. Monitor and record the pulse rate, noting whether the rhythm is regular or arrhythmic, and the volume is bounding, normal, or thready.
   - *Locate and record pulse at multiple sites.*
     The most common sites used to feel the pulse are the temporal, carotid, apical, brachial, radial, femoral, popliteal, and dorsalis pedis arteries. (Procedures 5.6 and 5.7 present the specifics on recording apical and radial pulses.)

3. **Do the following related to respiration:**
   - *Cite the average respiratory rate for various age groups.*
     As a rule, both the pulse and the respiratory rate respond to exercise and emotional upset. Table 5.3 presents a list of normal respiratory rates for patients in various age groups.
   - *Demonstrate the best way to obtain an accurate respiratory count.*
     Count the number of respirations for 30 seconds and then multiply by 2. This should be done immediately after taking the patient's pulse, while still holding the pulse point and without warning the patient, because the patient may inadvertently alter the respiratory rate if he or she is aware that breaths are being counted. (See Procedure 5.7, p. 130.)

4. **Do the following related to blood pressure:**
   - *Cite the approximate blood pressure range for various age groups.*
     Table 5.4 lists the normal blood pressure ranges for patients of various age groups.
   - *Specify physiologic factors that affect blood pressure.*
     Physiologic factors that affect blood pressure include the amount or volume of blood in circulation; the condition of the blood vessels, including the presence of atherosclerosis or arteriosclerosis; the degree of blood viscosity; and the condition of the myocardium.
   - *Differentiate between essential and secondary hypertension.*
     The cause of essential hypertension is unknown; it is diagnosed when a patient has a systolic reading higher than 140 mm Hg and/or a diastolic reading higher than 90 mm Hg. Secondary hypertension is caused by an underlying condition, such as renal disease, pregnancy, or a congenital heart defect.
   - *Interpret current hypertension guidelines and treatment.*
     AHA guidelines for the diagnosis and management of hypertension include a prehypertension category. Table 5.5 identifies the categories of normal, elevated, stage 1 hypertension, stage 2 hypertension, and hypertensive crisis. The goal of the AHA recommendations is to reduce the number of people who die each year from hypertension-related illness. Treatment includes a combination of weight management, sodium reduction, lifestyle changes, and the use of two or more antihypertensive and diuretic medications.
   - *Describe how to determine the correct cuff size for individual patients.*
     The proper size cuff must be used to obtain a correct blood pressure reading. To make sure the size is correct, the inflatable part (bladder) should cover about 80 percent of the circumference of the upper arm. (Table 5.6 presents the various sizes of blood pressure cuffs available.)
   - *Identify the different Korotkoff phases.*
     The Korotkoff phases are the categories of sounds heard during blood pressure measurement. These sounds are produced by vibrations of the arterial wall when the blood surges back into the vessel after it has been compressed by the blood pressure cuff. Phase I

Continued

SUMMARY OF LEARNING OBJECTIVES—*continued*

is the first sound heard as the cuff deflates and is the systolic reading; phase II is the swishing sound made by the movement of blood through the artery, although an auscultatory gap may occur in which sounds completely disappear; phase III involves distinct, sharp tapping sounds made as the blood rushes through the artery; in phase IV, the sound changes to a soft tapping, which becomes muffled and begins to grow fainter; and in phase V, sound completely disappears. The last sound heard is the diastolic reading.

- *Accurately measure and document blood pressure.*
  A sphygmomanometer is used with a stethoscope to hear the systolic over diastolic sounds. (Procedure 5.8 on p. 131 outlines the method for performing this skill.)

5. **Discuss and perform pulse oximetry.**
   Pulse oximetry measures the oxygen saturation of the blood in the peripheral blood vessels. If a patient has pneumonia, bronchitis, emphysema, or asthma, pulse oximetry will likely be performed. Procedure 5.9 on p. 133 describes the procedure for performing pulse oximetry.

6. **Accurately measure and document height and weight, use the body mass index scale, and convert kilograms to pounds and pounds to kilograms.**
   A patient's height and weight are anthropometric measurements that are recorded during the initial patient visit and periodically after that, depending on the patient's needs and the provider's preference. The scale should be kept in a private location. Variations in weight may indicate physical or emotional disorders, including diabetes, congestive heart failure, hormone abnormalities, depression, and eating disorders. (Procedure 5.10 on p. 133 describes the techniques for weighing a patient; the BMI is determined as indicated.)
   To convert kilograms (kg) to pounds (lb), multiply the number of kilograms by 2.2. To convert pounds to kilograms, divide the number of pounds by 2.2 kg, or multiply the number of pounds by 0.45 kg.

PROCEDURE 5.1   Obtain an Oral Temperature Using a Digital Thermometer

Task: Accurately determine and record a patient's oral temperature using a digital thermometer.

EQUIPMENT and SUPPLIES

- Patient's record
- Digital thermometer and probe covers
- Waste container

PROCEDURAL STEPS

1. Wash hands or use hand sanitizer.
   <u>PURPOSE</u>: To ensure infection control.
2. Assemble the needed equipment and supplies.
3. Greet the patient. Identify yourself. Verify the patient's identity with full name and date of birth. Explain the procedure to be performed in a manner that the patient understands. Answer any questions the patient may have about the procedure. Make sure the patient has not eaten, consumed any hot or cold fluids, smoked, or exercised during the 15 minutes before the temperature is measured.
   <u>PURPOSE</u>: Identification of the patient prevents errors, and explanations are a means of gaining implied consent and patient cooperation. The temperature will be inaccurate if hot or cold food or fluids have been consumed or if the patient has exercised within 15 minutes.

4. Prepare the probe for use as described in the directions (see the following figure). Make sure probe covers are always used.
   <u>PURPOSE</u>: To ensure infection control.

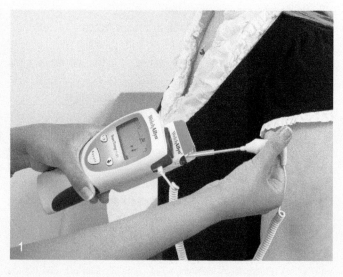

| PROCEDURE 5.1 | Obtain an Oral Temperature Using a Digital Thermometer—*continued* |

5. Place the probe under the patient's tongue (see the following figure) and instruct the patient to close the mouth tightly without biting down on the thermometer. Help the patient by holding the probe end, or the patient can hold the probe end if that is more comfortable.
   PURPOSE: Air seeping into the mouth interferes with an accurate body temperature reading.

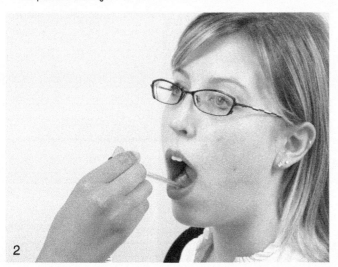

6. When a beep is heard, remove the probe from the patient's mouth and immediately eject the probe cover into an appropriate waste container.
   PURPOSE: The probe cover is contaminated and must be discarded in a waste container.
7. Note the reading on the display screen of the thermometer.
8. Document the reading in the patient's medical record (e.g., T: 97.7°F).
   PURPOSE: Procedures that are not documented are considered not done.
9. Wash hands or use hand sanitizer, and disinfect the equipment as indicated.
   PURPOSE: To observe infection control measures and Standard Precautions.

6/29/20XX 10:05 a.m. T: 97.7°F --------------- C. Ricci, CMA (AAMA)

| PROCEDURE 5.2 | Obtain an Axillary Temperature Using a Digital Thermometer |

Task: Accurately determine and record a patient's axillary temperature using a digital thermometer.

EQUIPMENT and SUPPLIES

- Patient's record
- Digital thermometer and probe cover
- Supply of tissues
- Patient gown as needed
- Waste container

PROCEDURAL STEPS

1. Wash hands or use hand sanitizer.
   PURPOSE: To ensure infection control.
2. Gather the needed equipment and supplies.
3. Greet the patient. Identify yourself. Verify the patient's identity with full name and date of birth. Explain the procedure to be performed in a manner that the patient understands. Answer any questions the patient may have about the procedure.
   PURPOSE: Identification of the patient prevents errors, and explanations are a means of gaining implied consent and patient cooperation.

4. Prepare the thermometer in the same manner as for oral use.
5. Expose the axillary region. If necessary, provide the patient with a gown for privacy.
6. Pat the patient's axillary area dry with tissues if needed.
   PURPOSE: To ensure an accurate reading. Do not rub the area because this may cause an elevated reading.
7. Place the probe tip into the center of the armpit, making sure the thermometer is touching only skin, not clothing.
   PURPOSE: To obtain the most accurate axillary reading; contact with clothing alters the reading.
8. Instruct the patient to hold the arm snugly across the chest or abdomen until the thermometer beeps (see the following figure).
   PURPOSE: To prevent air from leaking in and interfering with the temperature reading.

Continued

PROCEDURE 5.2 | Obtain an Axillary Temperature Using a Digital Thermometer—*continued*

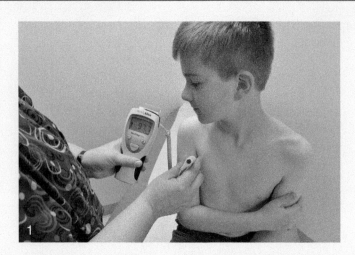

9. Remove the thermometer, note the digital reading, and dispose of the cover in the waste container.
10. Disinfect the thermometer if indicated.
    PURPOSE: To ensure infection control.
11. Wash hands or use hand sanitizer.
12. Document the reading in the patient's medical record (e.g., T: 97.6°F [A]).
    PURPOSE: Procedures that are not recorded are considered not done.

6/29/20XX 10:05 a.m. T: 98.2°F (A) --------------------------------
-- C. Ricci, CMA (AAMA)

PROCEDURE 5.3 | Obtain a Rectal Temperature of an Infant Using a Digital Thermometer

Task: Accurately determine and record a patient's rectal temperature using a digital thermometer.

EQUIPMENT and SUPPLIES

- Patient's record
- Digital thermometer and probe covers
- Disposable gloves
- Waste container

PROCEDURAL STEPS

1. Wash hands or use hand sanitizer.
   PURPOSE: To ensure infection control.
2. Assemble the needed equipment and supplies. Make sure that the red probe is used.
3. Greet the patient. Identify yourself. Verify the patient's identity with full name and date of birth. Explain the procedure to be performed in a manner that the patient's parent or caregiver understands. Answer any questions about the procedure.
   PURPOSE: Identification of the patient prevents errors, and explanations are a means of gaining implied consent and cooperation.
4. Have the parent or caregiver undress the infant.
5. Put on disposable gloves.
   PURPOSE: To ensure infection control.
6. Prepare the probe for use as described in the directions. Make sure probe covers are always used. Lubricate 2 inches of probe.
   PURPOSE: To ensure infection control.

7. Gently insert the thermometer probe $\frac{1}{2}$ inch for infants (this would change to $\frac{5}{8}$ inch for children and 1 inch for adults). Remain with the patient at all times, and hold the thermometer in place until a beep is heard.
8. Remove the probe, and immediately eject the probe cover into an appropriate waste container.
   PURPOSE: The probe cover is contaminated and must be discarded in a waste container.
9. Note the reading on the display screen of the thermometer.
10. Remove soiled gloves and discard them into an appropriate waste container.
11. Wash hands or use hand sanitizer, and disinfect the equipment as indicated.
    PURPOSE: To observe infection control measures and Standard Precautions.
12. Document the reading in the patient's medical record.
    PURPOSE: Procedures that are not documented are considered not done.

6/29/20XX 2:10 p.m. T: 100.7°F (R) --------------------------------
-- C. Ricci, CMA (AAMA)

| PROCEDURE 5.4 | Obtain a Temperature Using a Tympanic Thermometer |

Task: Accurately determine and record a patient's temperature using a tympanic thermometer.

EQUIPMENT and SUPPLIES

- Patient's record
- Tympanic thermometer
- Disposable probe covers
- Alcohol wipes
- Waste container

PROCEDURAL STEPS

1. Wash hands or use hand sanitizer.
   PURPOSE: To ensure infection control.
2. Gather the necessary equipment and supplies.
3. Greet the patient. Identify yourself. Verify the patient's identity with full name and date of birth. Explain the procedure to be performed in a manner that the patient understands. Answer any questions the patient may have about the procedure.
   PURPOSE: Identification of the patient prevents errors, and explanations are a means of gaining implied consent and patient cooperation.
4. Clean the probe with an alcohol wipe if indicated. Place a disposable cover on the probe (see the following figure).
   PURPOSE: To ensure a clean surface and prevent cross-contamination.

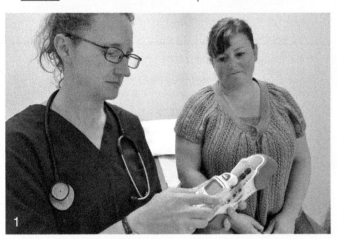

5. Insert the probe into the ear canal far enough to seal the opening. Do not apply pressure. For children younger than age 3, gently pull the earlobe down and back (see the first of the following figures); for patients older than age 3, gently pull the top of the ear (pinna) up and back (see the second of the following figures).
   PURPOSE: The external ear must be pulled gently to open the external auditory canal and expose the tympanic membrane for an accurate reading.

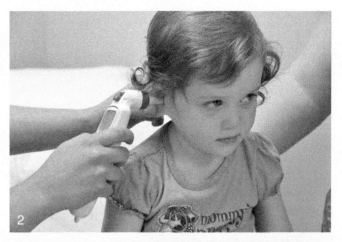

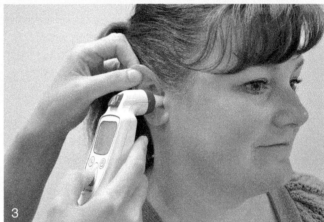

6. Press the button on the probe as directed. The temperature will appear on the display screen in 1 to 2 seconds.
7. Remove the probe, note the reading, and discard the probe cover into a waste container without touching it.
   PURPOSE: The probe cover is contaminated and must be discarded in a waste container.
8. Wash hands or use hand sanitizer and disinfect the equipment if indicated. See the manufacturer's manual for cleaning the probe tip. Many recommend cleaning the probe lens with alcohol wipes.
   PURPOSE: To ensure infection control.
9. Document the reading in the patient's medical record (e.g., T: 98.6°F [T]).
   PURPOSE: Procedures that are not recorded are considered not done.

7/11/20xx 2:20 p.m. T: 101.2°F (T) ------------------------------------
------------------------------------ C. Ricci, CMA (AAMA)

| PROCEDURE 5.5 | Obtain a Temperature Using a Temporal Artery Thermometer |

Task: Accurately determine and record a patient's temperature using a temporal artery thermometer.

EQUIPMENT and SUPPLIES

- Patient's record
- Professional temporal artery thermometer with probe covers
- Alcohol wipes
- Waste container

PROCEDURAL STEPS

1. Wash hands or use hand sanitizer.
   PURPOSE: To ensure infection control.
2. Gather the necessary equipment and supplies.
3. Greet the patient. Identify yourself. Verify the patient's identity with full name and date of birth. Explain the procedure to be performed in a manner that the patient understands. Answer any questions the patient may have about the procedure.
   PURPOSE: Identification of the patient prevents errors, and explanations are a means of gaining implied consent and patient cooperation.
4. Remove the protective cap on the probe. Depending on the facility's infection control procedures, disposable covers can be used on the scanner, or it can be cleaned by lightly wiping the surface with an alcohol wipe.
   PURPOSE: To ensure infection control.
5. Push the patient's hair up off the forehead to expose the site. Gently place the probe on the patient's forehead, halfway between the edge of the eyebrows and the hairline, at the center of the face (just above the nose).
   PURPOSE: This places the probe directly over the temporal artery.
6. Depress and hold the SCAN button, and lightly glide the probe sideways across the patient's forehead to the hairline just above the ear (see the following figure). As you move the sensor across the forehead, you will hear a beep, and a red light will flash.
   PURPOSE: This verifies that the scanner is recording temperatures as it moves across the surface of the temporal artery.

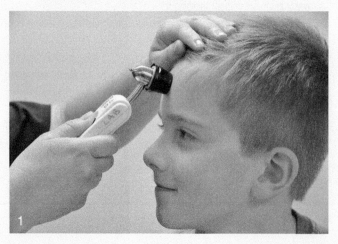

7. Keeping the button depressed, lift the thermometer, and place the probe behind the ear lobe (see the following figure). The thermometer may continue to beep, indicating that the temperature is rising.
   PURPOSE: To continue scanning of the temporal artery until the highest temperature is recorded on the thermometer.

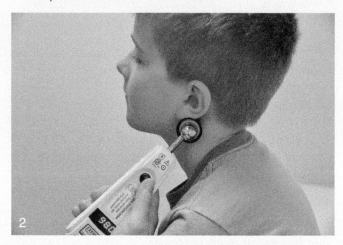

8. When scanning is complete, release the button and lift the probe. Note the temperature recorded on the digital display. The scanner automatically turns off 15 to 30 seconds after release of the button.
9. If a probe cover was used, eject it directly into a waste container. Disinfect the thermometer if indicated and replace the protective cap.
   PURPOSE: To ensure infection control. Depending on the facility's infection control procedures, disposable covers can be used on the scanner, or it can be cleaned between patients with a disinfectant wipe.
10. Wash hands or use hand sanitizer.
11. Document the reading in the patient's medical record (e.g., T: 101.6°F [TA]).
    PURPOSE: Procedures that are not recorded are considered not done.

8/1/20XX 11:20 a.m. T: 101.6°F (TA) ---------- C. Ricci, CMA (AAMA)

PROCEDURE 5.6 Obtain an Apical Pulse

Task: Accurately determine and record the patient's apical heart rate.

EQUIPMENT and SUPPLIES

- Patient's record
- Watch with a second hand
- Patient gown as needed
- Stethoscope
- Alcohol wipes

PROCEDURAL STEPS

1. Wash hands or use hand sanitizer and clean the stethoscope earpieces and diaphragm with alcohol wipes.
   PURPOSE: To ensure infection control and to follow Standard Precautions.
2. Greet the patient. Identify yourself. Verify the patient's identity with full name and date of birth. Explain the procedure to be performed in a manner that the patient understands. Answer any questions the patient may have about the procedure.
   PURPOSE: Identification of the patient prevents errors, and explanations are a means of gaining implied consent and patient cooperation.
3. If necessary, assist the patient in disrobing from the waist up and provide the patient with a gown that opens in the front.
   PURPOSE: To expose the chest and provide privacy and warmth.
4. Assist the patient into the sitting or supine position.
   PURPOSE: To allow easier access to the apical site at the apex of the heart.
5. Hold the stethoscope's diaphragm against the palm of your hand for a few seconds.
   PURPOSE: To warm the diaphragm, promoting patient comfort.
6. Place the stethoscope at the left midclavicular line at the fifth intercostal space over the apex of the heart (see the following figures). Do not touch the bell end of the stethoscope.
   PURPOSE: This is the point of maximum contractile strength, where the heartbeat can be heard best. Touching the bell end of the stethoscope may interfere with the sound.

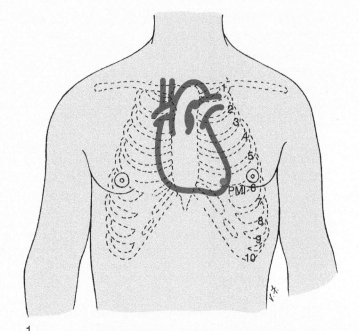

1

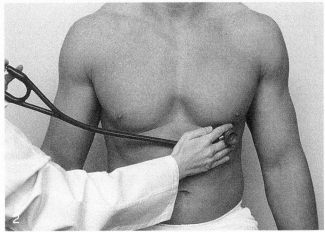

Continued

| PROCEDURE 5.6 | **Obtain an Apical Pulse**—*continued* |

7. Listen carefully for the heartbeat. Count the pulse for 1 full minute. Note any irregularities in rhythm and volume.
   PURPOSE: The apical pulse is always measured for 1 full minute to obtain the most accurate reading.
8. Help the patient to sit up and dress.
9. Disinfect the stethoscope with an alcohol wipe.
   PURPOSE: To ensure infection control.

10. Wash hands or use hand sanitizer.
11. Document the reading in the patient's medical record (e.g., AP: 96), and record any arrhythmias.

3/3/20XX 4:10 p.m. AP: 93 irregular ------------ C. Ricci, CMA (AAMA)

| PROCEDURE 5.7 | **Assess the Patient's Radial Pulse and Respiratory Rate** |

Task: Accurately determine and document a patient's radial pulse rate, rhythm, and volume and respiratory rate, rhythm, and depth.

Note: Respirations should be assessed immediately after the radial pulse, while the medical assistant is appearing to take the pulse, so the patient does not artificially alter breathing patterns.

EQUIPMENT and SUPPLIES

- Patient's record
- Watch with a second hand

PROCEDURAL STEPS

1. Wash hands or use hand sanitizer.
   PURPOSE: To ensure infection control.
2. Greet the patient. Identify yourself. Verify the patient's identity with full name and date of birth. Explain the procedure to be performed in a manner that the patient understands. Answer any questions the patient may have about the procedure.
   PURPOSE: Identification of the patient prevents errors, and explanations are a means of gaining implied consent and patient cooperation.
3. Place the patient's arm in a relaxed position, palm at or below the level of the heart.
   PURPOSE: The patient's radial artery is more easily palpated when the patient is relaxed and in this position.
4. Gently grasp the palm side of the patient's wrist with your first two or three fingertips approximately 1 inch below the base of the thumb (see the following figure).
   PURPOSE: This position puts your fingertips directly over the radial artery. Press firmly (but do not press too hard, or you will occlude the artery and feel nothing).

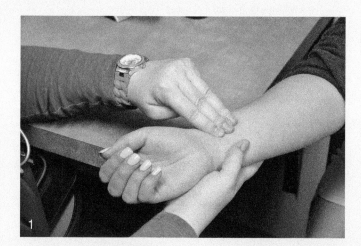

5. Count the beats for 1 full minute using a watch with a second hand.
   PURPOSE: Counting for 1 full minute allows you to obtain an accurate count, including any irregularities in rhythm and volume. Once you become more adept at taking a pulse, you can reduce this to 30 seconds and multiply that number by 2 to record the patient's heart rate.
6. While counting the beats, also assess the rhythm and volume of the patient's pulse.

PROCEDURE 5.7   Assess the Patient's Radial Pulse and Respiratory Rate—*continued*

7. While continuing to hold the patient's arm in the same position used to count the radial pulse, observe the rise and fall of the patient's chest (see Fig. 5.12). If you have difficulty noticing the patient's breathing, place the arm across the chest to detect movement.
   PURPOSE: The respiratory count may be altered if the patient is aware that you are counting his or her breaths; placing the arm across the chest allows you to feel or see the rise and fall of the chest wall.
8. Inhalation and exhalation make up one complete breathing cycle, or respiration. Count the respirations for 30 seconds and multiply by 2.
   PURPOSE: Counting for 30 seconds allows you to obtain an accurate count and determine any irregularities in rhythm or depth or unusual breathing patterns. If respirations are abnormal in any way, count for 1 full minute.

9. While counting, also assess the rhythm and depth of the patient's respirations.
10. Release the patient's wrist.
11. Wash hands or use hand sanitizer.
    PURPOSE: To ensure infection control.
12. Document both the radial pulse and respiration counts in the patient's health record. In a paper record the pulse is recorded immediately after the temperature and respirations after the pulse recording (e.g., P: 72, regular, thready R: 18, regular, normal).
    PURPOSE: Procedures that are not recorded are considered not done.

5/6/20XX 8:35 a.m. P: 72 regular, 1+ R: 18, regular, normal ------------
---C. Ricci, CMA (AAMA)

PROCEDURE 5.8   Determine a Patient's Blood Pressure

Task: Perform a blood pressure measurement that is correct in technique, accurate, and comfortable for the patient.

EQUIPMENT and SUPPLIES

- Patient's record
- Sphygmomanometer
- Stethoscope
- Antiseptic wipes/alcohol wipes

PROCEDURAL STEPS

1. Wash hands or use hand sanitizer.
   PURPOSE: To ensure infection control.
2. Assemble the equipment and supplies needed. Clean the earpieces and diaphragm of the stethoscope with alcohol wipes.
   PURPOSE: For infection control and to follow Standard Precautions.
3. Greet the patient. Identify yourself. Verify the patient's identity with full name and date of birth. Explain the procedure to be performed in a manner that the patient understands. Answer any questions the patient may have about the procedure.
   PURPOSE: Identification of the patient prevents errors, and explanations are a means of gaining implied consent and patient cooperation.
4. Select the appropriate arm for application of the cuff (no mastectomy on that side, no injury or disease). If the patient has had a bilateral mastectomy, the blood pressure should be taken using a large thigh cuff with the stethoscope over the popliteal artery.
   PURPOSE: The pressure of the cuff temporarily interferes with circulation to the limb.
   CAUTION: If a female patient has had a mastectomy, the blood pressure should never be taken on the affected side. Compressing the arm may cause complications. If she has had a bilateral mastectomy, another site, such as the popliteal artery, must be used, which requires use of a thigh cuff.

5. Seat the patient in a comfortable position with the legs uncrossed and the arm resting, palm up, at heart level on the arm of a chair or a table next to where the patient is seated.
   PURPOSE: To expose the brachial artery; also, to promote patient relaxation and ensure a true reading. Crossed legs may increase the blood pressure, and positioning of the arm above heart level may cause an inaccurate reading.
6. Roll the sleeve to about 5 inches above the elbow, or have the patient remove the arm from the sleeve.
   PURPOSE: Tight clothing prevents an accurate reading.
7. Select the correct cuff size.
   PURPOSE: An incorrect cuff size prevents accurate measurement of blood pressure. The cuff should fit comfortably around the patient's arm, and the bladder should be located over the brachial artery between the lines designated on the cuff. Pediatric, normal adult, and large adult cuff sizes should be available. Thigh cuffs may be needed for obese patients.
8. Palpate the brachial artery at the antecubital space in both arms. If one arm has a stronger pulse, use that arm. If the pulses are equal, select the right arm.
   PURPOSE: A stronger pulse is easier to measure; the right arm is the universal arm of choice.
9. Center the cuff bladder over the brachial artery with the connecting tube away from the patient's body and the tube to the bulb close to the body (see the following figure).
   PURPOSE: Pressure must be applied directly over the artery for an accurate reading. The cuff and its tubing should not touch the stethoscope. Noise from the tubing can interfere with a correct reading.

Continued

| PROCEDURE 5.8 | Determine a Patient's Blood Pressure—*continued* |

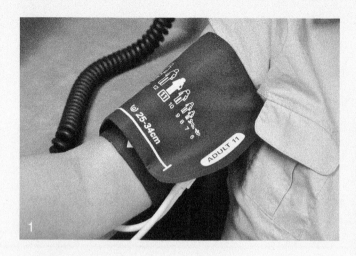

15. Close the valve and squeeze the bulb to inflate the cuff, rapidly but smoothly, to 30 mm Hg above the palpated systolic level, which was previously determined (see the following figure).

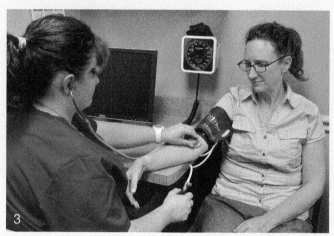

10. Place the lower edge of the cuff about 1 inch above the palpable brachial pulse, normally located in the natural crease of the inner elbow, and wrap it snugly and smoothly.
    <u>PURPOSE</u>: To help ensure an accurate reading. The cuff should be high enough on the arm that the stethoscope does not touch it and so that cuff sounds do not interfere with listening to the blood pressure sounds. A loose cuff results in an inaccurate reading.
11. Position the gauge of the sphygmomanometer so that it is easily seen.
    <u>PURPOSE</u>: An aneroid gauge should show the needle within the zero mark.
12. Palpate the radial pulse, tighten the screw valve on the air pump, and inflate the cuff until the pulse can no longer be felt. Make a note of the point on the gauge where the pulse could no longer be felt. Mentally add 30 mm Hg to the reading. Deflate the cuff and wait 15 seconds.
    <u>PURPOSE</u>: The point where the radial pulse is no longer felt provides an estimate of the systolic pressure. Pumping the cuff above that level ensures that phase I of the Korotkoff sounds will be heard.
13. Insert the earpieces of the stethoscope turned forward into the ear canals.
    <u>PURPOSE</u>: With the earpieces in this position, the openings follow the anatomic line of the ear canal and the blood pressure will be accurately heard.
14. Place the stethoscope's diaphragm over the palpated brachial artery for an adult patient or the bell for a pediatric patient. Press firmly enough to obtain a seal but not so tightly that the artery is constricted. Only touch the edges of the stethoscope head.
    <u>PURPOSE</u>: Forming a seal around the head of the stethoscope aids listening for blood pressure sounds. Placing your fingers directly over the stethoscope head will cause interference with the sound.

16. Open the valve slightly and deflate the cuff at a constant rate of 2 to 3 mm Hg per heartbeat.
    <u>PURPOSE</u>: Careful, slow release allows you to listen to all sounds.
17. Listen throughout the entire deflation; note the point on the gauge at which you hear the first sound (systolic), the last sound (diastolic), and until the sounds have stopped for at least 10 mm Hg.
18. Do not reinflate the cuff once the air has been released. Wait 30 to 60 seconds to repeat the procedure if needed.
    <u>PURPOSE</u>: Not allowing the blood to refill in the brachial artery results in inaccurate readings.
19. Remove the cuff from the patient's arm.
20. Remove the stethoscope from your ears and document the systolic and diastolic readings and the arm used as BP systolic/diastolic (e.g., BP: 120/80 R arm).
    Note: It is recommended that the blood pressure be checked and documented in each arm during the initial assessment of the patient and then bilaterally periodically after that for patients with hypertension.
    <u>PURPOSE</u>: Procedures that are not recorded are considered not done.
21. Clean the earpieces and the head of the stethoscope with an alcohol wipe and return both the cuff and the stethoscope to storage.
22. Wash hands or use hand sanitizer.
    <u>PURPOSE</u>: To ensure infection control.

5/19/20XX 11:00 a.m. BP: 124/82 ⊕ arm sitting, -
- C. Ricci, CMA (AAMA)

PROCEDURE 5.9   Perform Pulse Oximetry

Task: Assess the adequacy of oxygen levels (or oxygen saturation) in the blood using a pulse oximeter.

EQUIPMENT and SUPPLIES

- Patient's health record
- Pulse oximeter and probe of the appropriate size

PROCEDURAL STEPS

1. Wash hands or use hand sanitizer.
   PURPOSE: Standard Precautions must be followed to prevent the spread of disease.
2. Assemble the equipment.
3. Greet the patient. Identify yourself. Verify the patient's identity with full name and date of birth. Explain the procedure to be performed in a manner that the patient understands. Answer any questions the patient may have about the procedure.
   PURPOSE: An informed patient is more cooperative.
4. Turn on the monitor and attach the probe to the finger (preferred) or earlobe so it is flush with the skin.

5. The light-emitting diode (LED) should be placed on top of the nail. If the patient is wearing nail polish or has artificial nails, these may have to be removed to get a strong pulse signal.
   PURPOSE: To measure the pulse and oxygen saturation level.
6. Sanitize the patient probe and the external portion of the monitor with an aseptic cleaner.
   PURPOSE: To follow Standard Precautions.
7. Wash hands or use hand sanitizer.
   PURPOSE: To ensure infection control.
8. Document the oxygen saturation percentage and pulse in the patient's health record. Include date, time, and if the patient is receiving supplemental oxygen record the amount in liters.
   PURPOSE: Procedures that are not documented are considered not done.

PROCEDURE 5.10   Measure a Patient's Weight and Height

Task: Accurately weigh and measure a patient as part of the physical assessment procedure.
Note: Make sure the scale is located in an area away from traffic to maintain the patient's privacy.

EQUIPMENT and SUPPLIES

- Balance beam scale with a measuring bar
- Paper towel
- Patient record

PROCEDURAL STEPS

1. Wash hands or use hand sanitizer.
   PURPOSE: To ensure infection control.
2. Greet the patient. Identify yourself. Verify the patient's identity with full name and date of birth. Explain the procedure to be performed in a manner that the patient understands. Answer any questions the patient may have about the procedure.
   PURPOSE: Identification of the patient prevents errors, and explanations are a means of gaining implied consent and patient cooperation.
3. Have the patient remove his or her shoes. Place a paper towel on the scale platform. Check to see that the balance bar pointer floats in the middle of the balance frame when all weights are at zero.
   PURPOSE: A floating pointer indicates that the scale is properly adjusted and in balance.
4. Help the patient onto the scale. Make sure the patient has removed any heavy objects from pockets and is not holding anything such as a jacket or purse.

5. Move the large weight into the groove closest to the patient's estimated weight. The grooves are calibrated in 50-lb increments. If you choose a groove that is more than the patient's weight, the pointer will immediately tilt to the bottom of the balance frame. You then must move it back one groove (see the following figure).

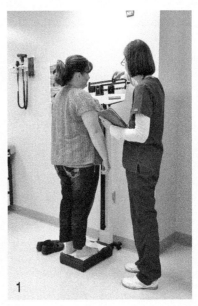

1

Continued

PROCEDURE 5.10   **Measure a Patient's Weight and Height**—*continued*

6. While the patient is standing still, slide the small upper weight to the right along the pound markers until the pointer balances in the middle of the balance frame.
   <u>PURPOSE</u>: The pointer floats between the bottom and the top of the frame when both lower and upper weights together balance the scale with the patient's weight.
7. Leave the weights in place.
8. Ask the patient to step off the scale and move the height bar to a point above the patient's height. Extend the bar and ask the patient step back on the scale. On some scales, the patient may need to turn with his or her back to the scale.
9. Adjust the height bar so that it just touches the top of the patient's head (see the following figure).

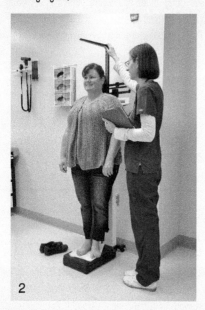

10. Leave the elevation bar set.
    <u>PURPOSE</u>: To maintain the height recording while protecting the patient from possible injury.

11. Assist the patient off the scale. Make sure all items that were removed for weighing are given back to the patient.
12. Read the weight scale. Add the numbers at the markers of the large and small weights, and document the total to the nearest quarter of a pound in the patient's health record (e.g., Wt: 136½ lb).
13. Read the height. Read the marker at the movable point of the ruler, and document the measurement to the nearest quarter of an inch on the patient's medical record (e.g., Ht: 5′ 6½″) (see the following figure).

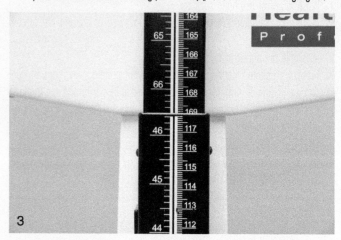

14. Use the patient's weight and height to determine the BMI if the EHR program does not do it automatically.
15. Return the weights and the measuring bar to zero.
16. Remove the paper towel and dispose of it in the waste container. Wash hands or use hand sanitizer.
17. Document the results in the patient's health record.
    <u>PURPOSE</u>: Procedures that are not documented are considered not done.

5/26/20XX 11:07 a.m. Wt: 136½ lb, Ht: 5′6½″ --------------------
-- C. Ricci, CMA (AAMA)

PHYSICAL EXAMINATION

SCENARIO

Chris Isaacson, CMA (AAMA), works for Walden-Martin Family Medical (WMFM) Clinic. He is responsible for initial patient interviews, taking medical histories, and documentation. Chris struggles with gathering the information needed from some patients. They do not always respond openly and honestly. Chris is also responsible for assisting with physical examinations. His duties include preparing and maintaining the examination room and equipment; getting the patient ready for specific physical examinations; and gowning, draping, and positioning the patient as needed. Because Chris assists with examinations, he must be familiar with the physical examination procedure and the order in which the provider needs various pieces of medical equipment. Throughout the physical examination process, Chris needs to be aware of proper body mechanics.

While studying this chapter, think about the following questions:

- How can Chris learn to develop helping relationships so that the patient's medical history is as comprehensive as possible?
- Would it help if Chris displayed greater sensitivity to diverse populations?
- Would using active listening techniques and attending to the patient's nonverbal behaviors better enable Chris to develop therapeutic communications skills?
- How can Chris's supervisor help him become a better communicator and demonstrate comprehensive and accurate documentation in patients' health records?
- What equipment does Chris need to gather before the provider enters the examination room, to make sure the examination goes smoothly and without interruption?
- What examination and treatment positions should Chris be familiar with, and when should the various positions be used?
- What measures can Chris take to protect himself from injury when lifting heavy items or assisting with the transfer of patients?

LEARNING OBJECTIVES

1. Describe the components of the patient's medical history and how to collect the history information.
2. Do the following related to understanding and communicating with patients:
   - Discuss how to successfully understand and communicate with patients and display sensitivity to diverse populations.
   - Demonstrate therapeutic communication feedback techniques to obtain information when gathering a patient history.
   - Obtain and document patient information.
   - Respond to nonverbal communication when interacting with patients.
   - Compare open-ended and closed-ended questions.
3. Do the following related to the patient interview:
   - Discuss the patient interview.
   - Identify barriers to communication and their impact on the patient assessment.
   - Detect a patient's use of defense mechanisms and the resultant barriers to therapeutic communication.
   - Demonstrate professional patient interviewing techniques.
4. Discuss the use of therapeutic communication techniques with patients across the life span.
5. Compare and contrast signs and symptoms.
6. Document patient care accurately in the medical record.
7. Do the following related to the physical examination:
   - Outline the medical assistant's role in preparing for the physical examination.
   - Summarize the instruments and equipment the provider typically uses during a physical examination.
8. Identify the principles of body mechanics and demonstrate proper body mechanics.
9. Outline the basic principles of gowning, positioning, and draping a patient for examination; also, describe how to position and drape a patient in different examining positions while remaining mindful of the patient's privacy and comfort.
10. Describe the methods of examination and give an example of each one.
11. Outline the sequence of a routine physical examination. Also, prepare for and assist in the physical examination of a patient, correctly completing each step of the procedure in the proper sequence.

VOCABULARY

auscultate (AW skuhl tayt) To listen with a stethoscope.

bruit (broot) An abnormal sound or murmur heard on auscultation of an organ, vessel (e.g., carotid artery), or gland.

chief complaint A statement in the patient's own words that describes the reason for the visit.

chronologic (kron ih LOJ ic) Arranged in the order of time.

clarification (klar i fi KAY shuhn) Allows the listener to get additional information.

clubbing Abnormal enlargement of the distal phalanges (fingers and toes) associated with cyanotic heart disease or advanced chronic pulmonary disease.

colonoscopy (kohl uh NOS kuh pee) A procedure in which a fiberoptic scope is used to examine the large intestine.

congruence (kun GROO uhns) Agreement; the state that occurs when the verbal expression of the message matches the sender's nonverbal body language.

correlate (CORE uh layt) To establish an orderly relationship or connection.

demographic (dem uh GRAF ik) Statistical data of a population. In healthcare this includes the patient's name, address, date of birth, employment, and other details.

electrocardiogram (ECG, EKG) A record or recording of electrical impulses of the heart produced by an electrocardiograph.

emphysema (em fuh ZEE mah) Thinning and eventual destruction of the alveoli; usually accompanies chronic bronchitis.

extension The process of stretching out; increasing the angle of a joint.

familial (fah MIL ee uhl) Occurring in or affecting members of a family more than would be expected by chance.

flexion The process of decreasing the angle of a joint.

gait The manner or style of walking.

history of present illness (HPI) Describes the signs and symptoms from the time of onset.

holistic (hoh LIS tik) Considering the patient as a whole; includes the physical, emotional, social, economic, and spiritual needs of the person.

inconspicuous (in kuhn SPIK yoo uhs) Not noticeable or prominent.

judicious (joo DISH uhs) Using good judgment; being discreet, sensible.

manipulation Movement or exercise of a body part by means of an externally applied force.

murmur An abnormal sound heard during auscultation of the heart that may or may not have a pathologic origin; it is associated with valve disease or a congenital heart defect.

nodules (NOD jools) Small lumps, lesions, or swellings that are felt when the skin is palpated.

palpation (pal PAY shuhn) The use of touch during the physical examination to assess the size, consistency, and location of certain body parts.

patient portal A secure online website that gives patients 24-hour access to personal health information using a username and password.

perineal (pair ih NEE uhl) Pertaining to the area between the vaginal opening and the rectum (perineum).

peripheral neuropathy (puh RIF er uhl noo ROP uh thee) A problem with the function of the nerves outside the spinal cord; symptoms include weakness, burning pain, and loss of reflexes; a frequent complication of diabetes mellitus.

rapport (ra POR) A relationship of harmony and accord between the patient and the healthcare professional.

sclera (SKLER uh) The white part of the eye that forms the orbit.

signs Objective findings determined by a clinician, such as a fever, hypertension, or rash.

symmetry (SIM ih tree) Similarity in size, form, and arrangement of parts on opposite sides of the body.

symptoms Subjective complaints reported by the patient, such as pain or nausea.

transillumination (trans ih LOO muh nay shun) Inspection of a cavity or organ by passing light through its walls.

trauma (TRAW muh) A physical injury or wound caused by external force or violence.

turgor (TUR ger) Referring to normal skin tension; the resistance of the skin to being grasped between the fingers and released. Turgor decreases with dehydration and increases with edema.

Medical assistants are directly involved in gathering information from patients about their health. It is important to remember that a healthy state is more than the absence of disease. The assessment process should be a reflection of the entire patient, not just a report about signs and symptoms. Individual lifestyles and environmental factors can be the cause of disease and should be considered when information is gathered about the patient's **chief complaint**. For example, if a patient smokes or works in a stressful occupation, he or she may be more prone to hypertension. Health professionals should consider all patient factors when gathering information about the patient's health status. The method of analyzing all factors that may contribute to the development of disease is based on a **holistic** perspective. Holistic patient care recognizes that illness is the result of many factors, not just physical ones.

As the first step in treating a disease process, the provider must determine the patient's medical diagnosis. A *differential diagnosis* considers which one of several diseases may be producing the patient's symptoms. The possible causes for a set of symptoms are considered in order to arrive at a diagnosis. For example, if a patient presents with moderate to severe knee pain, the provider might consider causes such as an injury or arthritis. A differential diagnosis is based on information gathered from the patient about symptoms; contributing family, personal, and social histories; and a complete physical examination. Multiple causes are not ruled out in a differential diagnosis because it is possible for patients to be sick with more than one thing at once. Once the provider has considered all the possible factors, he or she comes up with a working diagnosis and begins treatment. A working diagnosis is also called a *clinical diagnosis.* The clinical diagnosis is arrived at after taking a detailed history and doing a comprehensive physical examination, but before any laboratory tests or x-rays, diagnostic testing is done. For the patient with knee pain, after gathering detailed patient information and conducting a comprehensive physical examination, the provider decides that the clinical diagnosis is arthritic changes in the joint. The provider orders x-rays and a magnetic resonance image (MRI) of the knee to confirm the clinical diagnosis. The final diagnosis is determined after all diagnostic studies are completed.

However, patient care does not start with the physical examination; it begins when the patient first contacts the office. Even before the examination, the medical assistant has the opportunity to interact with the patient to ensure that he or she feels comfortable during the process and that all of the necessary information is obtained.

Interviewing patients, assisting with examinations, and preparing documentation are important responsibilities for a medical assistant. You must know the components of a medical history and the techniques for interviewing patients, because these will help the provider diagnose and treat the patient. The more complete the medical history, the better able the provider will be to treat the patient.

A medical assistant must also know how to best assist the provider during the physical examination. Understanding what supplies and instruments are needed will make the visit go more smoothly for both the patient and the provider. During a complete physical exam, the patient is placed in various positions to facilitate examination. It is often the medical assistant's responsibility to assist the patient into the correct position and drape him or her for modesty.

MEDICAL HISTORY

Collecting the History Information

A new patient is asked to complete a health history form. This form is useful for diagnosing and treating the patient. This self-history also allows the patient to be more involved in the process. The form may be mailed to the patient's home before the appointment or may be completed in the office during the first visit. Some healthcare facilities use electronic forms. These can be emailed to the patient before the first appointment and incorporated into the patient's electronic health record (EHR) when the completed form is emailed back. The patient may also be able to complete the form online through a **patient portal**. If a paper form is used, it can be scanned into the patient's EHR after it is completed.

If you are responsible for taking a portion of the medical history, conduct the interview in a private area, free of distractions and where others cannot overhear hear anything. Patients will not talk freely where they may be overheard or interrupted. Legally and ethically, the patient has the right to privacy, and access to the patient's health record is permitted only for healthcare workers directly involved in the patient's care or individuals the patient has specified on his or her Health Insurance Portability and Accountability Act (HIPAA) release form.

Listen to the patient. Do not express surprise or displeasure at any of the patient's statements. Remember, you are not there to pass

judgment but to collect medical data. The medical assistant should document the information in an organized manner, exactly as given by the patient, without opinion or interpretation. The documentation should include the following:

- Purpose of the patient's visit, written as the chief complaint (CC)
- Patient's vital signs (VS)
- Height and weight
- Pain; documented using a scale of 1 to 10, with 1 being the least amount of pain and 10 being the greatest amount

In some facilities, the provider takes the medical history during the patient's initial visit. The provider **correlates** the physical findings in the examination with the information in the history. The complete medical history and the physical examination are the starting point and foundation of all patient-provider contacts. EHR systems incorporate the patient's history and physical examination data directly into the health record (Fig. 6.1).

Components of the Medical History

Medical history forms vary, depending on the provider's preference, the practice specialty, and the EHR system used in the facility. The most commonly used medical history forms include these components:

- *Database:* The record of the patient's **demographic** information, along with history, physical examination, and initial laboratory findings. As new information is added, it becomes part of this database.
- *Chief complaint (CC):* The purpose of the patient's visit. Generally, this is documented in the patient's own words.
- **History of present illness (HPI):** The medical assistant should gather as much information about the health problem as possible and document it concisely in **chronologic** order.
- *Past history (PH)* or *past medical history (PMH):* A summary of the patient's previous health. It includes dates and details about the patient:
  - Usual childhood diseases (UCD or UCHD)
  - Major illnesses
  - Surgeries
  - Allergies
  - Accidents
  - Immunization record

Allergy Documentation

Each medical practice has a policy on how to document a patient's allergies. In a paper record they typically are written in red ink or identified by a colored sticker so that they can be easily seen by all healthcare workers. EHR systems have methods for including allergy information on all pertinent screens in the patient's record.

Included in the patient's medication history should be a record of frequently used over-the-counter (OTC) medications, including supplements and currently prescribed drugs.

- *Family history (FH):* Details about the patient's parents and siblings and their health; if they are deceased, the age and cause of death.

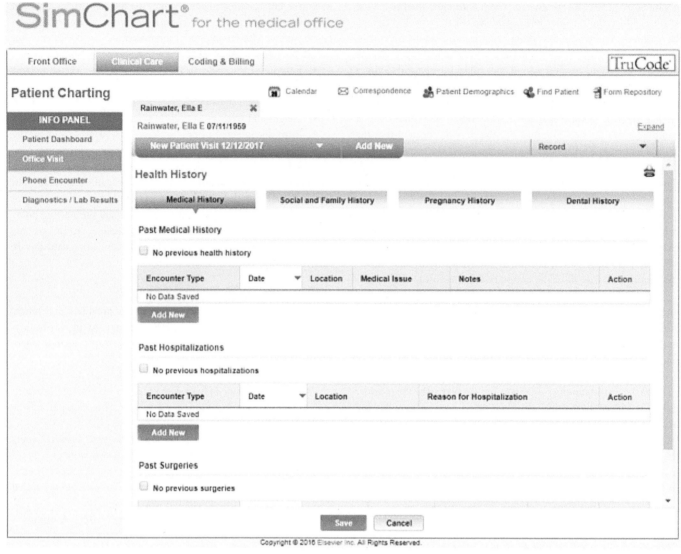

FIGURE 6.1 Example of an electronic health record (EHR) system.

This information is important because certain diseases and disorders have **familial** or hereditary tendencies.

- *Social history* (SH): This section includes information about the patient's lifestyle:
  - Whether he or she feels safe at home
  - Use of tobacco, alcohol, or recreational drugs
  - Sleeping and exercise habits
  - Typical diet
  - Education and occupation
  - Dental care history
  - For female patients, their last menstrual period (LMP), pregnancy history, and method of birth control if sexually active

It may be important to note the patient's cultural and religious background, because these factors could influence certain lifestyle and dietary choices. This information helps the provider to plan treatment for the patient or to determine causative factors for disease. It also provides a holistic picture of the patient's health. To meet the requirements of Meaningful Use (see Chapter 2), providers are required to collect information on allergies, patient history, safety at home, and alcohol use.

- *Systems review* (SR) or *review of systems* (ROS): These questions provide a guide to the patient's general health and help detect conditions other than those covered under the present illness. Often a patient may think certain health problems are irrelevant and may fail to mention them. However, these problems may help the provider determine the cause of the disorder currently being explored. A systems review is obtained through a logical sequence of questions about the state of health of body systems, beginning with the head and proceeding downward (Fig. 6.2). The provider typically completes this section of the medical history while conducting the physical examination.

UNDERSTANDING AND COMMUNICATING WITH PATIENTS

To provide high-quality patient care, we must communicate effectively with the patient and provide a warm, caring environment. Positive

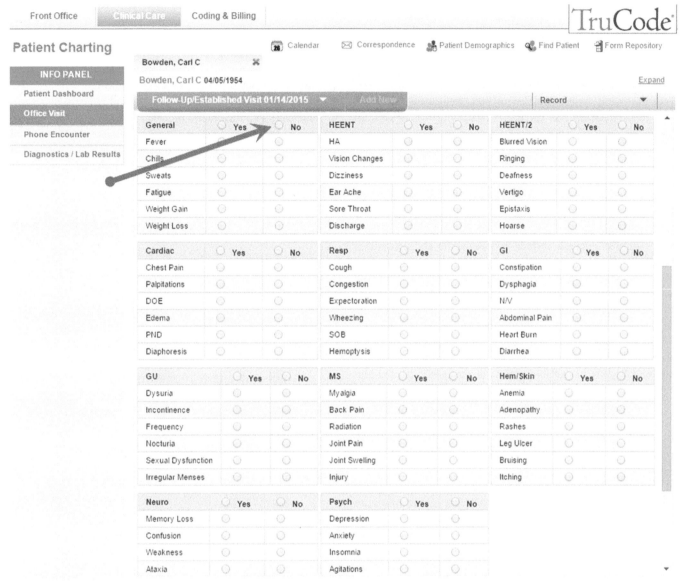

FIGURE 6.2 Example of review of systems (ROS) questions in an electronic health record.

reactions and interactions with the patient are vital. A medical assistant must always remember that each patient is an individual with certain anxieties. These anxieties often cause people to act and react in different ways; therefore, effective verbal and nonverbal communication with each patient is essential.

Healthcare professionals accept the responsibility of developing helping relationships with their patients. The interpersonal nature of the patient–medical assistant relationship means that the focus should be on the patient's needs. A medical assistant can bring out either a positive or a negative response simply by the way he or she treats and interacts with patients. You are usually the first person with whom the patient communicates; therefore, you play a vital role in therapeutic patient interactions (see Procedure 6.1, p. 162).

Another important aspect of communicating with patients is an awareness of self-boundaries. When working in healthcare, it is important to develop a solid professional relationship with our patients. By establishing realistic self-boundaries, that relationship can be protected. It is important to keep the focus on the patient. When you work with patients who are seen frequently, it is easy to start to think of them as friends. With a friend you are likely to share personal information that is not appropriate to share with a patient. Patients may feel that they cannot share important health-related information because you are their friend and it would be embarrassing to share that information with a friend.

Self-boundaries can also be thought of as professional boundaries. You need to treat patients with respect and keep the relationship professional. Be friendly to patients and always keep the focus on the patient.

Sensitivity to Diverse Patient Groups

Most healthcare facilities have a diverse patient population. The diversity could be based on race, age, culture, religion, or physical qualities, such as being deaf or hard of hearing. Whatever the origin of the diversity, practicing respectful patient care is extremely important. *Empathy* is the key to creating a caring, therapeutic environment. Empathy is different from sympathy. A medical assistant who is empathetic respects the individuality of the patient and attempts to see the person's health problem through his or her eyes. The medical assistant also recognizes the effect of all holistic factors on the patient's well-being. Empathetic sensitivity to diversity requires you to examine your own values, beliefs, and actions; you cannot treat all patients with care and respect until you first recognize and evaluate personal biases. We think and act a certain way for many reasons. The first step in understanding the process is to evaluate your individual value system. Why do you have certain attitudes or beliefs about the worth of individuals or things?

Many factors influence the development of a value system. Value systems begin as learned beliefs and behaviors. Families and cultural influences shape the way we respond to a diverse society. Other factors that influence reactions include socioeconomic and educational backgrounds. To develop therapeutic relationships, you must recognize your own value system to determine whether it could affect how you interact with patients. Preconceived ideas about people because of their race, religion, income level, ethnic origin, sexual orientation, or gender can act as barriers to the development of a therapeutic relationship. You cannot treat your patients empathetically unless you can connect with them in some way. Personal biases or prejudices are huge barriers to the development of therapeutic relationships (Fig. 6.3).

Regardless of the type of healthcare facility you work in, you will care for a wide variety of patients. The medical assistant should take the initiative to learn about the cultures represented in the healthcare practice. Some points to consider about diverse groups include the following:

- Patients of Asian backgrounds may have been raised in a culture that considers it extremely rude to establish eye contact. Americans view an unwillingness to establish eye contact as a sign of distrust or embarrassment; however, for people from Japan or China, lack of eye contact may be a way of demonstrating respect.
- Personal space may be an issue for patients from diverse backgrounds. If a patient appears very uncomfortable with touch or lack of personal space, attempt to accommodate him or her as much as possible during the office visit.

- Research has shown that older people face unique communications problems in the healthcare environment. The healthcare facility should have tools available to help patients with hearing or vision issues. When caring for an aging individual, it is important to focus patient teaching and information on the patient, rather than the family member who may be present.
- Patients may use their religious beliefs and values to understand and cope with their health problems. However, using religion to guide healthcare decisions may result in a conflict with the provider's recommendations. Healthcare workers may need to find a balance between respect for a patient's beliefs and the delivery of high-quality healthcare.

CRITICAL THINKING APPLICATION   **6.1**

Honestly evaluate your personal biases. What do you find unacceptable in people? Do you prejudge an individual based on his or her affiliation with a particular group or because of a certain lifestyle decision? Do these biases create barriers to the development of therapeutic relationships? If so, how can you get beyond these barriers?

Consider the following scenarios, and discuss them with your classmates:

- While you are conducting a patient interview, the patient informs you that he has tested positive for the human immunodeficiency virus (HIV). Do you think this will affect your therapeutic relationship?
- You are responsible for recording an in-depth interview on a homeless person with very poor hygiene. Will this cause a problem with your professional manner?
- Your office manager tells you that an inmate of the county prison is being brought in this afternoon for an examination. Do you think his status will affect your interaction with the patient?
- You are attempting to interview a 20-year-old patient who brought her two young children with her to the office today. She is a single mother who is pregnant with her third child and receives public assistance. What do you think? Will you have difficulty being empathetic?

Therapeutic Techniques

Communication is an interactive process involving the sender of the message, the receiver, and feedback. Feedback is a crucial component to confirm that the message was received. The message can be sent by a number of methods:

- Face-to-face communication
- Telephone
- Email
- Letter

Feedback lets us know that the receiver got the message and how he or she interpreted it. This completes the communication cycle by providing a means for us to know exactly what message the patient received and whether it requires **clarification**.

For example, as a medical assistant, one of your responsibilities will be to provide patient education on how to prepare for diagnostic studies. Let's say you have to explain to an older adult patient how to prepare for a **colonoscopy**. You provided a detailed explanation

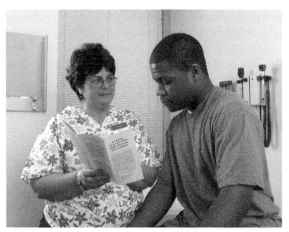

FIGURE 6.3 Respectful patient care.

of the preparation procedure and a handout explaining the step-by-step process. How do you really know whether the patient understands? You ask the patient to provide feedback by explaining the process back to you. As a member of the healthcare team, you must become an effective communicator. You will play a vital role in collecting and documenting patient information. If your methods of communication are faulty, the quality of patient care may be seriously impaired.

Active Listening Techniques

Hearing is a physical act. Someone speaks, and we hear what the person has said. Listening is something we consciously choose to do. Active listeners go beyond hearing the patient's message to concentrating, understanding, and listening to the main points. Active listening techniques encourage patients to expand on and clarify the content and meaning of their messages. These techniques are very useful communication tools when a patient is agitated or upset. They help the medical assistant clarify the important details of the patient's chief complaint.

Three processes are involved in active listening: restatement, reflection, and clarification. *Restatement* is simply paraphrasing or repeating the patient's statements with phrases such as, "My understanding of what you are saying is …" or "You are telling me the problem is …"

Reflection involves repeating the main idea of the conversation while also identifying the sender's *feelings*. For example, if the mother of a young patient is expressing frustration about her child's behavior, a reflective statement identifies that feeling with the response, "It sounds like you are frustrated about …" Or if a patient who has been newly diagnosed with insulin-dependent diabetes shows anxiety about administering injections, an appropriate reflective statement recognizes the patient's feelings: "You appear anxious about …" Reflective statements clearly demonstrate to patients that you are not only listening to their words; you also are concerned and are attending to their feelings.

Clarification seeks to summarize or simplify the sender's thoughts and feelings and to resolve any confusion in the message. Questions or statements that begin with "Give me an example of …" or "Explain to me about …" or "So what you're saying is …" help patients focus on the chief complaint and give you the opportunity to clear up any misconceptions before documenting patient information.

Listening is not a passive role in the communication process; it is active and demanding. You cannot be preoccupied with your own needs, or you will miss something important. For the duration of the patient interview, no one is more important than this particular patient. Listen to the way things are said, the tone of the patient's voice, and even to what the patient may not be saying out loud but is saying very clearly with body language (see Procedure 6.1).

Nonverbal Communication

Experts say that more than 90% of communication is nonverbal. Much of what we communicate to our patients is conveyed through the use of body language. Our nonverbal actions, such as gestures, facial expressions, and mannerisms, are learned behaviors that are greatly influenced by our family and cultural backgrounds. The body naturally expresses our true feelings.

Most of the negative messages communicated through body language are unintentional. It is important to remember while conducting patient interviews that nonverbal communication can seriously affect the therapeutic process.

The purpose of observing nonverbal communication is to become aware of the message conveyed by these behaviors rather than the words. This enables you to adapt your behavior to these feelings. You can deliberately select your response, either verbal or nonverbal, to have a favorable effect on others. The favorable effect may consist of the following:

- Providing emotional support
- Conveying that you care
- Defusing the patient's fear or anger
- Providing an invitation to release pent-up feelings by talking about the situation that aroused the feelings

Table 6.1 lists some nonverbal behaviors by patients that may indicate anxiety, frustration, or fear.

TABLE 6.1 Observations of Nonverbal Communication in Patients

AREA	OBSERVATION	INDICATION
Breathing patterns	Rapid respirations, sighing, shallow thoracic breathing	Anxiety, boredom, pain
Eye patterns	No eye contact, side-to-side movement, looking down at the hands	Anxiety, distrust, embarrassment
Hands	Tapping fingers, cracking knuckles, continuous movement, sweaty palms	Anxiety, worry, fear
Arm placement	Folded across chest, wrapped around abdomen	Anxiety, worry, fear, pain
Leg placement	Tension, crossed or tucked under, tapping foot, continuous movement	Frustration, anger

Helpful Listening Guidelines

- Listen to the main points in the discussion.
- Respond to both verbal and nonverbal messages.
- Be patient and nonjudgmental.
- Do not interrupt.
- Never intimidate the patient.
- Use active listening techniques: restatement, reflection, and clarification.

Your tone of voice can put a patient at ease. Your facial expression and the ease and confidence of your movements demonstrate a sincere interest to the patient. Therapeutic use of space and touch are also important ways of sending nonverbal messages to your patients. You should establish eye contact, sit in a relaxed but attentive position, and avoid using furniture as a barrier between you and the patient. Give the patient your undivided attention and let your body language inform each patient that you are interested in his or her medical problems (Fig. 6.4 and Procedure 6.2 on p. 163).

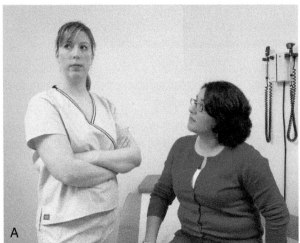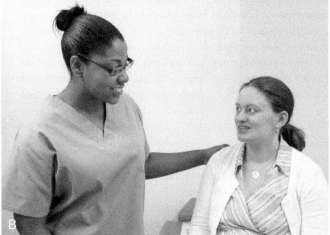

FIGURE 6.4 **(A)** Ineffective nonverbal language. **(B)** Therapeutic nonverbal language.

The key to successful patient interaction is **congruence** between verbal and nonverbal messages. Although choosing the correct words is very important, less than 10% of the message received is verbal; therefore, to be seen as honest and sensitive to the needs of your patients, you must be aware of your nonverbal behavior patterns. The nonverbal message the patient receives from the medical assistant's listening behavior should be "You are a person of worth, and I am interested in you as a unique individual."

Nonverbal Language Behaviors

Nonverbal behavior — your body language — can have either a positive or a negative effect on patient interactions. Positive nonverbal behaviors enhance the patient's experience in the healthcare setting. Communication experts recommend the following:

- When gathering a health history, lean toward the patient to show interest.
- Face the patient squarely and at eye level to make the process more comfortable and to demonstrate sensitivity and empathy.
- Eye contact is essential for therapeutic communication unless the patient is from a culture that discourages this.
- A closed posture (crossed arms or legs) may indicate disinterest.
- Be sensitive to the patient's personal space when possible. Maintain a comfortable distance from the patient, at least an arm's length, when conducting the interview.
- Be careful with body gestures, such as hand and arm movements. Gestures, such as nodding your head when the patient talks, can display interest, but too much body movement can be distracting.
- Your tone of voice should reflect your interest in the patient. Speaking too quietly or too loudly can detract from therapeutic communication.
- Continually observe the patient's body language during the interview; watch for signs of confusion, boredom, worry, and so on so that you can respond appropriately.
- Documenting in an EHR can be distracting to both the medical assistant and the patient. Remind yourself to look at the patient frequently and use encouraging body language to maintain a personal interaction.

Open-Ended Questions or Statements

An *open-ended question* or statement asks for general information or states the topic to be discussed, but only in general terms. This communication tool is used in various ways:

- To begin the interview
- To introduce a new section of questions
- Whenever the person introduces a new topic

It is an effective method of gathering more details from the patient about the chief complaint or health history. Consider these examples:

"What brings you to the doctor?"
"How have you been getting along?"
"You mentioned having dizzy spells. Tell me more about that."

This type of question or statement encourages patients to respond in a manner they find comfortable. It allows patients to express themselves fully and provide comprehensive information about their chief complaint.

Closed-Ended Questions

Direct, or *closed-ended*, *questions* ask for specific information. This form of questioning limits the answer to one or two words – in many cases, yes or no. Use this form of question when you need confirmation of specific facts, such as when asking about past health problems. Here are some examples:

"Do you have a headache?"
"What is your birth date?"
"Have you ever broken a bone?"

INTERVIEWING THE PATIENT

The *interview*, or gathering of the patient's medical history, is the first and most important part of data collection. The medical history identifies the patient's health strengths and problems and is a bridge to the next step in data collection, the physical examination performed by the provider. At this point, the patient knows everything about his or her own health status and you know nothing. Your interview skills help to collect the necessary information and build **rapport** for a successful working relationship.

Consider the interview a type of contract between you and your patient. The contract consists of spoken and unspoken language and addresses what the patient needs and expects from the healthcare visit. The patient interview consists of three stages: the initiation or introduction, the body, and the closing.

Preparing the Appropriate Environment

- *Ensure privacy:* Make sure the room you use is unoccupied for the entire time allowed for the interview. The patient needs to feel sure that no one can overhear the conversation or interrupt.
- *Prevent interruptions:* Inform your co-workers of the interview and ask them not to interrupt you during this time. You need to concentrate on the patient and establish rapport. An interruption can destroy in seconds what you have spent many minutes building up.
- *Prepare comfortable surroundings:* Conducting the interview in comfortable surroundings reduces the patient's anxiety. Keep the distance between you and the patient at arm's length. Arrange chairs so that you and the patient are comfortably seated at eye level and the desk or table does not act as a barrier between you.
- *Take **judicious** notes:* Note taking should be kept to a minimum while you try to focus your attention on the person. Note taking during the interview has disadvantages, such as breaking eye contact and shifting your attention away from the patient, which diminishes the patient's sense of importance. However, it is important to write down pertinent details as you are interviewing, because you may forget important facts if you do not note them at the time of the discussion. With experience, you will develop a personal type of shorthand that you can use during the interview process. If using an EHR medical history template, efficiently open boxes and choose the appropriate data, maintaining eye contact and using active listening techniques periodically throughout the interview.

The initiation of the interview is the time to introduce yourself, to identify the patient, and to determine the purpose of the interview (Fig. 6.5). If you are nervous about how to begin, remember to keep it short. The patient probably is nervous, too, and is anxious to get started. Address the patient by his or her last name and give the reason for the interview – for example, "Mr. Coleman, my name is Stacey, and I am a certified medical assistant who works with Dr. Perez. I have some questions to ask you about your health history."

After the brief introduction, move on to the body of the interview. This is when you use various therapeutic communication techniques to determine the following:

- The reason the patient is seeking healthcare
- The patient's perception of the problem
- The characteristics of the problem
- The patient's expectations of care

During this time, use active listening skills, meaningful silence, congruent verbal and nonverbal communication, and a combination of open-ended and closed-ended statements and questions to gather the details of the patient's history and current health problem (Table 6.2).

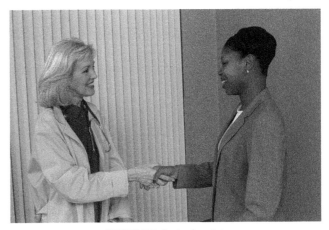

FIGURE 6.5 Greeting the patient.

TABLE 6.2   Therapeutic Communication Techniques

TECHNIQUE	VALUE
Open-ended questions and statements	Encourage the patient to respond in more detail
Direct or closed-ended questions	Ask for specific information; usual reply is yes or no
Active listening	Nonverbally communicates your interest in the patient
Silence	Nonverbally communicates your acceptance of the patient and willingness to wait until the patient is ready to answer
Establishing guidelines	Informs the patient of what to expect during the interview
Acknowledgment	Shows the importance of the patient's role and respect for autonomy
Restating	Checks your interpretation of the patient's message for validation
Reflecting	Shows the patient your acknowledgment of his or her feelings
Summarizing	Helps the patient separate relevant from irrelevant material; provides clarity to the interview

Conclude the interview by summarizing the results of your interaction. The closing of the interview should clarify the patient's chief complaint, the purpose of the visit, and the patient's expectations of care. This is the patient's opportunity to add any additional details or to explain further the characteristics of the health problem.

Interview Barriers

Providing Unwarranted Assurance

Mrs. Miller says to you, "I know this lump is going to turn out to be cancer." The typical reply is almost automatic: "Don't worry, I'm sure everything will be fine." This type of answer indicates that her anxiety is insignificant and denies her the opportunity to further discuss her fears. A reflective response, such as "You sound really worried about …" acknowledges her feelings and demonstrates empathy and a willingness to listen to her concerns.

Giving Advice

Mrs. Thompson has just finished talking to the provider. She looks at you and says, "Dr. Rowe says I need surgery to get rid of these gallstones. I just don't know. What would you do?" If you tell her how you would handle the situation, you may have shifted the accountability for decision making from her to you, and she has not worked out her own solution. Does this woman really want to know what you would do? Probably not. You could respond to her question by saying, "Based on what the doctor told you, what do you think you should do?" or "Do you need further information to make your decision?" If the patient continues to question the provider's recommendations, the medical assistant should encourage further discussion with the provider.

Using Medical Terminology

You must adjust your vocabulary to fit the patient. The more the patient understands what is happening and how to manage the problem, the better the outcome. Misinterpreted communication is the most common error in patient care. One of the biggest problems for the patient is understanding medical terminology. Closely observe the patient's body language while he or she receives instructions or patient education. If the patient shows signs of not understanding the procedure, ask the patient to repeat back to you the information or instructions. This demonstration–return demonstration form of providing feedback ensures that the patient completely understands what is happening. It also gives the medical assistant the opportunity to clarify any misconceptions.

Leading Questions

During the interview, you ask the patient, "You don't smoke, do you?" By asking questions in this manner, you indicate the preferred answer. Telling you that he or she does smoke would surely meet with your disapproval. Keep your questions positive. A better way of asking would be "Have you ever smoked?" or "Do you use tobacco?"

Talking Too Much

Some medical assistants associate helpfulness with verbal overload. The patient may let the interviewer talk at the expense of his or her own need to explain what is wrong. Always remember that when interviewing a patient, you should listen more than you talk. Pay close attention to the patient's body language to make sure you are giving the patient ample opportunity to discuss the health problem.

Defense Mechanisms

Many individuals respond to anxiety-provoking situations by automatically relying on defense mechanisms. Defense mechanisms are used consciously or unconsciously to block an emotionally painful experience. It is understandable that patients facing a traumatic diagnosis or a difficult treatment feel the need to protect themselves from the reality of the situation. Ensuring compliance with treatment becomes an issue if the patient is in denial, projecting feelings onto the healthcare

worker, or repressing the need for treatment or diagnostic follow-up. The medical assistant must be sensitive to patients' use of defense mechanisms. Consistently applying therapeutic communication techniques to interactions with patients will help to overcome the defense mechanisms.

Defense Mechanisms

Patients may use defense mechanisms to protect themselves from a situation they cannot manage psychologically. Defense mechanisms may hide any of a variety of thoughts or feelings: anger, fear, sadness, despair, or helplessness. A patient who uses defense mechanisms can be difficult to deal with. If the medical assistant is aware of the patient's need for psychological protection, he or she may be able to find a way to provide care for the patient while maintaining a therapeutic relationship. For example, Mrs. Alicia Simone, a 48-year-old patient, has just been told she has breast cancer. The following are defense mechanisms she might display to protect herself from the psychological reality of her disease.

- *Denial:* The patient completely rejects the information. Example: "I couldn't possibly have breast cancer. You must be mistaken."
- *Suppression:* The patient is consciously aware of the information or feeling but refuses to admit it. Example: "I don't think the test is accurate. My mammograms are always normal."
- *Reaction formation:* The patient expresses her feelings as the opposite of what she really feels. Example: If she is angry at the medical assistant for insisting that a biopsy be scheduled, she may express the opposite emotion — "I appreciate your trying to help me, but I just can't come to the hospital that day."
- *Projection:* The patient accuses someone else of having the feelings that she has. Example: If the patient is angry about the diagnosis, she may say to the medical assistant, "You don't have to lose your temper about this," even though the medical assistant's demeanor is completely professional.
- *Rationalization:* The patient comes up with various explanations to justify her response. Example: "I think the results are wrong. I didn't follow the directions for the tests like I should have, and besides, there's no history of breast cancer in my family."
- *Undoing:* The patient tries to reverse a negative feeling by doing something that indicates the opposite feeling. Example: If the patient feels angry and violated about the diagnosis but she finds those feelings unacceptable, she may say, "Don't worry, dear, I'm not upset with you for telling me about this."
- *Regression:* The patient reverts to an old, usually immature behavior to vent her feelings. Example: Perhaps instead of discussing the diagnosis and the need for treatment, she just storms out of the office. Or she may say, "I can't possibly schedule a procedure without discussing this with my mother."
- *Sublimation:* The patient redirects her negative feelings into a socially productive activity. Example: Mrs. Simone eventually becomes an active member of a local support group for women recovering from breast cancer.

CRITICAL THINKING APPLICATION 6.2

Mr. Gonzales, a 48-year-old patient recently diagnosed with hypertension, did not show up today for his follow-up appointment. Chris calls to find out why he failed to keep the appointment, and the patient tells Chris he forgot to come, even though an appointment reminder call was made yesterday. He also tells Chris he has not been taking his medicine and does not understand why it is so important for him and his wife to meet with the dietitian. Is this patient using defense mechanisms? How should Chris respond? What communications skills might promote a therapeutic relationship?

Communication Across the Life Span

The key to effectively communicating with patients is using an age-specific approach. Given the age and developmental level of your patient, how can you best interact with the person and with significant family members?

For example, Tasha, a 2-year-old patient, is scheduled for a physical examination. How can you best interact with her and her father to ensure that the history phase of the visit is complete and accurate? Therapeutic use of nonverbal language is essential to interacting with children of all ages. Getting down on the child's level, establishing eye contact, and using a gentle but firm voice are ways of gaining the child's confidence and cooperation. Children fear the unknown, so explaining all procedures with language that the child understands is important. At the same time, the medical assistant must communicate with the child's caregiver so that he or she can contribute to the intake process (Fig. 6.6). The following are some important guidelines for obtaining the health history of a child:

- Make sure the environment is safe and attractive.
- Do not keep children and their caregivers waiting any longer than necessary because children become anxious and distracted quickly.
- Do not offer a choice unless the child can truly make one. If part of the treatment requires an injection, asking the child whether she would like her shot now is most likely to get an automatic "No!" However, giving her a choice of stickers after the injection is appropriate.
- Praising the child during the examination helps reduce anxiety and boosts self-esteem. When possible, direct questions to the child so that he or she feels like part of the process.

- Involving the child in the examination by permitting him or her to manipulate the equipment may help relieve anxiety. If possible, use your imagination and make a game of the assessment or the procedure.
- A typical defense mechanism seen in sick or anxious children is regression. The child may refuse to leave the mother's lap or may want to hold a favorite toy during the procedure as a comfort measure. Look for signs of anxiety, such as thumb sucking or rocking during the assessment, and encourage caregivers to be involved in the process to help make the child feel as safe as possible.
- Listen to parents' concerns and respond truthfully to questions (Fig. 6.7).

Older children may also have difficulty during the health visit (Fig. 6.8). To help school-aged children gain a sense of control, give them the opportunity to make certain decisions about treatment. For example, Heather, a 13-year-old patient with diabetes, could be given the choice of having her father present during the visit. Or if she requires an insulin injection, she could choose the site of the injection or perhaps administer the medication herself. This gives the medical assistant an opportunity to observe her technique and allows Heather to exert her independence.

Privacy is an important issue to consider with older children, especially adolescents. During the physical examination, respect privacy

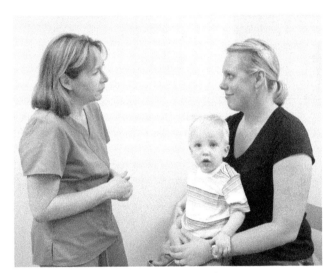

FIGURE 6.7 Responding to parental concerns.

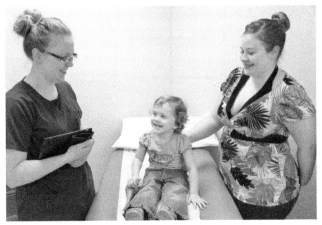

FIGURE 6.6 Interacting with a parent and child.

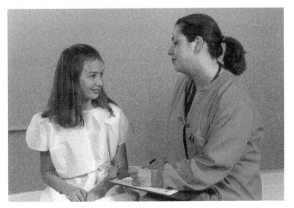

FIGURE 6.8 Interacting with a school-aged child.

by keeping body exposure to a minimum and adequately preparing the child for procedures and positions. In addition, older children want to know what is going on during the examination, what to expect, and what the findings mean; therefore, keeping them informed in a language they can understand is important. Teen patients should always be encouraged to ask questions, which should be answered as completely and clearly as possible. Take every opportunity to teach your patients, regardless of their age, about their disease and to share information about significant wellness factors.

Patient education is extremely important when interacting with adult patients. Using language that the adult patient understands and involving the patient in treatment decisions as much as possible are essential to developing a helping relationship with your older patients. Adults are bombarded by multiple responsibilities, which means that stress-related health problems are not unusual in these patients. Get to know your adult patients and emphasize preventive healthcare when possible.

CRITICAL THINKING APPLICATION   6.3

Toby Anderson, a 52-year-old, was recently diagnosed with hypertension and prescribed Lotensin twice a day for treatment. He is being seen today for follow-up measurement of his blood pressure. Mr. Anderson is 45 pounds overweight and was given information about a reduced-calorie, low-sodium diet 1 month ago, but he has not lost any weight. He tells Chris that he has been having side effects from the medication. He is sitting with his arms across his chest, tapping his foot and occasionally cracking his knuckles. Communication factors Chris should consider include the following:

- What nonverbal language is Mr. Anderson using, and how should Chris interpret it?
- Mr. Anderson tells Chris he is not following "that crazy diet" and never will. What therapeutic communication skills can Chris use to get more information out of Mr. Anderson and to reinforce the provider's recommendations?
- During the discussion, Mr. Anderson tells Chris he stopped taking the Lotensin because of the side effects. What communication techniques and therapeutic body language can Chris use to emphasize the need for Mr. Anderson to take his medicine as prescribed?

ASSESSING THE PATIENT

After the interview is complete, the patient is escorted to an examination room and prepared for the physical examination. During the examination, the healthcare provider methodically checks all the body's systems. For each system, the provider mentally compares the system with established norms. Normal and abnormal findings are documented in the patient's health record. The physical examination typically starts with the head and progresses downward to the feet. However, the order may vary, depending on the provider's specialty.

Signs and Symptoms

All the signs and symptoms are documented in the health record. To better understand the examination procedure, the medical assistant must know the difference between a sign and a symptom.

Subjective findings, or **symptoms,** are perceptible only to the patient; they are what the patient feels and can be interpreted only by the

patient. For example, only the patient experiences and can describe his or her discomfort, pain, nausea, or dizziness. Symptoms of the greatest significance in identifying a disease are called *cardinal symptoms.* For example, crushing chest pain and difficulty breathing are cardinal symptoms of a possible heart attack.

Assessing Pain

Pain is difficult to assess. We typically rely on the patient's report of symptoms to determine his or her level of pain. Some questions you can ask to evaluate the patient's perception of pain are as follows:

- Where is the pain located? Is it associated with any particular movement?
- Can you describe how it feels? Is it constant or intermittent? Does anything relieve the pain?
- When was the onset of the pain? Did something cause the pain to start?
- Are you taking any medication to relieve the pain? What is it, and how often are you taking it? Is it effective? When was your last dose?
- Does pain affect your daily activities?
- On a scale of 1 to 10, with 10 being the highest level of pain, where would you rate your pain (Fig. 6.9)?

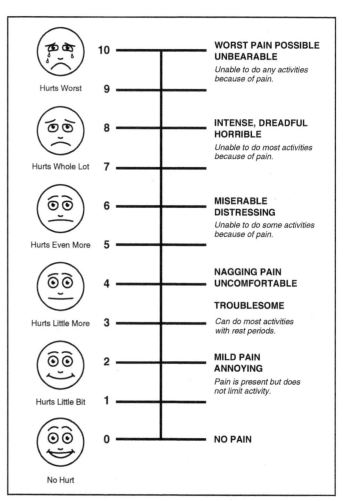

FIGURE 6.9 Wong-Baker faces pain scale.

Objective findings, or **signs**, can be observed or measured by the provider or medical assistant. They are the indicators of health or disease that a provider detects when examining a patient. The provider feels, sees, hears, or measures the signs that often are associated with a certain disease or abnormal condition. For example, a mass that a provider palpates, or feels, in the patient's abdomen is an objective finding and a sign of an abnormal condition. In addition, objective data can be measured and recorded, and repeat measurements can be taken to confirm the presence of or changes in the sign. The patient's temperature, pulse, respirations, and blood pressure are objective signs the medical assistant measures and regularly records.

DOCUMENTATION

Various methods can be used for documentation, depending on the healthcare provider's preference or the facility's EHR system. However, certain documentation procedures have been standardized to meet the legal requirements for maintaining medical records accurately and concisely. Complete, accurate documentation is one of the primary responsibilities of a medical assistant.

Documentation Guidelines

- Check the name on the record and make sure the information being documented is recorded on the correct form in the correct patient's health record or, with an EHR system, that the correct information is recorded using the correct system prompts. Confirm the patient's identity by checking his or her birth date.
- The month, day, and year must precede the entry; many facilities also require the time of the documentation.
- All unusual complaints, symptoms, or reactions must be noted in detail. Include complete information about the onset (when the problem started), duration (how long episodes last), and frequency (how often episodes occur) of each reported sign and symptom.
  Example: Pt reports night cough, which started 2 days ago, lasts approximately 10 minutes, and occurs 3–4 times per night.
- Describe objective data, such as the presence of a wound, using correct anatomic medical terminology.
  Example: Observed wound on left distal anterior leg approximately 2 cm long and 1 cm wide.
- If the patient reports pain, record the quality and intensity of the pain using a pain scale of 1 to 10.
  Example: Pt c/o dull pain at wound site, a 4 on a scale of 1–10.
- If the patient's comments are entered in the patient's own words, enclose them in quotation marks.
  Example: Pt states, "I fell against a stone foundation while cutting the grass and slashed my leg."
- Document the complete medication history, including both prescription and OTC medications taken on a regular basis, the last dose taken of the medication, its effectiveness, and any other pertinent details.
  Example: Pt reports taking 2 ibuprofen tablets for pain with moderate relief; last dose taken 45 minutes ago.
- Record details about the previous history of the current CC.
  Example: Pt reports having a similar cough 3 weeks ago.
- When entering information in the medical record, sign the entry, including the appropriate initials after your name (e.g., CMA).
- Learn to be observant and to note anything that seems pertinent.
- Use accurate abbreviations, symbols, and terminology (Table 6.3).
- Review your documentation immediately after completion so that you can detect errors while the information is fresh in your mind.
- The electronic record system will automatically track any corrections made to the original documentation entry.

TABLE 6.3   Medical Abbreviations

ABBREVIATION	DEFINITION	ABBREVIATION	DEFINITION
abd	abdomen	BOM	bilateral otitis media
ABG	arterial blood gases	BP	blood pressure
ac	before eating	BUN	blood urea nitrogen
ACLS	advanced cardiac life support	bx	biopsy
ad lib	as desired	c̄	with
AFP	alpha-fetoprotein	C&S	culture and sensitivity
AKA	above the knee amputation	CA	cancer
ASAP	as soon as possible	CABG	coronary artery bypass graft
ASHD	atherosclerotic heart disease	CAD	coronary artery disease
BE	barium enema	CBC	complete blood count
bid	twice a day	CC	chief complaint
BM	bowel movement	CHF	congestive heart failure
BMR	basal metabolic rate	CHO	carbohydrate

Continued

TABLE 6.3   Medical Abbreviations—*continued*

ABBREVIATION	DEFINITION	ABBREVIATION	DEFINITION
CNS	central nervous system	Hx	history
c/o	complains of	I&D	incision and drainage
COPD	chronic obstructive pulmonary disease	I&O	intake and output
CPK	creatinine phosphokinase	IG	immunoglobulin
CPR	cardiopulmonary resuscitation	lytes	electrolytes
CSF	cerebrospinal fluid	MI	myocardial infarction
CT	computed tomography	NG	nasogastric
CVA	cerebrovascular accident	NKA	no known allergies
CXR	chest x-ray	NPO	nothing by mouth
DAT	diet as tolerated	N/V	nausea and vomiting
dc	discontinue	p	after
D&C	dilation and curettage	PE	pulmonary embolism
DDx	differential diagnosis	prn	as needed
DM	diabetes mellitus	pt	patient
DNR	do not resuscitate	PE	physical examination
DVT	deep vein thrombosis	PT	physical therapy
Dx	diagnosis	q	every
ECG	electrocardiogram	RBC	red blood cells
EENT	eyes, ears, nose, throat	R/O	rule out
FBS	fasting blood sugar	ROM	range of motion
f/u	follow up	R/T	related to
FUO	fever of unknown origin	Rx	treatment
fx	fracture	$\overline{s}$	without
GC	gonorrhea	SOB	shortness of breath
GI	gastrointestinal	s/s	signs and symptoms
GTT	glucose tolerance test	STI	sexually transmitted infection
GU	genitourinary	STAT	immediately
HCT	hematocrit	Sx	symptoms
Hgb	hemoglobin	Tx	treatment
HIV	human immunodeficiency virus	UA	urinalysis
h/o	history of	URI	upper respiratory infection
HPI	history of present illness	UTI	urinary tract infection
hs	at bedtime or hour of sleep	VS	vital signs
HTN	hypertension	WNL	within normal limits

- If documenting in a paper record:
  - Do all charting in black ink except for noting allergies in red ink; never use pencil.
  - Write in a clear, legible manner.
  - Do not leave any blank spaces on the paper record, and do not skip lines between documentation entries.
  - Never scribble, erase, or use whiteout on an error. For legal purposes, it is crucial that the corrected error be readable.
  - Correct the error by drawing one line through it. Write "error" above the corrected word or words and date and initial the correction. Then write in the correction.
  - If details are omitted, add information by documenting after the last entry. Record "late entry," include date and time of note, and document the omitted information.

PHYSICAL EXAMINATION

The purpose of a physical examination is to determine the patient's overall state of well-being. All major organs and body systems are checked during a physical examination. As the provider examines the entire body, he or she interprets the findings. By the time the examination has been completed, the provider has formed an initial diagnosis of the patient's condition. Often laboratory and other diagnostic tests are ordered to supplement the provider's clinical diagnosis. The results of these tests are used to do the following:

- Refine the patient's diagnosis
- Help the provider plan or revise treatment for the patient
- Evaluate and maintain current drug therapy
- Determine the patient's progress

Before the examination, the medical assistant has the opportunity to make sure the patient feels comfortable during the examination process and that all the necessary medical information has been obtained. The medical assistant's duties include preparing and maintaining the examination room and equipment, preparing the patient, and assisting the provider during the physical examination.

Preparing the Examination Room

The medical assistant is responsible for making sure the examination room is ready for any procedure that might be performed during the physical examination. The area should be as comfortable as possible for the patient and free of any potential dangers, such as contaminated equipment or unlocked drug cabinets. You should prepare the examination room as follows:

- Check the area at the beginning of each day and between patients to make sure it is completely stocked with equipment and supplies and that all equipment is functioning properly. You must understand how to take care of and operate all equipment and instruments, and you should refer to operation manuals supplied by manufacturers as needed.
- Regularly check expiration dates on all packages and supplies; discard expired materials.
- Make sure the room is private, well lit, and at a comfortable temperature for the patient during the physical examination.

- Clean and disinfect the area daily and between patients to prevent the spread of infection and to ensure patients' comfort. When the patient leaves the room, discard the used exam table paper. Using disinfectant wipes, clean the table and any other potentially contaminated surface. When the table dries, replace the exam table paper.
- Arrange drapes, gowns, and all other patient supplies before the patient enters the room so that they are ready for use.
- To save time, prepare the instruments and equipment needed for the examination, arranging them for easy access, before the provider enters the room.
- Make sure the examination room has all materials required for observing Standard Precautions, including gloves, a sink with soap, paper towels, biohazard waste containers, sharps containers, and impervious gowns and face guards. Sharps containers are replaced when they are two-thirds full, as indicated by Standard Precautions.

Assisting the Patient

Getting the patient ready for the examination includes taking care of paperwork before the patient enters the examination room and performing related clinical skills.

- Make sure the health record is complete and that any needed consent forms have been signed; document current medications and allergies; identify any medications that need refills. The medical assistant is not responsible for obtaining informed consent, but he or she should review the paperwork to make sure that informed consent forms were reviewed by the provider and that the patient signed the forms.
- Introduce yourself, verify the patient's identity, and address the patient by his or her preferred name, making sure to show respect at all times. Pay close attention to the patient's nonverbal language to make sure he or she understands what to expect.
- Obtain specimens (e.g., urine, blood) if the provider has preordered them or if this practice is part of the office policy.
- Measure and record the patient's height, weight, body mass index (BMI), and vital signs.
- Conduct the initial investigation into the reason for the visit and explain the examination procedure to the patient. Be prepared to answer the patient's questions and ease any fears. If needed, refer the patient's questions to the provider.
- Ask whether the patient needs to empty his or her bladder before the examination, because a full bladder may interfere with the examination and may be uncomfortable for the patient.
- Help the patient physically prepare for the examination. Explain to the patient what clothing should be removed and in what direction to put on the gown (open to the front or to the back, depending on the type of examination); provide a drape to ensure the patient's privacy, and help as needed.
- Assist the patient into and out of various examination positions as needed.
- Throughout this sequence of events, explain what is happening, and consistently maintain the patient's privacy and confidentiality.
- Help the patient with dressing as needed after the examination.

Assisting the Provider

The medical assistant should be prepared to help the provider complete the physical examination as comprehensively and efficiently as possible. During the examination, the provider may expect the medical assistant to do the following:

- Hand him or her instruments and equipment as requested, and provide supplies as needed.
- Alter the position of the light source to better illuminate the area being examined and turn lights on and off during specific phases of the examination.
- Position and drape the patient during different phases of the examination.
- Assist in collecting and properly labeling specimens such as urine, Pap test specimens, and throat cultures.
- Conduct any diagnostic tests preordered by the provider, including hearing and visual screenings.
- Conduct follow-up diagnostic procedures as ordered, including an **electrocardiogram (ECG, EKG)**, urinalysis, and phlebotomy.
- Document patient data in the health record, completing all forms required.
- Schedule postexamination diagnostic procedures, such as mammography, x-ray examination, or colonoscopy.

Supplies and Instruments Needed for the Physical Examination

The instruments typically used during the physical examination are shown in Fig. 6.10. They enable the provider to see, feel, inspect, and listen to parts of the body. All equipment must be in good working order, properly disinfected, and readily available for the provider's use during the examination. The instruments most frequently used for a physical examination are described in Table 6.4. Physical examinations typically are performed from the head to the feet; the instruments are listed in the order in which the provider typically would request them.

PRINCIPLES OF BODY MECHANICS

Medical assistants should use proper body mechanics consistently throughout the work environment when sitting or standing, lifting or carrying objects, pushing or pulling, or transferring patients. Without consistent application of correct anatomic alignment, injuries, especially lower back injuries, easily occur.

Proper body alignment begins with good posture. Maintaining posture requires a combination of muscle efforts. Good posture keeps the spine balanced and aligned while a person is sitting or standing. A person in good body alignment can maintain balance without undue strain on the musculoskeletal system.

When reaching for an object, avoid twisting or turning; instead, move the feet to face the object needed; this prevents undue strain on the lumbar region. Do not cross the legs while sitting because this interferes with circulation to the legs and feet. When sitting, keep the popliteal area (behind the knees) free of the edge of the chair. Pressure in this area interferes with circulation and may damage nerves behind the knees. Do a mental check of your posture regularly. Hold the head erect, the face forward and the chin slightly up, the

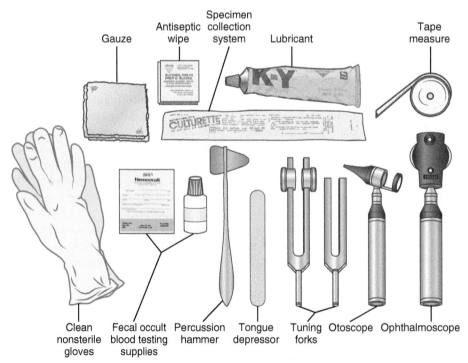

FIGURE 6.10 Instruments for the physical examination.

TABLE 6.4 Instruments Needed for the Physical Examination

INSTRUMENT	USE
Ophthalmoscope	To inspect the inner structures of the eye. It consists of a stainless-steel handle containing batteries and an attached head, which has a light, magnifying lenses, and an opening through which the eye is viewed.
Tongue Depressor	A flat, wooden blade used to hold down the tongue when the throat is examined.
Otoscope	To examine the external auditory canal and tympanic membrane. It has a stainless-steel handle containing batteries or is part of a wall-mounted electrical unit. The head of the otoscope has a light that is focused through a magnifying lens; it should be covered with a disposable ear speculum. The light also may be used to illuminate the nasal passages and throat.
Tuning Fork	Aluminum, fork-shaped instrument that consists of a handle and two prongs (Fig. 6.11). The prongs produce a humming sound when the provider strikes them against his or her hand. Tuning forks are available in different sizes, and each size produces a different pitch level. A tuning fork is used to check the patient's auditory acuity and to test bone vibration. A tuning fork can also be used to test for diabetic **peripheral neuropathy**.
Tape Measure	A flexible ribbon ruler that is usually printed in inches and feet on one side and in centimeters and meters on the reverse side. Measurements may be used to assess length and head circumference in infants, wound size, etc.

Continued

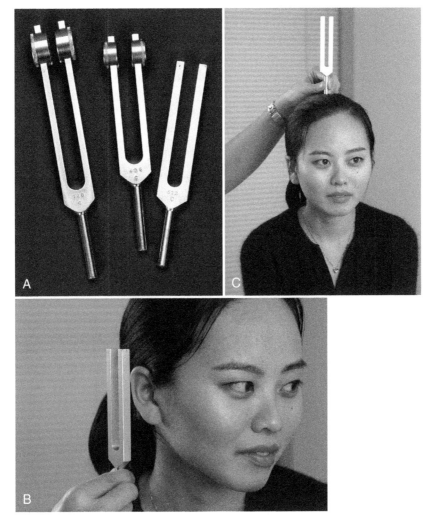

FIGURE 6.11 Tuning forks.

TABLE 6.4	Instruments Needed for the Physical Examination—*continued*
INSTRUMENT	USE
Stethoscope	A listening device used when certain areas of the body are **auscultated**, particularly the heart and lungs. This instrument is available in many shapes and sizes. All have two earpieces that are connected to flexible rubber or vinyl tubing (Fig. 6.12). At the distal end of the tubing is a diaphragm or bell (many have both); when it is placed securely on the patient's skin, it enables the provider to hear internal body sounds.
Reflex Hammer	Sometimes called a percussion hammer. This stainless-steel instrument has a hard rubber head that is used to strike the tendons of the knee and elbow to test the neurologic reflexes.
Gloves	Gloves protect the healthcare worker and the patient from microorganisms. According to Standard Precautions, gloves must be worn whenever the potential exists for contact with any body fluid, broken skin or wounds, or contaminated items.
Additional Supplies	Gauze, cotton balls, cotton-tipped applicators, disposable tissues, specimen containers, fecal occult blood test cards, Pap test supplies for female patients, lubricating jelly for vaginal and rectal examinations, and laboratory request forms should be easily accessible during the examination.

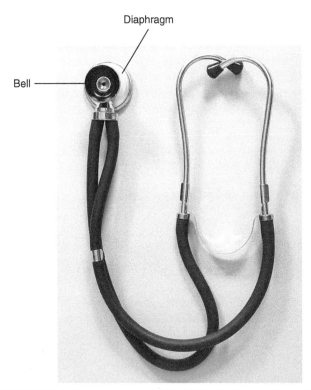

FIGURE 6.12 Stethoscope. (Modified from Ball JW, et al: *Seidel's guide to physical examination,* ed 8, St Louis, 2015, Mosby.)

Safe Lifting Techniques

- Always get help if the load is too heavy.
- Maintain correct body alignment, with the legs spread apart for a broad base of support.
- Do not reach for items; clear barriers out of the way and get as close as possible to what needs to be lifted.
- Bend at the knees with the feet shoulder width apart and keep the back straight. Use the major muscle groups of the arms and legs rather than the weaker ones of the back to help lift a heavy item (see Fig. 6.13).

Transferring a Patient

Patients may need assistance in moving from a chair to the examination table or back again. Patients can be transferred in multiple ways, but all should focus on correct body mechanics. If the patient is in a wheelchair, move the chair at a 45-degree angle toward the footrest that extends from the bottom of the exam table (Fig. 6.15), lock the wheels, and lift the footrests of the wheelchair out of the way. Explain the procedure to the patient and ask for his or her assistance.

If one side of the patient is weaker than the other, always provide support on the weak side. Support the patient close to your body on the strong side, with one hand under the axillary region and the other either grasping the patient's hand or holding the forearm. When bending, always bend at the knees and maintain the back's three natural curves, allowing the leg muscles to help in lifting. Give the patient a signal and lift as the patient assists. Help the patient step up onto the footrest with the strong leg first, then pivot. Ease the

abdominal muscles contracted up and in, the shoulders relaxed and back, the feet pointed forward and slightly apart, and the weight evenly distributed to both legs, with the knees slightly bent. Always be on the alert for poor body mechanics that may cause injury (Figs. 6.13 and 6.14).

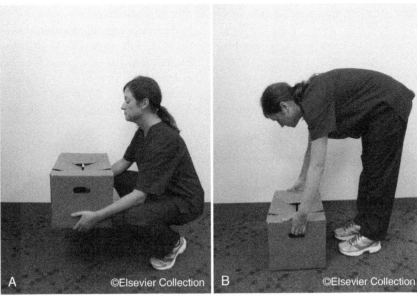

FIGURE 6.13 **(A)** Proper lifting technique. **(B)** Improper lifting technique.

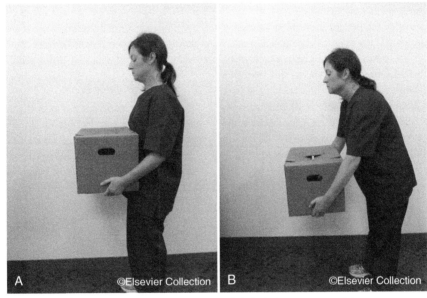

FIGURE 6.14 **(A)** Carrying an item close to the body. **(B)** Improper carrying technique.

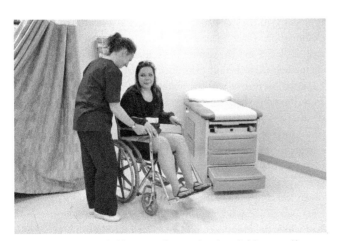

FIGURE 6.15 Wheelchair at a 45-degree angle at the end of the exam table.

patient down onto the table, bending your knees while keeping your back aligned. Make sure the patient is comfortable and safely positioned on the table.

Use a gait belt as needed to help transfer patients, prevent injury to yourself, and safeguard patients from falling. A gait belt is a safety device that is used to help transfer a patient from a wheelchair to the exam table or to help a patient walk. The gait belt helps you support the patient while keeping your body in proper alignment to prevent back injuries. A gait belt should be used if the patient is weak and at risk of falling. Follow these steps to use a gait belt:

- Place the belt around the individual's waist over clothing with the buckle in front.
- Insert the belt through the teeth of the buckle and pull it tight to lock it.

- The belt should be tight, with just enough room to place your fingers under it.
- Grip the belt tightly, bend your knees, and keep your back straight.
- Ask the patient to assist you; then lift, using your arm and leg muscles.
- Avoid twisting or turning as you help the patient stand.
- Keep your body close to the patient with your knees in front of his or hers at all times to stabilize the patient and prevent falls.
- Complete the transfer without bending or twisting your body; encourage the patient to bear as much weight as possible and to gently sit down on the table.
- After transferring the patient, remove the gait belt for the provider's examination, and replace it to help transfer the patient back to the wheelchair after the provider is finished.
- If the patient should start to fall during a transfer, do not try to stop the fall because you may be injured; use the gait belt to help guide the patient to the floor as gently as possible.

You may need to remain with the patient until the examination has been completed to ensure his or her safety. If the provider prefers that the patient be in a supine position, place one arm across the patient's shoulders and the other under the knees, and smoothly lower the patient's upper body to the table while raising the legs. Use the same pivoting techniques with proper body mechanics to help transfer the patient from the examination table back to the locked wheelchair. If the patient must hold onto you, have the person hold your waist or shoulders, not your neck (see Procedure 6.3, p. 164).

ASSISTING WITH THE PHYSICAL EXAMINATION

Positioning and Draping the Patient for the Physical Examination

Various patient positions are used to facilitate a physical examination. The medical assistant instructs the patient and assists the patient into these positions, ensuring as much ease and modesty as possible. The medical assistant may also help the patient maintain the position during the examination with as little discomfort as possible. Do not place a patient into a position that is uncomfortable or that compromises the patient's privacy until it is necessary to complete that part of the examination. Never leave the patient's side if he or she is in a position that could result in a fall.

Draping the patient with a sheet protects the individual from embarrassment and keeps the patient warm. However, the sheet must be positioned so that it allows complete visibility for the examiner and does not interfere with the examination. During the general examination, each part of the body is exposed one portion at a time. For gynecologic and rectal examinations, the sheet is positioned on the diagonal across the patient, or in a diamond shape, to provide maximum comfort for the patient while allowing the provider to perform the examination.

The following sections describe a number of the positions used during medical examinations.

Fowler Position

In the Fowler position, the patient sits on the examination table with the head of the table elevated 90 degrees. This position is useful for examinations and treatments of the head, neck, and chest, and for patients who have difficulty breathing while lying down. Drape placement varies, depending on the type of physical examination done and the need to maintain the patient's modesty (see Procedure 6.4, p. 165).

Semi-Fowler Position

The semi-Fowler position is a modification of the Fowler position. The head of the table is positioned at a 45-degree angle instead of at a full 90-degree angle. This position is useful for postoperative examinations, for patients with breathing disorders, and for patients suffering from head **trauma** or pain (see Procedure 6.4). The drape or gown should cover the entire patient from the nipple line down.

Supine (Horizontal Recumbent) Position

In the supine position, the patient lies flat with the face upward and the lower legs supported by the table extension (see Procedure 6.5, p. 166). This position is used for examination of the front of the body, including the heart, breasts, and abdominal organs. The patient's gown should open down the front, and the drape should be placed over any exposed area that is not being examined.

Dorsal Recumbent Position

In the dorsal recumbent position, the patient lies face upward, with the weight distributed primarily to the surface of the back. This is accomplished by flexing the knees so that the feet are flat on the table. This position relieves muscle tension in the abdomen and may be used for examination or inspection of the rectal, vaginal, and **perineal** areas. It may also be used if the patient experiences back discomfort when lying supine. This position can be used for digital examination of the vagina and rectum, but it is not used if an instrument such as a speculum is needed. To ensure the patient's privacy, it is important to keep the patient completely draped, with the drape in a diamond shape, until the provider is present (see Procedure 6.5).

Lithotomy Position

The patient should not be placed in the *lithotomy* position until the provider is in the examination room and is ready for this part of the examination. Place the patient on his or her back with the knees sharply flexed and the arms at the sides or folded over the chest; have the patient slide the buttocks down to the bottom edge of the table. Support the feet in stirrups placed wide apart and somewhat away from the table, with the stirrup arms extended to match the length of the patient's legs. If the heels are too close to the buttocks, the possibility of leg cramps increases, and it is more difficult for the patient to relax the abdominal muscles. Make sure the stirrups are locked in place. Place a drape diagonally over the patient's abdomen and knees. The drape must be long enough to cover the knees and touch the ankles and wide enough to prevent the sides of the thighs from being exposed. The provider lifts the drape away from the pubic area when the examination begins (see Procedure 6.6, p. 167). The lithotomy position is used primarily for vaginal examinations that require the use of a speculum and for Pap tests.

Sims Position

The Sims position is sometimes called the *left lateral position*. The patient is placed on the left side; the left arm and shoulder are drawn back behind the body so that the body's weight is predominantly on the chest. The right arm is flexed upward for support. The left leg is slightly flexed, and the buttocks are pulled to the edge of the table. The right leg is sharply flexed upward. The drape extends diagonally from under the arms to below the knees. The provider can raise a small portion of the sheet from the back of the patient to expose the rectum sufficiently. The remaining portion of the sheet covers the patient's chest area and thighs. This position is used for rectal examinations, for instillation of rectal medication, and for some perineal and pelvic examinations (see Procedure 6.7, p. 168).

Prone Position

In the prone position, the patient lies face down on the table on the ventral surface of the body. This is the opposite of the supine position and is another of the recumbent positions. The drape should cover from the middle of the back to below the knees, with the gown opening in the back (see Procedure 6.8, p. 168). This position is used for examination of the back and for certain surgical procedures.

Knee-Chest Position

For the knee-chest position, the patient rests on the knees and the chest with the head turned to one side. The arms can be placed under the head for support and comfort, or they can be bent and placed at the sides of the table near the head. The thighs are perpendicular to the table and slightly separated. The buttocks extend up into the air, and the back should be straight. The patient will need assistance to assume the knee-chest position correctly. Most patients have difficulty maintaining this position, so they should not be placed into it until it is required. The medical assistant must remain next to the patient for assistance and support the entire time the knee-chest position is needed. If the correct knee-chest position cannot be obtained, the patient may have to be placed in a knee-elbow position. This position puts less strain on the patient and is easier to maintain. These positions are used for proctologic examination and for sigmoid, rectal, and occasionally vaginal examinations. The patient's gown should open in the back, and a fenestrated (opening) drape or a single sheet should be draped diagonally over the patient's back at the sacral area (see Procedure 6.9, p. 169).

Trendelenburg Position

The Trendelenburg position is rarely used in the ambulatory care setting, but it may be needed if a patient has severe hypotension. This position can be achieved only if the examination table separates so that the legs can be elevated higher than the head (Fig. 6.16).

CRITICAL THINKING APPLICATION   **6.4**

Determine the correct patient position and method of gowning and draping for the following examinations:
- Insertion of a rectal suppository
- Annual Papanicolaou (Pap) test
- Examination of the back
- Patient with dyspnea
- Breast examination

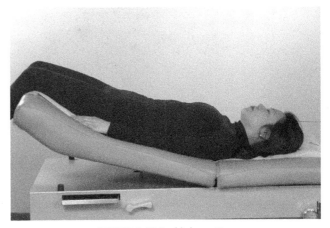

FIGURE 6.16 Trendelenburg position.

Methods of Examination

Examinations are performed as both a routine confirmation of wellness and a means of diagnosing disease. Healthcare providers use six methods to examine the human body:
- Inspection
- **Palpation**
- Percussion
- Auscultation
- Mensuration
- **Manipulation**

All six are part of a complete physical examination.

Inspection

During the *inspection*, the examiner uses observation to detect significant physical features or objective data. This method of examination ranges from focusing on the patient's general appearance (general state of health, including posture, mannerisms, and grooming) to more detailed observations, including body contour, **gait**, **symmetry**, visible injuries and deformities, tremors, rashes, and color changes. Inspection will be done before palpation or percussion so that there will be no changes made to the appearance of the skin.

Palpation

In **palpation**, the examiner uses the sense of touch (Fig. 6.17A). A part of the body is felt with the hand to determine its condition or the condition of an underlying organ. Palpation may involve touching the skin or performing a firmer exploration of the abdomen for underlying masses. With this technique, the provider is assessing the following:

- Temperature
- Vibration
- Consistency
- Form
- Size
- Rigidity
- Elasticity
- Moisture
- Texture
- Position
- Contour

Palpation is performed with one hand, both hands (bimanual), one finger (digital), the fingertips, or the palmar aspect of the hand. A pelvic examination is done bimanually, whereas an anal examination is performed digitally. Do not confuse palpation with *palpitation*, which is a throbbing pulsation felt in the chest.

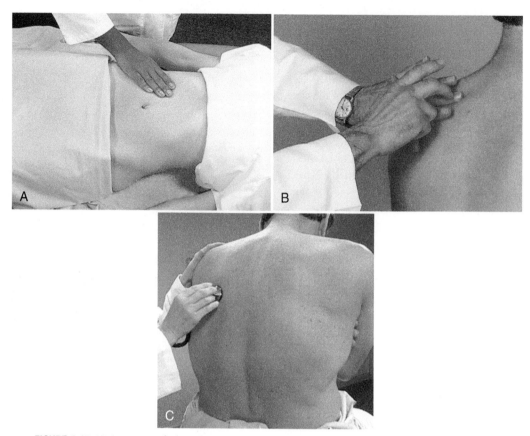

FIGURE 6.17 **(A)** Demonstration of palpation. **(B)** Demonstration of percussion. **(C)** Demonstration of auscultation. (From Ball JW, et al: *Seidel's guide to physical examination,* ed 8, St Louis, 2015, Mosby.)

Percussion

Percussion involves tapping or striking the body, usually with the fingers or a small hammer. This will cause sounds, vibratory sensations, or involuntary reactions. Percussion can help to determine the position, size, and density of an underlying organ or cavity. The examiner both hears and feels the effect of percussion. It is helpful in determining the amount of air or solid matter in an underlying organ or cavity. The two basic methods of percussion are direct percussion and indirect percussion. *Direct percussion* is performed by striking the body with a finger or a reflex hammer. With *indirect percussion*, which is used more frequently, the provider places his or her hand on the area and then strikes the placed hand with a finger of the other hand (see Fig. 6.17B). Both a sound and a sense of vibration are evident. The examiner assesses the sound in terms of pitch, quality, duration, and resonance.

Auscultation

For *auscultation*, the provider uses a stethoscope to listen to sounds from the body. Auscultation is a complex method of examination because the provider must distinguish between a normal sound and an abnormal sound (see Fig. 6.17C). It is particularly useful for evaluating sounds originating in the lungs, heart, and abdomen, such as a **murmur**, a **bruit**, and bowel sounds.

Mensuration

Mensuration is the process of measuring. Measurements that are recorded include the following:

- Height and weight
- Size and depth of a wound
- Extent of **flexion** or **extension** of an extremity
- Size of the uterus during pregnancy
- Pressure of a grip
- Length and diameter of an extremity

Measurements are taken with a flexible tape measure, a circular wound measurement device (Fig. 6.18), or a specialized piece of equipment (e.g., a goniometer, which is used to measure joint angles) and usually are recorded in centimeters.

Manipulation

Manipulation is the passive movement of a joint to determine the range of extension or flexion of a part of the body. Insurance and industrial reports often request this information in detail. For example, a patient involved in a work-related accident that caused joint damage may have to perform assisted range-of-motion (ROM) exercises to the joint, with subsequent measurements of joint flexion and extension to demonstrate improvement or lack thereof.

Examination Sequence

The physical examination sequence is fairly standard; however, variations may occur, depending on the provider's specialty, the reason for the examination, and the provider's preference. Patients are more cooperative and less anxious if they understand what is expected of them. Start by giving the patient a brief explanation of the examination process. Many healthcare facilities provide the option for patients to

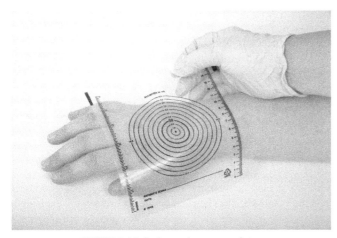

FIGURE 6.18 Circular wound measurement device.

have a chaperone present during physical examinations. Assemble all supplies and instruments needed for the examination before the provider enters the room. As the provider proceeds with the examination, make sure the patient remains unexposed by adjusting the drape and gown as needed. During the examination, the medical assistant assists the provider by handing him or her the correct instruments and needed supplies. When the provider begins the examination, the medical assistant should keep conversation to a minimum and remain **inconspicuous.**

The examination usually starts with the patient seated at the end of the exam table, or in the Fowler position, if the patient needs support. If the provider uses reflected light, the light source should be behind the patient's right shoulder. If illuminated instruments are used, standard overhead lights are sufficient. Take care not to shine a light directly into the patient's eyes; this can be done by turning on lights while they are directed away from the patient and carefully moving the light toward the area.

Chaperones During Physical Examinations

It is becoming common for chaperones to be present during physical examinations. Having a third person in the exam room provides protection for both the patient and the provider. A medical assistant may be asked to be a chaperone.

A chaperone can reassure the patient about the professional character of the healthcare facility. The patient has the right to refuse having a chaperone present in the room, but most are accepting. When the chaperone is another health professional, such as a medical assistant, she or he can serve two purposes: as a chaperone and as an assistant to the provider.

If a healthcare facility is going to have chaperones present, there should be a written policy that describes the role of the chaperone. This policy should allow for a private conversation between the patient and the provider.

General Appearance

The provider starts the physical examination by observing the patient's appearance, using an inspection technique. The general appearance explains whether the patient appears well and in good health (e.g.,

note whether the patient appears disoriented or in distress, well-nourished or undernourished, and answers questions with ease or confusion).

The patient's gait often provides important information. The patient may limp, walk with the feet wide apart, have a shuffle step, or have difficulty maintaining his or her balance. Posture also is checked for indications of pain, stiffness, or difficulty with limb movement. The provider notes body build and proportions. Any *gross* (immediately obvious) deformities are recorded. Sometimes abnormalities in height or body proportion may be caused by hormonal imbalances. If the medical assistant notices any of these or the patient reports any complaints, these should be documented in the patient's health record, along with the vital signs, before the provider begins the examination.

Speech

Speech may reveal a pathologic condition. Some basic speech defects include *aphonia,* the inability to speak because of loss of the voice, which is commonly seen with severe *laryngitis* or overuse of the voice; *aphasia,* the loss of expression by speech or writing because of an injury or disease of the brain; and *dysphasia,* lack of coordination and failure to arrange words in proper order, usually caused by a brain lesion. With *motor aphasia,* the patient knows what he or she wants to say but cannot use muscles properly to speak; for example, this may be noted as slurred or incoherent speech that might occur after a cerebrovascular accident (CVA). In *sensory aphasia,* the patient pronounces words easily but uses them inaccurately, as in jumbled speech. Speech is also assessed in well-child checkups. A delay in speech development can indicate an issue (e.g., a neurologic deficit or possible autism spectrum disorder) and the need for a referral.

Skin

The condition of the skin can be a reflection of the patient's nutritional status and hydration level. If dehydration is suspected, skin **turgor** is checked by pinching the skin on the posterior surface of the hands. The tissue is observed to see how quickly it returns to the normal location. A delay indicates a decrease in tissue fluid, confirming the diagnosis of dehydration. Extreme dryness, scaling, extended time for wound healing, or frequent breaks in the skin may indicate systemic disease.

Fingernails and toenails often give some indication of a person's health. Brittle, grooved, or lined nails may indicate local infection or systemic disease. **Clubbing** of the fingertips is associated with some congenital heart or lung diseases. Spooning of the nail is seen in some patients with severe iron-deficiency anemia. *Beau lines,* deep grooved horizontal lines, appear after an acute illness but grow out and disappear. The provider may refer a patient with skin disorders to a dermatologist for diagnosis and treatment.

Head

Once the provider makes the overall observations of the patient's general condition, the physical examination typically begins with the head and face and moves downward to the feet. The face reflects the patient's state and tells the provider a great deal about how the patient handles stress and illness. The skull, scalp, and face are palpated for size, shape, and symmetry. The distribution or lack of hair and hair texture may indicate hormonal changes. Excessive hair, especially facial hair in females, indicates a hormonal imbalance. As the head is palpated, the provider assesses possible **nodules**, masses, or signs of trauma.

Eyes

The pupils are checked for reaction by shining a light into one eye at a time. If the pupils constrict equally and smoothly to a light stimulus, the provider documents "PERRLA" (which means the pupils are equal, round, react to light, and accommodation). The **sclera** is checked for color, which ranges from white to pale yellow. If the eye is inflamed, it will be evident in the sclera. A sclera with a yellow tone indicates liver disease. Movements of the eyes are tested by having the patient follow the provider's finger. If eye movement is within average range, "extraocular movement (EOM) intact" is documented. The *ophthalmoscope* is used to examine the interior of the eye, including the retina and intraocular vessels. Some diseases, such as diabetes mellitus and hypertension, damage the blood vessels of the retina.

Ears

The ears are examined with an otoscope covered with a disposable speculum. The external ear is checked first for inflammation of the external auditory canal or for *cerumen* (earwax). The *tympanic membrane* (eardrum) is examined and should appear pearly gray. Scars on the eardrum are frequently the result of earlier, chronic ear infections or perforations. The color of the eardrum is important to the diagnosis because it may indicate fluids such as blood or pus behind the eardrum in the middle ear. The patient may be asked to swallow several times to allow observation of movement of the tympanic membrane, which occurs because of pressure changes in the eustachian tube. The eustachian tube equalizes air pressure between the middle ear and the throat. The ability of the tympanic membrane to move is crucial to the hearing process.

Nose and Sinuses

The mucosa of the nasal cavity is examined for color and texture. The sinuses cannot be seen, but the frontal and maxillary sinuses may be examined by firm palpation over the area and by **transillumination**. When disorders of the eyes, ears, nose, and throat are observed, and the provider believes that the condition warrants the attention of a specialist, the patient is referred to an ophthalmologist or an otorhinolaryngologist (ear, nose, and throat specialist).

Mouth and Throat

The mouth, or oral cavity, is usually thought of in terms of oral hygiene and dental care. Dental hygiene includes the condition of the teeth, how the patient cares for the teeth and gums, and whether the teeth of the upper and lower jaws meet properly (occlude) for chewing. Healthy gums are pale pink, glossy, and smooth and do not bleed when pressure from a tongue depressor is applied. The palatine tonsils are usually visible. The provider may use a tongue depressor and a piece of gauze to grasp the tongue to examine it carefully. The floor of the mouth is examined by both inspection and palpation for enlarged lymph nodes, salivary gland function, and ulcerations. The insides of the cheeks and the gum line are also examined for any abnormal marks or color. The provider may use the otoscope light to help with the examination.

Neck

The neck is examined for ROM by having the patient move the head in various directions. The thyroid gland is given special attention for symmetry, size, and texture. The provider manually palpates the thyroid area while the patient swallows several times because this action elevates the thyroid lobes. The carotid artery is palpated and auscultated for possible bruits. The lymph nodes are palpated. *Lymphadenopathy* (enlargement of the lymph nodes) can occur if the patient has an infection of the face, head, or neck.

Chest

While the patient is still in the sitting position, the chest, heart, and lungs are examined. The chest is examined for symmetric expansion. A tape measure may be used, especially if variation exists between the upper and lower chest expansion. A patient with a history of **emphysema** may have a barrel-shaped chest. The provider may use percussion to determine the density of lung tissues.

Placing a stethoscope on the patient's back, the examiner auscultates lung sounds. The patient is asked to take deep, regular breaths. This may produce slight dizziness, but the patient should be assured that it is only the result of the deep respirations and will rapidly pass. The provider notes the types of respirations and the presence of lung sounds in all lobes.

Because considerable concentration is required to interpret heart sounds, the provider must have complete silence when listening to the patient's heart. In patients with heart disease, the provider may spend an extended time listening to heart sounds. If lung or heart abnormalities are found, the provider typically orders further diagnostic tests, including blood analysis, x-ray evaluation, and an ECG. Once the results of these studies have been analyzed, the provider may refer the patient to a *cardiologist* for treatment of a heart condition, or a *pulmonologist* or a respiratory care specialist for treatment of a breathing disorder.

Abdomen

For the abdominal part of the examination, the patient is lowered to the dorsal recumbent or supine position, and the drape is lowered to the pubic hairline. The gown is raised to just under the breasts. The patient's arms may be placed at the side, or the hands may be crossed over the chest or under the head. Relaxation of the abdominal muscles is needed for the abdominal examination. To assist in this goal and to promote patient comfort, a small pillow can be placed under the head and knees. The provider auscultates the abdomen in all quadrants to confirm the presence of complete bowel sounds and palpates the abdomen for any abnormalities. The provider also may use percussion to determine the density, position, and size of underlying abdominal organs.

Reflexes

The patient's reflexes are checked with the patient sitting, in the Fowler position, or supine. While the patient is sitting, the biceps are checked with the patient's arm flexed and supported by the examiner. The knee jerk (patellar reflex) and the ankle jerk (Achilles reflex) are checked using tapotement (a tapping or percussing movement) with either the fingers or the reflex hammer. The plantar reflexes (Babinski reflex and Chaddock reflex) are tested with the patient in an upright or a supine position.

Breasts and Testicles

Careful breast examination is part of the physical examination for every female, even if she is asymptomatic. The breasts are examined both by inspection and by palpation with the patient in the supine position. The arm on the side that is being examined is bent and tucked under the head. Breast cancer is the most common malignancy in women, and early detection is the key to successful treatment. This is a good opportunity to discuss and reinforce the consistent use of monthly breast self-examination (BSE). For male patients who have reached puberty or are 14 years of age or older, the provider performs a testicular examination. The testicular self-examination (TSE) is an important self-examination for all males to perform each month because testicular carcinoma is a major health risk that has a high cure rate if discovered early.

CRITICAL THINKING APPLICATION   **6.5**

Alice Greenbaum, a 68-year-old patient of Dr. Walden, is scheduled for an annual physical examination, including a breast check and Pap test. Mrs. Greenbaum appears anxious and asks Chris whether the gynecologic examination is necessary. How should Chris answer this patient? What might help to ease the patient's fears and prepare her for the examination?

Rectum

The rectal examination usually follows the abdominal examination or may be part of the examination of the genitalia. Preserving the patient's comfort and dignity is vital. For this part of the examination, the provider needs gloves and water-soluble lubricating jelly (e.g., K-Y Jelly). The examination light should be directed at the perineal area during the examination.

Fecal occult blood test specimens are often collected at the time of the digital rectal examination. If this is a procedure the provider performs, be sure to include the necessary collection folder with the examination equipment. Patients diagnosed with gastrointestinal (GI) disorders may be referred to a gastroenterologist. Procedure 6.10 on p. 170 presents the steps for assisting with the physical examination.

CLOSING COMMENTS

Medical assistants play a vital role in the physical examination process. Having good communication skills helps in all aspects of the physical examination. Being familiar with the supplies needed and making sure that they are available in the examination room makes the process more efficient. Using good body mechanics helps to protect you and your patient. Using what you have learned in this chapter will help to make you a valued medical assistant.

Patient Coaching

The physical examination process is an excellent time for the medical assistant to assess the need for patient education. This assessment should be performed to identify the best ways to meet the patient's needs. When identifying these needs, consider the following:
- The information the patient needs to know
- How to convey the information so that the patient understands it
- How the patient will use the information
- Whether any community resources are available that might help the patient understand and learn more about health problems or treatment protocols

Develop a plan to teach the patient. Think about the different modalities available, such as pamphlets, pictures, DVDs, demonstrations, websites, and community resources. The more interesting the information, the more fun it is to teach the patient and the more enjoyment the patient will get out of learning. Many facilities keep patient education files that contain handouts on a wide range of health issues. The medical assistant should always review teaching plans with the provider and follow the provider's direction in patient education.

Legal and Ethical Issues

The medical history is a confidential record that can be shared only with healthcare personnel directly involved in the patient's care. Data provided to you by the patient or that you read in the patient's health record are confidential; you must not share any of this information with anyone. The consequences for disclosing private information to individuals not involved in the patient's care can be very serious and can result in the loss of your job, court-imposed fines, and even imprisonment.

In addition to maintaining patient confidentiality, consistently implementing correct documentation procedures is crucial for medical practices. The medical record is considered a legal document, and court cases can be won or lost based on the clarity and completeness of staff documentation. It is essential that medical assistants document all patient information in a factual, nonjudgmental manner.

Patient-Centered Care

The ability to communicate effectively is crucial to the role of the professional medical assistant and allows for excellent customer service. Effective communication includes the use of all of the therapeutic tools discussed in this chapter. The professional medical assistant should do the following:
- Watch for nonverbal behaviors to verify congruence between what the patient states verbally and demonstrates via body language.
- Modify communication methods as needed to meet the needs of a diverse patient population.
- Use restatement, reflection, and clarification to gather pertinent and comprehensive patient information.
- Use electronic communication appropriately and effectively.

Professional Behaviors

Courteous and respectful care is the hallmark of professional medical assistant behavior. Many times, the physical examination process requires patients to expose very private parts of their bodies, which can make them feel quite uncomfortable. Safeguarding the patient's privacy as much as possible with adequate gowning and draping helps prevent undue exposure and embarrassment for patients during the examination process. Treating patients with thoughtful consideration goes a long way in making them feel more comfortable with physical examination procedures.

SUMMARY OF SCENARIO

Chris has met with the office supervisor and reviewed essential techniques for gathering patient information. Therapeutic communication includes demonstrating respectful patient care, using active listening skills, observing nonverbal behaviors, and using a combination of both open-ended and closed-ended questions to gather the best possible detail about the patient's chief complaint. The supervisor gave Chris a variety of information on meeting the needs of a diverse patient population and also gave him suggestions on how to develop empathetic, helping relationships with patients.

Chris has also taken responsibility for making sure that exam rooms are fully supplied and equipment is in working order. He is able to place patients in all of the appropriate positions during the examination and run the vision and screening tests ordered by the providers. He is also aware of using correct body mechanics when working at the healthcare facility.

SUMMARY OF LEARNING OBJECTIVES

1. **Describe the components of the patient's medical history and how to collect the history information.**

   The medical history consists of the patient's database, past medical history, and family and social histories, in addition to the review of systems. A new patient should fill out a health history form, either online through a patient portal, electronically, or on paper.

2. **Do the following related to understanding and communicating with patients:**

   - *Discuss how to successfully understand and communicate with patients and display sensitivity to diverse populations.*

     Developing a professional helping relationship with patients is the responsibility of all healthcare workers. The helping relationship involves consistent application of respectful patient care that recognizes the impact of a patient's anxieties on interactions and responses to treatment. (See Procedure 6.1.)

     Sensitivity to diverse populations includes the use of empathetic communications and an awareness of the impact of individual value systems and personal prejudices on patient interactions.

   - *Demonstrate therapeutic communication feedback techniques to obtain information when gathering a patient history.*

     The linear communication model illustrates communication as an interactive process between the sender and the receiver of the message, with feedback as a crucial part of the process. Active listening techniques, which include restatement, reflection, and clarification, help the medical assistant go beyond hearing the message to actually listening and appropriately responding to the patient's main point. (Refer to Procedure 6.1.)

   - *Obtain and document patient information.*
     Refer to Procedure 6.1.

   - *Respond to nonverbal communication when interacting with patients.*
     Approximately 90% of patient interactions occur through nonverbal language. The key to successful patient interaction is congruence between verbal and nonverbal messages. (Refer to Procedure 6.2 and Table 6.1.)

   - *Compare open-ended and closed-ended questions.*
     Open-ended questions ask for general information and should be used to begin the interview, to introduce a new section of questions, or wherever the person introduces a new topic. Closed-ended questions are more direct and limit the answer to one or two words, typically yes or no.

3. **Do the following related to the patient interview:**

   - *Discuss the patient interview.*
     The interview should be considered a contract between you and your patient. Ask a variety of open-ended and closed-ended questions and conclude the interview by summarizing the results of your interactions.

   - *Identify barriers to communication and their impact on the patient assessment.*
     Certain communication styles can be misleading or can restrict the patient's response. The medical assistant must be careful to avoid using such faulty techniques as inappropriately providing reassurance, giving advice, using medical terminology without clarification, asking leading questions, and talking too much. These behaviors interfere with the process of gathering complete data during the interview and are obstacles to developing rapport with the patient.

   - *Detect a patient's use of defense mechanisms and the resultant barriers to therapeutic communication.*
     Patients use defense mechanisms to protect themselves in emotionally challenging situations. A medical assistant must consistently apply nonjudgmental therapeutic communication skills to maintain professional relationships.

   - *Demonstrate professional patient interviewing techniques.*
     The patient interview is divided into the introduction, the body, and the summary, or closing. Throughout the interview, the medical assistant should use professional interviewing techniques, such as empathetic patient care, sensitivity to patient diversity, active listening skills, appropriate nonverbal communication, attention to the interview environment, avoidance of communication barriers, and the framing of questions and statements in an open or closed manner, depending on the information needed and the patient's communication behaviors.

4. **Discuss the use of therapeutic communication techniques with patients across the life span.**
   Therapeutic communication techniques vary according to the patient's age and developmental level. A medical assistant should be aware

of how to interact most effectively with various age groups, including young children, adolescents, adults, elderly patients, and family members. Age-specific application of interview styles enables clear communication between the health professional and the patient.

5. **Compare and contrast signs and symptoms.**

   Subjective findings are symptoms; they are perceptible only to the patient. *Objective findings* are *signs;* they can be observed and/or measured by the provider or medical assistant.

6. **Document patient care accurately in the medical record.**

   The ability to document accurately and completely is an essential skill for all medical assistants. Documentation should describe the patient's chief complaint, identify all pertinent signs and symptoms, and demonstrate correct use of medical terminology, with appropriate abbreviations. Any error in the health record must be corrected according to legally approved methods.

7. **Do the following related to the physical examination:**

   - *Outline the medical assistant's role in preparing for the physical examination.*

     Before the examination, the medical assistant has the opportunity to interact with the patient to ensure that he or she feels comfortable during the examination process and that all necessary medical information has been obtained. The medical assistant's duties include preparing and maintaining the examination room and equipment; preparing the patient by conducting the initial interview and measuring vital signs; assisting the provider with positioning and draping; and providing instruments and supplies as needed during the physical examination.

   - *Summarize the instruments and equipment the provider typically uses during a physical examination.*

     Instruments and supplies typically used in a physical examination include ophthalmoscope, otoscope, tongue depressor, reflex hammer, various tuning forks, stethoscope, sphygmomanometer, thermometer, tape measure, scale, examination light, disposable gloves, biohazard container, specimen bottles, laboratory requisitions, fecal occult blood test supplies, patient gown, drapes, and lubricating gel.

8. **Identify the principles of body mechanics and demonstrate proper body mechanics.**

   Proper body alignment begins with good posture. When reaching for an object, avoid twisting or turning; instead, move the feet to face the object needed. Do not cross the legs while sitting, and keep the popliteal area free of the edge of the chair. Hold the head erect, the face forward, and the chin slightly up, the abdominal muscles contracted up and in, the shoulders relaxed and back, the feet pointed forward and slightly apart, and the weight evenly distributed to both legs, with the knees slightly bent.

   Good body mechanics principles include maintaining balanced posture, bending the knees while maintaining the back's three natural curves, and using leg muscles to help lift. Move the wheelchair close to the examination table, lock the wheels, and lift the foot rests of the

wheelchair out of the way. Provide patient support close to your body on the patient's strong side. Place the wheelchair at a 45-degree angle next to the foot rest at the end of the table, and with one hand under the axillary region and the other grasping the patient, help the patient step up onto the foot rest with the strong leg; then help the patient pivot into a sitting position on the table. Use a gait belt as needed to assist in patient transfer. (Refer to Procedure 6.3.)

9. **Outline the basic principles of gowning, positioning, and draping a patient for examination; also, describe how to position and drape a patient in different examining positions while remaining mindful of the patient's privacy and comfort.**

   The patient should be instructed on whether to wear the gown open in the front or the back, depending on the type of examination to be done. The position assumed by the patient during the examination depends on the part of the body to be examined or the procedure to be done.

   Possible patient positions include *Fowler's position,* in which the patient sits straight up, and *semi-Fowler's position,* in which the patient's torso is elevated 45 degrees; the *dorsal recumbent position,* in which the patient lies on the back with the legs bent; the *supine position,* in which the patient lies flat on the back; the *lithotomy position,* in which the patient's buttocks are at the bottom of the table and the legs are positioned in stirrups; the *prone position,* in which the patient lies on the stomach; *Sims position,* in which the patient lies on the left side with the limbs flexed so that the weight of the body is tilted forward; and the *knee-chest position,* in which the patient is on the knees with the buttocks elevated and the weight of the body tilted downward toward the chest. Trendelenburg position, in which the patient's head is lower than the legs, is not typically used in the ambulatory care setting. Draping requires constant attention to maintaining the patient's privacy throughout the examination while assisting the provider with exposure of the area being examined. The general rule is to cover all exposed body parts until the point in the examination when the provider must evaluate that particular area. Procedures 6.4 through 6.9 outline the steps for positioning and draping patients.

10. **Describe the methods of examination and give an example of each one.**

    The examiner uses *inspection* to detect significant physical features, such as the patient's general appearance. With *palpation,* the sense of touch is used to feel the brachial pulse before a blood pressure reading is taken. *Percussion* involves tapping or striking the body to elicit sounds or vibratory sensations, as in percussion of the chest to detect fluid in the lungs. A stethoscope is used to *auscultate* or listen to the lungs and heart. *Mensuration* is the process of measuring the patient's height and weight. *Manipulation* is the passive, assisted movement of a joint to determine the range of extension or flexion.

11. **Outline the sequence of a routine physical examination. Also, prepare for and assist in the physical examination of a patient, correctly completing each step of the procedure in the proper sequence.**

Continued

The examination sequence depends on the type of examination and the provider's preference. The provider typically begins the examination by noting the patient's general health appearance, nutrition status, speech, breath odor, skin condition, and reflexes. The physical examination begins at the head and proceeds down through the body. Any abnormalities are noted and may be further investigated with diagnostic tools after the examination has been completed.

Prepare the examination room and the patient; complete the initial patient interview and measure and record vital signs; gather the needed equipment and place it in the order of use; gown and drape the patient as needed; provide patient instruction and check for understanding throughout the process; assist during the examination by handing the provider instruments, managing changes in lighting, collecting samples as ordered, and conducting diagnostic procedures as ordered; assist the patient when the examination is complete, including helping the patient dress, scheduling further diagnostic tests as ordered, and answering the patient's questions. Complete the documentation, disinfect the examination room and equipment, and restock supplies to ready the room for the next patient. Procedure 6.10 presents the steps for assisting with the physical examination.

PROCEDURE 6.1   Obtain and Document Patient Information

Task: Use restatement, reflection, and clarification to obtain patient information and document patient care accurately.

EQUIPMENT and SUPPLIES

- History form or EHR system with the patient history window opened
- If using a paper form, a red pen for recording the patient's allergies and a black pen to meet legal documentation guidelines
- Quiet, private area

Directions: Complete this procedure with another student playing the role of the patient. To make the experience more realistic, choose a student about whom you know very little. To maintain the student's privacy, he or she does not have to share any confidential information.

PROCEDURAL STEPS

1. Greet the patient. Identify yourself. Verify the patient's identity with full name and date of birth. Explain your role.
   PURPOSE: To make the patient feel comfortable and at ease.
2. Take the patient to a quiet, private area for the interview, and explain why the information is needed.
   PURPOSE: A quiet, private area is necessary to protect confidentiality and prevent interruptions. An informed patient is more cooperative and therefore more likely to provide useful information.
3. Complete the history form by using therapeutic communication techniques, including restatement, reflection, and clarification. Make sure all medical terminology is adequately explained. A self-history may have been mailed to the patient before the visit. If so, review the self-history for completeness.
   PURPOSE: Therapeutic communication techniques help the medical assistant gather complete information; the self-history is designed to save time and to involve the patient in the process.
4. Speak in a pleasant, distinct manner, remembering to maintain eye contact with your patient.
   PURPOSE: Positive nonverbal behaviors create a friendly, caring atmosphere.
5. Remain sensitive to the diverse needs of your patient throughout the interview process.
   PURPOSE: Incorporate awareness of your personal biases into treating all patients with respect despite their diverse backgrounds.
6. Record the following statistical information:
   - Patient's full name, including middle initial
   - Address, including apartment number and ZIP code
   - Marital status
   - Sex (gender)
   - Age and date of birth
   - Telephone numbers for home, cell, and work
   - Insurance information if not already available
   - Employer's name, address, and telephone number
7. Record the following medical history:
   - Chief complaint
   - Present illness
   - Past history
   - Family history
   - Social history
   PURPOSE: The provider needs this information to make an accurate assessment and diagnosis. The provider usually completes the review of systems (ROS) during the preexamination interview.
8. Ask about allergies to drugs and any other substances and record any allergies in red ink on every page of the history form, on the front of the patient record, and on each progress note page; in the EHR, enter allergy information where designated.
   PURPOSE: The presence of an allergy may alter medication and treatment procedures.
9. If using a paper form, record all information legibly and neatly, and spell words correctly. Print rather than writing in cursive. Do not erase, scribble,

PROCEDURE 6.1 Obtain and Document Patient Information—*continued*

or use whiteout. Do not leave any blank spaces or skip lines between documentation entries. If you make an error, draw a single line through the error, write "error" above it, add the correction, and initial and date the entry. If recording the information in the patient's EHR, accurately locate each box; errors in the EHR should be corrected and are automatically tracked within the system.

PURPOSE: To maintain a medical record that is understandable and defensible in a court of law.

10. Thank the patient for cooperating, and direct him or her back to the reception area.

11. Review the record for errors before you pass it to the provider or exit the EHR health history area.

12. Protect the integrity of the health record and the confidentiality of patient information. Safeguards mandated by the Health Insurance Portability and Accountability Act (HIPAA) include the following:
    - Passwords to secure access to all EHRs
    - Computer monitor shields to protect patient information if data are left on the screen
    - Turning monitors away from patient traffic areas to prevent accidental release of information
    - Securing all medical records

    PURPOSE: Patient information may be legally and ethically shared only with a member of the healthcare team who is directly providing care to the patient.

PROCEDURE 6.2 Respond to Nonverbal Communication

Task: Observe the patient and respond appropriately to nonverbal communication.

Scenario: Monique Jones is a new patient with the CC of intermittent abdominal pain with alternating diarrhea and constipation. Ms. Jones has experienced this discomfort for several months and appears frustrated. She is sitting on the end of the exam table with her arms wrapped around her abdomen. She sighs frequently and refuses to maintain eye contact. What is her nonverbal behavior telling you, and how can you establish therapeutic communication with this patient?

EQUIPMENT and SUPPLIES

- Patient's record

Directions: Complete this procedure with another student playing the role of the patient. To make the experience more realistic, choose a student about whom you know very little. To maintain the student's privacy, he or she does not have to share any confidential information.

PROCEDURAL STEPS

1. Greet the patient. Identify yourself. Verify the patient's identity with full name and date of birth. Explain your role.
   PURPOSE: To make the patient feel comfortable and at ease.

2. Ask the patient the purpose of her visit and the onset, duration, and frequency of her symptoms. Pay close attention to her body language to determine whether what she is telling you is congruent with her body language.
   PURPOSE: Nonverbal language naturally expresses the patient's true feelings. Closely observing body language will help you reach more accurate conclusions about the patient's information.

3. Use restatement, reflection, and clarification to gather as much information as possible about the patient's CC. Make sure all medical terminology is adequately explained.
   PURPOSE: Therapeutic communication techniques help the medical assistant gather complete information; using feedback techniques and making sure the patient understands medical terms can help to relieve anxiety.

4. Speak in a pleasant, distinct manner, remembering to maintain eye contact with your patient.
   PURPOSE: Positive nonverbal behaviors create a friendly, caring atmosphere. Remain sensitive to the diverse needs of your patient throughout the interview process.

5. Continue to observe nonverbal patient behaviors, and select the appropriate verbal response to demonstrate your sensitivity to her discomfort, frustration, and anxiety.
   PURPOSE: Displaying sensitivity to and awareness of the patient's nonverbal body language demonstrates your concern for the patient and can help defuse the patient's concerns.

PROCEDURE 6.3 Use Proper Body Mechanics

Task: Safely transfer a patient from a wheelchair to an examination table using proper body mechanics.

EQUIPMENT and SUPPLIES

- Patient's record
- Wheelchair
- Examination table with pull-out footrest
- Gait belt

PROCEDURAL STEPS

1. Wash hands or use hand sanitizer.
   PURPOSE: Hand sanitization is an important step for infection control.
2. Greet the patient. Identify yourself. Verify the patient's identity with full name and date of birth. Explain the procedure to be performed in a manner that the patient understands. Determine how much assistance the patient will need to transfer from the wheelchair to the examination table. Do not proceed if you think you will need additional help.
   PURPOSE: To promote the patient's cooperation during the transfer and prevent personal injury.
3. Place the wheelchair at a 45-degree angle toward the footrest at the base of the examination table (see Fig. 6.15).
4. Lock the brakes on the wheelchair and move the footrests of the wheelchair out of the way (see the following figure).
   PURPOSE: Never transfer a patient into or out of a wheelchair until the brakes are locked on both sides of the chair.

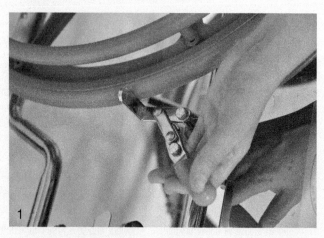

5. Place the gait belt around the patient's waist over clothing with the buckle in front. Insert the belt through the teeth of the buckle and pull it tight to lock it. The belt should be tight with just enough room to place your fingers under it.
6. Request that the patient place both feet flat on the floor with the hands on the armrests.
   PURPOSE: This position helps you grasp the gait belt; the patient can use the wheelchair armrests to help push herself or himself into an upright position, and feet flat on the floor help with patient stability.
7. Stand directly in front of the patient with your feet apart, back straight, and knees bent (see the following figure).

PURPOSE: This position helps you maintain good body mechanics during the transfer.

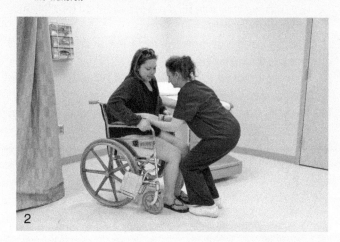

8. Slide your fingers under the gait belt on opposite sides of the patient's waist.
9. Instruct the patient at the count of 3 to push off from the armrests while you at the same time grasp the gait belt and, using your leg muscles, straighten your knees so that the patient is in a standing position.
   PURPOSE: This position allows the patient to assist as much as possible while you are using the large muscles of your legs to help lift the patient.
10. Ask the patient to step up onto the footrest at the bottom of the exam table, and assist the person in pivoting and sitting down on the examination table. Remove the gait belt until the provider has completed the examination (see the following figure).

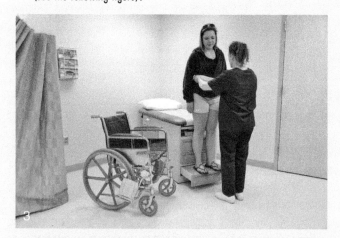

11. After the examination is complete, place the wheelchair at an angle next to the exam table and lock the wheels. Replace the gait belt. Make sure the patient is positioned at the edge of the table.
    PURPOSE: To prepare for transfer back to the wheelchair.
12. Place yourself directly in front of the patient with your back straight and your knees bent. Slide your fingers under the gait belt on opposite sides of the patient's waist.

PROCEDURE 6.3   Use Proper Body Mechanics—*continued*

13. Grasp the gait belt on both sides at the waist. Instruct the patient at the count of 3 to push off from the examination table and, using your leg muscles, straighten your knees so that the patient is in a standing position on the footrest of the examination table.
14. Maintaining your hold on the gait belt, ask the patient to step down. Pivot the person so that she or he can slowly sit in the wheelchair; at the same time, bend your knees but keep your back straight.
15. Remove the gait belt. Replace the wheelchair footrests and unlock the brakes on the wheelchair.

PROCEDURE 6.4   Fowler and Semi-Fowler Positions

Task: Position and drape the patient for examinations of the head, neck, and chest, or position and drape patients who have difficulty breathing when lying flat.

EQUIPMENT and SUPPLIES

- Patient's record
- Examination table
- Table paper
- Patient gown
- Drape
- Disinfectant wipes
- Gloves

PROCEDURAL STEPS

1. Wash hands or use hand sanitizer.
   PURPOSE: Hand sanitization is an important step for infection control.
2. Greet the patient. Identify yourself. Verify the patient's identity with full name and date of birth. Explain the procedure to be performed in a manner that the patient understands. Answer any questions the patient may have about the procedure.
   PURPOSE: To promote the patient's understanding and cooperation during the examination.
3. Give the patient a gown. Explain what clothing must be removed for the examination being done and whether the gown should open in the front or the back. Provide assistance as needed. Give the patient privacy while changing. Knock on the examination room door before reentering to make sure the patient has completed undressing and gowning.
4. For the Fowler position, elevate the head of the bed 90 degrees. Patients who feel more comfortable can sit at the end of the table. Extend the footrest as needed for patient comfort. The patient may be more comfortable in the semi-Fowler position. In this modification of the Fowler position, the head of the table is elevated 45 degrees. The semi-Fowler position may be used for postoperative follow-up or for patients with a fever, head injury, or pain. It also is a comfortable, supportive position for patients with breathing disorders (see Figure 1).

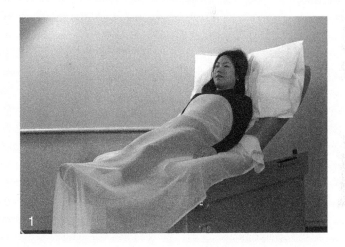

5. Drape the patient according to the type of examination and the required patient exposure.
   PURPOSE: Draping the patient provides warmth and privacy while giving the provider access to the examination site.
6. After the examination has been completed, assist the patient as needed to get off the table and get dressed.
7. Put on gloves and use disinfectant wipes to clean the exam table and all potentially contaminated surfaces. Dispose of used gloves and examination table paper according to facility policies. Pull clean paper over the table.
   PURPOSE: To ensure infection control and to prevent the transmission of pathogens from one patient to another.
8. Wash hands or use hand sanitizer.
9. Follow up with the provider's orders regarding scheduling of diagnostic studies, collection of specimens, or scheduling of future appointments.

PROCEDURE 6.5   Supine (Horizontal Recumbent) and Dorsal Recumbent Positions

Task: Position and drape the patient for examinations of the abdomen, heart, and breasts in the horizontal recumbent (supine) position and exams of the rectal, vaginal, and perineal areas in the dorsal recumbent position.

EQUIPMENT and SUPPLIES

- Patient's record
- Examination table
- Table paper
- Patient gown
- Drape
- Disinfectant wipes
- Gloves

PROCEDURAL STEPS

1. Wash hands or use hand sanitizer.
   <u>PURPOSE:</u> Hand sanitization is an important step for infection control.
2. Greet the patient. Identify yourself. Verify the patient's identity with full name and date of birth. Explain the procedure to be performed in a manner that the patient understands. Answer any questions the patient may have about the procedure.
   <u>PURPOSE:</u> To promote the patient's understanding and cooperation during the examination.
3. Give the patient a gown. Explain the clothing that must be removed for the examination being done and whether the gown should open in the front or in the back. Provide assistance as needed. For the horizontal recumbent position, the gown should be open in the front. Give the patient privacy while changing. Knock on the examination room door before reentering to make sure the patient has completed undressing and gowning.
4. Do not place the patient in the necessary positions until the provider is ready for that part of the examination.
   <u>PURPOSE:</u> To ensure the patient's privacy, comfort, and modesty.
5. Pull out the table extension that supports the patient's legs. For the horizontal recumbent (supine) position, help the patient lie flat on the table with the face upward (see the first of the following figures). For the dorsal recumbent position, have the patient lie flat on the back and flex the knees so the feet are flat on the table (see the second of the following figures). If needed, help the patient move down toward the foot of the table for the examination.

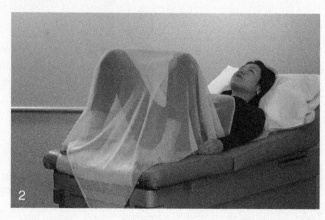

6. Drape the patient from nipple line to feet in the supine position, and diagonally with the point of the drape between the feet for the dorsal recumbent position.
   <u>PURPOSE:</u> Draping the patient provides warmth and privacy while giving the provider access to the examination site.
7. After the examination has been completed, assist the patient as needed to get off the table and get dressed.
8. Put on gloves, and use disinfectant wipes to clean the exam table and all potentially contaminated surfaces. Dispose of used gloves and examination table paper according to facility policies. Pull clean paper over the table.
   <u>PURPOSE:</u> To ensure infection control and to prevent the transmission of pathogens from one patient to another.
9. Wash hands or use hand sanitizer.
10. Follow up with the provider's orders regarding scheduling of diagnostic studies, collection of specimens, or scheduling of future appointments.

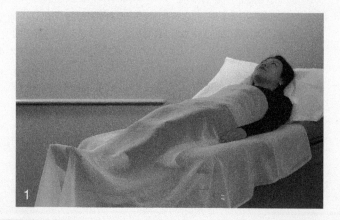

PROCEDURE 6.6 | Lithotomy Position

Task: Position and drape the patient primarily for vaginal and pelvic examinations and Pap tests.

EQUIPMENT and SUPPLIES

- Patient's record
- Examination table
- Table paper
- Patient gown
- Drape
- Disinfectant wipes
- Gloves

PROCEDURAL STEPS

1. Wash hands or use hand sanitizer.
   <u>PURPOSE:</u> Hand sanitization is an important step for infection control.
2. Greet the patient. Identify yourself. Verify the patient's identity with full name and date of birth. Explain the procedure to be performed in a manner that the patient understands. Answer any questions the patient may have about the procedure.
   <u>PURPOSE:</u> To promote the patient's understanding and cooperation during the examination.
3. Give the patient a gown. Instruct the patient to undress from the waist down with the gown open in the back. If the provider also will be doing a breast examination, the patient should undress completely and put on the gown so that it opens in the front. Provide assistance as needed. Give the patient privacy while changing. Knock on the examination room door before reentering to make sure the patient has completed undressing and gowning.
4. Do not place the patient in the lithotomy position until the provider is ready for that part of the examination.
   <u>PURPOSE:</u> To promote the patient's privacy, comfort, and safety.
5. Pull out the table extension that supports the patient's legs, and help the patient lie face upward on the table. Pull out the stirrups, adjust their extension length for the patient's comfort, and lock them in place.
6. Reinsert the table extension, and have the patient move toward the foot of the table with her buttocks on the bottom table edge. Gently place the patient's legs in the stirrups, checking for comfort. Some offices may stock cloth or paper stirrup covers to protect the patient and make the position more comfortable. The patient's arms can be placed alongside the body or across the chest (see Figure 1).

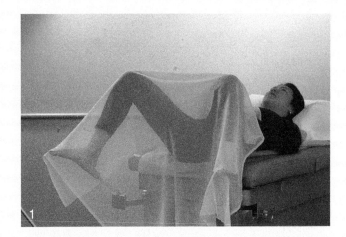

7. Drape the patient diagonally, with the point of the drape between the feet. The drape should be large enough to cover the patient from the nipple line to the ankles and wide enough so the patient's thighs are not exposed.
   <u>PURPOSE:</u> To provide warmth and privacy for the patient while giving the provider access to the examination site.
8. After the examination has been completed, assist the patient as needed to get off the table and get dressed.
9. Put on gloves and use disinfectant wipes to clean the exam table and all potentially contaminated surfaces. Dispose of used gloves and examination table paper according to facility policies. Pull clean paper over the table.
   <u>PURPOSE:</u> To ensure infection control and to prevent the transmission of pathogens from one patient to another.
10. Wash hands or use hand sanitizer.
11. Follow up with the provider's orders regarding scheduling of diagnostic studies, collection of specimens, or scheduling of future appointments.

| PROCEDURE 6.7 | Sims Position |

Task: Position and drape the patient for examination of the rectum, instillation of rectal medication, perineal examination, and some pelvic examinations.

EQUIPMENT and SUPPLIES

- Patient's record
- Examination table
- Patient gown
- Table paper
- Drape
- Disinfectant wipes
- Gloves

PROCEDURAL STEPS

1. Wash hands or use hand sanitizer.
   PURPOSE: Hand sanitization is an important step for infection control.
2. Greet the patient. Identify yourself. Verify the patient's identity with full name and date of birth. Explain the procedure to be performed in a manner that the patient understands. Answer any questions the patient may have about the procedure.
   PURPOSE: To promote the patient's understanding and cooperation during the examination.
3. Give the patient a gown and explain what clothing must be removed for the examination being done. Tell the patient that the gown should open in the back. Provide assistance as needed. Give the patient privacy while changing. Knock on the examination room door before reentering to make sure the patient has completed undressing and gowning.
4. Do not place the patient in the Sims position until the provider is ready for that part of the examination.
   PURPOSE: To promote the patient's privacy, comfort, and safety.
5. Help the patient turn onto the left side; the left arm and shoulder should be drawn back behind the body so that the patient is tilted onto the chest. Flex the right arm upward for support, slightly flex the left leg, and sharply flex the right leg upward. Help the patient move the buttocks to the side edge of the table (see Figure 1).

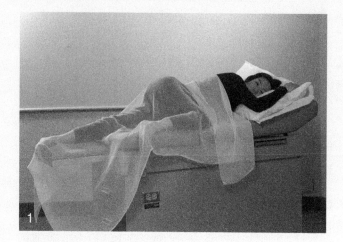

6. Drape the patient diagonally in a diamond shape, with the point of the diamond dropping below the buttocks. Make sure the drape is large enough to prevent exposure of the patient.
   PURPOSE: Draping the patient provides warmth and privacy while giving the provider access to the examination site.
7. After the examination has been completed, assist the patient as needed to get off the table and get dressed.
8. Put on gloves and use disinfectant wipes to clean the exam table and all potentially contaminated surfaces. Dispose of used gloves and examination table paper according to facility policies. Pull clean paper over the table.
   PURPOSE: To ensure infection control and prevent the transmission of pathogens from one patient to another.
9. Wash hands or use hand sanitizer.
10. Follow up with the provider's orders regarding scheduling of diagnostic studies, collection of specimens, or scheduling of future appointments.

| PROCEDURE 6.8 | Prone Position |

Task: Position and drape the patient for examination of the back and for certain surgical procedures.

EQUIPMENT and SUPPLIES

- Patient's record
- Examination table
- Patient gown
- Table paper
- Drape
- Disinfectant wipes
- Gloves

PROCEDURAL STEPS

1. Wash hands or use hand sanitizer.
   PURPOSE: Hand sanitization is an important step for infection control.
2. Greet the patient. Identify yourself. Verify the patient's identity with full name and date of birth. Explain the procedure to be performed in a manner that the patient understands. Answer any questions the patient may have about the procedure.

PROCEDURE 6.8   Prone Position—*continued*

PURPOSE: To promote the patient's understanding and cooperation during the examination.

3. Give the patient a gown, and explain what clothing must be removed for the examination being done. Tell the patient that the gown should open in the back. Provide assistance as needed. Give the patient privacy while changing. Knock on the examination room door before reentering to make sure the patient has completed undressing and gowning.
4. Do not place the patient in the prone position until the provider is ready for that part of the examination.
   PURPOSE: To promote the patient's privacy, comfort, and safety.
5. Pull out the table extension, and help the patient lie down on his or her stomach (see Figure 1).

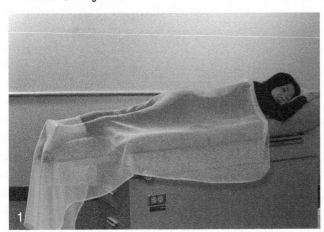

6. Drape the patient over any exposed area that is not included in the examination. For female patients, the drape should be large enough to cover from the breasts to the feet so that the patient is not exposed accidentally if she is asked to roll over.
   PURPOSE: Draping the patient provides warmth and privacy while giving the provider access to the examination site.
7. After the examination has been completed, assist the patient as needed to get off the table and get dressed.
8. Put on gloves and use disinfectant wipes to clean the exam table and all potentially contaminated surfaces. Dispose of used gloves and examination table paper according to facility policies. Pull clean paper over the table.
   PURPOSE: To ensure infection control and to prevent the transmission of pathogens from one patient to another.
9. Wash hands or use hand sanitizer.
10. Follow up with the provider's orders regarding scheduling of diagnostic studies, collection of specimens, or scheduling of future appointments.

PROCEDURE 6.9   Knee-Chest Position

Task: Position and drape the patient for examinations of the back and rectum and for certain surgical procedures.

EQUIPMENT and SUPPLIES

- Patient's record
- Examination table
- Table paper
- Patient gown
- Drape
- Disinfectant wipes
- Gloves

PROCEDURAL STEPS

1. Wash hands or use hand sanitizer.
   PURPOSE: Hand sanitization is an important step for infection control.
2. Greet the patient. Identify yourself. Verify the patient's identity with full name and date of birth. Explain the procedure to be performed in a manner that the patient understands. Answer any questions the patient may have about the procedure.

PURPOSE: To promote the patient's understanding and cooperation during the examination.

3. Give the patient a gown and explain what clothing must be removed for the examination being done. Tell the patient that the gown should open in the back. Provide assistance as needed. Give the patient privacy while changing. Knock on the examination room door before reentering to make sure the patient has completed undressing and gowning.
4. Do not place the patient in the knee-chest position until the provider is ready for that part of the examination.
   PURPOSE: To promote the patient's privacy, comfort, and safety.
5. Pull out the table extension if necessary. Help the patient lie down on his or her back and then turn over into the prone position. Ask the patient to move up onto the knees, spread the knees apart, and lean forward onto the head so that the buttocks are raised. Tell the patient to keep the back straight and turn the face to either side. The patient should rest his or her weight on the chest and shoulders (see Figure 1).

Continued

PROCEDURE 6.9   Knee-Chest Position—*continued*

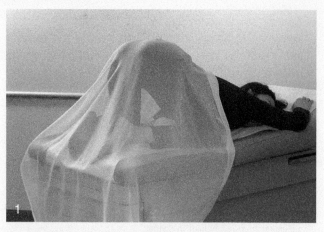

6. If the patient has difficulty maintaining this position, an alternative is to place weight on bent elbows with the head off the table.
7. Drape the patient diagonally so that the point of the drape is on the table between the legs.

PURPOSE: Draping the patient provides warmth and privacy while giving the provider access to the examination site.

8. After the examination has been completed, assist the patient as needed to get off the table and get dressed.
9. Put on gloves and use disinfectant wipes to clean the exam table and all potentially contaminated surfaces. Dispose of used gloves and examination table paper according to facility policies. Pull clean paper over the table.
PURPOSE: To ensure infection control and to prevent the transmission of pathogens from one patient to another.
10. Wash hands or use hand sanitizer.
11. Follow up with the provider's orders regarding scheduling of diagnostic studies, collection of specimens, or scheduling of future appointments.

PROCEDURE 6.10   Assist Provider With a Patient Exam

Task: Aid the provider in the examination of a patient by preparing the patient and the necessary equipment and ensuring the patient's safety and comfort during the examination.

EQUIPMENT and SUPPLIES

- Patient's record
- Stethoscope
- Gauze
- Ophthalmoscope
- Pen light
- Scale with height measurement bar
- Tuning fork
- Tongue depressor
- Biohazard waste container
- Cotton balls
- Examination light
- Laboratory request forms
- Percussion hammer
- Specimen bottles and laboratory requisitions
- Lubricating gel
- Gloves
- Patient gown
- Sphygmomanometer
- Drapes
- Otoscope with disposable speculum
- Thermometer
- Cotton-tipped applicators
- Tape measure
- Fecal occult blood test supplies
- Disinfectant wipes
- Table paper

PROCEDURAL STEPS

1. Check the examination room at the beginning of each day and between patients to make sure it is completely stocked with equipment and supplies and that the equipment functions properly.
PURPOSE: The room must be ready for patient services.
2. Check expiration dates on all packages and supplies regularly, and discard expired materials.
PURPOSE: To ensure the patient's safety.
3. Prepare the examining room before and between patients according to acceptable medical rules of asepsis.
PURPOSE: The room must be aseptically clean to prevent the spread of infection.
4. Wash hands or use hand sanitizer.
PURPOSE: Hand sanitization is an important step for infection control.
5. Locate the instruments for the procedure. Set them out in order of use within reach of the provider and cover them until the provider enters the examination room.
PURPOSE: To promote time management and ensure that all needed equipment and supplies are ready.

PROCEDURE 6.10 | **Assist Provider With a Patient Exam**—*continued*

6. Greet and identify the patient, introduce yourself, and determine whether the patient understands the procedure. If the patient does not, explain what to expect. Refer any unanswered questions to the provider.
   PURPOSE: To promote the patient's understanding and cooperation during the examination.

7. Review the medical history with the patient and investigate the purpose of the visit. Review current medications and document any changes or prescription refills needed. Document the interview results.
   PURPOSE: To verify that all information is current and complete.

8. Measure and record the patient's vital signs, height, weight, and body mass index (BMI). Instruct the patient on how to collect a urine specimen, if ordered, and hand the patient a properly labeled specimen container. Obtain blood samples for any tests ordered.
   PURPOSE: To gather data needed before the examination begins.

9. Hand the patient a gown and drape. Explain what clothes should be removed for the examination and whether the gown should open in the front or the back. Help the patient with undressing as needed (most patients prefer to undress in privacy). Knock on the door before reentering the room to protect the patient's privacy.
   PURPOSE: To assist the patient in preparing for the examination and to safeguard the patient's privacy, comfort, and safety.

10. Assist the patient as needed in sitting at the foot of the examination table; place the drape over the patient's lap and legs. If the patient is an older adult, confused, or feeling faint or dizzy, do not leave him or her alone.
    PURPOSE: To provide for the patient's warmth and privacy and to prevent a fall or injury.

11. Place the patient's paper health record in the designated area, or make sure the computer is ready for the provider to log in and access the patient's electronic health record (EHR). Be careful to safeguard patient confidentiality during this step of the procedure.

12. Assist during the examination by handing the provider instruments as needed and by positioning and draping the patient.

13. When the provider has completed the examination, allow the patient to rest for a moment, then help the patient from the table. Assist with dressing, if necessary. Use proper body mechanics if assistance in transfer is needed.
    PURPOSE: To ensure the patient's stability and safety and to protect yourself from injury.

14. Return to the patient, and ask whether he or she has any questions. Give the patient any final instructions, and schedule tests as ordered by the provider or the next appointment.
    PURPOSE: To clarify instructions, eliminate any misunderstandings, and allow the patient to discuss any concerns. If the patient's misunderstandings or concerns are beyond your scope of experience or skill, arrange for the provider to speak with the patient again.

15. Put on gloves, and dispose of used supplies and linens in designated biohazard waste containers. Dispose of exam table paper. Use disinfectant wipes to clean the examination table and any other potentially contaminated surface. Disinfect all equipment.
    PURPOSE: To prevent cross-contamination with any potential infectious materials.

16. Remove the gloves, discard them in the biohazard waste container, and wash hands or use hand sanitizer.
    PURPOSE: To ensure infection control.

17. Cover the exam table with fresh paper, replace used supplies, and prepare the room for the next patient.

7

PATIENT COACHING

SCENARIO

Suzanne Peterson, CMA (AAMA), has worked for Walden-Martin Family Medicine (WMFM) Clinic for 5 years. Her favorite part of her job is coaching patients on health topics, diagnostic tests, and treatment plans. Her patients know they can contact Suzanne if they have questions between appointments. Suzanne answers the questions she can and also talks with the providers for other questions. She feels that it is very important for patients to understand how to self-manage their conditions and to know when to contact their providers.

Over the years, Suzanne has seen the role of the medical assistant expand. She has learned the importance of screening patients during the initial interview. The information that she enters into the electronic health record is then used to collect data on how well the clinic provides patient care. She has also learned the importance of patient care coordinators. She hopes WMFM Clinic implements a care coordinator program soon.

While studying this chapter, think about the following questions:

- What are basic concepts of teaching and learning? What are the domains of learning? How can a medical assistant adapt coaching to patients?
- What are types of disease prevention coaching?
- What are types of health maintenance coaching?

- What coaching should a medical assistant do for common diagnostic tests?
- What coaching can be done for treatment plans?
- What is the medical assistant's role with coordination of care, navigation, and community resource referrals?

LEARNING OBJECTIVES

1. Describe the medical assistant's role as a coach.
2. List and describe the stages of grief; also, discuss how the health belief model helps to explain what factors influence a person's health beliefs and practices.
3. Describe the three domains of learning.
4. Explain how a medical assistant can adapt coaching to the patient.
5. Describe the teaching-learning process.

6. Discuss how a medical assistant can coach on disease prevention.
7. Describe how a medical assistant can coach on health maintenance and wellness, including different types of self-exams and screenings.
8. Describe how a medical assistant can coach on diagnostic procedures and treatment plans.
9. Describe care coordination and patient navigation, develop a list of community resources, and facilitate referrals.

VOCABULARY

adherence (ad HEER ehns) The act of sticking to something.
anhedonia (an hee DOE nee ah) The inability to feel or experience pleasure during a pleasurable activity.
cessation (se SAY shuhn) Bringing to an end.
compliance (kuhm PLIE ahns) The act of following through on a request or demand. Patient compliance sounds negative, thus patient adherence is now being used.

patient navigator A person who identifies patients' barriers, works closely with the healthcare team and patients, and guides the patients through the healthcare system; may also be called *care coordinator*.

Healthcare is changing, and the role of the medical assistant is changing too. Some of the current challenges in healthcare include the following:

- Pressure to reduce cost
- Shorter primary care provider visits, yet an increased need for data collection to incorporate patient interviews and outcome measurements (e.g., test results)
- Patients leaving the facility not understanding what they were told
- An unwillingness on the part of patients to adhere to treatment plans (e.g., not taking medication or not taking it correctly, not making lifestyle changes that would improve their health)

Many experts have researched ways to reduce these challenges. Several studies have examined patient medication **adherence** or **compliance.** *Medication adherence* means patients are taking the right dose at the right times as prescribed by the provider. Research has shown that medication adherence with chronic diseases is low. This leads to the progression of the disease and more medical visits for the patient. Ultimately, nonadherence to medication is increasing the cost of healthcare.

Why is it that patients do not take their medication correctly? This question has been a focus of many studies. Common reasons include the following:

- Forgetfulness and confusion on how to take it
- Side effects and cost of the medication
- Feeling it is not helping

Research has shown that many patients are confused after seeing their providers. Patients do not always understand the treatment plan designed to manage their conditions. Confusion about medication and home care is prevalent. Many patients are not able to manage their disease adequately between provider visits; thus, their condition worsens. To solve this problem, ambulatory care facilities are moving toward coaching and care coordination. This chapter focuses on the medical assistant's role in coaching and care coordination.

COACHING

Coaching provides patients with skills, knowledge, support, and confidence to manage their disease between provider visits. One study found that coaching by medical assistants increased the patients' compliance with medication regimens and lifestyle changes. Coaching is extremely valuable for patients. The medical assistant can coach patients in many areas, including the following:

- *Disease prevention:* Provide patients with information on preventing the disease or the spread of disease. Medical assistants can provide information on hygiene practices, recommended vaccines, and nicotine **cessation.**
- *Health maintenance:* Provide patients with information on routine screenings and show patients how to do self-exams (e.g., foot, breast, and oral self-exams).
- *Diagnostic tests:* Instruct patients prior to diagnostic tests. This can include special preparation (e.g., fasting and bowel cleansing preparations).
- *Treatment plans:* Instruct patients on home care and follow-up as ordered by the provider. Research has shown that coaching

can help patients understand information from the visit. It can ensure patients understand how they need to proceed and addresses any concerns before patients leave the facility. Coaching educates patients on self-management of diseases, thus increasing compliance with the treatment plans.

- *Specific needs:* Patients have unique concerns. These can include personal, family, social, financial, and culture-related issues. By listening and asking questions, the medical assistant can help address their specific needs. By closely working with the patient, the medical assistant can provide emotional support and create a bond with the patient. This bond helps the patient feel comfortable. With encouragement, the patient may be more willing to call the medical assistant with questions and concerns between visits.
- *Community resources:* By listening to patients and by asking questions, the medical assistant can identify patients' unique needs. Patients have many needs that affect their health. For instance, if a patient has a limited income, does the patient purchase the prescribed medication, or food? Community resources exist to address many needs, including low-cost medications, food banks, transportation, medical supplies, assisted living, and so on.

This chapter provides information on specific aspects of patient education required for these coaching areas. But first, let's examine health beliefs and practices and how to adapt education to patients' needs.

MAKING CHANGES FOR HEALTH

Often, healthcare professionals see patients who do not comply with the treatment plan. They may not take the prescribed medication, or maybe they do not make the recommended lifestyle changes. If the diagnosis is life-threatening or life-changing, grief and loss can occur. Other times, patients may not perceive the change as necessary. The following sections examine theories that may explain why patients do not comply with the treatment plan.

Stages of Grief

Elisabeth Kübler-Ross studied people's reactions to death and dying. She found that people experienced similar stages. Over the years, these stages have been applied to grief and loss. When a patient and the family get a life-threatening or life-changing diagnosis, they can feel grief and loss. People go through the stages of grief in their own way and at their own pace (Table 7.1). This process can take weeks to months. Patients may not be open to making the recommended changes. Healthcare professionals may view this as the patient not wanting to comply with the treatment plan. Sometimes a patient has to accept a diagnosis before compliance occurs. It is important for the medical assistant to adapt interactions to help with the stages of grief.

CRITICAL THINKING APPLICATION   **7.1**

Suzanne has seen many patients dealing with grief. Why might a patient who is grieving not adhere to a treatment plan?

TABLE 7.1   Stages of Grief and Dying

STAGE	DESCRIPTION	ADAPTIVE INTERACTIONS
Denial	Refuses to accept the fact (i.e., diagnosis or prognosis). May refuse to discuss the diagnosis. May not remember the health coaching. Denial is a defense mechanism that allows the person to ignore what is happening.	Provide handouts that explain the disease and treatment. Encourage family member(s)' support with the treatment. Provide online and community resources (i.e., support groups).
Anger	Anger can be directed at self or others. Anger can surface at unrelated times and be directed toward unrelated issues.	Use therapeutic communication techniques (e.g., reflection) to acknowledge the patient's feelings about the issue. Recognize the real cause of the anger.
Bargaining	Attempts to bargain with the higher power the person believes in (i.e., God). Sometimes the patient will bargain with the provider to make lifestyle changes at a later time.	Work with the healthcare team regarding the bargaining requests. Help provide opportunities where the patient can make decisions.
Depression	People feel sadness, fear, and uncertainty. They may grieve the loss of their health or independence. They may dread the change that is occurring.	Encourage the use of community and healthcare resources to help ease the change process for the patient and family members.
Acceptance	Has come to terms with situation.	Provide coaching on aspects of the disease and self-care management.

Health Belief Model

The health belief model helps explain what factors influence a person's health belief and practices. The first part of this model deals with a person's perception of his or her chance of developing a disease. Some examples include the following:

- Jess is in her 20s and has lost her mother, sister, and grandmother to breast cancer. She feels her chance of developing breast cancer is significant.
- Sam has an older brother with heart disease that is being managed by medication, diet, and exercise. Sam blames the disease on his brother's stressful job. Sam does not have a stressful job, so he feels he will not get heart disease. Even

though Sam receives education on a heart-healthy lifestyle, he ignores the information.

The second part of this model deals with a person's perception of the severity of the disease. A person's perception is influenced by the following:

- Personal factors (e.g., age, gender, race, employment)
- Social factors (e.g., peers, personality, family)
- Perceived threats of the disease
- Cues to action (e.g., mass media campaigns, social media, advice from family, friends, and healthcare providers and professionals)

In the prior examples, Jess has lost three family members to breast cancer. She perceives breast cancer as being a severe disease. Sam, on the other hand, may not perceive the severity of heart disease, because his brother's heart disease is being managed.

The third part of the model focuses on whether the person will take preventive action. A person weighs the benefits of and barriers to taking the preventive actions. For example, Jess may decide to have a double mastectomy as a preventive strategy. For many it may seem severe, but for Jess, she is willing to take such a preventive action. Sam, on the other hand, may not see the benefit of following a heart-healthy lifestyle. He may feel that he has to "give up" his current lifestyle and make changes.

Because a medical assistant coaches patients on preventive actions, it is important to remember the model. Start with identifying if the person perceives he or she is at risk for a disease. Exploring the patient's beliefs and educating the patient on the facts, in addition to getting rid of the myths, can be helpful. Discussing the severity of the disease or what the disease can lead to is the next important step. Finally, offering the patient help in eliminating or diminishing the barriers and helping the person see the benefits of the preventive action are important.

CRITICAL THINKING APPLICATION   7.2
Suzanne has had patients state they do not want to give up their lifestyle and follow the provider's recommendations for better health. How might a medical assistant address this issue with a patient?

BASICS OF TEACHING AND LEARNING
Domains of Learning

Learning is the process of gaining new knowledge or skills through instruction, experience, or study. We learn new information in three different ways or *domains*: cognitive, psychomotor, and affective. These domains are discussed in the coming sections.

Cognitive Domain

The *cognitive domain* of learning involves the mental processes of recall, application, and evaluation. We learn new information by listening to what is said and by reading written words. Many experts believe we have three ways to store memories:

- *Sensory stage:* For a memory to be created, we must pick up something from our senses (e.g., touch, hearing, sight). Our senses are constantly picking up perceptions. Many will be forgotten in a split second. We will pay attention to just a few, and they will move to the short-term memory. The deciding factor between what is forgotten and what moves into the short-term memory is based on its importance to us.

- *Short-term memory:* This is our temporary working memory. If nothing is done with the memory, it will fade within 30 seconds. The short-term memory can only handle about seven units of information at once. By chunking information into meaningful units or attaching it to something we already know, we can increase the amount in our short-term memory.
- *Long-term memory:* The more we use short-term memories, the quicker they enter our long-term memory. We can add endless memories to our long-term memory, but without use (recall), those memories can fade.

Our goal for patient education is to put the information into patients' long-term memory. Not everything we tell the patient will be picked up and remembered. We hope the important information will be. The following tips can be used to help patients remember critical information:

- *Present the information at an appropriate level for the patient.* Most studies show that patient education literature should be at a sixth-grade reading level. According to the US National Library of Medicine's website MedlinePlus, patient educational materials should be between a seventh- and eighth-grade reading level. If the patient's primary language is not English, then a lower reading level is needed.
- *Build on the patient's prior knowledge about the topic.* Start by finding out what the patient knows about the topic. Clarify any inaccurate information and then provide new information that builds on the existing knowledge.
- *Present information in small chunks, in a clear well-organized manner.* Do not overwhelm the patient; keep to the facts and keep it simple. For complex topics, meeting with the patient over several days may help the patient to retain the information.
- *Provide the information in two different ways* (e.g., verbally discuss it and provide a written handout) (Fig. 7.1).
- Tell the patient "this is important to remember" and repeat important information several times during the session. Be aware that if everything is "important to remember," nothing will be remembered. Do not overuse this strategy.
- *Have the patient teach back the information you provided.* This allows you to check what the patient recalls and if it is accurate. Teaching back also helps the patient remember the information even more.

Table 7.2 provides strategies to use for the cognitive domain. The *barriers* or reasons learning does not occur effectively are also listed. These barriers are important for the medical assistant to limit if possible.

Psychomotor Domain

The *psychomotor domain* is the "doing" domain. We learn new skills and procedures by watching demonstrations and assisting with something. Many people would prefer to attempt a skill versus reading about it or discussing it. They learn best through the psychomotor domain. Table 7.2 provides some barriers to the psychomotor domain.

Some tips to help patients remember critical information include the following:

- Provide written step-by-step directions for the patient to follow and then take home.

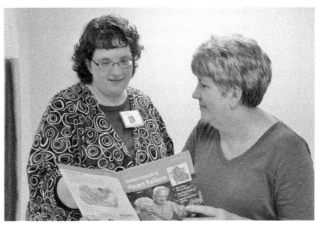

FIGURE 7.1 Provide patients with handouts to take home.

TABLE 7.2	Strategies to Use and Barriers for the Three Domains of Learning			
DOMAIN	INVOLVES	TEACHING STRATEGIES TO USE	BARRIERS TO LEARNING	STRATEGIES TO ADAPT TO BARRIERS
Cognitive	Learning new concepts and information	Discussion, written information, online videos, computer instruction	Memory or cognition issues; language barriers	Keep it simple. Provide easy-to-read handouts. Use an interpreter and provide handouts in the patient's primary language if possible.
Psychomotor	Learning new skill or procedure	Demonstration and return demonstration	Tremors and paralysis; sensory limitations (e.g., visual impairment, hearing impairment)	Use adaptive equipment, such as a magnifying glass and a magnifier for syringes.
Affective	A change in attitude or emotions that will influence the person's behavior	Discussion, role-play, and simulations	Anxiety, denial, pain, fatigue, or stress, cultural customs, previous experience, and poor coping skills	Provide analgesics as ordered by the provider, help to minimize barriers, provide home instructions, and include additional family member(s) if possible.

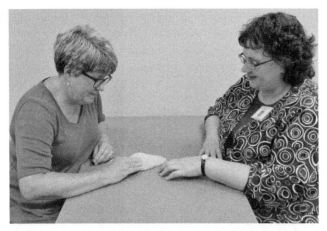

FIGURE 7.2 Having a patient do a return demonstration or "teach back" the skill allows the medical assistant to check the patient's knowledge and skills for accuracy.

- Give timely feedback on the person's performance.
- Have the patient "teach back" the skill to check for accuracy (Fig. 7.2).
- Repeated practice doing the skill helps with recall and retention of the steps.
- Make sure to use the equipment and supplies the patient will be using at home.

Affective Domain

The *affective domain* is the "feeling" domain. It includes our feelings, emotions, values, and attitudes. Our emotions and values are very important. They affect our motivation, confidence, and priorities. When our personal values conflict with the new information presented, a barrier to learning can occur. Pain is another example of an affective barrier. If you are instructing a patient on wound care and he is in pain, he may not remember what you said. Additional barriers to the affective domain are listed in Table 7.2.

Make sure that you address (as much as you can) any affective domain barriers prior to educating a patient. If another family member accompanied the patient, it can be helpful to instruct both the patient and the family member (Fig. 7.3). Written home instructions should also be given.

Adapting Coaching to the Patient

When coaching patients, it is important to recognize that they are individuals. One way of presenting new information to a patient may not work for another patient. It is important for the medical assistant to consider the barriers to learning and possible ways to help the patient overcome those barriers. It is also important for the medical assistant to remember the patient's developmental level and possible cultural diversity issues that may impact learning.

Developmental Level

As we grow and develop, our thought processes and behaviors change. We learn differently. We can understand more complex concepts than when we were younger. It is important for the medical assistant to consider the person's developmental level when coaching. For instance, young children are concrete thinkers. What you say is what they believe you will do. For example, if you say, "I am going to take

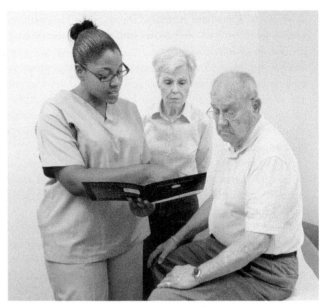

FIGURE 7.3 Teaching the family member along with the patient can provide the patient with more support.

your blood pressure," a 2-year-old child would have no idea what you are going to do. If you say, "I am going to give your arm a hug," then the child may have a better understanding of what you are going to do. Coaching techniques you use for teens will be different from those you use with older adults. Also, referencing materials as you talk can be helpful to the patient.

Erikson's psychosocial developmental stages can be useful when considering the developmental level of patients. Understanding the goal of each stage can help a medical assistant to coach patients in that age group. Table 7.3 provides coaching tips based on the developmental stages.

CRITICAL THINKING APPLICATION   7.3

In the family practice environment, Suzanne sees patients of all ages. Explain why the methods she uses with 2-year-old children should differ from those she uses when working with teens. What strategies could she use when coaching both of these populations?

Cultural Diversity

Culture is the set of behaviors, ideas, and customs shared by a specific group of people, which distinguishes the members from other people. Some characteristics of a culture group may include its language, religious beliefs, geographic origin, ethnicity, history, sexual orientation, and socioeconomic class. Culture can be learned from prior generations and passed on to future generations. It is dynamic and evolving. Our culture frames and shapes how we feel about our health and the world around us. Factors affected by a person's culture that healthcare professionals should consider include the following:

- Role of the family and community: Who makes the healthcare decisions? Who pays for the healthcare? Who needs to be present during healthcare discussions?

TABLE 7.3	Erikson's Psychosocial Development Stages With Coaching Tips	
DEVELOPMENT STAGE	**GOALS OF STAGE**	**COACHING TIPS**
Trust versus mistrust (age range 0–1.5 years [*infancy*])	Must develop trust, with the ability to mistrust should the need arise.	Use a calm, soothing voice, hold child securely. Involve the parent(s) as much as possible. Keep routines consistent as much as possible (if it is time for the infant to eat, allow the child to eat unless eating/drinking is restricted for a medical reason).
Autonomy versus shame and doubt (age range 1.5–3 years [*toddler*])	Must explore and manipulate things in their "world" to develop autonomy and self-esteem.	Use simple, familiar words. Allow child to handle equipment and make choices. Use play to teach the child.
Initiative versus guilt (age range 3–6 years [*preschool*])	Encourage to try new activities. Must assume responsibilities and learn new skills. Will make child feel purposeful and increase self-esteem.	Use familiar words and simple explanations and demonstrations. Allow the child to handle equipment and make choices. Explain a procedure as the child would sense it (e.g., how it feels, looks).
Industry versus inferiority (age range 6–12 years [*school age*])	Must seek to finish tasks. Recognition for accomplishments is important.	Use engaging simple tools to communicate information (videos, gaming software, and pamphlets). Encourage discussion, questions, and making choices. Use concrete terms (with pictures and diagrams) when explaining procedures.
Identity versus role confusion (age range 12–18 years [*adolescence*])	To know whom you are as a person and how you fit into the world around you. Creates a meaningful self-image.	Provide privacy and independence. Encourage responsible decision making. Encourage discussion and questions. Address how a procedure might affect the adolescent's appearance. Promote honest discussion about lifestyle issues.
Intimacy versus isolation (age range 18–25 years [*young adult*])	Can vary. Develops friendships; takes on commitments.	Identify motivating factors. Find out what they know about the topic; correct any inaccuracies. Build on prior information. Listen to their concerns and provide resources as needed.
Generativity versus stagnation (age range about 25–60 years [*middle adulthood*])	Achieve a balance between the concern for the next generation (having a family) and being self-absorbed.	
Ego integrity versus despair (age range 60 or older [*late adulthood*])	Reflect on one's life and come to terms with it instead of regretting the past.	Communicate with dignity and respect. Use simpler language. Speak clearly. Allow time to respond. Find out what they know about the topic; correct any inaccuracies. Build on prior information. Listen to their concerns and provide resources as needed.

- Religion: What are the beliefs about illness? Will the person's religious beliefs affect adherence to the treatment?
- Views on health, wellness, death, and dying
- Views on complementary therapies (e.g., chiropractic care, massage) and *alternative therapies* (other practices used in place of conventional medicine)
- Views on gender roles and relationships
- Beliefs related to food, diet, illness and health
- Beliefs regarding sexuality, fertility, and childbirth

In the United States, disease conditions are seen as more of a scientific situation. Science plays a major role in medicine. Many other cultures take more of a *holistic* approach. A holistic view focuses on the interrelationship among the physical, mental, social, and spiritual aspects of the person's life. A holistic approach is broader than a scientific approach to health and illness.

Many cultures have similar practices, such as:
- *Coining* and *spooning*: Rubbing a silver coin or spoon vigorously on the skin. These practices leave red marks on the skin. Do not confuse the marks with signs of abuse.
- *Cupping*: Applying suction to the skin, which can leave marks. Do not confuse these marks with signs of abuse.
- *Acupressure*: Applying firm pressure on specific points on the body.
- *Acupuncture*: Inserting fine needles into *acupuncture points* (specific sites on the body).

It is important to remember that not every member of the same culture has the same health beliefs. Differences are typically seen between the generations. The healthcare professional should not assume patients have specific health beliefs. Being aware of possible cultural beliefs and practices of a group is important. It can help the medical assistant ask related questions to identify a patient's beliefs and practices.

Cultural Differences

African Americans
- Extended family and church play important roles.
- May have a key family member who must be consulted on healthcare decisions.
- Older members may look at their health as being up to God's will, although younger members seek health screening and treatments as needed.

Cambodians
- Good health means the person is balanced; believe in the balance of hot and cold.
- Illness may be seen as punishment for sins in a past life.
- Typically use traditional healing practices before seeking conventional medicine. May use herbs, cupping and coining, acupuncture and acupressure.
- They may not be interested in preventive care and screenings.

Chinese
- May use acupuncture, massage, and herbs, seeking care from traditional practitioners for less severe illnesses.
- Respectful of elders, teachers, and healthcare professionals. May affect how a person interacts and discusses health topics with the healthcare professional. The person may not ask questions or discuss concerns.

Hispanics/Latinos
- May have strong family and religious beliefs. Family is respected and plays an important role. May view an illness as God's will.
- May use home remedies or folk healer's advice over conventional medicine.
- Sickness is caused by a person having too much heat or cold. Foods and herbs are used to bring back the balance. (Heat and cold are not temperature related.) Cold diseases have more unseen symptoms, such as a chest cold and an earache. Hot diseases have more visible symptoms, such as vomiting, fever, and sore throat.
- Males often answer questions and give consent. Make sure to address the patient also. Friendliness and respectfulness are very important.

Hmong
- Lack words in native language for medical terms and some body organs.
- May seek care from folk medicine doctors and shaman.
- Herbs, massage, coining or spooning, and cupping can be used.
- Accessories may be worn around wrists, necks, or ankles for health or religious reasons.

- Respecting older family members is very important. Often oldest male in the family is the decision maker. Extended family is very important.
- Eye contact is considered rude.
- Touching the head of a child is not accepted. The head is considered sacred.

Native Americans
- May place a lot of value in family and spiritual beliefs.
- State of health occurs when living in total harmony with nature. Illness is the imbalance between the person and nature.
- May use a traditional tribal medicine person.
- Often avoid direct eye contact out of respect and concern for the loss of one's soul.

Russians
- May view healthcare with some mistrust, based on past experience.
- May not be used to asking questions and participating in a discussion with a provider.
- Some practice home remedies and bonki. *Bonki* is practiced by pressing glass cups against the person's shoulders to ease the symptoms. Bruising can occur, which should not be confused with abuse.
- Family likes to receive news about patient's condition and prognosis and may not give bad news to the patient. This lessens the person's anxieties and promotes calmness.

Somali
- Believe that individuals do not prevent illness, which is only done through prayer and living a life according to their religion.
- Use traditional spiritual healers.
- May not take medication if they feel healthy.
- Healthcare decisions are made by the family, and the father gives consent for procedures.
- Male and female circumcisions are performed; being uncircumcised means the person is unclean.

Vietnamese
- Illness is often explained by mystical beliefs.
- Health is the balance between the hot and cold poles that govern the bodily functions.
- Use alternative therapies, such as acupuncture, coining, spooning, and cupping.

CRITICAL THINKING APPLICATION   7.4

In the family practice environment, Suzanne sees patients from a variety of cultures. If you worked in a similar place, what would you do if you noticed red circles on a child's back? You are unsure as to what caused the circles.

Communication Barriers

Coaching patients with communication barriers can be a challenging process. Hearing, vision, and language barriers are common in healthcare. It is estimated that 2% of people in the United States have a visual impairment, 3% have a hearing impairment, and 9% have limited English proficiency. It is important to overcome these barriers when coaching patients.

For healthcare agencies accepting federal funds, the Civil Rights Act requires that all patients have equal access to services. People with vision, hearing, or speech impairments use different ways to communicate. The Americans with Disability Act requires effective communication with patients who have impairments. This may mean offering a qualified medical interpreter or other interpretation services free of charge. Large-print materials and written instructions are also required. Translated written materials are needed for non-English-speaking patients.

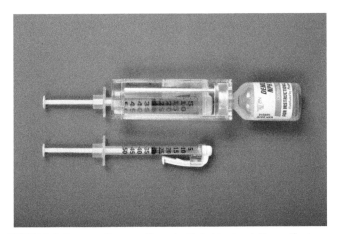

FIGURE 7.4 Syringe magnifiers are used by people with visual impairments. The magnifiers increase the size of the calibration markings on the syringes.

The following sections provide tips for communicating with patients. It is important to listen to patients concerning what works best for them.

Patients Who Have Impaired Vision. When working with patients who have impaired vision, it is important to ensure the room has adequate light. Position the patient so he or she does not have to look directly toward the light source. Make sure the patient is wearing glasses or contacts if needed. When teaching a patient with impaired vision, the following are important:

- Consider the impact of color contrast and glare on the materials used. Use a large black and white font (>14 point font) or electronic copy that can be enlarged. Use bold markers for handwritten information.
- Ask the patient how he or she prefers the information. Provide the patient with large-print directions or brochures.
- Have adaptive equipment available or information on resources for such equipment. For instance, you need to show a patient how to draw up insulin using a syringe. Having a syringe magnifier can help the patient see the calibration markings on the syringe (Fig. 7.4).
- Face the patient directly. Make eye contact. Use a normal tone of voice.
- Gestures and other nonverbal cues are not as helpful with visual impairments.
- Encourage the patient to use his or her own magnification aids.

Patients Who Have Impaired Hearing. When teaching a patient with impaired hearing, the following are important:

- Face the person when speaking.
- Determine if the person has better hearing in one ear over the other. Position yourself so your voice is close to that side.
- If the patient has a hearing aid, encourage the patient to use it.
- Use a low-pitched voice, and speak clearly, slowly, and distinctly. Pause between sentences or phrases. Speak naturally; do not shout. Limit medical terms.
- Say the person's name before you begin a conversation.
- Keep your hands away from your face when talking.
- If an interpreter is present, look at the patient, not the interpreter.
- Limit extra noises in the environment.

- Attempt to rephrase or find a different way to say something if the patient has difficulty understanding a phrase.
- Provide important information in writing.
- Have the person repeat back important information.

Patients Who Have Language Barriers. When teaching a patient who has a language barrier, the following are important:

- Address the patient by his or her last name (e.g., Mrs. Martinez, Mr. Nguyen).
- Be respectful and courteous.
- Use simple phrases. If medical terminology must be used, make sure to define it for patients.
- Use an interpreter or an interpretation service. Focus on the patient and not on the interpreter.
- Use translated materials.
- Pictures and models can be helpful during the coaching session.

Teaching-Learning Process

Teaching opportunities vary greatly in ambulatory care. Sometimes a patient wants to know what a certain medication is for. Other times, the medical assistant needs to coach a patient on a diagnostic test.

Always take a moment to look over any information you provide to patients. Make sure you know the content before you review it with the patient. Providing information that conflicts with the handout will confuse the patient.

The medical assistant should start the coaching process by finding out what the patient knows about the topic. A simple way to do this is by asking a few questions, such as, "Have you had an ultrasound before? If so, what do you remember about it?" This helps the medical assistant identify what the patient knows. From there the medical assistant can begin teaching.

Other coaching sessions will be lengthy because more complex topics are being taught. These coaching sessions should be well planned so the time is used efficiently. Using the teaching-learning process requires the following steps:

- *Assessing the learning needs*: What does the patient need to learn? How ready is the patient for learning? What are the patient's motivations and concerns? What is the patient's learning style? It is important to identify the patient's *learning goals* or the main reason for learning the content.
- *Determining teaching priorities*: It is important to prioritize what the patient needs to learn first. When there is a lot of content to learn, the medical assistant must prioritize the most important topics and address those. Other topics will be addressed on another day. To determine the priorities, ask what information does the patient need to maintain his or her health until the next meeting?
- *Planning the teaching process:* When planning, determine what teaching aids and strategies will be used. The teaching strategies and aids used must be appropriate for the content being taught. For instance, demonstrating how to give an injection and having the patient give a return demonstration will be more useful than just discussing the steps of giving an injection.
  - *Teaching aids* are materials that will be used. These can include brochures, online resources, health-related apps, videos, posters, models, and drawings. Be sure to consider the patient's individual needs (e.g., primary language, developmental level, barriers to learning). For patients with lower reading levels or English as a second language, using more pictures can be helpful.

- *Teaching strategies* are ways the information will be given. For skills, demonstration and role-play with demonstration are effective strategies. Discussion, videos, and internet sites can be helpful for teaching about a disease, diagnostic tests, or treatment.
- *Implementing the teaching process*: It is important to start with the basics and build from there. Keep the information simple, focused, and appropriate for the individual patient. Reinforce important information. If teaching a skill, make sure to have the equipment available that the patient will use at home. This will promote the patient's comfort with the task.
- *Evaluating the patient's learning*: After teaching important points, have the patient summarize what you stated. Keeping the patient involved will help him or her to retain more information. Throughout the teaching session, make sure to ask the patient for feedback on if he or she understands what you are discussing. Instead of just saying, "Do you understand?" Ask specific questions to evaluate the patient's learning; for example, "What are four symptoms of low blood sugar?" Summarize the important points at the end of the teaching session. Answer any questions the patient may have. Identify areas in which the patient needs more information. If there will be more than one session, summarize what will occur during the next meeting
- *Documenting the teaching-learning process*: It is important to document the content taught to the patient, how the patient responded, evidence that the patient learned the content, handouts given, and any plans for follow-up. Make sure to include the provider's name and any adaptations you made to individualize the teaching/learning experience. Evidence may include statements such as, "Pt safely and accurately walked 20 feet using the walker." "Pt stated six signs and symptoms of hypoglycemia."

Tips on Patient Education Materials

Guidelines to follow if you are responsible for developing or ordering educational supplies include:
- The material should be written in lay language at a sixth- to eighth-grade level to promote understanding.
- Good pictures can help patients understand the information.
- Information should be well organized and clearly described.
- All material should be checked for accuracy. (Providers will request to approve the information ahead of time.)
- Handouts should be attractive and professional.
- Copies should be available in languages other than English when possible and in large print for visually impaired clients.
- Do not use disease information literature from medical and pharmaceutical companies that includes advertising of their products. (This type of information can create confusion, if the patient is not using the product advertised.)

COACHING ON DISEASE PREVENTION

Medical assistants coach patients of all ages on disease prevention. It is important to help patients understand ways to prevent diseases in their lives (see Procedure 7.1, p. 191). Common disease prevention coaching by age group includes the following:

- School-age children: Teaching about handwashing and cough etiquette.
- Teens and adults: Teaching about ways to prevent sexually transmitted infections (STIs) and the risks of using cigarettes, smokeless tobacco, and e-cigarettes.
- All age groups: Coaching patients and parents on the vaccines recommended for that specific age (see Procedure 7.1, p. 191). Childhood immunization schedules can be found on the website for the Centers for Disease Control and Prevention (CDC), https://www.cdc.gov/vaccines/schedules/downloads/child/0-18yrs-child-combined-schedule.pdf. Common adult vaccines usually include the following:
- Influenza yearly
- Tetanus and diphtheria (Td) every 10 years and substitute tetanus, diphtheria, and acellular pertussis vaccine (Tdap) once.
- Recombinant zoster vaccine (RZV), Shingrix, two doses for adults age 50 or older; or Zoster vaccine live (ZVL), Zostavax, one dose for adults age 60 or older.
- 13-Valent pneumococcal conjugate vaccine (PCV13), one dose usually after age 65 unless given before based on the patient's health.
- 23-Valent pneumococcal polysaccharide vaccine (PPSV23 or PPSV), one to two doses, depending on patient's health
- Additional vaccines can be given based on the situation (e.g., traveling or job related); adulthood immunization schedules can be found on the CDC's website, *https://www.cdc.gov/vaccines/schedules/downloads/adult/adult-combined-schedule.pdf*

Cough Etiquette

- When coughing or sneezing, turn away from others and cover your mouth and nose with a tissue. If a tissue is not available, cough or sneeze into your elbow or upper sleeve.
- Discard the tissue in the nearest waste container.
- Sanitize hands with an alcohol-based hand sanitizer or wash hands.

How to Prevent Sexually Transmitted Infections

- Abstinence (not having any type of sex) is the most reliable way to prevent STIs.
- Long-term mutual monogamy (an agreement to be sexually active with just one person) with an uninfected partner is also a reliable way to prevent STIs.
- Reducing the number of partners reduces the risk. All partners need to be tested.
- Use latex condoms, although they are not 100% effective.
- Avoid sharing underwear and towels.
- Wash after intercourse.
- Avoid anyone with a genital rash, sore, discharge, or other symptoms.
- Get vaccinated for hepatitis B and human papillomavirus (HPV).

Health Risks Associated With Cigarettes, Smokeless Tobacco, and E-Cigarettes

Tobacco smoke contains more than 7000 chemicals, of which 250 are harmful and at least 69 can cause cancer. One in five deaths are related to smoking. According to the Centers for Disease Control and Prevention (CDC), smokers are more likely to develop heart disease, lung cancer, and strokes. Smoking can cause problems in all parts of the body (see Chapter 25).

Secondhand smoke causes lung cancer, strokes, low-birth-weight babies, and heart disease. Children exposed to secondhand smoke have increased risks of sudden infant death syndrome (SIDS), ear infections, bronchitis, pneumonia, colds, and asthma.

Quitting has numerous health advantages for the smoker:
- Blood pressure and heart rate begin to return to normal.
- Within a few hours, carbon monoxide levels in the blood decline.
- Within a few weeks, circulation improves and abnormal respiratory systems (e.g., cough, wheezing) decrease.
- One year after quitting smoking, the cardiovascular risks decrease sharply.
- Two to 5 years after quitting, the risk for stroke returns to nonsmoker level.
- Five years after quitting, the risk of cancer of the esophagus, bladder, throat, and mouth is cut in half.
- Ten years after quitting, the lung cancer risk decreases by 50%.

The CDC reports that at least 28 cancer-causing chemicals have been found in smokeless tobacco (e.g., chew and dip). Smokeless tobacco can cause cancer of the mouth, pancreas, and esophagus.

According to the US surgeon general, e-cigarettes heat liquids to form an aerosol that is then inhaled. Many people call this *vaping*. The liquids typically contain nicotine, flavorings, and other additives. E-cigarettes are considered tobacco products because they contain nicotine that comes from tobacco. The nicotine makes e-cigarettes addictive. The additives can pose health risks.

There are many resources available to help smokers quit, including online resources (*https://smokefree.gov*) and the National Cancer Institute's Smoking Quitline at 1–877–44U–Quit. Local resources are usually available. Healthcare providers can discuss medications that can be helpful.

From the Centers for Disease Control and Prevention (CDC). *https://www.cdc.gov/tobacco/infographics/health-effects/index.htm#smoking-risks*; Office of the US Surgeon General: Know the risks. *https://e-cigarettes.surgeongeneral.gov/*. Accessed October 21, 2018.

CRITICAL THINKING APPLICATION 7.5

Suzanne has seen many patients who smoke. Describe how a medical assistant should discuss cessation with a patient who uses nicotine.

COACHING ON HEALTH MAINTENANCE AND WELLNESS

Often with health maintenance and wellness, the provider establishes standing orders for specific education to be given based on the patient's history or age. When the medical assistant rooms a patient, a health history is obtained, and screening questions are asked. Based on the patient's answers, the medical assistant may need to provide coaching on specific topics per the provider's standing orders. For instance, a patient states she smokes 1 pack of cigarettes daily. The provider's standing order for smokers requires the medical assistant to provide information on the hazards of tobacco use and resources for quitting. Another example would be a patient who is turning 45. Because colon cancer screenings typically start at age 45, the provider's standing order would be to provide this information to the patient.

The following sections discuss self-exams that can be taught to patients and the screenings that are commonly done. The medical assistant completes some screenings, whereas others require the medical assistant to educate the patient on the tests to be performed.

Self-Exams

The purpose of self-exams is to identify changes in one's body. Sometimes these changes can be the first sign of a disease. Self-exams are typically done monthly. To help maintain a person's health, the early diagnosis of a disease such as cancer is important.

Breast Self-Exam

Breast cancer can affect both females and males, though males are at a lower risk. Breast cancer is the second most common cancer in females after skin cancer. The risk of breast cancer increases with age. About one in eight women will have invasive breast cancer. Typically, the survival rate is higher the earlier the cancer is diagnosed.

According to the American Cancer Society, research has not shown a benefit for patient or provider breast exams when women are also getting mammograms. It is recommended for women with an average risk of breast cancer to start having yearly mammograms between ages 45 and 50. It is important for all women to know what is normal with their breasts. Any abnormality should be reported to their provider. Some providers still recommend a monthly breast self-exam (BSE) to be done after the menses (discussed in Chapter 27).

Testicular Self-Exam

According to the American Cancer Society, males at any age can develop testicular cancer. About 50% of those diagnosed are between 20 and 34 years of age. It is estimated that 1 in 263 males will get testicular cancer. If the cancer is found early (before it has spread), there is a good chance of a cure. The American Cancer Society recommends that providers perform a testicular exam as part of a routine physical exam. Some providers recommend that after puberty (around age 15) males should do a monthly testicular self-exam (TSE) after a shower (discussed in Chapter 26).

Skin Self-Exam

Skin cancer is the most common type of cancer in the United States. The three most common types of skin cancer are basal cell, squamous cell, and melanoma. Basal cell and squamous cell carcinomas are curable. Melanoma is more dangerous and can cause death. These three types of skin cancers are caused by overexposure to ultraviolet (UV) light. UV exposure comes from the sun, tanning beds, and sun lamps. UV rays are an invisible kind of radiation that penetrates and changes skin cells.

Certain people have more risk than others for skin cancer. Experts recommend monthly skin self-exams. It is important to watch for changes in moles. To remember how moles may change, use the ABCDE rule (Table 7.4). Any change in moles, including in the size, shape, color, elevation, or symptom (e.g., bleeding, itching, or crusting), should be reported immediately (Fig. 7.5).

When doing the monthly skin check, start at the scalp and work toward the soles of the feet. Use mirrors to exam the back of the ears and the back. Many people miss mole changes on the back of their ears. When examining hands and feet, make sure to check between the fingers and toes and to check the nail beds. Check all skin surfaces. Document the location of the moles and their appearances. Any changes seen, or any suspicious-looking mole, should be reported to the provider immediately.

TABLE 7.4 Early Warning Signs of Malignant Melanoma: ABCDE Rule	
Asymmetry	One half of the mole does not match the other half.
Border	The edges of the mole are blurred or irregular.
Color	The mole is not the same color throughout and has shades of tan, brown, black, red, white, or blue
Diameter	The mole is larger than 6 mm, about the size of a pencil eraser or pea; but it could be smaller.
Evolving	The mole changes over time.

Risk Factors for Skin Cancer

- Skin that is lighter than normal skin color; burns, freckles, or reddens easily; becomes painful in the sun
- Family or personal history of skin cancer
- History of sunburns (especially early in life) or indoor tanning
- Exposure to sun through work or play
- Green or blue eyes
- Red or blond hair
- Certain types and a large number of moles

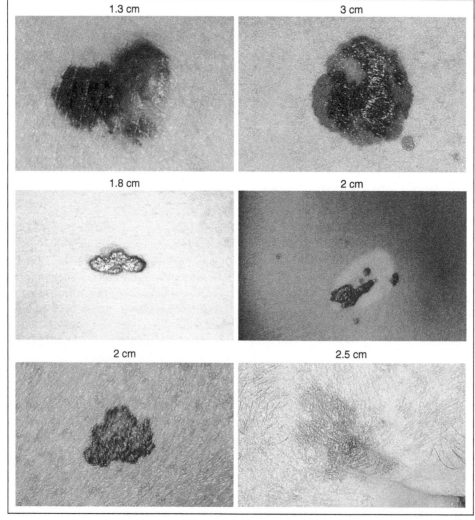

FIGURE 7.5 Malignant melanomas. Note the presence of the ABCDE characteristics. (From Rothrock J: *Alexander's care of the patient in surgery,* ed 14, St Louis, 2011, Mosby.)

Oral Cancer Self-Exam

Oral cancer includes cancer of the lips, tongue, throat, salivary glands, pharynx, larynx, and sinuses. Most oral cancers occur after age 40. It is estimated that more than 40,000 new cases of oral cancer are diagnosed yearly with almost 9,000 related deaths. Early detection is important for oral cancer. Here are some facts about oral cancer:

- Men get oral cancer twice as often as women.
- Using tobacco, drinking alcohol, or having oral human papillomavirus (HPV) are risk factors for oral cancer.
- About 25% of those with oral cancer had no risks.

Oral cancer screening is routinely done by the dentist and should occur every 6 months. It is important for people to do a monthly oral cancer self-exam. Any changes in appearance or sores that do not heal should be reported to the dentist immediately. According to the American Dental Hygienists Association, an oral cancer self-exam consists of looking for lumps and color changes and then feeling for lumps and swelling. To do an oral cancer self-exam, follow these steps:

- Check the head and neck for lumps, bumps, or swelling. Is one side of the face larger than the other?
- Check the skin on the face for changes. Is there a color change? Are there sores, moles, or growths?
- Check for any lumps or tenderness in the neck.
- Check the upper and lower lip for sores and color changes. After the visual inspection, feel for any changes in texture or lumps.
- Check the inner cheek for any color changes (red, white, or dark patches). Then palpate the cheeks with a thumb on the outside and a finger inside. Are any lumps found?
- Check the roof of the mouth for lumps and color changes. Feel for any lumps.
- Check the floor of the mouth using your tongue for any lumps or color changes. Examine all angles. Feel the tongue with a finger for any lumps or tenderness.

Symptoms of Oral Cancer

- White or red patches in the mouth or on the gums, tongue, or lips
- Numbness or pain in the mouth; pain with chewing or talking
- Long-term hoarseness or sore throat
- Swelling in the jaw area or constant earache
- Bleeding in the mouth or a long-term sore
- Feeling of a lump or something stuck in the throat

Regular Screenings

Medical assistants in primary care typically need to talk with patients about the recommended regular screenings for different diseases. Suggested times for screenings are based on an adult with an average risk. If a patient has family members with the disease, that person may have a higher than normal risk. This means the patient may need to be screened earlier and more often than other adults. Regular preventive screenings are summarized by age in Table 7.5 and include the following:

- *Blood pressure:* Patients at higher risk include African Americans, those who are overweight, and those with previously higher than normal blood pressure readings.

- *Bone density:* This screening provides information on the strength of the patient's bones and if the patient has osteoporosis. Women have a higher risk than men, and it increases with age.
- *Cholesterol:* Adults with a family history of high cholesterol levels or who have high cholesterol need more frequent testing.
- *Colorectal cancer screening:* The American Cancer Society recommends that regular screening start at age 45. Screening can either be stool based or visual exams (Table 7.6).
- *Dental exam:* The American Dental Association recommends a dental exam and cleaning yearly. Dental health can affect the overall health of the body.
- *Dilated eye exam:* It is important to have a dilated eye exam if a person has a risk of eye disease (e.g., glaucoma). The CDC recommends dilated eye exams for the following individuals:
  - Patients with diabetes (recommended annually)
  - African American patients age 40 years or older (recommended every 2 years)
  - Patients older than 60 years of age (recommended every 2 years)
  - Patients with a family history of glaucoma (recommended every 2 years)
- *Lung cancer screening:* Patients who are 55 to 80 years old, have a history of heavy smoking, and are currently smoking or quit in the previous 15 years should be screened for lung cancer. (Heavy smoking means smoking one pack of cigarettes a day for 30 years or two packs for 15 years.)
- *Mammogram:* This x-ray of the breasts helps to identify breast cancer. The American Cancer Society recommends women ages 40 to 44 have the option to have annual mammograms. Women ages 45 to 54 should have annual mammograms, and those age 55 years or older should have mammograms every 2 years.
- *Pap test:* This test is used to identify cervical cancer.
- *Prostate cancer:* Risk factors include being 50 years old or older, being African American, exposure to Agent Orange, and having a father, brother, or son who had prostate cancer. No specific test exists for prostate cancer. The digital rectal exam (DRE) and the prostate-specific antigen (PSA) test are used. The provider may offer either test after age 50. Frequency is based on the patient's history.
- *Blood glucose test:* Adults should be screened for Type 2 diabetes mellitus every 3 years or sooner, depending on their medical history.

CRITICAL THINKING APPLICATION   7.6

Suzanne has seen more providers ordering the fecal immunochemical test (FIT) over the guaiac fecal occult blood test. What are the advantages of the FIT test?

One-Time Screenings

The medical assistant may also need to coach patients on one-time screening as indicated by the provider. People are recommended to have the following screenings at least once, unless a person's risk is greater than average:

- *Abdominal aortic aneurysm:* Males between 65 and 75 years of age who have smoked at one time in their lives should receive

TABLE 7.5   Preventive Recommendations

	AGE 18–39	AGE 40+
Blood Pressure	Every 3–5 years	Age 40+: every year
Bone Density		Age 65+: Females: every 2 years
Cholesterol	Every 5 years	
Stool-based Tests (gFOBT, FIT, iFOBT)		Age 45–75: annually Age 75+: individual decision
Stool-based Test (MT-sDNA [Cologuard])		Age 45–75: every 3 years Age 75+: individual decision
Colonoscopy		Age 45–75: every 10 years Age 75+: individual decision
Dental exam	Yearly	
Dilated eye exam		Age 60+: every 2 years
Lung Cancer Screening		Age 55–80: those who meet the criteria: annual low-dose computed tomography (LDCT)
Mammogram		Age 45–54: every year Age 55 or older: every 2 years
Pap Test	Females age 21–29: every 3 years Age 30–65: every 3 years or every 5 years if having an HPV test Over 65: individual decision	
Prostate Cancer (DRE or PSA test)		Males age 50+: individual decision
Blood Glucose Test	Every 3 years or more frequent if patient has hypertension or obesity	

From Healthfinder.gov. *https://healthfinder.gov/HealthTopics/Category/doctor-visits*; the American Cancer Society. *https://www.cancer.org.*

this screening. This population has the highest risk of having an abdominal aortic aneurysm (AAA).

- *Human immunodeficiency virus (HIV) screen (blood test):* People 15 to 65 years old need to get an HIV test at least once in their lifetime. All pregnant women need to be tested. People with a high risk for HIV should have testing annually, if not more often. High-risk factors include multiple sexual partners, sexual partners who have or may have HIV, and those who use injectable illegal drugs.
- *Hepatitis C:* This condition is passed through blood from an infected person. A person with risk factors should be tested. Risk factors for hepatitis C include the following:
  - Born between 1945 and 1965
  - History of a blood transfusion or organ transplant before 1992
  - Use of injected illegal drugs
  - Has chronic liver disease, HIV, or AIDS

Additional Screenings

When rooming patients, medical assistants have to perform different screenings. Either the patient's age or the patient's responses will trigger the need for the screening. Screenings have increased throughout the years. This is due to increased data collection requirements and

focusing on prevention and quality patient care. Common screenings include the following:

- *Alcohol misuse screening:* Drinking in moderation means that females have no more than one drink a day and males have no more than two drinks per day. (An alcoholic drink is classified as a 12-oz bottle of beer, a 5-oz glass of wine, or a 1.5-oz shot of liquor.) Drinking more than the recommended daily amount may lead to health issues.
- *Nicotine or tobacco screening:* Various tools are used. Tools typically focus on whether or not tobacco products are used, how much is used per day, the history of use, and quitting behaviors (e.g., strategies used in the past or thoughts of quitting).
- *Drug abuse screening:* Various tools are used. Tools focus on prescription drug use for nonmedical reasons and illegal drug use. Tools are designed differently, but it is important to identify any history of or recent drug abuse. Common signs of drug abuse include the following:
  - Poor hygiene; changes in eating and sleeping patterns
  - Loss of interest in favorite things
  - Very energetic, talking fast, very sociable
  - Tired, sad, nervous, agitated, and bad moods
  - Missing school, work, or appointments

TABLE 7.6 Common Colorectal Cancer Screenings

TEST	TESTING FREQUENCY	DESCRIPTION	PATIENT PREPARATION
Guaiac fecal occult blood test (gFOBT)	Age 45–75: every year Age 75–85: individual decision based on health of the person and prior screening history	A fecal specimen is examined for occult or hidden blood, which may indicate gastrointestinal (GI) bleeding. Intestinal bleeding may be an indicator of colon cancer. Stool samples are collected by the patient and returned to the medical laboratory for testing.	For 7 days prior to the test must not take vitamin C supplements, aspirin, or nonsteroidal anti-inflammatory medications (e.g., ibuprofen, naproxen, and indomethacin). Many foods can create false positives. For 3 days before the test, do not eat red meat and raw fruits or vegetables (e.g., horseradish, turnips, broccoli, melons, and radishes).
Fecal immunochemical test (FIT) (also called immunochemical fecal occult blood test [iFOBT])	Age 45–75: every year Age 75–85: individual decision based on health of the person and prior screening history	A fecal specimen is examined for human hemoglobin protein, which may indicate GI bleeding and cancer. Stool samples are collected by the patient and returned to the medical laboratory for testing.	No dietary restrictions are required.
Multi-targeted stool DNA test (MT-sDNA [Cologuard])	Age 45–75: every 3 years Age 75+: individual decision *Used in place of the gFOBT and FIT*	A fecal specimen is examined for blood. Computer analysis looks at the DNA in the stool, checking for cancer and precancerous cells. Positive results should lead to a colonoscopy. Stool samples are collected by the patient and returned to the medical laboratory for testing.	No patient preparation is required.
Colonoscopy	Age 45–75: every 10 years Age 75+: individual decision	An endoscopy is inserted through the anus and used to visualize the colon.	Usually clear liquids the day before the test. No red liquids allowed. Laxatives and/or enema(s) are used to clean the bowel. May have food and fluid restrictions prior to the test.
Computed tomography (CT) colonography or virtual colonoscopy	Age 45–75: every 5 years	A small tube is inserted into the rectum. The lower colon is inflated with gas. CT images are taken of the colon and rectum.	
Flexible sigmoidoscopy	Age 45–75: every 5 years or every 10 years with yearly FIT	A sigmoidoscope is inserted into the rectum and most of the sigmoid colon. Requires patient dietary and colon preparation.	

- Spending money excessively
- Slowed reaction time, paranoid thinking
- *Intimate partner violence screening*: This screening covers domestic abuse. It is important to remember that both males and females can be victims of domestic abuse. Many psychological and health problems come from violence, including substance abuse, obesity, depression, brain trauma, pregnancy complications, and chronic pain. Intimate partner violence includes controlling behaviors, physical abuse, sexual abuse, and emotional or verbal abuse.
- *Elderly safety screening*: These screening tools focus on how safe the older person feels at home. The tools screen for abuse and neglect.
- *Functional status screening*: Several tools are available for primary care providers to use for older patients. By using a functional status screening tool, the provider obtains information on the patient, such as the following:

- Physical functions with daily activities (e.g., grooming, bathing, walking, and eating)
- Psychological health (e.g., mood and anxiety)
- Role function (e.g., employed or volunteer)
- Social function (e.g., interacting with others or isolating self)

- *Depression screening*: Several tools are used to screen for depression. The screening tools ask questions related to moods, thoughts, and feelings. The number of questions will vary depending on the tools. For instance, the Patient Health Questionnaire–2 (PHQ-2) asks two questions that focus on the frequency of depressed mood and **anhedonia** over the previous 2 weeks. If the patient screens positive, then the Patient Health Questionnaire–9 (PHQ-9) is given to see if the patient meets the criteria for a depressive disorder (Fig. 7.6). (The first two questions of the PHQ-9 are the two questions on the PHQ-2 tool.)

PATIENT HEALTH QUESTIONNAIRE-9 (PHQ-9)

Over the <u>last 2 weeks</u>, how often have you been bothered by any of the following problems? *(Use "✓" to indicate your answer)*	Not at all	Several days	More than half the days	Nearly every day
1. Little interest or pleasure in doing things	0	1	2	3
2. Feeling down, depressed, or hopeless	0	1	2	3
3. Trouble falling or staying asleep, or sleeping too much	0	1	2	3
4. Feeling tired or having little energy	0	1	2	3
5. Poor appetite or overeating	0	1	2	3
6. Feeling bad about yourself — or that you are a failure or have let yourself or your family down	0	1	2	3
7. Trouble concentrating on things, such as reading the newspaper or watching television	0	1	2	3
8. Moving or speaking so slowly that other people could have noticed? Or the opposite — being so fidgety or restless that you have been moving around a lot more than usual	0	1	2	3
9. Thoughts that you would be better off dead or of hurting yourself in some way	0	1	2	3

FOR OFFICE CODING <u> 0 </u> + _____ + _____ + _____

=Total Score: _____

If you checked off <u>any</u> problems, how <u>difficult</u> have these problems made it for you to do your work, take care of things at home, or get along with other people?

Not difficult at all	Somewhat difficult	Very difficult	Extremely difficult
☐	☐	☐	☐

FIGURE 7.6 Example of a depression screening tool: Patient Health Questionnaire–9 (PHQ-9).

• *Peripheral neuropathy screening*: Screening questions focus on loss of feeling or a "pins and needles" sensation in the feet and hands. Besides asking the patient screening questions, the medical assistant may also need to do a monofilament foot test and coach the patient on foot care (discussed in Chapter 23).

Types and Signs of Elder Abuse and Neglect

• *Physical abuse*: Fractures, rope marks, cuts, bruising, dislocations, broken glasses, giving too little or too much medication, bleeding, and sudden changes in the person's personality or behavior
• *Sexual abuse*: Unexplained sexually transmitted infections, bruising in the genital region, and reports from the older person
• *Emotional abuse*: Not communicating, withdrawn, agitated, and symptoms that mimic dementia
• *Neglect*: Malnutrition, dehydration, lack of proper living conditions, and failing to treat health problems
• *Abandonment*: Leaving the person in a public place
• *Financial abuse*: Stealing from the older person, forging signatures on financial transactions, and any other illegal action that represents a financial loss for the older person

COACHING ON DIAGNOSTIC TESTS

It is important for the medical assistant to provide the necessary teaching for diagnostic and laboratory tests ordered for patients. For tests to be completed, the patient needs to be prepared. Some tests require fasting, whereas others do not. The medical assistant needs to provide answers to these questions:

• What is the test?
• Where does the patient need to go for the test? When is the test scheduled?
• Does the test require fasting? If so, for how long? If no foods or beverages can be consumed, does this include water?
• Should patients continue or stop taking their medications? This may require a discussion with the provider.

It is important to give patients the correct answers. Tables 7.7 and 7.8 provide information on common imaging procedures and medical laboratory tests. Remember, patient preparation may vary based on the facility.

CRITICAL THINKING APPLICATION   7.7
Sometimes Suzanne has a patient who refuses to follow the preparation steps for a diagnostic test. How might you handle this situation?

TABLE 7.7 Common Patient Instructions for Imaging Procedures

PROCEDURE	DESCRIPTION	COMMON PATIENT INSTRUCTIONS
X-ray	X-ray particles pass through the body, and an image is recorded. Many different types of x-rays.	Provide overview of test and why it is being done. Screen for pregnancy. X-rays are painless, although some body positions may be uncomfortable. Patients may be asked to hold the breath during the procedure to get a clear x-ray.
Computed tomography scan (CT scan, CAT scan)	Uses x-rays to create pictures of cross sections of the body. Several types of CT scans exist; each may have different preparations. Patient will lie on a narrow table that slides into the center of the CT scanner. The x-ray beam will rotate around the patient, creating separate images (slices) of the body.	Provide overview of test and why it is being done. May require an intravenous (IV) or oral contrast medium. If so, • Check allergies (contrast medium and iodine). • Check if patient has kidney disease or is on dialysis. • Nothing by mouth (NPO) for 4–6 hours before test. • Address if medications need to be stopped. • IV contrast medium may cause a slight burning feeling and a metallic taste in the mouth; flushing can occur.
Magnetic resonance imaging (MRI)	Uses powerful magnets and radio waves to create images of the body. Does not use radiation. Several types of MRIs exist; may have different preparations. Patient will lie on a table. The machine makes loud noises. No metal is allowed in the room.	Provide overview of test and why it is being done. May require contrast (see CT scan contrast medium information). May require being NPO for 4–6 hours Must identify if patient is claustrophobic (afraid or anxious of close spaces). Due to strong magnets, must screen for artificial heart valves, brain aneurysm clips, heart pacemaker or defibrillator, cochlear (inner ear) implants, recent artificial joint, vascular stents, or history of working with metal. Must remove all metal from patient including removable dental work (e.g., plates).
Mammography	An x-ray picture of the breasts used to find tumors. The breast will be compressed on a flat surface for the x-ray.	The patient should not use any perfume, deodorant, powders, or ointments on the arms or breast on the day of the test. These products may interfere with the results of the x-ray. The patient will need to undress from the waist up. All jewelry from the neck and chest area needs to be removed. Screen for pregnancy, breastfeeding, or if the patient has had a breast biopsy.
Positron emission tomography (PET) scan	Imagining test that uses an IV radioactive substance (tracer) to identify disease in the organs and tissues. Patient will lie on a table that slides into the tunnel shaped PET scanner.	May require patient to be NPO for 4–6 hours (with exception of water) before the scan. Medications may be held (check with the provider). IV tracer will be given, which may cause a sharp sting. Afterward the patient needs to rest for 1 hour. During the test, the patient must lie still to prevent blurry images. Screen for claustrophobia, pregnancy, and allergies to contrast medium and iodine.
Ultrasound (US)	Uses high-frequency sound waves to create the image of the organs and structures.	May require special preparation based on the type of US done. Patient will need to expose the area. A clear, water-based gel is applied to the skin, and a transducer (handheld probe) moves over the area.

COACHING ON TREATMENT PLANS

Many facilities have the medical assistants meet with the patients after the providers finish. The medical assistants review the treatment plan with the patients. They answer any questions, explore any issues the patients may have, and provide additional instructions. As mentioned, this type of coaching has been shown to increase patients' compliance with the treatment plans. Additionally, it provides patients with a lifeline should they have questions or concerns at home.

Medical assistants coach patients on treatments to do at home. These could include taking medications, caring for casts and splints, applying hot or cold therapy, and using assistive devices (discussed in Chapter 20). Besides these treatments, the medical assistant may also need to help coordinate the patient's care for additional treatments such as physical, occupational, or massage therapies. This section focuses on common treatments and important information for patients to know.

Medication Administration at Home

It is important for patients to know how to take medications at home. This includes the following questions:

• When should the patient take the medications and how should he or she take them?

TABLE 7.8	Patient Instructions for Common Medical Laboratory Tests	
TEST	**USE**	**COMMON PATIENT PREPARATION**
Creatinine	Used to monitor kidney health and disease.	May need to fast overnight. May need to refrain for eating meat for a period of time, as it could increase the creatinine level.
Glucose tests	Used to determine the blood glucose level.	For a fasting glucose test, the patient needs to be NPO (with exception of water) for at least 8 hours. Other glucose tests may require fasting and eating at specific times.
Lipid profile	Used to monitor cholesterol levels and treatment.	May require NPO (with exception of water) prior to the test.
Pap test	Used to screen for cervical cancers and some uterine or vaginal infections.	Do not schedule the test during the menstrual period. For 48 hours prior to the test: • Refrain from sexual intercourse. • Do not use vaginal creams or foams. For 24 hours prior to the test: • Do not douche or tub-bathe.

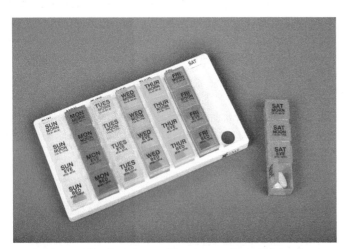

FIGURE 7.7 Daily medication boxes can help patients remember to take their medications.

• Do the medications need to be taken on an empty stomach?
• Can they be taken with the other medications?
• Do they need to be taken at bedtime?

Some patients are on a lot of medications. It is important that the medications are taken correctly. When updating the patient's current medications list, it is common to find discrepancies. The patient can be taking the medication differently than how it was ordered. Any discrepancy found needs to be communicated to the provider.

The medical assistant may coach the patient on the proper ways to take medication. Sometimes the medical assistant may need to help patients find ways to remember to take medications. Many patients use medication boxes that they, a family member, or a pharmacy set up. The boxes typically are arranged for 7 days a week with one or more boxes per day (Fig. 7.7). The medications are placed in each box based on the administration time. Some have boxes for morning, noon, and night medications.

If patients are receiving injections at home, they will need to know how to safely dispose of the needles. Patients can dispose of needles in biohazard sharps containers. These containers are available at local pharmacies and medical supply stores. An internet search can identify local sites that take biohazard sharps containers from patients. Some drug companies have mail-back programs for specific medications. (For more information, visit *https://safeneedledisposal.org.*)

Discarding Medications at Home

It is important to encourage patients to discard expired, unwanted, or unused medications. This will help prevent misuse and theft. To get rid of controlled substances, take the medications in their original prescription bottles to a medicine take-back facility. Usually, Drug Enforcement Administration (DEA) representatives are available to take control of the controlled substances. Another option is to contact a DEA-authorized collector. The DEA's website has more information on both programs (*https://www.deadiversion.usdoj.gov*).

If these programs are not available, some medications are labeled with specific disposal instructions. Many times, the label recommends flushing controlled substances down the sink or toilet. The website for the Food and Drug Administration (FDA) contains a complete list of medications that can be discarded by flushing (*www.fda.gov*).

If the label does not indicate flushing, then mix the medications in an unpalatable substance (dirt, used coffee grounds, or kitty litter). Place the mixture in a plastic bag. Seal and discard it in the household trash. Make sure all personal information and the prescription number have been scratched out on empty pill bottles.

CARE COORDINATION

Care coordination provides personalized patient- and family-centered care in a team-based environment. Advantages of care coordination include the following:

- Greater efficiency with providing patient care
- Reduced costs
- Greater patient care
- Individualized patient guidance and services
- Encourages patients to focus on goals and self-management
- Reduces hospital emergency department visits and readmissions
- Ensures the patient's needs and preferences for healthcare services are met

The care coordinator communicates between the patient and the healthcare team. Care coordinators ensure patients get timely care and do not fall through the cracks. In the ambulatory care setting, care coordination can be set up in different ways. It has been shown to be successful in primary and specialty care areas. The overall goals include:

- Help patients understand why and what services are needed
- Schedule and sequence appointments
- Provide instructions and directions to patients
- Ensure that test results are available to the providers during patient appointments
- Communicate the patient's needs and concerns to providers

A **patient navigator** (also called a *patient advocate*) has been described as a type of care coordinator. The navigator program was established at the Harlem Hospital Center in 1990. The goal was to assist cancer patients in accessing quality healthcare. Based on the success of patient navigators, the Patient Navigator, Outreach and Chronic Disease Prevention Act of 2005 funded additional positions. Today, patient navigators typically guide chronically ill patients through the healthcare system. They identify patients' financial, cultural, physical, and emotional barriers. Then, they work closely with the healthcare team and the patients to ensure barriers are eliminated and patients get timely care.

In the ambulatory care setting, medical assistants can be care coordinators. A person must have strong interpersonal skills to be successful as a care coordinator. The medical assistant must listen to the patient and family to identify their needs and concerns. The care coordinator must be compassionate yet provide firm guidance with patients who are difficult.

Possible areas involved with care coordination can include the following:

- Interview patients to identify their needs and barriers to wellness and healthcare.
- Provide patients with resources based on their needs and barriers.
- Schedule and sequence appointments.
- Make sure the required information is communicated to and from specialty departments.
- Assist with reducing language barriers by identifying bilingual providers and translators.
- Discuss special needs patients have with their healthcare team.
- Identify community resources, which may include the following:
  - Transportation and medical equipment
  - Adult daycare, assistive living, and long-term care
  - Educational programs and support groups
  - Low-cost medication programs
  - Low-cost preventive screening and immunizations

Procedure 7.2 on p. 192 describes the process of creating a current list of community resources and referring patients or family members.

CLOSING COMMENTS

It is an exciting time to become a medical assistant. The medical assistant's role is changing to meet healthcare needs. Studies have shown that medical assistants play an important role in coaching and helping patients comply with treatment and lifestyle changes. It is important for the medical assistant to coach the patient in a manner that helps the patient understand and retain the information. Adapting the coaching to the patient's communication barriers, developmental stage, and cultural practices will help the patient complete the treatment plan.

Patient Coaching

With the advances in technology, patient education materials are no longer available just on paper. Apps can help providers explain procedures and diseases to patients. YouTube links and other websites provide videos and information on diseases, procedures, and treatments.

When you use patient education materials from apps and online sites, it is important to use only provider-approved sites. The information must be current and from a reputable source. Possible online websites for patient education materials include the following:

- National Institutes of Health (NIH) from the US Department of Health and Human Services (*https://www.nih.gov/health-information*)
- Centers for Disease Control and Prevention (CDC) (*https://www.cdc.gov/*)
- MedlinePlus from the US National Library of Medicine (*https://medlineplus.gov/*)
- American Diabetes Association (ADA) (*http://www.diabetes.org/*)
- American Heart Association (AHA) (*https://www.heart.org/en/health-topics*)
- Drugs.com (*https://www.drugs.com/*)
- Mayo Clinic (*https://www.mayoclinic.org/*)
- Cleveland Clinic (*http://my.clevelandclinic.org/health/*)
- Stanford Health Care (*http://healthlibrary.stanford.edu/resources/bodysystems/*)
- Familydoctor.org from the American Academy of Family Physicians (*https://familydoctor.org/*)

Legal and Ethical Issues

After coaching a patient on a topic, it is important for the medical assistant to document the teaching. The medical assistant should indicate what the provider ordered for coaching, materials used, and general topics taught. The medical assistant should also document an evaluation statement regarding the learning.

Evaluating a patient's learning can be done through several methods, including asking the patient questions regarding the content or having the patient teach back the skill or content. The purpose of the evaluation is to determine if the patient accurately understood the information or skill. The evaluation method and the patient's response should be documented in the medical record for legal purposes.

Patient-Centered Care

Just by the design, care coordination helps provide patients with individual assistance. Patients who feel well cared for and who feel comfortable talking with their healthcare team stay with their provider. It is estimated that care coordination will increase in popularity in the coming years. This model of care will also promote exceptional customer service in healthcare.

Professional Behaviors

When coaching patients, the medical assistant must observe the patient's nonverbal and verbal communication. It is important for the medical assistant to listen to the patient and be open to questions from the patient. If the medical assistant does not know the answers to questions or if the questions are outside the medical assistant's scope of practice, the provider should be notified.

SUMMARY OF SCENARIO

During Suzanne's yearly review with her supervisor, she mentions that she is interested in becoming a care coordinator. She and the supervisor discuss how the program might assist the providers and patients. Suzanne agrees to research the role and bring a proposal to her supervisor in the coming weeks. The supervisor would then take it to the provider meeting and discuss the care model with all of the WMFM providers. Both Suzanne and her supervisor are excited to pursue changes in the practice and to continue to provide patients with the best possible care.

SUMMARY OF LEARNING OBJECTIVES

1. **Describe the medical assistant's role as a coach.**

   Coaching provides patients with skills, knowledge, support, and confidence to manage their disease between provider visits. The medical assistant can coach patients in many areas, including disease prevention, health maintenance, diagnostic tests, treatment plans, specific needs, and community resources.

2. **List and describe the stages of grief; also, discuss how the health belief model helps to explain what factors influence a person's health beliefs and practices.**

   The stages of grief include denial (refuses to accept the fact), anger at one's self or others, attempts to bargain, depression, and acceptance. Table 7.1 described adaptive interactions for each stage.

   The first part of the health belief model deals with a person's perception of his or her chance of developing a disease. The second part of this model deals with a person's perception of the severity of the disease. The third part of the model focuses on whether the person will take preventive action. A person weighs the benefits and barriers of taking the preventive actions.

3. **Describe the three domains of learning.**

   We learn new information in three different ways, or *domains*: cognitive, psychomotor, and affective. The *cognitive domain* of learning involves mental processes of recall, application, and evaluation. The *psychomotor domain* is the "doing" domain. We learn new skills and procedures by watching demonstrations and assisting with something. The *affective domain* is the "feeling" domain. It includes our feelings, emotions, values, and attitudes. Our emotions and values are very important.

4. **Explain how a medical assistant can adapt coaching to the patient.**

   It is important for the medical assistant to consider the barriers to learning and possible ways to help the patient overcome those barriers. It is also important for the medical assistant to remember the patient's developmental level. Erikson's psychosocial developmental stages are described in Table 7.3. Understanding the goal of each stage can help a medical assistant to coach patients in that age group. Learning about cultural differences can help the medical assistant ask related questions to identify a patient's beliefs and practices. Besides developmental levels and cultural differences, the medical assistant may also need to adapt to communication barriers, including impaired vision, impaired hearing, and language barriers. Review the related sections in the chapter for more information on each of these areas.

5. **Describe the teaching-learning process.**

   The medical assistant should start the coaching process by finding out what the patient knows about the topic. From there the medical assistant can begin teaching. For lengthy coaching situations, the medical assistant should plan so the time is used efficiently. Using the teaching-learning process requires the following steps:
   - Assessing the patient's learning needs
   - Determining teaching priorities
   - Planning the teaching process
   - Implementing the teaching process
   - Evaluating the patient's learning
   - Documenting the teaching-learning process

6. **Discuss how a medical assistant can coach on disease prevention.**

   Medical assistants coach patients of all ages on disease prevention. These topics can include hand washing and cough etiquette; STI prevention; the risks of cigarettes, smokeless tobacco, and e-cigarettes; and vaccines recommended for specific age groups.

7. **Describe how a medical assistant can coach on health maintenance and wellness, including different types of self-exams and screenings.**

   Often with health maintenance and wellness, the provider establishes standing orders for specific education to be given based on the patient's history or age. Based on the patient's answers to the health history and screening questions, the medical assistant may need to provide coaching on specific topics per the provider's standing orders. The medical assistant can provide coaching on self-exams, including breast, testicular, skin, and oral cancer. Besides self-exams, the medical assistant can provide coaching on regular screenings, on-time screenings, and additional screenings, such as tobacco screening and alcohol misuse screening.

8. **Describe how a medical assistant can coach on diagnostic procedures and treatment plans.**

It is important for the medical assistant to provide the necessary teaching for diagnostic and laboratory tests ordered for patients. For tests to be completed, the patient needs to be prepared.

Many facilities have the medical assistants meet with the patients after the providers finish. The medical assistants review the treatment plan with the patients. They answer any questions, explore any issues the patients may have, and provide additional instructions.

9. **Describe care coordination and patient navigation, develop a list of community resources, and facilitate referrals.**

Care coordination provides personalized patient- and family-centered care in a team-based environment. The care coordinator communicates between the patient and healthcare team. A patient navigator (also called a *patient advocate*) has been described as a type of care coordinator. Patient navigators typically guide chronically ill patients through the healthcare system. They identify patients' financial, cultural, physical, and emotional barriers. Then, they work closely with the healthcare team and the patients to ensure barriers are eliminated and patients get timely care. Procedure 7.2 on p. 192 describes the process of creating a current list of community resources and referring patients or family members.

PROCEDURE 7.1 Coach a Patient on Disease Prevention

Tasks: Coach a patient on the recommended vaccinations for his or her age. Adapt coaching for the patient's communication barrier and developmental life stage. Document the coaching in the patient's health record.

Scenario: You are working with Dr. David Kahn. You need to room Charles Johnson (date of birth [DOB] 03/03/1958), and his record indicates he has not been seen in several years. Charles has significant hearing loss, and he communicates by signing. His wife interprets for him. You look in his health record and see that he is due for influenza, Td, and recombinant zoster (shingles) vaccines. Per the provider's request (order), you need to coach adult patients on potential vaccines they are due for during the initial rooming process.

Directions: Role-play this scenario with two peers.

EQUIPMENT and SUPPLIES

- Vaccine Information Statements (VIS) (available at *http://www.immunize.org/vis/*)
- Patient's health record

PROCEDURAL STEPS

1. Wash hands or use hand sanitizer.
   PURPOSE: Hand sanitization is an important step for infection control.
2. Greet the patient. Identify yourself. Verify the patient's identity with full name and date of birth. Explain what you will be doing.
   PURPOSE: It is important to identify the patient in two different ways to ensure that you have the correct patient. Explaining the procedure can make the patient feel more comfortable and helps to reduce anxiety.
3. Arrange the chairs so the patient can see both you and the person signing. Speak slowly. Pause as needed to allow person signing to finish with the last statement. Look at the patient when communicating.
   PURPOSE: The medical assistant must focus on the patient and not the person signing or the interpreter. Speaking slowly and pausing allows the person to sign what you are saying.

4. Use simpler language when talking. Speak clearly. Communicate with dignity and respect. Allow time for the patient to respond. Listen to the patient's concerns.
   PURPOSE: When working with older patients, it is important to treat them with respect and dignity. Listening is important.
5. Ask the patient if he has received vaccines somewhere else over the past few years.
   PURPOSE: It is important to verify that the health record is accurate.
   Scenario Update: *The patient has not seen any healthcare providers over the past few years. The only vaccines received were given at this facility.*
6. Describe the vaccines that are due. Use the VIS for each vaccine as you coach the patient on the purpose of the vaccine.
   PURPOSE: The VIS is written for patients and describes the vaccine, disease(s) it prevents, and adverse reactions (side effects).
   Scenario Update: *The patient knows the shingles vaccine is not covered and costs more than $200. He refuses the shingles vaccine, and he does not believe in getting the influenza vaccine. He is interested in getting the Td vaccine.*

Continued

PROCEDURE 7.1   Coach a Patient on Disease Prevention—*continued*

7. Ask the patient which vaccines he is interested in getting. If he refuses, be respectful of his choice. Any reason he gives for the refusal should be communicated to the provider.
   PURPOSE: Patients have the right to refuse. Any treatment refused must be communicated to the provider.
8. Document the coaching in the patient's health record. Include the provider's name, what was taught, how the patient responded, and any vaccines refused.
   PURPOSE: It is important to document the procedure in the health record to show it was done.

07/16/20XX 1305 Per Dr. Kahn's order, instructed pt on the RZV, influenza, and Td vaccines. Pt stated he was not interested in the influenza vaccine or the RZV. He also stated his insurance wouldn't cover the RZV, and he didn't have the money to pay for it. He is interested in receiving the Td vaccine. Reviewed the Td VIS (07/15/20XX) with the patient. Pt stated he understood and would call if he had any issues. Due to pt's hearing impairment, pt's wife interpreted for pt during the visit._____ Suzanne Peterson CMA (AAMA)

PROCEDURE 7.2   Develop a List of Community Resources and Facilitate Referrals

Tasks: As a patient navigator, develop a current list of community resources that meet the patient's healthcare needs. Discuss the resources with the patient and facilitate referrals to the chosen resources.

Scenario 1: Robert Caudill (DOB 10/31/1940) was just diagnosed with dementia. He currently lives with his daughter, Ruby, who works full time. Ruby is feeling overwhelmed with being his only caregiver and realizes that she needs to find someone to care for her father while she is working.

Scenario 2: Leslie Green (DOB 08/03/03) just tested positive for pregnancy. She does not feel that she has a support system to help her make decisions.

Scenario 3: Ella Rainwater's husband of 30 years died suddenly 1 month ago. Ella (DOB 07/11/1959) stated that she feels alone and has no one to talk to. Her daughter feels that Ella needs the support of others who have gone through the same thing.

Directions: Role-play these scenarios with two peers.

EQUIPMENT and SUPPLIES

- Computer (with internet) or a telephone book
- Paper and pen
- Community Resource Referral Form or other referral form
- Patient's health record

PROCEDURAL STEPS

1. Using the scenarios, identify the possible types of community resources that would assist each patient or family. Identify three different types of resources (e.g., medical equipment, support group) that would meet each patient's needs.
   PURPOSE: A variety of community resources are available for patients and families who are dealing with chronic illnesses and death. Such resources range from daycare, meals, transportation, medical equipment, assistive living, support groups, to reduced costs for medications.
2. Using the internet or the phone book, identify two local resources for each of the three kinds of resources (i.e., find two assistive living resources, two medical equipment suppliers, etc.). Make a list of six resources for the patient and family. Include the following:

a. Organization's name
b. Address and contact information
c. Summary of the services provided
d. Cost and other relevant information
PURPOSE: As the patient navigator or care coordinator, it is important for you to provide patients and families with the contact information for various community resources. This information can help the family find the best solution for the situation.

3. *Role-play the scenario indicated by the instructor.* Provide the patient or family member with the list of six resources. Describe the services offered and any costs.

4. Allow the patient or family member time to review the services. Answer any questions.
   PURPOSE: It is important that the patient and family members understand the services available.

5. Use professional, tactful verbal and nonverbal communication as you work with the patient or family member.
   PURPOSE: Patients and family members are more apt to respond positively to assistance if the medical assistant's communication is professional, empathetic,

PROCEDURE 7.2 Develop a List of Community Resources and Facilitate Referrals—*continued*

and tactful. Talking down to patients or acting superior are unprofessional behaviors that negatively impact the working relationship with patients.

6. *Role-play making the community referrals.* Have the patient or family member decide on two or more services they are interested in. Complete the referral document. Have the patient provide any additional information required on the form. Call the community resource agency and provide the referral information to the representative (a peer).

Note: Some community referrals (e.g., support groups) will require the patient to make contact and not the healthcare professional.

PURPOSE: The referral document is used by many organizations to capture the patient's preferences and to help process the referral.

7. Document the patient education and the referrals in the health record.

PURPOSE: It is important to document all patient interactions and referrals in the health record.

8

NUTRITION AND HEALTH PROMOTION

SCENARIO

Kayla Smith, registered medical assistant (RMA), has been working at Walden-Martin Family Medical (WMFM) Clinic for 4 years. She enjoys working with the patients and the providers. Kayla's supervisor is impressed with her motivation, patient care skills, and attention to detail. Kayla was asked to mentor John O'Neill, a medical assistant student from a local college.

John needs to complete a 190-hour practicum at WMFM Clinic. John has an interest in nutrition, because his mother is a registered dietitian. He is eager to see how Kayla works with patients who face the need for dietary changes. He hopes he will have the opportunity to observe her and then assist with the teaching process before doing it by himself.

While studying this chapter, think about the following questions:

- Why are carbohydrates, fat, protein, minerals/electrolytes, vitamins, fiber, and water important to the body?
- What are the special dietary needs of those with diabetes, cardiovascular disease, hypertension, cancer, and lactose sensitivity?
- What are the special dietary needs for a person with allergies and celiac disease?

- How should a medical assistant coach patients regarding special dietary needs?
- How can a medical assistant show awareness of a patient's concerns regarding a dietary change?

LEARNING OBJECTIVES

1. Describe metabolism.
2. Describe dietary nutrients, including carbohydrates, fiber, protein, fat, minerals and electrolytes, vitamins, and water.
3. Explain current dietary guidelines.
4. Describe how to read a food label.
5. Describe the different types of medically ordered diets.
6. Identify the special dietary needs for weight control, diabetes mellitus, cardiovascular disease, and hypertension.

7. Identify the special dietary needs for those with food allergies, celiac disease, and lactose intolerance.
8. Identify special dietary needs for those with various conditions, including pregnancy and lactation, epilepsy, HIV and AIDS, and cancer.
9. Instruct a patient on dietary changes while demonstrating awareness of others' concerns.

VOCABULARY

amino acids (ah MEE noe) Released during the digestion of protein foods in the intestines; carried by the blood to cells, where they are used to make proteins. Used for growth, maintenance, and repair of cells; they also transport nutrients.

anaphylaxis (an ah fah LAK sis) A rapidly progressing, life-threatening allergic reaction; characterized by hives, swelling of the mouth and airway, difficulty breathing, wheezing, and loss of consciousness.

antioxidant (an tee OK si dahnt) Synthetic or natural substance found in food and supplements; may prevent or delay some types of cell damage.

coaching Providing information in a supportive environment that allows people to grow, change, or improve their situation.

enriched Nutrients are added back into a food after they were lost during food processing.

enzymes (EN zimes) Special proteins that speed up the chemical reaction in the body.

fatty acids Result when fats are broken down; used by the body for energy and tissue development.

fortified Nutrients are added to a food; these nutrients were never originally in the food.

glucagon (GLOO kah gon) A hormone produced by the alpha cells in the pancreas; works on the liver to release glycogen and thereby prevent dangerously low blood glucose levels.

glucose Results when carbohydrates are broken down; main sugar found in the blood and used as the main source of energy.

insulin (IN suh lin) A hormone produced by the beta cells in the pancreas; moves glucose into the cells so it can be used for energy.

metabolism (me TAB oh lizm) The chemical process that occurs within a living organism in order to maintain life.

recommended dietary allowance (RDA) Average daily level of food intake needed to meet the nutrient requirements of most healthy people.

registered dietitian (die eh TISH an) A credentialed healthcare professional who is trained in nutrition and is able to apply the information to the dietary needs of healthy and ill patients.

regular diet The food and drink a person typically consumes when there are no dietary limitations.

Nutrition is a field of study that examines the substances in food that help us grow and stay healthy. Nutrition can also be defined as the intake of food for the body's dietary needs. It is important to eat a healthy and balanced diet. *Nutrients* are the chemicals in food that the body uses for energy, growth, and development. Nutrients include water, protein, carbohydrate, fat, vitamins, and minerals.

A medical assistant helps the provider by **coaching** patients on dietary changes. It is important to be aware of nutrients and the different types of diets commonly ordered in the ambulatory care environment. This chapter discusses metabolism and the nutrients essential for growth and development. Dietary requirements, along with medically ordered diets, are also discussed.

METABOLISM

Metabolism is the process the body uses to obtain or make energy from the food eaten. Metabolism has two phases:

- *Catabolism*: The process of breaking down molecules into smaller molecules, resulting in energy being released
- *Anabolism*: The process of smaller molecules being used to build larger molecules with the use of energy

For example, you eat a piece of chocolate candy with peanuts. It is broken down by **enzymes** in the intestines. The enzymes break down the proteins into **amino acids**, the fats into **fatty acids**, and the complex *carbohydrates* into simple sugars (e.g., **glucose**). These substances are absorbed by the blood and brought to the cells. In the cells, other enzymes catabolize or break down these substances, and energy is released. The energy released can be used or stored by the body. The small molecules created from catabolism are used to create larger molecules as the body repairs tissues and performs other functions. This process requires energy and is called *anabolism*. Every action of the body, involuntary or voluntary, requires energy.

Many times, metabolism is thought of as what influences our bodies to gain or lose weight. This is where calories come in. A *calorie* is a unit that measures how much energy is in a particular food. People use calories or the energy at different rates. Some people eat a lot of food and do not put on any weight, whereas others feel they look at food and gain weight. The number of calories a person burns each day is affected by the following factors:

- How much the person exercises
- The amount of fat and muscle on the person's body
- The person's *basal metabolic rate* (BMR), or the rate the body burns calories while the person is at rest

The BMR can play a role in a person's tendency to gain weight. For example, two people eat and exercise the same amount, but they have two different BMRs. The person with the lower BMR would have a greater tendency to gain more weight. Remember, the body stores unused calories as fat.

Variables That Affect the Basal Metabolic Rate (BMR)

- *Genetics*: Some people are born with a higher metabolism.
- *Gender*: Males have a higher density of lean muscle mass with a lower body fat percentage. This causes a higher BMR.
- *Age*: BMR decreases with age.
- *Weight*: The heavier an individual, the higher the BMR.
- *Body surface area*: This relates to a person's height and weight. The larger the body surface area, the higher the BMR.
- *Body fat percentage*: The lower a person's body fat percentage, the higher his or her BMR.
- *Diet*: Starvation and low-calorie diets can decrease the BMR.
- *Body temperature*: A higher body temperature results in an increased BMR.
- *External temperature*: The colder the external temperature, the more the body has to provide additional heat to maintain the body's temperature. This increases the BMR.
- *Thyroxin*: Produced by the thyroid gland, thyroxin can increase the BMR.
- *Exercise and lean muscle tissue*: Exercise will create lean muscle tissue, which increases the BMR.
- *Drugs*: Certain drugs (e.g., caffeine) can increase the BMR.

DIETARY NUTRIENTS

Nutrients in food, such as carbohydrates, can provide energy. Nutrients can also supply materials to build and repair tissues (e.g., proteins and amino acids). Lastly, nutrients can regulate metabolic processes. Some nutrients have only one purpose, whereas others have several jobs in the body. A combination of different foods is necessary to promote health. With a little planning, all the body's needs can be met by a well-balanced diet.

Nutrients can be classified into two different groups. *Essential nutrients* cannot be made by the body and must be in the food eaten. *Nonessential nutrients* are created by the body and do not need to be in food. For example, vitamin D is created from sun exposure on the skin, so it does not need to be consumed. Foods can also be described as:

- *Nutrient rich* (also called *nutrient dense*): Foods high in nutrients (e.g., vitamins, minerals, complex carbohydrates, healthy fats, and lean protein) and low in calories.
- *Non-nutrient rich:* Foods lacking vitamins, minerals, and fiber. They provide "empty calories" and can cause people to gain weight.

Carbohydrates

Carbohydrate is a nutrient found in our diet. Carbohydrates are used for energy and to regulate protein and fat metabolism. This nutrient encompasses a broad range of simple sugars, starches, and fiber.

Simple Sugars

There are many types of simple sugars. Nutrient-rich foods containing simple sugars include:

- Fruits and vegetables, which contain fructose and glucose
- Milk and milk products, which contain lactose

Non-nutrient-rich foods and food additives containing simple sugars include desserts (cookies, cakes), candy, soda, and syrups, white sugar (*sucrose*), honey, molasses, corn syrup, and high-fructose corn syrup.

During digestion, most sugars (except lactose from milk) break down into fructose and glucose. Lactose breaks down into glucose and galactose. Simple sugars are rapidly absorbed and quickly raise blood glucose levels. They provide a quick source of energy.

Starches

Starches are called *complex carbohydrates*. Examples of food sources of complex carbohydrates include:

- *Nutrient-rich starches:* Legumes (e.g., split peas, beans [kidney, black, garbanzo, and pinto]), starchy vegetables (e.g., corn, green peas, and potatoes), and whole grains (e.g., oats, barley, quinoa seeds, and brown rice)
- *Non-nutrient-rich starches:* White bread, crackers, and white rice

Complex carbohydrates are digested in the intestine before being absorbed. They break down into simple sugars and become a source of energy.

The glucose from the simple sugars and starches raises the blood glucose level. With the help of **insulin**, glucose is moved out of the bloodstream and into cells; it is then used for energy. Some glucose is stored in the liver and muscles as *glycogen*. The body uses the stored glycogen in between meals and during strenuous exercise. As the blood glucose levels start to drop, **glucagon** works on the liver to release the stored glycogen. Glycogen is released back into the blood and raises the blood glucose level.

It is important to remember that excessive carbohydrates can be converted into fat. Smart carbohydrate dietary choices include the following:

- Eat a variety of whole grains, fruits, vegetables, legumes, and low-fat or nonfat dairy products.
- At least half of all grains eaten should be whole grains.
- Limit processed foods in your diet, especially those with added sugar, salt, and fat.
- Eat enriched refined grains, if eating refined grains.

Whole Grains and Refined Grains

Foods made from wheat, oats, cornmeal, rice, and barley are grain products. Grains are divided into whole grains and refined grains:

- *Whole grains:* Use the entire grain kernel (e.g., bran, germ, and endosperm); they include whole-wheat flour, cracked wheat (bulgur), whole cornmeal, oatmeal, and brown rice.
- *Refined grains:* Are milled, and the bran and germ are removed to create a finer texture and longer shelf life. Examples include white flour, degermed cornmeal, white rice, and white bread. During the milling process, dietary fiber, iron, and many B vitamins are removed. For this reason, most refined grains are **enriched**. This means certain B vitamins and iron are added back to the grains. Fiber is not added back into the product.

Glycemic Index. The *glycemic index* (GI) is a numeric index used to indicate how much a carbohydrate food raises the blood glucose level. The foods are ranked from 0 to 100. Carbohydrates that are rapidly digested, absorbed, and considerably raise the blood glucose level are considered high GI foods ($\geq$70). Low GI foods ($\leq$55) produce a smaller change in the blood glucose level. The goal is to eat more low GI foods to reduce the risk of type 2 diabetes mellitus and heart disease. Low GI foods can also help maintain weight loss. Table 8.1 provides examples of the GI of some common foods.

Fiber

Fiber is different from simple sugars and starches. It cannot be digested by the body and thus it does not raise the blood glucose level. Fiber helps a person feel full and can help with weight management. There are two types of fiber: soluble fiber and insoluble fiber.

Soluble fiber dissolves in water and forms a gel-like substance. Soluble fiber helps:

- Soften the stool
- Lower the blood glucose level by slowing sugar absorption

TABLE 8.1 Glycemic Index (GI) for Foods	
PER SERVING	**GI**
Bagel, white frozen	72
Bread, whole wheat	71
Tortilla, wheat	30
Gatorade	78
Instant oatmeal	83
Skim milk	32
Apple	39
Banana	62
Watermelon	72
Peanuts	7

- Lower the low-density lipoprotein (LDL, or bad cholesterol) level by binding to fatty acids

Examples of soluble fiber foods include the following:

- Nutrient-rich: Legumes, oats, barley, fruits (e.g., avocados, apples, and citrus fruits) and carrots
- Non-nutrient rich: Processed and refined goods

Insoluble fiber bulks up the stool and helps to prevent constipation. Examples of insoluble fiber include the following:

- Nutrient-rich: Whole grains (whole wheat and brown rice), vegetables (corn, broccoli, green beans, cauliflower, and potato with skins), nuts and seeds, popcorn, and prunes
- Non-nutrient rich: Processed and refined goods

Fiber supplements are usually taken to reduce constipation. They can help a person be "regular." The active ingredient in the supplements can vary between natural and synthetic soluble fiber. Consider the following:

- Metamucil contains *psyllium* husk, a natural substance that contains about 70% soluble fiber and 30% insoluble fiber.
- Citrucel contains *methylcellulose*, a semisynthetic soluble fiber.
- Fibercon contains calcium *polycarbophil*, a synthetic soluble fiber.

It is important to drink plenty of water when taking fiber supplements. Some fiber supplements have been shown to lower blood pressure, blood glucose, and the risk of heart disease.

CRITICAL THINKING APPLICATION 8.1

Kayla wants to help John review carbohydrates. She asks him to list two foods from each category: simple sugars, starches, and fiber. What foods would you list?

Protein

Protein is a nutrient in our diet. Proteins are broken down into amino acids. Amino acids can be used as a source of energy in the absence of carbohydrates. Amino acids are also used to make proteins to help the body do the following:

- Break down food (e.g., enzymes)
- Grow and repair body tissues (e.g., connective tissue, hair, nails, muscles)
- Perform other functions (e.g., those related to hemoglobin, antibodies, and hormones)

Protein and amino acids are considered the building blocks of life. The body needs several amino acids in large enough amounts to maintain good health. Protein malnutrition is seen around the world. This can lead to *kwashiorkor*. A lack of dietary protein can cause growth failure, loss of muscle mass, anemia, edema and potbelly, skin depigmentation and hair loss, weakening of the circulatory and respiratory systems, decreased immunity, and death.

Amino acids are classified into three groups:

- *Essential amino acids*: Cannot be made by the body, thus must come from food eaten throughout the day
- *Nonessential amino acids*: Can be made by the body from essential amino acids or in the normal breakdown of proteins
- *Conditional amino acids*: Usually not essential, except in times of illness and stress

Foods that have all the essential amino acids to support the body are called *complete proteins*. Foods that are considered complete proteins are fish, meat, poultry, dairy products, quinoa seeds, buckwheat, chia seeds, and eggs. Foods that do not contain all the essential amino acids are called *incomplete proteins*. Nuts, legumes, grains, and vegetables are examples of incomplete proteins.

Smart protein choices include the following:

- Choose lean or low-fat meat and poultry.
- Eat seafood rich in omega-3 fatty acids, such as salmon, trout, herring, Pacific oysters, and Atlantic and Pacific mackerel.
- Limit processed meats (e.g., ham, sausage, and deli meats), which contain added salt (sodium).
- Eat unsalted nuts and seeds to keep sodium intake low.

Omega-3 Fatty Acids

Omega-3 fatty acids are a group of polyunsaturated fatty acids found in fish (e.g., salmon, herring, halibut, and mackerel) and some nuts and seeds. These fatty acids play a role in reducing blood cholesterol, heart disease risk, inflammation, and depression. Omega-3 fatty acids also increase the effectiveness of anti-inflammatory and antidepressant drugs.

CRITICAL THINKING APPLICATION 8.2

Kayla wants to help John review proteins. She asks John to list six foods that contain proteins. What foods would you list?

Fat

Fat is an important nutrient in our diet. Fats provide 9 calories per gram, whereas carbohydrates and proteins provide only 4 calories per gram. The body uses fat for the following:

- A source of energy. If glucose is not available for energy, the body will break down fat and the resulting ketones are used for energy.
- Healthy skin and hair.
- Vitamin absorption. Vitamins A, D, E, and K are fat soluble.
- Insulation (cushion) for organs and to keep the body warm.
- Brain development, controlling inflammation, and blood clotting. Linoleic and linolenic acid, which are essential fatty acids, are used for these processes.

Fat is required in the diet. Table 8.2 describes the types of fats found in foods. Diets low in fats can cause cold sensitivity, increased infections, and amenorrhea in women. Long-term fat deficiency can lead to metabolic problems and fat-soluble vitamin deficiency.

Triglycerides are another type of fat in the body. Our livers make triglycerides from the calories we do not use. Triglycerides are also found in foods.

Cholesterol is a waxy, fat-like substance. It is used to make hormones, vitamin D, bile acids, and cell membranes. Cholesterol is created in the liver and dietary cholesterol is found in animal-based foods (e.g., egg yolks, meat, shellfish, and cheese). Cholesterol is carried in the blood by the following lipoproteins:

- *High-density lipoprotein* (HDL): Considered "good" cholesterol. It helps move the cholesterol from the tissues to the liver. The

TABLE 8.2   Types of Fats

TYPE	DESCRIPTION	IMPACT ON CHOLESTEROL	FOUND IN
Saturated fats	Solid at room temperature	Increase the LDL level	Butter, cheese, whole milk, ice cream, cream, fatty meats; processed coconut oil, palm oil
Unsaturated fats	Liquid at room temperature; two kinds: monounsaturated and polyunsaturated	Decrease the LDL level	Monounsaturated: olive and canola oil Polyunsaturated: safflower, sunflower, corn, and soy oil
Trans fatty acids	Also called *hydrogenated fats* and *trans fats*; created when hydrogen is added to vegetable oils during food manufacturing	Increase LDL and decrease HDL levels	Foods made with hydrogenated and partially hydrogenated oils; margarine, commercially prepared baked goods

liver helps remove cholesterol from the body. A low level of HDL increases the risk of heart disease.

- *Low-density lipoprotein* (LDL): Considered "bad" cholesterol. It moves cholesterol to tissues, including arteries. Most of the cholesterol in the blood is in LDL. The higher the LDL level in the blood, the greater the risk for heart disease. LDL can be lowered through diet, exercise, and medications. Using unsaturated fats can help lower the LDL level.

Triglycerides

Triglycerides are stored in the fat cells and have the following characteristics:
- Are used for energy when carbohydrates are limited
- Absorb vitamins and other nutrients
- Contain essential fatty acids, which are important for growth and development

A person's triglyceride level is usually checked with the cholesterol levels. High triglyceride levels increase one's risk for heart disease and stroke. There are other reasons for high triglyceride levels, including poorly controlled type 2 diabetes mellitus, liver disease, kidney disease, and hypothyroidism.

The best ways to lower the triglyceride level is to do the following:
- Cut back on calories and lose weight.
- Avoid sugary and refined food; choose monounsaturated fats over saturated fats.
- Limit the amount of alcohol consumed, and exercise daily.
- Medications can also be ordered to help reduce the triglyceride level.

CRITICAL THINKING APPLICATION   8.3
Kayla wants to help John review the three types of fats. She asks John to describe unsaturated fats, saturated fats, and trans fatty acids. How would you describe them?

Minerals and Electrolytes

Minerals are naturally occurring inorganic substances (e.g., iron, zinc, and calcium). Minerals needed by the body are divided into two

categories: major and trace. *Major minerals*, or macrominerals, are needed in larger amounts. *Trace minerals*, or microminerals, are needed in smaller amounts in the body.

Electrolytes are minerals in the body fluid that have an electrical charge. They are found in the blood, urine, and other body fluids. Electrolytes come from the foods we eat and fluids we drink (Table 8.3). Too little or too much water in the body, vomiting, diarrhea, sweating, and kidney problems can change our electrolyte levels. A provider will order laboratory tests to measure a patient's electrolyte levels.

CRITICAL THINKING APPLICATION   8.4
Kayla asks John how he would explain the difference between minerals and electrolytes. How would you respond?

Vitamins

Vitamins are organic substances needed by the body in very small amounts for specific roles. There are 13 vitamins required by the body. It is important to get the **recommended dietary allowance (RDA)** of each vitamin. A deficit of a vitamin can lead to disease.

Vitamins are either water soluble or fat soluble (Table 8.4). Water-soluble vitamins dissolve in water. These include vitamins B and C. Any unused water-soluble vitamins leave the body through the urine. Vitamin B_{12} is an exception, because the liver stores the vitamin for years. Water-soluble vitamins need to be taken in daily. Fat-soluble vitamins are vitamins A, D, E, and K. These vitamins are absorbed more easily with the presence of fat in the diet. They can build up in the body, reaching toxic levels, so typically supplements are not needed.

CRITICAL THINKING APPLICATION   8.5
Kayla and John are reviewing vitamins that patients commonly take. John asks Kayla to explain the difference between water-soluble and fat-soluble vitamins. How would you explain the difference?

TABLE 8.3   Examples of Major and Trace Minerals

CATEGORY	MINERAL	ROLE IN THE BODY	FOUND IN
Major minerals (*macrominerals*)	Calcium	For healthy teeth and bones; muscle and nerve function, blood clotting, blood pressure regulation, immune system health	Milk products, canned fish (e.g., salmon), **fortified** soy milk, greens (e.g., broccoli), legumes
	Potassium	For proper muscle and nerve function, fluid balance	Milk, fresh fruits and vegetables, whole grains, legumes, meats
	Sodium		Table salt, processed foods, condiments
	Chloride	For proper fluid balance; stomach acid	Table salt, processed foods, tomatoes, celery, and olives
	Phosphorus	For healthy teeth and bones; important in the acid-base balance system	Meat, poultry, fish, eggs, milk, processed foods, soda pop
	Sulfur	Found in body proteins	Meats, poultry, fish, eggs, legumes, nuts
	Magnesium	Needed to make proteins; for muscle and nerve function and immune system health	Nuts, legumes, seeds, seafood, chocolate, and leafy green vegetables
Trace minerals (*microminerals*)	Iron	Part of hemoglobin found in red blood cells, used for energy metabolism	Meats, fish, poultry, shellfish, egg yolks, legumes, dark leafy greens, iron-enriched or fortified foods
	Zinc	Used for making proteins, taste perception, wound healing, immune system health, production of sperm, normal growth	Vegetables, poultry, fish, meats
	Iodine	Found in thyroid hormone, which is involved with metabolism, growth, and development	Seafood, iodized salt, milk products
	Selenium	**Antioxidant**	Seafood, grains, and meats
	Fluoride	Involved with healthy teeth and bones	Fish, tea, and drinking water
	Chromium	Used in the metabolism of carbohydrates and fats; also aids in insulin action and glucose metabolism	Brewer's yeast, beef, liver, eggs, chicken, wheat germ, potatoes
	Copper	Helps to form red blood cells; involved with keeping the blood vessels, nerves, immune system, and bones healthy; aids in iron absorption	Shellfish, whole grains, beans, nuts, liver, dark leafy greens, dried fruits, yeast, and cocoa

TABLE 8.4   Fat- and Water-Soluble Vitamins

CATEGORY	VITAMIN	RECOMMENDED DIETARY ALLOWANCE FOR ADULTS	ROLE IN THE BODY	FOUND IN	EFFECT(S) OF DEFICIENCY	TOXIC?
Fat-Soluble Vitamins	Vitamin A	700–900 mcg	Antioxidant; helps form and maintain healthy teeth, bones, mucous membranes, soft tissue, and skin.	Dark-colored fruits and leafy vegetables, egg yolks, fortified milk products, liver, beef, fish	Night blindness	Yes, can cause liver toxicity
	Vitamin D	15–20 mcg	Bone growth; made by the body after being in the sun	Fatty fish (e.g., salmon, herring), fish liver oils, fortified cereals, fortified milk products	Bone pain, muscle weakness	Yes, *hypercalcemia* (elevated blood calcium levels) and kidney problems

Continued

TABLE 8.4   Fat- and Water-Soluble Vitamins—*continued*

CATEGORY	VITAMIN	RECOMMENDED DIETARY ALLOWANCE FOR ADULTS	ROLE IN THE BODY	FOUND IN	EFFECT(S) OF DEFICIENCY	TOXIC?
	Vitamin E (tocopherol)	15 mg	Antioxidant; helps form red blood cells and use vitamin K	Avocado, dark green and dark leafy vegetables (e.g., spinach, broccoli, and asparagus); safflower, corn, and sunflower oils; papaya, mango, wheat germ, seeds, nuts	Hemolytic anemia, neurologic deficits	Yes, hemorrhagic toxicity can occur with supplement use
	Vitamin K	90–120 mcg	Blood clotting; made in the intestine	Cabbage, cauliflower, cereals, dark green and dark leafy vegetables, fish, liver, eggs, beef	Bleeding	No toxic effects reported
Water-Soluble Vitamins	Thiamine (vitamin B_1)	1.1–1.2 mg	Used for nervous system, muscle function, and carbohydrate metabolism	Eggs, enriched flour, lean meats, legumes, nuts, seeds, organ meats, peas, whole grains	Beriberi, usually in alcoholics	No toxic effects reported
	Riboflavin (vitamin B_2)	1.1–1.3 mg	Works with other B vitamins; important for growth and red blood cell production	Milk, mushrooms, spinach, almonds, lamb	Riboflavin deficiency	No toxic effects reported
	Niacin (vitamin B_3)	14–16 mg	Used in digestive process and skin and nerve functions; treats low HDL and high LDL cholesterol and triglyceride levels	Avocados, eggs, enriched breads and cereals, lean meats, fish, poultry, legumes, nuts, and potato	Pellagra, digestive issues	Niacin-containing supplements should be taken as provider indicates
	Pantothenic acid (vitamin B_5)	5 mg	Involved with metabolism, hormone and cholesterol production, and needed for growth	Avocados, broccoli, egg yolks, legumes, milk, yeast, organ meats, potatoes, and whole grains	Vitamin B_5 deficiency	No toxic effects reported
	Pyridoxine (vitamin B_6)	1.3–1.7 mg	Helps form red blood cells and maintain brain function; also used for protein metabolism	Avocado, banana, legumes, meat, nuts, poultry, and whole grains	Cracks around mouth, depression, rash	No toxic effects reported
	Biotin (vitamin B_7)	30 mcg	Used for fat and carbohydrate metabolism; also used in the production of hormones and cholesterol	Chocolate, legumes, milk, nuts, organ meats (e.g., liver, kidney), pork, egg yolks, and yeast	Hair loss, cheilitis, glossitis	No toxic effects reported

TABLE 8.4 Fat- and Water-Soluble Vitamins—*continued*

CATEGORY	VITAMIN	RECOMMENDED DIETARY ALLOWANCE FOR ADULTS	ROLE IN THE BODY	FOUND IN	EFFECT(S) OF DEFICIENCY	TOXIC?
	Folate (vitamin B$_9$, folic acid)	400 mcg	Works with vitamin B$_{12}$ to help form blood cells; important in pregnancy to prevent spina bifida	Asparagus, broccoli, beets, brewer's yeast, legumes, enriched breads and cereals, green leafy vegetables, oranges, peanut butter	Anemia, diarrhea	Caution with high doses, limited data on toxicity
	Cobalamin (vitamin B$_{12}$)	2.4 mcg	Important for protein metabolism, the formation of red blood cells, and the maintenance of the central nervous system	Meat, eggs, fortified foods, milk products, organ meats, poultry, and shellfish	Pernicious anemia, confusion	No toxic effects reported
	Vitamin C (ascorbic acid)	75–90 mg	Antioxidant; promotes healthy gums and teeth; helps absorb iron; maintains healthy tissue and promotes wound healing	Citrus fruits, tomatoes, broccoli, cabbage, cauliflower, potatoes, spinach, strawberries	Scurvy	Kidney stones, excess iron absorption, gastrointestinal disturbances

mcg, Micrograms; *mg,* milligrams; *RDA,* recommended daily allowance.
Some information was obtained from the Vitamins Food and Nutrition Board, Institute of Medicine, National Academies. *https://www.nal.usda.gov/sites/default/files/fnic_uploads//DRI_Vitamins. pdf* Accessed March 30, 2019.

Antioxidants

When our body uses oxygen to burn food for energy, free radicals are formed. Free radicals are also formed due to environmental influences (e.g., water and air pollution, cigarette smoke, fried foods). Excessive free radicals can affect our health by attacking cells' DNA and blood vessels. This increases the risk for cardiovascular disease, strokes, arthritis, cataracts, and other degenerative diseases.

Antioxidants protect cells from free radicals and limit the damage free radicals can do to the cells. Antioxidants are powerful and beneficial for us. Antioxidants include vitamins A, C, and E, beta-carotene, lycopene, lutein, and selenium.

Water

Drinking water every day is important for a person's health. Water is the basis for the fluids in the body. It makes up more than two-thirds of the body's weight. Without water, we would become dehydrated and die within a few days. All cells and organs need water to function and survive. Water plays important roles in the body, including the following:

- Keeps the body temperature normal with perspiration
- Lubricates and cushions joints (e.g., saliva, fluid around joints)
- Helps to prevent and relieve constipation by moving food through the intestines
- Protects the spinal cord, brain, and other sensitive tissues
- Gets rid of waste products in the body through urine, sweat, and stool

Our need for water increases in hot weather, when we are more active, or when we have a fever, diarrhea, or vomiting. The recommended daily intake of water for healthy men is about 13 cups; the recommendation for healthy women is 9 cups. The individual need for water is based on a person's weight, age, activity level, and certain medical conditions.

Water and Diseases

Some patients are placed on fluid restrictions. This means they can only have a certain amount of fluids a day. The provider will indicate the maximum amount of fluids to be consumed daily. It is important to limit fluids that act like a diuretic (e.g., alcohol and caffeinated beverages), because they pull fluid from the body and increase the risk of dehydration. Conditions that may require fluid restrictions include the following:

- Heart problems, including congestive heart failure
- Kidney problems, such as those that might affect patients on dialysis and those with end-stage renal disease
- Adrenal insufficiency and corticosteroid treatment

Some diseases and conditions require more fluids/water to be consumed. People with postural orthostatic tachycardia syndrome (POTS) need to drink at least 2 to 3 liters of water a day to maintain their blood pressure. Other conditions, such as diabetes insipidus, diabetes mellitus, and Addison disease, may cause patients to excrete more urine and thus put them more at risk for dehydration.

DIETARY GUIDELINES

For over a century, the US Department of Agriculture (USDA) has provided food guides to the public. Some of the more recent guides include the following:

- 1992: Food Guide Pyramid, which showed the five basic food groups, with fats and sugars making up the tip of the pyramid
- 2005: MyPyramid Food Guidance System, which continued with the pyramid design but added physical activity and oils
- 2011: MyPlate, which was introduced along with the 2010 Dietary Guidelines for Americans

MyPlate

MyPlate focuses on making healthy food choices because everything eaten matters (Fig. 8.1). Some of the key messages with these dietary guidelines include the following:

- Fill half the plate with fruits and vegetables. Vary the color and type of fruits and vegetables.
- Make half of the grains each day whole grains.
- Vary the types of proteins eaten.
- Move to low-fat or fat-free milk and yogurt.
- Drink and eat less saturated fat, sodium, and added sugars.

MyPlate consists of five food groups, along with oil (Table 8.5). Oil contains required nutrients, so the USDA addresses it. Oil is usually consumed in nuts, fish, cooking oil, and salad dressing. Most children need between 3 to 6 teaspoons, and adults need from 5 to 7 teaspoons, depending on gender and age.

The MyPlate website (*www.choosemyplate.gov*) offers numerous online resources for individuals and professionals. Tip sheets, food plans, and other resources provide additional information. MyPlate is very flexible for cultural foods.

Dietary Guidelines

The USDA publishes Dietary Guidelines every 5 years. The guidelines are for individuals 2 years or older. The focus is on disease prevention and health promotion. The current dietary guidelines focus on overall eating patterns, health, and the risk of chronic disease.

Key recommendations from the 2015–2020 Dietary Guidelines for Americans include those listed with MyPlate, in addition to the following:

- Limit foods with saturated and trans fats, added sugars, and sodium.
- Less than 10% of daily calories should come from saturated fats (e.g., butter, whole milk, fatty meats, coconut oil, and palm oil).
- Individuals age 14 or older should consume fewer than 2300 milligrams (mg) of sodium a day.
- Limit the alcohol consumed to one drink per day for women and two drinks for men.
- Incorporate physical activity (e.g., aerobic, muscle-strengthening, and bone strengthening activities) into the week.

READING FOOD LABELS

Knowing how to read a food label is important when making healthy food selections. The food label contains the nutritional information and the ingredient list. The government has required food manufacturers to include certain information on the food label. The amounts for "Trans Fat" and "Added Sugars" are some of the newer additions to the food label.

Food labels provide nutritional facts. This information is presented in both the quantity (e.g., grams [g] or milligrams [mg]) and as a percentage. The percentage reflects the *% Daily Value* (DV). This is the percentage of the nutrient in a single serving in terms of the daily recommended amount based on a 2000-calorie diet. You will see this description at the bottom of the list of nutrition facts. Remember that if you are eating fewer than 2000 calories daily, these percentages will be different for you.

When reading the nutrition facts (Fig. 8.2), start at the top and work down:

- Check the calories per serving. If you eat the entire container and it consists of two servings, you need to double the calories.
- Check the amount of fat. Limit the saturated fat intake and avoid trans fats.
- The amounts listed for cholesterol, sodium, total carbohydrates, and added sugars are also numbers to consider. Choose foods with low amounts of these nutrients.
- Examine the dietary fiber, protein, vitamin D, calcium, iron, and potassium. Make sure you are getting enough of these beneficial nutrients.

Ingredient lists on foods are also important to understand (Fig. 8.3). The ingredients are listed in descending order, starting with the one that weighs the most and ending with the one that weighs the

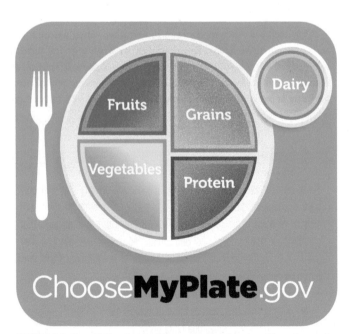

FIGURE 8.1 Choose MyPlate. (From the US Department of Agriculture. *https://www.choosemyplate.gov.*)

TABLE 8.5 Food Groups with Serving Amounts for MyPlate

FOOD GROUP	WHAT COUNTS?	RECOMMENDED DAILY AMOUNTS[a]			
		CHILDREN 2–8 yr	CHILDREN 9–18 yr	WOMEN 19–51+ yr	MEN 19–51+ yr
Dairy	*1 cup equivalent:* 1 cup milk, yogurt, soymilk, almond milk, coconut milk 1½ oz natural cheese 2 oz processed cheese	2–2½ cups	3 cups	3 cups	3 cups
Proteins	*1 oz equivalent:* 1 oz meat, poultry, or fish ¼ cup cooked beans 1 egg 1 tablespoon peanut butter ½ oz nuts or seeds	2–4 oz	5–6½ oz	5–5½ oz	5½–6½ oz
Vegetables	*1 cup equivalent:* 1 cup raw or cooked vegetables or vegetable juice 2 cups raw leafy greens	½ cup	2–3 cups	2–2½ cups	2½–3 cups
Fruits	*1 cup equivalent:* 1 cup fruit or 100% fruit juice ½ cup dried fruit	1–1½ cups	1½–2 cups	1½–2 cups	2 cups
Grains	*1 oz equivalent:* 1 slice of bread 1 cup dry cereal ½ cup cooked rice, pasta, or cereal (at least half should be whole grains)	3–5 oz	5–8 oz	5–6 oz	6–8 oz

[a]The amount required is based on the individual's gender and age and the amount of exercise he or she does. This table shows ranges; for more specific information, go to *https://www.choosemyplate.gov.*

Nutrition Facts

2 servings per container
Serving size 1 1/2 cup (208g)

Amount per serving
Calories 240

	% Daily Value*
Total Fat 4g	**5%**
Saturated Fat 1.5g	**8%**
Trans Fat 0g	
Cholesterol 5mg	**2%**
Sodium 430mg	**19%**
Total Carbohydrate 46g	**17%**
Dietary Fiber 7g	**25%**
Total Sugars 4g	
Includes 2g Added Sugars	**4%**
Protein 11g	
Vitamin D 2mcg	10%
Calcium 260mg	20%
Iron 6mg	35%
Potassium 240mg	6%

* The % Daily Value (DV) tells you how much a nutrient in a serving of food contributes to a daily diet. 2,000 calories a day is used for general nutrition advice.

FIGURE 8.2 Nutrition facts. (From the US Food and Drug Administration. *https://www.fda.gov/Food/IngredientsPackagingLabeling/LabelingNutrition/ucm537159.htm.*)

Food Label #1	Food Label #2
Ingredients: semolina (wheat), durum flour (wheat), eggs, partially hydrogenated oil, niacin, ferrous sulfate, thiamin mononitrate, riboflavin. **Contains: Wheat, Eggs.** **Manufactured in a facility that uses tree nuts and eggs.**	**Ingredients:** grapes, corn syrup, high fructose corn syrup, fruit pectin, and citric acid.

FIGURE 8.3 Ingredient list on food labels.

least. There are several reasons a person may look at the ingredient list:

- To look for trans fats: Even if the nutrition information indicates 0 grams trans fats, the product may still contain less than 0.5 gram of trans fats per serving. Look for ingredients such as "hydrogenated" or "partially hydrogenated oil." This indicates the presence of trans fats. So even if the nutrition information indicates 0 grams of trans fats, you may quickly reach your daily limit if you eat more than one serving.
- To avoid certain ingredients: Some people try to avoid ingredients such as high fructose corn syrup and certain food colorings.

- To identify allergens: More than 160 foods have been found to be allergens. The government has identified eight allergens that make up about 90% of all food allergy reactions. Laws regulating food labeling require manufacturers to indicate if any of these top allergens are in the food product. Advisory statements, such as "May contain peanuts" or "Made in a factory that also processes tree nuts," are optional and not required by law. (More information on allergens will be presented later in the chapter.)

MEDICALLY ORDERED DIETS

Patients may need to change their diet for a variety of reasons:
- Preparation for a procedure
- Dental problems
- Illness
- A condition that requires dietary changes (e.g., allergy, hypertension)

If the dietary change is also a lifestyle change (e.g., for diabetes or hypertension), the provider may refer the patient to a **registered dietitian**. The registered dietitian can provide in-depth coaching and counseling on dietary changes.

For other dietary changes or to review a person's knowledge of a specific diet, the medical assistant may be involved. When the provider orders a specific test or a particular diet, the medical assistant may need to coach the patient on the new diet. As with other coaching, it is important for the medical assistant to provide the patient with a reference handout to take home. This will help guide the patient on the dietary changes. Learning about different medically ordered diets is important for the medical assistant.

Clear Liquid Diet

A clear liquid diet is made up of foods and beverages that are liquid at room temperature. Clear means you need to see through the liquids. Examples of foods included on a clear liquid diet include the following:
- Water, tea, coffee, sport drinks, and clear soda
- Popsicles and juice without pulp
- Soup broth and gelatin (Jell-O)

Clear liquid diets are ordered for only a short time because they do not contain adequate nutrition. A clear liquid diet may be used when a person experiences diarrhea, vomiting, or nausea. It is commonly ordered after surgery and as part of the preparation for intestinal procedures. If a person is undergoing an intestinal procedure, red or pink clear liquids are not allowed because they could be mistaken for blood in the intestine.

Full Liquid Diet

A full liquid diet is made up of foods and beverages that are liquid at room temperature. Unlike the clear liquid diet, the full liquid diet includes milk products. Foods included in a full liquid diet include the following:
- Clear liquids (see clear liquid diet)
- Strained creamy soups
- Milk, milkshakes, pudding, plain yogurt, custard, and ice cream
- Liquid supplements
- Sugar, honey, syrups, butter, margarine

Some providers will allow cooked, refined cereals (e.g., cream of rice), baby food strained meats, and potatoes pureed in soup on a full liquid diet. This diet is a step above a clear liquid diet and below a **regular diet**.

Full liquid diets are ordered for only a short time because they do not contain adequate nutrition. A full liquid diet may be used before or after surgery, as part of the preparation for tests or procedures, and if a person has difficulty chewing or swallowing.

CRITICAL THINKING APPLICATION   **8.6**

Kayla and John are working with Janine Butler. Janine needs to undergo an intestinal procedure and needs to be on clear liquids for 2 days. Janine states, "I was on a full liquid diet last year for a procedure. What is the difference between a clear liquid diet and a full liquid diet?" How would you answer this question?

Soft and Mechanical Soft Diets

A soft diet is a transition between a liquid diet and a regular diet. The foods on this diet are soft in texture, low in fiber, and easy for a person to digest. The soft diet eliminates food that is hard to chew and swallow (Table 8.6).

This diet is used for patients recovering from surgery or a lengthy illness. It can also be used for people with chewing or swallowing problems due to illness or dental issues.

Mechanical soft diets consist of foods that have been prepared for easier chewing and swallowing using household tools (e.g., grinder, blender, and knife). Typically, there are no limitations (e.g., spicy, gassy, and fried) to mechanical soft diets. Mechanical soft diets are used for the following groups:
- Those recovering from head, neck, or mouth surgery
- Those who have difficulty swallowing (*dysphagia*), poor fitting dentures, no teeth
- Those who are too ill to chew

Bland Diet

A bland diet includes foods that are soft and low in fiber. This diet eliminates foods that are spicy, fried, or raw and beverages that contain caffeine or alcohol. Citrus juices and foods may also be eliminated. The foods included in a bland diet are similar to those incorporated into a soft diet.

TABLE 8.6	**Soft Diet**
FOODS ELIMINATED	**FOODS INCLUDED**
• Raw fruits and vegetables • Chewy or crispy breads • Tough meats • Broccoli and cauliflower • Fried, greasy foods • Highly seasoned or spicy foods • Nuts and seeds	• Grains: soft breads, crackers, white rice pasta • Fruits and vegetables: soft cooked, canned (no skin) • Milk products: milk, yogurt, cottage cheese, ice cream, pudding • Protein: tender meat, poultry, and fish; eggs, tofu, smooth peanut butter

A bland diet is ordered to help treat gastroesophageal reflux disease (GERD), ulcers, nausea and vomiting, diarrhea, and gas. It can also be used after stomach or intestinal surgery.

Weight Control Diet

When trying to achieve or maintain a healthy weight, a person needs to find the balance between the number of calories eaten and the number used. Extra calories eaten and not used will result in a weight gain. For people to lose 1 to 2 pounds per week, they need to reduce their caloric intake by 500 to 1000 calories a day or increase their exercise to burn more calories. Identifying the calories consumed is an important step in achieving a healthy weight. Food diaries, apps, and trackers are available to help gauge food intake and activity.

Nutritional tips for patients trying to achieve a healthy weight include the following:

- Commit to a lifestyle change. Identify resources for information and support.
- Track foods eaten and beverages drunk, along with physical exercise.
- Set realistic goals, knowing that slips will occur.
- Eat healthy meals. They should be low in saturated fat, trans fat, cholesterol, salt, and added sugar. Eat lean meats, fish, poultry, beans, eggs, and nuts. Include fruits (especially whole fruits), vegetables, whole grains, and fat-free or low-fat milk products.
- Control portion sizes. *Portion size* is the amount of food we eat. *Serving size* is a standard measurement of food (e.g., 1 cup or 1 oz). Many foods that come as a single portion actually contain multiple servings. For instance, a serving size of potato chips is 1 oz. The 3-oz potato chip bag is a single portion, but three servings. Another example is bread. You use two pieces of bread for a sandwich (portion size), but a serving is one slice. Most people overestimate serving sizes. It is best to measure the food or use a quick estimate method (Table 8.7).

TABLE 8.7 Quick Methods to Estimate Portion Size

AMOUNT OF FOOD	APPROXIMATE SIZE
3 oz of chicken and lean beef	Deck of cards
1 medium potato	Computer mouse
½ cup cooked pasta	Tennis ball
1 oz of cheese	Two dice
1 medium size fruit	Tennis ball
1 cup fruit or cooked vegetables	Baseball
1 oz of nuts	Handful
1 oz of chips or pretzels	Two handfuls (13–16 chips)
1 cup	Woman's fist
1 tablespoon (tbs)	First joint of thumb
1 teaspoon (tsp)	Fingertip

CRITICAL THINKING APPLICATION 8.7

Kayla and John are working with Amma Patel. Kayla is explaining the weight control diet that Dr. Perez ordered for Amma. They are discussing serving size and portions. Amma states she is confused by the difference. How might you explain the difference between these two concepts? Provide an example for Amma.

Portion Size and Obesity

In some cases, portion sizes and serving sizes are the same. Over the years many portion sizes have changed. Some experts attribute the growing obesity epidemic in the United States to this change. In the 1950s the dinner plate was 9 inches in diameter; today it is 11 to 12 inches. Some restaurants use even larger plates. With the plate change, the average portion of food also has increased. Restaurants have increased the amount of food they serve, and more Americans are eating out. With the increase in portions, *portion distortion* is occurring. The size of restaurant portions is causing Americans to rethink what the "normal" portions of food should be. Here are some examples of portion changes since the 1990s:

- Bagels have increased by 3 inches and added 210 calories.
- Muffins have increased by 3.5 oz and added 290 calories.
- Cheeseburgers have increased in size and added almost 260 calories.
- Soda size has increased by 13.5 oz and added almost 170 calories.

As these examples show, the increase in portion sizes has led to an increase in the number of calories. Remember, the calories consumed and not used turn into fat.

Information from the National Heart, Lung, and Blood Institute, *https://www.nhlbi.nih.gov/health/educational/wecan/eat-right/distortion.htm.* Accessed September 25, 2018.

Obesity

According to a study from 2015 to 2016, the prevalence of obesity in adults has increased to 39.8%, which is up from 10 years earlier. Obesity affects over 93.3 million adults in the US according to the Centers of Disease Control and Prevention (CDC). Obesity-related diseases (e.g., heart disease, type 2 diabetes, stroke, and certain types of cancer) are some of the leading causes of death in the US.

Childhood obesity remained stable over the past 10 years and affects about 18.5% of children. The prevalence of childhood obesity is higher in children after age 6 than in earlier years of life.

People are considered overweight or obese when they weigh more than what is considered a healthy weight for their height. The Body Mass Index (BMI) is a screening tool for obesity. Chapter 5 discusses the BMI. If a person's BMI is less than 18.5, that person is considered underweight. A BMI higher than 18.5 but less than 25 is considered normal; a BMI higher than 25 but less than 30 is consider overweight; and a BMI 30 or higher is considered obese.

Treatment for obesity includes:

- *Dietary changes*: Cutting calories, making healthier choices, restricting certain foods, and meal replacements
- *Exercise and activity*: Exercising 150 to 300 minutes a week.
- *Behavior changes*: Trying to eliminate the obstacles to managing weight (e.g., high-risk situations). Recording diet and exercise patterns. Counseling and support groups can be helpful.
- *Prescription weight-loss medications* (Table 8.8)
- *Vagal nerve blockade*: An implanted device sends electrical impulses to the vagus nerve, telling the brain when the stomach is empty or full.
- *Weight-loss surgery*: Also called *bariatric surgery*; it helps the person feel fuller sooner. Common weight-loss surgeries include the following:
  - *Gastric bypass surgery*: A small pouch is created at the top of the stomach, and the rest of the stomach is stapled shut. The small intestine is cut, with one end attached to the new pouch, thus bypassing the duodenum. The other end, which is attached to the stomach, is attached to another section of the intestine. Patients may have issues with iron and calcium absorption. Vitamin B_{12} supplements must be taken.
  - *Laparoscopic adjustable gastric band* (LAGB): A band is placed on the upper part of the stomach, creating a small pouch that helps to restrict food. A small port is implanted below the skin, and fluid can be injected into the band to adjust the size of the pouch outlet.
  - *Gastric sleeve*: A small pouch is created in the stomach, and about 67% of the stomach is removed. The person feels full sooner.

Diabetic Eating Plans

People with diabetes mellitus need to monitor their carbohydrate intake. Remember that carbohydrates are broken down into glucose in the body. Insulin moves the glucose from the blood into the cells.

For people with diabetes, the body either does not make enough insulin or does not respond to the insulin produced. As a result, their blood glucose levels are high. In the absence of insulin, the body metabolizes fat and uses the ketones for energy. Ketones build up in the body. (Too many ketones can lead to ketoacidosis, a life-threatening condition.) See Chapter 23 for more information on the treatments for type 1 and type 2 diabetes.

Over the years, several different diabetic eating plans have been created for people with diabetes mellitus. You may hear of patients being on diet plans such as the exchange list system. This diet plan grouped similar foods that had the same amount of carbohydrate, protein, fat, and calories. Each food item had a measurement (e.g., 1 cup) to indicate how much could be eaten for that exchange. Three main groups were given in the plan: carbohydrate, meat, and fat.

The American Diabetes Association (*www.diabetes.org*) encourages the following diabetes meal plans: the Glycemic Index approach, the "Create Your Plate" method, and carb counting. The GI was explained earlier in this chapter. Eating lower GI foods helps one to maintain a more stable blood glucose level.

The "Create Your Plate" method uses a 9-inch dinner plate (Fig. 8.4). To follow this meal plan, do the following:

- Fill half of the plate with nonstarchy vegetables (e.g., beans, broccoli, carrots, salad greens, and peppers).
- Split the remaining unfilled side of the plate in half. One small half is filled with a protein (e.g., lean meat, poultry, and fish).
- The other small half is filled with a grain and starch vegetable (e.g., brown rice, potato, squash, green peas, and corn).
- Complete the meal with a serving of fruit, a serving of dairy (milk product), and a nonsweetened beverage.

Carb counting, or carbohydrate counting, is a meal planning tool used by people with diabetes mellitus. Using this method, a person keeps track of the amount of carbohydrates eaten each day. Carbohydrates are measured in grams. This system may give some people better control of their diabetes, but it is a learning process. The person

TABLE 8.8	Weight Loss Medications		
MEDICATION	**CLASS**	**ACTION**	**COMMON SIDE EFFECTS**
Xenical, Alli (orlistat)	Lipase inhibitors	Prevents some of the fat consumed from being absorbed in the intestines	Oily spotting, loose stools, difficulty controlling stools, stomach pain, headache
Belviq (lorcaserin)	Serotonin receptor agonists	Increases the feeling of fullness so less food is consumed	Constipation, dry mouth, excessive tiredness, back pain, headache, dizziness, anxiety
Qsymia (phentermine and topiramate)	Anorectic (phentermine), anticonvulsants (topiramate)	Reduces the appetite and causes a person to feel fuller longer after eating	Headache, dizziness, numbness and burning in hands and feet, decreased sensation, excessive tiredness, dry mouth, thirst
Contrave (naltrexone–bupropion)	Opiate antagonist (naltrexone), antidepressant (bupropion)	Reduces hunger and helps control cravings	Drowsiness, anxiety, dry mouth, headache, stomach pain, vomiting, loss of appetite, excessive sweating, constipation
Saxenda (liraglutide)	Incretin mimetics	Helps the pancreas release the right amount of insulin when the blood glucose is high.	Headache, constipation, heartburn, cough, tiredness, difficulty urinating

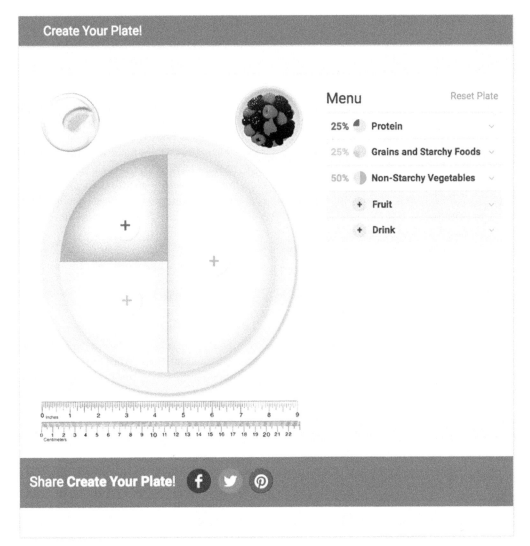

FIGURE 8.4 Create Your Plate! method recommended by the American Diabetes Association.

needs to identify which foods contain carbohydrates and how to estimate the number of grams. The total grams are calculated over the day. Some people with type 1 diabetes may need to adjust the amount of insulin they take for a specific meal based on the amount of carbohydrates they will consume.

Low-Sodium Diet

Sodium is essential to our bodies because it helps to regulate fluid balance. The Food and Drug Administration (FDA) recommends that healthy adults consume no more than 2300 milligrams (mg) of sodium per day. Patients with high blood pressure, heart disease, or kidney disease are usually on reduced sodium diets. Excessive sodium in a person's diet can lead to increased blood pressure, thus increasing the risk for heart disease and stroke.

If a patient is on a reduced sodium diet, the provider will usually refer him or her to a registered dietitian. The dietitian will help educate the individual on the sources of sodium. Typically, alternative lower sodium foods are discussed. Reading labels is also an important skill for those on reduced sodium diets.

Foods High in Sodium

- Processed meats (e.g., deli meats, bacon, frankfurters, and sausage)
- Frozen dinners and ready-to-eat cereals
- Canned foods (e.g., soups, vegetables, and vegetable juice)
- Salted nuts and peanut butter
- Buttermilk, cheese, and processed cheese products
- Quick breads and salted crackers
- Prepackaged mixes for potatoes, rice, and pasta
- Olives, pickles, sauerkraut, pickled vegetables, and spaghetti sauce
- Soy sauce, seasoning salt, marinades, ketchup, mustard, and salad dressings
- Instant puddings and cakes
- Chips and pretzels

Dietary Approaches to Stop Hypertension

Dietary Approaches to Stop Hypertension (DASH) is a flexible eating plan recommended for those with hypertension and cardiovascular disease. The goal of the plan is to reduce the blood pressure and the LDL and triglyceride levels. Table 8.9 indicates foods included and omitted on the DASH eating plan.

CRITICAL THINKING APPLICATION   8.8

Kayla and John are working with Al Neviaser, who has hypertension. Dr. Martin has ordered the DASH eating plan instructions for Mr. Neviaser. John explains to Mr. Neviaser that high salt foods make the blood "salty" and more water is needed in the bloodstream to bring the "salty" level down. The extra water in the blood increases the blood pressure. Mr. Neviaser asks which foods he should stay away from. Give 10 foods that are high in salt (sodium).

Heart-Healthy Diet

The diet and lifestyle recommendations of the American Heart Association (AHA) closely resemble the DASH diet and the MyPlate guidelines. The AHA incorporates a focus on exercise, along with a healthy diet. The following are the AHA's recommendations:

TABLE 8.9 Dietary Approaches to Stop Hypertension (DASH) Eating Plan

INCLUDED IN THE DASH PLAN	OMITTED OR LIMITED IN THE DASH PLAN
• Fruits and vegetables • Low-fat or fat-free dairy foods • Whole grains • Poultry and fish • Beans, nuts, and vegetable oils • Foods high in potassium, calcium, magnesium, protein, and fiber • Foods low in salt (sodium)	• Foods high in saturated fat, total fat, and cholesterol • Red meats • Sugar-sweetened beverages and sweets • High-salt (sodium) foods • Full-fat dairy foods • Tropical oils (coconut, palm, kernel, and palm oil)

• Limit sugary drinks, sweets, fatty meats, and salty or highly processed foods.

• Read labels and select products with the lowest amounts of sodium, added sugar, and saturated fats. Eat fewer than 2400 mg of sodium a day to lower blood pressure. To lower the blood pressure even further, sodium can be reduced to 1500 or 1000 mg per day.

• Be physically active. Balance the calories you burn during exercise with the calories you consume to maintain your weight. Include 150 minutes of moderate physical activity or 75 minutes of vigorous physical activity or a combination of both each week. Break up exercise into 10-minute sessions if needed. To lower blood pressure or cholesterol, 40 minutes of aerobic exercise of moderate to vigorous intensity three to four times a week is recommended.

• Drink alcohol in moderation. Women should have only one drink and men should have only two drinks per day.

• Table 8.10 lists the adult servings for each food group. These are based on a 2000-calorie per day diet.

Low-Protein Diet

The body uses protein for tissue repair, growth, healing, and the ability to fight infection. When protein is broken down in the body, the waste products (e.g., urea and ammonia) are eliminated in the urine. People with liver and kidney disease are often prescribed a low-protein diet. They limit or restrict foods that contain high amounts of protein. Their bodies cannot clear the protein waste products. They can have nausea, headaches, fatigue, and a bad taste in the mouth. Eating a low-protein diet helps to prevent worsening of their disease. Remember, protein cannot be eliminated from the diet. It plays an essential role in the body.

Foods high in protein include milk products (e.g., yogurt and cheese), peanut butter, nuts (e.g., almonds, pistachios, and cashews), quinoa, lentils (e.g., soybeans, kidney beans, and chickpeas), meat, fish, poultry, and eggs. Foods with small amounts of protein include vegetables and starches (e.g., breads, cereals, and pastas). Fruits, sugars, and fats have trace amounts of protein.

High- and Low-Fiber Diets

A prior section of the chapter discussed fiber as a carbohydrate. The provider may order a low-fiber or restricted-fiber diet. This type of

TABLE 8.10 American Heart Association's Eating Healthy Recommendations

FOOD GROUP	DAILY AMOUNTS	HEALTHY RECOMMENDATIONS
Dairy	3 servings or 3 cups	Use low-fat (1%) and fat-free options
Proteins	1–2 servings or 5.5 oz	Eat skinless poultry, seeds, legumes, nuts, lean meat, eggs, and nonfried fish. Avoid fatty meats.
Vegetables	5 servings or 2.5 cups	Eat canned, dried, fresh, and frozen vegetables. Eat a variety of vegetables.
Fruits	4 servings or 2 cups	Eat canned, dried, fresh, and frozen fruits. Eat a variety of fruits.
Whole grains	3–6 servings or 3–6 oz	Eat barley, brown rice, millet, oatmeal, popcorn, and whole wheat bread, crackers, and pasta.
Oils	3 tablespoons	Use polyunsaturated and monounsaturated oils. Use canola, olive, peanut, safflower, and sesame oil. Avoid partially hydrogenated oils, tropical oils, and excessive calories.

Information from the American Heart Association. *https://www.heart.org/en/healthy-living/healthy-eating/eat-smart/nutrition-basics/what-is-a-healthy-diet-recommended-serving-infographic.*

diet limits the type of vegetables, grains, and fruits eaten. Limiting fiber and the residue (e.g., peels, nuts, and seeds) makes the stools smaller and lessens the irritation on the intestinal lining. Possible reasons for a low-fiber diet include the following:

- Narrowing of the intestine due to a tumor
- During a flare-up of an intestinal disease (e.g., irritable bowel syndrome, Crohn's disease, and diverticulitis)
- After intestinal surgery
- Prior to an intestinal procedure (e.g., radiation and colonoscopy)

The provider can also order a high-fiber diet. This diet adds more bulk to the stools. High-fiber diets are used for the following reasons:

- Reduces constipation and may lower the risk of hemorrhoids
- Lowers cholesterol levels
- Helps control blood glucose levels
- Used for weight loss

Elimination Diet and Food Allergies

A food allergy occurs when the immune system overreacts to a protein in the food. The immune system makes IgE antibody in response to the protein. This causes the person to quickly experience the allergy symptoms. Symptoms may include itching, hives, nausea and vomiting, diarrhea, difficulty breathing (e.g., tightness in the throat, coughing, wheezing) or **anaphylaxis**.

As earlier indicated, eight allergies make up about 90% of the food allergy reactions. These eight food allergens can be hiding in ingredient lists under other names. Some examples are listed here:

- Milk (e.g., cream, casein, ghee, galactose, lactalbumin, lactose, and whey)
- Eggs (e.g., albumin, eggnog, ovalbumin, and ovomucin)
- Fish (e.g., cod, bass, flounder)
- Crustacean shellfish (e.g., crab, lobster, shrimp)
- Tree nuts (e.g., almonds, cashews, filberts, hazelnuts, marzipan, nut meal)
- Peanuts (e.g., peanut butter, peanut flour)
- Wheat (e.g., emmer, einkorn, durum, kamut, modified wheat starch, wheat bran, wheat germ)
- Soybeans (e.g., edamame, miso, soya, tempeh, tofu)

It is important to realize that parts of these foods are used in other foods. For instance, milk proteins (e.g., whey and casein) and milk sugar, lactose, appear in some surprising food, medications, and hygiene products. Some examples include chicken broth, deli meats, hot dogs, French fries, shampoos and conditioners, dry powder medication inhalers (e.g., Advair Diskus, Flovent Diskus, and Serevent Diskus) and some medications (e.g., alprazolam, cetirizine hydrochloride, lorazepam, Viagra, and Xanax). Reading ingredient lists is critical for those with allergies.

When people suspect a food allergy, the elimination diet can be used. People remove the suspicious foods from their diet. They may need to track what they eat and how they feel. Slowly they add the suspicious foods back into their diet, one food at a time. This process helps identify the allergen. In some cases, a cross-reactivity may occur, and the person will have additional food allergies. An allergist can help identify additional food and environmental allergies.

Cross-Reactivity With Allergens

Another issue faced by those with food allergies is cross-reactivity. This means that the protein in the allergic food is similar to that in other foods. The person's immune system cannot tell the proteins apart and thus reacts to similar foods. Cross-reactivity can occur with foods and nonfood items. For instance, a person with a latex allergy could also be allergic to avocados, bananas, chestnuts, and kiwi.

Oral allergy syndrome (also called *pollen-food syndrome*) is caused by cross-reacting allergens found in pollens, raw foods, and tree nuts. Symptoms include itchy mouth and ears, scratchy throat, and swollen lips, mouth, tongue, and throat. Typically, the symptoms disappear when the food is out of the mouth. Some common cross-reactions include the following:

- Ragweed pollen: cucumber, banana, melons, potatoes, and zucchini
- Grass pollen: celery, melons, oranges, peaches, and tomatos
- Birch pollen: pitted fruit (e.g., plum, pear, peach, and apple), kiwi, carrot, celery, almond, and hazelnut

Gluten-Free Diet

People with celiac disease are put on a gluten-free diet. Gluten is a protein found in the following products:

- Barley and malt products (e.g., flavoring and vinegar)
- Rye
- Triticale (wheat and rye crossbred hybrid)
- Wheat (e.g., durum flour, farina, graham flour, spelt, semolina, and kamut)

Gluten is commonly found in breads, cereals, pastas, cakes, cookies, and other foods. It causes inflammation in the small intestine of people with celiac disease. Removing gluten from the diet helps to control the symptoms.

The FDA regulates the gluten-free food labeling claim. This is a voluntary claim that manufacturers may opt to use. If they use the label, they are accountable for using the claim in a truthful way.

Lactose-Intolerance Diet

Lactose intolerance, or sensitivity, is not an allergy. Lactose is the main sugar found in dairy products. Lactose is broken down by lactase, an enzyme created by the small intestine. If a person's small intestine does not produce enough lactase, the lactose moves into the large intestine. The bacteria in the large intestine break down the lactose, causing bloating, cramps, diarrhea, nausea, and gas. Treatment for lactose intolerance or sensitivity involves avoiding milk products or using an oral enzyme replacement supplement.

NUTRITIONAL NEEDS FOR VARIOUS POPULATIONS

Nutritional needs change throughout life. Our needs for calories, vitamins, minerals, and protein change as we grow and develop. With pregnancy and breastfeeding, the needs increase. With disease conditions, the needs change. We have already discussed different diets and conditions treated with those eating plans. Table 8.11 describes the nutritional needs by age groups. (Eating disorders are discussed in Chapter 22.)

TABLE 8.11	Nutritional Needs by Age Groups
AGE	**NUTRITIONAL NEEDS**
Infancy to 2 years	Birth to 6 months of age: Breast milk or formula is given. If an infant cannot tolerate milk-based formulas, other types of formulas are available, including soy formula. Some formulas are available by prescription only. Six months of age: The child is started on soft, pureed solid foods. Usually, infant cereals, fruits, and vegetables are first introduced. One year of age: The child is transitioned to whole milk, and pureed foods are gradually replaced with easy-to-eat foods. It is important to offer foods from each food group.
2 to 12 years	Age 2: The child should eat several dairy products, fruits, vegetables, meats, breads, pasta, cereals, and beans. As the child grows and develops, more foods can be added to his or her diet. Portion sizes also grow.
12 to adulthood	Adolescents experience rapid growth periods, which require more energy. Teens may need encouragement to consume dairy products (e.g., milk) instead of soda. The growth spurts require calcium for strong bones. Females who have started their menses should eat foods high in iron to replace the iron lost in menstrual blood.
Older adults	As a person grows older, the metabolism decreases, and the caloric needs also decrease. Special nutritional concerns of the older adult include the following: • Difficulty chewing and swallowing, which can be related to poor-fitting dentures. • Decrease in eating due to changes in the senses (e.g., taste, smell) • Lack of a well-balanced diet (e.g., limited income, loneliness, and lack of initiative to cook for oneself)

Pregnancy and Lactation

During pregnancy, it is important to eat a healthy diet. The first trimester can be difficult with nutrition. Depending on the mother's morning sickness, eating a balanced diet can be tricky. Many providers recommend eating small, frequent meals to combat morning sickness. Dry crackers and toast are also encouraged. Eating low-odor protein foods can also help. Avoiding triggers such as spicy foods and certain smells are important in managing morning sickness.

Providers usually recommend a daily prenatal vitamin and mineral supplement to ensure adequate folic acid and prevent spina bifida. Consuming alcohol during pregnancy is not recommended. Despite the saying "eating for two," the daily caloric intake only needs to increase by 300 calories for the second and third trimester of most pregnancies.

Women who are pregnant or breastfeeding should avoid eating raw fish or fish high in mercury. Two to three servings of seafood per week are recommended during pregnancy and when breastfeeding. According to the FDA, examples of the best choices of seafood to eat include salmon, cod, tilapia, catfish, haddock, lobster, perch, squid, trout, shrimp, and light canned tuna. Mercury, which can be toxic to the nervous system, can be found in higher levels in marlin, orange roughy, bigeye tuna, swordfish, shark, king mackerel, and tilefish from the Gulf of Mexico. Consumption of locally caught fish and white albacore tuna intake should be limited to no more than 6 ounces per week.

With lactation or breastfeeding, the mother needs to eat a healthy diet, and a vitamin supplement may be recommended. It is important to get adequate vitamins and minerals, which are passed to the baby in the breast milk. The mother also needs to drink additional water to maintain her milk volume.

Epilepsy

Some patients with epilepsy follow a ketogenic diet. This diet consists of very-low-carbohydrate, high-fat, and adequate protein foods. Some people have also used this type of diet to lose weight. Without carbohydrates, the body metabolizes fat, and the ketones are used for energy. It is important to monitor kidney function when a person is on a ketogenic diet.

HIV and AIDS

When a person has HIV or AIDS, it is important to eat a well-balanced diet. Making sure the immune system is nutritionally supported is critical. People with this disease can struggle with several issues, including nausea, diarrhea, constipation, and poor appetite. The provider may order medications to help with the nausea. Drinking extra fluids will help with both diarrhea and constipation issues. Restricting milk products with diarrhea and increasing fiber intake with constipation can help. A poor appetite can cause weight and nutrient loss. Frequent small meals, nutritional supplements (e.g., Ensure), and light exercise may help. A provider may encourage a daily vitamin and mineral supplement. With unintended weight loss, additional "healthy" calories should be added to the diet.

Cancer

Patients undergoing radiation and chemotherapy can experience issues that affect eating. The treatments can harm fast-growing cells in the lining of the mouth, lips, and intestinal tract. Patients may have mouth sores that cause pain and swallowing problems. Taste and smell changes can occur. The treatments can cause appetite changes, diarrhea or constipation, fatigue, dry mouth, nausea, vomiting, and weight gain or loss. Good nutrition is critical for people to regain their strength and to heal after the treatments. A registered dietitian is commonly involved with the team of healthcare professionals caring for patients undergoing treatment.

Nutritional tips for patients undergoing cancer treatments include the following:

- Eat a soft, bland diet.
- Eat six to eight small meals a day instead of three meals. Attempt to eat high-calorie, high-protein snacks (e.g., hard-cooked eggs, peanut butter, nuts, supplements, trail mix, and canned chicken).
- Take only sips of liquids during meals. Drink most of the liquids between meals. Drink 8 to 10 cups of liquid a day to prevent constipation. Water, prune juice, and warm liquids are helpful.
- To reduce mouth dryness and sores, limit caffeine and alcohol; keep the mouth clean using water or a mild mouth rinse; avoid tart, acidic or salty foods; eat lukewarm, cold, soft, and creamy foods; and use anesthetic rinses prior to eating.
- Avoid foods with strong odors and those that are overly sweet, spicy, greasy, or fried.
- Eat small bites and chew the food well. Eat dry foods (e.g., crackers, toast).
- In addition, use a straw and/or a small spoon, and puree food as needed. Suck on hard candies and ice chips to soothe the mouth and prevent mouth dryness.

CRITICAL THINKING APPLICATION   8.9

Kayla and John are working with Noemi Rodriguez, who is currently undergoing chemotherapy. She was not able to see her oncologist today, and she had a very sore mouth after the last treatment. List some nutritional tips for patients undergoing cancer treatments.

INSTRUCTING PATIENTS ON DIETARY CHANGES

When a patient needs a dietary change, the provider will give the order to the medical assistant. The provider will tell the medical assistant what type of diet the patient needs to be on. If the diet is only for a short period of time, the provider will indicate the time period. Sometimes the dietary change is related to a procedure. The provider will order the diagnostic procedure, and the medical assistant should be knowledgeable about the dietary changes required for that procedure.

Before meeting with the patient for coaching, it is important for the medical assistant to gather any brochures or information needed. Remember, it is a good idea to send the patient home with written instructions on dietary changes. If the patient does not understand English, use an interpreter service and make sure brochures are in the patient's primary language.

Lastly, before meeting with the patient, the medical assistant should look over the brochure. It is important to be knowledgeable about the content you are explaining to the patient. Reading the brochure aloud as a way of instructing the patient is not professional. The patient may feel you do not know what you are talking about.

When a medical assistant instructs a patient on a dietary change, it is important to know why people eat what they do and to understand how cultural dietary traditions relate to illness, as described in the following section. Procedure 8.1 on p. 214 details the process of coaching a patient regarding a dietary change.

Showing Awareness of a Patient's Concerns

Being aware means being alert and understanding what you are perceiving. When working with patients, we first need to be aware of the patient's concerns before we can show that we are aware. It is important to be accurate in our perception of the patient's concerns. If our perceptions are incorrect, we could say or behave in a way that is insensitive to the patient.

Chapter 2 in the main text discusses therapeutic communication techniques. Let's review a few ways a medical assistant can show awareness of the patient's concerns:

- *Reflection:* The medical assistant puts words to the patient's emotional reaction, which acknowledges the person's feelings; for example, "It sounds like you are unsure of this new way of eating."
- *Restatement or paraphrasing:* The medical assistant rewords or rephrases a patient's statement to check the meaning and interpretation. This shows you are listening and understanding the patient. You might say, for example, "What I am hearing is that you really like your family traditions for holiday meals."
- *Summarizing:* This allows the medical assistant to recap and review what was said; for example, "If I understand how you feel about this new eating plan ..."

Remember that a medical assistant can also show awareness by using positive and open, nonverbal behaviors. These nonverbal behaviors could be used when working with a patient on a dietary change:

- *Position:* The medical assistant should be at the level of the other person and angled toward the patient. For example, if the patient is sitting, then the medical assistant should be sitting also.
- *Arms and posture:* The medical assistant should be poised with his or her arms to the side. This is an open, positive nonverbal behavior that shows interest in the other person.
- *Facial expression:* The medical assistant should be smiling. Refrain from rolling your eyes, yawning, or frowning. These can be perceived as showing boredom or rudeness.
- *Gestures and touch:* The medical assistant should use small gestures and an appropriate light touch on the hand of the patient, depending on the situation.
- *Mannerisms:* The medical assistant should focus on the patient. It is not appropriate to look at your watch, phone, or the clock. This gives the patient the feeling you are bored or impatient.

Awareness of Others' Concerns

When working with patients regarding a dietary change, it is important to understand the factors that can affect what we eat:

- *Cost*: How much money we have affects what foods we purchase. It can be expensive to purchase fresh fruits and vegetables, fish, and lean cuts of meat. Less expensive options are available, but they may not have the same taste or appeal.
- *Convenience*: With busy lifestyles, people sometimes choose what is easiest and quickest. This usually includes eating out or take-home meals.
- *Background*: Our background can influence the foods we eat. Some cultures have healthier diets than others. It can be helpful for people to modify cultural dishes by cutting the salt, fat, and sugar, without giving up the taste.
- *Emotional comfort*: Some people may eat when they are happy or when they are sad. Usually under these conditions, the food choices are not the healthiest. Some people stop eating when they are emotional.
- *Routine*: People eat what they always eat out of habit, personal preference, and availability. People may also eat with certain activities, like viewing a sports event, driving, or watching television. These habits are difficult to break.

It is important for the medical assistant to get to know what the patient is eating and why. This helps when coaching a patient on a dietary change. For instance, knowing your patient has a limited food budget is helpful when coaching him or her on healthier choices. You might be able to share ideas on healthy foods that are less costly or places to shop that are cheaper.

CLOSING COMMENTS

Patient Coaching

Good nutrition is important for a person's health and well-being. For many people, changing their diet can be difficult and uncomfortable. It is important for the medical assistant to be sensitive to the change that the patient is asking about. Educating the patient about the benefits of making a dietary change may make the transition easier. Compliance with the diet increases if the person meets certain conditions:

- Can modify special foods and not give them up completely
- Has support from family and friends
- Can slowly transition to the new diet, though this might not always be possible

The medical assistant is an important team member when there is a need to help patients transition to a new diet. It is important for the medical assistant to be familiar with the dietary changes required for common procedures and diagnoses.

Legal and Ethical Issues

After the medical assistant coaches a patient on a dietary change, it is important to document the teaching in the health record. The documentation should reflect the provider ordering the teaching, the general topics taught, and how the patient's learning was evaluated. If the medical assistant provided the patient with written materials, this should also be noted in the documentation.

Patient-Centered Care

As medical assistants work with patients from various cultures, it is also important to know more about those cultures. Many cultures have dietary traditions that influence how they respond to illness. In some cultures, food is considered a cure for illness. For instance, in the Mexican culture, when people are sick, they are out of balance in that they have too much heat or cold. To correct this balance, the person needs to eat foods of the opposite quality. It is important to be sensitive to these cultural practices. If the dietary change conflicts with the cultural practice, it is important to talk with the provider. A referral to a registered dietitian may provide the patient with extra support and information.

Cultural Diets

- Asian diets include whole grains (e.g., millet and rice), fruits, vegetables, legumes, nuts, and seeds. Fats are derived largely from vegetable oils (peanut or sesame oils). Dairy products are not traditionally eaten. Protein sources include broiled or stir-fried fish and seafood, egg whites, tofu, and nuts.
- Latin American diets include food from plant sources at each meal. This can include maize (corn), potatoes, fruits, vegetables, whole grains, beans, and nuts. Poultry, fish, and dairy typically are consumed daily. Meat and eggs are eaten weekly.
- Mediterranean diets include whole grains, fresh fruits and vegetables, and all types of legumes (e.g., beans, lentils, and peas) daily. Olive oil is used. Fish, poultry, and eggs are consumed weekly and meat monthly.
- Mexican diets include corn or flour tortillas, cabbage, legumes, squash, tomatoes, corn, and potatoes daily. Cheeses are eaten, but milk is not regularly consumed. Protein sources typically are fish, beef, poultry, lamb, and many types of beans.

Professional Behaviors

When working with patients who are making dietary changes, it is important to be respectful of the patient. It is easy to tell a patient what to eat and what not to eat, but that might not be the best way to approach the situation. A medical assistant may want to start by finding out the patient's favorite foods. What foods does the patient typically eat at meals? Are any health beliefs related to that food? Learning about the patient's diet can then help the medical assistant coach the patient.

If the medical assistant feels the patient needs additional dietary support, talking with the provider is important. The provider can refer the patient to a registered dietitian for additional assistance.

SUMMARY OF SCENARIO

John really enjoyed working with Kayla for his practicum. He learned a lot from her as she worked with patients. His favorite part of the experience was the patient education, in which he was able to observe and participate. Kayla also learned from John during the experience. Because of his interest in nutrition, John was able to share with Kayla what he knew about current dietary trends.

John hopes to obtain a medical assistant job in a practice like the one where he did his practicum. He feels that the family practice environment will allow him to use many of the skills he learned in school. He will also have a lot of experience talking to patients about dietary changes.

SUMMARY OF LEARNING OBJECTIVES

1. **Describe metabolism.**
   Metabolism is the process the body uses to obtain or make energy from the food eaten. Catabolism and anabolism are the two phases of metabolism.

2. **Describe dietary nutrients including carbohydrates, fiber, protein, fat, minerals and electrolytes, vitamins, and water.**
   - Carbohydrates are used for energy and to regulate protein and fat metabolism. Simple sugars, starches, and fiber are carbohydrates. Desserts, milk products, breads, and fruits are some examples of carbohydrates.
   - Proteins break down into amino acids; both are considered building blocks for the body. Essential amino acids must come from food eaten, whereas nonessential amino acids are made in the body. Meat, poultry, dairy products, eggs, and nuts are sources of protein.
   - Fat provides a source of energy when carbohydrates are not available. Saturated fats are solid at room temperature and should be limited in the diet. Unsaturated fats are liquid at room temperature. Monounsaturated and polyunsaturated fats are two types of unsaturated fats. Trans fatty acids or trans fats are created during the food manufacturing process and are considered unhealthy.
   - Minerals in the body are called electrolytes. Some examples include calcium, potassium, sodium, sulfur, iron, and iodine.
   - Vitamins can be either fat or water soluble. Vitamins A, D, E, and K are fat soluble, and B vitamins and vitamin C are water soluble. A deficit of a vitamin can lead to a disease.
   - Water is the basis for the fluids in the body. Our bodies need water to function and survive.

3. **Explain current dietary guidelines.**
   The US Department of Agriculture publishes Dietary Guidelines every 5 years. The guidelines are for individuals 2 years or older. Key recommendations from the 2015–2020 Dietary Guidelines for Americans include those listed with the MyPlate regimen, in addition to the following:
   - Limit foods with saturated and trans fats, added sugars, and sodium.
   - Less than 10% of daily calories should come from saturated fats (e.g., butter, whole milk, fatty meats, coconut oil, and palm oil).
   - Individuals age 14 or older should consume fewer than 2300 milligrams (mg) of sodium a day.
   - Limit alcohol consumed to one drink per day for women and two drinks for men.
   - Incorporate physical activity (e.g., aerobic, muscle-strengthening, and bone strengthening activities) into the week.

4. **Describe how to read a food label.**
   Food labels provide nutritional facts. This information is presented in both the quantity (e.g., grams [g] or milligrams [mg]) and as a percentage. The percentage reflects the % Daily Value (DV). This is the percentage of the nutrient in a single serving in terms of the daily recommended amount, based on a 2000-calorie diet. Refer to the section in the chapter for additional steps in reading food labels.

5. **Describe the different types of medically ordered diets.**
   Clear liquid diet: Made up of foods and beverages that turn to liquid at room temperature.
   Full liquid diet: Made up of clear liquids and milk products.
   Soft and mechanical soft diet: Made up of foods soft in texture, low in fiber, and easy to digest. Mechanical soft diets are prepared for easier chewing.
   Bland diet: Consists of foods that are soft and low in fiber and eliminates foods that are spicy, fried, and raw. Citrus foods, caffeine, and alcohol are eliminated.
   Weight control diet: Can help people lose or maintain weight. Control of portion sizes is very important on the weight control diet.
   Diabetic eating plans: Used for people with diabetes, who need to monitor their carbohydrate intake. There are several diabetic eating plans, including the glycemic index approach, the "Create Your Plate" method, and carb counting.
   Low-sodium diet: Helps to lower the blood pressure and also used to address kidney disease. DASH is used for hypertension and cardiovascular disease.
   Heart-healthy diet: Consists of limiting sugary, salty, and highly processed foods. Limiting the consumption of saturated fats, trans fats, and added sugar is also important.
   Low-protein diet: Used for people with liver and kidney disease.
   High- and low-fiber diets: Limit or add fiber to the diet. A high-fiber diet helps with constipation and weight loss. Low-fiber diets are used during a flare-up of an intestinal disease.
   Elimination diet: Removes suspicious allergens from the diet. Slowly they are reintroduced to find the allergens.
   Gluten-free diet: Used for people with celiac disease. Wheat, barley, and rye foods are removed from the diet.

Continued

214   **UNIT TWO**   FUNDAMENTALS OF CLINICAL MEDICAL ASSISTING

SUMMARY OF LEARNING OBJECTIVES—*continued*

Lactose-intolerance diet: Involves avoiding milk products or using oral enzyme replacement supplements.

6. **Identify the special dietary needs for weight control, diabetes mellitus, cardiovascular disease, and hypertension.**

Weight control: When trying to achieve or maintain a healthy weight, a person needs to find the balance between the number of calories eaten and the number used. Extra calories eaten and not used will result in a weight gain. For people to lose 1 to 2 pounds per week, they need to reduce their caloric intake by 500 to 1000 calories a day or increase their exercise to burn more calories.

Diabetes mellitus: People with diabetes mellitus need to monitor their carbohydrate intake. The American Diabetes Association recommends the following diabetes meal plans: the glycemic index approach, the "Create Your Plate" method, and carb counting.

Cardiovascular disease and hypertension: Sodium is essential to our bodies because it helps to regulate fluid balance. The Food and Drug Administration (FDA) recommends that healthy adults consume no more than 2300 milligrams (mg) of sodium per day. Patients with high blood pressure, heart disease, or kidney disease are usually on reduced sodium diets. Excessive sodium in a person's diet can lead to increased blood pressure, thus increasing the risk for heart disease and stroke. Dietary Approaches to Stop Hypertension (DASH) is a flexible eating plan recommended for those with hypertension and cardiovascular disease. The goal of the plan is to reduce the blood pressure and the LDL and triglyceride levels.

7. **Identify the special dietary needs for those with food allergies, celiac disease, and lactose intolerance.**

Food allergies: When people suspect a food allergy, the elimination diet can be used. People remove the suspicious foods from their diet. They may need to track what they eat and how they feel. Slowly they add the suspicious foods back into their diet, one food at a time. This process helps identify the allergen.

Celiac disease: People with celiac disease are put on a gluten-free diet. Gluten is a protein found in the following products: barley, malt products, rye, triticale, and wheat.

Lactose intolerance: Treatment for lactose intolerance or sensitivity involves avoiding milk products or using an oral enzyme replacement supplement.

8. **Identify special dietary needs for those with various conditions, including pregnancy and lactation, epilepsy, HIV and AIDS, and cancer.**

Pregnancy and lactation: A healthy diet is recommended, along with a daily prenatal vitamin and mineral supplement. Consuming alcohol during pregnancy is not recommended. Despite the saying "eating for two," the daily caloric intake only needs to increase by 300 calories for the second and third trimesters of most pregnancies. Women who are pregnant or breastfeeding should avoid eating raw fish or fish high in mercury.

Epilepsy: Some patients with epilepsy follow a ketogenic diet. This diet consists of very-low-carbohydrate, high-fat, and adequate protein foods.

HIV and AIDS: It is important to eat a well-balanced diet. The provider may order medications to help with nausea. Drinking extra fluids will help with both diarrhea and constipation issues. Restricting milk products with diarrhea and increasing fiber intake with constipation can help. Frequent small meals, nutritional supplements (e.g., Ensure), and light exercise may help. A provider may encourage a daily vitamin and mineral supplement.

Cancer: Many patients undergoing cancer treatment may have changes in their appetite. Good nutrition is critical for people to regain their strength and to heal after the treatments. Refer to the section for more nutritional tips for patients undergoing cancer treatment.

9. **Instruct a patient on dietary changes while demonstrating awareness of others' concerns.**

When a medical assistant instructs a patient on a dietary change, it is important to know why people eat what they do and to understand how cultural dietary traditions relate to illness. When working with patients regarding a dietary change, it is important to understand the factors that can affect what we eat: cost, convenience, background, emotional comfort, and routine. It is important for the medical assistant to get to know what the patient is eating and why. This helps when the medical assistant is coaching a patient on a dietary change. Procedure 8.1 details the process of coaching a patient regarding a dietary change.

PROCEDURE 8.1   **Instruct a Patient on a Dietary Change**

Tasks: Instruct a patient according to a patient's special dietary needs. Show awareness of the patient's concerns regarding the dietary change. Document in the health record.

Scenario: You are working with Dr. Angela Perez, a family practice provider. She just finished seeing Al Neviaser (date of birth [DOB]: 6/21/1968). Dr. Perez orders that the patient be given Heart-Healthy Diet instructions.

| PROCEDURE 8.1 | Instruct a Patient on a Dietary Change—*continued* |

EQUIPMENT and SUPPLIES

- Patient's health record
- Heart-healthy diet brochure

PROCEDURAL STEPS

1. Using the scenario, role-play the situation with a peer. Assemble supplies needed for the provider's order. Ensure that the patient can read and understand the written materials. Verify the order if you have any questions.
   PURPOSE: Using written materials is helpful when instructing a patient on a dietary change.

2. Greet the patient. Identify yourself. Verify the patient's identity with full name and date of birth. Explain the order from the provider. Answer any questions the patient may have about the procedure.
   PURPOSE: It is important to identify the patient in two different ways to ensure that you have the correct patient. Explaining the order can make the patient feel more comfortable and helps to reduce anxiety.

3. Position yourself at the same level as the patient. Angle yourself toward the patient. Have a poised position.
   PURPOSE: This position shows positive nonverbal behaviors to the patient. Being at the same level as the patient and angling toward the patient show openness.

4. Accurately instruct the patient on the new diet. Use the written materials as you discuss the new eating plan.
   PURPOSE: The information taught to the patient should match what is in the written materials. Any inaccuracies will confuse the patient.

5. Use words that the patient can understand. Refrain from jargon and medical terminology. Use professional verbal and nonverbal communication.
   PURPOSE: Jargon and medical terminology can confuse patients. Unprofessional nonverbal behaviors, such as rolling your eyes, checking the clock, or yawning, are disrespectful to the patient.

Scenario Update: After going over the heart-healthy eating plan, Mr. Neviaser states he is not sure this diet is for him. He likes his red meat and does not like to eat fish. He does not have a lot of money to buy expensive fresh fruits and vegetables.

6. Using therapeutic communication techniques (e.g., reflection, restatement, and summarizing), show the patient you are aware of his concerns.
   PURPOSE: By using therapeutic communication techniques, the medical assistant can show awareness of the patient's concerns.

7. Based on the patient's concerns, provide food alternatives that would meet the eating plan requirements.
   PURPOSE: The medical assistant can show awareness of the patient's concerns by providing alternative food choices that would meet the patient's requirements.

8. Evaluate the patient's understanding of the teaching by asking him to summarize the eating plan or describe a day's worth of meals. Answer any questions the patient may have.
   PURPOSE: It is important to check the patient's understanding of what was taught. Having the patient provide information back to the medical assistant is a better evaluation of understanding than asking, "Do you understand?"

9. Document the instruction in the patient's health record. Include the order, instructions given, written materials provided, and the patient's feedback.
   PURPOSE: Documenting indicates the instruction was provided to the patient.

11/04/20XX 0923 Per Dr. Perez's order, the pt and his wife were instructed on a heart-healthy diet. Pt indicated he did not eat fish and was concerned about the cost of fresh foods. Alternative healthy proteins and inexpensive food options were discussed with the patient. The pt and his wife were able to describe a day's worth of heart-healthy meals. Pt was encouraged to call with any additional questions. _____ Kayla Smith, RMA

9

SURGICAL SUPPLIES AND INSTRUMENTS

SCENARIO

Tom Anderson, CMA (AAMA), works for Walden-Martin Family Medical (WMFM) Clinic. Tom enjoys assisting with the minor surgical procedures performed in the office. Tom is also responsible for maintaining stock supplies in the minor surgery room, including solutions and medications, and for cleaning, maintaining, and inspecting the surgical instruments. Because no procedures are scheduled for today, Tom plans to compile an inventory of supplies and equipment and perform routine maintenance activities.

While studying this chapter, think about the following questions:

- What solutions and medications should be available in the surgical area of a medical office?
- What are the typical instruments used in minor surgical procedures?
- How are surgical instruments identified and classified?
- How should surgical instruments be cared for and handled before, during, and after a surgical procedure?
- What types of sutures and needles are used in minor surgical procedures?

LEARNING OBJECTIVES

1. Describe typical solutions and medications used in minor surgical procedures.
2. Summarize methods for identifying surgical instruments used in minor office surgery, and then identify some surgical instruments.
3. Outline the general classifications of surgical instruments.
4. Identify drapes and different types of sutures and surgical needles.
5. Describe the care and handling of surgical instruments.

VOCABULARY

abscess Localized collection of pus, which may be under the skin or deep in the body, that cause tissue destruction.

anesthetic (an ehs THET ik) An agent that causes partial or complete loss of sensation.

cannula (KAN yuh la) A rigid tube that surrounds a blunt trocar or a sharp, pointed trocar, which is inserted into the body; when the trocar is withdrawn, fluid may escape from the body through the cannula, depending on the insertion site.

caustic (KAW stik) Capable of burning, corroding, or destroying living tissue.

curettage (kyoo reh TAHZH) The act of scraping a body cavity with a surgical instrument, such as a curette.

dilation (die LAY shuhn) The opening or widening of the circumference of a body orifice with a dilating instrument.

diluent (dye LU ent) A liquid substance that dilutes or lessens the strength of a solution or mixture; it is added to vials of powdered medications to create a solution of the drug for injection.

dissect To cut or separate tissue with a cutting instrument or scissors.

fornix (FORE niks) A recess in the upper part of the vagina caused by protrusion of the cervix into the vaginal wall.

impervious (im PUR vee uhs) Not permitting penetration.

infection Invasion of body tissues by microorganisms, which then multiply and damage tissues.

obturator (OB tuh rayt oar) A metal rod with a smooth, rounded tip that is placed in hollow instruments to reduce injury to body tissues during insertion.

patency (PAT en see) Open condition of a body cavity or canal.

pathogen A disease-causing organism.

permeable (PUR mee uh buhl) Allowing for penetration.

spore A thick-walled, dormant form of bacteria that is very resistant to disinfection measures.

stylus (STIE luhs) A metal probe that is inserted into or passed through a catheter, needle, or tube used for clearing purposes or to facilitate passage into a body orifice.

transient (TRAN zee uhnt) Not lasting, enduring or permanent; transitory.

vasoconstriction (vay zoh kuhn STRIK shuhn) Contraction of the muscles causing the narrowing of the inside tube of the vessel.

Office surgery is restricted to the management of minor problems and injuries. The medical assistant is expected to prepare the patient and the sterile field, assist the provider as needed, take care of the patient after the procedure, properly disinfect the area, and document appropriately. Some medical assistants are employed in outpatient surgical facilities and are expected to assist with procedures that once were performed in hospitals. Although these more difficult operations may involve complete gowning and gloving with surgical masks and caps, the two surgical chapters in this text limit discussion and descriptions to the routines necessary to prepare for and assist in minor surgery only. This chapter includes a discussion of surgical supplies and instruments, the care and handling of instruments, and the different types of surgical sutures and needles, and sterilization procedures. The next chapter presents preparation of the sterile field, specific minor surgical procedures, and care of the patient.

MINOR SURGERY ROOM

When minor surgery is routinely performed, a minor surgery room that is separate from the other examining rooms may be used. Recovery rooms and family waiting areas may also be available and are common in the larger surgery centers. The minor surgery room in a provider's office, often called the *procedure room,* should be near a workroom with a sink and an autoclave. In some facilities, the sink and autoclave will be located in the procedure room. Cabinets with countertops serve as a side or back table during surgical procedures. Regardless of the setup, it should be easy to disinfect the area, and it should remain uncluttered to allow for easy access to the patient and necessary supplies.

Surgical supplies, wound care equipment, medications, and biopsy containers are stored in the cabinets. The exam table should be easy to adjust. In addition, the room should have bright lighting, a Mayo stand for instruments, vital signs equipment, and possibly an electrocardiograph (ECG) machine as part of the standard equipment (Fig. 9.1).

SURGICAL SOLUTIONS AND MEDICATIONS

Procedure room supplies include the standard solutions and medications used in minor surgery and dressing changes. Although the

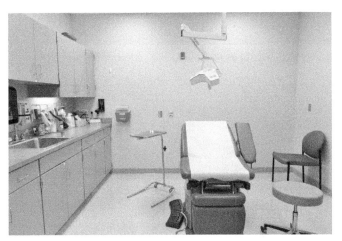

FIGURE 9.1 Typical surgical procedure room in an ambulatory care setting.

solutions and medications listed here are basic, every healthcare facility has preferred items and methods of applying them. The medical assistant is responsible for their care and for maintaining up-to-date supplies.

Sterile water is kept in two forms. Multiple-dose or single-use vials are used as a **diluent** for medications. Larger containers of sterile water are for irrigating wounds or rinsing instruments that have been in a chemical disinfectant solution.

Sterile normal saline solution is also stocked in two sizes. The small vial is used for injection (e.g., 0.9% Sodium Chloride Injection USP single-dose vials, Bacteriostatic 0.9% Sodium Chloride Injection USP multiple-dose vials). A larger plastic container of sterile saline (e.g., 0.9% Sodium Chloride Irrigation USP) is used for cleaning, rinsing, and irrigating wounds. These commercially prepared products are ordered from a medical supply company.

Before surgery, the surgical site on the patient must be disinfected with an antiseptic skin cleansing preparation. This will reduce the number of **pathogens.** Although it is not possible to remove all microorganisms from the skin, using an antiseptic cleanser will remove most of the **transient** and pathogenic microorganisms. Resident flora will also be reduced. Research indicates that chlorhexidine gluconate products (Hibiclens) and povidone-iodine (Betadine) are safe and effective antiseptics.

The provider's hands and those of the medical assistant should be scrubbed to reduce the chances of wound contamination, even though the hands will be covered by sterile gloves. Surgical scrub preparations should:

- be effective against bacterial **spores**
- work to reduce transient bacteria
- show evidence of persistent activity on the skin
- work despite the presence of organic matter, such as blood or wound drainage

Research has shown that the use of a hand sanitizer can be as effective as an extensive surgical scrub.

Even minor surgical procedures require the use of **anesthetics,** which either are injected locally at the site of the procedure or may be applied topically to the skin. For patients who find injections of a local anesthetic painful or traumatic, the provider may first apply a topical anesthetic. Topical anesthetics come in many forms, including sprays, gels, lotions, swabs, and foams. Immediately after applying the topical anesthetic, the provider injects the local anesthetic around the surgical area.

Another topical anesthetic is an ethyl chloride spray, a vapocoolant that controls pain associated with minor surgical procedures (e.g., lancing boils, incision and drainage of small **abscesses**), by causing freezing of the affected area. Because ethyl chloride is highly flammable, it should never be used in the presence of electrical cauterizing equipment. In addition, petroleum jelly must be applied to the surrounding areas to protect them from the cooling action of the spray. Ethyl chloride spray has a short duration of action, so all equipment must be prepared, and the provider must be ready to perform the procedure before the spray is applied.

Local anesthetics are injected into the subcutaneous tissue. These produce a temporary numbing at the site of injection by blocking the generation and conduction of nerve impulses. Many different types of local anesthetics are available, but all share the same suffix, *-caine* such as lidocaine (Xylocaine), procaine (Novocain), chloroprocaine (Nesacaine), and bupivacaine (Sensorcaine). Local anesthetics are purchased in multiple-dose vials of 30 to 50 mL and in various strengths, such as 0.5%, 1%, and 2%. They begin acting relatively quickly, within 5 to 15 minutes; the duration of action depends on the type of anesthetic, but they usually last 1 to 3 hours. When highly vascular areas are involved, local anesthetics containing epinephrine may be used. Epinephrine causes **vasoconstriction** at the site, which keeps the anesthetic in the tissues longer, prolonging its effect. It also minimizes bleeding. However, epinephrine is not used in areas where decreased circulation may cause problems with healing, such as fingertips or toes.

All tissues removed or biopsied are sent to the pathology laboratory for analysis. A 10% formalin solution typically is used to preserve excised tissue for specimens. Specimen bottles are purchased with preservatives included and should be part of the supplies prepared for a surgical procedure, if a biopsy is to be done. The provider places the specimen in the container. The medical assistant is responsible for accurately labeling the container with:

- patient's name and date of birth
- medical history number
- date of collection
- type of specimen

Sometimes the provider may want to use topical silver nitrate ($AgNO_3$) solution or coated applicator sticks to stop localized bleeding, such as with *epistaxis* (nosebleed) or capillary bleeding at the site of a wound. The applicators must be kept in lightproof containers. The applicator sticks are convenient for use in the mouth or nose.

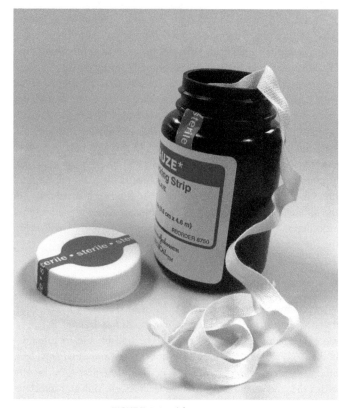

FIGURE 9.2 Iodoform gauze strips.

Additional Surgical Supplies

- Sterilized gauze squares or strips saturated with petroleum jelly or petrolatum — used to pack wounds
- Sterilized iodoform gauze strips, ¼ inch to 2 inches wide and impregnated with iodoform iodine (Fig. 9.2) — used to pack abscesses to act as a wick to draw out the infection; also used as a local antibacterial agent
- Surgical sponges — used to absorb blood and protect tissues during surgery
- Syringes and needles — used to inject local anesthetics and irrigate wounds
- Sterile dressing and bandaging materials

CRITICAL THINKING APPLICATION   **9.1**

Tom is ready to do an inventory of supplies in the minor surgery room. What solutions, medications, and miscellaneous supplies should he make sure are on hand for the busy surgical schedule planned for next week?

SURGICAL INSTRUMENTS

The medical assistant must know which instruments are used for each procedure and should be able to identify and understand the function of the surgical instruments preferred by the provider. Instruments have clearly identifiable parts and can be visually differentiated from one another. The basic components are the handle, the closing mechanism, and the part that comes in contact with the patient,

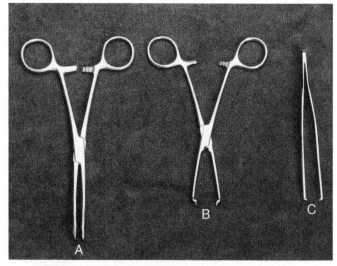

FIGURE 9.3 (A) and **(B)** Ring-handle forceps. **(C)** Spring-handle thumb forceps.

commonly called the *jaws*. Many instruments can have either straight or curved tips, depending on the operator's preference and the task to be performed.

Instruments have either ring handles (finger rings) (Fig. 9.3A–B) or spring handles (Fig. 9.3C); these sometimes are called *thumb-handled* or *thumb grasp* instruments. Scissors are an example of a ring-handled instrument; forceps (tweezers) have spring handles. Some instruments have a hinge-type mechanism called a *box lock*.

Ratchets resemble gears and are located just below or next to the ring handle (see Fig. 9.3A–B). They are used to lock an instrument into position. Most ratchets can be closed at three or more positions, depending on the thickness of the tissue or materials being grasped.

The inner surfaces of the jaws on some instruments have ridged teeth, called *serrations*; both ring-handled and thumb-type instruments may have them. These serrations may be crisscross, horizontal, or lengthwise (Fig. 9.4). Serrations prevent small blood vessels and tissue from slipping out of the jaws of the instrument.

Instrument tips or jaws may be plain tipped or toothed (Fig. 9.5A–B). Tissue forceps usually are toothed instruments and are identified by the number of intermeshing teeth (e.g., 1 × 2, 2 × 3, 3 × 4). Allis forceps (Fig. 9.5C) are used to grasp delicate, soft tissues, so the teeth are finer, shallower, and more rounded. Other forceps have teeth that are sharper and deeper. Still others have sharp, hooklike, single or double teeth, such as a tenaculum (see Fig. 9.13C). Toothed instruments commonly have ratchets for locking into towels or human tissues. Instrument tips may also be either straight or curved, depending on their use.

An instrument can be named for its use (e.g., splinter forceps, for removing splinters) or after the person or people who developed it (e.g., Mayo-Hegar needle holder). Many general instruments are identified by the part of the body on which they are used (e.g., rectal speculum and nasal speculum).

Thousands of surgical instruments have multiple names. The same instrument may have two or three different names, depending on the provider identifying it or the part of the country in which the practice is located. For example, a provider may ask for a clamp or forceps when he or she wants a Kelly hemostat. It is important to learn the provider's preference in terminology. Learn to recognize the distinctive parts of instruments and the reasons for each part, and you will quickly build a working knowledge of hundreds of instruments.

CLASSIFICATIONS OF SURGICAL INSTRUMENTS

Surgical instruments are generally classified according to their use, and most belong to one of four groups:
- Cutting
- Grasping
- Retracting
- Probing and dilating

Cutting and Dissecting Instruments

Cutting and dissecting instruments, which are used for cutting, incising, scraping, punching, and puncturing, include scissors (Table 9.1), scalpels, chisels, elevators, curettes, punches, drills, and needles. Instruments with a sharp blade or surface can cut, scrape, or **dissect** (Figs. 9.6 and 9.7).

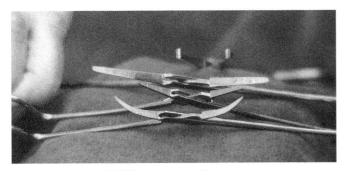
FIGURE 9.4 Instruments with serrations.

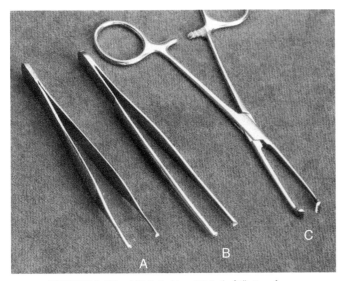
FIGURE 9.5 **(A)** and **(B)** Toothed jaws. **(C)** Teeth of Allis tissue forceps.

TABLE 9.1	Scissors
INSTRUMENT	DESCRIPTION
Lister bandage scissors	• Blunt probe tip • Easily inserted under bandages with relative safety • Used to remove bandages and dressings
Operating scissors	• 5 to 6 inches long • Curved or straight blade tips • Used to cut and dissect tissue
Suture scissors	• Blade has beak or hook to slide under sutures • Used to remove sutures

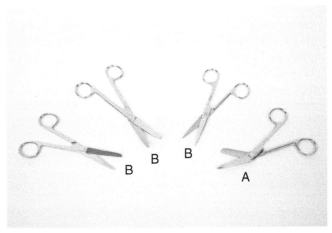
FIGURE 9.6 Scissors. **(A)** Lister bandage scissors. **(B)** Operating scissors.

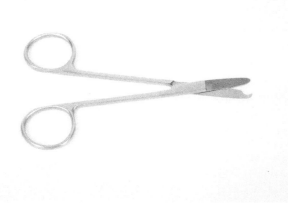

FIGURE 9.7 Suture scissors.

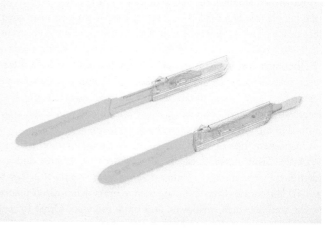

FIGURE 9.8 Disposable scalpels.

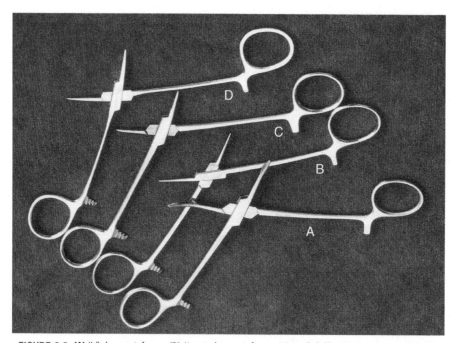

FIGURE 9.9 (A) Kelly hemostatic forceps. **(B)** Mosquito hemostatic forceps. **(C)** Needle holder. **(D)** Smooth-tip needle holder.

Disposable Scalpels

Most scalpels used in minor procedures are disposable (Fig. 9.8), with different handle sizes and types of blades already attached to the handles. However, stainless steel, reusable scalpel handles can be used. A variety of blades can be used, which must be attached to the handle using forceps and sterile technique. After the procedure, the handles are sterilized, and the blades are discarded in a sharps container. Once used, disposable scalpel/blade units are also discarded in a sharps container.

- *Handles:* No. 3 is the standard handle; No. 3L and No. 7 are used in deeper cavities.
- *Blades:* No. 15 is commonly used; Nos. 10, 11, and 12 are used for specialty incisions.

Grasping and Clamping Instruments

Clamping instruments are used for many different tasks. Many have a sharp tooth or teeth and are used to retract, hold, and manipulate

fascia. The most common clamping instruments are hemostats, which originally were designed to stop bleeding or to clamp severed blood vessels. Some clamping instruments are used to grasp other instruments or sterilized materials. Sometimes hemostats and other clamping instruments are used interchangeably. Table 9.2 lists the most common grasping and clamping instruments (Figs. 9.9 to 9.13).

Retractors

Retracting instruments hold tissue away from the surgical wound (incision). Depending on the provider's preference, handheld skin hooks and Senn retractors are used to retract during most minor surgical procedures.

Senn Retractor (Fig. 9.14)

- Flat end is a blunt retractor.
- Three-prong end may be sharp or dull.
- Used to retract small incisions or to secure a skin edge for suturing.

TABLE 9.2	Grasping and Clamping Instruments
INSTRUMENT	**DESCRIPTION**
Hemostatic forceps	• Jaws may be fully or partly serrated, without teeth • May be curved or straight • Used to clamp small vessels or hold tissue • Mosquito forceps (4 inches) are smaller and used for very small vessels • Kelly forceps (6 to 7 inches) are larger
Needle holder	• 4 to 7 inches long • Jaws are shorter and stronger than hemostat jaws • Jaws may be serrated or may have a groove in the center • Used to grasp a suture needle firmly
Splinter forceps	• Design and construction vary • Fine tip for foreign object retrieval
Plain thumb (dressing) forceps	• Manufactured in lengths from 4 to 12 inches • Varying types of serrated jaws but no teeth • Used to insert packing into or remove objects from deep cavities
Towel clamp	• Various lengths from 3 to 6½ inches • May have sharp or atraumatic (dull-edged) tips • Used to hold drapes in place during surgery
Allis tissue forceps	• Available in different lengths and jaw widths • Used to grasp tissue, muscle, or skin surrounding a wound
Toothed tissue forceps	• Manufactured in 4- to 18-inch lengths • Pincher grip • Used to grasp tissue, muscle, or skin surrounding a wound
Foerster sponge forceps	• Used to hold gauze squares to sponge the surgical site • Used as transfer forceps to arrange items on a sterile tray • Straight or curved, with or without serrations
Bozeman sponge forceps	• Designed to hold sponges or dressings • Capable of reaching the cervix through the vagina • Used to swab the area or apply medication
Tenaculum forceps	• Very sharp, pointed tips • Used to hold tissue (e.g., the cervix) while a tissue specimen is obtained or to lift the cervix so that the fornix can be seen

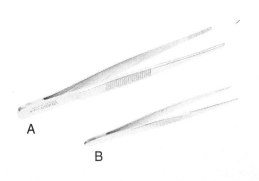

FIGURE 9.10 (A) Plain-thumb (dressing) forceps. **(B)** Splinter forceps.

Probes and Dilators

Probes and dilators are used both for surgery and for examinations. Probes can be used to search for a foreign body in a wound or to enter a fistula. Dilators are used to stretch a cavity or opening for examination or before inserting another instrument to obtain a tissue specimen. Table 9.3 lists the most common probes and dilators (Figs. 9.15 and 9.16).

SPECIALTY INSTRUMENTS

Although all instruments fall into the same four categories as the surgical instruments just discussed, the following instruments are organized into specialty groupings. Presenting the instruments in this manner makes it easy to see how the instruments relate to particular examinations. In addition to recognizing the name and use of each instrument, the

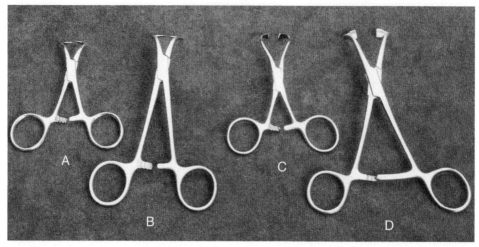

FIGURE 9.11 **(A)** Small sharp towel forceps. **(B)** Large sharp towel forceps. **(C)** Small atraumatic towel forceps. **(D)** Large atraumatic towel forceps.

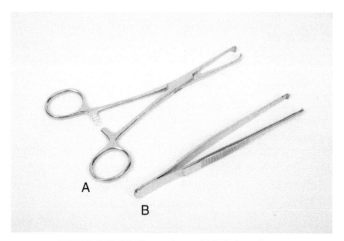

FIGURE 9.12 **(A)** Allis tissue forceps. **(B)** Toothed tissue forceps.

medical assistant must organize and set out the instruments needed for each particular examination in what is called a *tray setup*.

Gynecologic Instruments

Table 9.4 describes the common gynecologic instruments used in an office setting (Figs. 9.17 and 9.18).

Ophthalmologic and Otolaryngologic Instruments

Table 9.5 describes the common ophthalmologic and otolaryngologic instruments used in an office setting (Figs. 9.19 and 9.20).

Biopsy Instruments

Table 9.6 describes the common biopsy instruments used in an office setting (Fig. 9.21).

Genitourinary Instruments

Table 9.7 describes the common genitourinary instruments used in an office setting (Fig. 9.22).

DRAPES, SUTURES, AND NEEDLES

Disposable surgical drapes are available in several different materials and sizes. These typically have an opening (*fenestrated*) for the

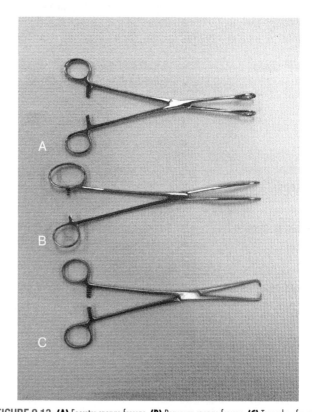

FIGURE 9.13 **(A)** Foerster sponge forceps. **(B)** Bozeman sponge forceps. **(C)** Tenaculum forceps.

operative site (Fig. 9.23). The drape is placed over the operative area, using sterile technique, after the patient's skin preparation has been completed. If a fenestrated drape is not available, multiple nonfenestrated drapes can be used to create a sterile field around the surgical site.

Sutures

The word *suture* is used as both a noun and a verb. As a noun, it refers to a surgical stitch or to the material used to close a wound. As a verb, it refers to the act of stitching. The primary purpose of a suture is to hold the edges of a wound together until natural healing occurs.

A suture may also be used as a *ligature*. This is a strand of suture material used to tie off a blood vessel or to strangulate tissue. If a ligature is used to tie off an internal tubular structure, it must last permanently or long enough for the structure itself to disintegrate. The ideal suture material has certain characteristics:

- Easy to handle and makes a secure knot
- Does not cause a localized tissue reaction and is nonallergenic
- Has adequate strength without cutting through tissue
- Can be sterilized

The provider will request a certain type of suture based on the specific properties of the suture material, such as rate of absorption, size of the suture, and type of needle. Both natural and synthetic suture materials are available. Sutures may be classified as either absorbable or nonabsorbable. Many different suture materials are available, each having its advantages and disadvantages. Suture materials

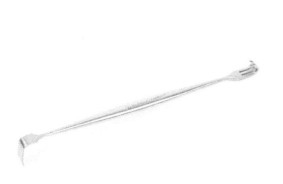

FIGURE 9.14 Senn retractor.

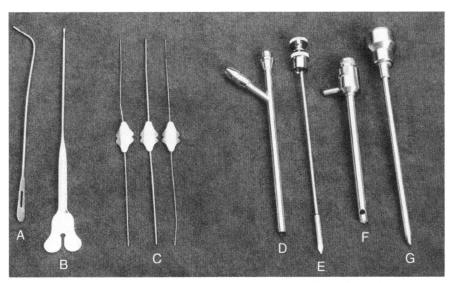

FIGURE 9.15 (A) Probe. **(B)** Grooved dilator. **(C)** Lacrimal duct probes. **(D)** Double-ended cannula. **(E)** Sharp trocar. **(F)** Canula. **(G)** Blunt-tip obturator.

TABLE 9.3	Probes and Dilators
INSTRUMENT	**DESCRIPTION**
Probes	• Lengths range from 4 to 12 inches; available with or without bulbous tip • May be smooth or may have a grooved director • Used to find foreign bodies embedded in dermal tissue or muscle or to trace a wound tract
Trocars and obturators	• Available in various sizes • Consist of a sharply pointed **stylus (obturator)** contained in a **cannula** • Used to withdraw fluids from cavities or for draining and irrigating with a catheter
Specula	• Most common dilator used • Valves are spread apart, dilating the opening • Used to open or distend a body orifice or cavity • The most common of these is the vaginal speculum used during gynecologic examinations (see Fig. 9.16C). Vaginal specula can be stainless steel (reusable) or plastic (disposable) and can also have a light source for illumination.

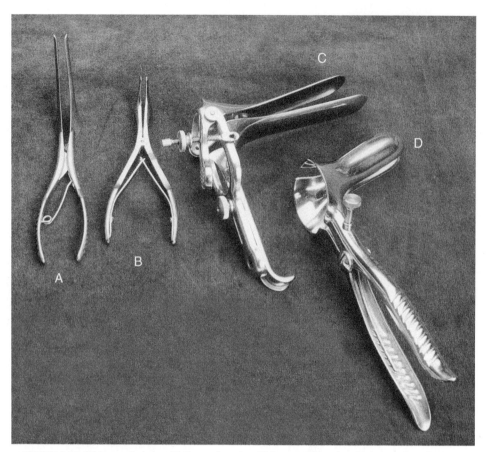

FIGURE 9.16 **(A)** Long nasal speculum. **(B)** Short nasal speculum. **(C)** Graves vaginal speculum. **(D)** Anal speculum, self-retaining.

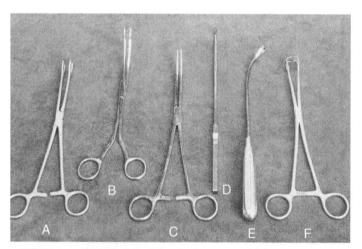

FIGURE 9.17 **(A)** Foerster sponge forceps. **(B)** Placenta forceps. **(C)** Bozeman uterine dressing forceps. **(D)** Endocervical curette. **(E)** Sims uterine curette. **(F)** Schroeder uterine vulsellum forceps.

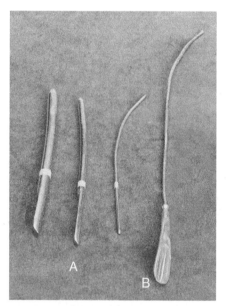

FIGURE 9.18 **(A)** Uterine dilators. **(B)** Sims uterine sounds.

commonly used in minor surgical procedures are described in the following paragraphs (Fig. 9.24).

Absorbable Sutures

Absorbable sutures are dissolved by the body's enzymes during the healing process. They are used when deep incisions or lacerations require inner layers of sutures to close the wound. Absorbable suture material is also used in areas where suture removal is difficult (e.g., oral surgery). Catgut (sheep, cattle, or pig intestine) was once the absorbable suture material of choice, but it has largely been replaced in recent years by synthetic absorbable suture material (e.g., Vicryl). Other synthetic absorbable suture materials include Dexon, PDS, and Maxon. These materials remain stable longer than natural catgut (up to 11 weeks), allowing the wound to heal completely before absorption occurs.

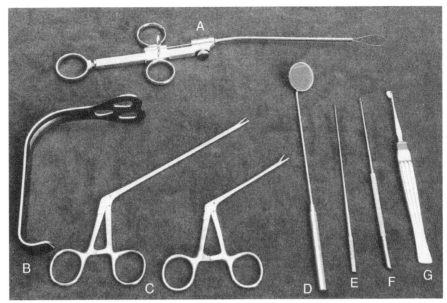

FIGURE 9.19 **(A)** Krause nasal snare. **(B)** Metal tongue depressor. **(C)** Long and short alligator forceps. **(D)** Laryngeal mirror. **(E)** Ivan metal applicator. **(F)** "Buck" ear curette. **(G)** Sharp ear dissector.

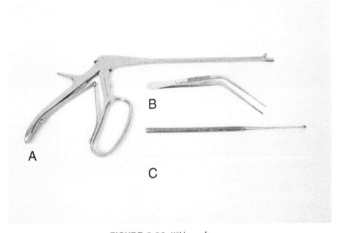

FIGURE 9.20 Wilde ear forceps.

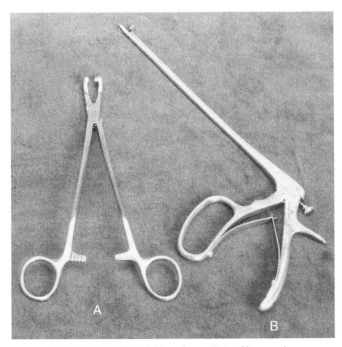

FIGURE 9.21 **(A)** Cervical biopsy forceps. **(B)** Rectal biopsy punch.

TABLE 9.4	Gynecologic Instruments
INSTRUMENT	**DESCRIPTION**
Placenta forceps	• Used to remove tissue from the uterus
Endocervical curette	• Smaller than the uterine curette • Used in the same way as the uterine curette
Sims uterine curette	• Available in several sizes • Hollow and spoon shaped; used for scraping • Used to remove polyps, secretions, and bits of placental tissue
Schroeder uterine vulsellum forceps	• Very sharp, pointed tips • Used to hold tissue (e.g., the cervix) while a tissue specimen is obtained or to lift the cervix so that the **fornix** can be seen
Hegar uterine dilators	• Available in sets • Double or single ended • Used to dilate the cervix for **dilation** and **curettage**
Sims uterine sounds	• Used to check the **patency** of the cervical os or the urethral meatus

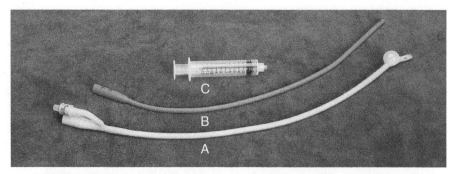

FIGURE 9.22 **(A)** Foley catheter with inflated balloon. **(B)** Red Robinson catheter. **(C)** 12-mL Luer-Lok syringe.

TABLE 9.5	Ophthalmologic and Otolaryngologic Instruments
INSTRUMENT	**DESCRIPTION**
Krause nasal snare	• Wire loop at the tip that can be tightened • Used to remove polyps from the nares
Metal tongue depressor	• Used to depress the tongue for oral examinations
Hartmann "alligator" ear forceps	• 3½-inch shaft; made in a variety of styles • Action of the jaw similar to that of an alligator's jaws • Used to remove foreign bodies or polyps
Laryngeal mirror	• Made in various sizes • May have a nonfogging surface • Used for examination of the larynx and postnasal area
Ivan laryngeal metal applicator	• 6 to 9 inches long with curved end for use in throat or postnasal areas • Holds cotton in place with its roughened end; used to swab or sponge throat or postnasal tissue • Used to remove foreign bodies embedded in the pharynx
"Buck" ear curette	• Manufactured in various sizes • Available as disposable curettes in many different sizes • Has a stainless steel loop at the end • Made with sharp or blunt scraper ends • Used to remove foreign matter from the ear canals
Sharp ear dissector	• Used to remove debris from the ear canal
Wilde ear forceps	• Angled, with serrated tips • Provides easier access to the ear canal and nasal cavities • Used for packing after ear or nasal procedures • Can be used to remove foreign bodies

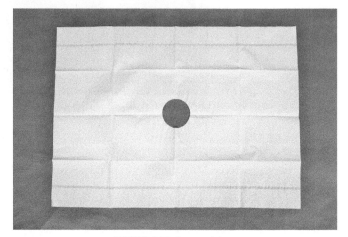

FIGURE 9.23 Fenestrated drape.

TABLE 9.6	Biopsy Instruments
INSTRUMENT	**DESCRIPTION**
Cervical biopsy forceps	• Available with or without teeth • Used to obtain cervical specimens for diagnostic examination
Rectal biopsy punch	• Available in different lengths and styles • Manufactured with interchangeable stems • Used through a proctoscope or sigmoidoscope
Silverman biopsy needle	• Manufactured with a split cannula • Stylus is removed, and cannula is inserted to retrieve the specimen • Needle biopsy can eliminate the need for surgical incision

Nonabsorbable Sutures

Nonabsorbable suture material is left in place until healing is complete. It frequently is used in minor surgical procedures performed in the medical office because most of the suturing required is superficial. It can be used in areas where sutures can be easily removed after healing has taken place. Silk is a common nonabsorbable suture material because it is strong and easy to tie. It is treated with a coating to prevent tissue drag and flaking. Polyester fiber sutures (e.g., Dacron and Prolene) are among the strongest nonabsorbable sutures, along with surgical steel. These fine filaments are braided and have great

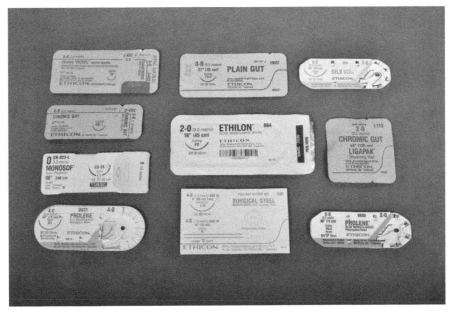

FIGURE 9.24 Suture packets labeled according to size, type, length, and type of needle point and shape.

TABLE 9.7	Genitourinary Instruments
INSTRUMENT	**DESCRIPTION**
Foley catheter with inflated balloon	• Manufactured in sizes 8 to 32 French with a double rubber lining toward the tip (each French unit is equal to 1.32 mm; the higher the number, the larger the lumen) • After insertion, sterile solution is injected into the inner lining (inflating the balloon) to hold it in the bladder • Used as an indwelling catheter
Red Robinson catheter	• Soft rubber urethral catheter in sizes 8 to 32 French • Inserted temporarily into the bladder for drainage or to obtain a specimen
Coudé-tip catheter	• Slightly curved catheter tip • Designed to allow it to navigate past obstructions in the urinary tract, such as a swollen prostate in men
12-mL Luer-Lok syringe	• Typically used to inject sterile saline into a catheter to inflate the balloon at the tip of an indwelling catheter • Used for injecting amounts greater than 5 mL

strength. Nylon suture is strong and has a high degree of elasticity. It is used primarily for skin closure. Due to its elasticity and stiffness, many knots must be used because the knots tend to untie if placed incorrectly.

Suture Sizing and Packaging

Suture material is available in a variety of diameters and lengths. The diameter of the suture strand determines its size; the smaller gauges are numbered below 0 (pronounced *aught*), and the larger gauges are identified with numbers above 0. For instance, 2-0 suture is thinner than size 0, which is thinner than size 2. The sizes from 6-0 to 2-0 are used most frequently in the medical office. The length of the suture material may vary, with strands precut in 18-, 24-, 54-, and 60-inch lengths.

Suture Sizes[a]	
SUTURE SIZE	**DIAMETER**
6-0	0.07 mm
5-0	0.10 mm
4-0	0.15 mm
3-0	0.20 mm
2-0	0.30 mm
0	0.35 mm
1	0.40 mm
2	0.50 mm

[a]Sutures are sized according to the U.S. Pharmacopoeia (USP) scale.

Needles. Surgical needles are chosen according to the area in which they are to be used and the depth and width of the desired suture. They are classified according to shape, which may be straight or curved. Most sutures are applied with curved needles because they allow the provider to penetrate the surface and then come back up on the other side. The sharper the curve of the needle, the deeper the provider can pass it into the tissue. The point of a needle can be a taper or a cutting edge. A taper is used on delicate tissues. The cutting-edge needle is used on the skin. It lacerates the skin as the needle is passed through. This is advantageous on tougher tissues, such as connective tissue.

Needles are manufactured with the suture material attached, or *swaged*, to the needle. These atraumatic needles do not have an eyelet and cause the least amount of trauma as they are passed through the tissue. Manufacturers package suture strands with the suture needle attached in peel-apart sterile, disposable packages. These may be obtained as single, individually packed, or multipack sutures in a variety of needle types and sizes with a wide range of suture materials and lengths. The most common needle type for minor skin repair is the curved, cutting-edge, swaged needle (Fig. 9.25).

Other Closure Materials

Surgical staples can also be used for skin closure. They are made of stainless steel or titanium and are available in different sizes. Surgical staples are applied (Fig. 9.26) and removed (Fig. 9.27) with specific staple instruments.

Another technique for wound closure is the use of Steri-Strips, which are self-adhesive tapes that are placed over the wound, pulling the wound edges together. Using a tincture of benzoin prior to the application of Steri-Strips can help them remain in place longer. Tincture of benzoin is applied parallel to the edges of the wound. Care should be taken so that it does not go into the wound because it can cause a burning pain. The compound becomes tacky, and the Steri-Strips stay on longer. Steri-Strips can be used to support a wound if there is potential tension at the site, or for superficial wounds. Frequently, small, clean lacerations may be closed with Steri-Strips (Fig. 9.28). These strips reduce the chance of infection and do not leave suture scars. Steri-Strips are used on areas of the body that are protected from movement and stress. They often are used on the face. A medical assistant can place Steri-Strips as ordered by the provider. They are placed on the wound in the same sequence and at the same intervals as interrupted sutures and are left in place until they fall off or the wound heals.

Tissue adhesives, similar to glue, can also be used for superficial wounds. Examples of tissue adhesives are Histoacryl, Dermabond, and SurgiSeal. Tissue adhesives form a strong bond across wound edges, allowing normal healing to occur below. Skin adhesives are also an alternative to sutures. They are frequently used for closure of facial lacerations, especially in pediatric patients, because they are effective for wound closure without requiring the use of needles and sutures.

Advantages of Tissue Adhesive

- Saves time during wound repair
- Creates a flexible, water-resistant protective coating for the wound
- Eliminates the need for suture removal
- Results in better cosmetic outcomes because there is no scarring from suture entry
- May also be used on larger wounds for which subcutaneous sutures are needed
- Especially helpful in pediatric patients or individuals afraid of needles

SURGICAL ASEPSIS AND PREPARATION OF SURGICAL INSTRUMENTS

Asepsis is the condition of being free of **infection** or infectious material. *Medical asepsis* is the reduction of microorganisms and the prevention of the transfer of microorganisms. This creates an environment that is clean but not *sterile* (i.e., free of microorganisms). The principles of medical asepsis are implemented to prevent reinfection of a patient

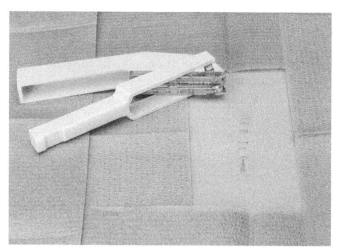

FIGURE 9.26 Disposable skin stapler.

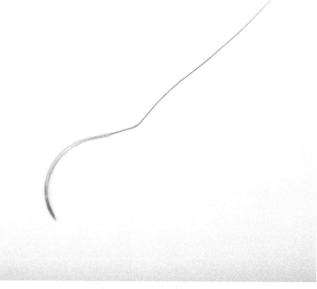

FIGURE 9.25 Swaged suture needle.

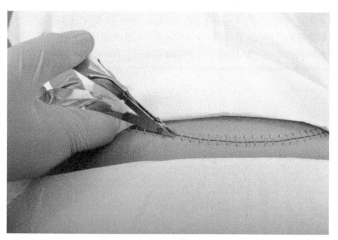

FIGURE 9.27 Surgical staple remover.

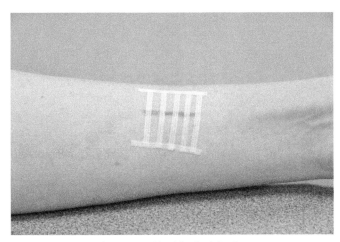

FIGURE 9.28 Wound closed with Steri-Strips.

and cross-infection of another patient or medical personnel. To prevent cross-contamination, potential microorganisms and pathogens must be isolated by following standard blood and body fluid precautions and by sanitizing, disinfecting, and/or sterilizing objects as soon as possible after they become contaminated.

Surgical asepsis is the complete destruction of microorganisms. This technique is mandatory for any procedure that invades the body's skin or tissues, such as surgery. In surgical asepsis, everything that comes in contact with the surgical site must be sterile, including surgical gowns, drapes, instruments, and the gloved hands of the surgeon and surgical assistants. Any time the skin or a mucous membrane is punctured or pierced, as in venipunctures or injections, surgical aseptic techniques must be practiced. Urinary catheterizations, biopsies, and dressing changes on open wounds are performed using sterile technique. In the next section we will discuss how to prepare instruments to be used in surgically aseptic procedures.

Care and Handling of Instruments

Because instruments are expensive, and the success of the procedure depends on their quality, the medical assistant must properly care for each instrument to maximize its life and ensure that every part is in safe working order.

Instruments that are not disposable are made of fine-grade stainless steel. The term *stainless* usually is taken too literally. Although stainless steel does resist rust and keeps a fine edge and tip longer, even the best stainless steel may develop water spots and stains. Proper hardness and flexibility are important. Inexpensive instruments that are chrome plated may be too brittle or too soft. In addition, mistreatment of chrome-plated instruments can cause tiny breaks in the finish, which may become a source of contamination or may tear the provider's gloves.

All instruments should be carefully examined when they are purchased. Scissors should be tested to see whether they shear the full length of the blades completely to the tip. If the scissors cut a piece of cloth cleanly and do not chew at any point, even at the tip, they are functioning correctly. Teeth and serrations should be checked to see whether they intermesh completely and whether the jaws are even on the sides and tip. Each instrument should be felt over its entire surface for any rough areas that may tear or snag the provider's gloves or act as a future source of contamination. Box locks and hinges must work freely but should not be too loose. Thumb- and spring-handled instruments must have the correct tension and meet evenly at the tips. After inspection, instruments should be sanitized and checked again for possible faulty workmanship before sterilization.

Under no circumstances should instruments be bundled together or allowed to become entangled. Do not mix stainless steel instruments with others made of different metals, including chrome-plated instruments, because this may cause electrolysis and result in etching. If an instrument is accidentally dropped, it may be permanently damaged. If scissors are dropped with the blades partly open, there may be a nick at the point where the blades cross. Any damaged or malfunctioning instrument must be disposed of to prevent complications during a surgical procedure.

After a surgical procedure, contaminated instruments should be placed in a basin of disinfectant solution. Heavier instruments should be on the bottom of the basin and lighter, more delicate instruments on top. Always unlock each instrument before immersing it in the chemical decontaminant to permit sanitization of the entire surface area. Never allow blood or other substances to dry on an instrument because they will be difficult to remove. If immediate sanitization and disinfection are not possible, the instruments should be rinsed well and placed in a cold-water solution with a blood solvent and mild detergent. It is best to use a detergent that has a neutral pH, is low sudsing, and can be rinsed off easily. The manufacturer's recommendations for the correct dilution and time of immersion of the various sanitizing agents, disinfectants, and blood solvents must be strictly followed for the chemicals to be effective.

When the surgical procedure is completed, the receiving basin for instruments should be transferred from the surgical area to the disinfection and sterilization room. It is important to remove used instruments from the patient's view as soon as possible. After sanitization is complete, instruments should be rinsed thoroughly and either washed by hand or washed mechanically using an ultrasonic device. Some delicate instruments, such as microsurgical and lensed instruments, should be washed by hand with a mild, low-sudsing, neutral-pH detergent solution, and a soft brush.

All instruments should be cleaned while submerged to prevent the airborne spread of microorganisms. Throughout the sanitization process, the medical assistant should wear heavy utility gloves to prevent possible exposure to contaminants. Some clinical policies require the medical assistant to wear disposable gloves under utility gloves for added protection from contaminants. Instruments then should be rinsed, dried with a lint-free cloth, and inspected for proper functioning before they are packed for sterilization.

Mechanical washing, such as with an ultrasonic device, can be used for most instruments and is an especially good method for sanitizing sharp instruments to prevent injuries (Fig. 9.29). In an ultrasonic cleaning unit, the instruments are immersed in a cleaning solution and the device produces sound waves that clean contaminants from the instruments' surfaces. Some units then rinse and dry the instruments, leaving them ready for the sterilization process. However, manufacturers' guidelines should be followed for rubber and plastic materials.

After sanitization and inspection, the instruments are ready for the sterilization process. Commercially prepared, disposable packs are available for most minor surgical procedures. They save time and eliminate the need for sanitization, disinfection, and sterilization of reusable stainless-steel instruments, but they may also be too costly for individual practices.

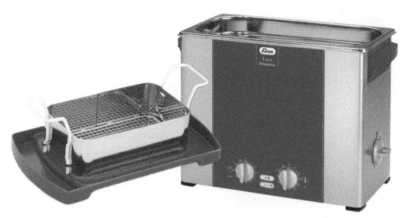

FIGURE 9.29 Elmasonic E ultrasonic cleaner unit. (Courtesy Tovatech, South Orange, NJ.)

CRITICAL THINKING APPLICATION   9.2

Tom is preparing instrument and supply packs for specific procedures performed by Dr. Martin. One of the packs he is preparing for the autoclave is for removal of a nasal polyp. Based on your understanding of typical and specialty instruments and supplies, what items should Tom include in the instrument pack?

Sterilization

Before an instrument or piece of equipment can be used in a surgical procedure, it must first be sanitized, then disinfected, and finally sterilized to remove all forms of microorganisms. It is essential that you understand the concepts of sanitization and disinfection before learning sterilization methods. Written sanitization, disinfection, and sterilization procedures should be in place for each workplace.

Utility Room

To ensure proper sterilization for surgical aseptic procedures, an area should be set aside for just this purpose. The area should be divided into two sections, one dirty and one clean. The dirty section is used for receiving contaminated instruments and other materials at the end of surgical procedures. This area should have a sink, receiving basins, proper sanitizing and disinfecting agents, brushes, utility gloves, autoclave wrapping paper or cloth, autoclave envelopes and tape, sterilizer indicators, and gloves. Designated biohazard waste containers are needed for gloves worn when handling contaminated items. Personal protective equipment (PPE) for sanitization, disinfection, and autoclave procedures includes:

- Fluid-resistant gloves to prevent contact with contaminants
- A laboratory coat or impervious gown, if needed, to protect against splashes
- A face shield and/or goggles if a splash hazard exists
- Heat-resistant autoclave gloves for unloading

The clean section of the utility room should be reserved for receiving the sterile items after they have been removed from the autoclave. Clear, clean plastic bags in which to store sterile packs may be kept in the clean area. Both areas should be spotlessly clean and well organized.

Instruments and other items used in ambulatory surgery, examination, or treatment must be carefully cleaned before proceeding with the steps of disinfection or sterilization. *Sanitization* is the cleansing process that removes organic material and reduces the number of microorganisms to a safe level. This cleansing process removes debris, such as blood and other body fluids, from instruments or equipment. Sanitization should be completed immediately after instruments are used. This should occur in a separate workroom or area or on the "dirty" side of the utility room to prevent cross-contamination of clean instruments and equipment. If it is not possible to sanitize instruments immediately after a procedure, rinse them under cold water immediately after the procedure and place them in a low-sudsing, rust-inhibiting, enzyme-containing detergent solution. Blood and debris must be removed so that later disinfection with chemicals and/or sterilization can penetrate to all the instruments' surfaces. Never allow blood or other substances that can coagulate or dry on an instrument.

The medical assistant should always wear utility gloves while performing sanitization to prevent possible personal contamination with potentially infectious body fluids that may be present. When you are ready to sanitize instruments, drain the soaking solution and rinse each instrument in cold, running water.

Clean all sharp instruments at one time, when you can concentrate on preventing injury to yourself. Open all hinges and scrub serrations and ratchets with a small scrub brush or toothbrush. Rinse the instruments in hot water and then check carefully that they are in proper working order before they are disinfected or sterilized. Generally, these instruments are then left out to air dry, but they may be hand dried with a microfiber towel to prevent spotting. Follow facility policy as to how instruments should be dried.

Disinfection is the process of killing pathogenic organisms or rendering them inactive. Many types of disinfecting agents are available, and they have varying degrees of effectiveness. It is important to follow the manufacturer's guidelines on how to use each product properly and to understand its advantages and disadvantages and possible sources of error. Disinfectants are used on equipment that cannot be sterilized (e.g., blood pressure cuffs and stethoscopes); on countertops and other physical surfaces in the healthcare facility; and for soaking instruments and equipment before sterilization. It is important to wear proper protective equipment when using disinfectants because they are generally strong enough to damage human tissue and will often leave burns if allowed prolonged contact with the skin.

CRITICAL THINKING APPLICATION   **9.3**

The office manager tells Callie she needs to review the office policy and procedures manual on sanitization, disinfection, and sterilization methods. Why is this important to accomplish before Callie starts performing sterilization procedures? What information in this manual would be most important to Callie as she starts this new position? Why?

Autoclave

Sterilization can be achieved by moist heat, dry heat, ultraviolet or ionizing radiation, or gas, or with chemicals. Medical facilities typically use the autoclave method, which uses moist heat and pressure to achieve sterilization. Steam under pressure in the autoclave (Fig. 9.30) is an excellent method of sterilization because it kills all pathogens and **spores**.

Pressurized steam is fast, convenient, and dependable. The pressure allows for heat higher than the boiling point. Steam from a pot of boiling water on a stove is about 212° F (100° C). We know that spores can survive temperatures of up to 240° F (115° C) for 4 hours. In an autoclave, the steam is contained within a chamber and is under 15 pounds per square inch (psi) of pressure. This pressure allows the steam to reach 250° F (121° C). No organism can last at that temperature for more than 15 minutes. When steam enters the autoclave chamber, it simultaneously heats and wets the object, coagulating the proteins present in all living organisms. When the cycle is complete, and the chamber has cooled, the steam condenses and explodes the cells of microorganisms, thus destroying them. To be effective, the steam moisture must come in contact with all surfaces being sterilized. Steam under pressure is capable of much faster penetration of fabrics and textiles than dry heat, but its use has definite limitations if the proper techniques are not followed.

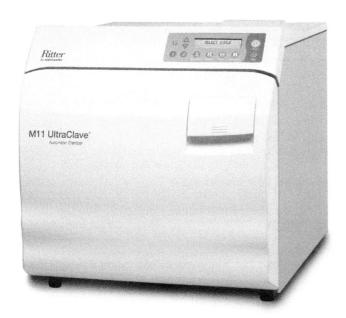

FIGURE 9.30 Steam autoclave. (Courtesy Midmark Corp., Dayton, OH.)

The recommended temperature for sterilization in an autoclave is 250° to 255° F (121° to 123° C). Follow the guidelines that come with the autoclave; in general, unwrapped items are sterilized for 20 minutes, small wrapped items for 30 minutes, and large or tightly wrapped items for 40 minutes. Processing time starts *after* the autoclave reaches normal operating conditions of 250° F (121° C) and 15 pounds per square inch (psi) pressure. There are different autoclave cycles for different materials; ambulatory care facilities do not autoclave liquids or dressing material, so the most used cycle will be the gravity cycle, which is used to sterilize stainless steel instruments. In the *gravity ("fast exhaust") cycle,* the autoclave fills with steam and is held at a set temperature for a set period. When the cycle is complete, a valve opens, and the chamber rapidly returns to atmospheric pressure. Drying time may be added to the end of the cycle.

Incorrect operation of an autoclave may result in superheated steam. If steam is brought to too high a temperature, it is literally dried out, and the advantage of a higher heat is diminished. Wet steam is another cause of incomplete sterilization. Wet steam results from failing to preheat the chamber, which causes excessive condensation in the interior of the chamber. Condensation is necessary, but too much prevents the sterilization process from being completed properly. It can be compared with taking a hot shower in a cold bathroom, which results in heavily steamed mirrors, walls, and towels. If packs become too saturated to dry during the drying cycle, the packs pick up and absorb bacteria from the air or any surface on which they are placed after removal from the autoclave. Placing cold instruments in a hot chamber also increases condensation. Other causes of wet steam include opening the door too wide at the end of the cycle or allowing a rush of cold air into the chamber. Overfilling the water reservoir may produce this same effect (Table 9.8).

The main cause of incomplete sterilization in the autoclave is the presence of residual air. Without the complete elimination of air, an adequately high temperature cannot be reached. Air and steam do not mix. Because air is heavier than steam, it pools wherever possible. One tenth of 1% (0.1%) residual air trapped around an instrument prevents complete sterilization. This is especially dangerous in older autoclaves that do not have a chamber thermometer separate from the pressure gauge. Adequate chamber pressure does not guarantee a proper chamber temperature. Table 9.9 provides tips for improving autoclave techniques.

Wrapping Materials. Maintaining the sterility of the autoclaved package depends completely on the wrapper and method of wrapping (see Procedure 9.1, p. 235). The wrapping material must be **permeable** to steam but **impervious** to contaminants. Acceptable wrapping materials for autoclaving should allow the steam to penetrate and also prevent pathogens from entering during storage and handling. A wrapper should not be used if it is torn or has a hole in it.

The types of wrapping material used for instruments that are to be autoclaved are disposable double-ply autoclave paper and peel-apart polypropylene bags (Fig. 9.31). Multiple layers of autoclave paper are recommended to maintain the integrity of sterilization during handling and storage of autoclaved instrument packs. Double-layered autoclave paper provides these multiple layers of protection for surgical instruments from contamination and saves time because wrapping is done only once.

TABLE 9.8   Common Factors Influencing the Effectiveness of Sterilization

CAUSES	POTENTIAL PROBLEM
Improper sanitization of instruments	Protein and salt debris may prevent direct contact with pressurized steam and heat in the autoclave.
Improper packaging	Prevents penetration of the sterilizing agent; packing material may melt.
Wrong packaging material for the method of sterilization Excessive packaging material	Reduces penetration of the steam and heat.
Improper loading of the sterilizer Overloading	Increases heat-up time and decreases penetration of pressurized steam and heat to the center of the sterilizer load.
No separation between packages, even without overloading	May prevent or reduce thorough contact of the sterilizing agent with all the items in the chamber.
Improper timing and temperature Incorrect operation of the sterilizer	Insufficient time at proper temperature to kill organisms.

Adapted from CDC: Infection Control. *https://www.cdc.gov/infectioncontrol/guidelines/disinfection/sterilization/sterilizing-practices.html.* Accessed October 6, 2018.

CRITICAL THINKING APPLICATION   9.4

Tom is processing instruments and trays when he notices that one of his co-workers never places gauze squares around the tips of sharp instruments before wrapping a pack. He also notices that not all of the packs are labeled properly. What is the significance of Tom's observation? How should he handle this situation? Why?

Wrapping Instruments. The method used to wrap instruments for autoclave sterilization must allow the pack to be opened without becoming contaminated. The rules for protecting package contents include the following:

- Discard autoclave paper that is torn or has holes.
- Wrap all hinged instruments in the open position to allow full steam penetration of the joint.
- Place a gauze square around the tips of sharp instruments to prevent them from piercing the wrapping material.
- If a number of instruments are to be placed on a stainless-steel tray for wrapping, first place a double-folded towel on the tray, and then position the instruments. This helps to protect them.
- Polypropylene is a plastic capable of withstanding autoclaving but is resistant to heat transfer. Therefore, materials in a polypropylene pan take longer to autoclave than the same materials in a stainless-steel pan.
- When using sterilizing bags, insert the handles of the instruments into the end of the bag that will be opened first to ensure that the grasping end of the instrument can be reached easily when the bag is opened.

TABLE 9.9   Tips for Improving Autoclave Techniques

PROBLEM	CAUSES	CORRECTION
Damp autoclave paper	Clogged chamber drain; items removed from chamber too soon after cycle; improper loading	Remove strainer; free openings of lint. Allow items to remain in sterilizer an additional 15 min with door slightly open. Place packs on edge; arrange for least possible resistance to flow of steam and air.
Stained autoclave paper	Dirty chamber	Clean chamber with mild detergent solution; never use strong abrasives, such as steel wool; rinse thoroughly after cleaning.
Corroded instruments	Poor sanitization; residual soil; exposure to hard chemicals (e.g., iodine, salt, and acids); inferior instruments	Improve sanitization process; do not allow soil to dry on instruments — sanitize first. Do not expose instruments to hard chemicals; if exposure occurs, rinse immediately. Use only top-quality instruments.
Spotted or stained instruments	Mineral deposits on instruments; residual detergents from cleaning; mineral deposits from tap water	Wash with soft soap and detergent with good wetting properties. Rinse instruments thoroughly with distilled water.
Instruments with soft hinges or joints	Corrosion or soil in joint; instrument parts out of alignment	Clean with warm, weak acid solutions (e.g., 10% nitric acid solution); rinse thoroughly. Have instrument realigned by qualified instrument repair professional.
Steam leakage	Worn gasket; door closed improperly	Replace gasket; reopen door and shut carefully; have serviced if unable to close door properly.
Chamber door does not open	Vacuum in chamber (check chamber pressure gauge)	Turn on controls to start steam pressure; wait until equalized, then vent and open door.

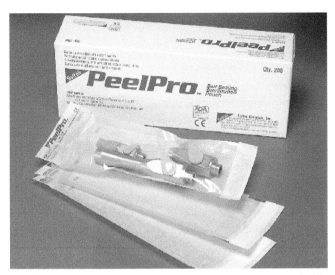

FIGURE 9.31 Sterilization pouches with sterilization indicators on the outside and inside of the envelope. The puncture-resistant, tinted plastic front is safety sealed to an autoclave paper backing. (Courtesy Practicon Dental, Greenville, NC.)

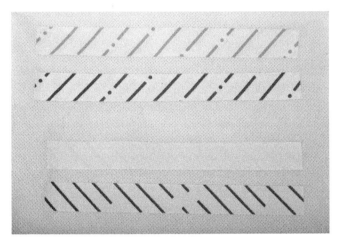

FIGURE 9.32 Autoclave tape.

- When using two-ply autoclave paper, use specialized autoclave tape to seal the package.
- Label each pack according to the instrument contents and sterilization date and write your initials. Use a permanent marker; never use a ballpoint pen.

Whether you are wrapping one item or many items together on a tray as a surgical pack, the procedure is the same; be sure the wrapper is large enough to cover the items to be sterilized.

Sterilization Indicators. Sterilization is achieved only when steam reaches the optimum temperature for a designated length of time and has penetrated to the center of the articles. Sterilization indicators must be used routinely to determine whether all microorganisms have been destroyed. The two basic types of sterilization indicators are chemical indicators (e.g., autoclave tape) and biologic indicators.

Chemical Sterilization Indicators. Autoclave tape, a commonly used sterilization indicator, contains a chemical dye that changes color when exposed to steam (Fig. 9.32). The tape is not an absolute

indication that the proper sterilization time, temperature, and steam have been maintained. It merely indicates that a high temperature was reached while the article was in the autoclave. The tape strip must completely change color (colors vary by manufacturer) or reveal the word "autoclaved" to show effective operation. The main function of autoclave tape, besides holding the wrapping material together, is to verify at a glance that the package was autoclaved. Other chemical indicators are placed inside the instrument packages to verify steam and heat penetration of the wrapping. Some instruments are autoclaved unwrapped, such as stainless-steel vaginal specula. A chemical indicator should be placed in the autoclave with unwrapped instruments in an area most difficult for steam to access, such as under the tray or between the instruments.

Biologic Sterilization Indicators. The healthcare facility should have a policy for how frequently the autoclave is tested using biologic sterilization indicators. The Centers for Disease Control and Prevention (CDC) recommends that this procedure should be performed weekly. Spore strip indicators have been replaced by rapid-readout biologic indicators that use ampules of *Bacillus stearothermophilus*, which is destroyed at 250° F (121° C). The ampule is placed in the center of the largest pack that is autoclaved in the facility to determine the accuracy of the autoclave and autoclave procedures in destroying all microbes. On completion of the cycle, the ampule is sent to a laboratory for analysis of any type of microbial growth. If tests show that microbes are present in the sample, then a report is sent to the facility notifying it that the autoclave, or possibly its sterilization procedures, are not effective in achieving sterilization. Results from the biologic indicator testing must be documented. Failed tests must be investigated, and the causes resolved.

Quality Assurance Records for Office Sterilization. Every office should have specific protocols to follow for quality assurance evaluations of the autoclave, including regular maintenance. This is done at specified intervals, depending on the volume and frequency of autoclave use. A log must be kept of the type of control test done, when it was performed, and the testing results. If the testing results indicate that sterilization was inadequate, a report must be made and filed. The report should identify the nature of the problem and how and when it was corrected. The report also should contain proof of correction by indicating the date and time of a first, subsequent, and successful sterilization run.

Loading the Autoclave. Prepare all packs and arrange the load in a way that allows maximum circulation of steam and heat (see Procedure 9.2, p. 237). Articles should be resting on their edges and should not be crowded. Placing the packs in stainless steel racks prevents packing of the autoclave too tightly. Instruments may be autoclaved unwrapped if they do not need to be sterile when used later. For example, although vaginal specula do not need to be sterilized for use (the vagina is a body cavity that is naturally open to the external environment), they must be sanitized and sterilized to prevent cross-contamination among patients. They can be placed, unwrapped, on a perforated stainless-steel tray in the autoclave and then stored in a clean area for future use.

Unloading Guidelines. When the autoclave's sterilization cycle is complete, release the pressure according to the manufacturer's guidelines. Once the pressure gauge reads "0," stand behind the door and, with heat-resistant gloves, open the door approximately ¼ inch. Allow the load to dry for at least 15 minutes (this time varies according to the type of autoclave and the size of the load). Packs can act as a sponge, attracting outside moisture and microorganisms. Touching a wet pack allows microorganisms on your hands to penetrate the wrappings, making the contents of the pack nonsterile. Dry, wrapped packs may be removed with clean, dry hands, but it is safer to wear heat-resistant gloves to reduce the possibility of burns from the hot instruments inside the packs. If possible, allow all packs to cool in the autoclave with the door open. Place the packs on a dry, dust-free surface inside an enclosed cupboard or drawer for storage. Do not place the packs on cold surfaces, because hot packs may cause condensation, and moisture will contaminate the contents.

Guidelines for Unloading an Autoclave

- Stand behind the door when opening it to prevent accidental steam burns.
- Slowly open the door only a crack, allowing the items to cool for 15 to 20 minutes before removing them.
- If for any reason the integrity of the sterilization process is in question, the load should be considered contaminated and autoclaved again. Reasons for concern include:
  - Any load that fails to convert a sterilization indicator strip (autoclave tape)
  - Any loads processed after a biologic test indicates that the autoclave is not working properly

---

Shelf Life of Sterilized Packs. The CDC no longer identifies specific time limits for the shelf life of sterilized packs. The general recommendation is that as long as the sterilized items are stored so that the packaging material remains intact and undamaged, then the pack is considered sterile. All sterile packs should be stored on dry, dust-free, covered shelves or in drawers. Some facilities continue to date every sterilized package and use shelf-life practices, such as first in, first out; other facilities have switched to event-related practices. With event-related practices, items remain sterile until some event causes contamination (e.g., a pack becomes wet or packing material is torn). The quality of the packaging material, storage conditions, and how much the packs are handled all affect the possibility of contamination. Therefore, sterile packs should be inspected before they are used to verify the integrity of wrapping material. Any package that is wet, torn, dropped on the floor, or damaged in any way should be sanitized, disinfected, wrapped in new autoclave paper or placed in new autoclave pouches, and autoclaved again.

CRITICAL THINKING APPLICATION   9.5
Tom discovers a number of packages of paper-wrapped sterile instruments that appear to have water marks on them. The indicator tape shows that they have been autoclaved. What should he do with these packs? Why?

Chemical Sterilization

In the medical office, chemical sterilization is used for instruments that cannot be exposed to the high temperatures of steam sterilization. The sterilizing chemical solution must be mixed exactly according to the instructions on the bottle. The solution must be marked with the date of preparation and expiration. Materials to be sterilized must be submerged in this chemical bath with a closed lid for 8 hours or longer. Items are removed with sterile forceps and must be rinsed with water to remove all traces of the chemical before the items are used on a patient. You must avoid skin contact with the sterilizing solution because it is very **caustic**.

The use of chemicals for sterilization is not very practical in the ambulatory facility. The instruments or equipment cannot be wrapped during processing in the liquid chemical. Once they are removed from the liquid, they are no longer considered sterile. In addition, because of the caustic nature of the chemicals, instruments must be rinsed with water after removal from the chemical fluid. This water is typically not sterile. However, high-level chemical disinfectants do have a place in health care. They can be used on instruments (e.g., endoscopes) that would be damaged by autoclaving. Because of the limitations of using liquid chemicals for sterilization, their use should be restricted to reprocessing critical devices that are heat sensitive and incompatible with other sterilization methods.

CLOSING COMMENTS

Patient Coaching

Patients may have questions about the instruments the provider will use, and the medical assistant can help allay patients' fears by answering these questions. Explaining the patient preparation for the procedure, how the procedure will be performed, and what to expect afterward helps make the procedure go more smoothly and encourages the patient to follow the provider's advice and orders.

Legal and Ethical Issues

It is important for patient health that medical assistants ensure that all instruments used in procedures are sterile. The sterilization process begins with sanitization. No short cuts should be taken when prepping instruments for sterilization. It might be easier to overlook the damaged sterilization pack, but using instruments from that pack could lead to an infection, which in turn could lead to a lawsuit.

Professional Behaviors

Performing medical assistant duties responsibly and accurately is crucial in the surgical area of the ambulatory care setting. The provider relies on the medical assistant to have the appropriate supplies and instruments available before a procedure begins. To achieve this goal, the medical assistant must have a working knowledge of the typical instruments and supplies used in the facility, in addition to an understanding of the types of instruments needed for each procedure. Medical assistants must make sure tasks are completed according to the facility's policies and procedures so that they are able to assist the provider and protect the patient.

SUMMARY OF SCENARIO

Tom has worked for the providers at Walden-Martin Family Medical Clinic for 2 years and is familiar with their preferences in surgical solutions, local anesthetics, and suture materials, in addition to the typical instruments used in the practice. He also has worked hard to update the policies and procedures manual to include standards for instrument care so that other medical assistants in the office will know how instruments should be sanitized, disinfected, inspected, and prepared for the autoclave. Tom realizes he needs to continue his education in surgical procedures and takes advantage of professional workshops on the topic. Tom consistently attempts to stay up to date on surgical advances and also the medications and instruments used at WMFM.

SUMMARY OF LEARNING OBJECTIVES

1. **Describe typical solutions and medications used in minor surgical procedures.**

   Solutions used in minor surgery include sterile water for mixing with medications or rinsing instruments; sterile saline for injection or wound irrigation; antiseptic skin cleansers (e.g., Hibiclens and Betadine) for site preparation; and local anesthetics, including topical applications, in addition to lidocaine, Nesacaine, or Sensorcaine injectables. These local anesthetics may come packaged with or without epinephrine. The provider also may use topical silver nitrate to control local bleeding.

2. **Summarize methods for identifying surgical instruments used in minor office surgery, and then identify some surgical instruments.** Refer to Tables 9.1 through 9.7.

3. **Outline the general classifications of surgical instruments.**

   Surgical instruments are classified according to their use as cutting, grasping, retracting, probing, or dilating tools. The components of the instrument include the type of handle, the closing mechanism, and the jaws. Instrument tips may be either straight or curved and toothed or not toothed. The instruments used in minor surgical procedures depend on the type of procedure and the provider's preference. Specialty instruments are used in specialty practices (e.g., gynecology, ophthalmology, otolaryngology) and for particular procedures (e.g., biopsies).

4. **Identify drapes and different types of sutures and surgical needles.**

   Surgical drapes come in various sizes and materials. They are placed over the operative area after the skin preparation has been completed. There is typically an opening (fenestrated) for the operative site.

   Suture material is available as absorbable (for internal sutures) and nonabsorbable (for skin closure). Dexon, PDS, and Maxon are popular absorbable materials; nonabsorbable sutures can be made of silk or nylon, or staples can be used. Tissue adhesives, similar to glue, can also be used for superficial wounds. Suture materials range in size from smaller gauges (i.e., below 0 [aught] for finer tissues) to thicker gauges (above 0) and are available in various lengths. Surgical needles are either straight or curved. Most needles are manufactured with swaged suture material.

5. **Describe the care and handling of surgical instruments.**

   Surgical instruments are expensive and must be cared for properly to maintain function and maximize durability. Instruments must be examined when purchased for proper working order and possible faults with mechanisms. Stainless steel instruments should be kept separate from other metal types. Each instrument must be cleaned according to the manufacturer's guidelines, unlocked, and disinfected immediately after use. Most instruments can be cleaned with an ultrasonic washer, which helps prevent injuries.

PROCEDURE 9.1   Wrap Instruments and Supplies for Sterilization in an Autoclave

Task: Place dry, inspected, and sanitized supplies and instruments inside appropriate wrapping materials for sterilization and storage without contamination.

EQUIPMENT and SUPPLIES

- Dry, inspected, and sanitized instruments
- Double-ply autoclave paper
- Autoclave tape
- Sterilization strip
- Waterproof, felt-tipped pen
- Gloves (if part of office policy)

PROCEDURAL STEPS

1. Wash or sanitize your hands. Collect and assemble already inspected, sanitized instruments to be wrapped. Gloves may be worn.
2. Place the double-ply autoclave paper on a clean, flat surface.
3. Place the instruments diagonally at the approximate center of the double-ply autoclave paper. Make sure the size of the square is large enough for the items (see the following figure).
   PURPOSE: Each of the four corners must fold over and completely cover the instruments, with a few extra inches of overlap for folding.

Continued

PROCEDURE 9.1   Wrap Instruments and Supplies for Sterilization in an Autoclave—*continued*

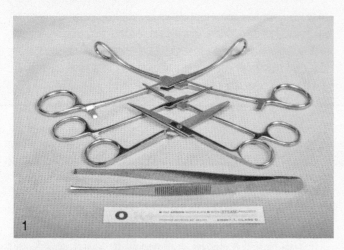

4. Open any hinged instruments. If the instrument is sharp, its teeth or tip should be shielded with cotton or gauze.
   <u>PURPOSE</u>: To prevent puncture of the package or injury to the operator.
5. Place a sterilization strip in the center of the pack to check for sterilization standards.
   <u>PURPOSE</u>: To ensure that the autoclave is reaching effective levels of heat and pressure to destroy all microorganisms.
6. Bring up the bottom corner of the wrap and fold back a portion of it.
   <u>PURPOSE</u>: This folded-back flap is the only part of each wrapper corner that can be touched when a sterile package is opened (see the following figure).

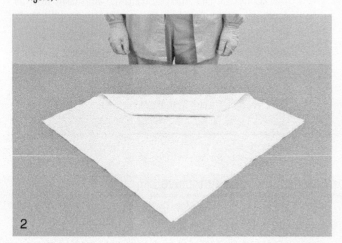

7. Repeat the previous step with each corner, making sure to turn back a portion each time (see the following figures).

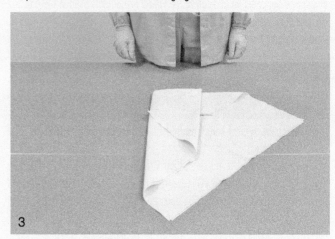

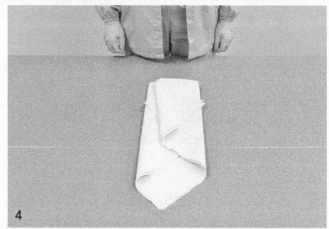

PROCEDURE 9.1 | **Wrap Instruments and Supplies for Sterilization in an Autoclave**—*continued*

8. Fold the last flap over (see the following figure).

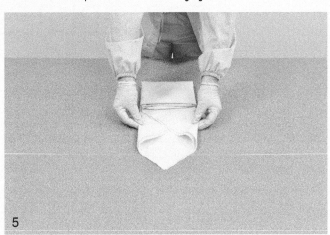

9. Secure with autoclave tape (see the following figure) and label the package with the date, including the year, contents, and your initials.
   PURPOSE: So that staff members will know what is in the pack, when it was autoclaved, and who performed the task.

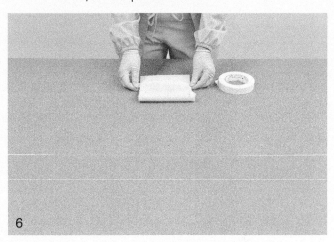

PROCEDURE 9.2 | **Operate the Autoclave**

Task: Sterilize properly prepared supplies and instruments using the autoclave.

EQUIPMENT and SUPPLIES

- Autoclave
- Wrapped items ready to be sterilized
- Heat-resistant gloves

PROCEDURAL STEPS

Note: The specific instructions for operating an autoclave may vary based on the model number and manufacturer. Refer to the instructions that accompany the autoclave to be sure the appropriate steps are followed.

1. Check the water level in the reservoir and add distilled water as necessary.
   PURPOSE: Too much or too little water may alter the effectiveness of the equipment. Tap water leaves lime deposits in the chamber.
2. Turn the control to "Fill" to allow water to flow into the chamber. The water flows until you turn the control to its next position. Do not let the water overflow.
3. Load the chamber with wrapped items, spacing them for maximum circulation and penetration.
   PURPOSE: To ensure sterilization of all items.
4. Close and seal the door.
   PURPOSE: The door must be closed, or the heated water in the chamber evaporates.
5. Turn the control setting to "On" or "Autoclave" to start the cycle.

6. Watch the gauges until the temperature gauge reaches at least 121° C (250° F) and the pressure gauge reaches 15 pounds of pressure.
   PURPOSE: The proper temperature and pressure must be reached before sterilization can begin.
7. Set the timer for the desired time.
8. At the end of the timed cycle, turn the control setting to "Vent."
   PURPOSE: This releases the steam and pressure. The water at the bottom of the chamber drains back into the reservoir. Newer autoclaves automatically perform this step.
9. Wait for the pressure gauge to reach zero.
10. Standing behind the autoclave door, carefully open the chamber door ¼ inch.
    PURPOSE: To allow steam to escape faster. Be careful to prevent accidental burns.
11. Leave the autoclave control at "Vent" to continue releasing heat.
    PURPOSE: To dry the items faster.
12. Allow complete drying of all articles.
13. Using heat-resistant gloves, remove the items from the chamber and place the sterilized packages on dry, covered shelves or open the autoclave door and allow the items to cool completely before removal and storage.
14. Turn the control knob to "Off" and keep the door slightly ajar.
    PURPOSE: To allow the inside of the autoclave to dry completely.

10 ASSISTING WITH SURGICAL PROCEDURES

SCENARIO

Callie Casper, CMA (AAMA), works for the Walden-Martin Family Medical (WMFM) Clinic. Callie was hired to work as an administrative medical assistant at the front desk, but one of the clinical medical assistants unexpectedly quit, and the office manager has offered Callie the position. Callie is excited about this opportunity, especially the chance to work with Dr. Angela Perez, but she is also concerned about her skill level in sterile procedures. At least she is familiar with a number of the patients, most of the staff, and the types of outpatient surgeries performed in the facility. Surgical asepsis and assisting with surgery were her favorite topics when she was in her medical assisting program. However, before she can assist with surgeries, Callie must demonstrate her ability to set up a sterile field without contaminating the site. She also must show that she can perform wound care skills, including applying sterile dressings and changing bandages.

While studying this chapter, think about the following questions:

- What are common surgical procedures performed in an ambulatory care facility?
- What is the medical assistant's role in preparing the patient, equipment, and room for a surgical procedure?
- What are the crucial steps Callie must follow to set up and maintain a sterile field?
- What techniques must Callie follow to prepare for and assist with a surgical procedure?
- Why is it important that Callie understand and be prepared to answer patients' questions about the process of wound healing?
- What bandaging techniques should Callie be prepared to perform?

LEARNING OBJECTIVES

1. Summarize common minor surgical procedures.
2. Detail the medical assistant's role in minor office surgery when it comes to preparation of the patient and the room. Also, explain how to perform skin prep for surgery.
3. Outline the rules for setting up and maintaining a sterile field; explain how to perform the following procedures related to sterile techniques:
   - Open a sterile pack and create a sterile field
   - Transfer sterile instruments and pour solutions into a sterile field
   - Perform a two-person sterile tray setup
   - Apply sterile gloves without contaminating them
4. Discuss how to assist the provider during surgery and demonstrate how to assist with a minor surgical procedure and suturing.
5. Summarize postoperative instructions and explain how to remove sutures and surgical staples.
6. Explain the process of wound healing.
7. Explain how to properly apply dressings and bandages to surgical sites.

VOCABULARY

approximated (uh PROK si may ted) Near, close together.
cicatrix (SIK uh triks) Early scar tissue that appears pale, contracted, and firm.
hemostasis (hee muh STAY sis) The stoppage of bleeding.

plume Vapor, smoke, and particle debris produced by laser procedures.
vigilance (VIJ uh lahns) Keen watchfulness to detect danger.

Common surgical procedures that are routinely performed in the primary care facility include suturing, cyst removal, incision and drainage (I&D) of abscesses, and collection of biopsy specimens. The medical assistant should be proficient in:

- explaining each of these procedures to the patient
- preparing the patient and the room
- assisting the provider with the surgery
- applying a sterile dressing and bandage after the procedure is finished

Each surgical procedure requires appropriate skin preparation and draping with a *fenestrated* drape. This is a surgical drape with an opening in the center. The size of the opening depends on the size of the surgical field. The opening is placed directly over the surgical site after the site has been prepared (or "prepped," as it is called in healthcare practice). A minor surgery tray is opened, and a sterile field is created on a Mayo stand. Sutures, scalpels, and any other instruments needed are added to the field, according to the provider's preference. An injectable and/or a spray local anesthetic should also be ready for the provider's use, with the needed injection supplies.

After achieving suitable local anesthesia, the provider opens the skin with an incision. If a cyst is being removed, the provider dissects around it and usually tries to "deliver" it from the wound intact. If the procedure is an I&D, foul matter will start oozing from the wound immediately after the skin is incised. The wound is drained completely and flushed with copious amounts of sterile saline solution. If the procedure is a biopsy, a small amount of tissue is removed and placed in a specimen container with preservative. The specimen container must be carefully labeled with the appropriate patient information, the date, and specifics about the specimen type and location. It then is sent to the laboratory, where it is examined microscopically for changes or abnormalities.

SURGICAL PROCEDURES

Electrosurgery

Electrosurgery is also known as *electrocautery.* An electrosurgical unit (ESU) uses high-frequency current to cut through tissue and coagulate blood vessels. A small probe with an electric current running through it is used to *cauterize* (i.e., burn or destroy) the tissue. This process seals blood vessels, minimizing cellular oozing and bleeding. Electrosurgery may be used to destroy granulations and small polyps or to take a tissue sample for pathology examination. The loop electrosurgical excision procedure (LEEP) uses a wire loop heated by electric current to remove cells and tissue as part of the diagnosis and treatment of abnormal or cancerous conditions of the uterine cervix.

Necessary components are the ESU's power source, the grounding cable and pad, and the active electrode (i.e., a pencil-like instrument with a tip and cord). The grounding pad is a gel-covered adhesive electrode that provides a safe return path for the electrosurgical current. Electrode tips are disposable and are used according to the type of procedure performed. The two most commonly used tips are the needle and flat designs.

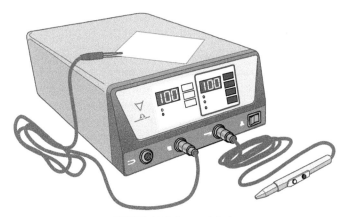

FIGURE 10.1 Electrosurgical unit.

Holding the pencil-like instrument, the provider touches the tissue with the tip and activates the electric current with a switch on the instrument. The electric current is delivered to the tissues, and tissue is vaporized at the site of contact, or a specimen can be removed for pathology (Fig. 10.1).

Laser Surgery

Laser is an acronym for *l*ight *a*mplification by *s*timulated *e*mission of *r*adiation. Because a laser beam is so small and precise, it can be used to safely treat specific tissue with minimal damage to surrounding tissues and limited scar formation. Lasers were first used in medicine to treat diseases of the retina, and they now are used for many procedures, including:

- excision of lesions
- cauterization of blood vessels
- removal of warts or moles
- cosmetic surgical procedures

Several types of lasers are used, including the carbon dioxide, yttrium-aluminum-garnet (YAG), and pulsed dye lasers. Each laser has a specific use. The color of the laser light beam is directly related to the type of surgery performed.

A medical assistant must be specially trained about lasers before assisting with laser surgery. Laser equipment requires very careful handling, care, and maintenance. Laser light destroys tissue and can harm the patient, the provider, and you if handled improperly. The medical assistant should complete a full laser safety program before assisting in laser procedures. Once trained, the medical assistant's role during laser surgery includes:

- Protecting the patient's eyes from the potential damaging light of the laser
- Observing the surgical field through safety goggles for possible contamination
- Keeping wet sponges ready
- Removing any flammable items from the laser's path
- Assisting with suctioning of the **plume** to maintain a clear visual field
- Providing a basin of sterile normal saline solution and a filled irrigating syringe
- Watching each application of the laser beam and anticipating the need for protective supplies, special equipment, or instruments

---

Important Tips About the Grounding Pad

- Carefully inspect the pad, cable, and skin before the procedure.
- Place the pad close to the operative site.
- The pad must be tight against the patient's skin.
- Apply the pad to a fleshy area, such as the thigh.
- Do not place the pad over a bony area.
- Do not place the pad over body hair.
- Do not place the pad over metal implants or a pacemaker.
- Carefully inspect the pad site on the skin after the procedure for signs of burns.

Microsurgery

Microsurgery involves the use of an operating microscope to perform delicate surgical procedures. One of its major uses is in ophthalmologic surgery. It also is used in otologic, rhinologic and sinus, laryngologic, neurosurgical, microvascular, gynecologic, and genitourinary procedures. A medical assistant must acquire a basic knowledge of the operation and care of a microscope before becoming qualified to assist in these types of procedures.

The basic components of an operating microscope are the light source, eyepieces (also called the *oculars*), lenses, and cord. Accessory pieces include assistant and observer lenses, cameras, video recorders, television monitors, and printers. These are all valuable for documentation and teaching purposes. Disposable sterile drapes and handle covers are used on the microscope during surgical procedures.

Surgical microscopes are expensive, delicate instruments that require extreme care in handling and cleaning. All lenses and cords should be carefully inspected before and after each use.

Endoscopic Procedures

An endoscope is a medical device consisting of a miniature camera mounted on a flexible tube with an optical system and a light source that is used to examine the area inside an organ or a cavity. Many types of endoscopes are used, and they are named according to the organs or areas they are used to explore, such as the urinary bladder, bronchus, larynx, colon (Fig. 10.2), stomach, uterus, abdomen, and

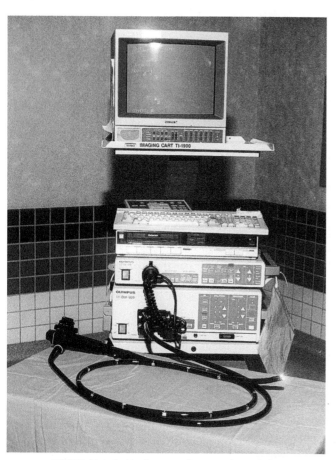

FIGURE 10.2 Flexible colonoscope with monitor and video recorder.

various joints. Small instruments can be used to take samples of suspicious tissues through the endoscope.

Direct visualization with an endoscope is used for diagnostic purposes or to perform surgical procedures. Endoscopes may be rigid (e.g., laparoscope or hysteroscope), semirigid, or flexible (e.g., colonoscopes, bronchoscopes, gastroscopes). All are delicate and expensive and require extreme care in handling to protect them from damage.

Accessory equipment used with endoscopes includes fiberoptic light cables and light source; irrigators for solution instillation and suction; and a camera, monitor, printer, and video recorder. The fiberoptic light cable consists of hundreds of glass fibers. It is important to protect it from being bent, dropped, kinked, squashed, or smashed. The light source can become very hot and must be kept out of contact with the patient, the provider, the staff, and any flammable material, such as surgical draping. All equipment must be checked before and after use. Always follow the manufacturer's recommendations for use, care, and maintenance of equipment. Endoscopic instruments would be damaged by the high temperature and steam under pressure in autoclaves. Special care must be taken in sanitizing and using high-level disinfectants after each procedure to destroy pathogenic organisms and prevent cross-contamination to subsequent patients.

Cryosurgery

Cryosurgery involves the use of a very-low-temperature probe to destroy tissue by freezing it on contact. The probe's temperature is usually below 4° F (−20° C). This cold temperature is achieved by circulating liquid nitrogen through the tip of the probe. A local anesthetic is usually administered before cryosurgery. Cryosurgery is used to treat cancers of the skin and warts. In many situations, cryosurgery is less invasive than traditional surgery and therefore generally has fewer associated complications. Cryosurgery often is performed in an ambulatory setting or in an outpatient surgery center.

ASSISTING WITH SURGICAL PROCEDURES

Surgery performed in a medical office is restricted to the management of minor problems and injuries. The medical assistant is expected to assist with preparing the patient and setting up the sterile field. The following procedures must be used without exception when assisting with minor surgery. Individual facilities may have specific guidelines for some of these procedures; however, the theory behind sterile technique is universal, regardless of where you work.

Preparation of the Patient

Whether minor surgery is performed because of an unforeseen accident or is a planned, elective procedure, the patient needs both psychological and physical support. A patient facing a surgical procedure may be concerned about pain, disfigurement, and the possible diagnosis. An injured patient may feel anxious about medical bills or possible loss of employment. Because surgery is a frightening experience, the medical assistant must take the time, both preoperatively and at the time of surgery, to help the patient deal with fears and anxieties. The best way to help is to make sure that the patient understands the details of the procedure, that all questions are answered by the provider, and that the patient has the opportunity to talk about the procedure and voice any concerns.

Questions should be answered directly, but you should answer only the questions that are within your scope of knowledge and the policies of the office. If you cannot answer a question, assure the patient that you will relay it to the provider before the procedure and then be sure to do so. What may seem to be a minor or unimportant question to you may be a very frightening concern to the patient. The minor surgery room can be intimidating, so unless the patient is sedated, try to make conversation with him or her while you prepare for the provider's arrival.

Preoperative preparation may include:

- blood and urine tests
- completion of a consent form
- gathering of the current history concerning any recent illnesses
- medications and allergies

Patient preparations before surgery may include a shave prep, cleansing enemas, food intake restrictions, special bathing, and administration of a sedative medication. On the day of surgery, the patient is instructed to empty the bladder and undress and gown as requested. The vital signs are recorded in preparation for the procedure.

Preoperative Instructions

When office surgery is planned, certain procedures are followed before the appointment. These include:

- Having the necessary consent forms ready to sign
- Giving the patient the necessary preoperative instructions, such as medications to be used and special skin-cleansing instructions
- Telling the patient to bring a relative or friend to drive him or her home after the surgery
- Instructing the patient to leave jewelry and other valuables at home
- Calling the patient the day before the scheduled surgery to confirm any special instructions

Informed Consent

The provider must have the patient's written informed consent before sedating medication is given and surgery begins. To sign an informed consent form permitting the provider to legally perform the surgery, the patient must understand:

- what procedure will be performed
- why it should be done
- the potential risks and benefits of the surgery
- alternative treatments (including no treatment)
- possible risks of any alternative treatment

This legal requirement is not met simply by having the patient sign a consent form; a discussion must occur, during which the provider gives the patient or the patient's legal representative enough information to enable the person to decide whether to proceed with the proposed surgical treatment. After this discussion, the patient either consents to or refuses the surgery. The patient then signs or refuses to sign the consent form. The discussion must be fully documented in the patient's health record. A copy of the signed form must also be included in the patient's record. Sometimes the patient will sign the form directly on the electronic record. Treatment may not exceed the scope of the consent form.

The patient must not be under the influence of any sedative medication at the time he or she signs the consent form. An interpreter must be used if the patient does not understand English. This condition must *never* be violated.

CRITICAL THINKING APPLICATION   **10.1**

Callie is preparing a patient for a biopsy of a suspected cancer of the skin. The consent form has been signed and is in the chart. While Callie is chatting with the patient during completion of the final setup for the procedure, it becomes clear the patient thinks she is having a "skin tag" removed from her back. What action should Callie take, if any? What is the significance of what the patient said in this situation?

Positioning

Have the patient disrobe sufficiently to expose the surgical site completely so that accidental contamination does not occur during the procedure. Clothing may also act as a tourniquet or may make applying a proper dressing or bandage difficult. In addition, the patient's clothing may be stained by the skin prep solution or may interfere with adequate site preparation.

The patient needs to be positioned as comfortably as possible for the procedure. An uncomfortable position can be held for only a limited time, and the patient may have to move, perhaps in the middle of a procedure, if you have not ensured his or her comfort from the beginning. When deciding on the correct position, consider where you and the provider will stand or sit, where the instruments will be placed, and where other needed equipment will be located. If the patient has an open wound, wear gloves to assist the patient into position. If there is active and profuse bleeding, wear an impermeable gown and gloves. If there is danger of blood and body fluid contamination to your face or eyes, wear a face shield.

Skin Preparation

The human skin is a reservoir of bacteria, but it cannot be sterilized without the risk of damaging cells and tissues. The goal of adequate skin preparation for a surgical procedure is to reduce the number of transient flora so that transfer of harmful organisms at the incision site is limited. Cleansing the patient's skin before surgery with surgical soap and an antiseptic and shaving the area if needed is called a *skin prep* (see Procedure 10.1, p. 252). Sometimes the patient may be instructed to repeatedly cleanse the surgical area with bacteriostatic or antiseptic soap several days before the surgery. Disposable skin prep trays and electric razors should be available in the ambulatory facility.

Preparation of the Room

If you are to assist in a minor surgical procedure, study the provider's care preferences, review the procedure, and note the materials needed. Next, prepare the room and gather the supplies to be used. Sterile supplies are opened just before the procedure. Opened materials that have been exposed longer than 1 hour, usually because of a delay, are considered nonsterile. Supplies should not be placed where they can be knocked over or dropped. Wrapped sterile supplies that fall to the floor must not be used. Make sure the patient and family members understand that they should not approach or touch the sterile field.

Sterile Technique

Accurately performing surgical aseptic technique requires a great deal of concentration and planning of all movements and procedural steps. The procedures covered in this chapter are for minor surgery, but they are the same techniques used during major surgery. To develop a sound knowledge of sterility and sterile technique, use the following memory aid: *Everything sterile is white and everything that is not sterile is black. There is no gray!* Sterile surfaces must *never* come in contact with nonsterile surfaces. If this occurs, the sterile surface immediately is considered contaminated or nonsterile. Constant **vigilance** and absolute honesty are essential for maintaining sterile techniques. When a sterile surface comes in contact with a nonsterile item, this is called a "break" in sterility or a "break" in the sterile field. During any procedure, everything must stop at this point and the "break" must be corrected immediately. This usually means the assistant must start over again at the very beginning of the procedure. Any break could lead to serious wound contamination, postoperative infection, and even death.

Before assisting with minor surgery, the medical assistant must perform a series of procedures to ensure surgical asepsis (see Procedures 10.2 to 10.5, pp. 253-259). These skills must be learned, practiced, and followed precisely to establish and maintain the sterile environment required during a surgical procedure. Surgical asepsis directly affects the health and well-being of the patient, the provider, and the office staff and must be practiced without fail.

CRITICAL THINKING APPLICATION   10.2

After completing a surgical scrub before assisting with a minor surgical procedure, Callie remembers that she forgot to lay out the practitioner's sterile glove package. She opens up the storage cabinet and quickly adds this to the collection of sterile supplies. Can she go ahead with putting on her sterile gloves? Why or why not?

Sterile Field

A sterile field is any sterile surface on which sterile items are placed. In the ambulatory facility, a sterile field most often is set up on a Mayo stand (Fig. 10.3). In surgery, a sterile field is created by draping

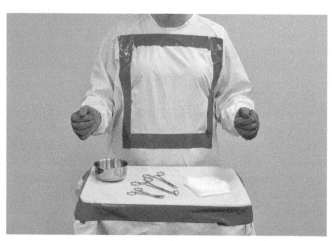

FIGURE 10.3 Sterile field *(red outline)*.

sterile towels (either disposable or from autoclaved packs) over a Mayo stand or table. The surgical site on the patient's skin is prepared and then draped with sterile towels or drapes so that it, also, becomes a sterile field.

Hands and hair are two of the greatest sources of contamination when a sterile field is set up. With practice, you will learn to know what may be touched with your hands and what must be touched only with sterile gloved hands. Hair that falls freely over the shoulders and forward gives off a cloud of bacteria with every movement. It must always be secured back and up, not touching the shoulders.

Rules for Maintaining a Sterile Field

- Talking should be kept to a minimum because air currents carry bacteria.
- Sterile team members should always face one another.
- Always keep the sterile field in your view. If you turn your back on a sterile field or lose sight of it, it is considered contaminated.
- Nonsterile body parts (e.g., hands or elbows) and items should never cross over the sterile field.
- Tables and trays are sterile only at table level; anything that falls below the edge of the Mayo tray is considered contaminated. A 1-inch border around the edge of the tray is considered contaminated, so anything placed on the tray within that 1-inch border is contaminated.
- Consider a sterile barrier contaminated if it has been wet, cut, or torn.
- Packages placed on a clean surface are contaminated on the outside, but the inside of the sterilized package may be used as a sterile field.
- Keep sterile gloved hands above waist level at all times; do not let hands drop below the waist.
- Never remove and then replace any item in the field (e.g., using sterile forceps to cleanse a wound), or the field is contaminated.
- The inside of a sterile package remains so if the package is peeled open properly; it should be opened the entire way, and the contents then tossed onto the field without crossing over the sterile area; a two-person transfer can be used, in which one person opens the sterile supplies and another, wearing sterile gloves, removes the contents from the package and places them on the sterile tray.
- If a sterile package falls to the floor, it must be discarded.
- If you are in doubt about the sterility of anything, consider it contaminated.

Assisting the Provider During Surgery

The provider ultimately is responsible for the patient. The medical assistant is responsible for ensuring that everything the assistant and the provider will use in caring for the surgical patient is accounted for, ready for use, and prepared in a safe and sterile manner (see Procedure 10.6, p. 260). Every team has preferences about the sequence it follows during routine minor surgery. Once a routine has been established, it should be followed in every case. Sample setups for various types of minor surgery are provided in Table 10.1.

The medical assistant sorts and places the scalpels, hemostats, scissors, tissue forceps, and retractors on the sterile field according to their sequence and frequency of use. Scalpels and sharp instruments

TABLE 10.1   Setups for Minor Surgeries

PROCEDURE	SIDE COUNTER	STERILE FIELD	COMMENTS	POSTOPERATIVE CARE
Suture repair	Local anesthetic, dressings and bandages, splints or guards, tape, drape, gloves, sterile normal saline solution	Syringe and needle, hemostats (three), scissors, sponges, suture material and needle, tissue forceps or skin hook, needle holder	If a patient arrives with a pressure dressing over a laceration, follow Standard Precautions. Do not remove the pressure dressing until the provider is ready to suture. If the patient's pressure cloth must be removed, have ample sterile dressings ready to apply immediately. Ask the patient the approximate length, depth, and exact location of the laceration. Follow the provider's directions regarding cleansing of the wound.	Clean lacerations in a moderately protected area; may not require a dressing. The patient is instructed to keep the area clean and dry. Some lacerations may be closed with Steri-Strips or a topical skin adhesive.
Needle biopsy	Specimen container with prepackaged fixative or preserving solution, laboratory form and label, local anesthetic, gloves	Biopsy needle, syringe and needle, sponges	A biopsy is the examination of tissue removed from the living body. Biopsies usually are done to determine whether a growth is malignant or benign; however, a biopsy may be done as a diagnostic aid in other diseases or infections. A needle biopsy may be done by aspiration with a needle and syringe or with a special biopsy needle. The specimen then is sent to a pathologist for either a cytologic or a histologic examination.	Usually no special dressing is required after a needle biopsy. An adhesive bandage strip (e.g., Band-Aid) often is sufficient.
Cyst removal	Local anesthetic, disinfectant (skin prep), laboratory form, dressing (size depends on site), gloves, drape, specimen container with prepackaged fixative or preserving solution	Kelly hemostats (two straight and two curved), dressing forceps (two), suture and needle, scissors, dissector (provider's choice), skin hook, syringe and needle, disposable scalpel with No. 11 or No. 15 blade, tissue forceps (two), Allis forceps, needle holder, sponges	A sebaceous cyst is a benign retention cyst of a sebaceous gland containing fatty substance from the gland. The cyst is attached to the skin and moves freely over the underlying tissue. For cosmetic reasons the provider makes the incision on the natural skin crease lines if possible.	See suture repair, earlier, or apply a small sterile dressing, depending on the size of the incision.

should be conspicuously placed so that they do not accidentally injure a team member. The provider enters the room after scrubbing and then puts on gloves. The provider drapes the patient with towels or a fenestrated drape as the medical assistant hands him or her the drapes, one at a time. Once the site has been draped, the Mayo stand with the sterile field is positioned below the site, and the medical assistant stands opposite the provider over the patient, ready to help as needed.

Passing Instruments

During a procedure, the medical assistant must protect the sterile field from contamination. Notify the provider if a break in sterile technique occurs, dispose of soiled sponges in the biohazard waste container, and anticipate the provider's need for instruments. The provider may request instruments or may use hand signals. As the team works together over time, the provider may not need to give any signals, because the assistant will be able to anticipate the instrument needed next during the procedure.

Instrumentation is logical; if the practitioner requests a suture, scissors will be needed next to cut the suture strand. In the case of sudden hemorrhage from a bleeding vessel, the provider will need an appropriately sized hemostat. While gaining experience, the assistant watches, listens, and learns to judge what will be needed or performed next. While wearing sterile gloves, pass instruments with a firm, purposeful motion so that the provider does not have to look up. Wait until you feel the provider grasp the instrument so that it does not drop onto the patient or the floor. Be careful that you and the provider are protected from injury. Pass the scalpel with the blade down and present the handle to the provider. Hold all instruments by their tips and pass the handle ends into the provider's palm or fingers (Fig. 10.4).

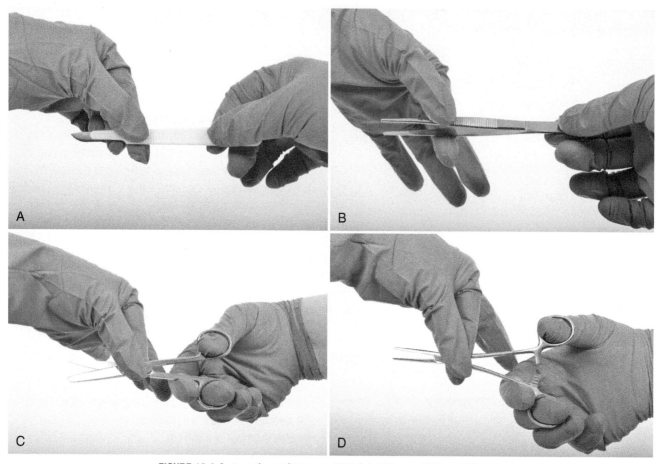

FIGURE 10.4 Passing sterile surgical instruments. **(A)** Scalpel. **(B)** Forceps. **(C)** Scissors. **(D)** Clamp.

CRITICAL THINKING APPLICATION   **10.3**

In passing the scalpel to the provider while assisting with an incision and drainage (I&D), Callie feels the blade slice through her glove. She quickly and secretly looks at it and notices a "very tiny" nick in her glove. Because this is a "dirty" procedure, she decides to say nothing and continues assisting with the procedure. Is her reasoning sound here? What is the best approach to handling this situation? Why?

Specimen Collection

If a specimen is collected during a procedure, it is placed in a sterile specimen cup or basin. Do not remove the specimen from the sterile field until the provider gives the order. The provider may want to examine the specimen again during the procedure. After the procedure is complete, place the specimen in an appropriate container, label it, and send it to the laboratory for analysis.

Completing the Surgical Procedure

At the conclusion of the procedure, the provider begins wound closure. The techniques and methods of tissue closure vary; all of them cannot be described or illustrated here. The two basic methods of suturing are the continuous running suture (Fig. 10.5A) and the interrupted suture (Fig. 10.5B), in which each knot is placed and tied one at a time, so that if one breaks, the others keep the wound closure intact.

The interrupted technique is used for most skin closures in a medical office.

The provider may prefer that the medical assistant place the needle in a needle holder and pass it, handle first. When the wound is closed, you may assist by cutting the suture and sponging the site. If an interrupted suture method is used, the first suture is placed at the midpoint of the incision. Then each side of the first suture is mentally divided in half again, and the next two sutures are placed at each of these midpoints. The rest of the sutures are placed using the same technique until the wound edges have been completely **approximated**. The provider may also choose to close a wound with surgical staples.

After the skin closure, the blood and iodine should be gently removed and the area blotted dry using sterile dry sponges. Care must be taken not to disturb the wound edges or sutures. Next, a sterile dressing is placed over the incision (see Procedure 10.7, p. 262), and a bandage is applied to support the dressing.

Postoperative Responsibilities

After caring for the patient, the medical assistant clears the sterile field, following Standard Precautions. Wear gloves until all contaminated materials have been properly removed and handled. Place disposable equipment and supplies in biohazard waste containers and/or sharps containers. The room should be checked for any blood spills or other contamination and disinfected appropriately. After completing this process, remove the contaminated gloves and sanitize your hands.

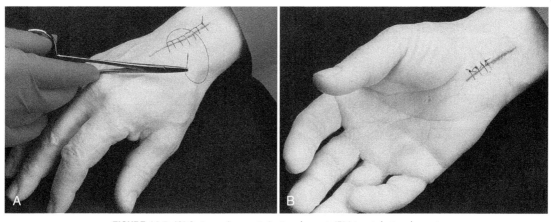

FIGURE 10.5 **(A)** Continuous (i.e., running) suture placement. **(B)** Interrupted suture placement.

Single-Assistant Preparation for Minor Surgery

1. Sanitize your hands and gather all supplies.
   - *Sterile side (Mayo tray):* Two towel packs, skin prep pack, patient drape pack, instrument pack, miscellaneous pack or packs, three glove packs, face shields, impermeable gowns
   - *Nonsterile side (side counter):* Syringes, suture material, anesthetic solutions, additional sponges, sterile dressings, bandages, transfer forceps, waste basin, sharps and biohazard waste containers, nonsterile gloves, face shields, and impermeable gowns
2. Verify that the informed consent has been signed and is in the patient's health record.
3. Identify the patient and escort him or her into the room.
4. Greet and converse with the patient.
5. Position the patient on the table.
6. Sanitize your hands.
7. Open the first towel pack.
8. Open the skin prep pack.
9. Pour the soap and antiseptic solutions.
10. Expose the site to be prepped.
11. Put on gloves and arrange prep items within the sterile field.
12. Place sterile towels at skin scrub boundaries using sterile technique.
13. Prep the patient's skin.
14. Discard skin prep materials in appropriate sharps/biohazard containers.
15. Discard gloves; sanitize your hands, following the guidelines for a surgical hand scrub (Procedure 10.2) if this procedure is part of the policy of the provider or the facility.
16. Open the table drape pack on the Mayo stand to create a sterile field.
17. Open the instrument pack or packs and transfer the instruments to the sterile field. Add the sterile syringe unit.
18. Add sterile items as requested.
    The provider joins you and converses with the patient.
19. Open the provider's glove pack (the provider now puts on gloves).
20. Open the patient drape pack (the provider now drapes the surgical site).
21. Cleanse and hold up the anesthetic vial for the provider to withdraw anesthetic with the sterile syringe (the provider now administers the anesthetic).
22. Repeat the surgical hand wash; reglove with a new glove pack.
23. Arrange the sterile field instruments and other materials for safety and in sequence; check the condition of each instrument.
24. Open the suture/needle pack per the provider's choice; load the first suture into the needle holder.
25. Place two gauze squares at the site.
26. Assist with the procedure.[a]
    - *For the provider:* Pass the instruments; maintain the field; anticipate his or her needs; and cut sutures.
    - *For the patient:* Retract tissue; sponge blood from the wound; apply the sterile bandage; and care for the specimen.
27. Help the patient sit up and dress if needed and monitor vital signs as instructed.
28. Record and prepare specimens.
29. Sanitize and disinfect the room; clear materials and discard in biohazard waste containers.
30. Document the procedure in the patient's health record.
31. Help the patient prepare to leave the office.
32. Sanitize, disinfect, and sterilize the equipment at the first available time.

[a]By law, the assistant may not clamp tissues, place sutures, or alter body tissues in any way.

Wear gloves while disinfecting the room, including the table, Mayo stand, side and back tables, any other equipment in the room, and the floor. Used instruments must be sanitized, disinfected, and resterilized for future use.

The provider and the medical assistant both document the surgical procedure in the patient's health record.

Postoperative Instructions and Care

The patient should be given time to rest after the surgery. If a sedative was administered, make sure the patient has recovered sufficiently to avoid injury after the surgery or during the trip home. If the patient was given a topical or local anesthetic, explain to him or her that the anesthesia effect will wear off and that some discomfort may be felt

POSTOP INSTRUCTIONS FOR _____

☐ Elevate your arm.
☐ Elevate your leg.
☐ Limit food intake to _____.
☐ Limit activity to _____.
☐ Do not bathe or shower.
☐ Sponge bath only.
☐ Change dressing as instructed.
☐ Call the office for fever, redness, pain, swelling, or bleeding.
☐ Take_____ every 4 hours as needed for pain.
☐ Return to school/work in _____days.
☐ Call the office tomorrow before _____ p.m.
☐ Your next appointment is on M T W Th F S_____ at _____.

FIGURE 10.6 An example of preprinted postoperative patient instructions.

at the operative site. Check with the provider whether pain medication needs to be prescribed. If medication has been prescribed, review the purpose of the medication and the directions for its use with the patient and his or her companion. Make a follow-up appointment before the patient leaves the office.

Postoperative care extends for the total recovery period, not just for the time of immediate care before the patient leaves the office. Most medical assistants are responsible for teaching patients to care for themselves at home after surgery. A postoperative patient may have trouble comprehending or remembering instructions. All instructions should be given to the patient in writing. They should be simple and easily understood by both the patient and caregivers. These instructions can be preprinted forms for each type of surgery, or a general form with checked boxes for particular postoperative instructions that apply specifically to the individual patient (Fig. 10.6).

Warning Signs

Explain to the patient the importance of calling the office if any questions come up or changes occur that cause the person concern. If the patient does not call within the next 24 hours, you should call the patient. Many patients tend to "ride it out" or say they did not want to disturb you. Never allow the postoperative patient to leave the office without the provider's knowledge and approval. Tell the patient to call the office immediately if he or she notes redness around the operative site, bleeding from the wound, fever, swelling, or increasing or severe pain. The wound should be kept clean and dry, and the patient should be taught how to change the dressing, if needed.

Follow-Up

If the healing process is a long one or if the wound becomes infected, the patient may return for follow-up care. If the wound requires a new dressing, follow Standard Precautions; wear gloves and other protective barriers as appropriate. If at any time you determine that the wound may be infected, stop and have the provider examine it. Generally, no bandaging material should be reused, including elastic bandage wraps.

Tape applied directly to a patient's skin is not a good dressing immobilizer. If tape is used, always keep it to a minimum. If tape is

holding a dressing in place, always remove it by pulling toward the wound. If it is adhering to a hairy area of the body, lift the outer tape edge with one hand and slowly and gently separate the underlying hair and skin from the tape with the thumb of your other hand. Peel the skin from the bandage, not the bandage from the skin. Never rapidly "rip" tape from the body, because this may injure the skin. If the tape is not irritating to the patient, it may be advisable to leave the tape in place until total healing has taken place.

When the wound has healed, the provider may ask the medical assistant to remove the patient's sutures or staples. The patient must return to the facility to have the sutures/staples removed (see Procedure 10.8, p. 264). When removing sutures or staples, it is important for medical assistants to alert the provider to any concerns they notice with the wound healing, and to document the procedure.

WOUND CARE

A wound can be intentional (e.g., from a surgical incision) or accidental, and it may be open or closed (Fig. 10.7). An open wound has an outward opening; the skin is broken, exposing the underlying tissues. A closed or nonpenetrating wound does not have an outward opening, but the underlying tissues are damaged, as in a hematoma, contusion, or bruise. Closed wounds usually are the result of some type of blunt trauma to the body. An aseptic (i.e., clean) wound is not infected with pathogens. Septic wounds are infected with pathogens.

Open wounds may be classified according to the appearance of their openings. An incised wound has a clean edge and is made with a cutting instrument. An incised wound may be the result of surgery, an accident, or a knife wound. A lacerated wound has torn or mangled tissues and is made by a dull or blunt instrument. A penetrating or puncture wound is caused by a sharp, slender object, such as a needle or an ice pick, and passes through the skin into the underlying tissues. A perforated wound is a penetrating wound that passes through to a body organ or cavity, such as a gunshot wound.

Wound Healing

All wounds go through a healing or repair process that has four phases. **Hemostasis** is the first phase. Blood vessels contract to control hemorrhage, and blood platelets form a network that acts as a glue to plug the wound. After a cascade of chemical reactions, fibrin is released into the wound and clotting begins. Fibrin continues to collect red blood cells (RBCs), and the clot dries into a scab.

The second, or inflammatory, phase focuses on destroying bacteria and removing debris. Special white blood cells (WBCs), called *macrophages,* arrive to clear away bacteria and dead tissue. Within 1 to 4 days the fibrin threads contract and pull the edges of the wound together under the scab. During this phase, edema, *erythema* (redness), heat, and pain can occur.

The third phase, *proliferation,* encompasses wound healing and new growth; this lasts 5 to 20 days. During this phase, the tissues repair themselves. New cells form, and the wound continues to contract and seal. If the wound is a clean surgical incision, complete contraction usually takes place and a **cicatrix** forms.

The final phase, the *remodeling* phase, extends from day 21 onward. Clean, shallow wounds may contract in the first two stages; large or mangled wounds require the time and cellular activity of this third phase to build a bridge of new tissue to close the gap of the wound. The cells produce a fibrous protein substance called *collagen* (i.e., connective tissue) that gives the wounded tissues strength and forms scar tissue. Scar tissue is not true skin; it usually is very strong, but it lacks the elasticity of normal skin tissue. There is no blood supply or nerves in scar tissue.

Several factors influence the healing process. People who are young, in good general health, and have adequate nutrition heal more rapidly. Adequate protection and rest of the injured area also enhance the healing process. Destruction or reinjury during the second phase can delay healing and increase scarring. Wounds are susceptible to infection because the normal skin barrier is broken. If debris is present in a wound as the result of the breakdown of various cellular components, this dead (i.e., necrotic) tissue acts as a culture medium for bacterial growth. Suppuration (i.e., pus) contains necrotic tissue, bacteria, dead WBCs, and other products of tissue breakdown. Necrotic tissue must be removed; the removal of debris is called *debridement,* which may occur naturally or may be performed surgically.

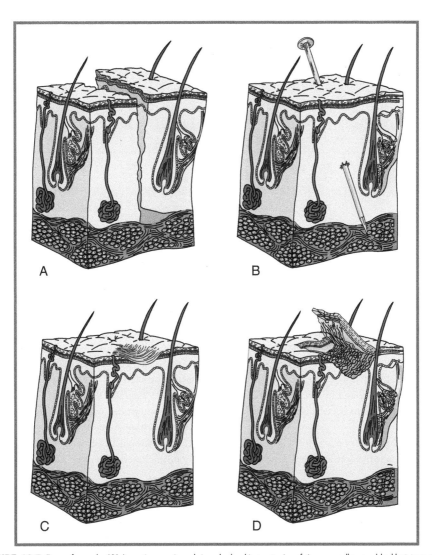

FIGURE 10.7 Types of wounds. **(A)** Laceration — a jagged, irregular breaking or tearing of tissues, usually caused by blunt trauma. **(B)** Puncture — piercing of the skin by a pointed object, such as a pin, nail, splinter, or bullet. **(C)** Abrasion — a superficial wound made by scraping of the skin. **(D)** Avulsion — tissue forcibly torn or separated, caused by accidents.   *Continued*

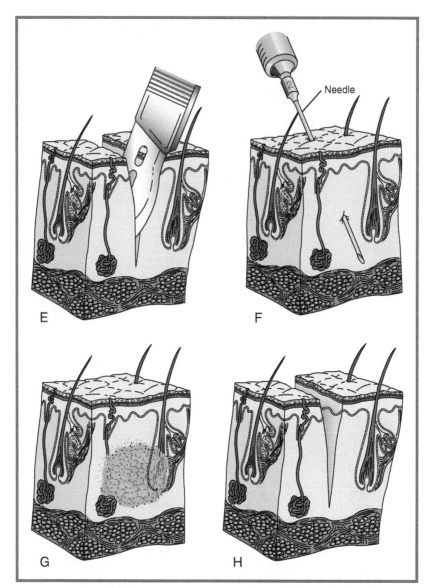

FIGURE 10.7, cont'd (E) Surgical incision — a neat, clean cut. **(F)** Hypodermic puncture — an injection under the skin. **(G)** Contusion — a closed nonpenetrating wound in which blood from broken vessels accumulates in tissues. **(H)** Incision — a neat, clean cut from sharp objects, such as glass, knives, or metal.

Sometimes the provider may prefer no dressing or bandage on small wounds. This is called *open wound healing*. Some advantages to open wound healing are:
- Air can circulate freely around the wound.
- The wound is not irritated or rubbed by a dressing.
- The wound stays dry, which inhibits bacterial growth, reducing the chance of infection.
- Sutures stay dry and hold together better.
- Any preexisting infection remains localized and is not spread by the dressing or bandage.

Dressings

A dressing is a sterile covering placed over a wound for the purposes of:
- Protecting the wound from injury and contamination
- Maintaining constant pressure to minimize bleeding and swelling
- Holding the wound edges together
- Absorbing drainage and secretions

A dressing usually consists of a strip of lubricated mesh gauze, a nonstick Telfa pad, or a clear dressing placed over a sutured wound. Gauze may be placed over nonadhering material, depending on the provider's preference. Body cavities or wounds that need to remain open for a time are dressed with long, thin packing material that often is impregnated with an antiseptic or a lubricant; this sometimes is called *packing*. A good dressing must be effective and comfortable and must remain in place. If the dressing covers a hairless area, it may be anchored with tape, but no tape should touch the wound.

Bandages

Bandages hold dressings in place and also help maintain even pressure, support the affected part, and help protect the wound from injury and contamination. Bandages can be gauze, cloth, or elastic cloth rolls and are bound by clips, tape, or ties. Dressings and bandages frequently appear easy and simple to apply; however, special skill is required to use different types of bandaging techniques. Bandages

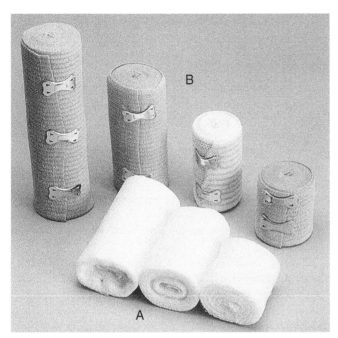

FIGURE 10.8 **(A)** Wrinkled crepe-type roller bandages (e.g., Kling). **(B)** Elastic roller bandages (e.g., Ace).

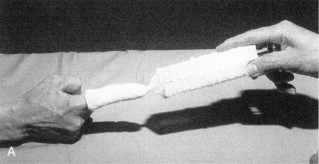

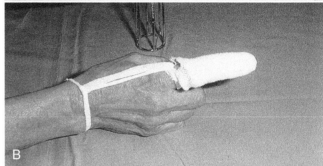

FIGURE 10.9 **(A)** Tube gauze is applied with even tension and is twisted at the fingertip before the next layer is applied. **(B)** A tube gauze bandage has been applied and secured by tying at the wrist.

that are too loose fall off, whereas those that are too tight may compromise circulation and further harm the patient.

Plain roller gauze is seldom used. It is difficult to handle, has no elasticity, and tends to bind. It also tends to slip because it does not adhere to itself. Wrinkled crepe–type roller bandages (e.g., Kling) are preferred because they easily conform to various shapes of the body and adhere to themselves (Fig. 10.8A). If the bandage is to cover a wound, it should always be applied over a sterile dressing.

Plain elastic cloth bandages or elastic roller cloth bandages with adhesive backing (e.g., Ace) (see Fig. 10.8B) make flexible, secure covers. When an elastic roller bandage is applied as a pressure bandage, especially to the lower limbs, it is essential to keep the bandage consistent in spacing and tension to ensure even pressure. Even, gentle pressure stimulates circulation and healing. Uneven pressure causes constriction points that can create pressure sores, ulcers, or edema. Roller bandages usually are applied from the distal to the proximal part of the area, because they are more even and snug if they are wrapped from a smaller to a larger circumference. Elevate the limb while you are bandaging and work with the roller facing upward, close to the patient's skin. Elastic bandages are excellent for bandaging the hand and wrist and the foot and ankle.

Remember: CSMT When Bandaging

When applying bandages, you should assess the following:

- **C**olor: Should be the same as the opposite extremity; report any bluish or white fingers or toes
- **S**ensation: Should be able to feel fingers/toes; report any numbness
- **M**ovement: Should be able to move fingers/toes
- **T**emperature: Should be the same as the opposite extremity; report any cool/cold fingers/toes

Seamless tubular gauze bandage, with or without elastic, is a superior material for covering round, narrow surfaces such as fingers or toes. It can be used as a dressing if the gauze material is sterile; it can also be used as a bandage. A tubular gauze bandage is applied with a cage-like applicator (Fig. 10.9). Work with the open circle of the applicator toward the patient. Hold the applicator in the dominant hand and control the tension flow with your fingers as the applicator is gradually rotated and the material slides off. Tubular dressing may be applied with or without slight pressure. Beyond the tip of the bandaged part, give the applicator a full half-turn, place the applicator again over the part, and repeat the process, being careful not to create a tourniquet effect when you reverse the applicator. When the desired thickness of the bandage is reached, cut the gauze and anchor the final gauze application with tape or by tying at the wrist.

CLOSING COMMENTS

Assisting with minor surgery can be challenging and rewarding. There are many things to remember, but the key piece is to always maintain sterile technique. Whether it is in handling instruments, setting up trays, or assisting the provider, sterile technique must be followed to protect our patients.

Patient Coaching

The best time for a medical assistant to instruct the patient in aseptic techniques to be used at home is during an aseptic procedure. Patient education includes the purpose and importance of hand washing; using disposable tissues to cover the nose and mouth when coughing or sneezing and properly disposing of used tissues; the differences between sterile and clean dressings and bandages; and step-by-step instructions on how to change a dressing properly and dispose of contaminated items.

Legal and Ethical Issues

Many minor surgical procedures previously performed in the hospital are now being done in a medical office, surgery center, or clinic. As insurance companies continue to recognize the cost-effectiveness of performing minor surgical procedures in these settings, the role of the medical assistant continues to expand.

Patients should have absolute assurance that they are being taken care of in an aseptic atmosphere and under the most stringent aseptic conditions. This assurance is just as important for the protection of the office staff as it is for the patient. Allowing the provider to assume that the correct aseptic techniques have been used in the preparation of equipment and allowing him or her to use contaminated equipment on a patient can result in claims of malpractice and charges of battery. Absolute, uncompromising honesty on the part of the assistant builds self-respect and contributes to professional achievement and satisfaction.

To have a good understanding of the subject, you must become familiar with the various techniques of sanitization, disinfection, and sterilization. Ignorance or carelessness can be dangerous and is inexcusable before the law.

The medical assistant must know what procedure is scheduled and whether the patient has been informed about the procedure. In the surgical setting, the medical assistant must realize the full extent of his or her role as the patient's advocate and the physician's agent.

Confirm that the provider has explained the procedure to the patient and that the patient fully understands all aspects of the procedure to be performed. This means that when the patient signs the informed consent for surgery, he or she is fully informed. Legal action can result if complications arise because of failure to complete consent forms. The surgical procedure is expedited when the patient is given instructions and knows what to expect. Increasing the patient's understanding ensures greater compliance with presurgical preparations, and the patient is more likely to follow instructions and advice after surgery.

The medical assistant must practice perfect aseptic technique. A break in technique may invite infection and possible legal action. It is the medical assistant's duty to protect the patient. A major responsibility of the medical assistant is to adhere strictly to aseptic technique and to correct immediately any break in technique.

Patient-Centered Care

A medical assistant's duty may include calling the patient the day before surgery to confirm the scheduled surgical procedure and appointment time. Explaining the procedure and what to expect during and after surgery prepares the patient and helps calm the person's fears or concerns. Lying still during surgery is important, and eating a light meal the night before should be encouraged. Bathing before coming to the office helps reduce the number of bacteria on the skin, and the patient should wear comfortable, loose clothing. Sometimes in the course of general conversation, the medical assistant can pick up hints of concerns the patient may have and can direct the conversation into a discussion of these concerns.

Patients should be informed that they may need someone to accompany them home. A bandage is applied after surgery, and it must be kept clean and dry. The patient may have some pain, and the provider probably will prescribe some type of analgesic. After the procedure is complete, make sure the patient makes an appointment for a return visit and examination. Patients should also be encouraged to call the office immediately if they suspect an infection or have a sudden increase in pain at the surgical site.

Professional Behaviors

Accountability is a crucial part of the medical assistant's professional responsibilities. An accountable individual recognizes if an error has been committed and does everything possible to correct his or her mistake. Personal accountability and discipline are the primary concerns in surgical asepsis. Often the assistant is alone when performing a surgical aseptic procedure; if contamination occurs, no one may know except the medical assistant. If there is any doubt about the sterility of the surgical field, instruments, or supplies, or if sterile technique is broken in any way, it is the assistant's responsibility to begin the procedure again. There is no room for compromise.

SUMMARY OF SCENARIO

Callie is finding her clinical medical assisting position at the Walden-Martin Family Medical Clinic rewarding, exciting, and challenging. She enjoys coming to work every day and has learned all aspects of her position much more quickly than most of her peers. Callie frequently reads the latest information on new developments in minor surgery practice. Her concern for her patients' well-being makes her stand out, and the providers constantly get positive comments on her level of professionalism.

Callie has made a few errors in sterile technique since starting the clinical assistant position, but she has learned from each situation and has never covered up a mistake. Whenever she realized that she did not follow procedure, she has discussed the issue with her supervisor and with Dr. Perez. In this way, errors can be corrected, if possible, and she most likely will not make the same or similar mistakes again.

Callie is a team player who consistently tries to anticipate the needs of the provider and patient both before and during surgery. Her cooperative, supportive manner is appreciated by everyone on the clinical staff.

SUMMARY OF LEARNING OBJECTIVES

1. **Summarize common minor surgical procedures.**

   Typical minor surgical procedures include incision and drainage (I&D) of a cyst; electrosurgery, which uses high-frequency current to cut through tissue and coagulate blood vessels; laser surgery, which uses tiny light beams to safely treat specific tissues with minimal damage to surrounding tissues and limited scar formation; microsurgery, which involves the use of an operating microscope to perform delicate surgical procedures; endoscopic procedures, which use a fiberoptic instrument with a miniature camera mounted on a flexible tube to examine the area within an organ or cavity and which are named according to the organs or areas they explore; and cryosurgery, which is the use of extreme cold to destroy tissues such as warts and skin lesions.

2. **Detail the medical assistant's role in minor office surgery when it comes to preparation of the patient and the room. Also, explain how to perform skin prep for surgery.**

   The medical assistant is responsible for preparing the patient for surgery; performing the physician's preoperative orders; confirming that the patient has signed an informed consent form; making sure all the patient's questions and concerns have been addressed; assisting with positioning of the patient; performing skin preparation if ordered; and preparing the room for the procedure.

   Refer to Procedure 10.1 for the steps in performing a skin prep for surgery. A surgical hand scrub is done to lower the number of transient flora on the practitioner's hands so that the risk of wound contamination is reduced (see Procedure 10.2).

3. **Outline the rules for setting up and maintaining a sterile field; explain how to perform the following procedures related to sterile techniques:**

   Sterile surfaces must never come in contact with nonsterile surfaces. If this occurs, the sterile surface immediately is considered contaminated. The rules for maintaining a sterile field include (1) keep talking to a minimum; (2) maintain sight of the sterile field; and (3) never cross over the sterile field. Anything that falls below the edge of the Mayo tray and within a 1-inch border surrounding the tray is considered contaminated. A sterile barrier that is wet, cut, or torn is contaminated. Sterile gloved hands must be kept above waist level at all times. An item is never removed from and then again put into the field. A sterile package should be opened the entire way and the contents tossed onto the field without crossing over the sterile area. If a sterile package falls to the floor, it must be discarded. If any doubt exists about sterility, the field must be considered contaminated and the process must start all over again.

   - *Open a sterile pack and create a sterile field*
     Refer to Procedure 10.3.

   - *Transfer sterile instruments and pour solutions into a sterile field*
     Refer to Procedure 10.3.
   - *Perform a two-person sterile tray set-up*
     Refer to Procedure 10.4.
   - *Put on sterile gloves without contaminating them*
     Refer to Procedure 10.5.

4. **Discuss how to assist the provider during surgery and demonstrate how to assist with a minor surgical procedure and suturing.**

   The physician is responsible for the patient; however, the medical assistant is responsible for ensuring that everything the assistant and the physician will use in caring for the surgical patient is accounted for, ready to use, and prepared in a safe and sterile manner. Refer to Procedures 10.6 and 10.7.

5. **Summarize postoperative instructions and explain how to remove sutures and surgical staples.**

   If medication is prescribed, review the purpose of the medication and directions for its use with the patient and his or her companion and make a follow-up appointment. The patient should be taught to care for himself or herself at home after surgery and should receive both verbal and written instructions. Explain to the patient the importance of calling the office if any questions arise or if he or she notes redness around the operative site, bleeding from the wound, fever, swelling, or increasing or severe pain. If the patient does not call within the next 24 hours, the medical assistant should call the patient.

   Refer to Procedure 10.8 for the steps in removing sutures and surgical staples.

6. **Explain the process of wound healing.**

   All wounds go through a healing or repair process that has three phases. The lag phase occurs first when the blood vessels contract to control hemorrhage, platelets form a fibrin network, and a clot dries into a scab. Proliferation is a new growth period during which tissues repair themselves. During the final, or remodeling, phase, a bridge of new tissue is built to close the gap of the wound. Collagen gives the wounded tissues strength and forms scar tissue. Wounds are classified by the way they repair themselves: either by first intention, with clean, straight edges that heal quickly, or by granulation (or second intention), as in tissues that are severely damaged and are left open or fail to close.

7. **Explain how to properly apply dressings and bandages to surgical sites.**

   Refer to Procedure 10.7.

PROCEDURE 10.1   Perform Skin Prep for Surgery

Task: Prepare the patient's skin and remove hair from the surgical site to reduce the risk of wound contamination.

EQUIPMENT and SUPPLIES

Disposable skin prep kit, or collect the following:
- Gauze
- Cotton-tipped applicators
- Soap
- Gloves
- Electric clippers
- Two small bowls
- Antiseptic or antiseptic swabs (e.g., Betadine swabs)
- Sterile normal saline solution
- Optional: cotton balls, nail pick, scrub brush
- Sterile drape
- Biohazard waste/sharps containers
- Patient's record

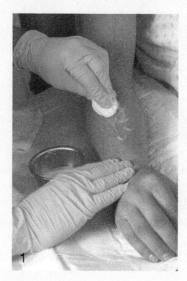

PROCEDURAL STEPS

1. Wash hands or use hand sanitizer.
   PURPOSE: To follow Standard Precautions.
2. Greet the patient. Identify yourself. Verify the patient's identity with full name and date of birth. Explain the procedure to be performed in a manner that is understood by the patient. Answer any questions the patient may have on the procedure.
   PURPOSE: To ensure cooperation and demonstrate awareness of possible patient concerns.
3. Ask the patient to remove any clothing that might interfere with exposure of the site and provide a gown if needed.
4. Assist the patient into the proper position for site exposure. Provide a drape if necessary to protect the patient's privacy.
5. Expose the site. Use a light if necessary.
6. If hair is present, the area may need to be shaved. Put on gloves and shave the required area with electric clippers.
   PURPOSE: Hair should be removed before any invasive procedure to limit the potential for infection; follow Standard Precautions regarding sharps.
7. While wearing gloves, open the skin prep pack and add the soap to the two bowls.
8. Start at the incision site and begin washing with the soap on a gauze sponge in a circular motion, moving from the center to the edges of the area to be scrubbed (see the following figure).
   PURPOSE: A circular motion from inside to outside drags contaminants away from the incision site.

9. After one complete wipe, discard the sponge and begin again with a new sponge soaked in the antiseptic solution.
   PURPOSE: After one circular sweep, the sponge is contaminated with skin bacteria and debris.
10. Repeat the process, using sufficient friction for 5 minutes (or follow office policy for the length of time required for a particular prep).
11. Rinse the area with sterile normal saline solution (see the following figure).

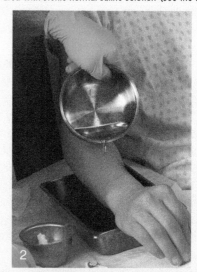

12. Dry the area, using the same circular technique with dry sponges. The area may be dried by blotting with a sterile towel.
13. Paint on the antiseptic with the cotton-tipped applicators or gauze sponges, using the same circular technique and never returning to an area that has already been painted.
14. Place a sterile drape and/or towel over the area.
15. Answer all the patient's questions to relieve anxiety about the upcoming surgical procedure.
16. Document completion of the skin prep in the patient's health record.

PROCEDURE 10.2 | Perform a Surgical Hand Scrub

Task: Scrub the hands with surgical soap, using friction, running water, and a disposable sterile brush to sanitize the skin before assisting with any procedure that requires surgical asepsis.

EQUIPMENT and SUPPLIES

- Sink with foot, knee, or arm control for running water
- Surgical soap in a dispenser
- Towels (sterile towels if indicated by office policy)
- Nail file or orange stick
- Sterile disposable brush

PROCEDURAL STEPS

1. Remove all jewelry.
   PURPOSE: Jewelry harbors bacteria and is not permitted in surgical asepsis.
2. Roll long sleeves above the elbows.
3. Inspect your fingernails for length and your hands for skin breaks.
4. Turn on the faucet and regulate the water to a comfortable temperature, being careful to stand away from the sink to prevent contamination of clothing from contact with the sink or counter top.
5. Keep your hands upright and held at or above waist level (see the following figure).
   PURPOSE: Water running from the unscrubbed area above the elbow down to the hands can carry bacteria back onto the hands. All areas below the waist are considered contaminated during all surgical procedures.

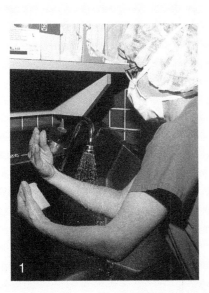

6. Clean your fingernails with a file, discard it (in most situations you will drop the file into the sink and discard it later to prevent contamination by lowering your hands and/or touching a waste receptacle), and rinse your hands under the faucet without touching the faucet or the inside of the sink basin (see the following figure).

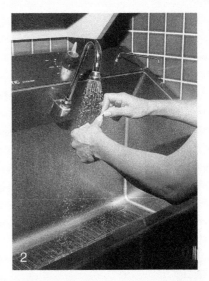

7. Allow the water to run over your hands from the fingertips to the elbows without moving the arm back and forth under the water.
   PURPOSE: Water running from the elbow down to the hands can carry bacteria back onto the hands.
8. Apply surgical soap from the dispenser to the sterile brush (or use a prepared disposable brush) and start the scrub by scrubbing the palm of the hand in a circular fashion.
9. Continue from the palm to the base of the thumb, then move on to the other fingers, scrubbing from the base, along each side, and across the nail, holding the fingertips upward and remembering to rub between the fingers (see the following figure). After the fingers have been completely scrubbed, clean the posterior surface of the hand in a circular fashion and then proceed to the wrist. The scrub process should take at least 5 minutes for each hand and arm.
   PURPOSE: The surfaces of the fingers have four sides that all need to be thoroughly cleaned.

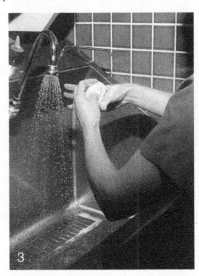

Continued

PROCEDURE 10.2   Perform a Surgical Hand Scrub—*continued*

10. Do not return to a clean area after you have moved to the next part of the hand.
    <u>PURPOSE</u>: Once an area has been scrubbed, it is considered surgically clean, and rubbing that area again contaminates it.

11. Wash the wrists and forearms in a circular fashion around the arm while holding your hands above waist level (see the following figure).

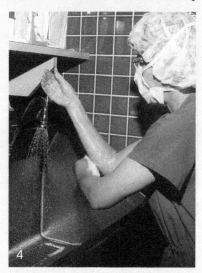

12. Rinse the arms and forearms from the fingertips upward, holding the fingers up, without touching the faucet or the inside of the sink basin (see the following figure).
    <u>PURPOSE</u>: Keep the fingers higher than the rest of the arm to prevent contamination from water running downward from the elbow. Touching the dirty faucet and/or basin causes contamination.

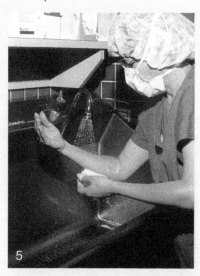

13. Apply more solution without touching any dirty surface and repeat the scrub on the other side, remembering to wash and use friction between each finger with a firm, circular motion.

14. Scrub all surfaces, being careful not to abrade your skin. The second hand and arm should take at least 5 minutes.

15. Rinse thoroughly, keeping your hands up and above waist level. Discard the scrub brush without lowering the arms below the waist (see the following figures).

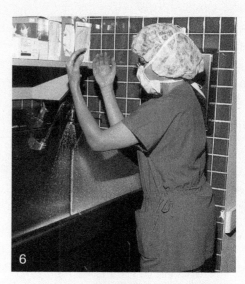

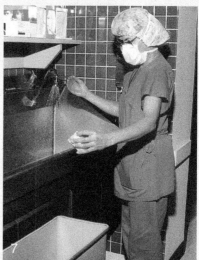

16. Turn off the faucet with the foot, knee, or forearm lever, if available.
    <u>PURPOSE</u>: To prevent clean hands from touching the contaminated faucet handles.

17. Dry your hands with a sterile towel, being careful to keep the fingers pointing upward and your hands above the waist. Do not rub back and forth, dragging contaminants from the dirtier area of the upper arm down toward the hands (see the following figures). Use the opposite end of the towel for the other hand.
    <u>PURPOSE</u>: To keep your clean hands from touching the part of the towel that comes in contact with your forearms, which are not as clean as your hands. If you are to gown and glove for a procedure, you must use a sterile towel.

PROCEDURE 10.2 Perform a Surgical Hand Scrub—*continued*

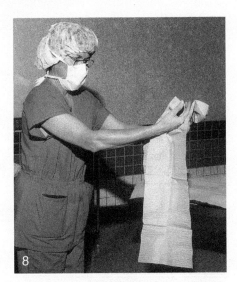

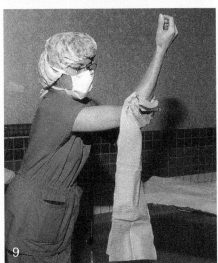

18. Using a patting motion, continue to dry the forearms. Discard the towel and keep your hands up and above waist level (see the following figure).

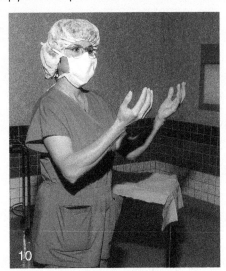

PROCEDURE 10.3 Prepare a Sterile Field, Use Transfer Forceps, and Pour a Sterile Solution Into a Sterile Field

Tasks: Open a sterile instrument pack using correct aseptic technique and create a sterile field; move sterile items on a sterile field or transfer sterile items to a gloved team member; pour a sterile solution into a sterile stainless steel bowl or container sitting at the edge of a sterile field.

EQUIPMENT and SUPPLIES

- A sterile instrument pack wrapped with autoclave paper that, when opened, will serve as a sterile table drape or field
- Mayo stand or countertop
- Disinfectant and gauze sponges or disinfectant wipes

- Sterile item to move or transfer
- Sterile wrapped transfer forceps
- Bottle of sterile solution
- Sterile bowl or container
- Sink or waste receptacle

Continued

PROCEDURE 10.3 | **Prepare a Sterile Field, Use Transfer Forceps, and Pour a Sterile Solution Into a Sterile Field**—*continued*

PROCEDURAL STEPS

1. Check that the Mayo stand or countertop is dust free and clean. If it is not, disinfect and allow to air dry.
   PURPOSE: Although some areas cannot be sterile, steps must be taken to keep contamination to a minimum; moisture on a tray contaminates the pack.

2. Wash your hands or use hand sanitizer and make sure they are completely dry. If you will be assisting with a surgical procedure immediately after opening the sterile pack, perform the surgical hand scrub as explained in Procedure 10.2.
   PURPOSE: To reduce the number of transient flora on your hands and forearms; moisture on your hands contaminates the pack.

3. Gather supplies. Check the label of the ordered solution. Check the solution name and the expiration date.

4. If using an autoclaved pack, check the indicator tape for a color change.
   PURPOSE: Autoclave indicator tape changes color after the sterile processing cycle.

5. Open the outside cover (see the following figure). Position the package so that the outer envelope flap is at the top and with the tab facing you.
   PURPOSE: This positions the pack for correct opening so that you do not have to cross over the sterile pack to open it.

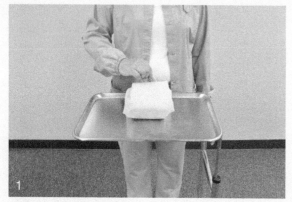

6. Open the outermost flap (see the following figure). Next, open the first flap away from you. You can cross over the uncovered portion of the Mayo stand because it is not sterile. Do not cross over the pack.

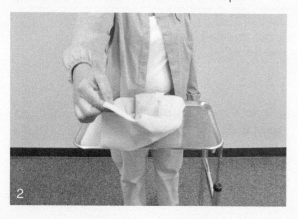

7. Open the second corner, pulling to side (see the following figure).
   PURPOSE: To prevent contamination of the sterile field.

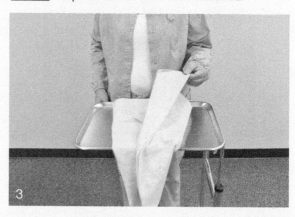

8. Be careful to lift the flaps by touching only the small, folded-back tab and without touching or crossing over the inner surface of the pack or its contents. Open the remaining two corners of the pack (see the following figure).

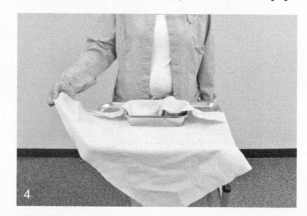

9. You now have a sterile drape as a sterile field from which to work and for the distribution of additional sterile supplies and instruments (see the following figure).

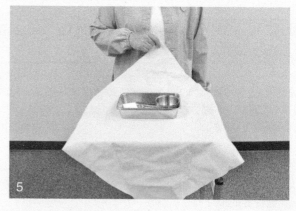

10. Open a package containing sterile transfer forceps (see the following figure). Using sterile technique, handle the sterile forceps by the ring handle only. Always point the forceps tips down.

PROCEDURE 10.3	Prepare a Sterile Field, Use Transfer Forceps, and Pour a Sterile Solution Into a Sterile Field—*continued*

PURPOSE: If the tips are turned upward, any solution encountered will run onto the nonsterile area, and then back down over the sterile end when the tips are turned down again, thus contaminating the forceps.

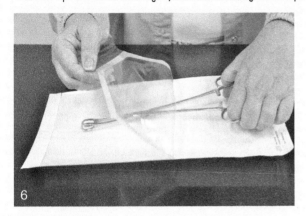

6

11. Grasp an item on the sterile field with the sterile forceps, points down, and move it to its proper position for the procedure, making sure not to cross the sterile field with the hand or contaminated end of the forceps (see the following figure).

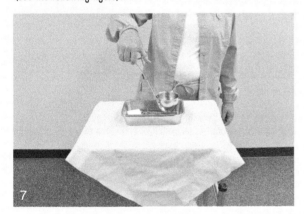

7

12. Set the forceps aside after one-time use.
    Note: The sterile bowl should be placed, using sterile transfer forceps, near one edge of the field and the perimeter of the 1-inch barrier.
13. Check the label of the ordered solution when first obtaining the solution.
    PURPOSE: Always perform the three label checks before administering any solution or medication.

14. Check the label of the solution for the second time. Place your hand over the label and lift the bottle.
    Note: If the container has a double cap, set the outer cap on the counter inside up and then proceed.
15. Lift the lid of the bottle straight up and then slightly to one side; hold the lid in your nondominant hand facing downward.
    PURPOSE: Air currents carry contaminants that could settle on the inside of the lid.
16. Pour away from the label without allowing any part of the bottle to touch the bowl and without crossing over the sterile field (see the following figure).
    PURPOSE: Spills down the side of the bottle can stain the label or make it unreadable. The bottle exterior is not sterile, so it cannot pass over the sterile field.

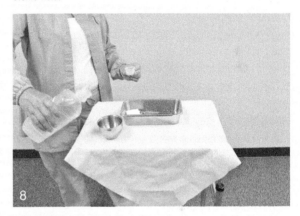

8

17. If the container does not have a double cap, before pouring the solution into the sterile container, pour off a small amount of the solution into a waste receptacle.
    PURPOSE: To rinse any contaminants off the bottle lip.
18. Tilt the bottle up to stop the pouring while it is still over the bowl.
    PURPOSE: Solutions spilled on the sterile field may contaminate the field.
19. Check the label of the solution for the third time. Replace the cap (or caps) off to the side, away from the sterile field, being careful not to touch and therefore contaminate the internal surface of the lid.

PROCEDURE 10.4   Two-Person Sterile Tray Setup

Task: Perform a sterile tray setup for a cyst removal.

EQUIPMENT and SUPPLIES

- Sterile drape
- Sterile gloves
- In a sealed autoclave pouch: needle holder, operating scissors, tissue forceps, hemostatic forceps
- Suture material with needle
- Sterile 4 × 4s
- Disposable scalpel

Note: This procedure involves two people. One person will act as the nonsterile person, and the other will have on sterile gloves and will place the items on the sterile tray.

PROCEDURAL STEPS

Nonsterile Person

1. Check that the Mayo stand or countertop is dust free and clean. If it is not, disinfect and allow to air dry.
   PURPOSE: Although some areas cannot be sterile, steps must be taken to keep contamination to a minimum; moisture on a tray contaminates the pack.

2. Wash your hands or use hand sanitizer and make sure they are completely dry. If you will be assisting with a surgical procedure immediately after opening the sterile pack, perform the surgical hand scrub as explained in Procedure 10.2.
   PURPOSE: To reduce the number of transient flora on your hands and forearms; moisture on your hands contaminates the pack.

3. Place the package containing the sterile drape on a flat surface near the Mayo stand/tray. Check the integrity of the outer package. Open the package without touching the barrier field.

4. Pick up the barrier field, by the corner, as you move away from table and allow it to unfold without touching anything else. Drape over the Mayo stand.
   PURPOSE: This maintains the sterility of the barrier field creating the sterile field on the Mayo stand.

5. Inspect the sterile pack for holes and tears; discard if seen and start over. Slowly pull the sides of the peel pack of sterile 4 × 4s away from each other. Maintain control of the item inside the package by opening only far enough for a sterile person to grab the item. Allow the sterile person to take the 4 × 4s. Inspect the package for holes and tears and indicators before the sterile person places the item on the sterile field. Inspect and discard the wrapper.
   PURPOSE: By inspecting the package after the item has been removed, you can ensure that it is truly sterile.

6. Slowly pull the sides of the peel pack of suture away from each other. Maintain control of the item inside the package by opening only far enough for the sterile person to grab the item. Allow the sterile person to take the suture package. Inspect the package for holes and tears and indicators before the sterile person places the item on the sterile field. Inspect and discard the wrapper.

7. Slowly pull the sides of the peel pack of a scalpel away from each other. Maintain control of the item inside the package by opening only far enough for the sterile person to grab the item. Allow the sterile person to take the scalpel. Inspect the package for holes and tears and indicators before the sterile person places the item on the sterile field. Inspect and discard the wrapper.

8. Slowly pull the sides of the peel pack of instruments away from each other. Maintain control of the items inside the package by opening only far enough for the sterile person to grab the items. Allow the sterile person to take all of the instruments. Inspect the package for holes and tears and indicators before the sterile person places the items on the sterile field. Inspect and discard the wrapper.

Sterile Person

1. Wash your hands or use hand sanitizer and make sure they are completely dry. If you will be assisting with a surgical procedure immediately after opening the sterile pack, perform the surgical hand scrub as explained in Procedure 10.2.
   PURPOSE: To reduce the number of transient flora on your hands and forearms; moisture on your hands contaminates the pack.

2. Remove an item from a peel pack and maintain sterile technique.

3. After the nonsterile person has indicated that the peel pack has not been compromised, place the item on the sterile tray. Repeat for all items. Arrange items on the sterile tray.

4. Maintain sterility of sterile field and sterile supplies.

PROCEDURE 10.5	Put on Sterile Gloves

Task: Put on sterile gloves correctly before performing sterile procedures.

EQUIPMENT and SUPPLIES

- Pair of packaged sterile gloves in your size

PROCEDURAL STEPS

1. Perform the surgical hand scrub as explained in Procedure 10.2 before putting on sterile gloves.
2. Open the glove pack, being careful not to cross over the open area in the middle of the pack. Remember, a 1-inch area around the perimeter of the glove wrapper is considered not sterile.
   PURPOSE: The open glove pack is a sterile field.
3. Glove your dominant hand first.
   PURPOSE: This sets up your dominant hand to do the more difficult step, which is to put on the second glove.
4. With your nondominant hand, pick up the glove for your dominant hand with your thumb and forefinger, grabbing the edge of the folded cuff closest to you, which is the inside of the glove, being careful not to cross over the other sterile glove (see the following figure).
   PURPOSE: The inside of the glove will be next to your skin and is considered not sterile.

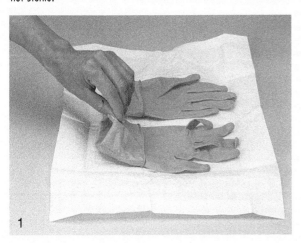

5. Lift the glove up and away from the sterile package.
   PURPOSE: To prevent accidental contamination from touching the glove on the 1-inch area around the perimeter of the glove wrapper.
6. Hold your hands up and away from your body and the sterile field (containing the other glove). Slide the dominant hand into the glove (see the following figure).

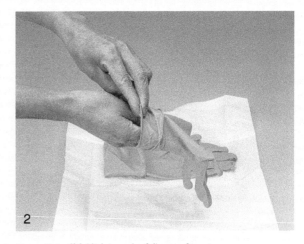

7. Leave the cuff folded (see the following figure).
   PURPOSE: You will unfold the cuff later.

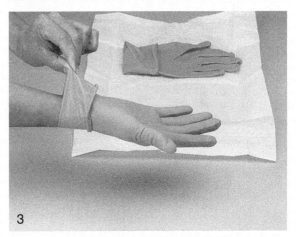

8. With your gloved dominant hand, pick up the second glove by slipping your gloved fingers under the cuff, extending the thumb up and away from the glove (thumbs up position), so that your gloved fingers touch only the outside of the second glove (see the following figure).
   PURPOSE: Sterile surfaces must always touch sterile surfaces.

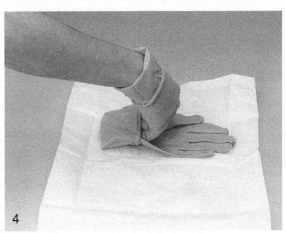

Continued

PROCEDURE 10.5   **Put on Sterile Gloves**—*continued*

9. Slide your nondominant hand into the glove without touching the exterior of the glove or any part of the gloved hand (see the following figures).

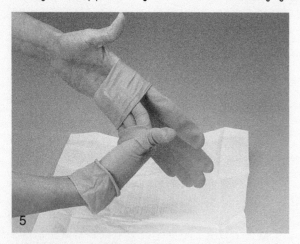

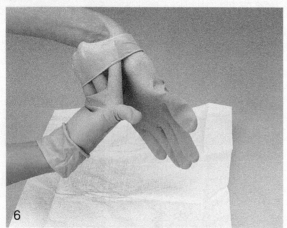

10. Still holding your hands away from you, unroll the cuff by slipping the fingers into the cuff and gently pulling up and out. Do not touch your bare

arm or the internal surface of the glove with any part of the sterile glove (see the following figure).

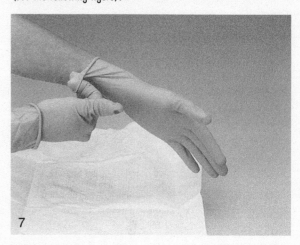

11. Now, slip your gloved fingers up under the first cuff and unroll it, using the same technique (see the following figure).

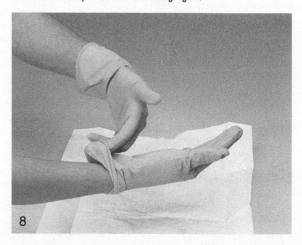

PROCEDURE 10.6   **Assist With Minor Surgery**

Tasks: Maintain the sterile field and pass instruments in a prescribed sequence during a surgical procedure that involves making a surgical incision and removing a growth.

EQUIPMENT and SUPPLIES

- Open patient drape pack on the side counter
- Mayo stand covered with a sterile drape
- Packaged sterile gloves (two pairs)
- Needle and syringe for local anesthetic medication
- Vial of local anesthetic medication
- Sterile drape
- Disposable scalpel with No. 15 blade
- Tissue forceps
- Skin retractor

- Three hemostats
- Needle holder
- Supply of sterile gauze sponges
- Biohazard waste container
- Sharps container
- Needle with suture material
- Specimen cup
- Laboratory requisitions
- Patient's record

PROCEDURE 10.6   **Assist With Minor Surgery**—*continued*

PROCEDURAL STEPS

1. Prep the patient's skin with surgical soap and antiseptic solution as explained in Procedure 10.1. Explain the prep procedure to the patient.
   <u>PURPOSE</u>: To ensure infection control and to demonstrate awareness of possible patient concerns.
2. Perform the surgical hand scrub as explained in Procedure 10.2.
3. Instruct and prepare the patient for the procedure. Explain what will occur, what the patient should do during the procedure, how long the procedure will take, and what the patient will sense (e.g., feel, smell). Set up the sterile field with instruments and supplies (see the following figure)

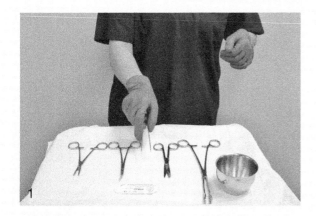

4. Position the Mayo stand near the patient and the operative site, making sure the patient understands not to touch the sterile field (see the following figure).
   <u>PURPOSE</u>: To prevent contamination of supplies and provide easy access for the provider.

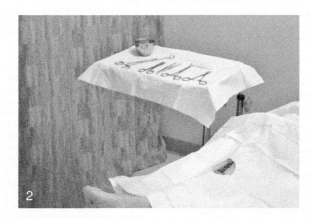

5. Put on sterile gloves using surgical technique.
6. Grasp the patient drape by holding one edge or corner in each hand (see the following figure).

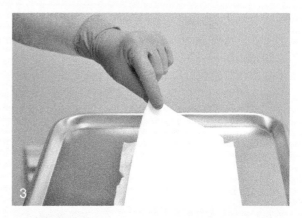

7. Drape the surgical site without touching any part of the patient or the operating area with your gloved hands.
8. If the provider requests medication, such as a local anesthetic, a second circulating assistant holds the vial of local anesthetic so that the provider can read the label. The provider withdraws the desired amount using sterile technique (see the following figure).
   <u>PURPOSE</u>: The vial of local anesthetic medication must be held by the second assistant away from the sterile field to prevent crossing over the field with a nonsterile item. The medication label must be checked before a medication is dispensed or administered.

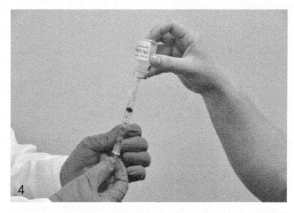

9. The provider injects the local anesthetic and waits a few minutes for it to take effect.
10. Position yourself across from the practitioner. Arrange the sterile field. Check the placement location on the Mayo stand (see the following figure).

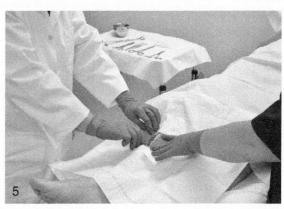

Continued

PROCEDURE 10.6   Assist With Minor Surgery—*continued*

11. Keep all sharp equipment conspicuously placed on the sterile field.
    <u>PURPOSE</u>: Sharp instruments that are not clearly visible may injure a team member.
12. Pass the scalpel, blade down and handle first, to the provider, or the provider will reach for it. The provider will take the scalpel with the thumb and forefinger in the position ready for use (see the following figure).
    <u>PURPOSE</u>: To protect the practitioner and yourself from injury.

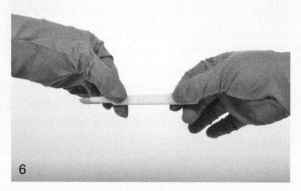

13. Pick up a tissue forceps by the tips and pass it to the provider to grasp a piece of the tissue to be excised (see the following figure).

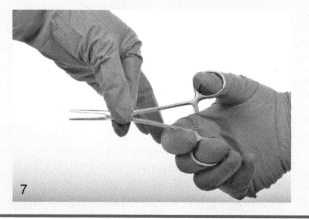

14. Dispose of soiled sponges in the biohazard waste container, being careful to keep your hands above your waist and to avoid touching any nonsterile items.
15. Hold clean sponges in your hand to pat or sponge the wound as needed.
16. Safely position the specimen (if any) where it will not be disturbed in a sterile container on the sterile field.
17. If there is a bleeding vessel or if a hemostat is requested, pass the hemostat in the manner described in step 13.
18. Continue to sponge blood from the wound site.
19. Retract the wound edge, as needed, with a skin retractor.
20. Continue to monitor the sterile field and assist the provider as needed.
21. Pass the needle and suture material to close the wound and apply a sterile dressing as requested (see the following figure).

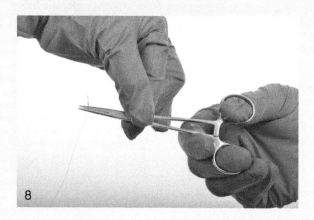

22. Monitor the patient and provide assistance as needed.
23. When the provider is finished, clean the surgical site using sterile technique.
24. Collect the specimen using Standard Precautions, place it in a labeled specimen cup, and send it to the laboratory with the proper requisitions.
25. Wash your hands or use hand sanitizer. Document the procedure, wound condition, and patient education on wound care.

PROCEDURE 10.7   Apply a Sterile Dressing

Tasks: Perform a dressing change. Apply a sterile dressing while maintaining aseptic technique. Instruct and prepare the patient for the procedure. Explain the rationale for the procedure.

EQUIPMENT and SUPPLIES

- Gloves
- Biohazard waste container
- Sterile water or hydrogen peroxide (optional)
- Disposable ruler
- Culture swab
- Lab requisition, label, and plastic specimen bag for transport
- Sterile gloves

- Antiseptic swabs
- Sterile dressing and ABD pad
- Tape
- Mannequin with a wound
- Patient's record

Provider's Order: Change dressing and apply a sterile dressing. Culture wound drainage.

PROCEDURE 10.7 Apply a Sterile Dressing—*continued*

Scenario: Dr. Walden ordered a dressing change. You are to apply a sterile dressing after you obtain a culture of the wound drainage. As you are beginning the procedure, the patient asks you questions regarding PPE and the reason for the wound culture. You need to explain the rationale for wearing PPE and why a wound culture is obtained.

Directions: Role-play the scenario with a peer. The peer will be the patient, and you are the medical assistant. After the role-play, the rest of the procedure is done on a mannequin.

PROCEDURAL STEPS

1. Wash your hands or use hand sanitizer. Assemble supplies on Mayo stand/ tray and place biohazard waste container within easy reach.
   PURPOSE: To follow Standard Precautions.
2. Greet the patient. Identify yourself. Verify the patient's identity with full name and date of birth. Verify the patient's allergies.
3. Instruct and prepare the patient for the procedure. Explain the procedure to be performed in a manner that is understood by the patient. Explain what will occur, what the patient should do during the procedure, how long the procedure will take, and what the patient will sense (e.g., feel, smell). Answer any questions the patient may have on the procedure.
   PURPOSE: To ensure cooperation and demonstrate awareness of possible patient concerns.
   Scenario update: The patient questions why you need to change gloves so much during the procedure. She also asks why the wound culture needs to be done.
4. Based on the patient's comments, explain the reason for changing your gloves during the procedure and also for the wound culture.
   PURPOSE: Demonstrates empathy and appropriate nonverbal communication while addressing the patient's questions and concerns.
   Scenario update: The rest of the steps are done on a mannequin.
5. Put on gloves. Loosen tape on old bandage from edges to the middle, toward the wound. Remove bandage and dressing, one at a time. If dressing is stuck, use a small amount of sterile water or hydrogen peroxide to loosen.
   PURPOSE: To follow Standard Precautions.
6. Check for drainage on the dressing and bandage. Note the color of the drainage. Measure any drainage using a disposable ruler, then discard everything in the biohazard waste container.
7. Assess the wound. If present, count the sutures or staples. Check if they are intact. Check the wound for signs of infection.
8. If the wound is open and/or redness or drainage is present:
   a. Culture the wound using a sterile swab (if ordered). Place in a culture transfer tube. Squeeze the tube to release formalin to preserve the specimen.
   b. Concisely and accurately report the relevant information (any issues with the wound or wound closures) to the provider. Ask the provider to check the wound before redressing.

9. Remove gloves and place in a biohazard waste container.
10. Wash your hands or use hand sanitizer.
11. Open and arrange sterile supplies in the order they will be used. Apply the principles of sterile technique.
12. Put on sterile gloves. State that the nondominant hand will be nonsterile and the dominant hand will be sterile.
13. With the nondominant hand, pick up the antiseptic swab container. With the dominant hand, grasp an antiseptic swab without touching the package. Clean from the center of the wound to the edge; use one roll of the swab and discard in waste container. Start with new swab where you left off with the previous swab. Continue until all the exudate is removed.
    PURPOSE: By cleaning from the center of the wound to the edge you prevent contamination of the open wound.
14. With the dominant hand, remove the sterile dressing without touching the package. Place the sterile dressing material over the wound and cover the wound completely.
15. With the dominant hand, place an ABD pad over the dressing as a bandage.
16. Remove and discard the sterile gloves. Secure the bandage with tape.
17. Provide patient education as needed for wound care.
18. Complete the lab requisition for the culture. Put on gloves. Label the culture tube and place the culture tube in the plastic specimen bag for transport to the lab.
19. Clean up the area. Discard all biohazard waste in biohazard waste containers. Discard all other waste in the regular waste containers. Disinfect the tables.
20. Remove gloves and dispose of them appropriately. Wash hands or use hand sanitizer.
21. Using the patient's health record, document wound appearance, number of intact sutures or staples (if present), the culture obtained, wound care performed, and the patient education provided.
22. In the following written response section, discuss the implications for failing to comply with CDC regulations in healthcare settings.

10/12/20XX 2:15 p.m.: Dressing change completed to wound on ⊕ mid-forearm. Area slightly inflamed, mod amt serosanguineous drainage noted. Site cleansed and sterile dressing applied. Pt instructed on home wound care and to notify provider if drainage changes, inflammation increases, or fever occurs. _____ Callie Casper, CMA (AAMA)

WRITTEN RESPONSE QUESTIONS

You fail to wear gloves when changing a patient's dressing. During the procedure you get blood on your hands. Discuss the implications for failing to comply with CDC regulations in healthcare settings. Answer the following questions:

1. How might your action (i.e., not wearing gloves) affect the patient's health and safety?
2. How might your action (i.e., not wearing gloves) affect your health and safety?

PROCEDURE 10.8 | Remove Sutures and/or Surgical Staples

Task: Remove sutures and/or surgical staples from a healed incision using sterile technique and without injuring the closed wound.

EQUIPMENT and SUPPLIES

Sterile suture removal kit containing the following:
- Suture removal scissors
- Gauze
- Thumb dressing forceps
- Steri-Strips or adhesive bandage strips (e.g., Band-Aids)
- Skin antiseptic swabs (e.g., Betadine swabs)
- Surgical staple remover with 4 × 4-inch gauze
- Biohazard waste/sharps container
- Sterile gloves
- Patient's record

PROCEDURAL STEPS

1. Wash your hands or use hand sanitizer. Assemble the necessary supplies.
2. Greet the patient. Identify yourself. Verify the patient's identity with full name and date of birth. Explain the procedure to be performed in a manner that is understood by the patient. Answer any questions the patient may have on the procedure. Instruct the person to lie or sit still during the procedure.
   PURPOSE: To ensure cooperation during the procedure.
3. Position the patient comfortably and support the sutured area.
4. Place dry towels under the site.
5. Check the incision line to make sure the wound edges are approximated and there are no signs of infection, such as inflammation, edema, or drainage.
   PURPOSE: Sutures or staples should not be removed unless the site is completely healed with the wound edges together; infection at the site will interfere with the healing process; removing sutures or staples before the site is completely healed may result in the wound edges separating.
6. Put on gloves. Using antiseptic swabs, cleanse the wound to remove exudate and destroy microorganisms around the sutures or staples. Clean the site from the inside out, starting at the top of the wound and working your way down. Use a new swab if the step must be repeated. Remove gloves and discard.
   PURPOSE: Dried exudate on sutures or staples may make removing them without traumatizing the wound more difficult. Cleansing the wound reduces the possibility of wound infection.
7. Open the suture or staple removal pack while maintaining the sterility of the contents.
8. Place sterile gauze next to the wound site.
   PURPOSE: To receive the removed sutures or staples.
9. Put on sterile gloves.
10. Remove the sutures or staples.

To Remove Sutures
   a. Grasp the knot of the suture with the dressing forceps without pulling.
   b. Cut the suture at skin level.
   c. Lift, do not pull, the suture toward the incision and out with the dressing forceps.
   d. Place the suture on the sterile gauze sponge and check that the entire suture strand has been removed.
      PURPOSE: Suture fragments left in a wound may cause irritation and/or infection and may prolong the healing process.
   e. If any bleeding occurs, blot the area with a sterile gauze sponge before continuing.
   f. Continue in the same manner until all sutures have been removed.

To Remove Staples
   a. Gently place the bottom jaw of the staple remover under the first staple (see the following figure).

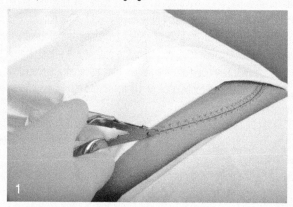

   b. Tightly squeeze the staple handles together.
   c. Carefully tilt the staple remover upward until the staple lifts out of the wound.
   d. Place the removed staple on a 4 × 4-inch gauze square.
   e. Continue the process until all staples have been removed.
11. Remove the gauze holding the sutures or staples. Dispose of sutures in the biohazard waste container. Dispose of staples in the biohazard sharps container.
12. The provider may apply or may have you apply Steri-Strips or an adhesive bandage strip for added support, strength, and protection.
13. Instruct the patient to keep the wound edges clean and dry and not to place excessive strain on the area.
14. Document the procedure, wound condition, number of sutures or staples removed, whether a dressing or bandage was applied, and the instructions on wound care given to the patient.
   PURPOSE: A procedure that is not documented was not done.

07/30/20XX 10:20 a.m.: Pt in for suture removal. The edges of the wound are well approximated with 5 intact sutures. There is no sign of infection. The site was cleaned with Betadine and 5 sutures were removed. Pt instructed on home wound care and to notify provider if drainage changes, inflammation increases, or fever occurs _____ Callie Casper, CMA (AAMA)

PRINCIPLES OF ELECTROCARDIOGRAPHY

11

SCENARIO

Renee Thomas, CMA (AAMA), is a Certified Medical Assistant at Walden-Martin Family Medical (WMFM) Clinic. According to her manager, over the time that she has been at WMFM Clinic, she has excelled. Because of Renee's professionalism and attention to detail, her manager, Sue, has asked her to mentor a new employee, Eva Ning.

Eva Ning, RMA, just graduated from a local medical assistant program. She really enjoyed the hands-on learning with the skills. During her practicum, she worked in a cardiology department for 6 weeks and really enjoyed the experience. Now that she has graduated, she looks forward to learning on the job.

Eva and Renee will spend a month with each provider. This month they are working with Dr. David Kahn, who sees many older patients. Renee tells Eva that they will be doing a lot of cardiac tests and treatments. Eva looks forward to learning from Renee and Dr. Kahn.

While studying this chapter, think about the following questions:
- What are the components of the ECG tracing?
- Where are the electrodes placed on the body for a 12-lead ECG?
- How can a medical assistant obtain a clear ECG?
- What are the different types of artifacts? Why does each type of artifact occur? What can the medical assistant do to prevent the artifact?
- What are other types of ECG tests?

LEARNING OBJECTIVES

1. Review the structures and functionality of the cardiovascular system.
2. Use correct electrocardiography (ECG) terminology.
3. Discuss ECG waves, segments, and intervals.
4. Describe the medical assistant's role in a resting 12-lead ECG.
5. Describe the bipolar (standard) leads, augmented leads, and chest (precordial) leads.
6. Prepare a patient for an ECG and obtain an electrocardiogram.
7. Troubleshoot artifacts in an ECG.
8. Identify abnormal rhythms in an ECG tracing.
9. Discuss additional ECG tests.

VOCABULARY

arrhythmia (ah RITH mee ah) An abnormal heart rate or rhythm.

artifact A substance, structure, or event that does not naturally occur in a situation. Examples include interference, or electrical "garbage," on an ECG, or crystals, lint, or contamination of a staining technique.

bipolar Having two poles or electrical charges.

caliper A pocket-sized tool used for measuring the height and width of the ECG waves and intervals.

dextrocardia (dek stro KAHR dee ah) The heart is located on the right side of the chest and the apex is pointing to the right.

echocardiography (ECHO) (eck oh KAR dee ah gruh fee) The use of ultrasonic waves directed through the heart to study the structure and motion of the heart. The visual record produced is called an echocardiogram.

electrocardiogram (ECG, EKG) (ee leck troh KAR dee ah gram) A record or recording of electrical impulses of the heart as produced by an electrocardiograph.

electrodes Adhesive patches that conduct electricity from the body to the ECG machine wires.

ion (AHY ons) An electrically charged atom, or the smallest component of an element.

unipolar Having one pole or electrical charge.

Heart disease is the leading cause of death in the United States. Medical assistants in primary and specialty areas often care for patients with heart disorders. All medical assistants must:

- Understand the cardiovascular system
- Recognize early symptoms of potential disorders
- Coach patients on cardiac tests and treatments ordered by providers
- Accurately perform cardiac tests
- Identify and troubleshoot problems when performing tests

The heart is a complex organ. Electrical impulses move through the heart, and the cells react by contracting. The contracting cells result in contraction of the chambers. The contractions cause the blood to move through the heart and out to the arteries. To monitor the heart's function, both the electrical and mechanical activities of the heart can be assessed. When a provider needs to assess the electrical activity of the heart, an **electrocardiogram** is commonly ordered.

Electrocardiography is a painless test. **Electrodes** are placed on the body, and wires connect the electrodes to the ECG machine (*electrocardiograph*). Electrical impulses from the heart make their way to the surface of the skin. Think of what occurs when you throw a rock into a lake. Waves are created, and they eventually make their way to the shore. The electricity from the heart eventually makes its way to the surface of the skin. The electrodes pick up the electricity, and the electricity moves into the machine. The electrocardiograph creates a record of the impulses, which is called an *electrocardiogram* (ECG, EKG).

A medical assistant performs the electrocardiography. The provider reads and interprets the ECG to identify any abnormalities in the electrical conduction in the heart. It is important for the medical assistant to:

- Know the normal function of the heart
- Perform the procedure accurately
- Identify problems during the ECG procedure and take appropriate actions

The chapter begins with a review of the cardiovascular system. The components of the ECG and the process of obtaining an ECG follow the review.

CARDIOVASCULAR SYSTEM REVIEW

Heart Structure

The heart is divided into four chambers. Two atrial chambers receive blood from the body. Two ventricular chambers pump blood out to the body. The septum divides the right and left sides of the heart.

The tricuspid valve is found between the right atrium and the right ventricle (Fig. 11.1). The pulmonary valve is between the right ventricle and the pulmonary artery. The bicuspid, or mitral, valve is found between the left atrium and left ventricle. The aortic valve is between the left ventricle and the aorta. When the valves open, blood moves to the next chamber, or out of the heart through the arteries. The mechanical action of the heart and valves can be assessed by **echocardiography (ECHO)**.

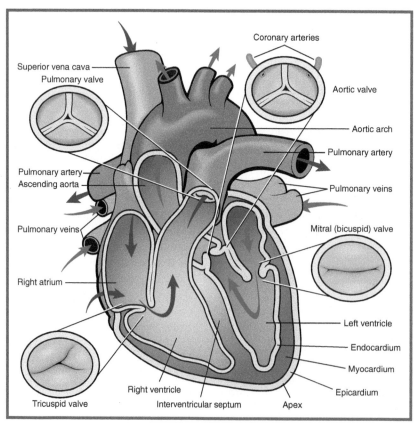

FIGURE 11.1 Chambers and valves of the heart. (From Damjanov I: *Pathology for the health-related professions*, ed 4, St Louis, 2012, Saunders.)

The heart wall has three layers: the epicardium, the myocardium, and the endocardium. Cardiac muscle fibers in the myocardium are electrically linked together, forming "one unit." A myocardial cell forms a strong connection to the next cells through special junctions called *intercalated discs*. These discs allow electricity to flow freely from one cell to the next. The intercalated discs are responsible for the cell-to-cell communication that is required for coordinated muscle contraction. The intercalated discs help the muscle fibers form one unit that contracts all at once, instead of a little at a time. The one-unit approach is important, because the atria and ventricles need to contract in an appropriately timed and coordinated effort.

Blood Flow

The right atrium receives deoxygenated blood from these structures:
- Superior vena cava (blood comes from the head, neck, and upper extremities)
- Inferior vena cava (blood comes from the thorax, abdomen, pelvis, and lower extremities)
- Coronary sinus (blood from the coronary veins)

When the right atrial chamber contracts, the tricuspid valve (atrioventricular [AV] valve) opens. Blood empties from the right atrium into the right ventricle. When the ventricles contract, the deoxygenated blood in the right ventricle passes through the opened pulmonary valve (semilunar [SL] valve) and moves into the pulmonary artery. The pulmonary artery brings the blood to the lungs. In the lungs, the blood picks up oxygen (O_2) and gives up carbon dioxide (CO_2). The pulmonary vein brings the oxygenated blood back to the left atrium. When the left atrial chamber contracts, the blood is pushed past the opened mitral (or bicuspid) valve (AV valve). The blood empties into the left ventricle. When the ventricles contract, the blood in the left ventricle moves through the opened aortic valve (SL valve) and into the aorta. The aorta transports oxygenated blood to the body. The first arteries to split off the aorta are the left and right coronary arteries. These arteries bring the oxygenated blood to the heart muscles.

A complete heartbeat, or *cardiac cycle,* can be divided into diastole and systole phases. During the *diastole* phase, the heart is at rest and the atria fill with blood. The *systole* phase occurs when the heart is contracting.

CRITICAL THINKING APPLICATION   **11.1**

Renee wants to help Eva review the cardiovascular structures before they see their first patient of the day. She asks Eva to describe the blood flow through the heart, starting with the superior vena cava and the inferior vena cava. Describe the blood flow.

Heart's Conduction System

The electrical cells make up the conduction system of the heart. These cells are found throughout the myocardium. They can respond to and transmit electrical impulses to neighboring cells. The conduction system is composed of five structures:
- *Sinoatrial* (SA) *node:* The SA node is called the "pacemaker of the heart" (Fig. 11.2). It is located in the posterior superior wall of the right atrium. The cardiac cells in the SA node generate the impulse. An impulse from the SA node starts each heartbeat.

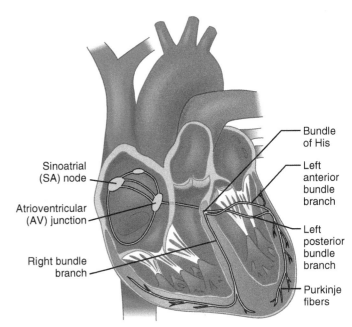

FIGURE 11.2 Cardiac conduction system.

When the SA node discharges the impulse, it travels in many directions through the heart muscle. Nearby atrial cardiac cells slowly pick up the impulse. The impulse also moves quickly across special bands of tissue called *intermodal tracts. Bachmann's bundle,* a specialized intermodal tract, takes the impulse to the left atrium. Other intermodal tracts take the impulse quickly to the AV node.
- *Atrioventricular* (AV) *node:* The AV node is located at the base of the interatrial septum. When the impulse reaches the AV node, it moves very slowly through the node. This slowdown allows the atrial chambers to finish contracting, moving the blood into the ventricular chambers.
- *Bundle of His* (or *AV bundle*): The bundle of His is located in the upper interventricular septum. When the impulse leaves the AV node, it moves to the bundle of His.
- *Right and left bundle branches:* The bundle branches are located in the lower interventricular septum. After the impulse passes through the bundle of His, it enters the right and left bundle branches. The right bundle branch brings the impulse to the right ventricle. The left bundle branch brings the impulse to the left ventricle.
- *Purkinje fibers:* The bundle branches split into many Purkinje fibers. The Purkinje fibers transmit the impulse quickly and efficiently to the ventricular cardiac cells. This helps the ventricular chambers to contract.

The cardiac cells cycle through three states, or steps, in the same sequence for each impulse.
- *Polarized state:* Before the impulse hits the cardiac cell, the cell is in the resting state, or *resting potential*. The inside of the cardiac cell is negatively charged. Outside of the cell is positively charged. There is no electrical activity seen on the ECG during the polarized state.
- *Depolarized state:* When the impulse hits the cardiac cell, large amounts of positively charged sodium **ions** move into the cell. A small amount of potassium ions moves outside of the cell. The

movement of sodium and potassium changes the cell's charge to positive. The change, also called *action potential*, allows the impulse to move through the cell. *Depolarization* (when the impulse hits the cell) causes electrical activity on the ECG.

- *Repolarized state*: After the impulse passes over the cell, the sodium and potassium ions move back to their original locations. This causes the cell's charge to change back to a negative charge. This recovery phase is called the *repolarized state*. Electrical activity (less than the depolarized state) can be recorded during the repolarized state.

Remember that the impulse occurs first and very soon after the contraction starts. These are two very distinct activities yet appear very closely together. The electrical activity from the depolarized state and the repolarized state is recorded on the ECG. The contractions are mechanical actions and are not recorded on the ECG. An echocardiogram (ECHO) can be used to gather information on the mechanical action of the heart.

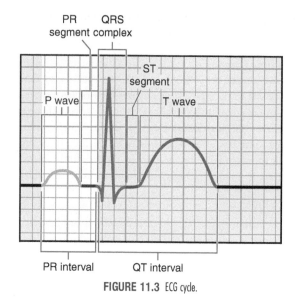

FIGURE 11.3 ECG cycle.

CRITICAL THINKING APPLICATION   11.2

Renee, knowing they have ECGs scheduled for today, asks Eva to list the conduction system structures in order and briefly describe polarization, depolarization, and repolarization. List the conduction system structures in order and then describe polarization, depolarization, and repolarization.

ECG TRACING

The medical assistant must obtain a clear ECG tracing for the provider to read or interpret. Knowing what a normal ECG looks like will help the medical assistant distinguish between normal rhythms, abnormal rhythms, and **artifact.** Abnormal rhythms and artifact will be discussed later in the chapter. This section will focus on the ECG tracing.

ECG Terminology

To understand the ECG tracing, it is important to understand the common terminology used:

- *Isoelectric line*: A straight line that is also called the *baseline*. It represents a period of time with no electrical activity.
- *Deflection:* Any movement away from the baseline in the tracing. The deflections reflect the heart's electrical flow. Upward movement is called a *positive deflection*. Downward movement is a *negative deflection*.
- *Wave:* A deflection from the baseline.
- *Complex:* A form made up of many waves (e.g., QRS complex).
- *Segment:* A part of a line between two points (e.g., the ST segment starts at the end of the S wave and ends at the start of the T wave).
- *Interval:* A period of time between two points or events. During an interval, many waves can occur.

Each deflection in the ECG tracing corresponds to a part of the cardiac cycle. The ECG cycle consists of waveforms that are labeled: P, Q, R, S, T, and U (Fig. 11.3). The Q, R, and S waves are usually grouped together and called the *QRS complex*. In the next section, each part of the ECG is discussed in more detail.

ECG Waves and Segments

The *P wave* is the first deflection in the tracing. It is created from the electrical impulses moving through the right and left atria. The P wave appears as a small, rounded hill. The first part of the P wave reflects the impulse moving from the SA node to the AV node in the right atrium. The second part of the P wave reflects the impulse in the left atrial chamber. Electricity given off when the atrial cells are depolarized creates the P wave. Thus, the P wave represents *atrial depolarization*. During the P wave, the atrial chambers contract and the blood moves into the ventricles (Table 11.1).

The *PR segment* follows the P wave and appears as an isoelectric line. The electrical impulse moves slowly through the AV node. This electricity is not picked up on the ECG tracing. The PR segment is the time between the end of the atrial depolarization and the start of the ventricular depolarization. During the PR segment, the atrial chambers finish contracting.

The *QRS complex* is the next wave in the tracing. The impulse moves from the AV node through the remaining conduction system structures. The electricity given off from the impulse moving down the septum and around the outer walls of the ventricles creates the QRS complex. The electricity from the activity in the ventricles masks the repolarization electricity given off from the atrial cells as they recover. The QRS complex activity can be summarized as ventricular depolarization and atrial repolarization. During the QRS complex, the ventricles start contracting and the blood moves into the arteries.

Each wave in the QRS complex is different. The Q wave is a negative deflection and represents interventricular septal depolarization. The large, triangular-shaped R wave reflects the depolarization of most of the ventricular walls. The S wave is the final depolarization of the ventricular walls. Not all of these three waves may be seen. The positive and negative deflections of these waves can be different in the 12 *leads*, or pictures, of the ECG.

The *ST segment* follows the last wave in the QRS complex and ends at the start of the T wave. The *J point* is the point where the QRS complex ends and the ST segment starts. The ST segment is an isoelectric line. There is no electrical activity in the heart during

TABLE 11.1   Summary of ECG Waves and Segments

WAVES	APPEARANCE	SUMMARIZED	CONDUCTION SYSTEM	MECHANICAL ACTION
P wave	Small "hill" (positive deflection seen on lead II)	Atrial depolarization	Impulse moves from the SA node (pacemaker) to the AV node.	Atrial chambers contract; blood moves into the ventricles.
PR segment	Isoelectric line		Impulse moves slowly through AV node; electricity is not picked up on tracing.	
QRS complex	(See below)	Ventricular depolarization; atrial repolarization (hidden)	AV node to the bundle of His to the right and left bundle branches to the Purkinje fibers.	Ventricular chambers contract, pushing blood out of the heart.
Q wave	Negative deflection	Interventricular septal depolarization; atrial repolarization (hidden)		
R wave	Positive triangular deflection	Ventricular depolarization; atrial repolarization (hidden)		
S wave	Any downward deflection following the R wave			
ST segment	Isoelectric line			
T wave	Positive deflection (upright and rounded in lead II)	Ventricular repolarization		
U wave	Usually not seen.	Purkinje fibers are repolarized		

AV, Atrioventricular; *SA,* sinoatrial.

this segment. (Remember, the impulse moving through the conduction system finished in the QRS complex.) During the ST segment, the ventricles finish contracting.

Repolarization causes electrical activity that creates the remaining waves. The *T wave* follows the ST segment and appears as a smooth, rounded, asymmetric waveform. The electrical activity from ventricular repolarization creates the T wave.

The *U wave* may follow the T wave, but in many cases it is not seen. The U wave is created from the repolarization of the Purkinje fibers. A U wave may also appear if the patient has hypercalcemia, hypokalemia, or digoxin toxicity.

CRITICAL THINKING APPLICATION   11.3

Before doing the ECGs scheduled for today, Renee reviews the waveforms with Eva. She asks Eva the following questions regarding the ECG tracing:
- What shows atrial depolarization?
- What shows ventricular depolarization?
- What shows ventricular repolarization?

ECG Intervals

An *interval* is a period of time from a start point to an end point. It is not a wave. If you need to define what occurs during an interval, you would simply summarize the activities that happen for each wave and segment during the interval period of time.

The *PR interval* starts at the beginning of the P wave and ends at the start of the Q wave. It represents atrial depolarization. The *QT interval* starts at the beginning of the Q wave and extends to the end of the T wave. During the QT interval, the atrial chambers move from repolarization to the polarized state. The ventricular chambers depolarize and then move into the repolarized state.

CRITICAL THINKING APPLICATION   11.4

Eva is confused about the PR interval and the QT interval. How might Renee describe these two intervals?

12-LEAD ECG

One of the most common ECG procedures in the ambulatory care setting is a resting 12-lead ECG. The medical assistant is responsible for:
- Assembling the supplies and equipment needed
- Preparing the patient for the test
- Performing the test

Before the medical assistant finishes the procedure, the ECG tracing must be examined for artifact. If any artifact is present on the tracing, the medical assistant must problem-solve the situation. Ultimately, the goal is to give the provider a clear ECG.

For a resting 12-lead ECG, the patient rests on the exam table. Ten electrodes are placed on the body. Lead wires attach to the electrodes and connect to the ECG machine (electrocardiograph). The 10 electrodes and lead wires pick up the electrical impulse from the surface of the body and carry it to the ECG machine (Fig. 11.4). The machine creates the ECG tracing.

A more in-depth discussion of electrode placement and artifact is presented later in the chapter. For now, it is important to have an idea of where the electrodes are placed on the body. An electrode is placed on each of the arms and legs. The right leg electrode is considered the ground electrode and is required for a clear ECG tracing. Six electrodes are placed on the chest.

Using the 10 electrodes and lead wires, the ECG machine creates 12 images, or pictures, that are called *leads*. Each lead picture looks different. Think of a photographer moving around a person, taking 12 pictures. Each picture looks different because of the change of the photographer's angle. For each lead, the picture is created differently. It is important for the medical assistant to know what electrodes and lead wires create the leads when troubleshooting unclear tracings. The three types of leads – bipolar, augmented, and precordial – are discussed in the following sections.

CRITICAL THINKING APPLICATION   11.5
Robert Caudill is scheduled for an ECG today. When he arrives, Eva discusses the procedure. Robert asks what "12 lead" stands for. How would you answer his question?

Bipolar (or Standard) Leads

The **bipolar** (standard) leads are named leads I, II, and III. They use the arm electrodes and the left leg electrode to create pictures of the vertical (or frontal) plane of the heart. (Remember, the right electrode is used as a ground and is important for all leads.)

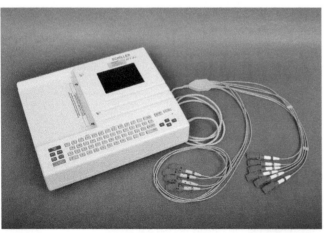

FIGURE 11.4 ECG machine.

The bipolar leads are created from a measurement of current traveling from a negative pole to the positive pole (Fig. 11.5):
- Lead I: Right arm (RA) to left arm (LA)
- Lead II: Right arm (RA) to left leg (LL)
- Lead III: Left leg (LL) to left arm (LA)

If you join the end points (positive poles) of these three leads, you get a triangle. This triangle is known as *Einthoven's triangle*.

It is important to know which two electrodes create each lead when troubleshooting problems with the ECG tracing. If a lead has artifact, the medical assistant must check the two electrodes and the lead wires that create the lead.

CRITICAL THINKING APPLICATION   11.6
As Eva and Renee perform an ECG, they find artifact on a few leads. For the following leads, which electrodes should be checked in each situation?
- Lead II is unclear.
- Leads I and III are unclear.
- Leads II and III are unclear.

Augmented Leads

Augmented leads also provide information on the vertical (frontal) plane of the heart. These **unipolar** leads are *augmented*, or increased in size, on the tracing. Augmented leads use the right arm (RA), left arm (LA), and left leg (LL) electrodes.

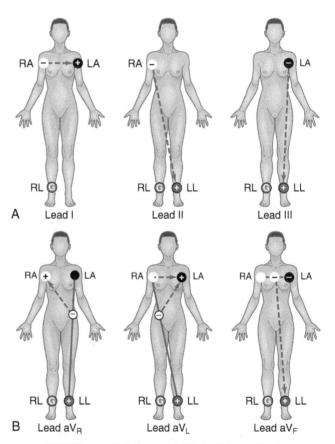

FIGURE 11.5 (A) Bipolar, or standard, leads. (B) Augmented leads.

Each augmented lead uses all three extremity electrodes (RA, LA, and LL) to create the picture. Midpoint between two of the electrodes is the negative pole. The current is measured as it moves from the negative pole to the positive pole (Table 11.2).

If the medical assistant identifies artifact on an augmented voltage–right arm (aVR) lead, all three electrodes and lead wires should be checked. (Check the RA, LA, and LL electrode and lead wires.)

Chest (or Precordial) Leads

The chest (precordial) leads are also unipolar leads. Each is a positive pole. The precordial leads provide information on the horizontal (front to back) plane of the heart. The six precordial leads are labeled V_1, V_2, V_3, V_4, V_5, and V_6 (Fig. 11.6).

The six leads are numbered the same as the precordial lead wires (i.e., V_1 through V_6). If one of the leads is unclear, the medical assistant should refer to the related lead wire and electrode. For instance, with artifact on V_4, the medical assistant will check the V_4 electrode and lead wire.

ECG SUPPLIES AND EQUIPMENT

The medical assistant needs to be familiar with the supplies and equipment used for ECGs. It is important to monitor the expiration dates of ECG supplies. Using expired supplies can cause unclear ECG tracings.

Thermal ECG Paper

ECG machines with printers use special ECG paper. The paper can be either **Z**-fold paper or 8.25 × 11-inch paper. A special heat-sensitive coating on the paper allows the tracing to be "burnt" onto the paper. Tips for handling the ECG paper include:

- Store in a dry, cool, dark location.
- Do not expose to heat, bright light, or ultraviolet (UV) light source.
- Do not expose to alcohol, adhesives, cleaners, or solvents.
- Do not store with vinyl, shrink wrap, or plastics.

The ECG paper is universally created with small and large boxes. The small box is 1 × 1 mm, and the large box is 5 × 5 mm. The large box is made up of 25 small boxes (5 rows and 5 columns) (Fig. 11.7). It has a thicker border than the small boxes. When the provider analyzes the tracing, the height and the width of the wave forms are measured with a **caliper** (Fig. 11.8). The small and large boxes can help in the interpreting process.

TABLE 11.2	Augmented Voltage Leads
LEAD	**MEASURES CURRENT TRAVEL TOWARDS POSITIVE POLE**
aVR (augmented voltage – right arm)	Right arm
aVL (augmented voltage – left arm)	Left arm
aVF (augmented voltage – left leg [foot])	Left leg

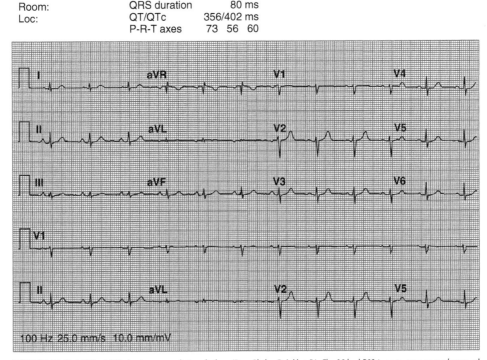

Female Caucasian	Vent. rate 77 bpm	Normal sinus rhythm	
Room:	PR interval 156 ms	Normal ECG	
Loc:	QRS duration 80 ms		
	QT/QTc 356/402 ms		
	P-R-T axes 73 56 60		

100 Hz 25.0 mm/s 10.0 mm/mV

FIGURE 11.6 A 12-lead ECG showing a normal sinus rhythm. (From Phalen T, Aehlert BJ: *The 12-lead ECG in acute coronary syndromes,* ed 3, St Louis, 2012, Mosby.)

The vertical lines measure the amplitude, or *voltage*, of the waveforms. Each small box is 0.1 mV (millivolt), and each large box is 0.5 mV. To determine the amplitude, count the small boxes vertically, starting at the baseline to the highest/lowest point of the wave.

The horizontal lines measure the time. When the paper speed (*chart speed*) is set at 25 mm/second, each small box is 0.04 second and each large box equals 0.2 second. To determine the width and time of the waveform, count the small boxes horizontally from the start to the finish of the wave. Multiply the number of small boxes by 0.04 to find the time.

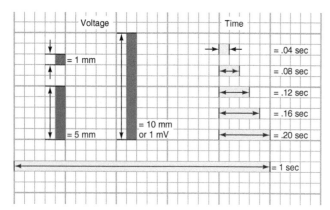

FIGURE 11.7 ECG paper.

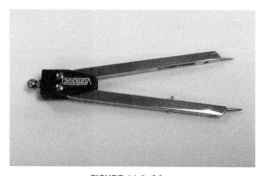

FIGURE 11.8 Caliper.

Electrodes

Electrodes are single-use disposable adhesive tabs that are placed on the skin. The skin is a poor conductor of electricity. The electrodes contain an electrolyte gel that helps pick up the electrical impulses. As the impulses make their way to the surface of the body, the electrolyte gel helps to conduct the impulses into the lead wires. For a resting 12-lead ECG, the most common type of electrode is the tab variety (Fig. 11.9A). The snap electrode is used more often for exercise stress tests and in hospital settings (Fig. 11.9B).

It is important to check the expiration date of the electrodes. If they are expired, the gel may be dried out and the conduction will be poor. Many operators' manuals for ECG machines recommend not mixing different manufacturers' electrodes.

Electrocardiograph

The lead wires may have a snap or a clip (also called an *alligator clip*; patient end adaptor) that attaches to the electrode. The lead wires merge into the patient cable that takes the electrical impulses to the electrocardiograph (ECG machine). In the machine, the impulses pass through an amplifier, which magnifies the impulses. A digital converter changes the analog signal into a digital signal. The digital signal can be printed off on special ECG paper, which will be discussed in the next section.

The features of ECG machines can vary greatly. The two types of ECG devices in ambulatory healthcare facilities include:
- *Box model ECG machine*: Usually has an LCD screen.
- *Computer-based ECG*: May have a touch screen and stress testing features. Can have its own computer device with preloaded software, or a facility can purchase software to add to any laptop computer.

Additional features commonly seen in both types of ECG devices:
- Interpretive software: Assists providers with reading the tracing.
- Bluetooth or Wi-Fi capacity: Allows the ECG to be sent to providers and printers and to be uploaded into an electronic health record (EHR).
- Thermal printers
- Spirometer

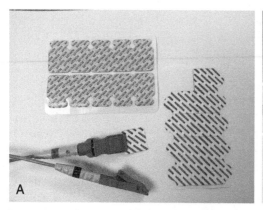
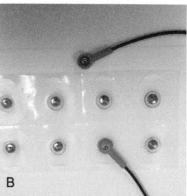

FIGURE 11.9 (A) The appearance of tab electrodes can vary, depending on the manufacturer. Alligator clips on the lead wires attach to the tab electrodes. (B) Snap electrodes use the snap adaptors on the lead wires.

TABLE 11.3 Common ECG Settings

SETTING	DESCRIPTION	NORMAL DEFAULT	REASON TO CHANGE SETTING
Chart speed	Regulates the speed of the paper during the recording. *Example:* 25 mm/s means 25 millimeters (25 small blocks) of tracing is printed in 1 second.	25 mm/s (second)	*For very fast heart rates:* Increase speed to 50 mm/s to get more defined waveforms. *For very slow heart rates:* Reduce rate to 5 or 10 mm/s to capture more waveforms on the paper.
Gain or sensitivity	Regulates the height (amplitude) of the tracing. *Example:* 10 mm/mV means 1 mV (millivolt) of electricity causes the recorder to move up 10 millimeters (10 small blocks).	10 mm/mV	*For very short waveforms:* Increase to 20 mm/mV, which doubles the height of the waves. *For very tall waveforms:* Reduce to 5 mm/mV, which reduces the wave height by half.

Settings and Calibration

ECG machines have settings that can be useful for obtaining a tracing. Many machines have filters to block disturbances. Filters can help to create a clearer tracing. Refer to the operator's manual when changing settings. Table 11.3 presents common settings. It is important to indicate on the tracing if any of the default settings were changed. Changes to the default settings will affect how the provider measures and interprets the tracing.

Most ECG machines automatically complete a self-test when the machine is turned on. Typically, the self-test examines the battery and the memory. Like many machines used in the healthcare setting, the ECG machine needs to be calibrated daily or per the facility's policy. The calibration results should be documented on the log flow sheet.

Maintenance of the Electrocardiograph

- The lead wires are not disposable; clean as indicated in the operator's manual.
- Handle the lead wires and patient cable with care. They should be stored in a loose coil. Tight coils or bending of the wires and cable can result in breakage of the fine wires inside the unit. This will cause artifact on the ECG and requires replacement of the cable.
- Clean the tracing stylus and the machine casing as indicated in the operator's manual.

When ECG machines are calibrated, the sensitivity, or gain, should to be checked. The machines usually print a calibration marking either at the beginning or at the end of the tracing. This marking is called the *standardization mark*. If the machine is set at 10 mm/mV, the standardization mark will be an upward rectangle that is 10 small boxes tall. If the gain is doubled, then the standardization mark also will be doubled in size (Fig. 11.10).

CRITICAL THINKING APPLICATION   11.7

The next day, Eva prepares to do an ECG on Charles Johnson. She turns on the machine to check to see if it has been set up correctly. She sees the following:
- Chart speed: 10 mm/s
- Gain: 10 mm/mV

Which of these settings is normal and which needs to be changed prior to the next ECG?

ECG PROCEDURE

Patient Preparation

Before the procedure is started, it is always important for the medical assistant to coach the patient on the procedure and the preparation required. The medical assistant should prepare the patient for an ECG by explaining that:
- Ten electrodes and wires are placed on the body.
- The machine will take 12 pictures of the electrical activity of the heart.
- The procedure is painless.
- The patient must be still and not talk during the time the pictures are being made (during the actual tracing).
- The patient should not use his or her cell phone or other electronic device during the procedure.
- The provider will need to look at the ECG pictures and then the patient will be notified of the results. (Remember, the medical assistant cannot tell the patient if it is normal or abnormal.)

The patient needs to remove all clothing above the waist and wear a gown that opens in the front. Cloth gowns or paper capes can be used. An electrode must be placed on each lower leg, so tights or pantyhose also must be removed. Socks and pants can be moved to allow application of the electrodes, so they can usually stay on (see Procedure 11.1, p. 284).

The patient should be in the supine position on the exam table. A pillow can be placed under the patient's head. The patient's legs and arms need to be supported on the table. It is important for the patient to be relaxed and comfortable during the procedure. If the patient is having chest pain or problems breathing, the head of the exam table may be elevated. Any change of position from the supine position must be noted on the ECG tracing. Any position change can create a change on the leads (pictures). The provider needs to be aware of it when reading the tracing.

Before placing the electrodes on the skin, it is important to prepare the skin. This helps the electrodes adhere and minimizes artifact, thus producing an accurate tracing. There are several techniques used to prepare the skin:
- Wipe the area with an alcohol pad to clean it. This helps to remove sweat and lotion that may prevent the electrodes from adhering to the skin.

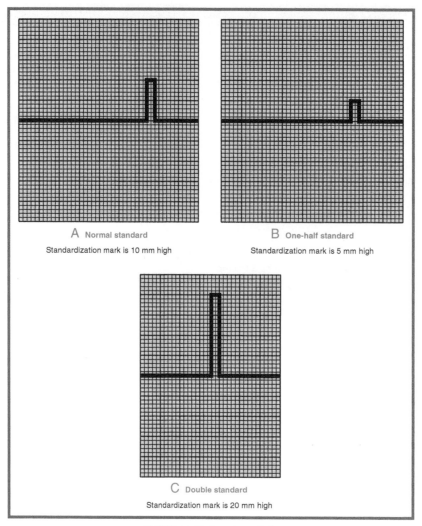

A Normal standard
Standardization mark is 10 mm high

B One-half standard
Standardization mark is 5 mm high

C Double standard
Standardization mark is 20 mm high

FIGURE 11.10 Sensitivity standards.

- Use a razor to shave chest hair. Obtain the patient's verbal consent before shaving the chest.
- Gently abrade the skin, using a gauze sponge, special gel, or special fine sandpaper tape (Fig. 11.11)

Applying Electrodes and Lead Wires

Apply electrodes to both arms and legs. The electrodes on the lower legs should be placed on the inner side, just above the ankles. If tab electrodes are used, have the tabs on the leg electrodes point toward the center of the person. All the other tabs can be facing the feet.

The placement of the arm electrodes may vary, depending on the ECG machine and manufacturer. For instance, many Schiller ECG machines indicate that the electrodes should be placed just above the wrists. Other machines indicate placement on the upper arms. Check the operator's manual for correct placement of the arm electrodes. Table 11.4 describes where to place the electrodes on the limbs and the chest (Fig. 11.12).

The lead wires are typically color coded and include an abbreviation on each wire. Colors may vary from manufacturer to manufacturer.

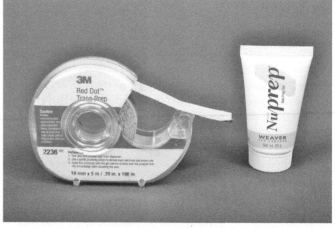

FIGURE 11.11 Special fine sandpaper tape and Nuprep skin prep gel are used to abrade the skin. This provides a better ECG tracing.

TABLE 11.4   Electrode and Lead Wire Placement

ELECTRODE	LEAD WIRE ABBREVIATION AND COLOR	PLACEMENT
Right arm	RA (white)	Placed just above the wrist or upper arm, indicated in the operator's manual
Left arm	LA (black)	
Right leg	RL (green)	Placed on the inner lower leg, just above the ankle
Left leg	LL (red)	
Chest V$_1$	V$_1$ (red)	Fourth intercostal space at the right sternal edge
Chest V$_2$	V$_2$ (yellow)	Fourth intercostal space at the left sternal edge
Chest V$_3$	V$_3$ (green)	Midway between V$_2$ and V$_4$
Chest V$_4$	V$_4$ (blue)	Fifth intercostal space on the midclavicular line
Chest V$_5$	V$_5$ (orange)	Same horizontal plane as V$_4$ at the left anterior axillary line or the midpoint between V$_4$ and V$_6$
Chest V$_6$	V$_6$ (purple)	Same horizontal plane as V$_4$ at the midaxillary line

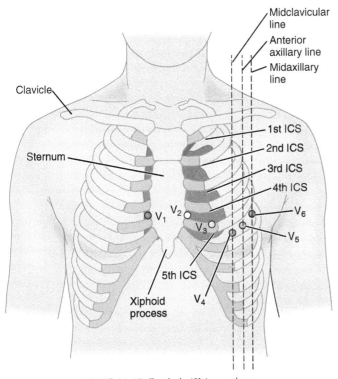

FIGURE 11.12 Chest leads. *ICS,* Intercostal space.

TABLE 11.5   Electrode Placement in Special Situations

CONDITION	ELECTRODE PLACEMENT
Dextrocardia	Place chest electrodes on the right side of the chest using the same intercostal spacing and landmarks. Switch the right and left limb lead wires (e.g., LA would be attached to the right arm electrode).
Amputated limb	Place electrode on the remaining part of the limb. Place the electrode on the opposite limb in the same location.
Casted limb	Place the electrode above the cast on the limb. Place the electrode on the opposite limb in the same location.
New surgical incision or wound	Place the electrodes near the correct area, but not on the incision or wound.

the normal location. The provider reading the tracing needs to take the placement into consideration.

Running the ECG Tracing

Once the lead wires are attached to the electrodes, the medical assistant enters the patient information into the ECG machine. In some facilities this may be done prior to bringing the patient into the room for the ECG. Typically, the patient's name, date of birth, and medical record number are entered. Facilities will have additional information that they require to be entered, such as the ordering provider's name and the provider reading the ECG.

After the information is entered, the medical assistant should remind the patient to remain still and not to talk during the procedure.

It is important to know and to use the abbreviations. One of the most common errors is to mix up the right and left limb lead wires. This can cause abnormal leads (pictures) and result in additional patient workup before the mistake is discovered. It is important to always double-check the placement of the lead wires.

In some cases, the electrodes may need to be placed in alternative locations. Table 11.5 identifies special situations. It is important to note on the ECG tracing any electrode placement deviation from

It usually takes a minute or less for the tracing to be created with a multichannel machine. Talking and movement will create artifact. If the patient is cold, a blanket can be used to cover him or her.

Prior to running the tracing, double-check that all the electrodes are attached and the lead wires are in the correct location. If the ECG machine has a screen, check the digital picture of the leads. Are they clear (without artifact)? If not, is the filter(s) on? Are the leads (pictures) an equal distance from each other? Is the baseline horizontal, or is it moving up and down like a roller coaster? Do not run the tracing until it is clear, and the baseline is horizontal. Problem-solve and fix the issue before running the tracing or redo the tracing if it was printed. Additional problem-solving strategies will be discussed later in this chapter. Once the tracing looks good on the screen, print it.

> ### Single- and Multiple-Channel ECG Machines
>
> ECG machines can be single or multiple channel. In *single-channel* models, the machine contains one amplifier channel and one recording stylet. The single-channel machines record one lead (picture) at a time. The medical assistant must manually switch to the next lead until the procedure is done. When these machines are used, the process of recording a tracing takes up to 3 to 5 minutes. Single-channel machines can use paper rolls or Z-fold paper. These small strips of paper need to be mounted (see the section Finishing the ECG).
>
> *Multichannel* machines monitor all 12 leads. This model has several stylets that allow for four groups of three leads to be traced every few seconds. With some machines, a fourth stylet traces one lead for the entire width of the page. Typically, the multichannel machines print the tracing on 8.25 × 11-inch paper or Z-fold paper.

Troubleshooting Artifact

Artifact is signal distortion or unwanted, erratic movement of the stylus caused by outside interference. The medical assistant needs to identify the type of artifact and then take actions to prevent the artifact. The leads can be viewed on the screen or after printing the ECG tracing. Carefully look for artifact. The following sections discuss the appearance and causes of the common types of artifact and ways to prevent them.

Wandering Baseline

Wandering baseline artifact is an upward and downward movement of the waveform (Fig. 11.13). The isoelectric lines shift locations. This artifact can be the result of:

- *Poor skin preparation*: Patient has oily skin or used lotion. The electrodes are falling off.
- *Old electrodes*: The electrodes are dirty or expired; or the gel on the electrodes is dried.
- *Placement of electrodes*: Electrodes are placed on bony areas.
- *Movement*: The movement of breathing can also be the cause of this artifact.

The medical assistant should:

- Clean the skin with alcohol and allow it to dry. Slightly abrade the skin with a gauze pad or fine sandpaper tape to help the electrodes stick to the skin.
- Replace the electrode with a new one. Ensure the electrodes are not expired and the gel is not dried.
- Make sure all electrodes and lead wires are firmly attached.
- Make sure the baseline filter is turned on (if it is a feature of the machine).

Somatic Tremor

Somatic tremor artifact appears as jagged peaks with irregular heights and spacing (Fig. 11.14). The causes include:

- *Involuntary movement*: Tremors from disease conditions (e.g., Parkinson's disease), shivering due to coldness
- *Voluntary movement*: Talking, chewing gum, supporting arms or legs because table is too small for the person

The medical assistant should:

- Help the patient relax. Cover the patient with a blanket if he or she is cold.
- Remind the patient to not move or talk during the tracing.
- Watch to see if there is a pattern with involuntary movements. Take the tracing when the movements lessen.
- Use a larger exam table for the procedure.
- If the machine has a muscle tremor filter, make sure it is turned on.

AC Interference

AC interference artifact appears as a series of small spikes that creates a thick-looking tracing (Fig. 11.15). The causes include:

- *Electrical interference*: Too many electrical devices in the area; patient cable and lead wires are wrapped closely together; electrical cord is under the exam table; and electrical outlet is improperly grounded. A cell phone in a patient's pocket or a smart watch may also cause interference.

The medical assistant should:

- Unplug the ECG machine.
- Unplug or remove nearby electrical devices (e.g., laptops, pagers, cell phones).
- Separate the lead wires so they do not overlap.

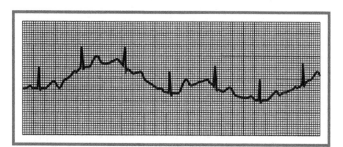

FIGURE 11.13 Wandering baseline artifact.

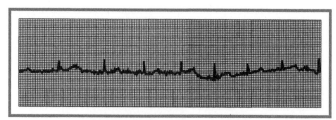

FIGURE 11.14 Somatic tremor artifact.

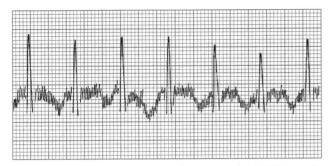

FIGURE 11.15 AC interference artifact. (From Urden L, Stacy K, Lough M: *Thelan's critical care nursing: diagnosis and management*, ed 7, St Louis, 2014, Mosby.)

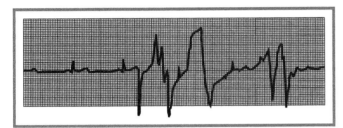

FIGURE 11.16 Interrupted baseline artifact.

- Move the table away from the wall or move to another room for the procedure.
- Ensure cell phones are not near the procedure area.

Interrupted Baseline

Interrupted baseline artifact (also called *intermittent signal artifact*) occurs when the tracing looks normal at the beginning, but then it disappears or goes all over when the electrical connection is interrupted (Fig. 11.16). The causes include:

- *Electrical connection is interrupted*: Due to a loose cable or lead wire, or a broken cable, clip, or lead wire.

The medical assistant should:

- Check that all electrodes and lead wires are attached.
- If a broken wire is suspected, a new cable will be needed.

CRITICAL THINKING APPLICATION   **11.8**

While Eva is performing Charles Johnson's 12-lead ECG, she notices that the tracing line looks thick. On closer inspection she finds that there are small, spiked lines that make the tracing look like a thick line. What is occurring? How might Eva troubleshoot the problem?

Evaluating an ECG Tracing

The provider reads the ECG, but the medical assistant must be able to determine abnormal rates and rhythms that might be life-threatening. This section will discuss how to determine the heart rate, evaluate the ECG tracing, and identify abnormal rhythms.

Rate

Many machines indicate the heart rate. The medical assistant can also calculate the rate from the ECG tracing. Methods used to calculate

TABLE 11.6	Sequence Method
NUMBER OF LARGE (5 mm) BOXES BETWEEN R WAVES	HEART RATE
1	300
2	150
3	100
4	75
5	60
6	50
7	43
8	37

a regular heart rate when the paper speed (chart speed) is 25 mm/second include:

- *Six second method*: Count the number of P waves in a 6-second strip (30 large boxes) and multiply by 10 (least accurate method).
- *1500 method*: Count the number of small boxes between two R waves or the two P waves. Divide the number into 1500.
- *Sequence method:* Count the number of large boxes between the R waves. By memorizing the numbers in Table 11.6, you will have a quick method to calculate the heart rate.

Analyzing an ECG Tracing

For most medical assistants, their job description states that they need to be able to perform ECGs. For some medical assistants, they may work as an ECG technician. In this position they may need to analyze an ECG tracing.

The ECG rhythm strip (lead II view) is evaluated from left to right. The following should be assessed:

- *Rate*: What is the rate?
- *Rhythm*: Is it regular or irregular? An irregular rhythm on an ECG tracing will have time differences between cardiac cycles. With a regular rhythm, each cardiac cycle occurs the same length of time apart.
- *Appearance of the segments, waves, and intervals*: Table 11.7 lists questions to consider when analyzing a tracing.

Identifying an Abnormal Rhythm

When performing an ECG, the medical assistant must identify if the patient has an **arrhythmia** that requires immediate care by the provider. If the medical assistant identifies a life-threatening arrhythmia, it is important to keep the patient hooked up to the ECG machine and to immediately get the provider.

Sinus Arrhythmias. A sinus rhythm is considered normal. The electrical activity begins in the SA node and goes through the rest of the conduction system. Atrial and ventricular depolarizations occur. With sinus arrhythmias, the electrical pathway is normal. The rate or rhythm of the heartbeat is altered. The alteration may come from the SA node firing too slowly or too quickly.

TABLE 11.7   Analyzing an ECG Tracing

TRACING FEATURE	NORMAL	QUESTIONS TO ADDRESS	TIMING (HORIZONTAL – LENGTH)
P wave	Largest in lead II; upright in all leads except aVR Voltage (vertical – height): less than 2.5 small boxes (0.25 millivolts)	• Is there one P wave before each QRS complex? • Is each P wave a positive deflection? • Are all the P waves similar in size and shape? • Is there more than one P wave per cardiac cycle?	>0.11 second
PR interval	From start of P wave to start of QRS complex	• Are the PR intervals the same size throughout the tracing?	0.12–0.2 second
QRS complex	Largest in lead II compared to leads III and I	• Is there a QRS complex without a previous P wave?	0.06–0.12 second
ST segment	On the baseline	• Is the ST segment lower or higher than the baseline? (Could be an indication of infarction or ischemia.)	Not usually measured
QT interval	From start of Q wave to end of T wave	• Are the QT intervals the same size throughout the tracing?	0.40 second

- *Sinus bradycardia*: The adult heart rate is below 60 beats per minute. This is a normal finding in well-conditioned athletes. It is abnormal in other individuals.
- *Sinus tachycardia*: The adult heart rate is above 100 beats per minute. This is normal in a person doing aerobic exercise. It is abnormal in a resting individual.

Atrial Arrhythmias. Atrial arrhythmias occur when there is a problem with the SA node starting the impulse. They can also occur due to a conduction problem in the atria.

- *Premature atrial contractions* (PACs): Occur when the atria contract sooner than they should. The P wave can be abnormally shaped, or an extra P wave can be seen. PACs can be seen in people who smoke or consume large amounts of caffeine. An occasional PAC is not abnormal. More than six PACs in a minute is considered abnormal.
- *Atrial flutter*: Occurs when the atria contract faster than the ventricles (up to 300 beats per minute). They become out of sync with the ventricles. Extra P waves are seen with regular QRS complexes. Atrial flutter can be caused by alcohol and stimulants (cocaine, caffeine, diet pills, and cold medications). It can also be caused by coronary heart disease, hypertension, cardiomyopathy, heart valve diseases, hyperthyroidism, obstructive pulmonary disease, and pulmonary embolism diseases. Atrial flutter is reversed with medication to slow the heart or with *cardioversion* (electrical shock).

Heart Block. A heart block occurs when there is a disruption or slowing of the electrical impulse through the heart. Heart block can be congenital or acquired. Heart disease, surgery, or medications can cause acquired heart block. There are three types of heart block, with third degree being the most severe:

- *First-degree heart block*: The impulse slows as it moves from the atria to the ventricles. This creates a longer PR segment. First-degree heart block may not cause symptoms. It may not require treatment.
- *Second-degree heart block*: The impulse slows or is blocked as it moves into the ventricles. When blocked, there is no QRS complex after the P wave, and the ventricles do not contract.

When the impulse slows, the PR segment is longer. This arrhythmia requires a pacemaker to help maintain the heart rate. Pacemakers will be discussed in a later section of this chapter.

- *Third-degree heart block*: The impulse does not reach the ventricles. As a backup system, special ventricular cells create an impulse that causes the ventricles to contract. On the ECG tracing, the P wave is faster than normal and the QRS complex is not coordinated with the P wave. This is a life-threatening arrhythmia and requires emergency treatment and a pacemaker.

Ventricular Arrhythmias. Ventricular arrhythmias are abnormalities in the ventricles. Most of the ventricular arrhythmias discussed are life-threatening rhythms.

- *Premature ventricular contractions* (PVCs): Occur when the ventricles contract sooner than they should. An impulse originating in the ventricles creates this abnormality. The QRS complex appears before a P wave. The P wave can also be absent. The T wave can be abnormally shaped, and a widened QRS complex can be seen (Fig. 11.17A–B). PVCs can be caused by tobacco, alcohol, epinephrine, and anxiety. They can also be caused by hypertension, coronary artery disease, and lung disease. Infrequent PVCs can be normal. More than six PVCs in a minute is abnormal and can lead to a life-threatening condition.
- *Ventricular tachycardia (V-tach)*: Occurs when the ventricles beat at a rapid rate (up to 250 beats per minute). It may be seen with multiple PVCs in a row. It may be a short run of fast beats or may last longer than 30 seconds (see Fig. 11.17C). V-tach is a life-threatening condition. If it is not reversed with drugs and/or cardioversion, it can become ventricular fibrillation.
- *Ventricular fibrillation (V-fib)*: Occurs when the ventricles quiver uncontrollably (see Fig. 11.17D). They are essentially ineffective at pumping any blood. The patient has no pulse, is not breathing, and is unresponsive. This is the most critical, life-threatening arrhythmia. Cardioversion with a defibrillator is necessary to restore normal function of the electrical conduction system.

- *Asystole*: Results in the absence of a heartbeat. A flat line appears on the tracing (see Fig. 11.17E.)

Implantable Device Rhythms. Implantable devices (e.g., pacemaker and implantable cardioverter-defibrillator) create abnormal waveforms on the ECG tracing. A pacemaker is used to treat some types of arrhythmias. It uses low-energy electrical pulses to assist the heart to beat at a normal rate. Pacemakers can change the ECG tracing. Fig. 11.18 shows a pacemaker rhythm strip. There are two types of pacemakers:

- Temporary pacemaker: Used in an emergency until the permanent pacemaker can be placed; also used for temporary conditions (e.g., heart attack and medication overdose).
- Permanent pacemaker: Surgically inserted into the chest or abdomen. Patients can use technology (e.g., smart phones) to transmit their pacemaker data to their provider.

An implantable cardioverter-defibrillator (ICD) can provide low-energy electrical pulses and high-energy pulses (Fig. 11.19). The high-energy pulses can treat life-threatening arrhythmias. ICDs are surgically implanted in the chest or abdomen. The ICD is programmed to meet the needs of the patient. Some ICD functions can be checked using technology such as pacemakers. ICD batteries can last 5 to 7 years.

Finishing the ECG

If the ambulatory care facility uses an EHR system and the ECG machine interfaces with the EHR software, then follow the procedure and upload the tracing to the patient's health record. The provider will read the tracing once it is uploaded.

An ECG must be read by the provider before it is filed in the paper medical record. If the tracing was done on small strips of ECG paper, the strips need to be mounted per the facility's procedures. Special 8.5 × 10-inch paper with adhesive strips is used to stick the ECG tracing strips. Once the strips are mounted, they can be given to the provider to read. If the ECG prints on 8.5 × 10-inch paper, it does not need to be mounted. It can be given to the provider immediately.

CRITICAL THINKING APPLICATION   **11.9**

The clinic uses an ECG machine that uploads the ECGs into patients' electronic health records. Based on what you have learned so far in your courses, why is this useful and efficient?

ADDITIONAL ECG TESTING

Exercise Stress Test

An exercise stress test records the ECG while the patient is exercising. The patient either walks on a treadmill with an incline or uses an exercise bike (Fig. 11.20). During the test, a continual ECG is recorded, and the blood pressure is monitored.

Why the test is ordered:
- The patient is starting an exercise program.
- The patient has angina that is getting worse.
- To evaluate the patient's heart after an angioplasty or bypass surgery.
- To evaluate heart rhythm changes with the stress of exercise.

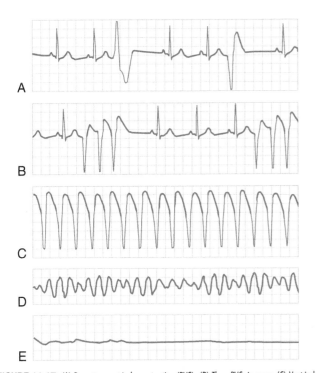

FIGURE 11.17 (A) Premature ventricular contraction (PVC). (B) Three PVCs in a row. (C) Ventricular tachycardia (V-tach). (D) Ventricular fibrillation (V-fib). (E) Asystole.

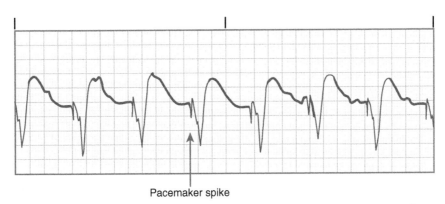

Pacemaker spike

FIGURE 11.18 Pacemaker rhythm strip. (From Lewis S, et al: *Medical-surgical nursing*, ed 9, St Louis, 2014, Mosby.)

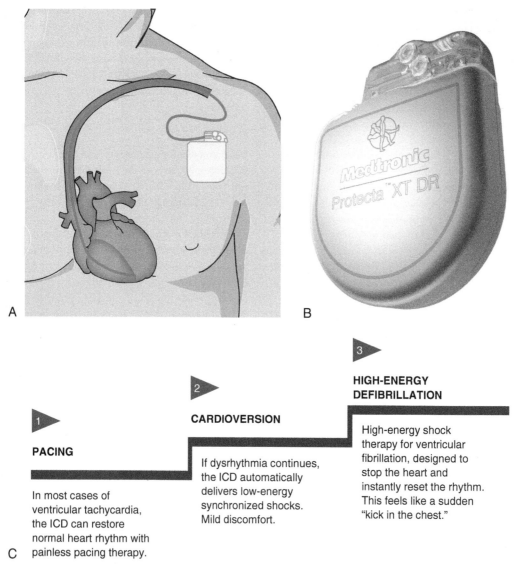

PACING

In most cases of ventricular tachycardia, the ICD can restore normal heart rhythm with painless pacing therapy.

CARDIOVERSION

If dysrhythmia continues, the ICD automatically delivers low-energy synchronized shocks. Mild discomfort.

HIGH-ENERGY DEFIBRILLATION

High-energy shock therapy for ventricular fibrillation, designed to stop the heart and instantly reset the rhythm. This feels like a sudden "kick in the chest."

FIGURE 11.19 Implanted cardioverter-defibrillator (ICD). (From Urden L, Stacy K, Lough M: *Thelan's critical care nursing: diagnosis and management,* ed 7, St Louis, 2014, Mosby.)

Preparation for the test:
- The patient should wear clothes and shoes for exercising.
- The provider will indicate what daily medications should be taken prior to the test.
- The patient should not take a dose of Viagra, Cialis, or Levitra for erectile dysfunction 48 hours before a stress test.
- The patient should not smoke or consume caffeine or alcohol 3 hours before the test.
- The patient signs a consent form prior to the test.

During the test:
- Electrodes and lead wires will be placed on the patient. A blood pressure cuff will be applied to the patient's arm.
- The patient will begin to exercise slowly, and gradually the exercise difficulty will increase.

- The provider should always be present during the test. If the patient has chest discomfort, dizziness, palpitations, or shortness of breath, the test will stop. Emergency supplies or a crash cart should be kept nearby in case of an emergency.

Nuclear Stress Test

The nuclear stress test shows the blood flow into the heart muscle during rest and activity. A radioactive substance (e.g., thallium or sestamibi) is injected into a vein using an intravenous line (IV). After 15 to 45 minutes of resting, a gamma camera is used to take images of the blood flow in the heart. Then the person either exercises or is given a vasodilating medication to dilate the coronary arteries. The radioactive substance is again injected, and the person rests. After the required rest period, the gamma camera is used to take additional

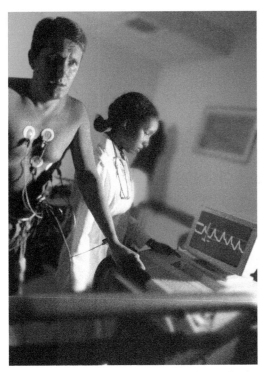

FIGURE 11.20 Exercise Stress Test. (Courtesy Stockbyte/Thinkstock.)

images of the blood flow through the coronary vessels. Throughout the test, the blood pressure and ECG are monitored.

Holter Monitor

A Holter monitor is used to monitor the heart over a 24- to 48-hour period while the patient goes about his or her normal activities. Sometimes patients experience a heart issue that cannot be picked up on a resting 12-lead ECG. Having a longer monitoring period can capture the abnormalities.

When placing electrodes for a Holter monitor, consult the operator's manual. There are many configurations for electrode placement. Different monitors use varying numbers of electrodes. Holter monitors typically use three to seven chest electrodes.

As with the resting 12-lead ECG, lead wires attach the electrodes to the small Holter monitor. The monitor runs on batteries and is small enough to fit into a pocket. The patient is given a journal and instructions on completing the journal. Procedure 11.2 on p. 285 describes the steps in applying a Holter monitor to a patient.

Patient Education for a Holter Monitor Test

• Wear the monitor continuously. The monitor will be removed during your appointment in 24 to 48 hours.
• While wearing the Holter monitor, avoid metal detectors, large magnets, high-voltage areas, x-rays, and electric blankets. Do not get the monitor wet (e.g., no bathing, showering, or swimming).

• Keep a detailed journal of the symptoms experienced. These symptoms could include chest pain, shortness of breath, palpitations or changes in the heartbeat, dizziness, or fainting. Document:
  • Date and time
  • Symptoms experienced
  • Activity being done at the time
• At the return visit, the provider will look at the tracing for abnormalities. The journal of timed activities will help the provider identify what is occurring.
• What to do if the electrodes or lead wires fall off.
• Who to contact in case of questions or if problems occur.

Cardiac Event Recorder

The cardiac event recorder is a portable, battery-powered ECG device. The recorder is activated by the patient when symptoms occur, and it records the ECG. Patients may wear a cardiac event recorder for 30 days. When symptoms occur only occasionally, it is difficult to capture the abnormality on a resting 12-lead ECG or a Holter monitor. The patient may also be asked to keep a journal, as with the Holter monitor. With the cardiac event recorder, the patient goes about his or her daily activities. The monitor can be removed during bathing and showering or swimming.

When patients experience symptoms, they push the recorder's activation button. An ECG is recorded and stored. The ECG can be sent to the provider via a phone or other technology. A provider will review the tracing. If there is an emergency, the patient will be called and told to go to the nearest emergency department.

There are two types of cardiac event recorders:

• *Looping memory monitor* (also called a *cardiac loop recorder*): A pager-sized monitor that connects to two chest electrodes by wires. The monitor continuously records the ECG. When the memory is full, it overwrites from the beginning (i.e., continues loop of recording). When a patient has symptoms, he or she activates the monitor. The ECG from prior to, during, and for a short while after the event is stored. It does not overwrite the stored ECGs.
• *Symptom event monitor* (also called a *post-event monitor*): Can be a handheld device or worn on the wrist. When symptoms are felt, the patient activates the monitor and places it on the chest. Small metal discs on the back of the monitor act as electrodes. The current ECG is recorded and stored. Unlike the looping memory monitor, the symptom event monitor cannot record and store the ECG prior to the symptoms.

Implantable Loop Recorder

The implantable loop recorder (also called a *loop recorder implant*) is a small recorder (under 2 inches) that looks like a flash drive. It is surgically implanted just under the skin in the upper left chest. It can be implanted in an ambulatory care facility.

Often the device is used for patients who have episodes of fainting, seizures, and palpitations, and other ECG tests have not been able to detect the abnormality. It also catches infrequent arrhythmias that can be missed with traditional ECG monitoring.

The device continuously records the ECG for 2 to 3 years. It records the ECG if the heart rate falls below or rises above the preset limits (set by the provider). The patient can also record the ECG if symptoms are experienced. The provider can download the saved ECG data at the next appointment.

Transtelephonic Monitoring

A transtelephonic monitor (TTM) is a small device that records a patient's ECG when the patient pushes the activation button. The TTM has four electrodes on the back of the device that can record a single lead. The ECG data is sent via phone to the base station at the provider's office. The signal is converted to a readable tracing that can be displayed on a monitor or printed out. There are two types of TTMs:

- *TTM with internal memory*: The ECG is recorded and stored when the patient pushes a button. The data can be transmitted by phone to the provider. This type of TTM is used for patients with infrequent arrhythmias.
- *TTM with no internal memory*: The TTM is placed over the heart, and the phone receiver is placed over the TTM. Once the activation button is pushed, the TTM records and immediately sends the live ECG to the provider via the phone line. The data is not saved in the device. This type of TTM is used for patients with pacemakers and internal cardioverter-defibrillators. It allows the provider to monitor the patient remotely.

Portable Handheld ECG Monitors

There are a variety of portable handheld ECG monitors on the market. Many produce a single lead. The ECG data can then be transferred to other devices using software, Bluetooth, smart phones, or USB ports. These devices are marketed to be used at home. A person can use the device and save ECG tracings. The tracings can then be reviewed by the person's provider at the next visit. The machines work differently; some having several electrode options. Finger contact, chest contact (bare skin just below the nipple), and regular chest electrodes can be used to create an ECG tracing.

CRITICAL THINKING APPLICATION   11.10

Monique Jones is Eva's last patient before lunch. As Eva is gathering Monique's history, Monique mentions that she has heart palpitations. She had heard about ECG monitors that could be used at home. She was able to order one off the internet and was able to capture her palpitation spell. She is here today to show the doctor her monitor results. Eva has never heard of such a thing. How might she respond to the patient?

CLOSING COMMENTS

Patient Coaching

For any cardiac procedures that patients need to undergo, it is important for the medical assistant to coach the patient on the required preparation. The medical assistant should instruct the patient what to expect during the test and then explain any follow-up required. Explaining procedures to patients can help to reduce the stress and confusion they experience.

Legal and Ethical Issues

When a medical assistant is performing an ECG, it is important that the electrodes and lead wires are placed on the patient correctly. If lead wires are switched, the ECG tracing may look abnormal. This can lead to more cardiac testing and additional provider visits. The medical assistant has a professional responsibility to perform ECGs accurately, so the patient receives the best possible care.

Patient-Centered Care

When a patient is undergoing cardiac testing to rule out or rule in a heart condition, it can be a stressful experience. It is important for the medical assistant to be sensitive to the patient's concerns and feelings. Questions from the patient and family members should be addressed, and any questions outside of the medical assistant's scope of practice should be directed to the provider.

The medical assistant should provide the patient with clear directions on the cardiac procedure being done. After the procedure, the medical assistant should let the patient know who will contact him or her about the test results. If possible, give the patient the timeline of when to anticipate the notification.

Professional Behaviors

Many times, patients may think that the medical assistant can read ECGs. They may ask the medical assistant if everything looks all right or if the ECG is normal. It is outside of the medical assistant's scope of practice to read ECGs. This is the role of the provider. The medical assistant should explain to the patient that the provider will read the ECG and the patient will be informed of the results. A medical assistant should refrain from adding in false hope comments, such as "I am sure the ECG will be normal." These types of comments may give the patient a false impression of the results, and the medical assistant's behavior is unprofessional.

SUMMARY OF SCENARIO

Renee is enjoying working with Eva. They have seen many different cardiac tests while working with Dr. Kahn's patients. Renee has found herself learning new things. If she does not have the answers to Eva's questions about cardiac tests, she looks up the information. She finds herself learning new information as a result.

Eva is really enjoying working with Renee and Dr. Kahn. She is feeling so much better performing ECGs. Her understanding of the ECG tracing and how to resolve artifact has greatly improved. She is also feeling more confident performing cardiac testing. She is hoping to be able to work with Dr. Kahn in the future, because she enjoys ECGs so much!

SUMMARY OF LEARNING OBJECTIVES

1. **Review the structures and functionality of the cardiovascular system.**

   The heart is divided into four chambers. Two atrial chambers receive the blood from the body. Two ventricular chambers pump blood out to the body. The septum divides the right and left sides of the heart. The tricuspid valve is found between the right atrium and the right ventricle. The pulmonary valve is between the right ventricle and the pulmonary artery. The bicuspid or mitral valve is found between the left atrium and left ventricle. The aortic valve is between the left ventricle and the aorta. When the valves open, blood moves to the next chamber, or out of the heart through the arteries.

   The conduction system is made up of the SA node, AV node, bundle of His, right and left bundle branches, and the Purkinje fibers. The cardiac cells cycle through the polarized, depolarized, and repolarized states.

2. **Use correct electrocardiography (ECG) terminology.**

   Common ECG terminology includes:

   - *Isoelectric line:* A straight line that represents a period of time with no electrical activity
   - *Deflection:* Any movement away from the baseline in the tracing
   - *Wave:* A deflection from the baseline
   - *Complex:* A form made up of many waves
   - *Segment:* A part of a line between two points
   - *Interval:* A period of time between two points or events

3. **Discuss ECG waves, segments, and intervals.**

   The components of the ECG tracing are:

   - P wave: Shows atrial depolarization; atrial chambers contract and the blood is pushed to the ventricles
   - PR segment: Isoelectric line; allows the atria to finish contracting
   - QRS complex: Shows ventricular depolarization; atrial repolarization also occurs during this time, though it is hidden. The ventricles contract, pushing blood out of the heart.
   - ST segment: Isoelectric line; allows the ventricles to finish contracting
   - T wave: Ventricular repolarization and atrial polarization

   The *PR interval* starts at the beginning of the P wave and ends at the start of the Q wave. It represents atrial depolarization. The *QT interval* starts at the beginning of the Q wave and extends to the end of the T wave. During the QT interval, the atrial chambers move from repolarization to the polarized state. The ventricular chambers depolarize and then move into the repolarized state.

4. **Describe the medical assistant's role in a resting 12-lead ECG.**

   The medical assistant is responsible for assembling the supplies and equipment needed, preparing the patient for the test, and performing the test. Before the medical assistant finishes the procedure, the ECG tracing must be examined for artifact. If any artifact is present on the tracing, the medical assistant must problem-solve the situation.

5. **Describe the bipolar (standard) leads, augmented leads, and chest (precordial) leads.**

   For a resting 12-lead ECG, three leads are bipolar, three are augmented, and the remaining six are precordial. The bipolar leads are created from a measurement of current traveling from a negative pole to the positive pole:

   - Lead I: Right arm (RA) to left arm (LA)
   - Lead II: Right arm (RA) to left leg (LL)
   - Lead III: Left leg (LL) to left arm (LA)

   Each augmented lead uses all three extremity electrodes (RA, LA, and LL) to create the picture. Midpoint between two of the electrodes is the negative pole. The precordial leads provide information on the horizontal (front to back) plane of the heart. The six precordial leads are labeled V_1, V_2, V_3, V_4, V_5, and V_6.

6. **Prepare a patient for an ECG and obtain an electrocardiogram.**

   Procedure 11.1 on p. 284 describes the process of obtaining an ECG.

7. **Troubleshoot artifacts in an ECG.**

   Wandering baseline artifact is an upward and downward movement of the waveform. The medical assistant should clean the skin, replace the electrode with a new one, make sure all electrodes and lead wires are firmly attached, and turn on the baseline filter.

   Somatic tremor artifact appears as jagged peaks with irregular heights and spacing. The medical assistant should help the patient relax and encourage him or her not to talk or move during the procedure.

   AC interference artifact appears as a series of small spikes that creates a thick-looking tracing. The medical assistant should unplug the ECG machine and other electrical devices. The lead wires should not overlap, and no cell phones should be near the patient.

   Interrupted baseline artifact (also called *intermittent signal artifact*) occurs when the tracing looks normal at the beginning, but then it disappears or goes all over when the electrical connection is interrupted. The medical assistant should check that all electrodes and lead wires are attached.

8. **Identify abnormal rhythms in an ECG tracing.**

   A sinus rhythm is considered normal. Alterations of the sinus rhythm include sinus bradycardia and sinus tachycardia. Atrial arrhythmias occur when there is a problem with the SA node starting the impulse. Atrial arrhythmias include PACs and atrial flutter. A heart block occurs when there is a disruption or slowing of the electrical impulse through the heart. Ventricular arrhythmias are abnormalities in the ventricles and include PVCs, V-tach, V-fib, and asystole.

9. **Discuss additional ECG tests.**

   This chapter discussed additional ECG tests, including exercise stress tests, nuclear stress tests, Holter monitors, cardiac event recorders, implantable loop recorders, transtelephonic monitoring, and portable handheld ECG monitors. See the chapter sections for more information on these tests.

PROCEDURE 11.1   Perform Electrocardiography

Tasks: Perform electrocardiography and routine maintenance on the machine. Document the procedure in the patient's health record. Show awareness of a patient's concerns and incorporate critical thinking skills when performing patient care.

EQUIPMENT and SUPPLIES

- ECG machine
- Disposable electrodes
- ECG paper
- Alcohol pads
- Razor (optional)
- Gauze pads (optional)
- Patient gown or paper cape
- Tissue
- Disinfecting wipes
- Gloves
- Waste container
- Patient's health record

PROCEDURAL STEPS

1. Wash hands or use hand sanitizer.
   PURPOSE: Hand sanitization is an important step for infection control.
2. Assemble equipment and supplies needed for the ECG procedure. Plug in and turn on the ECG machine. Verify that the standardization and chart/paper speed are correct.
   PURPOSE: Having the equipment ready helps reduce the patient's wait time.
3. Greet the patient. Identify yourself. Verify the patient's identity with full name and date of birth. Explain the procedure to be performed in a manner that is understood by the patient. Answer any questions the patient may have on the procedure.
   PURPOSE: It is important to identify the patient in two different ways to ensure that you have the correct patient. Explaining the procedure can make the patient feel more comfortable and helps to reduce anxiety.
   Scenario update: The patient states that she is really worried that something is wrong with her heart. She states that she is really nervous about having an ECG.
4. Using therapeutic communication techniques (e.g., reflection, restatement, and summarizing), show the patient you are aware of his concerns.
   PURPOSE: Using therapeutic communication techniques can be helpful to show patients you hear their concerns. It also always helps the medical assistant to clarify the patient's concerns.
5. Ask the patient to remove all clothing from the waist up, including undergarments, and put on the gown/cape so that the opening is in the front. Ask the patient if assistance is needed. If so, provide help. If not, leave the room and allow the patient time to change. When reentering the room, provide a courtesy knock on the door.
   PURPOSE: The patient needs to be undressed from the waist up for you to place the electrodes. Patients require privacy to change.

6. Assist the patient into a comfortable supine position on the exam table. Provide support for the legs and arms.
   PURPOSE: To reduce artifact on the tracing, the patient must be comfortable, and the extremities need to be supported.
7. Identify the locations for the ECG electrodes on the chest. Prepare the skin. If the patient has a hairy chest, get the person's permission prior to shaving the areas (optional). Wipe each spot with alcohol and allow it to dry. Fold the gauze pad over your index finger and briskly rub the site to abrade the skin (optional).
   PURPOSE: The alcohol will prepare the skin and help the electrode adhere to the skin.
8. Correctly apply the six chest electrodes. If using tab electrodes, the tabs should be pointed toward the waist.
   PURPOSE: Having the tabs face the core of the body will help reduce the tension on the lead wires when they are attached.
9. Identify the locations for the ECG electrodes on the extremities. Refer to the operating manual for the arm electrode position if needed. Wipe each spot with alcohol and allow it to dry. Correctly apply the four limb electrodes to nonbony areas. If using tab electrodes, the lower leg tabs should point toward the waist. The arm/wrist tabs should point toward the fingers.
   PURPOSE: The alcohol will prepare the skin and help the electrode adhere to the skin.
10. Attach the correct lead wire to each of the electrodes (see the following figure). The wires should follow the natural contour of the body and not overlap other wires.
    PURPOSE: Overlapping wires can cause artifact.

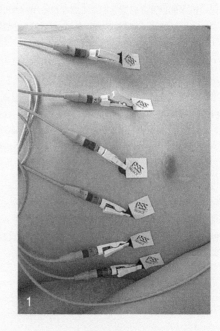

PROCEDURE 11.1   **Perform Electrocardiography**—*continued*

---

11. Enter the patient's data into the ECG machine. Identify any changes with the default settings, electrode position, or patient's position.
    <u>PURPOSE:</u> The ECG tracing needs to be labeled with the patient's identifying information. The provider must be aware of any changes in the procedure. Electrode position changes, chart/paper speed, and so on can change the appearance of the tracing.

12. Double-check that the lead wires are in the correct position and attached to the electrodes. Make sure each electrode is attached to the skin. Take any corrective action necessary.
    <u>PURPOSE:</u> The lead wires and electrodes must be in the correct spot and attached for the tracing to be accurate.

13. Instruct the patient to lie still and not to talk during the tracing. Tell the patient how long the tracing will take.
    <u>PURPOSE:</u> Talking and moving during the tracing will create artifact.

14. Verify that the filter(s) are on. Check the leads on the screen or monitor. Based on what is observed, use critical thinking skills and take any corrective action necessary. Run the tracing when the leads look clear and without artifact.
    <u>PURPOSE:</u> The filters will minimize the artifact. Checking the appearance of the leads helps to identify if corrective action is needed to minimize artifact.

15. Check the tracing for clarity, artifact, and abnormal life-threatening rhythms. Based on what is observed, use critical thinking skills and take any action necessary.
    <u>PURPOSE:</u> The provider will need a clear tracing. Life-threatening rhythms need to be identified and the provider needs to be told immediately.

16. Disconnect the lead wires and remove the electrodes. Wipe any residue from the patient's skin. Wash your hands or use hand sanitizer. Instruct the patient to get dressed. Ask the patient if assistance is needed. If so, help the patient to dress.
    <u>PURPOSE:</u> The medical assistant must be the one to remove the wires and electrodes.

17. Provide the patient with information about following up with the provider. Complete any necessary actions with the ECG (e.g., upload to the electronic health record, mount and route to the provider).
    <u>PURPOSE:</u> After tests, patients will want to know what the results are. The provider will need to read the tracing before any results are given to the patient.

18. Document accurately in the patient's health record. Indicate the provider ordering the test, what test was performed, how the patient tolerated the test, and what you did with the ECG tracing. You can also add any instructions you provided to the patient regarding follow-up.
    <u>PURPOSE:</u> Indicating who ordered the test and what was done is important for insurance reimbursement and for legal reasons.
    Scenario update: Perform routine machine maintenance by adding paper to the ECG machine or printer.

19. Review the operator's manual on how to change the paper. Gather the new ream of ECG paper (or roll).
    <u>PURPOSE:</u> The operator's manual will indicate how the paper should be added to the machine.

20. Open the machine. Remove the remaining paper and add the new paper per the steps in the manual.
    <u>PURPOSE:</u> It is important to remove the last few sheets of the old paper to make room for the new ream.

21. Put on gloves and disinfect the lead wires per the operator's manual. Disinfect the exam table. Clean up the work area. Remove the gloves. Wash your hands or use hand sanitizer.
    <u>PURPOSE:</u> For infection control purposes, it is important to disinfect the lead wires and exam table between each use.

08/06/20XX 1423 Per Dr. James Martin's order, a resting 12-lead ECG was performed. Pt tolerated the procedure well. Pt was instructed to call the clinic tomorrow for the ECG results. The ECG tracing was routed to Dr. Martin.
_____Eva Ning, RMA

PROCEDURE 11.2   **Apply a Holter Monitor**

Tasks: Apply a Holter monitor and coach a patient on the procedure. Document the procedure in the patient's health record.

EQUIPMENT and SUPPLIES

- Holter monitor, new batteries, flash memory card (if required), carrying case, and operator's manual
- Disposable electrodes
- Razor
- Sharps container
- Alcohol pads
- Gauze pads (optional)

- Cloth nonallergenic tape (optional)
- Journal
- Waste container
- Patient's health record

PROCEDURAL STEPS

1. Wash hands or use hand sanitizer.
   <u>PURPOSE:</u> Hand sanitization is an important step for infection control.

Continued

PROCEDURE 11.2   Apply a Holter Monitor—*continued*

2. Assemble equipment and supplies needed for the procedure. Insert flash memory card if required. Insert new batteries into the monitor (see the following figure). Consult the operator's manual for the required amount and placement of electrodes.
   PURPOSE: Having the equipment ready helps reduce the patient's wait time. New batteries will ensure accurate functioning.

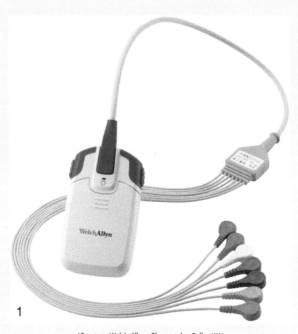

1

(Courtesy Welch Allyn, Skaneateles Falls, NY.)

3. Greet the patient. Identify yourself. Verify the patient's identity with full name and date of birth. Explain the procedure to be performed in a manner that is understood by the patient. Answer any questions the patient may have on the procedure.
   PURPOSE: It is important to identify the patient in two different ways to ensure that you have the correct patient. Explaining the procedure can make the patient feel more comfortable and helps to reduce anxiety.

4. Ask the patient to remove clothing from the waist up and to sit at the end of the exam table. Ask the patient if assistance is needed. If so, help. If not, leave the room and allow the patient time to change. When reentering the room, provide a courtesy knock on the door.
   PURPOSE: The patient needs to be undressed from the waist up for you to place the electrodes. Patients require privacy to change.

5. Identify the locations for the electrodes and prepare the skin for the electrodes. Shave the area if the patient has a hairy chest. Wipe the area with the alcohol pad and allow it to dry. Fold the gauze pad over your index finger and briskly rub the site to abrade the skin (see the following figure).
   PURPOSE: These techniques help the electrodes to better adhere to the skin, which creates a better tracing.

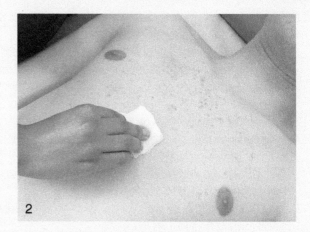

2

6. Snap the lead wire onto the electrode. Apply the electrodes to the sites as indicated by the manufacturer. Press firmly and make sure the entire electrode adheres completely to the skin (see the following figure).
   PURPOSE: Secure electrode attachment is necessary to produce an accurate tracing.

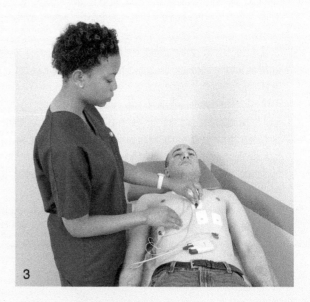

3

7. Loop and tape down the wires on the chest.
   PURPOSE: The tape will hold the wires in place and reduce the tension on the electrodes.

8. Attach the patient cable to the monitor if required. Turn on the recorder and set as indicated by the manufacturer. Enter the patient data as indicated.
   PURPOSE: Each manufacturer will have directions to operate the monitor.

9. Have the patient get dressed. Assist as needed.
   PURPOSE: Some patients may require assistance when hooked up to the monitor.

10. Coach the patient regarding making journal entries while wearing the monitor. Provide the required patient education.
    PURPOSE: It is important for the patient to keep a diary of what he or she is doing. The provider will check the ECG for abnormalities and then check what the patient was doing during the event.

PROCEDURE 11.2 Apply a Holter Monitor—*continued*

11. Assist the patient in scheduling a return appointment in 24 hours. Provide the patient with contact information should a question arise.
    PURPOSE: The patient will need to return in 24 hours for the monitor to be removed. Providing contact information will help reduce the patient's anxiety.

12. Document accurately in the patient's health record. Indicate the provider ordering the test, the procedure done, patient education provided, and return appointment.
    PURPOSE: Indicating who ordered the test and what was done is important for insurance reimbursement and for legal reasons.

08/06/20XX 1423 Per Dr. James Martin's order, a Holter monitor was applied. Pt was instructed how to complete the diary, and a contact number was provided if pt has additional questions. Pt verbalized what he was to write in the diary. Appointment was made for 08/07/20XX to remove the monitor.
_____ Eva Ning, RMA

12

MEDICAL EMERGENCIES

SCENARIO

Gabe Garcia, CMA (AAMA), has worked for Walden-Martin Family Medical (WMFM) Clinic for 4 years. He was hired right after he completed his medical assistant program. Gabe has learned a lot through the years. He has impressed his supervisor with his dedication, attention to detail, punctuality, and patient care skills. Gabe was just promoted to a medical assistant lead position. In this new position, Gabe has additional responsibilities. He will now oversee the crash carts in the clinic, and he will train staff on emergency procedures.

The current emergency procedures need to be revised, and the crash cart procedures need updating. Gabe is excited to take over his new responsibilities. He looks forward to what he will learn in this new role.

While studying this chapter, think about the following questions:
- How are emergencies handled in ambulatory care settings?
- What are common emergency equipment and supplies found in the ambulatory care settings?
- What are first aid actions for cold and heat illnesses, burns, poisonings, anaphylaxis, bites, and foreign bodies in the eye?
- What are first aid actions for diabetic emergencies?
- What are first aid actions for musculoskeletal emergencies?

- What are first aid actions for neurological emergencies, including vertigo, concussion, seizure, and stroke?
- What are first aid actions for respiratory emergencies, including hyperventilation, asthmatic attack, and choking?
- What are first aid actions for cardiovascular emergencies, including syncope, bleeding, shock, and heart attack?

LEARNING OBJECTIVES

1. Discuss emergencies in healthcare settings and possible roles each team member has during an emergency.
2. Describe emergency equipment and supplies.
3. Explain first aid procedures for environmental emergencies, including temperature-related emergencies, burns, poisonings, anaphylaxis, bites and stings, and foreign bodies in the eye.
4. Discuss diabetic emergencies and provide first aid for a patient in insulin shock.

5. Discuss musculoskeletal and neurological emergencies and provide first aid for a patient with seizure activity.
6. Discuss respiratory emergencies and provide first aid for a choking patient.
7. Discuss cardiovascular emergencies and provide first aid for a patient with a bleeding wound, fracture, or syncope; a patient in shock; and a patient in need of rescue breathing or cardiopulmonary resuscitation (CPR).

VOCABULARY

cardiopulmonary resuscitation (ri sus i TAY shun) (CPR) The application of manual chest compressions and ventilations (also called *rescue breathing*) to patients who are not breathing or do not have a pulse; also known as *basic life support* (BLS).

code A term used in healthcare settings to indicate an emergency situation and to summon the trained team to the scene.

concussion (kuhn KUSH uhn) A traumatic brain injury caused by a blow to the head.

endotracheal (en doe TRAY kee al) (ET) tube A catheter that is inserted into the trachea through the mouth; provides a patent airway.

erythema (er ee THEE mah) Redness.

intraosseous (in tra OS ee us) Within bone; route for delivery of fluids and medications through a needle inserted into the marrow of certain bones (e.g., humerus, tibia, and femur).

nasopharyngeal (nae zoe fah RIN jee ahl) airway (NPA) A soft flexible tube that is inserted in the nose and provides a patent airway; also known as a *nasal trumpet*.

necrosis (neh KROH sis) Tissue death.

patent (PAY tent) Open.

pocket face mask A device used to deliver a rescue breath.

pruritus (proo RIE tuss) Itching.

recovery position A position on the person's side that helps to keep the airway open and clear.

retractions (re TRAK shuns) The sucking in of tissues between the intercostal spaces and neck due to respiratory distress; classic sign of severe asthma.

standard of care The level and type of care an ordinary, prudent healthcare professional with the same training and experience in a similar practice would have provided under a similar situation.

triage (tree AHZH) To sort out and classify the injured; used in the military and emergency settings to determine the priority of a patient to be treated.

triaging flow map A written flow map to make triage decisions; based on answers to questions, the person moves through the map until a triage decision is made.

vasoconstriction Contraction of the muscles, causing narrowing of the inside tube of the vessel.

vertigo (VER ti goe) Sensation that causes someone to feel as though everything is spinning.

Emergencies happen everywhere. As a medical assistant, it is important for you to know how to handle emergencies because you may need to respond to one:

- *Outside of your job, in the community.* You may be one of the first people on the scene and need to provide first aid to the victims.
- *In the healthcare setting.* You may need to provide first aid as the provider assesses the injured person. Additional treatments, such as oxygen and medications, are provided in the healthcare setting.
- *Over the phone.* You may need to obtain information from someone involved in an emergency and provide first aid coaching. The medical assistant asks screening questions and provides the information to the provider. The provider instructs the medical assistant what to tell the caller.

This chapter starts by discussing emergencies in the healthcare setting and the medical assistant's role. Next, common emergency medical equipment, supplies, and medications are explained. Lastly, emergency conditions are described, along with the first aid procedures to perform.

EMERGENCIES IN HEALTHCARE SETTINGS

Every employee in a healthcare setting should know how to get help in an emergency. This process will vary. Healthcare facilities use special phrases for emergencies. For instance, "Code Blue Urgent Care" may indicate that an emergency is occurring in Urgent Care. Sometimes the **code** words indicate the age of the person. For instance, "Code Pink Family Practice" may mean that an emergency is occurring in Family Practice and "pink" indicates a child.

Once the call goes out for help, staff members respond to the scene. In small settings, most members of the staff may be needed. In large facilities, only certain staff members respond. Usually, medical assistants, licensed practical nurses (LPNs), registered nurses (RNs), and providers attend the emergency. Possible roles for each team member include:

- *Provider:* Assesses the patient, orders treatments and procedures, performs advanced procedures, may administer intravenous (IV) medications, and indicates when 911 needs to be called.
- *Nurse:* Registered nurses (RNs) administer intravenous (IV) medications and fluids. Licensed practical nurses (LPNs) may do the same if permitted by the state's scope of practice. RNs and LPNs assist with treatments and procedures, perform **cardiopulmonary**

resuscitation (CPR), call 911, and document the code activities as they occur.

- *Clinical medical assistant:* Assists with treatments and procedures, performs CPR, documents the code activities as they occur, and calls 911. He or she may hand supplies to staff members and assist with caring for the family (moving them to a private area away from the emergency).
- *Administrative medical assistant:* Performs CPR and hands supplies to the staff (in small agencies), calls 911, escorts the emergency responders to the patient, and assists with caring for the family.

Importance of Documentation

In a code situation, it is important that at least one team member document everything that occurs. This is a stressful job because many things are occurring during an emergency. There are several reasons why accurate documentation is critical.

- The information is used during the code. For instance, CPR was started, and the team member documented "1413 CPR initiated." As the code progresses, the provider may want to know when the CPR was started.
- Emergency responders will need to know what occurred during the code. (What medications were given? When were they given? How much was given?)
- The documentation will provide evidence that the **standard of care** was met in the treatments given to the patient. Many lawsuits have originated from emergencies. The lawyers review the documentation. They look for delays in emergency care and lack of appropriate treatment. Complete and accurate documentation may make a difference between a lawsuit surviving and being dismissed in favor of the healthcare team.

If you are new to codes and if given the option, perform a role other than documenting. Observe what occurs during a code as you complete your task. Study the code documentation form during noncode times. As you become more comfortable with codes, assist the documenter if you can. A second pair of eyes is always helpful. Lastly, become the documenter and have a seasoned team member assist you.

CRITICAL THINKING APPLICATION   12.1

Currently, the clinic does not have a procedure for documenting during code situations. The provider documents after the emergency. Gabe would like to discuss using a standard code form for all emergencies. A team member would be responsible for documenting during the code. Discuss the pros and cons of documenting during the code.

EMERGENCY EQUIPMENT AND SUPPLIES

The emergency supplies available at healthcare facilities will vary based on the size and location of the facility. Some practices have a small box that contains a few supplies and medications. Other practices place many crash carts throughout the building (Fig. 12.1). A *crash cart* is a rolling supply cart that contains emergency equipment.

The crash cart should be checked monthly. This can be done by the supervisor or by two qualified employees (e.g., medical assistants, LPNs, or RNs). Expiration dates on the supplies are checked. Old supplies are replaced with new supplies. All the equipment and supplies are inventoried. When the inventory is completed, a plastic lock (or locking tag) is placed on the cart. The crash cart is used only in emergencies. You should never break the lock and use something from the crash cart unless it is an emergency. The plastic locks should be kept safe and used only when the cart is inventoried monthly or after an emergency. Many of the locks are numbered, and the number is written on the inventory document. Keeping the locks safe minimizes the number of people going into the crash cart for nonemergency reasons.

This section will focus on the equipment and supplies typically found on a crash cart. The medical assistant should be familiar with the supplies and their location within the crash cart.

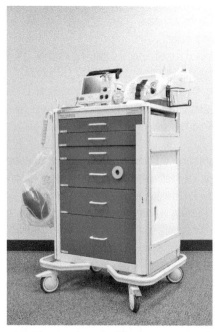

FIGURE 12.1 Crash carts are used in an emergency. The drawers should be labeled to allow speedy retrieval of supplies.

Oxygen and Airway Supplies

Oxygen and airway supplies are common items found on crash carts. If the patient needs oxygen, the provider will order oxygen to be applied via a mask or a nasal cannula. (Refer to Chapter 25 for additional information on oxygen delivery systems.)

If the patient has difficulty breathing or if an airway constriction may be occurring, the provider will insert a **nasopharyngeal airway** or an **endotracheal (ET) tube** to create a **patent** airway (Fig. 12.2). Providers also use the following to maintain airways:

- *Esophageal tracheal tubes*, which are placed in the trachea or esophagus
- *Laryngeal mask airways*, which are inserted through the mouth and advanced to the hypopharynx
- *Laryngeal tubes*, which are also inserted through the mouth and placed in the hypopharynx

Endotracheal Tube Intubation

The medical assistant should be aware of the equipment required during an ET tube intubation. During an endotracheal intubation, the provider will need the following:

- *Laryngoscope* with either a curved (MacIntosh) or straight (Miller) blade. The sizes of blades are indicated on the side or back of the blade (Fig. 12.3A). The medical assistant must hand the laryngoscope with the blade attached to the provider (Fig. 12.3B).
- ET tube in the appropriate size. Cuffed ET tubes come in a variety of sizes for adults and older children (e.g., 7.5, 8, and 8.5). Uncuffed ET tubes come in a variety of sizes for children (e.g., 2.5, 3, and 3.5) (Fig. 12.4). A syringe is used to inflate the cuff with air once it is in place.
- *Stylet* is a metal or flexible plastic wire inserted into the ET tube to create a firm, curved tube (see Fig. 12.4). After the ET tube is in place, the stylet is removed.
- Ambu-bag, which is attached to the ET tube and used to administer room air or oxygen (Fig. 12.5). An Ambu-bag can cover the mouth or be attached to an airway tube (e.g., endotracheal tube). Ambu-bags can come with oxygen tubing

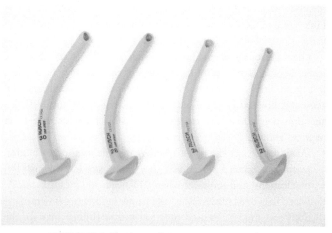

FIGURE 12.2 Nasopharyngeal airways come in a variety of sizes.

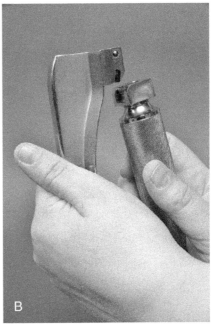

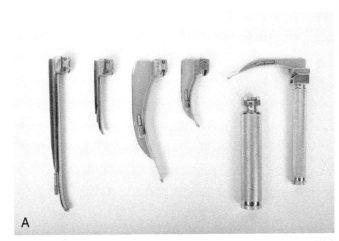

FIGURE 12.3 (A) *Left to right:* Two different sizes of straight blades and curved blades; adult laryngoscope handle and an assembled pediatric laryngoscope. A curved or straight blade must be attached to the laryngoscope handle. **(B)** To attach the blade, hold the blade parallel to the handle and attach.

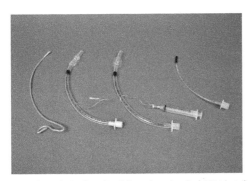

FIGURE 12.4 *Left to right:* A stylet is threaded into the endotracheal (ET) tube to help maintain the tube's curve. ET tubes for adults are cuffed (or have a balloon that is inflated using a syringe). ET tubes for children are uncuffed *(far right).* ET tubes come in a variety of sizes.

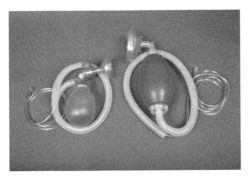

FIGURE 12.5 *Left to right:* Pediatric and adult Ambu-bags.

attached, which can be connected to an oxygen tank. Oxygen can be administered during the ventilation.

• Stethoscope. Once the tube is in place, a team member will provide ventilation with the Ambu-bag. The provider must ensure the ET tube is in the correct location by listening over the lung field for air movement. If the ET tube is in the wrong location, the abdomen will become bloated with air. The patient is then not being ventilated. (A provider will usually state that breath sounds are heard bilaterally. This is important to document on the code form. This verifies the ET tube is in the correct location.)

CRITICAL THINKING APPLICATION   12.2

Gabe has decided that the crash carts must be inventoried monthly. He will have two medical assistants inventory each cart. Gabe feels it is important that all medical assistants have an opportunity to inventory the crash cart at least every 4 months. Why would this be important for the medical assistants? Besides checking expiration dates, what else could they do to increase their skills and knowledge for emergencies?

Defibrillator

A *defibrillator* is a device that delivers an electrical shock to the heart muscle in an attempt to restore a normal heartbeat. The defibrillator's shock causes the heart to momentarily stop. When it restarts, the hope is the heart will beat at a normal rhythm. The quicker a defibrillator can be used, the better the person's chances of survival.

Typically, a defibrillator or an automated external defibrillator (AED) is used in healthcare facilities.

• A defibrillator consists of two handheld paddles that are placed on gel pads located on the patient's chest (Fig. 12.6). Gel pads are required to prevent burns. They provide better electricity conduction from the paddles to the patient. The provider indicates how many joules at which to set the machine, and someone announces "All clear" to ensure no one is touching the patient. The provider pushes the button to give the shock.

- An *automated external defibrillator* is a portable, lightweight machine (Fig. 12.7). Sticky pads that contain electrodes (sensors) are attached to the patient's chest. The AED checks the heart rate and determines if a shock is required. If a shock is needed, the AED gives audible directions to the user to administer a shock.

Medications

The medications in crash carts can vary. Common medications used in emergencies are listed in Table 12.1. Most crash carts and emergency

supply boxes include intravenous (IV) supplies. An IV is usually inserted into the hand, wrist, or arm of the patient. If an IV line cannot be inserted, the provider may insert an **intraosseous** needle that can be used to give IV fluids and medications (Fig. 12.8). The intraosseous needle can be inserted into the humerus, tibia, femur,

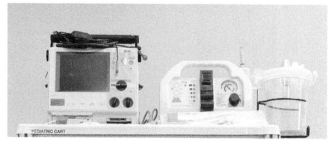

FIGURE 12.6 *Left to right:* The defibrillator usually sits on top of the crash cart. Other equipment, such as a suction machine, can also be found on the top of the crash cart.

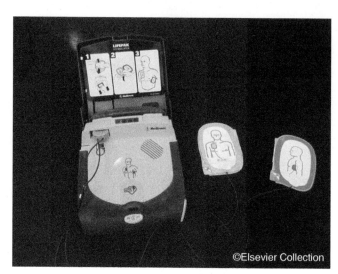

©Elsevier Collection

FIGURE 12.7 Automated external defibrillator.

TABLE 12.1	Common Medications Used in Emergencies	
MEDICATION	**ACTION**	**USED FOR**
amiodarone (Cordarone, Pacerone)	Slows the heart rate and allows blood to fill in the ventricular chambers.	Ventricular tachycardia, ventricular fibrillation
atropine	Increases the heart rate.	Bradycardia
calcium chloride	Increases the calcium levels in the serum.	Hyperkalemia and *hypocalcemia* (too little calcium in the blood)
diazepam (Valium)	Affects the chemicals in the brain.	Seizures, agitation
diphenhydramine (Benadryl)	Antihistamine that reduces the effects of histamine.	Allergic reactions, second-line drug for anaphylaxis (used after epinephrine has been given)
dopamine (Intropin)	Increases the stimulation of the heart muscle	Hypotension, heart failure
epinephrine (Adrenalin)	Increases the stimulation of the heart muscle; vasoconstrictor and bronchial relaxant	Anaphylaxis, cardiac arrest, severe asthma, bronchospasms
glucagon	Hormone that stimulates the liver to release glucose into the blood	*Hypoglycemia* (below-normal glucose in the blood)
lidocaine	Helps to restore the regular heart rhythm	Ventricular arrhythmias
magnesium	Electrolyte that helps maintain a normal heart rhythm	Arrhythmias
naloxone (Evzio, Narcan)	Blocks or reverses opioid medication effects	Opioid (narcotic) overdose
nitroglycerin	Vasodilator	Congestive heart failure, angina
sodium bicarbonate	Decreases the pH of the serum	Metabolic acidosis, *hyperkalemia* (excessive potassium in the blood)

sternum, or iliac crest. The provider must be specially trained to insert the intraosseous needle.

Administering IV medications is outside the scope of practice for the medical assistant. In many states, inserting an IV and giving IV fluids are also outside the medical assistant's scope of practice. The medical assistant may help by getting the required supplies and documenting what was given.

Other Supplies

Various other supplies can be found in the crash cart. Some items not already mentioned include:

- Personal protective equipment (PPE), such as gloves, a sharps disposal container, and a **pocket face mask**
- *Algorithms,* or step-by-step instructions for reference
- Clipboard with documents for charting the code
- Backboard, which is placed under the patient to provide a firm surface for compressions
- Extra batteries for the laryngoscope

Pediatric Supplies

In the 1980s, James Broselow, a family practice doctor working in an emergency department, came up with an idea for simplifying pediatric medication doses administered during emergencies. Medications for children are based on weight. Rescue personnel spent critical moments during emergencies calculating medication doses for children. Broselow's idea was to measure the child's length and come up with

a suggested dose. After much research, the Broselow tape was created (Fig. 12.9A).

A healthcare professional measures a child using the tape. The tape is placed from the top of the head to the child's heel. The length is measured as a specific color (see Fig. 12.9B). Based on the "color" of the child, the tape lists common medication dosages and emergency equipment sizes that should be used for that size of child. This system has sped up the response time for treating children during emergencies. It eliminates the use of reference guides and calculators for medication dosages.

Many ambulatory care settings that routinely see sick children use the Broselow tape. In addition to the tape, pediatric crash carts (Broselow ColorCode Carts) have been created (Fig. 12.10). Each color on the tape has a matching drawer. Each drawer contains the right-sized equipment for that size of child.

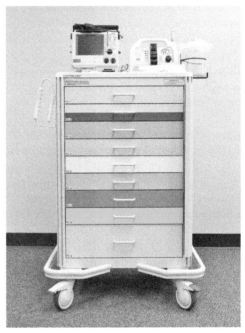

FIGURE 12.10 Each drawer in the Broselow ColorCode Cart is color coded.

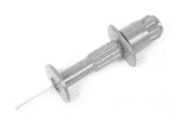

FIGURE 12.8 An intraosseous needle may be used to give IV fluids and medications in an emergency.

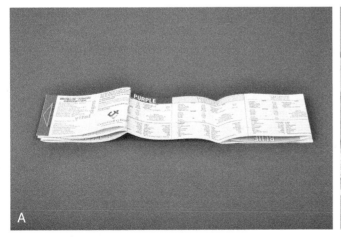
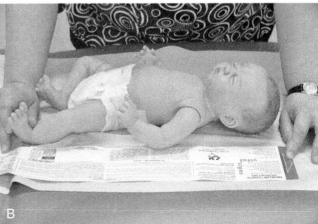

FIGURE 12.9 (A) Broselow tape. **(B)** Measure the child with the Broselow tape. Measure from the head to the heel and identify the color by the child's heel. This is the color to use during the emergency.

HANDLING EMERGENCIES

In the ambulatory care setting, many different types of emergencies can occur. Some of the more common emergencies include these:

- A patient who is being seen and treated has a life-threatening occurrence (e.g., an allergic reaction to a medication).
- A person (e.g., employee, visitor, or patient) has an accident or health issue that results in an emergency.
- A *walk-in patient* (a patient without an appointment) comes to the facility with a critical health issue.
- An individual calls about an emergency.

How these are handled can differ greatly among ambulatory care facilities. Factors that affect how emergencies are handled include:

- Facility's size and distance from emergency medical services
- Available equipment and supplies
- Providers' training and scope of practice
- Number and type of clinical care employees (medical assistants, licensed practical nurses, and registered nurses) and their scopes of practice

Some facilities only have minimal staff, whereas others have specific employees who respond to emergencies.

In small facilities, the medical assistant may be responsible for screening emergency calls and walk-in patients. The medical assistant must follow the facility's screening protocols. She or he cannot assess the patient or give advice. The information collected must be reported to the provider. The provider tells the medical assistant what should be done. Examples of screening questions are provided later in the chapter.

In larger facilities, registered nurses (sometimes called **triage** *nurses*) gather information from walk-in patients and emergency calls. Using a **triaging flow map** or triaging software, the nurse identifies how quickly the patient needs to be seen and where the patient needs to be seen (Fig. 12.11).

Sometimes patients come to the ambulatory healthcare setting with life-threatening conditions. The provider sees these patients immediately and assesses their conditions. The provider will order 911 to be called if needed. Treatment is provided as the team waits

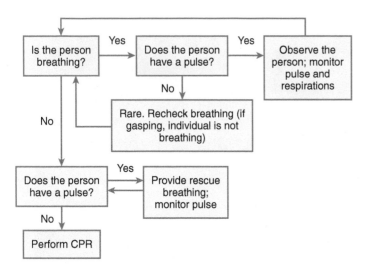

FIGURE 12.11 Example of a flow map. Similar flow maps can be used when triaging or treating emergencies.

for the emergency responders to transport the patient to the emergency department. The following sections explain the first aid given for different types of emergencies.

Environmental Emergencies

Environmental emergencies arise from an exposure to a harmful environmental agent rather than a traumatic injury or medical condition already present in the patient. For instance, the outdoor temperature can cause a life-threatening condition. A bite from certain reptiles can cause death if not treated immediately. A flying piece of metal in a factory can cause blindness. Many environment-related emergencies are severe enough that the affected person seeks medical care.

Temperature-Related Emergencies

Overexposure to hot or cold temperatures can cause mild to life-threatening issues. Environmental temperatures affect the body's temperature.

Cold-Related Conditions. Cold-related conditions include frostbite and hypothermia. In cold weather, our bodies tend to lose heat faster than we can produce it. This results in a lowered body temperature. Uncovered skin can result in injuries faster than covered skin. It does not take long for frostbite to occur. For instance, with a 10-mile-per-hour (mph) wind speed and a temperature of −5°F (−20.6°C), a person can get frostbite in 30 minutes. With the same wind speed and a temperature of −25°F (−31.7°C), a person can get frostbite in 5 minutes.

Possible screening questions for cold-related conditions include:

- What is the person's age?
- How long was the person exposed to the cold temperature?
- What symptoms does the person have? What color is the exposed skin?
- What is the person's medical history?

Table 12.2 describes frostbite and hypothermia. With severe hypothermia, an individual can develop arrhythmias. Medical attention is critical. Warming a patient with hypothermia too quickly can also lead to cardiac issues and additional tissue damage. Because of this, the emergency department gradually warms all patients with hypothermia.

Heat-Related Conditions. Heat injuries occur most often on hot, humid days. Heat-related conditions include cramps, exhaustion, and stroke (Table 12.3).

Possible screening questions for heat-related conditions include:

- What is the person's age?
- How long was the person exposed to the hot temperature?
- What symptoms does the person have? Is the person sweating? What does the skin look like? Is the person alert or confused?

It is important to treat heat-related illnesses immediately. An untreated condition can progress to become a more severe situation.

TABLE 12.2	Cold-Related Conditions	
CONDITION	**FROSTBITE**	**HYPOTHERMIA**
Description	Occurs when the skin and body tissues are exposed to cold temperatures. Susceptible areas include cheeks, nose, ears, fingers, toes, and chin.	Core body temperature drops to below 95°F (35°C). In severe hypothermia, the body temperature drops to 82° F (27.8°C), causing a life-threatening condition.
Etiology and Risk Factors	Caused by exposure to cold temperatures. Risk factors include: • Smoking or taking a beta-blocker medication (e.g., atenolol) • Having diabetes or poor blood circulation • High winds, wet clothes	Caused by exposure to cold temperatures or immersion in cold water for a long period of time. Risk factors include those for frostbite; also dehydration and exhaustion.
Signs and Symptoms	Pins-and-needles sensation followed by numbness; hard, pale, cold skin; aching or lack of feeling in area; blisters.	Slurred speech; slow, shallow breathing and weak pulse; clumsy, drowsy, confused, loss of consciousness; bright red, cold skin (seen in infants).
First Aid Procedures	• Move the person to a warmer location. • Remove all wet clothing and cover with warm dry clothing. • Observe for signs of hypothermia. • Seek medical care; if not available, then rewarm the area by soaking in warm water (104°–108°F [40°–42.2°C]) for 20–30 minutes. Do not rub the area. Apply sterile dressing to area. • Give the person a warm drink to replace lost fluids; do not give alcohol.	• Move the person to a warmer location. • Remove all wet clothing and cover with warm dry clothing. • Seek medical care. • Give the person a warm drink to replace lost fluids; do not give alcohol.

TABLE 12.3	Heat-Related Conditions		
CONDITION	**HEAT CRAMPS**	**HEAT EXHAUSTION**	**HEAT STROKE**
Description	Mild heat-related illness that causes muscle pains and spasms due to electrolyte imbalance. Usually occurs with strenuous activities or in those who sweat a lot.	Milder form of heat-related illness. Due to exposure to high temperatures and inadequate fluid and electrolyte replacement.	Most serious heat-related illness. Body is unable to sweat and thus cannot cool down.
Etiology and Risk Factors	Caused by prolonged heat exposure. With high humidity, sweat, which cools the skin, does not evaporate as quickly. Risk factors include: • Age (older adults and children age 4 and younger) • Fever, dehydration, heart disease, poor blood circulation • Mental illness, sunburn; using alcohol • Prescription drugs (e.g., antidepressants, anticonvulsants, antipsychotics, and diuretics)		
Signs and Symptoms	• Muscle pains or spasms in the abdomen, arms, or legs.	• Heavy sweating, muscle cramps • Cool, moist skin • Fast, weak pulse; fast, shallow respirations • Tired, weak, pale • Dizzy, headache, fainting • Nausea, vomiting	• Body temperature over 103°F (39°C) • Red, hot, dry skin • Rapid, strong pulse • Dizzy, throbbing headache, nausea • Confusion, unconsciousness
First Aid Procedures	• Rest for several hours in a cool place. • Drink cool electrolyte (sports) beverages to replace electrolytes lost. • Do not drink caffeinated or alcoholic beverages, which can cause dehydration.	• Move to a shady or air-conditioned area and rest. • Drink cool sports beverages. • Do not drink caffeinated or alcoholic beverages. • Take a cool shower or sponge bath.	• Move the person to a shady or air-conditioned area. • Spray or sponge the person down with cool water. • Seek medical attention immediately.

An effective way to lower the person's temperature is to apply cool, wet cloths and then fan the moist skin. This will lower the person's body temperature by the evaporation process.

Burns

Heat, freezing cold temperatures, chemicals, sunlight, radiation, and electricity can cause burns to the body tissue. Hot liquids, fires, and flammable products are the most common causes of burns. Breathing in smoke can also cause inhalation injuries. Table 12.4 describes the different degrees of burns.

Possible screening questions for burns include:
- What occurred? Where was the person burned? What caused the burn?
- What symptoms does the person have? What does the person's skin look like?
- If the face or chest is affected: Is the person experiencing any breathing issues?

Providers estimate the percent of total burn surface area (%TBSA) by using the rule of nines diagram (Fig. 12.12). Table 12.5 shows the difference between the rule of nines for an adult and for a child.

TABLE 12.4   Types of Burns

CONDITION	FIRST-DEGREE BURN	SECOND-DEGREE BURN	THIRD-DEGREE BURN	FOURTH-DEGREE BURN
Also Known As	Superficial burn	Partial-thickness burn	Full-thickness burn	Deep full-thickness burn
Description	Damage to epidermis	Damage to the epidermis and part of the dermis	Damage to the epidermis, dermis, and subcutaneous tissue	Damage beyond the subcutaneous tissue into the muscle and bone (not universally accepted)
Signs and Symptoms	Redness (erythema), tenderness, physical sensitivity No scar development	Redness, blisters, and pain. Possible scar development.	No pain because nerve endings are destroyed. Skin appears deep red, pale gray, brown, or black. Scar formation is likely.	
First Aid Procedures	For minor burns: • For unbroken skin, soak in cool water (not ice water) for at least 5 minutes. • Cover with sterile dressing. • (For second-degree burns 3 inches or larger or located on hands, feet, groin, buttock, or over joint — treat as major burn.)		For major burns: • Seek immediate medical attention (call 911). • Do not remove burned clothing stuck to skin. • Monitor breathing. Perform rescue breathing or CPR as needed. • Raise burned body part above heart level. • Separate burned fingers or toes with dry, sterile dressing.	

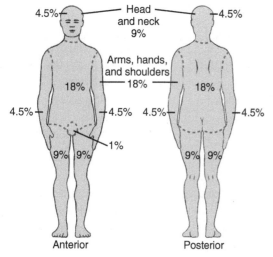

FIGURE 12.12 Rule of nines for adults. (From Callen JP, Greer KE, Saller AS, et al: *Color atlas of dermatology*, ed 3, Philadelphia, 2003, Saunders.)

TABLE 12.5   Rule of Nines for Adults and Children

AREA BURNED	ADULT	CHILD
Head and neck	9%	18%
Front of torso	18%	18%
Back	18%	18%
Arm, hand, and shoulder	9% (LA) 9% (RA)	9% (LA) 9% (RA)
Leg and foot	18% (LL) 18% (RL)	13.5% (LL) 13.5% (RL)
Genital	1%	1%
Total	100%	100%

LA, Left arm; *RA*, right arm; *LL*, left leg; *RL*, right leg.

Poisonings

Poison can enter the body through swallowing, inhaling, injecting, or absorbing it through the skin. Common poisons include:

- Medications (prescription or over the counter) taken in high doses
- Overdoses of illegal drugs
- Household products (e.g., laundry detergent, furniture polish, and cleaning products)
- Indoor and outdoor plants
- Pesticides and fertilizers
- Metals (e.g., mercury and lead)

American Association of Poison Control Centers are national poison resources with 55 centers around the country. This resource is available online (PoisonHelp.org) and via a hotline (1-800-222-1222). Medical assistants should have the phone number and website available for reference. If the medical assistant receives a call regarding a poisoning, the call must be handled according to the facility's protocols. Many times, the medical assistant must contact Poison Control while keeping the patient on the phone. The medical assistant then relays the information from Poison Control to the patient.

Signs and symptoms of poisoning can develop over time. They can also vary based on the poison. Some examples of symptoms include:

- Bluish lips, cough, difficulty breathing
- Heart palpitations, chest pain
- Confusion, dizziness, double vision, drowsiness, irritability, headache
- Nausea, vomiting, abdominal pain
- Numbness, tingling, seizures
- Unconsciousness, stupor, weakness, unusual odor

First aid includes checking and monitoring the person's airway, breathing, and pulse. If required, rescue breathing and cardiopulmonary resuscitation (CPR) are provided. Call 911 for medical help. If the person vomits, clear the airway. Monitor the person until help arrives. If poisoning is suspected, it is important to identify what the toxin is and how much was taken.

Do not have the person vomit unless you are instructed to do so by the Poison Control staff. If the person has swallowed a corrosive substance, it will cause additional injury as it is vomited. In this type of situation, a tube must be passed into the stomach to remove the substance. This is usually done in the emergency department.

Poisoning Facts

- Children younger than 6 years of age make up about half of the poisoning exposures reported.
- Children ages 1 to 2 have the greatest risk of poisoning.
- Cosmetics and personal care products, followed by cleaning products, are the most common substances involved in childhood poison exposures.
- About 20% of adult poisonings and 40% of teen poisonings are suspected suicides.
- Analgesics, followed by sedative/hypnotics/antipsychotic medications, are the top substances in adult poisonings.

From Poison Control. *http://www.poison.org/poison-statistics-national.* Accessed October 23, 2018.

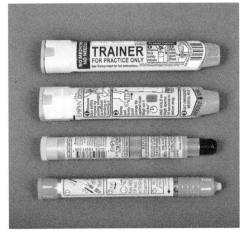

FIGURE 12.13 *Top to bottom:* Trainer that comes with the EpiPen, adult EpiPen, EpiPen Jr., and a generic adult epinephrine pen.

CRITICAL THINKING APPLICATION   12.4

Where might Gabe post the Poison Control numbers around the clinic? Describe places where this number will be useful.

Anaphylaxis

Anaphylaxis is a severe allergic reaction that can be life-threatening. Food, insect stings, and medications are the top allergens that cause anaphylaxis (Table 12.6). Allergic reactions that affect breathing are life-threatening.

First aid for severe allergic reactions includes:

- Do the 3Cs: Check the scene for safety. Call 911. Care for the victim.
- Give *epinephrine* (EpiPen) if the person has it available (Fig. 12.13).
- Stay with the individual and try to keep the person calm.
- If the person has a bee sting, scrape the stinger off the skin if it is visible. Use a fingernail or credit card to scrape it. Don't use tweezers, which can squeeze the stinger, releasing more venom.
- Monitor the individual's airway, breathing, and pulse. Perform rescue breathing or CPR if needed.
- Have the person lie flat and raise the feet 12 inches. Keep the person warm. This will help to prevent shock.

In the ambulatory care facility, if the medical assistant suspects the patient is starting to have an allergic reaction, he or she should immediately notify the provider. The provider will order epinephrine to be given and oxygen to be administered. Research has shown that epinephrine administered intramuscularly (IM) into the vastus lateralis absorbs quicker than that given IM in the deltoid or subcutaneously in the arm. If ordered, repeat every 5 to 10 minutes. Do not administer repeated injections in the same site, because **vasoconstriction** may cause tissue **necrosis**. The typical dose of epinephrine injectable solution (1 mg/mL) for anaphylaxis is:

- Children and adults (66 lb [30 kg] or more): 0.3 to 0.5 mg (0.3–0.5 mL)
- Children (under 66 lb [30 kg]): 0.01 mg/kg (0.01 mL/kg) with a maximum dose per injection of 0.3 mL

TABLE 12.6 Common Allergens and Anaphylaxis Symptoms

COMMON ALLERGENS	MOST COMMON ALLERGENIC FOODS	ANAPHYLAXIS SYMPTOMS
<ul><li>Animal dander</li><li>Insect bites and stings (especially bee stings)</li><li>Medicines</li><li>Plants</li><li>Pollens</li><li>Foods</li></ul>	<ul><li>Eggs</li><li>Fish</li><li>Milk</li><li>Tree nuts (hazelnuts, walnuts, almonds, Brazil nuts)</li><li>Peanuts (groundnuts)</li><li>Shellfish (crab, mussels, shrimp)</li><li>Soy</li><li>Wheat</li></ul>	<ul><li>Warm feeling, flushing</li><li>Shortness of breath</li><li>Dyspnea (difficulty breathing), wheezing</li><li>Throat tightening, difficulty swallowing</li><li>Cough</li><li>Anxiety</li><li>Pain or cramping</li><li>Vomiting or diarrhea</li><li>Unconsciousness</li><li>Shock</li><li>Palpitations, dizziness</li></ul>

The 3 Cs Are Important When Responding to Emergencies

If you are the first to arrive at the scene of an emergency, it is important to follow the 3 Cs:

- **Check** the scene of the emergency. Is it safe for you? Are there any toxic or electric hazards? What occurred? How many victims are involved? Where did it occur (so you can tell the 911 dispatcher)?
- **Call 911** or the local emergency number. Provide all the details you know.
- **Care** for the victims if it is safe to do so.

Always make sure you are safe before you assist others. If it is not safe for you, then wait for the emergency responders to arrive.

Insect Bites and Stings

Insect bites and stings can cause immediate skin reactions, including pain, burning, **erythema,** numbness, swelling, and **pruritus.** In some cases, the venom can cause severe illness and death. Some people have anaphylactic reactions to stings and bites (e.g., bee stings). Anaphylaxis symptoms were addressed in the prior section. If the medical assistant receives a phone call regarding a bite or sting, it is important to gather additional information for the provider, such as:

- What bit you?
- Do you have any allergies?
- How does the wound look? Describe the wound to me.
- Are you having any problems breathing? Any wheezing, shortness of breath, or difficulty breathing?
- Is there any swelling in the mouth or lips?

First aid for severe reactions includes all the steps indicated in the anaphylaxis section. Additional steps include removing any nearby constricting items, such as rings and clothing. The affected area may swell, and constricting items can cause additional problems. First aid for mild reactions includes:

- Move to a safe location.
- Remove the stinger if it is visible.
- Wash the affected area with soap and water.
- To reduce pain and swelling, apply a cool cloth and elevate the extremity.
- For pain, apply hydrocortisone or lidocaine cream to the area. An over-the-counter pain reliever can also be taken.
- Calamine lotion or a similar product can be applied to the area to reduce the pruritus.

Patients may also call for advice on removing ticks.

Removing Ticks

Ticks can spread diseases, including Rocky Mountain spotted fever, Powassan virus, *Babesia* infection, Lyme disease, and ehrlichiosis. If a person has a tick embedded, it needs to be removed. Wear gloves and use a fine-tipped pointed tweezers. Get as close to the head as possible. Do not squeeze the abdomen, because it may inject secretions into the person's body. Slowly pull the head out. Do not twist. Do not burn it or use petroleum jelly or nail polish. Once the tick is removed, place it in a container of rubbing alcohol to kill it. Clean the site with antiseptic soap and water. Apply an antibiotic ointment. Monitor the site for infections or other complications.

CRITICAL THINKING APPLICATION 12.5

Gabe realized that there were no patient education pamphlets in the exam rooms. He would like to talk with his supervisor about getting brochure racks for each room. His thought was to include procedures on home emergencies/first aid for patients. If you were Gabe, describe the talking points you could make to your supervisor in favor of placing patient education materials in the exam rooms.

Animal Bites

Patients who have animal bites will typically seek care or call their providers. It is important for the medical assistant to ask some screening questions before talking with the provider, such as:

- What type of animal bit you? Do you know the animal? If so, are the shots up to date?
- How does the wound look? Is it bleeding, dirty, or deep? Was it a puncture wound?
- Have you had the rabies vaccine series?
- When was your last tetanus vaccine?

Frequently, the bites are caused by domestic pets (e.g., dogs and cats). First aid for minor bites that only break the skin includes washing the area with soap and water. Then the person should apply over-the-counter antibiotic cream and cover the area with a clean bandage.

It is important to seek medical attention in the following situations:

- *For fang punctures:* For instance, cat bites. Bacteria are left deep in the puncture wound. Initially the wound may not look bad, but in a few hours the entire area could be hot and swollen.
- *For bleeding wounds*: Apply pressure with a clean cloth or bandage and seek help.
- *For dirty or deep wounds*: The person may require a tetanus vaccine booster if the last injection was given 5 or more years earlier.
- *For wounds that look infected*: The wound may look swollen, red, painful, or oozing.
- *For questions about the rabies risk*: Any wild or domestic mammal can get rabies and pass it on to people. Animals commonly seen with rabies include raccoons, skunks, bats, woodchucks (groundhogs), foxes, coyotes, cats, dogs, and cattle.

In the ambulatory care facility, the wound is examined, cleaned, and bandaged. The medical assistant should gather information on the patient's last tetanus booster. A tetanus immunization may be given. If there is a chance of rabies exposure, the provider will discuss the treatment options. Treatment for rabies can be costly, and the treatment time window is narrow. Table 12.7 describes the medications that can be given as treatment.

Foreign Body in the Eye

It is common for people with "something in the eye" to call or visit the ambulatory healthcare facility. This condition is known as a *foreign body in the eye*.

First aid for a foreign body in the eye is eye irrigation. Washing your hands before starting is important. Flush the eye with clean, warm water or with saline eye drops. Saline eye drops will be less irritating than water. If the foreign body cannot be removed through irrigation, the person should seek immediate medical care. It is important not to rub the eye, which may cause further damage.

In the ambulatory care facility, the medical assistant needs to ask the patient how the injury occurred. Further irrigation may be ordered after the provider examines the patient. It is important to check the date of the patient's last tetanus booster. The provider may order an updated tetanus booster, along with additional treatments.

Diabetic Emergencies

Diabetic emergencies occur when the person's blood glucose level is too low or too high. When a person eats carbohydrates (starches and sugars [e.g., breads, candy]), the blood glucose level rises. The pancreas makes insulin, and some people with diabetes mellitus must take insulin injections. Insulin is the only thing that moves the glucose out of the blood and into the cells, where it is used for energy. Without enough insulin, the blood glucose level rises. With too much insulin, the blood glucose level drops (Table 12.8).

If the blood glucose gets too high or too low, the person can go into a diabetic coma. Permanent brain damage and death can occur. If you come across an unresponsive person, check to see if the individual has a medical alert bracelet or necklace. (Some individuals have tattoos instead of wearing the medical alert jewelry.) The medical alert information may provide clues to what is occurring.

First aid for hypoglycemia includes:
- Test the blood glucose level if possible.
- *If the individual is conscious and able to swallow*: Give 4 ounces of fruit juice or regular (not diet) soda or three glucose tablets. Test the blood glucose every 15 minutes. If the blood glucose is under 70, give additional glucose. Continue until the glucose level is 70 or above (see Procedure 12.1, p. 310).
- *If the individual is unconscious*: Place the patient in the **recovery position** (Fig. 12.14). Call 911 and get medical help. Monitor

TABLE 12.7	Rabies Postexposure Treatment for Nonimmunized Individuals	
MEDICATION	**PURPOSE**	**ADMINISTRATION**
Rabies immune globulin (RIG)	Antibodies specifically for rabies. Provides rapid (immediate) passive immune protection against rabies.	Dose based on weight. Administer only once between day 0 (day of the bite) to day 7. Provider injects RIG around the bite wound if present. Remaining RIG is administered IM in the vastus lateralis or deltoid muscle (most distant from the wound). *If required, live virus vaccines (varicella, measles) must be either given with or spaced out 4 months after RIG.*
Rabies vaccine	Helps to provide long-term active immune protection against rabies.	Administer 1 mL IM in the deltoid muscle for adults and the vastus lateralis for children. Administer one dose on days 0, 3, 7, and 14. A fifth dose may be recommended on day 28 for immunocompromised individuals

TABLE 12.8	Diabetic Emergencies	
CONDITION	**INSULIN SHOCK**	**DIABETIC KETOACIDOSIS (DKA)**
Alternative Names	Severe *hypoglycemia* (low blood glucose); insulin reaction	Severe *hyperglycemia* (high blood glucose)
Why Does It Occur?	Imbalance between insulin and blood glucose. Too little glucose is in the blood because the individual: • Took too much insulin • Ate too few carbohydrates • Engaged in too much physical activity • Drank alcohol (may occur up to 2 days after drinking)	Imbalance between insulin and blood glucose. Too much glucose is in the blood because the individual: • Took too little insulin • Ate too many carbohydrates • Is ill, has an infection, trauma, or surgery • Used an illegal drug (e.g., cocaine, Ecstasy)
Symptoms	**Hypoglycemia** • Double or blurry vision • Fast pulse, palpitations • Irritable, aggressive, nervous • Headache, unclear thinking • Shaking, tired • Sweaty, cold skin • Hunger **Severe Hypoglycemia** • Disorientation, unconsciousness • Seizures • Shock • Diabetic coma and death	**Hyperglycemia** • Thirsty, hungry, stomach pain • Nausea, vomiting • Frequent urination • Fatigue • Shortness of breath • Very dry mouth • Rapid pulse **Diabetic Ketoacidosis** • Fruity odor on breath • Diabetic coma and death

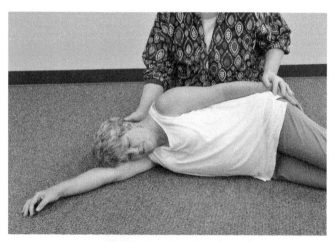

FIGURE 12.14 Recovery position.

How to Place a Person in the Recovery Position

- While kneeling at the person's side, place the lowermost arm next to the head with the palm facing up. Take the other arm and place it next to the person's side.
- Bend the lowermost leg up.
- You want to roll the person as one unit in case of head, neck, or spinal injuries. To do this, carefully slide one arm under the person's shoulder closest to you and the other under the arm and hip. Roll the person away from you and onto his or her side.
- Bend the top leg at the knee and place on top of the other knee. Place the upper arm near the person's hip.

the airway and pulse. Perform rescue breathing and CPR as needed. For an unconscious adult patient, glucagon 1 mL is given subcutaneously or IM (Fig. 12.15). Repeat dose in 15 minutes if patient is unconscious. (Children younger than 6 years of age get 0.5 mL.) Monitor the blood glucose. Once the patient is alert and able to swallow, give additional food (e.g., sandwich).

First aid for hyperglycemia includes:

- Call 911 and get medical help. Monitor the airway and pulse. Perform rescue breathing and CPR as needed.
- The patient will need IV fluids, insulin, and monitoring to bring down the blood glucose level.

Musculoskeletal Emergencies

Without a diagnosis, it is hard to tell if an injury is a strain, sprain, fracture, or dislocation. It is important always to treat the injury as a fracture until the provider diagnoses the injury. A few symptoms will indicate if the injury is more severe (e.g., dislocation), including:

- The person has difficulty or is not able to move the extremity normally.
- The extremity is deformed.
- Bone is exposed through the skin.
- There is heavy bleeding.

If a person has any of these symptoms or the injury was related to major trauma, call 911 and get medical help. Additional first aid steps involve:

- *For bleeding*: Apply pressure to the wound with a clean cloth or sterile bandage.
- *Immobilize the injured area*: Do not push the bone back. Do not move the area affected by the injury. Apply a splint beyond the joint above and the joint below the injury (Figs. 12.16 and 12.17).

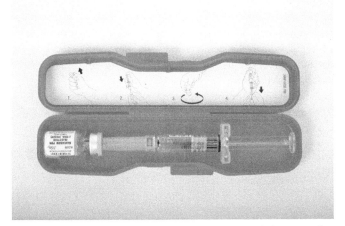

FIGURE 12.15 Glucagon is given to unconscious patients with diabetes. This hormone stimulates the liver to release glucose into the bloodstream, thus increasing the blood glucose level.

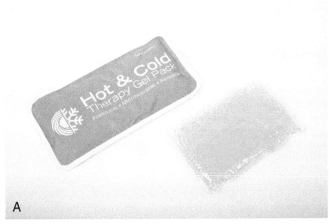

FIGURE 12.16 SAM Splint is a reusable splint that can conform to the extremity affected by the injury.

- *To limit swelling*: Apply a cold pack to the area. Make sure to cover the cold pack with a towel. Do not apply the cold pack directly on the skin (Fig. 12.18).
- *If the person is going into shock*: Make sure the person is lying down with the head slightly lower than the abdomen and elevate the legs. Monitor the person's breathing and pulse rate. Provide rescue breathing and CPR if needed.

Many times, patients will contact their provider regarding musculoskeletal injuries. The medical assistant should screen the patient and relay the information to the provider. Possible screening questions for musculoskeletal emergencies include:

- What happened?
- What does the injured body part look like? Is it deformed? Is it bleeding?
- Can the person move the injured part? Is there pain?
- How does the skin look over and near the injury?

Typically, the provider will need to examine the patient; then an x-ray will be taken before a final diagnosis is made. Depending on the diagnosis, the medical assistant may need to help apply a splint, cast, sling, or another device. Good patient education is required. The medical assistant should coach the patient on checking the circulation on the affected extremity. Coaching the patient on how to handle the protective device (e.g., cast, splint) while doing basic hygiene

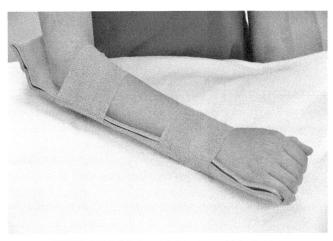

FIGURE 12.17 Splint beyond the joint, above and below the injury.

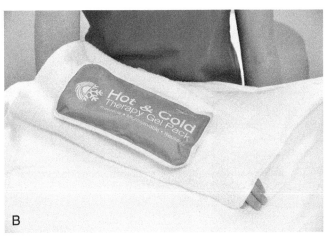

FIGURE 12.18 **(A)** A cold or hot pack cannot be applied directly to the skin. **(B)** Place a towel between the pack and the skin.

activities (e.g., showering) is important. Typically, musculoskeletal injuries require rest, ice, compression, and elevation (RICE).

First Aid and Applying a Splint

- Splint the body part in the position it is in. Do not attempt to readjust the area or straighten it.
- Use a commercial splint or create a splint. Use sticks, a board, or rolled up magazines, newspaper, or clothing as a splint.
- Make sure the splint extends below and above the injury.
- Secure the splint with ties (e.g., belt, cloth strips).
- Check the injured area for swelling, paleness, or numbness, which may indicate the ties are too tight. Loosen ties if needed.

Neurological Emergencies

Neurological emergencies can range from minor conditions, such as dizziness, to serious conditions, such as stroke. The medical assistant should know how to handle neurological emergencies.

Vertigo and Dizziness

Peripheral **vertigo** is caused by a problem in the inner ear (i.e., vestibular labyrinth, semicircular canals, and vestibular nerve). This issue affects the sense of balance. *Central vertigo* is caused by a brainstem or cerebellum disorder. It can be caused by certain drugs (e.g., aspirin, anticonvulsants, and alcohol), migraines, multiple sclerosis, stroke, and tumors.

With *dizziness*, people may feel lightheaded or lose their balance. Many people get dizzy if they move too quickly from a sitting or lying position to a standing position. Their blood pressure drops, causing dizziness. People may feel as if they will pass out. Usually dizziness resolves on its own, but it could be a symptom of another disorder.

First aid for vertigo and dizziness involves sitting or lying down. The affected person should gradually resume activities when the episode passes. In addition, he or she should avoid sudden position changes and bright lights and should drink more fluids. The patient should contact the provider if any of the following apply:

- This is the first episode of vertigo or dizziness.
- The episodes are increasing in number.
- The episodes are getting worse.

Concussion

A **concussion** is a traumatic brain injury caused by a blow to the head. Violently shaking the head can also cause a concussion. Concussions can occur with sports injuries, falls, physical assaults, and traffic accidents. Concussion symptoms may be slow to develop and could last for weeks. Symptoms include:

- Head pressure or headache
- Temporary loss of consciousness right after the incident
- Confusion, amnesia, disorientation, irritability, personality changes
- Dizziness, ringing in the ears
- Nausea and vomiting; taste and smell issues
- Slurred speech, delayed response to questions

- Listlessness, tiredness, sleep disturbances, concentration and memory issues
- Loss of balance, unsteady gait (walk)

First aid for moderate to severe head injuries involves immediately calling 911. Monitor the person until help arrives. Check the breathing and pulse. Provide rescue breathing and CPR as needed. If the person is breathing and has a pulse, treat the condition as a spinal injury. Stabilize the head and neck by placing your hands on both sides of the person's head. Prevent any movement of the head and keep the head in line with the spine until help arrives. If the person vomits, roll the person to the side and move the head, neck, and body as one unit. Moderate to severe head injuries are often seen in the emergency department.

Patients will call or come to ambulatory care facilities if they have a possible concussion or a mild head injury (see Procedure 12.2, p. 311). Possible screening questions include:

- What happened?
- Did the person lose consciousness? If so, for how long?
- Any bleeding?
- How is the person doing? Any vomiting? Are the pupils dilated, or is one larger than the other?
- Does the person remember what happened? Is the person confused or slurring his or her speech?

For mild head injuries, usually a person should seek medical treatment if these occur:

- Loss of consciousness lasting longer than 30 seconds after the initial injury
- Repeated vomiting
- Worsening headache
- Changes in behavior or coordination (irritable, stumbling, or falling)
- Changes in orientation and speech (disoriented, confused, or slurred speech)
- Neurological changes (seizures, visual disturbance, recurrent dizziness, difficulty with concentration, one pupil larger than the other or both pupils dilated)

The patient may need to undergo radiologic testing to check for skull fractures and internal bleeding. If there are no fractures, the provider will educate the patient about other symptoms that would require follow-up and postconcussion care. Athletes need to refrain from playing sports until the concussion symptoms are gone. Another hit on the head can cause additional damage.

CRITICAL THINKING APPLICATION   12.6

Gabe has a 12-year-old son who plays middle school football. Before the season started, Gabe and his wife had to sign an acknowledgment form discussing concussions. What are the benefits of informing parents of school athletes about concussion symptoms?

Seizures

A *seizure* is a sudden increase of electrical activity in one or more parts of the brain. *Epilepsy* is a disorder that causes recurring seizures. Seizures are classified based on how the abnormal brain activity begins. The three major classifications of seizures are:

- *Generalized onset seizure*: Affects both sides of the brain at the same time. Includes several types of seizures, such as tonic-clonic and absent. Symptoms may include jerking, rigid or twitching muscles, and staring spells.
- *Focal onset seizure*: Affects one area of the brain. This type of seizure used to be called a partial seizure. There are two subgroups of focal onset seizures:
  - *Aware seizure*: The person is awake and alert during the seizure.
  - *Impaired awareness seizure*: The person is confused during the seizure. This type of seizure was known as a complex partial seizure.
- *Unknown onset seizure*: When the seizure began is not known.

In most situations, seizures last 30 seconds to 2 minutes. Usually, they do not cause lasting issues. It is a medical emergency if the seizure lasts longer than 5 minutes or if a person has multiple seizures without becoming conscious between them.

Parents commonly call when their child has had a seizure. According to the facility's protocol, the medical assistant may need to ask some screening questions and relay the information to the provider. Possible screening questions for musculoskeletal emergencies include:

- What did the patient do during the seizure? How long was the seizure?
- Did the person lose consciousness?
- How is the patient now after the seizure?

If a person has a seizure in the healthcare facility, the medical assistant must also notify the provider immediately (see Procedure 12.3, p. 312). First aid for seizures focuses on the safety of the individual:

- Move the person to the floor and place the patient in the recovery position. Gently raise the chin to tilt the head back slightly to open the airway. Monitor the person's breathing and pulse. Perform rescue breathing after the seizure has stopped if the patient does not resume breathing. Provide CPR if needed.
- Protect the patient from harm. Clear the area of anything hard or sharp. Place a soft, folded towel under the head.
- Do not place anything in the patient's mouth.
- Remove any glasses and loosen any constrictive clothing around the neck (e.g., ties).
- Time the length of the seizure. Call 911 if the seizure lasts longer than 5 minutes.
- Stay with the person until he or she is fully awake and alert.

Cerebrovascular Accident

A cerebrovascular accident (CVA), also called a *stroke*, is a medical emergency. There are three types of strokes:

- *Ischemic stroke*: Occurs when the arterial blood flow to part of the brain is blocked. The brain cells start to die after a few minutes. This is the most common type of stroke. Two common types of ischemic stroke are:
  - *Thrombotic stroke*: A blood clot forms in an artery, blocking the blood to part of the brain.
  - *Embolic stroke*: A blood clot or other debris forms elsewhere in the body and moves into the brain arteries, blocking the blood flow.
- *Hemorrhagic stroke*: Occurs when an artery in the brain leaks or ruptures. The leaked blood puts pressure on the surrounding brain cells, causing damage. Two types of hemorrhagic stroke include:

- *Intracerebral hemorrhage*: The most common type of stroke; it occurs when a cerebral aneurysm ruptures.
- *Subarachnoid hemorrhage*: Bleeding occurs in the subarachnoid space, usually as a result of small aneurysms.
- *Transient ischemic attack (TIA)*: Also called a "mini-stroke" because it lasts for only a few minutes. The blood supply to a part of the brain is briefly blocked. Symptoms are similar to stroke symptoms but do not last as long (e.g., 1 to 24 hours).

The symptoms of a CVA relate to the part of the brain affected. The individual may not have all the symptoms. Possible symptoms of CVAs include:

- Confusion or mental changes; sudden severe headache
- Speech problems (difficulty forming words, difficult to understand, or using words that do not make sense)
- Numbness of the face, arm, or leg, usually on one side of the body
- Problem seeing in one or both eyes; facial drooping
- Trouble walking, lack of coordination or balance, or arm weakness

First aid for stroke-type symptoms involves getting help (calling 911) immediately. The emergency department (ED) is the best place for a patient to go. There is a small window of time during which clot-dissolving medications (e.g., a tissue plasminogen activator) can be given to help the body break down the clot that is blocking the artery. If a bleeding artery has caused the stroke, the ED providers can detect this on radiologic studies.

If a patient comes to the ambulatory care facility with stroke-like symptoms, it is important for the provider to see the patient immediately. Be ready to call 911 when the provider orders you to do so. Also, monitor the patient's vital signs for changes.

FAST

The American Stroke Association promotes FAST to spot stroke signs and encourages calling 911:

- **F**: Face drooping. Is one side of the face drooping or numb? Ask the person to smile to see if the smile is uneven or drooping on one side.
- **A**: Arm weakness. Is one arm weak or numb? Raise both arms and watch for an arm to drift downward.
- **S**: Speech difficulty. Is the person slurring his or her words? Is the person having problems speaking? Do the words not make sense, or are they hard to understand? Give the person a simple sentence to say and see if it is repeated correctly.
- **T**: Time to call 911. If the person is showing any of these symptoms, call 911 immediately. Let the emergency responders know you think it might be a stroke. Watch the person's respiration rate and pulse rate. Do not give the person anything to eat or drink. Have the person sit upright if possible.

American Stroke Association, *http://www.strokeassociation.org/STROKEORG/WarningSigns/Stroke-Warning-Signs-and-Symptoms_UCM_308528_SubHomePage.jsp*. Accessed October 23, 2018.

Respiratory Emergencies

Respiratory emergencies can create a number of different signs and symptoms. For example:

- *Skin*: Unusually moist, flushed, pale, bluish or ashen
- *Respirations*: Slow, rapid, deep, or shallow; trouble or no breathing
- *Audible breathing sounds*: Gasping, gurgling, high-pitched noises (e.g., whistling sound), wheezing
- *Patient complaints*: Shortness of breath, dizziness, lightheadedness, chest pain, tingling in extremities, fearful

It is important to get help immediately with respiratory emergencies. After calling 911, help the conscious individual into a comfortable position and monitor the respirations and pulse. Be ready to provide rescue breathing and CPR if required.

Common respiratory emergencies are discussed in the following sections. It is important for the medical assistant to recognize when a patient is having a respiratory emergency and get help immediately.

Hyperventilation

Hyperventilation, or overbreathing, is rapid and deep breathing. This leads to a low carbon dioxide level in the blood. This gas imbalance creates symptoms that can mimic those of a heart attack, thus increasing the person's anxiety, in addition to the hyperventilation. Symptoms of hyperventilation include:

- Dry mouth, belching, and bloating
- Lightheadedness, weakness, dizziness, and difficulty concentrating
- Shortness of breath and breathlessness
- Chest pain and heart palpitations
- Numbness and tingling in the arms or around the mouth
- Muscle spasms

Hyperventilation can be caused by many things, including panic attacks, stress, anxiety, bleeding, heart attack, drugs, and infections.

First aid treatments focus on raising the carbon dioxide level in the blood. This can be done by relaxing and using pursed lip breathing or slowly blowing out through the lips. A person should seek medical care if the hyperventilation episodes get worse. After diagnosing the condition, the provider may have the patient breathe slowly into a paper bag. This helps to restore the carbon dioxide and oxygen balances in the blood.

Asthmatic Attack

Asthma affects the airway and the lungs. During an asthmatic attack, the airway constricts, reducing the air moving into and out of the lungs. Mucus clogs up the airway, making airflow more difficult. Asthma causes wheezing, breathlessness, chest tightness, and coughing. Typically, asthmatic attacks occur at night or in the early morning hours.

If a patient or family member calls about an asthma attack, it is important to gather information quickly and talk with the provider. Possible questions to ask include:

- What symptoms is the person experiencing?
- Was medication given? What was the medication, and how much was administered?
- Did the medication ease the symptoms?
- Is the person having severe respiratory distress (e.g., unable to talk, blue lips, or **retractions**)? (This would be a medical emergency and calling 911 is critical.)

In the ambulatory healthcare setting, an asthmatic attack is an emergency. The provider needs to see the patient immediately. First aid actions for an asthmatic attack include:

- Helping the person into a comfortable sitting position. Usually sitting upright allows for easier breathing.
- Giving short-acting inhalers (e.g., albuterol), which will lessen the asthma attack within minutes.
- Monitoring the pulse oximetry and vital signs

Choking

Choking can occur in all age groups. Most choking cases relate to swallowing large pieces of food or doing an activity (e.g., running) while eating. Other causes are denture-related issues and eating too fast. Children under 5 tend to choke on candy, grapes, and large pieces of food. They are also more likely to put nonfood items in the mouth. Plastic, balloon pieces, coins, and buttons are extremely dangerous to children. Objects smaller than 1.75 inches (the diameter of a golf ball) can be caught in the throat and cause choking.

Any object caught in the throat is considered a foreign body obstruction. Signs of a partial airway obstruction include:

- Can still speak
- Forceful or weak coughing
- Labored, noisy, or gasping breathing
- Panicked appearance, extreme anxiety, or agitation

Signs of a total airway obstruction include:

- Clutching the throat with one or both hands
- Unable to breathe, cry, cough, or speak
- Bluish skin color (e.g., lips)

Do not give the person any liquids until the obstruction is cleared.

First aid for choking includes asking the individual if he or she is choking. If the person is forcefully coughing, stand by and see if the person can clear the airway without assistance. Procedure 12.4 on p. 312 describes the *abdominal thrusts* used on a conscious adult with a total airway obstruction. Treat children older than 1 year of age the same as adults (Fig. 12.19). If a person is pregnant or obese, wrap your arms around the person's chest. Place your fist in the middle of the breastbone between the nipples. Give firm, backward thrusts.

Conscious Choking Infant

Do the 3 Cs after gaining consent from the parent or guardians. Check the scene, call 911 (or have someone else call), and care for the infant. Hold the child with the head below the chest for the entire procedure. This allows gravity to help move the obstruction. Support the chin with your hand and the infant's body with your arm.

Have the child facing downward and give five back blows between the shoulder blades with the heel of your hand (see Fig. 12.19A). Flip the infant and place two or three fingers below the nipple line on the chest. Give five chest thrusts (see Fig. 12.19B). Do a mouth check, and insert a finger only to pull a loose object out. Doing a finger sweep is not recommended because it can push the item in farther. Continue until the object is out or the child becomes unconscious. If the child is unconscious, then place the child on a hard surface and begin CPR, starting with chest compressions.

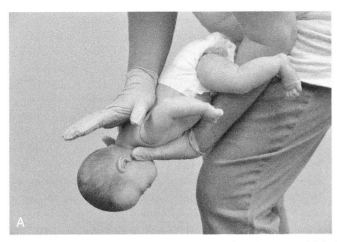
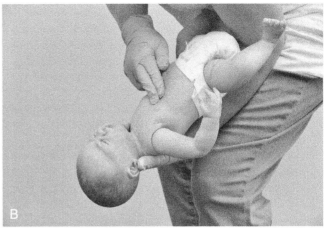

FIGURE 12.19 (A) Support the infant with your arm and thigh while giving back blows. **(B)** Chest thrusts are administered in the same position as for cardiac compressions.

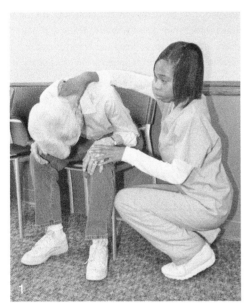

FIGURE 12.20 Placing the head between the legs helps to reduce the faint feeling.

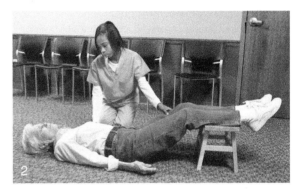

FIGURE 12.21 Elevate the legs about 12 inches using pillows, blankets, or a small stool.

Cardiovascular Emergencies

Syncope

Syncope means fainting, passing out, or having a temporary loss of consciousness. When people are about to faint, they may feel dizzy, nauseous, or lightheaded. The skin may be cold and clammy. People may experience a "black out" or "white out" in their visual field. Muscle control is lost. Fainting occurs when the blood pressure drops suddenly and the blood flow to the brain is reduced.

First aid actions for people who feel faint include having them sit and place their head between their knees (Fig. 12.20). For people who faint, position them on their back. Check their airway and make sure it is clear. Check for a pulse. If the pulse is not present, start CPR. Additional first aid actions include:

- Loosen any constrictive clothing.
- Raise the legs above the heart level (about 12 inches) (Fig. 12.21).
- Get help/call 911 if the person does not regain consciousness within 1 minute.

Possible Causes of Syncope

- Too hot
- Dehydrated and alcohol use
- Standing up too quickly
- Drop in blood glucose
- Certain medications: Diuretics, antihistamines, levodopa, calcium antagonists, angiotensin-converting enzyme (ACE) inhibitors, nitrates, antipsychotics, and narcotics
- Neurological conditions: Parkinson disease, postural orthostatic tachycardia syndrome (POTS), and diabetic neuropathy
- Heart problems
- Vasovagal syncope: Emotional stress, trauma, pain, reaction to the sight of blood, prolonged standing
- Carotid sinus syncope: Constriction of the carotid artery in the neck (occurs with turning the head, shaving, or wearing tight clothing around the neck)
- Situational syncope: Occurs during defecation, urination, and coughing

Bleeding

Bleeding can occur with and without trauma. First aid for bleeding involves stopping the bleeding and calling for help (see Procedure 12.5, p. 313). Nosebleeds are common in certain people. If a person has a nosebleed, have him or her sit upright and lean forward to prevent the person from swallowing the blood. Pinch the nostrils for 5 to 10 minutes, which helps to stop the bleeding. Continue to pinch the nostrils until the bleeding stops. The individual should refrain from blowing the nose for several hours to prevent rebleeding.

In the ambulatory care facility, always wear gloves and the required personal protective equipment (PPE) before assisting patients. Follow these steps to stop the bleeding:

- For bleeding wounds, remove any obvious debris. Do not remove any large objects embedded in the wound.
- Place a sterile gauze or clean cloth over the wound and press firmly to control the bleeding. Do not put direct pressure over an embedded object, an eye, or displaced organs.
- For severe bleeding, help the person lie down and cover him or her with a blanket. This will keep the person warm and conserve body heat.
- If the bleeding seeps through the gauze, apply another layer on top of the initial gauze. Do not move the initial gauze.
- To slow the bleeding or if the bleeding is spurting from an artery:
  - Elevate the bleeding extremity above the heart level. Hold direct pressure over the site.
  - If the bleeding does not stop with the elevation and direct pressure, apply pressure to the artery above the wound by pushing the artery against a bone. Continue to apply direct pressure on the wound. To see if the bleeding has stopped, slowly lift your fingers from the pressure point over the artery. Check to see if the wound is still bleeding. If so, continue to apply pressure. Do not hold pressure at the pressure point for longer than 5 minutes after the bleeding stops.

Shock

Shock occurs when the body is not getting enough blood flow. The vital organs (e.g., heart, brain) do not get enough oxygen and nutrients for the cells to function properly and survive. Organ damage can occur. Shock is a life-threatening condition. There are many types of shock, such as:

- *Cardiogenic shock*: Due to heart muscle damage caused by a *myocardial infarction* (also known as MI, heart attack); the heart cannot pump enough blood to the other organs.
- *Hypovolemic shock*: Due to heavy bleeding (i.e., accident or internal bleeding) or dehydration; blood volume is too low to provide nutrients and oxygen to the organs.
- *Anaphylactic shock*: Caused by a severe allergic reaction (*anaphylaxis*); blood pressure drops and the airway narrows. Not enough blood gets to the vital organs, and the narrowed airway prevents adequate oxygenation.
- *Septic shock*: Caused by a severe infection (severe sepsis) that affects the functioning of vital organs (e.g., heart, brain, kidneys). The blood pressure falls, and major organs can fail.
- *Neurogenic shock*: Due to a central nervous system injury (e.g., spinal cord injury). Leads to vasodilation (not enough blood can return to the heart) and low blood pressure.

Possible signs and symptoms of shock include:

- Anxiety, agitation, dizziness, feeling faint, lightheadedness, confusion, and unconsciousness
- *Cyanosis* (blue lips, fingernails) and shallow respirations
- Chest pain and a rapid, weak pulse
- Moist skin and *diaphoresis* (profuse sweating)
- Poor or no urine output

Shock requires immediate treatment for the person to have a chance of survival.

First aid actions for shock include calling 911 immediately. Check the person for responsiveness. Monitor the airway, breathing, and pulse. If needed, perform rescue breathing and CPR. If the person is breathing and has a pulse, monitor the vital signs at least every 5 minutes. If the person does not have any injuries to the head, neck or back, or legs, raise the legs 12 inches. This helps the blood to move back to the vital organs of the body. If the person has pain with raising the legs, keep him or her flat. Make sure the person's head is flat. Loosen clothing and provide the appropriate first aid for the person's injuries (see Procedure 12.6, p. 314).

If a person goes into shock in the ambulatory healthcare facility, the provider will order that 911 be contacted. Oxygen and IV fluids are given. The vital signs are monitored, and the person's legs are elevated. Based on the medications available and the person's blood pressure, the provider may give IV medications that will increase the blood pressure. The goals are to keep the blood pressure high enough to sustain life, and to get the patient to the emergency department as quickly as possible.

Myocardial Infarction

Myocardial infarction (MI) is more commonly known as *heart attack*. Coronary arteries that bring blood to the heart muscle are blocked by a clot or narrowed by plaque. When the blood flow to an area of the heart is limited or stopped, the heart cells die, and an MI occurs. Chest pain (*angina pectoris*), cold sweats, and heartburn are the most common symptoms. Chest pain can be described as mild or severe; sharp, burning, heaviness, squeezing, pressure; and constant or *intermittent* (comes and goes). Additional symptoms include:

- Upper body discomfort or pain in one or both arms, shoulders, neck, jaw, upper part of the abdomen, or back
- Arrhythmia, palpitations, tiredness without a reason, nausea, and vomiting
- Shortness of breath with activity or rest, cold sweats, dizziness, and lightheadedness
- Women may have back pain

First aid for a heart attack includes these measures:

- Have the person sit down and rest; keep the individual calm and loosen any tight clothing on the chest and neck area.
- Have the person take nitroglycerin if prescribed.
- Call 911 within 5 minutes of the onset of pain.
- Chew an aspirin (if not allergic).
- Monitor the person's respirations and pulse. Perform rescue breathing and CPR if needed (Figs. 12.22–12.24, Table 12.9, and Procedure 12.7 on p. 315).

If a patient arrives at the ambulatory care facility with chest pain or other MI-type symptoms, bring the patient to a procedure or exam room immediately. Notify the provider at once. Usually the provider will give these orders:

- One aspirin chewed and nitroglycerin administered sublingually
- Call to 911
- Vital signs, pulse oximetry, ECG, oxygen to be administered while waiting for the ambulance

The goals are to limit the damage to the heart muscle and transport the patient to the emergency department.

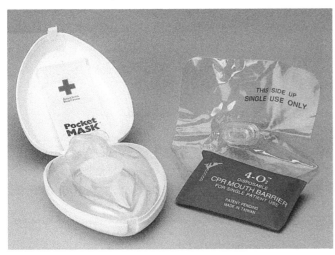

FIGURE 12.22 Rescue breathing mouth barriers.

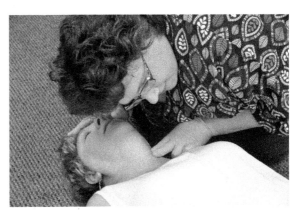

FIGURE 12.23 Use the head-tilt position to open an adult's airway while checking the carotid pulse.

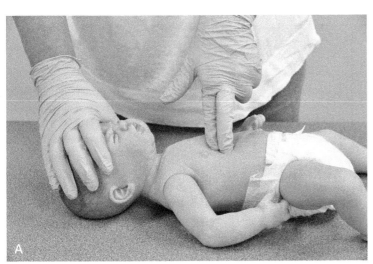

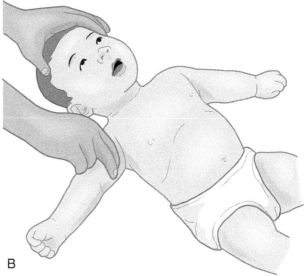

FIGURE 12.24 **(A)** Open an infant's airway by tilting the head to a neutral position. For chest compressions, place two fingers below the nipple line. **(B)** In an infant, check for a brachial pulse.

TABLE 12.9	Summary of Rescue Breathing and Cardiopulmonary Resuscitation Differences		
	ADULT	**CHILD**	**INFANT**
Check Responsiveness	Shout, "Are you all right?"		Tap infant's foot.
Open Airway	Head-tilt or if spinal injury is suspected, use the jaw thrust without head extension (see Fig. 12.23).	Tilt head slightly past the neutral position.	Tilt head to the neutral position (see Fig. 12.24A).
Assess Pulse	Feel for a carotid pulse near the middle of the throat (see Fig. 12.23).		Feel for brachial pulse on inside of upper arm (see Fig. 12.24B)
Give Rescue Breathing (Ventilation) Only	One rescue breath every 5–6 seconds; deliver each breath for 1 second.	One breath every 3 seconds; deliver each breath for 1 second.	
Chest Compression Hand Position	Heel of a hand is placed on the lower part of the chest (below the nipple line), and other hand is placed on top so that it overlaps the first hand.		Place two fingers just below the nipple line

Continued

TABLE 12.9   Summary of Rescue Breathing and Cardiopulmonary Resuscitation Differences—*continued*

	ADULT	CHILD	INFANT
Compressions	2–2.4 inches deep; 100–120 per minute	2 inches deep; 100–120 per minute	1.5 inches deep; 100–120 per minute
Compression-to-Ventilation Ratio	One or two rescuers: 30 compressions and two ventilations.	One rescuer: 30 compressions and two ventilations. Two rescuers: 15 compressions and two ventilations.	
Automated External Defibrillator (AED) Pads	Use only adult pads. Place one pad on the upper right chest and the second on the left side of the chest.	Use pediatric pads for children younger than 8 years; if not available use adult pads. If pads touch, place one on the back between the shoulder blades.	Use pediatric pads; if not available use adult pads. Place one pad on the chest and the other on the back.

Nitroglycerin and Angina

Nitroglycerin is used for *angina* (chest pain). It dilates the coronary arteries, allowing more blood to move into the heart muscle. Nitroglycerin can be given as an oral spray, a sublingual (SL) powder, or sublingual tablets.

- Do not shake the spray. Prime (or release a test spray) 5 to 10 times for new bottles, up to 5 times for bottles not used within 3 months, and 1 to 2 times for bottles that have not been used in more than 6 weeks. Prime the bottles away from everyone. When administering the dose, spray onto or under the tongue. One or two sprays can be taken at the start of the pain. Then, if the pain is not relieved in 5 minutes, give the third spray. Call 911 if the pain continues for an additional 5 minutes.
- Empty the pack of powder under the tongue. Allow the powder to dissolve without swallowing. Make sure the patient does not eat or rinse the mouth for 5 minutes.
- Tablets cannot be chewed or swallowed. Place a tablet under the tongue and let it dissolve. Usually it starts providing relief within 1 to 5 minutes. If the pain is not relieved in 5 minutes, give another tablet. If the pain continues after 5 minutes, give a third tablet. Call 911 if the pain is not relieved 5 minutes after taking the third tablet. (Do not give more than three tablets within 15 minutes.)

Nitroglycerin works fast. The patient may feel dizzy, lightheaded, or faint after taking the medication.

CRITICAL THINKING APPLICATION   12.7

Gabe is thinking of having a rescue breathing mouth barrier in each exam room and procedure room. He is also thinking of adding one to each of the first aid kits located in other parts of the clinic. Why is it important to make mouth barrier devices more available in the clinic?

CLOSING COMMENTS

Patient Coaching

Many ambulatory care facilities are coaching patients on what types of emergencies can be addressed in their facilities and what conditions need to be addressed in emergency departments. People seeking care in emergency departments for possible strokes, heart attacks, and other similar conditions will receive timely care, whereas such services in the ambulatory care facilities are limited and require the patient to be transported to the hospital. Educating patients through voice mail messages, websites, and flyers can help the public understand the limitations of ambulatory care services.

Legal and Ethical Issues

Lawsuits related to care provided during emergencies in healthcare settings are prevalent. Ambulatory care facilities need to have procedures in place to handle emergencies. Staff members need to be trained in handling emergencies. Many agencies have mock codes to help prepare staff. These are training events that allow staff members to practice their skills. Often after mock events, the supervisors assess how the training went. They identify processes and procedures that need refinement and additional training.

Another method of improving processes comes after a real-life code situation. Usually a few days after a code, the staff involved will gather to debrief or discuss what occurred. They will usually talk about:

- How the code progressed, from the time the patient had symptoms to the time the patient was transported to the emergency department
- What went well and what went not so smoothly
- Where more training is needed

These debriefings are extremely important after an emergency situation.

Patient-Centered Care

Medical emergencies are scary for patients and their families. We may be focused on providing emergency care, but we need to remember to communicate with the patient. Being sensitive to what patients are feeling is important. Remember to explain what you are doing. Ask the patient how he or she is doing.

Families of patients are often forgotten. In emergencies, often the family is moved to another room to allow more room for those helping with the code. It is helpful for the family to have a staff person wait with them. If this is not possible, then a staff person needs to report to the family and provide updates. It is important to remember that the rules of the Health Insurance Portability and Accountability Act (HIPAA) still apply in emergency situations.

Professional Behaviors

Code situations can be anxiety-inducing and stressful for staff members. It is important to talk through what occurred, taking confidentiality into account. Besides talking, it is critical to manage one's stress by maintaining a healthy diet and getting adequate sleep and exercise.

An employee assistance program (EAP) is also helpful after stressful code situations. EAP is a work-based program designed to help employees resolve issues. These issues can be personal (e.g., financial, marital, or involving substance abuse) and professional (e.g., communication issues with co-workers and stress-related issues). The EAP services are confidential and designed to help the employee's work performance. EAP counselors help employees to deal with the aftereffects of an emergency.

SUMMARY OF SCENARIO

Gabe has been in his new position for only 2 weeks. Already he has a list of concerns and possible solutions he wants to address with his supervisor. Gabe also wants to discuss forming an emergency response team. This team would respond when a code is called throughout the building.

He hopes to begin quarterly mock codes within the next 3 months. He wants to rotate the types of emergencies addressed by the mock codes. Gabe hopes that with additional training and more exposure to emergency supplies, the medical assistants will feel more comfortable with emergencies.

SUMMARY OF LEARNING OBJECTIVES

1. **Discuss emergencies in healthcare settings and possible roles each team member has during an emergency.**

   Healthcare facilities use special phrases for emergencies. Once the call goes out for help, staff members respond to the scene. In small settings, most members of the staff may be needed. In large facilities, only certain staff members respond. Usually, medical assistants, licensed practical nurses (LPNs), registered nurses (RNs), and providers attend the emergency. Refer to the section in the text for specific roles of each healthcare team member.

2. **Describe emergency equipment and supplies.**

   The emergency supplies available at healthcare facilities will vary based on the size and location of the facility. Some practices have a small box that contains a few supplies and medications. Other practices place many crash carts throughout the building. Equipment and supplies include:
   - Oxygen and airway supplies (includes endotracheal tube intubation supplies and equipment)
   - Defibrillator or an automated external defibrillator (AED)
   - Medications and IV supplies
   - Other supplies: Personal protective equipment, a sharps disposal container, pocket face mask, algorithms, clipboard with documents for charting the code, backboard, and extra batteries for the laryngoscope
   - Pediatric supplies

3. **Explain first aid procedures for environmental emergencies including temperature-related emergencies, burns, poisonings, anaphylaxis, bites and stings, and foreign bodies in the eye.**
   - Temperature-related emergencies: Tables 12.2 and 12.3 discuss first aid for temperature-related emergencies. Hypothermia and heat stroke are emergencies, and the person needs to be transported to the hospital.
   - Minor burns can be treated at home; however, people with major burns need to seek immediate medical attention.
   - First aid for severe allergic reactions and severe reactions related to bites and stings includes giving epinephrine and monitoring the patient's airway, breathing, and pulse.
   - First aid for poisonings includes monitoring the patient's airway, breathing, and pulse. Call 911. The Poison Control staff can be a resource.
   - First aid for a foreign body in the eye is to try to irrigate it out. Flush the eye with clean, warm water or with saline eye drops. Saline eye drops will be less irritating than water. If the foreign body cannot be removed through irrigation, the person should seek immediate medical care.

4. **Discuss diabetic emergencies and provide first aid for a patient in insulin shock.**

   First aid for hypoglycemia includes:
   - Test blood glucose if possible.
   - If the individual is conscious and able to swallow: Give 4 oz. of fruit juice or regular (nondiet) soda or three glucose tablets. Test blood glucose every 15 minutes. If the blood glucose is under 70, give additional glucose. Continue until the glucose level is 70 or above (see Procedure 12.1, p. 310).
   - If the individual is unconscious: Place the patient in the recovery position. Call 911 and get medical help. Monitor the airway and pulse. Perform rescue breathing and CPR as needed. For an unconscious adult patient, administer glucagon 1 mL, given subcutaneously or IM.

   First aid for hyperglycemia includes:
   - Call 911 and get medical help. Monitor the airway and pulse. Perform rescue breathing and CPR as needed.
   - The patient will need IV fluids, insulin, and monitoring to bring down the blood glucose level.

5. **Discuss musculoskeletal and neurological emergencies and provide first aid for a patient with seizure activity.**
   - First aid for major musculoskeletal injuries involves calling 911.

Continued

SUMMARY OF LEARNING OBJECTIVES—*continued*

- Other first aid actions include applying pressure for bleeding, immobilizing the injury, and applying a cold pack to minimize swelling.
- If the person goes into shock, make sure he or she is lying down with the head slightly lower than the abdomen and elevate the legs. Monitor the person's breathing and pulse rate. Provide rescue breathing and CPR if needed.
- First aid for vertigo and dizziness involves sitting or lying down.
- First aid for moderate to severe head injuries involves immediately calling 911. Monitor the person until help arrives. Provide rescue breathing and CPR as needed. If the person is breathing and has a pulse, treat the condition as a spinal injury. Stabilize the head and neck by placing your hands on both sides of the person's head.
- First aid for seizures focuses on the safety of the individual. Move the person to the floor and into the recovery position.
- First aid for stroke-type symptoms involves getting help (calling 911) immediately.

6. **Discuss respiratory emergencies and provide first aid for a choking patient.**
   - First aid treatments focus on raising the carbon dioxide level in the blood. This can be done by relaxing and using pursed lip breathing or slowly blowing out through the lips.

- First aid actions for an asthmatic attack include helping the person into a sitting position, giving short-acting inhalers, and monitoring the pulse oximetry and vital signs.
- Procedure 12.4 on p. 312 discusses first aid for choking.

7. **Discuss cardiovascular emergencies and provide first aid for a patient with a bleeding wound, fracture, or syncope; a patient in shock; and a patient in need of rescue breathing or cardiopulmonary resuscitation (CPR).**
   - Refer to Procedure 12.5 on p. 313 for first aid steps for a patient with a bleeding wound, fracture, or syncope.
   - First aid actions for shock include calling 911 immediately. Check the person for responsiveness. Monitor the airway, breathing, and pulse. If needed, perform rescue breathing and CPR. If the person is breathing and has a pulse, monitor the vital signs at least every 5 minutes. If the person does not have any injuries to the head, neck or back, or legs, raise the legs 12 inches.
   - Refer to Procedure 12.7 on p. 315 for the steps to provide rescue breathing and CPR and for using the AED.

PROCEDURE 12.1   Provide First Aid for a Patient in Insulin Shock

Task: Provide first aid to an individual with hypoglycemia.

Scenario: You are working with Dr. Martin, a family practice provider. Maude Crawford arrives for her appointment.

EQUIPMENT and SUPPLIES

- Sugary drink (4-oz fruit juice or regular soda) or three glucose tablets
- Patient's health record

PROCEDURAL STEPS

1. Wash hands or use hand sanitizer.
   PURPOSE: Hand sanitization is an important step for infection control.
2. Greet the patient. Identify yourself. Verify the patient's identity with full name and date of birth.
   PURPOSE: It is important to identify the patient in two different ways to ensure that you have the correct patient.
   Scenario update: Mrs. Crawford has diabetes and states that she thinks she has low blood sugar. She has blurry vision, tremors, and a headache. She asks you for something to eat. According to the facility's policy, you check her blood glucose level and it is 48 mg/dL.
3. Obtain a sugary drink or a fast-acting sugary food. Indicate how much to give to the patient.
   PURPOSE: Consuming a sugary food or drink will help to increase the blood glucose. Do not give a drink or food that contains fat or protein, which can slow the absorption rate.

Scenario update: After 15 minutes, her blood glucose level is 59 mg/dL. You notify the provider while a co-worker stays with the patient.
4. Describe follow-up care for the patient.
   PURPOSE: A blood glucose test should be done to find out how low the patient's level is. After 15 minutes of her eating/drinking the sugary food, the glucose test should be done. If her level is below 70 mg/dL, give her additional sugary food/drink and repeat the glucose test in 15 minutes. Continue until the blood glucose level is 70 or higher.
Scenario update: After 15 minutes, her blood glucose level is 82 mg/dL. You notify the provider.
5. Document the situation. Include the blood glucose levels, your actions, the provider who was notified, and the patient's response.
   10/04/20XX 1023 Pt c/o blurry vision, tremors, and a headache. She stated she thought she had low blood sugar. Four oz. of orange juice given to pt. After 15 minutes her blood glucose was 59 mg/dL. Dr. Martin notified and ordered additional orange juice and to recheck blood glucose until 70 mg/dL or more. Four oz. of orange juice given and after 15 minutes her blood glucose was 82 mg/dL. Provider notified. _____ Gabe Garcia, CMA (AAMA)

| PROCEDURE 12.2 | Incorporate Critical Thinking Skills When Performing Patient Assessment |

Tasks: Use critical thinking skills while performing a patient assessment regarding a neurological emergency.

Scenario: You are working with Dr. Martin, a family practice provider. Maude Crawford's daughter calls, concerned about her mother. She states that Maude fell and hit her head. She was "knocked out" for about a minute. She has been acting differently since the fall. You need to follow the "Emergency Phone Protocol" for your clinic.

Directions: Role-play the scenario with a peer. The peer will be the daughter, and you will be the medical assistant. The peer can make up information regarding the scenario. Your instructor will be the provider.

WMFM – Neurological Emergency Phone Protocol
Obtain the patient's name, date of birth, signs/symptoms, and the history of the situation. After call, document situation, symptoms, and action in the patient's health record.

With the following neurological concerns, send the patient to the emergency department via the ambulance immediately.
- Seizure lasting 3 or more minutes
- Passing out or fainting; dizziness or weakness that doesn't go away
- Sudden or unusual headache that starts suddenly
- Unable to see or speak; sudden confusion
- Neck or spine injury
- Injuries that cause loss of feeling or inability to move
- Head injury with passing out, fainting, or confusion

With the following concerns, schedule a visit for the same day. If no appointments are available, consult the triage nurse or the provider regarding the situation.
- Headache/migraine
- Nonemergent neurological concern

EQUIPMENT and SUPPLIES

- Patient's health record
- Paper and pen
- Emergency Phone Protocol for clinic

PROCEDURAL STEPS

1. Write five questions that can be asked to obtain additional information on the patient's signs and symptoms.
   PURPOSE: It is important to ask open and closed-ended questions to obtain information about the patient's condition.
2. Obtain the patient's name and date of birth.
   PURPOSE: Obtaining the patient's information is important for any patient-related phone call.
3. Write down the patient's information obtained.
   PURPOSE: Writing down the information will help when you discuss the situation with the provider and when you document the call.

4. Using critical thinking skills, ask appropriate questions to obtain information about the patient's condition.
   PURPOSE: Thoughtful questions related to the situation and the patient's condition must be asked to gather the appropriate information.
5. Follow the protocol to determine what actions to take.
   PURPOSE: Protocols are approved and signed by the providers. They need to be followed by the staff.
6. Instruct the caller on what should be done.
   PURPOSE: The caller needs clear directions on what to do.
7. Document the call in the patient's health record. Include the caller's name, the patient's condition (e.g., signs, symptoms, and concerns), name of the protocol used, information given to the caller, and the provider who was notified.
   PURPOSE: Legally it is important to document all patient interactions.

PROCEDURE 12.3   Provide First Aid for a Patient With Seizure Activity

Tasks: Provide first aid to an individual having seizure activity and document it in the health record.

Scenario: You are working with Dr. Martin, a family practice provider. Walter Biller arrives for his appointment.

EQUIPMENT and SUPPLIES

- Watch
- Folded towel, blanket, or coat
- Patient's health record
- Gloves and other personal protective equipment (as required)

PROCEDURAL STEPS

1. Wash hands or use hand sanitizer.
   PURPOSE: Hand sanitization is an important step for infection control.
2. Greet the patient. Identify yourself. Verify the patient's identity with full name and date of birth.
   PURPOSE: It is important to identify the patient in two different ways to ensure that you have the correct patient.
   Scenario update: While you are getting Mr. Biller's health history, he starts to have seizure activity.
3. Lower the patient to the floor and note the time when the seizure started. Gently raise the chin to tilt the head back slightly to open the airway.
   PURPOSE: The patient needs to be on the floor for his safety. It is important to time seizures.
4. Yell for help while moving the patient into the recovery position.
   PURPOSE: The recovery position will help to open up the person's airway. Yelling for help in the ambulatory care facility is reserved for emergencies. You need to notify the provider as soon as possible.

5. Check his pulse rate and respiration rate.
   PURPOSE: You need to make sure he is breathing and has a pulse. If not, rescue breathing and CPR must be started.
6. Put on gloves and other personal protective equipment as needed.
   PURPOSE: Wearing personal protective equipment will protect you if the patient vomits or becomes incontinent of urine or stool during the seizure.
7. Clear any hard or sharp items away from the patient. Place a soft folded towel, blanket, or coat under the patient's head.
   PURPOSE: It is important to protect the patient from harm.
8. Remove the patient's glasses (if on) and loosen any constrictive clothing around the neck. Stay with the person until he or she is fully awake and continue to monitor the respiration and pulse rates.
   PURPOSE: Tight clothing can restrict breathing.
9. Document the first aid measures you provided in the order that they occurred. In addition, document the seizure activity you witnessed, the length of the episode, and the provider notified.
   PURPOSE: Specifying the care provided, along with details of the seizure activity, will help the provider.
   10/05/20XX 1423 While rooming pt, he started to jerk his arms. He became unresponsive. Pt was moved to the floor and placed in the recovery position. P: 86 regular, thready; R: 18 regular, normal. Dr. Martin arrived. Pt's clothing was loosened. The seizure activity lasted for 4.5 minutes.
   _____ Gabe Garcia, CMA (AAMA)

PROCEDURE 12.4   Provide First Aid for a Choking Patient

Tasks: Provide first aid to a conscious adult who is choking. Document it in the health record.

Scenario: You are working with Dr. Martin, a family practice provider. As you return from lunch, you notice that an adult visitor is having an issue. It appears that she had been eating fast food and now she is holding her neck with both hands. She appears to be panicking.

EQUIPMENT and SUPPLIES

- Patient's health record
- Gloves
- Mannequin

PROCEDURAL STEPS

1. Approach the person and ask, "Are you choking?"
   PURPOSE: If the person can speak and is coughing forcefully, then let her cough and try to dislodge the obstruction. If the person is not able to speak, then assist the patient.
   Scenario update: She nods her head yes but cannot speak. She is standing.

2. Yell for help. Put on gloves if available. Stand behind the victim with your feet slightly apart. Reach your arms around the person's waist.
   PURPOSE: With an obstructed airway, the person may lose consciousness at any time. The rescuer must be prepared to lower the unconscious individual to the floor safely. If the person in distress is a child, the rescuer may need to kneel when providing assistance.
3. Make a fist and place it just above the person's navel. Make sure your thumb side is next to the person. Grasp the fist tightly with your other hand (see the following figure).
   PURPOSE: Correct hand position is important as you do abdominal thrusts.

PROCEDURE 12.4 **Provide First Aid for a Choking Patient—***continued*

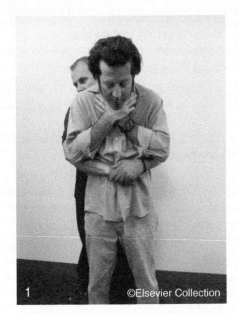

©Elsevier Collection

Scenario update: The next steps must be done on a mannequin.

4. With the correct hand position, make quick, upward and inward thrusts with your fist. Do 5 abdominal thrusts before doing back blows.
   PURPOSE: The fist should be placed in the soft tissue of the abdomen to avoid injury to the sternum or rib cage. If the person is supine, straddle and face the person's head. Push your grasped fist upward and inward.

5. Stand behind the person and wrap one arm around the person's upper body. Position the person so he or she is bent forward with the chest parallel to the ground.
   PURPOSE: This position helps objects to dislodge.

6. Use the heel of your other hand to give a firm blow between the shoulder blades. Check to see if the object dislodges. If not, continue by giving another 4 back blows.
   PURPOSE: Back blows can help dislodge the item.

7. Continue to give 5 abdominal thrusts followed by 5 back blows until the object is dislodged or the person loses consciousness.
   PURPOSE: Repeated abdominal thrusts and back blows can help dislodge the item.
   Note: If the person faints or loses consciousness, lower the person to the floor. Call 911 (or the local emergency number) or have someone else call. Begin CPR, starting with chest compressions. Check to see if the item is in the airway. Remove it only if it is loose.
   Scenario update: After two sets, she coughs out a piece of food. She can now talk.

8. Arrange for the person to be seen by the provider. Document the first aid measures you provided in the order that they occurred.
   PURPOSE: Specifying the care provided, along with details of the situation, will present the provider with a full picture of what happened.
   10/06/20XX 1223 Pt was found in reception room with her hands on her throat. She appeared to be panicky. She could not speak but indicated with a nod of her head that she was choking. After being given 2 sets of back blows and abdominal thrusts, she was able to cough out some undigested food. R: 22 regular, normal. Pt is alert. She agreed to see Dr. Martin immediately.
   _____ Gabe Garcia, CMA (AAMA)

PROCEDURE 12.5 **Provide First Aid for a Patient With a Bleeding Wound, Fracture, or Syncope**

Tasks: Provide first aid to an individual with a suspected fracture, a bleeding wound, and syncope. Document the first aid you provide.

Scenario: You are returning from lunch and see a person fall at the entrance of the healthcare facility. He is an older man and complains of pain in his right lower arm. His arm looks deformed and is bleeding. You call for help. A provider comes, and co-workers bring supplies. The provider tells you to care for the wound and splint the arm before moving the individual. You have a co-worker helping you.

EQUIPMENT and SUPPLIES

- Gloves
- Sterile gauze
- Bandage
- Splinting material (e.g., SAM Splint)
- Coban wrap or gauze roll

PROCEDURAL STEPS

1. Wash hands or use hand sanitizer if possible. Identify yourself to the patient. Obtain the patient's name and date of birth as you put on gloves.

PURPOSE: It is important to wear gloves when working with a wound. Obtaining the patient's name is important because the patient will be seen and you need to document the first aid provided.

2. Using sterile gauze, apply direct pressure over the wound to stop the bleeding. Make sure to immobilize the injured arm as you apply pressure. If possible, elevate the arm to help slow the bleeding. If the blood seeps through the gauze, apply another layer of gauze on the initial one. Continue with the direct pressure until the bleeding stops.
   PURPOSE: Applying pressure and elevating the arm will slow the bleeding.

Continued

PROCEDURE 12.5   Provide First Aid for a Patient With a Bleeding Wound, Fracture, or Syncope—*continued*

3. Once the bleeding has stopped, cover the dressing with a bandage. Remember to immobilize the injured arm as you work.

   PURPOSE: It is important to cover the wound with a bandage in case the bleeding restarts. Immobilizing a suspected arm is important until the splint can be applied.

   Scenario update: As you apply the bandage to the injured arm, the patient states he does not feel good. He says he feels dizzy and thinks he is going to pass out. Your peer takes over by supporting his arm, and the man faints. He is still breathing and has a pulse.

4. Position the patient on his back. Continue to check his respirations and pulse rates.

   PURPOSE: If the patient is not breathing or does not have a pulse, administer rescue breathing and begin CPR.

5. Loosen any constrictive clothing around the neck and chest. Raise the legs above the heart level (about 12 inches).

   PURPOSE: Raising the legs allows the blood to return to the vital organs.

   Scenario update: After a few minutes, he starts to come around. He jokes that blood makes him faint. As he is lying on his back talking with you, you need to splint his injured arm.

6. Use the splint material and shape it to the injured arm. Do not straighten the arm. Apply the splint beyond the joint above and the joint below the injury.

   PURPOSE: It is important to keep the arm in the same position until the provider examines the arm and x-rays are taken.

7. Use Coban or a gauze roll to secure the splint in place. Encourage the patient to hold the injured arm against his chest as he moves.

   PURPOSE: If the patient can hold the arm, this will reduce the pain.

8. Document the first aid measures you provided in the order they occurred. Note that the provider was at the scene.

   PURPOSE: Specifying the care provided, along with details of the seizure activity, will help the provider.

   10/07/20XX 1215 Pt fell at the clinic entrance. He c/o pain in his lower right arm. Dr. Martin ordered wound care and splinting of the arm before moving the pt. Using sterile gauze, applied direct pressure over the wound until the bleeding stopped. Wound was covered with a bandage while arm was manually immobilized. Pt stated he felt dizzy and fainted. P: 68 regular, thready; R: 16 irregular, normal. Pt was positioned on his back with his feet elevated. Within a few minutes patient came to and started talking. SAM Splint applied to right arm and Coban applied to hold the splint. Pt held arm while transferring into wheelchair. Pt to see Dr. Martin immediately. _____

   _____ Gabe Garcia, CMA (AAMA)

PROCEDURE 12.6   Provide First Aid for a Patient in Shock

Tasks: Provide first aid to an individual who is in shock. Document the first aid you provide.

Scenario: You are working with Dr. Julie Walden. The administrative medical assistant at the reception desk notifies you that Robert Caudill (date of birth [DOB] 10/31/1940) is here and looks very ill. You bring the patient and his wife immediately back to the procedure room, because it is the only available room. He asks to move to the exam table, and you assist him as he transfers to the table. You obtain his vital signs, which are P: 92, R: 26, BP 72/48, and T: 103.2.

EQUIPMENT and SUPPLIES

- Stethoscope
- Watch
- Pen
- Sphygmomanometer (blood pressure cuff)
- Pillows, blankets, or small stool to help elevate the feet
- Exam table

PROCEDURAL STEPS

1. Call for help. Monitor the patient's breathing and pulse until the provider arrives.

   PURPOSE: It is important to have the provider see the patient immediately.

   Scenario update: The provider examines the patient and suspects septic shock. You administer 2 L of oxygen per nasal cannula as the provider ordered. The triage RN inserts an IV and administers IV fluids. The provider directs another medical assistant to call 911.

2. Raise the patient's legs 12 inches.

   PURPOSE: Raising the person's legs helps the blood to return to the heart. Some tables will allow you to elevate the foot section. If this is not possible, use things such as pillows, blankets, or a small stool.

3. Make sure the patient's head is flat on the bed.

   PURPOSE: This helps the blood to flow to the head.

4. Loosen the person's clothing. Make sure the clothing does not restrict the neck and chest area.

   PURPOSE: Clothing that is tight can affect the breathing.

5. Obtain a pulse rate, respiration rate, and blood pressure. Continue to monitor the patient's airway, pulse rate, and respiration rate.

   PURPOSE: Monitor vital signs. If the person is not breathing, provide rescue breathing. If the person has no pulse, start CPR.

6. While monitoring the patient, speak calmly with him. Use a gentle tone of voice. Demonstrate calming body language (e.g., do not appear scared, rushed, or out of control).

PROCEDURE 12.6	**Provide First Aid for a Patient in Shock**—*continued*

PURPOSE: It is important to keep the patient calm during the crisis. Anxiety can be a symptom of shock.

7. Talk calmly with the patient's wife and explain what is occurring. Answer any questions the wife may have.
   PURPOSE: In an emergency, it is important to keep the family in the room updated on what is occurring. Depending on the emergency, sometimes a staff person will take the family members to another room.
8. Document the first aid measures you provided in the order they occurred. Indicate which provider examined the patient. In addition, document the administration of oxygen and the vital signs obtained.
   PURPOSE: Specifying the care provided, along with the vital signs, will help the provider and the emergency responders.

10/07/20XX 1525 P: 92 irregular, thready; R: 26 regular, shallow; BP: 72/48 RA lying; T: 103.2 (TA). Notified Dr. Walden. Pt resting on table with his wife at his side. _____ Gabe Garcia, CMA (AAMA)

10/07/20XX 1535 Administered 8 L of oxygen per mask per Dr. Walden's order. Raised legs about 12 inches, and head is flat. P: 98 irregular, thready; R: 32 regular, shallow; BP: 70/42 RA lying. _____ Gabe Garcia, CMA (AAMA)

PROCEDURE 12.7	**Provide Rescue Breathing, Cardiopulmonary Resuscitation (CPR), and Automated External Defibrillator (AED)**

Tasks: Perform rescue breathing and CPR. Use the AED machine.

Scenario: You are out jogging and find a person on the ground. No one is around.

EQUIPMENT and SUPPLIES

- AED machine with adult pads
- Barrier ventilation device
- Mannequin
- Gloves (if available)

PROCEDURAL STEPS

1. Check the scene for safety. Is it safe to approach and provide help to the victim?
   PURPOSE: It is important to look for toxic or electrical hazards. Also, look for other hazards that make the scene unsafe for you. If you find something, call 911 and wait for the emergency responders.
2. Check the person's response. Tap the individual on the shoulder and shout, "Are you all right?" Pause for a few moments for a response.
   PURPOSE: If the patient is responsive, the individual will talk, moan, move, or do something that indicates responsiveness.
   Scenario update: There is no response from the individual. A bystander comes up and you direct that person to find an AED machine.
3. Call 911 and answer the questions from the dispatcher.
   PURPOSE: The dispatcher needs to know what is occurring and the location of the emergency.
4. Put on gloves if available. Roll the person over if the person is face down. Roll the person as an entire unit, supporting the head, neck, and back. Open the airway and assess the respirations and the pulse for 5 to 10 seconds.
   Note: Occasional gasping is not considered breathing.

- Person is breathing and has a pulse: If no head, neck, or spinal injury is suspected, then place the patient in the recovery position.
- Person is not breathing and has a pulse: Give ventilations and monitor pulse.
- Person is not breathing and has no pulse: Give CPR starting with compressions.

PURPOSE: Before you initiate rescue breathing or CPR, you need to know if the person is breathing or has a pulse.

Scenario update: The individual has a weak pulse and is not breathing. (Use a mannequin for the following steps.)

5. Use a barrier device if available. Pinch the person's nose and give each rescue breath over 1 second. Watch for the chest to rise. Give the appropriate amount of ventilations for the person's age (see Table 12.9). Continue to monitor the pulse as you give rescue breaths.
   Note: For a situation in which a person had been choking, look in the mouth before giving a rescue breath. If you see the object, sweep it out with your finger. You can also provide nose ventilation, if the mouth is injured. Stoma ventilation must be done if the person has a stoma (in the throat area).
   PURPOSE: Adults get a rescue breath every 5 to 6 seconds. Children and infants get one every 3 seconds. If the chest does not rise, reposition and open the airway.
   Scenario update: When you check the pulse again, there is no pulse.
6. Place your hands at the correct location on the chest (see the first of the following figures). Bring your shoulders directly over the victim's sternum as you compress downward. Keep your elbows locked (see the second of the following figures).

Continued

PROCEDURE 12.7	Provide Rescue Breathing, Cardiopulmonary Resuscitation (CPR), and Automated External Defibrillator (AED)—*continued*

<u>PURPOSE</u>: The correct position will allow you to do the compressions at the depth they need to be.

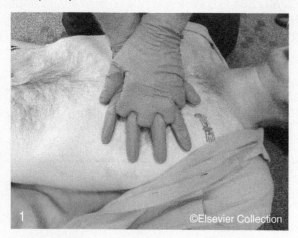

1   ©Elsevier Collection

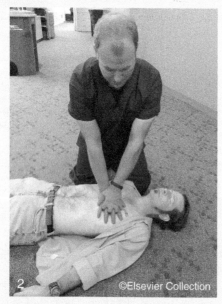

2   ©Elsevier Collection

7. Give 30 compressions at the appropriate depth (see Table 12.9). Give 100 to 120 compressions per minute.
   <u>PURPOSE</u>: The appropriate depth is required to help compress the chambers of the heart.
8. Give two ventilations and watch for the chest to rise. Continue with the cycle.
   <u>PURPOSE</u>: It is important to continue to provide ventilations and compressions until you are too exhausted, the person is breathing, an AED arrives, or emergency responders arrive.

Scenario update: After two cycles, a bystander brings an AED but does not know how to use it. The bystander also does not know CPR. You need to stop the CPR and use the AED.

9. Turn on the AED and follow the directions. Attach the AED pads to the individual's bare dry chest (see Table 12.9 and the following figure). Attach the pads to the machine if required.
   Note: Make sure to remove any medication patches and medication residue from the chest before applying the pads.
   <u>PURPOSE</u>: The pads need to be placed on the bare, dry chest for the AED to work correctly.

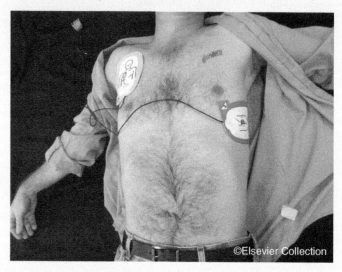

©Elsevier Collection

10. Have everyone stand back from the patient by announcing, "Stand clear." Push the analyze button and allow the machine to analyze the heartbeat.
    <u>PURPOSE</u>: "Stand clear" tells everyone to not touch the patient during this step.
11. Follow the prompts on the AED machine.
    • If a shock is advised, announce, "Stand clear" and make sure no one is touching the individual. Press the shock button. After the shock, do CPR for 2 minutes, starting with compressions. Continue following the prompts until the emergency responders arrive.
    • If a shock is not advised, continue doing CPR for 2 minutes, starting with compressions. Continue following the prompts until the emergency responders arrive.
    <u>PURPOSE</u>: The AED will prompt you as to what to do next.

PRINCIPLES OF PHARMACOLOGY

13

SCENARIO

Gabe Garcia, CMA (AAMA), has worked for Walden-Martin Family Medical (WMFM) Clinic for 3 years. He was hired right after he completed his medical assistant program. Gabe was asked to be Mark Allen's mentor for practicum. Mark has just completed all of his medical assistant courses at the local college and now needs 160 hours of practicum. He is excited to be working with Gabe.

Gabe works with several of the WMFM Clinic providers. He spends 1 to 2 hours a day working with prescription refills. Gabe also rooms patients, obtains their vital signs and history, and assist with injections. Mark will have a lot of great experiences with Gabe.

While studying this chapter, think about the following questions:

1. What are the sources and uses of drugs?
2. What is pharmacokinetics?
3. How does drug legislation affect the medical assistant practice?
4. What are the four names of a drug?
5. What information is contained in the different sections of the drug reference information?
6. How does a medical assistant prepare prescriptions for the provider to sign?

LEARNING OBJECTIVES

1. Describe the sources and uses of drugs.
2. Describe pharmacokinetics, including absorption, distribution, metabolism, and excretion.
3. Discuss drug action, including the factors that influence drug action, the therapeutic effects of drugs, and adverse reactions to drugs.
4. Explain drug legislation that is important in the ambulatory care setting. Also, discuss dietary supplements.
5. Describe the four types of drug names.
6. Describe various methods to access drug reference information.
7. Identify the classifications of medications, including the indications for use, desired effects, side effects, and adverse reactions.
8. Discuss the terminology used in drug reference information, including describing the differences among biologic half-life, onset, peak, and duration.
9. Discuss types of medication orders.
10. List the four parts of a prescription and the information required for all prescriptions; prepare prescriptions using prescription refill procedures; and define commonly approved abbreviations.
11. Describe common requirements for scheduled substances.
12. Discuss over-the-counter (OTC) medications and herbal supplements.

VOCABULARY

addiction A disease that occurs when a person cannot stop or limit the use of a drug, even after negative consequences have been experienced.

analgesic (an ahl JEE zik) A drug that reduces or eliminates pain.

antiarrhythmic (an tee ah RITH mik) A drug that prevents or alleviates heart arrhythmias.

antibiotic (an ti bie OT ik) A drug that destroys or inhibits the growth of bacteria.

anticoagulant (an tee koe AG yuh lant) A substance (i.e., medication or chemical) that prevents the clotting of blood.

anticonvulsant (an tee kahn VUL sahnt) A drug used to prevent or treat seizures.

antihistamine (an tee HIS tah meen) A drug that counteracts the effects of histamine.

anti-inflammatory (an tee in FLAM ah tor ee) A medication that prevents or reduces inflammation.

antimalarial (an tee mah LAR ee ahl) A drug used to treat or prevent malaria.

antiseptic (an ti SEP tik) A substance that inhibits the growth of microorganisms on living tissue (e.g., alcohol and povidone-iodine solution [Betadine]).

form Physical characteristics of a medication (e.g., tablet and suspension).

metabolites (muh TAB uh lites) Byproducts of drug metabolism

VOCABULARY—*continued*

National Provider Identifier (NPI) An identifier assigned by the Centers for Medicare and Medicaid Services (CMS) that classifies the healthcare provider by license and medical specialties.

psychiatrists Medical doctors who have been specially trained to diagnose and treat patients with mental, emotional, and behavioral conditions.

reconciling Comparing a document with another document to ensure that they are consistent.

side effects Unpleasant effects of a drug in addition to the desired or therapeutic effect.

therapeutic range Is reached when the blood concentration of a medication is high enough for the therapeutic effect to occur.

toxicity Harmful and deadly effects of a medication that can develop due to the buildup of medication or byproducts in the body.

Pharmacology is the study of the properties, actions, and uses of drugs. A *drug* is a chemical substance used to cure, treat, prevent, or diagnose disease. In the ambulatory care setting, medical assistants deal with medication, from history taking to administering medications. Medical assistants must have a general understanding of the classification of drugs. They need to know how to pronounce the medication names. They must know how to give medications, typical **side effects**, and the dose to give. New medications are continually being developed and released for patient treatment. Thus, medical assistants must stay updated on medications.

PHARMACOLOGY BASICS

Medications have been around for a long time. The first medications came from natural products found in our ancestors' living environment. Today, with advancing technology, most medications are created in a laboratory setting. These sources and others will be explained along with the uses of medications.

In addition, a basic description of how medication enters, moves through, and exits the body will be given. This knowledge will help the medical assistant identify patients who may be at risk for medication issues because of their age or a disease process.

Sources of Drugs

Drugs are either created from natural sources or made synthetically in a laboratory. Plants, animals, minerals, and microbiologic sources are natural sources of drugs.

Natural Sources of Drugs

Plants are the oldest source of drugs. Our ancestors found that different plants helped with different symptoms. Leaves, bark, stems, roots, and fruits have been used in medicinal preparations through the years. Some examples of medicinal plant sources include:

- Digitalis, an **antiarrhythmic** medication, comes from the purple foxglove flower.
- Nicotine comes from tobacco leaves.
- Quinidine, an **antimalarial** medication, comes from the bark of the cinchona tree.

Animals are also a source of medications. Natural substances are extracted from animal tissues and organs. Heparin, an **anticoagulant**, comes from pig intestines. Lanolin is found in topical preparations used to protect the skin. It comes from the sebaceous glands of sheep.

Other medications are developed with lactose and gelatin, which are from animals.

Minerals and microbiologic substances are other natural sources of medications. Examples of minerals include:

- Iron is used to treat iron-deficiency anemia.
- Iodine is an **antiseptic**.
- Zinc is used as a supplement and is found in topical pastes for wounds.

One microbiologic source is *Penicillium chrysogenum*. This is a fungus that creates penicillin.

Synthetic Sources of Drugs

Many medications originated in nature but have been recreated in the laboratory setting. For instance, insulin initially came from cattle and pigs. Many people developed allergies to the insulin. Now synthetic insulin is widely used. Biotechnology and genetic engineering techniques are continually being used to create new medications. With the help of technologic advances, individualized medications are also being produced. (Individualized medications will be discussed later in the chapter.) Synthetic medications are cheaper to produce because they are created in mass volumes. The quality of synthetic medications can also be controlled.

Uses of Drugs

When studying medications, it is important to identify the uses of drugs. Why are they being prescribed? What do they do in the body? Some medications may have more than one use. There are eight common uses of drugs:

- *Prevention*: Drugs used to prevent diseases. Example: vaccines are given, and the body creates antibodies to protect against specific diseases.
- *Treatment*: Drugs that relieve the symptoms while the body fights off the disease. Example: acetaminophen brings down a fever (*antipyretic*), while the body fights off a viral infection.
- *Diagnosis*: Drugs used to diagnose or monitor a condition. Example: contrast medium (radiopaque dye) is given to highlight organs on x-rays.
- *Cure*: Drugs that eliminate the disease. Example: amoxicillin, an **antibiotic**, is used to cure strep throat.
- *Contraceptive*: Drugs used to prevent pregnancy. Example: Depo-Provera is a contraceptive injectable medication.

- *Health maintenance*: Medications used to maintain or enhance health. Examples: vitamins and minerals.
- *Palliative*: Drugs that do not cure or treat the disease but improve the quality of life. Example: Morphine, an **analgesic**, is commonly used by patients with cancer.
- *Replacement*: Drugs used to increase the blood levels of naturally occurring substances in the body. Example: levothyroxine is used for patients with hypothyroidism.

CRITICAL THINKING APPLICATION   **13.1**

Gabe and Mark are discussing the basics of pharmacology and the eight common uses of medications. Gabe asks Mark which use would include taking an **antihistamine** for allergy symptoms. How would you answer this question?

Pharmacokinetics

Pharmacokinetics is the study of drug absorption, distribution, metabolism, and excretion in the body. Through pharmacokinetics, we understand when a medication starts to work in the body. We know how it moves through the body and what organs metabolize and excrete the drug from the body. Some of the patients you will be working with will have greater risks of side effects and **toxicity**. Understanding the basics of pharmacokinetics will help you identify those at greater risk for problems.

Absorption

Drugs can be administered in many ways. *Route* is the means by which a drug enters the body. Where a drug enters the body is considered the *site of administration*. *Absorption* is the movement of drug from the site of administration to the bloodstream. The following are commonly used routes:

- *Oral* (po): Medications taken by mouth.
- *Sublingual* (SL): Placed under the tongue to dissolve; absorbs quickly into the bloodstream.
- *Buccal*: Placed between the cheek and the gums dissolve and absorb quickly.
- *Intramuscular* (IM): Injected into the muscle. The greater the number of blood vessels in the muscle, the quicker the absorption.
- *Subcutaneous* (subcut): Injected just below the skin; moves into the capillaries or the lymphatic vessels and is brought to the bloodstream. This process is slower than the absorption of intramuscular drugs.
- *Intravenous* (IV): Injected directly in the bloodstream and has the fastest absorption rate.

The rate of absorption is influenced by the following factors:

- *Route*: Oral medications need to pass through the gastrointestinal (GI) tract. This takes time. IV medications are directly administered into the bloodstream and have virtually no absorption time. They start working faster than drugs given by other routes.
- *Blood flow to the absorption area*: Medication given by the sublingual and buccal routes is absorbed quickly into the bloodstream. These sites are rich with blood vessels. IM medications absorb quicker than subcut medications. The muscle tissue has more blood vessels than the subcutaneous tissue.

- *Ability of the medication to be absorbed*: Liquid medications are easier to absorb than solid medications. Solid medications need to be broken down before they absorb. Acidic medications are absorbed in the stomach. Base (or alkaline) medications are absorbed in the intestines.
- *Conditions at the site of the absorption*: Some medications must be taken with food, which can slow the absorption of the medication. Typically, medications taken on an empty stomach can be absorbed faster. The intestines provide more surface area than the stomach for the absorption of medications.

Distribution

Once the drug is absorbed into the blood, it rapidly circulates through the body (unless it has to go through the liver). During this time, the drug is brought to the body tissues. The movement of absorbed drug from the blood to the body tissues is called *distribution*. The speed of the drug's movement from the blood to the tissues varies greatly. Some drugs bind with proteins in the blood and move slowly into tissues. Some drugs accumulate in certain tissues. These tissues act as *reservoirs*, slowly releasing the drug into the bloodstream and keeping the blood levels from decreasing too rapidly. This process prolongs the effect of the drug. Circulation issues (e.g., peripheral artery disease) can also slow the distribution of medication.

For the medication to move into certain organs, it must be able to pass through the tissues. The blood-brain barrier allows only certain fat-soluble medications to pass into the cerebrospinal fluid and the brain. In comparison, the placental membrane allows most drugs to pass through from the mother to the baby in utero. This is why only certain medications are prescribed during pregnancy.

Routes Impact the Dose

Oral medications are absorbed in the stomach or in the intestines. The blood containing the absorbed digestive nutrients and drugs passes through the hepatic portal vein and the liver before it circulates to the rest of the body. In the liver, some of the drugs are chemically altered. Some of the active drug is lost during this first pass through the liver. This reduces the amount of drug in the circulating blood that can be used.

For instance, a person is having an allergic reaction and needs Benadryl. If the drug is to be taken orally, the person takes 50 mg. If it is to be given intravenously, 10 mg may be given. This is because all 10 mg gets into the bloodstream, whereas some of the 50 mg is lost as it passes through the liver before circulating through the body. It is important for a medical assistant to realize that doses (e.g., 10 mg) may vary based on the route used to give the medication.

Metabolism

Metabolism is a series of chemical processes whereby enzymes change drugs in the body. Metabolism is necessary so that medications can be cleared from the body. Active forms of drugs may be converted into water-soluble compounds, which are eventually excreted. Prodrugs can be changed into active forms of drugs.

Prodrugs

Prodrugs are medications that are administered in an inactive form. Through the normal metabolic processes, the medication is changed into an active form of a drug. The liver and the intestines are sites that can convert prodrugs to active forms of drugs. For instance, sulfasalazine (Azulfidine) is an **anti-inflammatory** drug that is used to treat ulcerative colitis. It is also a prodrug, since it is ingested in an inactive form. Bacteria in the colon change the drug into an active drug that is used by the body.

Most drug metabolism occurs in the liver. Younger children, older adults, and those with liver disease may have issues metabolizing medications. These populations could be at risk for drug toxicity. To prevent toxicity, the dose of medication is adjusted for at-risk populations.

Excretion

Excretion is the movement of **metabolites** out of the body. Most drugs are excreted through the large intestine and kidneys. The large intestine excretes the undigested drug products in the stool. The kidneys excrete metabolites in the urine. CLIA-waived urine drug screening test can detect certain metabolites.

Drugs can also be excreted in breast milk. This is critical information to have when a mother is breastfeeding her baby. As with pregnancy, only a limited number of drugs are safe with breastfeeding. Most drug references indicate if medications pass into the breast milk. Other ways drugs can be excreted are through sweat, exhaled air, and saliva.

Young children, older adults, and those with kidney disease are at risk for the buildup of metabolic drug byproducts in the body. These populations are at greater risk for symptoms of toxicity.

Drug Action

Drugs are chemicals that can cause changes in the cells. There are four main drug actions:

- *Depressing*: Slows down the cell's activity. For example, narcotic medications reduce the activity in the brain's respiratory center. This action slows the respiration rate.
- *Stimulating*: Increases the cell's activity. For instance, caffeine increases brain activity.
- *Destroying*: Kills cells or disrupts parts of cells. For example, chemotherapy medications destroy cancer cells.
- *Replacing substances*: Substances required by the body can be given as medications. For instance, patients with type 1 diabetes mellitus take insulin.

Factors Influencing Drug Action

One might think that a drug works the same for everyone. This is not so. Personal characteristics can cause minor differences in how a drug works from one person to another. Many factors influence drug action:

- *Age*: Infants and older adults have problems metabolizing and excreting medications. Their liver and kidneys are less effective. This can lead to possible drug accumulation and toxicity.
- *Body size*: A person's size affects the amount of drug needed. Children's dosages are calculated based on body weight. Thinner people require less medication than heavier people.
- *Gender*: Women have a higher proportion of body fat. Hormonal differences can affect metabolism. Women can react differently to some medications compared to men.
- *Genetics*: Genetic makeup can affect how a person responds to drugs. (This is discussed in more depth in the Pharmacogenomics section.)
- *Diseases:* Poor circulation, liver disease, and kidney disease can alter drug action.
- *Diet*: Certain foods can affect a drug's action. For instance, milk products can diminish the effects of tetracycline, an antibiotic.
- *Drug dosage, route, and timing of administration*: The greater the amount of drug taken, the greater the effect will be. The route will also affect drug action. Drugs absorb, distribute, and metabolize differently based on the administration route. Some drugs work better when taken with food, whereas others do not.
- *Mental state*: People with positive attitudes tend to do better than those with negative attitudes.
- *Environmental temperature*: In hot weather, heat relaxes blood vessels. This can speed up the distribution of medication, thus speeding up the drug's action.

Pharmacogenomics. Most medications are dosed as "one size fits all." Each person's genetic makeup affects how that person responds to medications. *Pharmacogenomics* or *pharmacogenetics* is the study of how genetic factors influence a person's metabolic response to a specific medication. Pharmacogenomics testing usually requires a small blood or saliva sample. The sample is analyzed to determine if a specific medication will be an effective treatment for a particular individual. Testing can determine the best dose of medication and if the person could have serious *adverse reactions* (unexpected or life-threatening reaction) from the medication. A different test is required for each medication. Pharmacogenomics is largely used in cancer treatments, but it is becoming more common in other areas of medicine.

Therapeutic Effects

Medications can have local or systemic effects. Medication effects that are seen at the site of administration are *local effects*. Medication effects that are seen throughout the body are *systemic effects*. Each medication has one or more *therapeutic effect* or desired effect. This is the intended action of the medication. For instance, the therapeutic effect of a pain reliever is to reduce pain.

Sometimes multiple doses are needed to achieve the therapeutic effect. Other times just one dose of medication can achieve the therapeutic effect. For some medications, the provider may prescribe a higher initial dose, called a *loading dose*. This helps to quickly increase the medication level in the blood. A loading dose helps the person achieve the **therapeutic range** sooner. A *maintenance dose* is the amount of medication needed to keep the blood levels within the therapeutic range. If the blood levels go beyond the therapeutic range, the person can experience signs and symptoms of toxicity. This is considered a *toxic dose* of medication. A *lethal dose* is the amount of medication that could kill a person.

TABLE 13.1   Common Adverse Reactions

ADVERSE REACTIONS	DESCRIPTION
Allergy	Drug allergy occurs when a person develops antibodies against a specific drug. When the drug is taken, the antibodies attack the antigens from the drug. Tissues are damaged during this process, and histamines are released. Histamines cause the allergic reactions.
Anaphylaxis	Extreme hypersensitivity to a specific drug (antigen) can cause life-threatening symptoms, including swelling of the mouth and airway, difficulty breathing, wheezing, loss of consciousness, and death.
Idiosyncrasy	A peculiar response to a certain drug. For instance, Benadryl causes drowsiness. When it is given to children, they often get extremely agitated.
Cumulative effect	For medications taken routinely, often the prior dose is not completely metabolized and excreted before the next dose is given. This can lead to a buildup of medication or byproducts that can produce toxic effects.
Toxicity	The harmful and possibly deadly effects of the medication that can develop due to the buildup of medication or byproducts in the body. People with liver or kidney disease, young children, older adults, and those who overdose are at risk for toxicity.
Drug interactions	When two or more drugs are taken, sometimes a drug-drug interaction can occur. The interactions can be helpful or harmful. Three types of drug interactions can occur: • *Antagonism*: One drug reduces or blocks the effect of another drug. Example: Naloxone is given for narcotic overdosage. • *Synergism*: The combined effect of two drugs used together is greater than the sum of each drug's effect (e.g., 1 + 1 > 2). Example of a harmful interaction: Alcohol has a synergistic effect on antidepressants. • *Potentiation*: A type of synergism; one drug increases the effect of the second drug. With L-dopa and carbidopa, one drug has no effect but increases the effect of the other drug (e.g., 0 + 1 > 1).
Tolerance	The need for a larger dose to get the same therapeutic or desired effect. Tolerance can be seen when taking narcotic pain medications and **anticonvulsants**.
Drug dependence	Strong psychological or physical need to take a certain drug. Withdrawal symptoms can be experienced when a person stops using a drug. Drug dependence can occur with or without **addiction**.

CRITICAL THINKING APPLICATION   13.2

Gabe and Mark are discussing therapeutic effect and loading dose. Gabe shares that patients sometimes get confused on how much medication to take when they are given two amounts, a loading dose and the regular amount. How might a healthcare professional instruct a patient who needs to take a loading dose?

Adverse Reactions

Most of the time when a medication is correctly administered, the therapeutic effect occurs. However, sometimes issues arise, and the person has problems with the medication. The person can experience an unexpected or life-threatening reaction, which is called an *adverse reaction*. Table 13.1 lists common adverse reactions.

Many experts and drug reference information will include side effects with adverse reactions. They may divide these into mild, moderate, and severe reactions. The side effects usually fall into the mild category. Severe adverse reactions are those that can cause disability, hospitalization, death, or birth defects.

Other reference information separates adverse reactions/events and side effects. Adverse reactions or events would be those that are life-threatening and may cause disability or birth defects. Side effects would be unpleasant effects of the drug, in addition to the desired

or therapeutic effect. They can be harmless or may cause injury. The most common side effects include symptoms of gastrointestinal (GI) distress, such as nausea, vomiting, constipation, and diarrhea.

DRUG LEGISLATION AND THE AMBULATORY CARE SETTING

In the ambulatory care environment, medications can be prescribed, administered, and dispensed.
- *Prescribe* means to order a medication as a treatment for a condition. Doctors (MDs [including **psychiatrists**], DOs, and dentists) and advanced practice professionals, including physician assistants (PAs), nurse practitioners (NPs), and certified nurse midwives (CNMs), can prescribe medications. State prescribing laws can vary for advanced practice professionals.
- *Administer* means to give a prescribed dose of medication to a patient. Medical assistants, nurses, and providers can administer medications. State laws related to medication administration by medical assistants can vary.
- *Dispense* means to give a supply of medication that the patient will take at a later time. In most scenarios, pharmacists dispense medications.

Federal and state legislation governs these three activities. The following sections will discuss these laws, the agencies responsible for overseeing the laws, and the laws' effect on medical assistants.

CRITICAL THINKING APPLICATION   **13.3**

At WMFM Clinic, pharmaceutical representatives drop off sample medications that are given to patients. Usually, the provider will give a few days' worth of samples to a patient to ensure the patient is tolerating the medication. If the patient has no issues, then he or she gets the prescription filled. Mark sees the provider bag up a few samples and attach directions to the bag. The provider gives the bag to Gabe and asks him to give it to the patient. Mark asks Gabe, "Who is dispensing the medication?" How would you answer this question?

Food, Drug, and Cosmetic Act

The Food, Drug, and Cosmetic Act of 1938 is enforced by the Food and Drug Administration (FDA). The FDA is a federal agency in the Department of Health and Human Services (HHS). The FDA is responsible for the safety, effectiveness, security, and quality of drugs, cosmetics, and food. Some of the areas overseen by the FDA include:

- *Foods*: Dietary supplements, bottled water, food additives, infant formula, and other food products
- *Drugs*: Prescription drugs (brand name and generic) and nonprescription (over-the-counter) drugs
- *Biologics*: Vaccines, blood, and blood products
- *Medical devices*: Medical equipment (from simple [tongue depressor] to complex [heart pacemaker]), dental devices, and surgical implants

---

Dietary Supplements

Dietary supplements are oral products that contain a "dietary ingredient." This ingredient can include a vitamin, mineral, amino acid, herb, or another substance that can supplement a person's diet. Dietary supplements come in many forms, including tablets, powders, energy bars, and liquids. Federal law does not require a dietary supplement to be proven safe, nor must any claims for it be proven truthful before the product appears on the market. The Food and Drug Administration (FDA) monitors the safety of such products after they are on the market.

The function of dietary supplements is to provide nutrients that are not obtained in the foods we eat and drink. Some examples of uses of dietary supplements include:

- Calcium and vitamin D for bone health and low vitamin D levels
- Folic acid in pregnancy to prevent spina bifida
- Iron for low iron levels
- Fiber for constipation

Before starting a dietary supplement, it is important to talk with the provider. Some medications may interact with dietary supplements. Some dietary supplements may work against medications. For instance, taking vitamin K promotes blood clotting, and Coumadin (warfarin) delays blood clotting.

Manufacturers must submit applications for new products to the FDA. Manufacturers must provide adequate data to show the safety and effectiveness of the product. The FDA must determine if drugs, devices, and products are safe and effective. Once this is determined, then the product is released to the general public.

The FDA monitors the safety of products released to the market. The FDA Adverse Event Reporting System (FAERS) is a computerized database that helps the FDA monitor drugs. It contains reports of adverse events reported to the FDA. MedWatch is the FDA's reporting program. It provides information on products overseen by the FDA. MedWatch is available to healthcare professionals (*www.fda.gov/safety/medwatch/*).

If the FDA determines a medication is unsafe, it will recall the medication. The medical assistant should remove any recalled medications from the stock and sample cabinets. (*Sample medications* come from pharmaceutical companies and are used for patients.) Concerned patients may contact their providers. The provider will determine what action to take for each patient.

Controlled Substances Act

The Controlled Substances Act (CSA), Title II of the Comprehensive Drug Abuse Prevention and Control Act of 1970, is a federal law. The Drug Enforcement Agency (DEA) is a federal law enforcement agency under the US Department of Justice. The DEA enforces the CSA. The DEA oversees the manufacturing, importation, possession, use, and distribution of illegal and legal controlled substances.

Under the CSA, controlled substances are divided into five schedules. These schedules are arranged from the greatest to the least abuse potential (Table 13.2). State statutes also address procedures related to scheduled medications. It is important for the medical assistant to know the schedule of commonly ordered medications. Some controlled substance prescriptions are handled differently. This will be discussed later in the chapter.

Compliance With the Controlled Substance Act

Providers prescribing controlled substances need a DEA registration number. Each provider has a unique number. The DEA number is good for 3 years. The medical assistant may need to assist the provider in renewing or obtaining a DEA number. This can be done at the DEA website at *www.deadiversion.usdoj.gov*. Additional state requirements may need to be met before a provider can prescribe controlled substances.

Controlled substances have a paper trail. This record starts with the manufacturer and ends when the medication is dispensed or administered. In some healthcare facilities, the in-house pharmacy handles the controlled substances that are administered. The provider gives the medical assistant a prescription for a patient. The medical assistant gives the pharmacist the prescription and, in return, gets the medication. (Please note that some state laws do not allow medical assistants to administer controlled substances.) With this scenario, the pharmacist is responsible for managing the paperwork for the controlled substances.

In healthcare facilities without pharmacies, providers must take the responsibility of ordering controlled substances from the manufacturer. The medical assistant must help the provider comply with the Controlled Substance Act. The following sections will discuss common compliance activities.

TABLE 13.2   Schedule of Controlled Substances

SCHEDULE	PSYCHOLOGICAL AND PHYSICAL DEPENDENCE	EXAMPLES
I	Highest potential for abuse; drugs with no currently accepted medical purpose.	Heroin, lysergic acid diethylamide (LSD), ecstasy
II/IIN (C–II)	High level of abuse; can lead to severe psychological or physical dependence	Schedule II narcotics: oxycodone (OxyContin, Percocet), fentanyl (Duragesic), codeine, morphine Schedule IIN stimulants: amphetamine (Adderall), methamphetamine (Desoxyn), methylphenidate (Concerta, Ritalin LA)
III/III N (C–III)	Moderate to low physical dependence or high psychological dependence	Schedule III narcotics: acetaminophen with codeine (Tylenol #2 or #3), buprenorphine (Suboxone) Schedule IIIN non-narcotics: ketamine, anabolic steroids (e.g., Depo-Testosterone)
IV (C–IV)	Low potential for abuse relative to substances in Schedule III	Schedule IV substances: alprazolam (Xanax), clonazepam (Klonopin), diazepam (Valium), lorazepam (Ativan)
V (C–V)	Lowest potential for abuse relative to substances listed in Schedule IV; contains limited quantities of certain narcotics	Schedule V substances: Robitussin AC, ezogabine (Potiga)

Storage. All controlled substances must be adequately safeguarded. They need to be kept in a locked cabinet or safe of substantial construction. Keys should be placed in a locked area accessible only to authorized persons. Controlled substances should be kept in their original containers.

Storage of Medications

- Store controlled substances in a different location than non-narcotic medications.
- Refer to package inserts for specific storage information.
- Store medications in a cool, dry location. Keep medications away from light, heat, or moisture.
- For refrigerated and frozen medications, keep temperature logs to ensure the appropriate temperature range is maintained.
- Medications with different lot numbers or expiration dates should not be combined or repackaged.
- Keep *stock medications* (purchased by department) separated from *sample medications* (given by pharmaceutical manufacturers for patients).
- Keep medications out of exam rooms. Lock medication cabinets at the end of the day.
- For information on vaccine storage, refer to Chapter 11 in the main text.

Inventory Records. It is important to keep an ongoing log of controlled substances received from manufacturers and administered to patients. Medications are tracked by the manufacturer, lot number, and expiration date. This information is found on the package. When a patient needs a controlled substance, the medical assistant must complete the log. The log typically requires:

- The medication information (name, dose, lot number, and expiration date)
- The ordering provider's name
- Information on the patient receiving the medication (name, date of birth, address, health record number, etc.)
- The name or initials of the healthcare professional administering the medication

The log must be kept separate from the patient's health record. The medication must also be documented in the patient's health record after it is administered.

Periodic **reconciling** of the log with the actual inventory count is important to identify missing medications. An inventory of all controlled substances must be done at least annually, unless required more often by law. Some states have special requirements for the inventory. It is important for the medical assistant to be knowledgeable about the special state requirements. The controlled substance inventory and log records need to be kept for 2 years. The records may be inspected by individuals authorized by the state attorney general.

Drug Destruction

Expired controlled substances are returned to the place from where they were received. For example, controlled substances that were sent by the manufacturer must be returned to the manufacturer, along with the required paperwork.

Sometimes a controlled substance must be destroyed in the healthcare facility. Examples of such situations are:

- Only part of the medication is used for the patient, and the extra amount must be destroyed.
- The patient refuses the medication after it has been opened and prepared.

• The medication is accidentally contaminated before it can be administered.

In these situations the controlled substance must be destroyed in the presence of two authorized persons (e.g., medical assistants, nurses). An entry on the waste log must be made. This information must include the date; the drug's name, strength, and quantity; the reason for destruction, and the signatures of both persons.

Discarding Medications in the Healthcare Facility

Discard medication that is expired, contaminated, unlabeled, or opened and not used. Some healthcare facilities have medication discarding programs to prevent medications from entering the city's water supply. Remember, if the medication is a controlled substance, two authorized employees must sign a waste log before the medication is discarded. Both employees must witness the disposal.

To discard medication, follow these steps if the facility has no other procedures in place:

• Return expired controlled substances to the place from which they were received (e.g., manufacturer), accompanied by the proper paperwork.
• Flush liquids down the sink.
• Flush pills down the toilet.
• Mix powdered medications with water and flush them down the toilet.
• Flush fluid from syringes down the sink and discard the syringe in a biohazard sharps container.

Theft and Diversion Reporting

Diversion of controlled substances means using the medication for personal reasons. If a medical assistant identifies that controlled substances are missing, it is important to notify the provider and supervisor. Many states and the DEA require any theft or loss to be reported to them within a given period of time. A report must be completed and filed by the deadline.

Medical Assistant's Role in Preventing Drug Abuse. By following these guidelines, the medical assistant can help prevent drug abuse.

• Carefully monitor patients who repeatedly call for prescription refills of controlled substances. Be aware that some patients will give *aliases* (false names).
• Request health records from other facilities for patients who report previous prescriptions for scheduled drugs.
• If the facility uses paper prescription pads, keep blank pads in a locked cabinet. They should be stored away from patient treatment areas.
• Never use prescription pads for notepads. Never use preprinted or presigned forms.
• Secure computers used for electronic health record (EHR) documentation to prevent patient access to prescription generation.
• Keep only a limited supply of controlled substances on hand.
• Keep accurate, complete records of controlled substances administered. Patients' records should contain information on prescribed and administered controlled substances.

DRUG NAMES

A single drug may have up to four names: chemical, generic, official, and brand. The drug is known by its chemical name until it receives FDA approval. The medical assistant should be familiar with the brand and generic names of common medications.

• *Chemical name:* Represents the drug's exact chemical formula. For example, the chemical name of ibuprofen is 2-(4-isobutylphenyl) propanoic acid.
• *Generic name:* Assigned by the US Adopted Names (USAN) Council. Similar medications are given similar-sounding generic names. All drugs need to have the generic name on the packaging. For example, ibuprofen is a generic name.
• *Official name:* Used to list the medication in the United States Pharmacopeia and the National Formulary (USP–NF). This book provides the standards (strength, purity, etc.) for drugs in the United States. In many cases, the official name is the same as the generic name. For example, ibuprofen is also the drug's official name.
• *Brand name:* Also called the *trade name.* The manufacturer assigns and registers the medication name. No other company can use that name. Usually the brand name begins with a capital letter and is followed by the registered sign (®). For example, brand names of ibuprofen include Advil and Motrin.

Generic Versus Brand Medications

If you ever walk through the pain medication aisle at a local store, you will see many bottles of ibuprofen products. Generally, the more expensive products are name brands, and less expensive products are generic products.

The company that initially created the medication will market it using a brand name. That company has sole rights to manufacture the medication until the patent expires. During this time, it is not uncommon for the price to be higher. The manufacturer may have spent years developing the medication before it went to market. Once the patent expires, other companies may create their own version of the medication. Some will market the medication under a brand name and others will use generic names.

When a company creates a medication, the company determines the appearance of the medication (e.g., color, size, and shape). It also comes up with the inactive ingredients or additives. This might be a color, sweetener, flavor, fillers, binders, and so on. For the active ingredient, the medication (i.e., ibuprofen), the company must comply with the FDA's regulations. The active ingredient must be of the same quality, purity, and amount as any other FDA-approved ibuprofen product of the same strength.

Most people do not notice a difference between generic and brand name medications. Other people do notice a difference. Their bodies may react to the inactive ingredients differently. This can affect their treatment for certain conditions. The provider can indicate if a generic medication can be used for prescriptions. This is important to keep in mind if you are assisting a provider by preparing prescriptions.

CRITICAL THINKING APPLICATION   13.4

Mark and Gabe are working with Janine Butler, a patient being seen for hypertension. While they are reviewing Janine's current medication list, she asks them what the difference is between generic and brand name medications. How might you answer this question?

DRUG REFERENCE INFORMATION

A medical assistant is obligated to become familiar with the drugs that are most frequently prescribed in the department. It is essential to know their indications, adverse reactions, administration routes, dosage, and storage. Using drug reference information can help the medical assistant learn about drugs. In the ambulatory care environment, drug reference information is available in both print and digital form.

With each drug (including drug samples and stock medications), the manufacturer includes a package insert. The package insert provides information about the medication, side effects, administration techniques, dosages, storage, and so on.

Drug handbooks provide condensed, more common information on the drugs. Many of these books are organized by the generic names of drugs.

An old classic, the *Physician's Desk Reference* (PDR), was a very large book that contained a comprehensive collection of package insert information. After publishing the 2017 version (the 71st edition), the company stopped printing the PDR. The drug reference information is available through its digital online products (*Prescribers' Digital Reference* [PDR]), its app, and other products that integrate with electronic health records. More information can be found on the website (*www.pdr.net*).

The digital drug reference information has a huge advantage over print information. Digital information can be updated more quickly and easily than the print information. The market for digital drug information has grown over the years. Digital drug reference information is available online, through apps, and with electronic health records.

- Online drug reference information is available from many sites. It is important for the medical assistant to use reliable websites. Government websites (e.g., *medlineplus.gov* and *www.fda.gov*) contain updated, reliable information. Sites that patients use may contain older information and can include medications that are not available in the United States.
- When selecting an app for drug reference information, be sure it is routinely updated. Read the reviews, and research the company providing the information. Only use reputable apps for drug reference information.
- Many electronic health record software programs incorporate drug reference information. This makes it easy for healthcare professionals to look up drug information.

Drug Classification

Drugs are grouped by classification or class. It is important for a medical assistant to be aware of the class of drugs. Oftentimes patients will ask what a specific medication is for, and the medical assistant

can provide that information. Table 13.3 provides a list of classifications of medications with descriptions.

Drug Terminology

Regardless of how drug reference information is obtained, it is important for the medical assistant to understand the terminology. The following terminology is typically found in drug reference information.

- *Names:* Usually the generic name is listed with the trade names. Some references may indicate if the trade name found is in the United States or Canada.
- *Description:* Describes the medication and its general use.
- *Boxed warning:* Also referred to as a *black box warning*. It addresses serious or life-threatening risks. This information also appears on the drug's label.
- *Dosage:* Specifies the route, dose, and timing of the medication; usually corresponds to an indication (disease or condition). May provide information on doses for different age ranges. *Maximum dosage* indicates the greatest amount of medication a person should have within a 24-hour period.
- *Indication:* Conditions or diseases for which the drug is used.
- *Dosage considerations:* Indicates recommended changes in dosages for special populations (e.g., patients with hepatic impairment, renal impairment).
- *How supplied:* Lists the **form** (e.g., chewable tablets, capsules) and the strength (e.g., 250 mg)
- *Administration:* Provides information on how the medication should be administered. Includes important administration techniques, such as information on shaking the medication, if it needs to be taken with food, and so on.
- *Contraindications:* Reasons or conditions that make administration of the drug improper or undesirable. For example, aspirin is contraindicated in patients with GI bleeding.
- *Precautions:* Indicates necessary actions or special care that needs to be taken when the patient is on the medication. May include information on laboratory tests, special populations (children and geriatric), pregnancy, breastfeeding, and so on.
- *Adverse reactions:* Also called *side effects* in some information. This section describes known undesirable experiences associated with the medication. Reactions may be divided into severe (life-threatening, serious reactions), moderate, and mild.
- *Interactions:* Includes medications, foods, and beverages that interact with the medication. These products may either increase or reduce the medication level in the blood. They may also increase the risk of adverse reactions if taken together with the drug.
- *Action:* How the drug provides therapeutic results in the body, or the use of the drug.
- *Pharmacokinetics:* Provides information on the absorption, distribution, metabolism, and excretion of the medication. Information on when the drug is at its highest level in the body or when the drug starts working may be included. Important terms for understanding the pharmacokinetics of a drug include:
  - *Biologic half-life:* The time it takes half of the drug to be metabolized or eliminated by normal biologic processes.
  - *Onset:* The time it takes for the drug to produce a response.

TABLE 13.3   Examples of Medication Classifications

CLASSIFICATION	DESCRIPTION	CLASSIFICATION	DESCRIPTION
Analgesic	Relieves pain	Contraceptive	Inhibits conception (prevents pregnancy)
Anesthetic	Produces local or general anesthesia	Corticosteroid	Reduces inflammation
Antacid	Neutralizes stomach acid	Decongestant	Relieves nasal and sinus congestion
Anti-Alzheimer	Treats dementia (Alzheimer)	Diuretic	Increases urinary output and lowers blood pressure
Antianxiety	Reduces anxiety and tension	Electrolyte	Maintains normal electrolyte level and proper functioning of the body systems
Antiarrhythmic	Treats heart arrhythmias		
Antibiotic	Treats bacterial infections	Erectile dysfunction agent	Facilitates an erection
Anticholinergic	Reduces smooth muscle spasms	Expectorant	Thins bronchial secretions, making it easier to cough up mucus
Anticoagulant	Decreases blood clotting ability		
Anticonvulsant	Reduces the frequency and severity of seizures	Hematopoietic	Promotes blood cell production
Antidepressant	Treats depression	Hemostatic	Clots blood
Antiemetic	Reduces nausea and vomiting	Hormone replacement	Replaces hormones or compensates for hormone deficiencies
Antifungal	Treats fungal infections		
Antigout	Reduces the uric acid in the body	Laxative	Promotes stools
Antihistamine	Relieves allergies by blocking the histamine action	Leukotriene receptor antagonist	Blocks the action of substances that cause asthma and allergic rhinitis
Antihyperglycemic	Reduces blood glucose level	Miotic	Drains excessive fluid from the eye, used for glaucoma
Antihypertensive	Lowers blood pressure		
Anti-inflammatory	Reduces inflammation	Muscle relaxant	Reduces pain
Antimigraine	Treats or prevents migraine headaches	Mydriatic	Dilates the pupil, used for ophthalmic procedures
Antineoplastic	Slows or stops the growth of cancer cells		
Antiplatelet	Prevents the function of platelets (formation of clots)	Osteoporosis agent	Promotes bone mineral density, used to treat osteoporosis
Antipsychotic	Alters the chemical actions in the brain	Proton-pump inhibitor	Reduces the acid produced in the stomach
Antitussive	Suppresses coughs	Sedative-hypnotic	Slows brain activity, allowing sleep
Antiviral	Treats viral infections	Stimulant	Stimulates the brain and body, makes the person more alert
Bronchodilator	Relaxes the smooth muscles of the bronchi		
Cholesterol-lowering agent	Reduces low-density lipoprotein and triglycerides in the blood while increasing the high-density lipoprotein	Tumor necrosis factor (TNF) inhibitor	Blocks the action of TNF, preventing inflammation in autoimmune disorders

- *Peak*: The time it takes for the drug to reach its greatest effective concentration in the blood.
- *Duration*: The time during which the drug is present in the blood at great enough levels to produce a response.

Table 13.4 provides drug information on the top 50 commonly prescribed medications. Please use drug reference information for additional information on these products.

Pregnancy and Lactation Labeling Rule

In 2015 the Pregnancy and Lactation Labeling Rule (PLLR) replaced the pregnancy risk letter categories (e.g., A, B, C, D, and X) with more comprehensive information. The goal is to provide the provider and patient with pregnancy and lactation information. This information can be used when discussing the risks versus the benefits of a medication. The FDA created the new system to help with patient-specific counseling and informed decision making for pregnant and breastfeeding mothers who need medication therapies. The system consists of three subcategories with detailed information about the following:

- *Pregnancy*: Includes information on the risks during pregnancy for the mother and baby, in addition to data on the risk of adverse developmental outcomes.
- *Lactation*: Includes information on the presence of the drug in breast milk, the effects on a breast-fed child, and the impact on milk production.
- *Females and males of reproductive potential*: Includes information about when pregnancy testing or contraception is required during drug therapy and data that suggest drug-associated fertility effects.

CRITICAL THINKING APPLICATION 13.5

Gabe mentions to Mark that he learned that the FDA had changed the pregnancy risk categories. Mark had not heard about this. Gabe further explains why. Describe how the changes provide more information to providers and patients.

TYPES OF MEDICATION ORDERS

A *medication order* refers to directions given by a provider for a specific medication to be administered to a patient. The medical assistant receives the information from the provider. The provider must give this information:

- Patient's name and health record number or date of birth (DOB) (e.g., Noemi Rodriguez DOB 11/04/1971)
- Medication name, dose, and route (e.g., Tylenol 1 g po)

The provider can give the order over the phone or in person. This type of order is called a *verbal order*. It is important for the medical assistant to write down the order and read it back to the provider. This process ensures the order was heard and recorded correctly. The provider can also give the medical assistant a *written order*. Usually, these are written on a prescription pad or in an electronic message. A written order only needs clarification from the provider if the medical assistant cannot read the order or has a question.

Text continued on p. 333

TABLE 13.4 Information on Commonly Prescribed Medications

GENERIC NAME	BRAND/TRADE NAME(S)	CLASS/ SCHEDULE	MEDICATION INFORMATION
hydrocodone/ acetaminophen (APAP)	Vicodin, Norco, Lortab	Analgesics (narcotic [opioids]) C–II	*Indication*: moderate to severe pain *Desired effects/action*: changes the way the brain and nervous system respond to pain *Side effects*: GI intolerance, difficulty urinating, anxiety, fuzzy thinking *Adverse reaction*: slowed breathing, chest tightness
oxycodone/ acetaminophen (APAP)	Percocet, Oxycet, Roxicet	Analgesics (narcotic [opioids]) C–II	*Indication*: moderate to severe pain *Desired effects/action*: changes the way the brain and nervous system respond to pain *Side effects*: GI intolerance, flushing, headache, mood changes *Adverse reaction*: slowed breathing, angina, hypersensitivity, seizures
tramadol	Ultram, Conzip	Analgesics (narcotic [opioids]) C–II	*Indication*: moderate to severe pain *Desired effects/action*: changes the way the brain and nervous system respond to pain *Side effects*: GI intolerance, difficulty sleeping, change in mood, dry mouth *Adverse reaction*: hallucinations, agitation, hypersensitivity, arrhythmias
memantine	Namenda	Anti-Alzheimer	*Indication*: Alzheimer disease *Desired effects/action*: reduces the brain chemicals that cause the dementia *Side effects*: GI intolerance, edema, weight loss, dizziness, anxiety, aggression *Adverse reaction*: angina, seizures, hypertension

Continued

TABLE 13.4   Information on Commonly Prescribed Medications—*continued*

GENERIC NAME	BRAND/TRADE NAME(S)	CLASS/ SCHEDULE	MEDICATION INFORMATION
alprazolam	Xanax	Antianxiety (benzodiazepines) C–IV	*Indication:* anxiety and panic disorders *Desired effects/action:* decreases abnormal excitement in the brain *Side effects:* drowsiness, headache, dizziness, GI intolerance, dry mouth, weight changes *Adverse reaction:* seizures, jaundice, depression, memory problems
clonazepam	Klonopin	Antianxiety (benzodiazepines) C–IV	*Indication:* seizures, panic attacks *Desired effects/action:* decreases abnormal excitement in the brain *Side effects:* drowsiness, coordination problems, joint pain, blurred vision, changes in sex drive *Adverse reaction:* hypersensitivity
diazepam	Valium	Antianxiety (benzodiazepines) C–IV	*Indication:* relieves anxiety, muscle spasms, and seizures *Desired effects/action:* produces a calming effect *Side effects:* GI intolerance, weakness, tiredness, drowsiness, dry mouth *Adverse reaction:* restlessness, frequent urination, blurred vision
digoxin	Lanoxin, Digitek, Cardoxin	Antiarrhythmics	*Indication:* congestive heart failure (CHF), atrial fibrillation *Desired effects/action:* helps the heart work better, controls heart rate *Side effects:* dizziness, drowsiness, visual changes (blurred, yellow), arrhythmias *Adverse reaction:* swelling of hands and feet, unusual weight gain, difficulty breathing *Assessment:* take apical pulse, hold if <60 in adults, <70 in children, and <90 in infants
cephalexin	Keflex	Antibiotics (cephalosporin)	*Indication:* bacterial infections (e.g., urinary tract, ear, and pneumonia) *Desired effects/action:* stops bacteria growth *Side effects:* GI intolerance, agitation, confusion, headache *Adverse reaction:* hypersensitivity, watery or bloody stools, hallucinations
azithromycin	Zithromax, Zithromax Z-Paks, Zmak	Antibiotics (macrolide)	*Indication:* bacterial infections (e.g., sexually transmitted infections, bronchitis, and pneumonia) *Desired effects/action:* stops bacteria growth *Side effects:* GI intolerance, headache *Adverse reaction:* hypersensitivity, mouth sores, arrhythmias, jaundice, dark-colored urine
amoxicillin	Amoxil, Moxtag	Antibiotics (penicillin)	*Indication:* bacterial infections (e.g., pneumonia, gonorrhea, ear, and throat) *Desired effects/action:* stops bacteria growth *Side effects:* GI intolerance *Adverse reaction:* hypersensitivity, seizures, jaundice
warfarin	Coumadin	Anticoagulants	*Indication:* prevents blood clots from forming *Desired effects/action:* decreases clotting ability of the blood *Side effects:* GI intolerance, loss of hair, chills *Adverse reaction:* hypersensitivity, infection, angina, jaundice, bleeding
gabapentin	Neurontin, Horizant	Anticonvulsants	*Indication:* seizures, postherpetic neuralgia, restless legs syndrome (RLS) *Desired effects/action:* decreases abnormal excitement in the brain; reduces seizures *Side effects:* drowsiness, blurred vision, anxiety, memory problems, weakness, GI intolerance *Adverse reaction:* hypersensitivity, seizures

TABLE 13.4	**Information on Commonly Prescribed Medications—***continued*		
GENERIC NAME	**BRAND/TRADE NAME(S)**	**CLASS/ SCHEDULE**	**MEDICATION INFORMATION**
duloxetine	Cymbalta	Antidepressant (selective serotonin and norepinephrine reuptake inhibitors [SNRIs])	*Indication:* major depressive disorder, generalized anxiety disorder, diabetic peripheral neuropathy, fibromyalgia, chronic pain *Desired effects/action:* increases the amounts of serotonin and norepinephrine in the brain; helps to maintain mental balance and stop pain signals in the brain *Side effects:* orthostatic hypotension *Adverse reaction:* suicidal thoughts, hepatotoxicity, seizures, glaucoma, hyponatremia
citalopram	Celexa	Antidepressant (selective serotonin reuptake inhibitors [SSRIs])	*Indication:* depression *Desired effects/action:* increases the amount of serotonin in the brain; helps to maintain mental balance *Side effects:* GI intolerance, frequent urination, weakness, joint pain, weight loss *Adverse reaction:* angina, shortness of breath, arrhythmias, hallucinations, coma, hypersensitivity, confusion, seizures, suicidal thoughts
escitalopram	Lexapro	Antidepressant (selective serotonin reuptake inhibitors [SSRIs])	*Indication:* depression, generalized anxiety disorder (GAD) *Desired effects/action:* increases the amount of serotonin in the brain; helps to maintain mental balance *Side effects:* GI intolerance, increased sweating, change in sex drive, flulike symptoms *Adverse reaction:* unusual excitement, hallucinations, confusion, arrhythmias, severe muscle stiffness, suicidal thoughts
sertraline	Zoloft	Antidepressant (selective serotonin reuptake inhibitors [SSRIs])	*Indication:* depression, obsessive-compulsive disorder (OCD), panic attacks, posttraumatic stress disorder (PTSD) *Desired effects/action:* increases the amount of serotonin in the brain; helps to maintain mental balance *Side effects:* GI intolerance, weight changes, difficulty falling asleep, change in sex drive, excessive sweating *Adverse reaction:* seizures, abnormal bleeding, arrhythmias, hypersensitivity, suicidal thoughts
trazodone	Oleptro	Antidepressant (serotonin modulators)	*Indication:* depression *Desired effects/action:* increases the amount of serotonin; helps to maintain mental balance *Side effects:* GI intolerance, weakness, headache, confusion, sweating, decreased coordination *Adverse reaction:* angina, fainting, seizures, coma, arrhythmias, suicidal thoughts
promethazine	Promethegan	Antihistamines	*Indication:* allergies, allergic conjunctivitis, anaphylaxis, sedation for procedures, motion sickness *Desired effects/action:* blocks histamine action *Side effects:* drowsiness, difficulty sleeping, ringing in ears, blurred vision, GI intolerance *Adverse reaction:* wheezing, slowed breathing, sweating, stiff muscles, decreased alertness
metformin	Glucophage, Fortamet, Glumetza, Riomet	Antihyperglycemics	*Indication:* type 2 diabetes mellitus *Desired effects/action:* reduces glucose absorption and increases body's response to insulin; controls the blood glucose level *Side effects:* GI intolerance, metallic taste in the mouth, flushing of the skin, nail changes *Adverse reaction:* angina, rash

Continued

TABLE 13.4 Information on Commonly Prescribed Medications—*continued*

GENERIC NAME	BRAND/TRADE NAME(S)	CLASS/ SCHEDULE	MEDICATION INFORMATION
valsartan	Diovan	Antihypertensive (angiotensin II receptor antagonists)	*Indication:* hypertension, heart failure, postmyocardial infarction (MI) *Desired effects/action:* prevents vasoconstriction, which lowers the blood pressure *Side effects:* headache, dizziness, flu symptoms, GI intolerance, blurred vision, mild itching *Adverse reaction:* hyperkalemia, arrhythmias
losartan	Cozaar	Antihypertensive (angiotensin II receptor antagonists)	*Indication:* hypertension, heart failure *Desired effects/action:* lowers the blood pressure *Side effects:* headache, dizziness, diarrhea, muscle cramps and pain, nasal congestion, cough, upper respiratory infections, sinusitis *Adverse reaction:* chest pain, difficulty swallowing, hoarseness
benazepril	Lotensin	Antihypertensive (angiotensin-converting enzyme [ACE] inhibitors)	*Indication:* hypertension *Desired effects/action:* causes vasodilation, lowering the blood pressure *Side effects:* cough, drowsiness, headache *Adverse reaction:* jaundice, difficulty breathing, lightheadedness, swelling, hoarseness
lisinopril	(no brand names)	Antihypertensive (angiotensin-converting enzyme [ACE] inhibitors)	*Indication:* hypertension, heart failure *Desired effects/action:* causes vasodilation, lowering the blood pressure *Side effects:* cough, dizziness, tiredness, GI intolerance, rash *Adverse reaction:* angina, lightheadedness, difficulty swallowing, hypersensitivity
atenolol	Tenormin	Antihypertensive (beta blockers)	*Indication:* hypertension, angina *Desired effects/action:* relaxes blood vessels and slows the heart rate, thus improving blood flow and decreasing blood pressure *Side effects:* dizziness, tiredness, depression, GI intolerance *Adverse reaction:* shortness of breath, swelling of legs and hands, weight gain, fainting
metoprolol	Lopressor	Antihypertensive (beta blockers)	*Indication:* hypertension, angina *Desired effects/action:* relaxes blood vessels and slows the heart rate, thus improving blood flow and decreasing blood pressure *Side effects:* dizziness, tiredness, depression, GI intolerance *Adverse reaction:* hypersensitivity, weight gain, arrhythmias
carvedilol	Coreg	Antihypertensive (beta blockers)	*Indication:* heart failure, hypertension *Desired effects/action:* relaxes blood vessels and slows the heart rate, thus improving blood flow and decreasing blood pressure *Side effects:* hyperglycemia, tiredness, weakness, dizziness, visual changes, joint pain, difficulty sleeping *Adverse reaction:* shortness of breath, swelling of arms and legs, arrhythmias
amlodipine	Norvasc	Antihypertensive (calcium channel blockers)	*Indication:* hypertension, angina *Desired effects/action:* relaxes the vessels so the heart does not have to pump as hard *Side effects:* GI intolerance, headache, swelling of legs and arms, tiredness, flushing *Adverse reaction:* more frequent or severe angina, fainting, arrhythmias
ibuprofen	Advil, Motrin, Midol	Anti-inflammatory drugs (nonsteroidal [NSAIDs])	*Indication for use:* osteoarthritis, rheumatoid arthritis, fever, pain *Desired effects/action:* stops the body's production of substances that causes pain, fever, and inflammation *Side effects:* GI intolerance, ringing in the ear *Adverse reaction:* weight gain, hypersensitivity, hoarseness, jaundice, bloody urine, stiff neck

TABLE 13.4 Information on Commonly Prescribed Medications—*continued*

GENERIC NAME	BRAND/TRADE NAME(S)	CLASS/ SCHEDULE	MEDICATION INFORMATION
clopidogrel	Plavix	Antiplatelets	*Indication:* used to prevent clots after a stroke, heart attack, or severe angina *Desired effects/action:* prevents platelets from collecting and forming clots *Side effects:* excessive tiredness, GI intolerance, nosebleed, dizziness *Adverse reaction:* hypersensitivity, bloody and tarry stools, coffee grounds–looking emesis, blood in urine, visual changes
aripiprazole	Abilify	Antipsychotics (atypical)	*Indication:* schizophrenia, bipolar disorder, major depressive disorder, Tourette disorder *Desired effects/action:* changes the actions of chemicals in the brain *Side effects:* GI intolerance, insomnia, headache, anxiety, trouble swallowing *Adverse reaction:* suicidal thoughts, stroke, compulsive behaviors, orthostatic hypotension, tardive dyskinesia
quetiapine	Seroquel	Antipsychotics (atypical)	*Indication:* schizophrenia, bipolar disorder *Desired effects/action:* changes the activity of certain substances in the brain *Side effects:* drowsiness, pain in joints, weakness, GI intolerance, difficulty concentrating and speaking *Adverse reaction:* seizures, visual changes, uncontrollable movements, arrhythmias
tiotropium	Spiriva	Bronchodilators	*Indication:* chronic obstructive pulmonary disease (COPD) *Desired effects/action:* prevents bronchospasms *Side effects:* dry mouth, GI intolerance, nosebleed, muscle pain, cold symptoms *Adverse reaction:* hypersensitivity reaction, paradoxical bronchospasm, glaucoma, urinary retention
albuterol	Ventolin HFA, Proventil HFA, Proair	Bronchodilators	*Indication:* bronchospasm (e.g., asthma) *Desired effects/action:* relaxes bronchial muscles and increases air flow to lungs *Side effects:* headache, dizziness, insomnia, cough, sore throat, nausea, vomiting, dry mouth *Adverse reaction:* paradoxical bronchospasm, cardiovascular effects, hypersensitivity, hypokalemia
atorvastatin	Lipitor	Cholesterol-lowering agent	*Indication:* hyperlipidemia, hypertriglyceridemia *Desired effects/action:* slows production of cholesterol in the body; decreases LDH and triglycerides; increases HDL *Side effects:* GI intolerance, joint pain, memory loss, confusion *Adverse reaction:* muscle pain, lack of energy, angina, weakness, hypersensitivity, dark-colored urine, jaundice
rosuvastatin	Crestor	Cholesterol-lowering agent	*Indication:* hyperlipidemia, hypertriglyceridemia *Desired effects/action:* slows production of cholesterol in the body; reduces LDH and triglycerides; increases HDL *Side effects:* headache, depression, muscle and joint pain, insomnia, GI intolerance *Adverse reaction:* muscle damage leading to acute renal failure and liver damage
simvastatin	Zocor	Cholesterol-lowering agent	*Indication:* hyperlipidemia, hypertriglyceridemia *Desired effects/action:* slows production of cholesterol in the body; reduces LDH and triglycerides; increases HDL *Side effects:* GI intolerance, memory loss, confusion, headache *Adverse reaction:* muscle pain, dark red urine, lack of energy, jaundice, hypersensitivity

Continued

TABLE 13.4   Information on Commonly Prescribed Medications—*continued*

GENERIC NAME	BRAND/TRADE NAME(S)	CLASS/ SCHEDULE	MEDICATION INFORMATION
methylprednisolone	Medrol	Corticosteroid (oral)	*Indication:* arthritis, certain cancers, allergies, asthma *Desired effects/action:* relieves inflammation symptoms *Side effects:* GI intolerance, increased hair growth, insomnia, acne *Adverse reaction:* swollen face and legs, visual problems, infection, black or tarry stool
fluticasone	Flonase nasal spray, Flovent HFA, Flovent Diskus	Corticosteroid (nasal and inhaled)	*Indication:* hay fever, allergies (nasal spray); asthma (inhaled) *Desired effects/action:* reduces inflammation and allergy reaction *Side effects:* headache, dryness in mouth, hoarseness or deepened voice *Adverse reaction:* reduced bone marrow density, immunosuppression, adrenal suppression, glaucoma, cataracts, hypersensitivity in individuals with milk allergy (Diskus)
furosemide	Lasix	Diuretics	*Indication:* hypertension *Desired effects/action:* causes the kidneys to increase the excretion of water and salt *Side effects:* frequent urination, blurred vision, headache, constipation, diarrhea *Adverse reaction:* ringing in the ears, loss of hearing, blisters, jaundice, hypersensitivity
hydrochlorothiazide (HCTZ)	Microzide, Oretic	Diuretics	*Indication:* hypertension *Desired effects/action:* causes the kidneys to increase the excretion of water and salt *Side effects:* frequent urination, diarrhea, loss of appetite, headache, hair loss *Adverse reaction:* joint pain, unusual bleeding, hypersensitivity, visual change
potassium	K-Tab, Klor-Con, K-Dur, Micro-K	Electrolyte	*Indication:* mineral supplement needed for certain diseases and medications (e.g., diuretic) *Desired effects/action:* proper functioning of the body systems *Side effects:* GI intolerance *Adverse reaction:* confusion, listlessness, gray skin, black stools
levothyroxine	Synthroid, Levothroid, Levoxyl	Hormone replacement (thyroid hormone)	*Indication:* hypothyroidism, pituitary TSH suppression *Desired effects/action:* replacement hormone; regulates body's energy and metabolism *Side effects:* reversible hair loss, dry skin, GI intolerance, headache, nervousness *Adverse reaction:* cardiac arrhythmias, angina, myocardial infarction, heart failure
montelukast	Singulair	Leukotriene receptor antagonists	*Indication:* asthma, exercise-induced bronchospasms *Desired effects/action:* blocks the action of substances that cause asthma and allergic rhinitis *Side effects:* headache, dizziness, heartburn, stomach pain, tiredness *Adverse reaction:* hypersensitivity, numbness in arms and legs, swelling of the sinuses
carisoprodol	Soma	Muscle relaxant C–IV	*Indication:* painful musculoskeletal conditions (e.g., strains, sprains, muscle injuries) *Desired effects/action:* reduces pain *Side effects:* drowsiness, clumsiness, tachycardia, GI intolerance *Adverse reaction:* difficulty breathing, fever, weakness, burning in the eyes, seizures
cyclobenzaprine	Flexeril	Muscle relaxant	*Indication:* painful musculoskeletal conditions (e.g., strains, sprains, muscle injuries) *Desired effects/action:* works on the brain and nervous system to allow muscle relaxation *Side effects:* GI intolerance, extreme tiredness, dry mouth *Adverse reaction:* hypersensitivity, angina

	BRAND/TRADE	CLASS/	
TABLE 13.4 **Information on Commonly Prescribed Medications—***continued*			
GENERIC NAME	**NAME(S)**	**SCHEDULE**	**MEDICATION INFORMATION**
esomeprazole	Nexium	Proton-pump inhibitors	*Indication:* gastroesophageal reflex disease (GERD), erosive esophagitis, *Helicobacter pylori* ulcers *Desired effects/action:* reduces the amount of stomach acid *Side effects:* headache, drowsiness, dry mouth, GI intolerance *Adverse reaction:* acute interstitial nephritis, *C. difficile*, bone fracture, systemic lupus erythematosus, cyanocobalamin (vitamin B_{12}) deficiency, hypomagnesemia
omeprazole	Prilosec	Proton-pump inhibitors	*Indication:* gastroesophageal reflux disease (GERD), ulcers, *H. pylori* *Desired effects/action:* reduces stomach acid *Side effects:* GI intolerance, headache *Adverse reaction:* hypersensitivity, dizziness, arrhythmias, muscle spasm
zolpidem	Ambien, Edluar, Zolpimist	Sedative — hypnotics C–IV	*Indication:* insomnia *Desired effects/action:* slows activity in the brain, allowing sleep *Side effects:* drowsiness, headache, dizziness, drugged feeling, unsteady walking, GI intolerance *Adverse reaction:* jaundice, hypersensitivity, light-colored stools, angina, blurred vision
methylphenidate	Concerta, Ritalin LA	Stimulants C–II	*Indication:* attention deficit hyperactivity disorder (ADHD), narcolepsy *Desired effects/action:* changes certain substances in the brain, allowing a person to concentrate and focus *Side effects:* nervousness, difficulty falling asleep, GI intolerance, restlessness, muscle tightness *Adverse reaction:* angina, arrhythmias, seizure, blurred vision

In addition to describing how medication orders are given to the medical assistant, they can be described by the type of order. The following are five types of medication orders.

- *Routine order:* Medication taken at a regular interval until it is canceled or expired. (Most non-narcotic routine orders expire in 12 months.) Examples: "Vitamin B_{12} 100 mcg IM monthly" and "Synthroid 75 mcg qam po."
- *Standing order:* Order applies to all patients who meet specific criteria. For departments, usually all providers agree collectively on standing orders and sign the order. Example: "For patients 18 years and older, with no allergy to acetaminophen and who have a temperature of 103°F or higher: give acetaminophen 650 mg po × 1 dose."
- *PRN order:* Medication that is given on an "as needed" basis for specific signs and symptoms. (It is important to indicate these symptoms when documenting the administered medication in the patient's health record.) Example: "Acetaminophen 325 mg, 2 tabs po q 4–6 hr prn pain."
- *Single order* or *one-time order:* Medication is administered one time. Example: "Acetaminophen 650 mg po × 1 dose."
- *Stat order:* Medication is administered one time right now. Example: "EpiPen 0.3 mg IM stat."

Prescriptions

A *prescription* is a written order by a provider to the pharmacist. It tells the pharmacist what medication and how much should be dispensed to the patient. There are four parts to a prescription: superscription, inscription, signature, and subscription. Fig. 13.1 describes the four parts of a prescription.

Medical Assistant's Role

In some ambulatory care facilities, medical assistants prepare prescriptions for providers to sign. Some such scenarios may include:

- A patient may request refills while the medical assistant is rooming the patient. The medical assistant may prepare the prescriptions, so the provider just needs to sign for the refills.
- A patient may call the department and request a refill on a medication. Using a medication refill protocol, the medical assistant needs to see if the patient can get a refill (Fig. 13.2). If the patient can, then the medical assistant prepares the prescription and has the provider sign it.

The prescription must be written in ink or be computer-generated. A medical assistant can prepare prescriptions for the provider to sign. The provider is responsible for ensuring the prescription meets federal and state laws and regulations. All prescriptions need to include this information:

- Date of issue (when it was written)
- Patient information (name and address are required; date of birth is helpful)
- Provider's full name and address
- Drug name (e.g., amoxicillin)
- Drug strength (e.g., 500 mg)

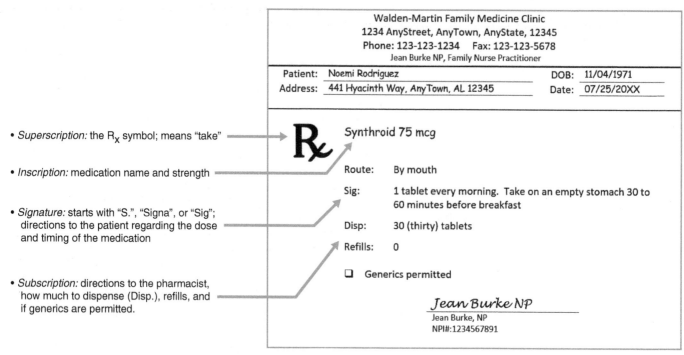

- *Superscription:* the R$_x$ symbol; means "take"

- *Inscription:* medication name and strength

- *Signature:* starts with "S.", "Signa", or "Sig"; directions to the patient regarding the dose and timing of the medication

- *Subscription:* directions to the pharmacist, how much to dispense (Disp.), refills, and if generics are permitted.

Walden-Martin Family Medicine Clinic
1234 AnyStreet, AnyTown, AnyState, 12345
Phone: 123-123-1234   Fax: 123-123-5678
Jean Burke NP, Family Nurse Practitioner

Patient: Noemi Rodriguez   DOB: 11/04/1971
Address: 441 Hyacinth Way, AnyTown, AL 12345   Date: 07/25/20XX

R$_x$ Synthroid 75 mcg

Route: By mouth

Sig: 1 tablet every morning. Take on an empty stomach 30 to 60 minutes before breakfast

Disp: 30 (thirty) tablets

Refills: 0

☐   Generics permitted

Jean Burke NP
Jean Burke, NP
NPI#:1234567891

FIGURE 13.1 Parts of a prescription.

Prescription Refill Protocol
Walden-Martin Family Medical Clinic

Description: A Certified Medical Assistant (CMA) can refill current hypertensive medications that fall within the guidelines of this protocol.

Step 1	Step 2	
For medications to be refilled, the following points need to be addressed.	Qualifying Medications	Prescription Refill
• Has the person seen the provider within the last year? • Is the prescription for a hypertensive, hyperlipidemia, or hyperthyroidism medication, a current prescription? • Is the person free of concerns or complications due to the medication? • Is it time for a refill? (The medical assistant must verify that it is time for a refill.) If the answers to the above questions are all YES, then proceed to Step 2. If any of the answers to the above questions are NO, then schedule the person for an appointment with the provider	amlodipine amlodipine/benazepril atenolol atenolol/Chlorthalidone benazepril captopril diltiazem enalapril felodipine fosinopril irbesartan isradiprine lisinopril losartan nifedipine quinapril ramipril	Extend the current prescription for 6 months. Instruct patient that in 6 months: • A visit to the provider will be required • Blood pressure reading will be required • Lab work may be required

FIGURE 13.2 Example of a prescription refill protocol. The medical assistant uses a protocol to determine what action to take with prescription refill requests.

- Dosage form (e.g., tablets)
- Quantity prescribed (e.g., 14 [fourteen]) – writing out the number prevents people from altering the prescription. This is especially important with controlled substances.
- Directions for use (e.g., take 1 tablet q 12 hr)
- Number of refills (e.g., Refills 0)
- **National Provider Identifier (NPI)** and signature of provider (a manual signature is required for controlled substances)
- Indicate if a generic is acceptable

If an electronic prescription is sent to the pharmacy and a paper copy is given to the patient, the copy should indicate that it is a copy ("Copy only – not valid for dispensing"). Procedure 13.1 on p. 340 indicates how to prepare prescriptions using a prescription refill procedure. Only facility-approved abbreviations should be used when preparing prescriptions and documenting in the patients' health records. Table 13.5 provides commonly approved abbreviations.

Once the prescriptions are prepared, they need to be given to the provider to sign. Either the provider or the medical assistant needs to document the refills in the patient's health record. The facility's policy will indicate who is responsible for the documentation.

Controlled Substance Prescriptions

For security reasons, the provider's DEA number should be used only on controlled substance prescriptions. It is not appropriate for the number to appear on non-narcotic prescriptions. The NPI is a national number that is unique to the provider. This number is found on prescriptions and may be used for tracking or treatment identification purposes.

The medical assistant needs to be aware of the special requirements for controlled substances. It is important for the medical assistant to stay updated on which frequently prescribed medications are controlled substances. Table 13.6 describes common requirements for scheduled substances.

CRITICAL THINKING APPLICATION   **13.6**

Mark and Gabe are working on prescription refills. A patient who just started taking a schedule 2 medication calls in for a refill. He says he was not happy that there were no refills on his original prescription. How might Gabe handle this type of call? What could he say to help the patient understand the situation?

OVER-THE-COUNTER MEDICATIONS AND HERBAL SUPPLEMENTS

Over-the-counter (OTC) medications and herbal supplements can affect medication treatment. It is important for the medical assistant to obtain a list of current prescription, OTC medications, and herbal supplements (Tables 13.7 and 13.8). Some patients may hesitate or may not want to share this information. They may not realize that OTC medications and herbal supplements can interfere with prescription medications. It is important for medical assistants to be professional and respectful when dealing with these situations. If they explain that sometimes the OTC medications and herbal supplements

react with prescription medications, patients may be more willing to share information on what they take.

CLOSING COMMENTS

Patient Coaching

With the frequency of opioid abuse, prescribing guidelines are changing. The Centers for Disease Control and Prevention (CDC) published "Guideline for Prescribing Opioids for Chronic Pain" (available at *https://www.cdc.gov/drugoverdose/pdf/Guidelines_Factsheet-a.pdf*). These guidelines help support providers who are working with patients with chronic pain. The medical assistant may need to coach patients on home care treatments. Opioids are not first-line or routine therapy for chronic pain. The medical assistant may need to coach the patient on the importance of using nonpharmacologic therapy and nonopioid pharmacologic therapy for chronic pain. For patients who receive opioid prescriptions, frequent follow-up is needed for the provider to evaluate the benefit and risk of the drug.

Legal and Ethical Issues

The magnitude of opioid abuse has increased dramatically, and it is currently considered a crisis. According to the CDC, in 2017 more than 70,230 people died from a drug overdose in the United States. About 67.8% of these deaths involved prescription or illicit opioid use. Many ambulatory care facilities have adopted procedures for specific controlled substance prescriptions. Before patients can get these prescriptions, they need to have a urine drug test. The urine drug test helps a provider assess what drugs the patient has taken. The provider expects the results to show the drug prescribed, but he or she also checks for other prescribed controlled substances and illicit drugs. In many cases, if the drug test shows evidence of illicit drug use or prescription-controlled substances not prescribed by the provider, the patient is referred for substance abuse counseling and treatment.

Patient-Centered Care

Many healthcare facilities require that patients receive a printout of their current medications at the end of each visit. When patients are taking a number of medications, it is important for the medical assistant to encourage these patients to carry a current medications list in their wallet or purse. This can be helpful in an emergency or when the patient needs to see a different provider.

Professional Behaviors

When working with prescription refills, it is important for the medical assistant to process the refill in a timely fashion. If the medical assistant procrastinates and does not process the refill, the patient may not have the medication when she or he needs it. Some medications need to be taken on a daily basis. If a dose is skipped, the patient may have serious consequences.

It is also important that the medical assistant honors what that patient was told. If the patient is told that the medication will be sent to a pharmacy by a specific time, it is important for the medical assistant to ensure this is done. If the medication is held up for some reason, the medical assistant should notify the patient about the delay.

TABLE 13.5 Commonly Approved Abbreviations

TYPE	ABBREVIATIONS	MEANING	TYPE	ABBREVIATIONS	MEANING
Routes and medication forms	subcut	subcutaneous		prn	as needed
	ID	intradermal		qh	every hour
	IM	intramuscular		q(2,3,4,6,8)h	every (2, 3, 4, 6, 8) hours (q2h = every 2 hours)
	IV	intravenous			
	NAS	nasal			
	po, PO	by mouth		qid	four times a day
	tinct	tincture		tid	three times a day
	ung.	ointment		bid	twice a day
	sol., soln	solution		qam	every morning
	cap	capsule		stat, STAT	immediately
	tab(s)	tablet(s)	**Medications**	ASA	aspirin
Measurements	C	Celsius		APAP	acetaminophen
	F	Fahrenheit		Fe	iron
	m	meter		K	potassium
	cm	centimeter		MOM	milk of magnesia
	mm	millimeter		NS	normal saline
	kg	kilogram		NSAID	nonsteroidal anti-inflammatory drug
	g	gram			
	mg	milligram		OTC	over-the-counter (drugs)
	mcg	microgram			
	L	liter		PPD	purified protein derivative (tuberculin skin test)
	mL	milliliter			
	gr	grain			
	gtt(s)	drop(s)	**Miscellaneous**	$\overline{aa}$	of each (used in prescriptions)
	lb	pound			
	fl oz	fluid ounce		aq	water
	oz	ounce		$\overline{c}$	with
	pt	pint		med	medicine
	qt	quart		NKA	no known allergies
	Tbs, tbsp	tablespoon		NKDA	no known drug allergies
	tsp	teaspoon			
Timing	ac	before meals		NPO	nothing by mouth
	pc	after meals		Pt, pt	patient
	ad lib	as desired		qs	quantity sufficient
	d	day		Rx	take
	AM, a.m.	morning		Sig	give the following directions
	PM, p.m.	afternoon			
	noc, noct	night		$\overline{s}$	without
	h, hr	hour		VO	verbal order
	min	minute		x	times
	$\overline{p}$	after			

TABLE 13.6	Special Requirements for Controlled Substances
SCHEDULE	**PRESCRIPTION SPECIFICS**
I	Not currently used for medical purposes.
II/IIN (C–II)	Written prescription manually signed by the provider or an electronic prescription that meets all DEA requirements for electronic prescriptions for controlled substances. No refills. In some cases, the prescription can be faxed to the pharmacy. The medication cannot be dispensed until the original prescription is given to the pharmacy.
III/III N and IV (C–III, C–IV)	Call-in prescriptions, written prescriptions, and electronic prescriptions are allowed. Faxed prescriptions must be manually signed by the provider prior to faxing. Prescription good for 6 months. No more than five refills are allowed.
V (C–V)	Phoned prescriptions, written prescriptions, e-prescriptions, and faxed prescriptions allowed. Prescription is good for 12 months (e.g., non-narcotic prescriptions). Refill quantity is up to the provider.

TABLE 13.7	Common Over-the-Counter (OTC) Medications			
MEDICATION: ***GENERIC NAME*** **(BRAND/TRADE NAME)**	**CLASSIFICATION**	**INDICATION AND DESIRED EFFECT**	**ADVERSE REACTION(S)**	**DRUG INTERACTION(S)**
aspirin *ibuprofen* (Advil, Motrin) *naproxen* (Aleve, Naprosyn)	Analgesics (nonsteroidal anti-inflammatory drugs [NSAIDs])	Inflammation and pain relief	GI bleeding, compromised renal function, tinnitus, diarrhea, and nausea	Antihypertensives, hyperglycemics, sulfa antibiotics, diuretics
acetaminophen (Tylenol)	Analgesic, antipyretic	Relief of pain and fever	Liver damage	Warfarin
pseudoephedrine (Sudafed)	Decongestant	Relief of nasal congestion caused by colds, allergies, and hay fever	Hypertension, vasospasm, arrhythmia, cerebrovascular accident	Antidepressant — monoamine oxidase inhibitors (MAOIs)
diphenhydramine (Benadryl)	Antihistamine	Cough, cold, allergy, and insomnia	Drowsiness, confusion, hallucinations, delirium	Acetaminophen with oxycodone, alprazolam, amitriptyline, metoprolol
dextromethorphan (Benylin and many DM cough and cold formulas)	Antitussive	Suppression of cough reflex	Dizziness, lethargy, nausea	Antidepressant — monoamine oxidase inhibitors (MAOIs)

TABLE 13.8	Commonly Used Herbal Supplements	
NAME	**USES**	**SIDE EFFECTS AND CAUTIONS**
Acai	Weight loss and antiaging; antioxidant	Little scientific information about the safety of acai; no scientific evidence to support use for any health-related purpose; might affect magnetic resonance imaging (MRI) results.
Aloe vera	Aloe gel is used for burns, frostbite, psoriasis, and cold sores. It can also be taken orally for osteoarthritis, bowel diseases, and fever.	Topical use of aloe gel is likely to be safe. More studies are needed to determine the safety of oral preparations. People with diabetes should be cautioned against using aloe, as it may lower blood glucose levels.

Continued

TABLE 13.8	Commonly Used Herbal Supplements—*continued*	
NAME	**USES**	**SIDE EFFECTS AND CAUTIONS**
Black cohosh	Relieve symptoms of menopause; treat menstrual irregularities and premenstrual syndrome; induce labor.	Headaches, gastric complaints, heaviness in the legs, weight problems; safety unknown for pregnant women or those with breast cancer.
Echinacea	Treat or prevent colds, flu, and other infections; believed to stimulate the immune system.	Most studies indicate echinacea does not appear to prevent colds or other infections; some people experience allergic reactions, including rashes, increased asthma, and anaphylaxis; gastrointestinal (GI) side effects.
Flaxseed	Flaxseed and flaxseed oil are used for constipation, diabetes, high cholesterol levels, cancer, and other conditions.	Few reported side effects; contains soluble fiber and is an effective laxative; both flaxseed and flaxseed oil can cause diarrhea. It is not recommended during pregnancy.
Garlic	Treat high cholesterol, heart disease, hypertension; prevent certain types of cancer, including stomach and colon cancer.	Some evidence indicates garlic can slightly lower blood cholesterol levels and may slow development of atherosclerosis; side effects include breath and body odor, heartburn, GI upset, and allergic reactions; acts as a mild anticoagulant (similar to aspirin); may increase the risk of bleeding; interferes with effectiveness of saquinavir, a drug used to treat human immunodeficiency virus (HIV) infection.
Ginger	Alleviate nausea associated with postoperative state, motion sickness, chemotherapy, and pregnancy; used for rheumatoid arthritis, osteoarthritis, and joint and muscle pain.	Short-term use can safely relieve pregnancy-related nausea and vomiting; also, may help with chemotherapy nausea and vomiting. Side effects most often reported are gas, bloating, heartburn, and nausea.
Asian ginseng	Support overall health and boost immune system; improve mental and physical performance; treat erectile dysfunction, hepatitis C, and menopause symptoms; lower blood glucose and control blood pressure.	Limited information available, more studies needed. May affect blood glucose levels and blood pressure; thus, patients should discuss this with their provider. May interact with certain medications, such as anticoagulants.
Ginkgo biloba	No conclusive evidence that it helps any health condition.	Side effects may include headache, stomach upset, and allergic skin reactions. Ginkgo may increase the risk of bleeding with pregnancy and in those on anticoagulants.
Green tea	Improve mental alertness, relieve digestive symptoms and headaches, promote weight loss; may have protective effects against heart disease and cancer.	Safe in moderate amounts; possible complications include liver problems with concentrated green tea extracts but not when used as a beverage. A specific green tea extract ointment is a prescription drug used for treating genital warts.
St. John's wort	Treat mental disorders and nerve pain; kidney and lung diseases, insomnia and wounds.	Some scientific evidence shows it helps treat mild to moderate depression; not effective in treating major depression. Side effects include photophobia (increased sensitivity to sunlight), anxiety, dry mouth, dizziness, GI symptoms, fatigue, headache, and sexual dysfunction. Can cause life-threatening reactions with certain medications. Drugs that can be affected include the following: • Antidepressants • Birth control pills • Cyclosporine (prevents rejection of transplants) • Digoxin (heart medication) • Some HIV and cancer medications • Warfarin and related anticoagulants

Modified from the National Center for Complementary and Alternative Medicine. *https://nccih.nih.gov/health/herbsataglance.htm.* Accessed September 23, 2018.

SUMMARY OF SCENARIO

Mark is enjoying working with Gabe. He is amazed at how much Gabe knows about medications that the providers commonly prescribe. Mark feels that he will never be as fluent with the medications as Gabe is. He even mentioned this to Gabe. His mentor laughed and said he felt the same way during his own practicum. Over the years, he has used drug reference materials to help him learn about medications. He has made it a practice to look up medications

he does not know. This helped him become more fluent. He assured Mark that if he was willing to read up on medications, he, too, will become fluent with them.

Mark is looking forward to administering medications with Gabe. Now that he understands how to use the drug reference materials, he will be working hard to learn the medications he encounters.

SUMMARY OF LEARNING OBJECTIVES

1. **Describe the sources and uses of drugs.**

   Drugs are either created from natural sources or made synthetically in a laboratory. Plants, animals, minerals, and microbiologic sources are natural sources of drugs. There are eight common uses of drugs: prevention, treatment, diagnosis, cure, contraceptive, health maintenance, palliative, and replacement.

2. **Describe pharmacokinetics, including absorption, distribution, metabolism, and excretion.**

   Pharmacokinetics is the study of drug absorption, distribution, metabolism, and excretion in the body. Absorption is the movement of drug from the site of administration to the bloodstream. The movement of absorbed drug from the blood to the body tissues is called *distribution*. Metabolism is a series of chemical processes whereby enzymes change drugs in the body. Excretion is the movement of the metabolites out of the body.

3. **Discuss drug action, including the factors that influence drug action, the therapeutic effects of drugs, and adverse reactions to drugs.**

   Drugs are chemicals that can cause changes in the cells. Four main drug actions are depressing, stimulating, destroying, and replacing substances. This chapter discussed the factors that influenced drug action, including age, body size, gender, genetics, diseases, diet, drug dosage, route, timing of administration, mental state, and environmental temperature. Each medication has one or more therapeutic effects or desired effects. This is the intended action of the medication. The person can experience an unexpected or life-threatening reaction, which is called an *adverse reaction*. Table 13.1 lists common adverse reactions.

4. **Explain drug legislation that is important in the ambulatory care setting. Also, discuss dietary supplements.**

   The Food, Drug, and Cosmetic Act is enforced by the Food and Drug Administration (FDA). The FDA is responsible for the safety, effectiveness, security, and quality of drugs, cosmetics, and food. The Controlled Substances Act (CSA), Title II of the Comprehensive Drug Abuse Prevention and Control Act of 1970, is a federal law. The DEA enforces the CSA. The DEA oversees the manufacturing, importation, possession, use, and distribution of illegal and legal controlled substances.

   Dietary supplements are oral products that contain a "dietary ingredient." This ingredient can include a vitamin, mineral, amino acid, herb, or another substance that can supplement a person's diet. The FDA monitors the safety of such products after they are on the market.

5. **Describe the four types of drug names.**

   The four types of drug names are:
   - *Chemical name*: Represents the drug's exact chemical formula.
   - *Generic name*: Assigned by the US Adopted Names (USAN) Council.
   - *Official name*: Used to list the medication in the United States Pharmacopeia and the National Formulary (USP–NF).
   - *Brand name*: Also called the *trade name*, used by one manufacturer.

6. **Describe various methods to access drug reference information.**

   Print drug references include package inserts and drug handbooks. Digital drug references include apps, products integrated with electronic health records, and online websites.

7. **Identify the classifications of medications, including the indications for use, desired effects, side effects, and adverse reactions.**

   Table 13.3 provides a list of classifications of medications with descriptions. Table 13.4 lists commonly prescribed medications and information on each, including the generic name, brand/trade name, class, schedule, indication, desired action, side effects, and adverse reactions.

8. **Discuss the terminology used in drug reference information, including describing the differences among biologic half-life, onset, peak, and duration.**

   The following terminology is typically found in drug reference information:
   - *Names:* Usually the generic name is listed with the trade names.
   - *Description:* Describes the medication and its general use.
   - *Boxed warning:* Addresses serious or life-threatening risks.
   - *Dosage:* Specifies the route, dose, and timing of the medication.
   - *Indication:* Conditions or diseases for which the drug is used.
   - *Dosage considerations:* Indicates recommended changes in dosages for special populations.
   - *How supplied:* Lists the form and the strength.
   - *Administration:* Provides information on how the medication should be administered.
   - *Contraindications:* Lists reasons or conditions that make administration of the drug improper or undesirable.

Continued

- *Precautions*: Indicates necessary actions or special care that needs to be taken when the patient is on the medication.
- *Adverse reactions*: Also called *side effects* in some information. This section describes known undesirable experiences associated with the medication. Reactions may be divided into severe (life-threatening, serious reactions), moderate, and mild.
- *Interactions*: Includes medications, foods, and beverages that interact with the medication. These products may either increase or decrease the medication levels in the blood.
- *Action*: How the drug provides therapeutic results in the body, or the use of the drug.
- *Pharmacokinetics*: Provides information on the absorption, distribution, metabolism, and excretion of the medication.

The differences among biologic half-life, onset, peak, and duration:

- *Biologic half-life*: Time it takes half of the drug to be metabolized or eliminated by normal biologic processes
- *Onset*: The time it takes for the drug to produce a response
- *Peak*: The time it takes for the drug to reach its greatest effective concentration in the blood
- *Duration*: The time during which the drug is present in the blood at great enough levels to produce a response

9. **Discuss types of medication orders.**

The provider can give the order over the phone or in person; this type of order is called a *verbal order*. The provider can also give the medical assistant a *written order* by using a prescription pad or in an electronic message. Besides describing medication orders by how they are given to the medical assistant, they can also be described by the type of order. Five types of medication orders are:

- *Routine order*: Medication is taken at a regular interval until it is canceled or expired.
- *Standing order*: Order applies to all patients who meet specific criteria.
- *PRN order*: Medication is given on an "as needed" basis for specific signs and symptoms.

- *Single order* or *one-time order*: Medication is administered one time.
- *Stat order*: Medication is administered one time right now.

10. **List the four parts of a prescription and the information required for all prescriptions; prepare prescriptions using prescription refill procedures; and define commonly approved abbreviations.**

There are four parts to a prescription: superscription, inscription, signature, and subscription. Fig. 13.1 describes the four parts of a prescription. All prescriptions need to include the date of issue; patient information; provider's full name and address; drug name, strength, and dosage form; quantity prescribed; directions for use; number of refills; NPI; and if a generic is acceptable.

Procedure 13.1 describes how to prepare prescriptions using a prescription refill procedure.

Table 13.5 provides commonly approved abbreviations regarding route, medication form, measurements, timing, and medications.

11. **Describe common requirements for scheduled substances.**

- *Schedule I*: Not used.
- *Schedule II*: Written prescription manually signed by the provider or an electronic prescription that meets all DEA requirements for electronic prescriptions for controlled substances. No refills.
- *Schedules III and IV*: Call-in prescriptions, written prescriptions, and electronic prescriptions are allowed. Faxed prescriptions must be manually signed by the provider prior to faxing. Prescription good for 6 months. No more than five refills are allowed.
- *Schedule V*: Phoned prescriptions, written prescriptions, e-prescriptions, and faxed prescriptions allowed. Prescription is good for 12 months (e.g., non-narcotic prescriptions). Refill quantity is up to the provider.

Also refer to Table 13.6.

12. **Discuss over-the-counter (OTC) medications and herbal supplements.**

Tables 13.7 and 13.8 provide information on the common OTC medications and herbal supplements.

PROCEDURE 13.1   Prepare a Prescription

Tasks: Prepare a prescription using a prescription refill protocol. Use approved abbreviations.

Scenario: You received a call from Noemi Rodriguez (DOB 11/04/1971). She is requesting refills on three of her prescriptions from Jean Burke, NP. She saw Jean Burke 10 months ago. Noemi has NKA. She is doing well with the prescriptions and has no concerns. You determine it is time for refills. Her prescriptions include Coumadin 5 mg, 1 tablet orally daily; Tenormin 50 mg, 1 tablet orally daily; and Plendil 5 mg, 1 tablet orally daily.

EQUIPMENT and SUPPLIES

- SimChart for the Medical Office (SCMO) or paper prescriptions and pen
- Prescription refill protocol (see Fig. 13.2)
- Drug reference book or online resource

PROCEDURAL STEPS

1. Using the scenario, look up the generic medication names using the drug reference book or online resource.
   <u>PURPOSE</u>: Generic names are typically used in the healthcare facility, though patients may give the brand name.

PROCEDURE 13.1 | Prepare a Prescription—*continued*

2. Read the prescription refill protocol. Compare the generic names to the list of medications given. Identify medications that meet the protocol.
   PURPOSE: All the criteria need to be met for the medical assistant to prepare prescriptions using the prescription refill protocol.
3. Prepare prescriptions for refill according to the protocol using SCMO or paper prescriptions.
   a. Using SCMO: Search for the patient. Verify the date of birth before selecting the patient. On the INFO PANEL, select Phone Encounter. Complete the fields on the Create New Encounter window and save. Check the box beside the No Known Allergy statement on the allergy screen and save. Select Order Entry from the Record dropdown list and select Add in the Out-of-office section (see the following figures).

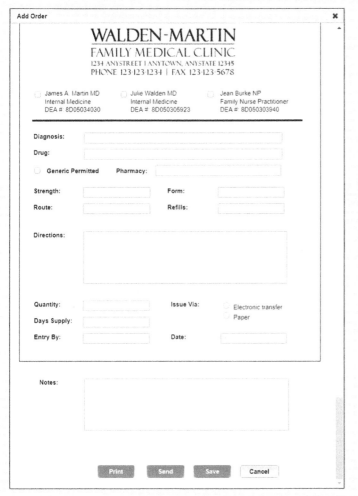

b. Using paper prescriptions: Add in the patient's complete name, date of birth, and address.
   PURPOSE: Most agencies using electronic health records require medical assistants to update the allergy screen when preparing refills. Prescriptions require the patient's name and address. If the DOB is available, add this to the prescription. An electronic health record will automatically add this information when it sends the prescription to the pharmacy.
4. Using the information in the scenario, complete the prescription information on either the paper prescription or in the SCMO fields. Use only approved abbreviations.
   PURPOSE: All information is required on the prescription for it to be accepted by the pharmacist and filled for the patient.
5. Complete any additional prescriptions as needed by the prescription refill protocol.
   PURPOSE: The patient requested refills on the medications indicated. Any medications that can be refilled should have prescriptions prepared for the provider.
6. Review the prescriptions for any errors. Void the prescription and redo if needed.
   PURPOSE: It is important to prepare accurate prescriptions. Any errors need to be fixed before giving the prescriptions to the provider.
   Note: After the provider signs the prescriptions and depending on the facility's policy, the medical assistant may need to document the refill in the health record. This cannot be done until the provider approves the prescriptions.

14

PHARMACOLOGY MATH

SCENARIO

Gabe Garcia, a certified medical assistant (CMA) through the American Association of Medical Assistants (AAMA), has worked for Walden-Martin Family Medical (WMFM) Clinic for 3 years. During his first year at WMFM Clinic, Gabe worked almost exclusively with a family practice provider who cared for older patients. Once the provider retired, Gabe switched providers. He is now working with both children and adult patients. He found himself administering more injections when working with the children than when working with the adults.

Gabe was asked to be Mark Allen's mentor for practicum. Mark has just completed all of his medical assistant courses at the local college and now needs 160 hours of practicum. He is excited to be working with Gabe. This week, Gabe will be working with Mark to review reading syringes and applying the math used for medication calculations.

While studying this chapter, think about the following questions:
- What are the parts of a drug label?
- What are the basic units of measure in the household system and the metric system?
- How can a person convert amounts between different measurement systems?
- How can a temperature be converted between Fahrenheit and Celsius?
- How are medication doses calculated?
- How does a person read the calibration markings on syringes?

LEARNING OBJECTIVES

1. Summarize the important parts of a drug label.
2. Discuss math basics, including writing numbers in healthcare and rounding numbers.
3. Define basic units of measure in the household system and the metric system, and convert between measurement systems.
4. Convert between Fahrenheit and Celsius temperatures.
5. Perform pharmacology calculations, such as quantity needed for a specific time period, number of tablets per dose, liquid medication doses, and pediatric doses.
6. Read the calibration markings on various types of syringes.

VOCABULARY

dosage May also be referred to as dose; the quantity of medication to be administered at one time.
exclusivity (ik skloo SIV i tee) The sole right to market an approved medication granted by the Food and Drug Administration (FDA); may occur with the patent.
patent (PAT ent) A grant from the government that gives a creator (or manufacturer) of an invention the sole right to produce, use, and sell the product for a set period of time.

product The number obtained by multiplying two or more numbers together.
scored tablet A tablet with a groove on the surface used for splitting it in half.
unit dose packaging A packaging method for drugs; holds a specified quantity of medication in a single-use container (e.g., syringe, blister pack).

Medical assistants are responsible for being absolutely certain that the medication they prepare and administer to a patient is exactly what the provider ordered. Although drugs often are delivered by the pharmacy or supplied by pharmaceutical representatives in **unit dose packaging**, the **dosage** ordered may differ from the dosage on hand. In this case, the medical assistant must be prepared to calculate the correct dose accurately before dispensing and administering the medication. There is never a margin of error in drug

calculations; even a minor mistake may result in serious complications for the patient. The medical assistant, therefore, must take meticulous care in calculating all drug dosages.

DRUG LABELS

The first step in safely calculating a drug dosage is to accurately read the label of the drug on hand to determine whether the provider's

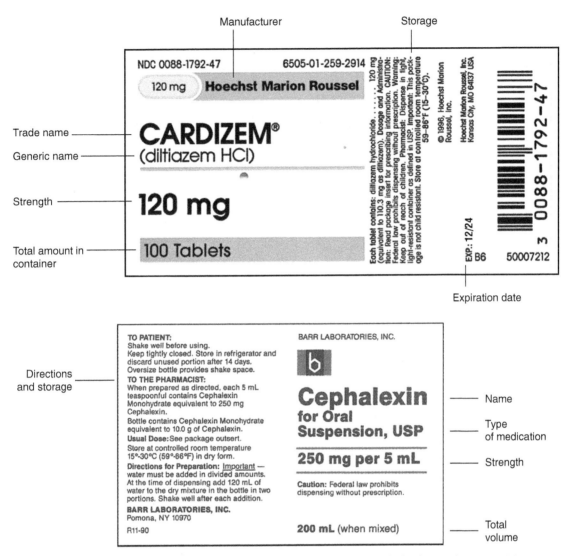

FIGURE 14.1 Drug labels. (From Brown M, Mulholland JM: *Drug calculations: process and problems for clinical practice*, ed 9, St. Louis, 2012, Mosby.)

order and the packaged drug are in the same system of measurement. The label shows the following information:

- *Brand name*: The manufacturer's name for the drug (e.g., Cardizem) (Fig. 14.1). The brand name is capitalized and typically in bold print. The brand name is copyright protected; therefore, it is followed by an ® symbol that indicates the US government has granted a Federal Registration Certificate for the drug.
- *Generic name*: The drug name used by all manufacturers who make that specific medication (e.g., diltiazem HCl, cephalexin) (see Fig. 14.1). The name is printed in lowercase letters and usually appears under the brand name in smaller print. If the patent and exclusivity have expired, only a generic name may be present on the label.
- *Strength*: The amount of drug in the unit dose (e.g., 200 mg, 180 mg/5 mL). In Fig. 14.1, each tablet of Cardizem is 120 mg. Cephalexin is a suspension (liquid) and the strength

or unit dose is 250 mg (of powdered medication) per 5 mL (of liquid).

- *Total amount or total volume:* Both liquid and solid medication labels indicate the amount of medication in the container.
- *Manufacturer:* The name of the manufacturer of the medication.
- *Directions and storage:* Instructions on how to take the medication and how to store the drug may be indicated on the label.
- *Expiration date:* Indicates when the drug can no longer be used.
- *Lot number:* Indicates the batch of drug the medication came from. The lot number is important to document when giving immunizations. Some agencies may require that lot numbers are documented for all medications administered.
- *National Drug Code (NDC):* A unique 10-digit number indicating the product. The NDC is required by federal law to be on all prescription and nonprescription medication packages and inserts in the United States.

Patents and Exclusivity

A **patent** is granted on a drug for 20 years from the date of filing for the patent. Patents are granted at any point in time along the development of a drug.

Exclusivity is granted by the Food and Drug Administration (FDA) to give exclusive marketing rights to the manufacturers of the drug when it earns FDA approval. This exclusive marketing right can vary from 3 to 5 years. If a medication has been on the market longer than 20 years or after the exclusive rights to the drug have expired, the generic name may be the only one listed (e.g., meperidine instead of Demerol, diazepam rather than Valium).

When preparing medications, it is important to compare the medication's name and strength with the provider's order. The medical assistant should also look at the expiration date. Preparing medications will be discussed in more detail in Chapter 15.

CRITICAL THINKING APPLICATION 14.1

Gabe and Mark are discussing the labels on vaccines. Mark asks Gabe why the lot numbers are important on vaccine vials. How would you answer this question?

MATH FOR MEDICATIONS

All medical assistants should be able to convert between units of measure. It is also important to be able to accurately calculate medication dosages. This section discusses different types of math problems that a medical assistant should be able to do. Please note that in some states, calculating medical dosages may be outside the legal scope of practice for medical assistants. State laws vary.

Math Basics for Medication

The following sections present guidelines for writing and calculating dosages. The medical assistant should always verify answers for dose calculations with a co-worker or the provider.

Healthcare Rules When Writing Numbers

With medications, it is important to be accurate in calculating and documenting amounts. There are four rules to follow when writing medication dosages in healthcare:

- Follow the number with the correct abbreviation for the unit of measure. Leave a space between the number and the abbreviation. Do not use a period with the abbreviations.
  - Correct examples: 2 mg, 10 mL, and 2 tabs
  - Incorrect examples: mg2, 10mL, and 2 tabs.
- Write a fraction of a dose as a decimal.
  - Correct examples: 0.2 mg and 0.5 mg
  - Incorrect examples: ⅕ mg and ½ mg
- If the dose is less than 1, place a zero to the left of the decimal point. This reduces the risk of misreading the dose as a whole number.
  - Correct examples: 0.75 mcg and 0.2 mL
  - Incorrect examples: .75 mcg and .2 mL
- Do not place a decimal point and a zero after a whole number. This can be easily misread, and the patient would be given an overdose of medication.

Hundred	Ten	One		Tenth	Hundredth	Thousandth
7	5	1	.	3	5	7

FIGURE 14.2 Place value.

- Correct examples: 2 mL and 5 mL
- Incorrect examples: 2.0 mL and 5.0 mL

Rounding Numbers

When calculating answers, sometimes the number needs to be rounded. The following steps describe the process for rounding a number:

1. Find the place value where you want to end up (Fig. 14.2). (Most answers in this chapter will be rounded to the nearest tenth, or one place after the decimal point.)
2. Look at the number to the right of the place value. If the number is
   - *4 or below*, drop the number(s) to the right of the place value
   - *5 or above*, add 1 to the rounded place value and drop the number(s) to the right of the place value

Let's practice rounding to the nearest tenth using the following examples:

- First example −569.365: In this example, 3 sits in the tenth-place value. The number to the right of the 3 is a 6. This means we need to add 1 to the 3, and then we can drop the 6 and 5. The answer is 569.4.
- Second example −339.926: In this example, 9 sits in the tenth-place value. The number to the right of the 9 is a 2. This means we just need to drop the 2 and 6. The answer is 339.9.

Rounding: Practice Problems

Directions: Round the following numbers to the nearest tenth. Write out as you would for a medication dose. (Remember: Add a zero before the decimal point if the answer is less than 1, and do not include a decimal point and a zero after a whole number.)

1. 2.467 = _____	2. .358 = _____	3. .98 = _____
4. 4.65 = _____	5. 45.234 = _____	6. 7.788 = _____

Roman Numerals

Sometimes a number might be written using Roman numerals. It is good for a medical assistant to be familiar with the Roman numeral system. In healthcare, you will see them written in lowercase letters. Sometimes a line may be written above the Roman numeral.

Roman Numerals

i = 1	vi = 6	$\overline{ss}$ = ½ or 0.5	**Examples:**
ii = 2	vii = 7	(for " ss": write out "one-	vss = 5½ or 5.5
iii = 3	viii = 8	half" in documentation	iiiss = 3½ or 3.5
iv = 4	ix = 9	notes to avoid errors)	
v = 5	x = 10		

CRITICAL THINKING APPLICATION   14.2
Mark is confused between the numbers 5 and 10 in the Roman numeral system. Come up with a way to remember the difference between these two, and share it with a classmate.

Household and Metric Equivalents

WEIGHT	FLUID	
2.2 lb = 1 kg	3 tsp = 1 Tbs	1 Tbs = 15 mL
16 oz = 1 lb	1 oz = 30 mL	1 oz = 2 Tbs
	1 tsp = 5 mL	1 oz = 6 tsp

Measurement Systems

In healthcare, both the household and metric systems are used. For instance, we weigh patients in pounds and tell a mother to give her son 1 teaspoon of medication before meals. Using the metric system is more accurate. The provider will use a child's weight in kilograms (kg) to calculate a medication dosage. The pharmacist will show the mother that 1 teaspoon is really 5 mL on the oral syringe. The oral syringe and plastic medicine cup are more accurate for measuring medications than the spoons used in the kitchen.

Household System

Sometimes we need to work within the household system as we solve problems. Other times we need to use both the metric and household measurement systems. Table 14.1 provides household measurement abbreviations.

There are many ways to set-up problems when converting between household and metric equivalents. The proportion method is one of the easiest techniques. In the proportion method, the cross-**products** are equal. This approach is easy if you remember three things:
1. Keep the information separate. The problem information is on one side of the equal sign and the equivalent information is on the other side.
2. Keep the labels in the same place. The labels should be in the exact same location on both sides of the equal sign.
3. Cross-multiply in the direction of the two numbers, then divide by the remaining number. You have your answer!

Household and Metric Problems: Proportion Method With Practice Problems

Problem: 15 Tbs = _____ mL

Solution for Problem

Step 1: Turn the problem into a fraction. It does not matter which number goes on the top or bottom, just keep the label with the number. Use x for the unknown (the blank answer line).

$$\frac{Problem}{15\,Tbs}{x\,mL}$$

Problem
$$\frac{15\,Tbs}{x\,mL}$$

Step 2: Add an equal sign and make a fraction on the opposite side. Fill in the labels. The labels need to be in identical locations on both sides of the equal sign.

Problem   Equivalent
$$\frac{15\,Tbs}{x\,mL} = \frac{Tbs}{mL}$$

Step 3: Using the Household and Metric Equivalents box, find the equivalent for Tbs and tsp. Fill in the numbers in the equivalent fraction. Make sure to put the right number in front of the correct label.

Problem   Equivalent
$$\frac{15\,Tbs}{x\,mL} = \frac{1\,Tbs}{15\,mL}$$

Step 4: Now solve for the unknown.

Using a calculator: Multiply in the diagonal direction of the two numbers (15 × 15), then divide by the number in the other direction (1), and the answer is x.

Problem   Equivalent
$$\frac{15\,Tbs}{x\,mL} = \frac{1\,Tbs}{15\,mL}$$
$$15 \times 15 = \underline{225}\,/1 = \underline{225}$$

To solve without a calculator: Multiply diagonally, and solve for x.
$$15 \times 15 = 1x$$
$$225 = 1x$$
$$\frac{225}{1} = \frac{1x}{1}$$
$$225 = x$$

Answer: 225 mL (Always make sure to label your answer.)

Practice Problems

Directions: Solve the following problems. Round your answers to the nearest tenth.

1. 11 oz = _____ lb
2. 90 mL = _____ oz
3. 8 tsp = _____ mL
4. 20 Tbs = _____ mL
5. 5.5 oz = _____ Tbs
6. 4 oz = _____ tsp
7. 23 lb = _____ kg
8. 28 kg = _____ lb
9. 56 oz = _____ lb

TABLE 14.1   Household Measurement Abbreviations

ABBREVIATION	MEANING
gtt, gtts	drop, drops
tsp	teaspoon
Tbs or tbsp	tablespoon
fl oz	fluid ounce
oz	ounce
qt	quart
pt	pint
lb	pound

Metric System

The metric system is commonly used in healthcare. We use it when measuring medications and wounds. A medical assistant should know how to use the metric system. Note these standards when using the metric system:

- Weight is measured in grams (g).
- Volume is measured in liters (L).
- Length is measured in meters (m).

Gram, liter, and *meter* are called root words. *Prefixes* are added to the front of root words to indicate the size of the unit. Fig. 14.3 lists the prefixes that can be added to the root words. Table 14.2 provides the metric measurements and equivalents commonly used in healthcare. Remember that a person cannot convert from base unit to base unit (i.e., gram to liter or meter to gram). A person can only convert within a base unit (i.e., centimeter to millimeter). Fig. 14.4 provides a memory tool for solving metric problems. There are many ways to do so.

TABLE 14.2   Metric Measurements and Equivalents Used in Healthcare

	VOLUME	LENGTH	WEIGHT
Units of Measure With Abbreviations	Liter (L) Milliliter (mL or ml) [Note: 1 cc = 1 mL Cubic centimeter (cc)]	Meter (m) Centimeter (cm) Millimeter (mm)	Gram (g) Kilogram (kg) Milligram (mg) Microgram (mcg)
Equivalents Commonly Used	1 L = 1000 mL 1 L = 1000 cc 1 mL = 1 cc (To avoid errors in documentation, use mL instead of cc.)	1 m = 100 cm 1 m = 1000 mm 1 cm = 10 mm	1 g = 1000 mg 1 g = 1,000,000 mcg 1 kg = 1000 g 1 mg = 1000 mcg

Size of the unit of measure	Prefixes	Size	Or another way to look at it!	Larger than the base unit
LARGE	Kilo (k)	1000 base units	1 kilo = 1000 base units	base unit
↓	BASE UNITS [Meter (distance), Liter (volume) or Gram (mass or weight)]			
	Centi (c)	0.01 base unit	100 centi = 1 base unit	Smaller
	Milli (m)	0.001 base unit	1000 milli = 1 base unit	than the
SMALL	Micro (mc)	0.000001 base unit	1,000,000 micro = 1 base unit	base unit

FIGURE 14.3 Prefixes of metric measurement.

Metric Problems: Proportion Method With Practice Problems

Problem: 17 g = _____ mg

Solution for Problem

Step 1: Turn the problem into a fraction. It does not matter which number goes on the top or bottom, just keep the label with the number. Use x for the unknown (the blank line).

Problem

$$\frac{17\ g}{x\ mg}$$

Step 2: Add an equal sign, and make a fraction on the opposite side. Fill in the labels. The labels need to be in identical locations on both sides of the equal sign.

Problem   Equivalent

$$\frac{17\ g}{x\ mg} = \frac{g}{mg}$$

Step 3: Using Table 14.2, find the equivalent for gram (g) and milligram (mg). Fill in the numbers in the equivalent fraction. Make sure to put the right number in front of the correct label.

Problem   Equivalent

$$\frac{17\ g}{x\ mg} = \frac{1\ g}{1000\ mg}$$

Step 4: Now solve for the unknown.

Using a calculator: Multiply in the diagonal direction of the two numbers (17×1000), then divide by the number in the other direction (1), and the answer is x.

Problem   Equivalent

$$\frac{17\ g}{x\ mg} = \frac{1\ g}{1000\ mg}$$

$$17 \times 1000 = \underline{17{,}000} / 1 = \underline{17{,}000}$$

To solve without a calculator: Multiply diagonally, and solve for x.

$$17 \times 1000 = 1x$$
$$17{,}000 = 1x$$
$$\frac{17000}{1} = \frac{1x}{1}$$
$$17000 = x$$

Answer: 17,000 mg (Always make sure to label your answer.)

Practice Problems

Directions: Solve the following problems. Do not round your answers.

1. 21 mL = _____ cc
2. 1.2 L = _____ cc
3. 2450 mL = _____ L
4. 2300 mm = _____ m
5. 87 cm = _____ mm
6. 458 cm = _____ m
7. 2.3 g = _____ mg
8. 1.3 kg = _____ g
9. 230 mcg = _____ mg

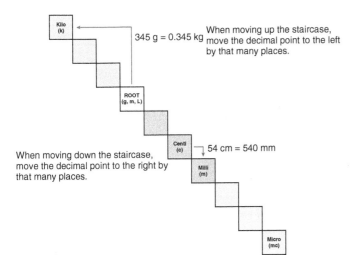

When moving up the staircase, move the decimal point to the left by that many places.

345 g = 0.345 kg

When moving down the staircase, move the decimal point to the right by that many places.

54 cm = 540 mm

FIGURE 14.4 Memory tool for solving metric problems.

CRITICAL THINKING APPLICATION   14.3

What unit of measure (e.g., liter, meter, or gram) would be used to measure the following?

1. Volume of urine
2. Length and width of a wound
3. Weight of a child

Temperature Conversion

Fahrenheit (°F) and Celsius (°C) are used in healthcare. A medical assistant should be able to convert between these two units of measure. To remember the steps for temperature conversion, use the memory tool presented in Fig. 14.5.

Temperature Conversions With Practice Problems

Problem: 102°F = _____ °C

Solution for Problem

Step 1: Subtract 32 from the Fahrenheit temperature.

$$102 - 32 = 70$$

Step 2: Divide the answer by 1.8, and round to the nearest tenth.

$$70/1.8 = 38.88889$$

Answer: 38.9°C

Problem: 25°C = _____ °F

Solution for Problem

Step 1: Multiply the Celsius number by 1.8.

$$25 \times 1.8 = 45$$

Step 2: Add 32 to the answer.

$$45 + 32 = 77$$

Answer: 77°F

Practice Problems

Directions: Solve the following problems. Round your answers to the nearest tenth.

1. 93.3°F = _____ °C
2. 42.9°F = _____ °C
3. 53°F = _____ °C
4. 103°C = _____ °F
5. 39.9°C = _____ °F
6. 88.2°C = _____ °F

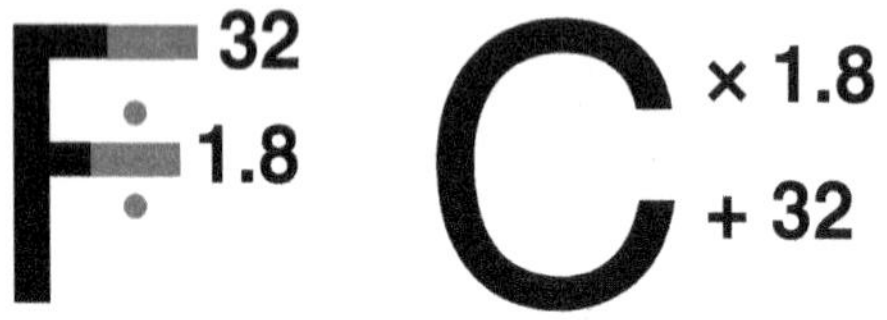

FIGURE 14.5 Memory tool for temperature conversions.

Amoxicillin 500 mg, 1 tab tid po x 10 days

| Medication name and size of the tablet | Daily dose (amount and timing) and number of days |

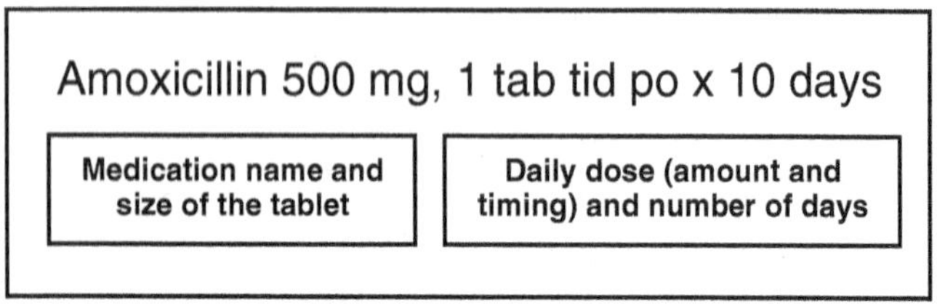

FIGURE 14.6 Medication order.

Solid Medication Doses

Quantity Needed for a Specific Time Period

It is not uncommon for patients to call their provider to request enough medication for a trip. It is important for the medical assistant to be able to calculate how many tablets a patient needs for a period of time.

Fig. 14.6 shows a medication order. The first part shows the name of the medication along with the tablet size (strength of each tablet). The last part of the order shows the following:

- How many tablets to take (*dose*) (e.g., 1 tab [tablet])
- The route (e.g., po [oral])
- How many times to take the medication during the day (e.g., tid [three times a day])
- How long to take the medication (e.g., 10 days)

Quantity Needed for a Specific Time Period With Practice Problems

Problem: Amoxicillin 500 mg, 1 tab tid po × 10 days. How many tablets would the patient need for the entire course of medication?

Solution for Problem

Step 1: Figure out the number of tablets per dose. (Use the abbreviation list if you need to; 1 tab equals 1 tablet.)

Step 2: Figure out the number of tablets taken throughout the day. Do this by multiplying the number of tablets per dose (1 tablet) by the number of times the medication is taken during the day (tid means 3 times a day).

1 tablet per dose
× 3 times a day (tid)
_____
3 tablets per day

Step 3: Figure out the number of tablets needed. Multiply the number of tablets per day by the number of days.

3 tablets per day
× 10 days
_____
30 tablets needed

Answer: 30 tablets needed

Practice Problems

Directions: Calculate the number of tablets the patient will need for the entire course of the prescription.

1. Prescription: XYZ medication 200 mg, 5 tabs tid × 6 days. How many tablets will the patient need?
2. Prescription: XYZ medication 250 mg, 3 tabs qid × 14 days. How many tablets will the patient need?
3. Prescription: XYZ medication 50 mg, 4 tabs bid × 10 days. How many tablets will the patient need?
4. Prescription: XYZ medication 70 mg, 4 tabs tid × 13 days. How many tablets will the patient need?

Number of Tablets per Dose

It is common for the provider to give medication orders without a tablet amount. For instance, the provider orders "Tylenol 975 mg po." The medical assistant must figure out how many tablets to give to the patient. To start, figure out the number of milligrams in each tablet, which will be indicated on the stock medication label. Once the tablet size is identified, the medical assistant can calculate the number of tablets required.

Number of Tablets per Dose: Proportion Method With Practice Problems

Problem: Order: Tylenol 975 mg po. Stock: Tylenol 325 mg per tablet. How many tablets should be given?

Solution for Problem

Step 1: Put the stock information into a fraction on one side. The location of the numbers does not matter. Make sure to add the labels. (Remember that 325 mg per tablet really means 325 mg in each tablet.)

$$\text{Stock}$$
$$\frac{325\,mg}{1\,tab}$$

Step 2: Add an equal sign, and make a fraction on the opposite side. Fill in the labels. The labels need to be in identical locations on both sides of the equal sign.

$$\begin{array}{cc} \text{Stock} & \text{Order} \\ \dfrac{325\,mg}{1\,tab} = & \dfrac{mg}{tab} \end{array}$$

Step 3: Fill in the order information. You do not know the number of tablets, so that is the unknown (x).

$$\begin{array}{cc} \text{Stock} & \text{Order} \\ \dfrac{325\,mg}{1\,tab} = & \dfrac{975\,mg}{x\,tab} \end{array}$$

Step 4: Now solve for the unknown.

Using a calculator: Multiply in the diagonal direction of the two numbers (1 × 975), then divide by the number in the other direction (325), and the answer is x.

$$\begin{array}{cc} \text{Stock} & \text{Order} \\ \dfrac{325\,mg}{1\,tab} & \dfrac{975\,mg}{x\,tab} \end{array}$$

$$1 \times 975 = \underline{975} \,/ 325 = \underline{3}$$

To solve without a calculator: multiply diagonally and solve for x.

$$1 \times 975 = 325x$$
$$975 = 325x$$
$$\frac{975}{325} = \frac{325x}{325}$$
$$3 = x$$

Answer: 3 tablets

Practice Problems

Directions: Calculate the number of tablets to give.
1. Order: ABC 120 mg po; stock: ABC 80 mg po **scored tablet**. How many tablets should be given?
2. Order: ABC 150 mg po; stock: ABC 30 mg po scored tablet. How many tablets should be given?
3. Order: ABC 105 mg po; stock: ABC 30 mg po scored tablet. How many tablets should be given?
4. Order: ABC 65 mg po; stock: ABC 130 mg po scored tablet. How many tablets should be given?

Number of Tablets per Dose: Formula Method

Problem: Order: Tylenol 975 mg po. Stock: Tylenol 325 mg per tablet. How many tablets should be given?

Solution for Problem

Setting Up the Problem

The set-up for the formula method is the following:

$$\frac{D\,(desired)}{H\,(on\,hand)} \times V\,(vehicle - tablet\,or\,liquid)$$

Step 1: D (desired) is 975 mg. H (on hand) is 325 mg. V (vehicle) is 1 tablet. Put the values into the formula method.

$$\frac{975\,mg}{325\,mg} \times 1\,tablet$$

Step 2: Multiply the problem. Then divide 975 by 325 to figure out the tablet amount.

$$\frac{975\,mg}{325\,mg} \times 1\,tablet = \frac{975}{325}$$

Answer: 3 tablets

It is important to double-check your answers. If the order is larger than the stock tablet, then you will be giving more than 1 tablet. If the order is smaller than the stock tablet amount, then you will be giving less than a tablet.

Liquid Medication Doses

When preparing a liquid medication, you will see two different units of measure on the bottle label. These two units include the weight of the powdered medications and the volume of liquid. The units typically used include the following:
- Weight of the powdered medication: units, g, mg, or mcg
- Volume of liquid: cc or mL

For instance, a bottle label states "50 mg/2 mL." This means that there are 50 mg of powdered medication in every 2 mL of liquid. If you want 50 mg of medication, then you would need to give 2 mL of liquid. Another example is 1500 mg/mL. This means that there are 1500 mg of powdered medicine in each milliliter of liquid. Remember that sometimes 1 mL is indicated by just "mL."

Liquid Medication Dose With Matching Labels

If the unit label of ordered medication is the same as the stock medication, then the units are considered to match. For instance, in the following box the ordered medication dose label was shown in milligrams (mg). The stock medication was 1300 mg/2 mL. The powdered medication label (mg) matches the label on the order.

Liquid Medication Dose With Matching Labels: Proportion Method With Practice Problems

Problem: Order: ABC medication 1500 mg. Stock: ABC medication 1300 mg/2 mL. How much medication (in milliliters) should be given?

Solution for Problem

Setting Up the Problem:

Make sure the label information is on the stock side of the equation. The order is on the opposite side. Remember, unit labels need to be in the same location on both sides of the equal sign.

Step 1: Put the stock information into a fraction. The location of the numbers does not matter. Make sure to add the labels.

$$\text{Stock}$$
$$\frac{1300\ mg}{2\ mL}$$

Step 2: Put the order information on the other side. Make sure the labels are in the exact same location.

$$\underset{\text{Stock}}{\frac{1300\ mg}{2\ mL}} = \underset{\text{Order}}{\frac{1500\ mg}{x\ mL}}$$

Step 3: Now solve for the unknown.

Using a calculator: Multiply the diagonal direction of the two numbers (2 × 1500), then divide by the number in the other direction (1300). Round your answer to the nearest tenth.

$$\underset{\text{Stock}}{\frac{1300\ mg}{2\ mL}} \quad \underset{\text{Order}}{\frac{1500\ mg}{x\ mL}}$$
$$2\times1500 = 3000/1300 = 2.3\ mL$$

To solve without a calculator: Multiply diagonally, and solve for x. Round your answer to the nearest tenth.

$$1300x = 1500\times2$$
$$1300x = 3000$$
$$\frac{1300x}{1300} = \frac{3000}{1300}$$
$$x = 2.3\ mL$$

Answer: 2.3 mL

Practice Problems

Directions: Solve the following problems. Round your answers to the nearest tenth.

1. Order: ABC 3200 units
   Stock: ABC 2800 units/mL
   How many milliliters will you give?
2. Order: ABC 230 units
   Stock: ABC 120 units/mL
   How many milliliters will you give?
3. Order: ABC 10 mg
   Stock: ABC 25 mg/3 mL
   How many milliliters will you give?
4. Order: ABC 45 mg
   Stock: ABC 125 mg/mL
   How many milliliters will you give?
5. Order: ABC 120 mg
   Stock: ABC 280 mg/mL
   How many milliliters will you give?
6. Order: ABC 500 mg
   Stock: ABC 1200 mg/2 mL
   How many milliliters will you give?

Liquid Medication Dose: Formula Method

Problem: Order: ABC medication 1500 mg. Stock: ABC medication 1300 mg/2 mL. How much medication (in milliliters) should be given?

Solution for Problem

Setting Up the Problem

The set-up for the formula method is the following:

$$\frac{D\ (desired)}{H\ (on\ hand)}\times V\ (vehicle-tablet\ or\ liquid)$$

Step 1: D (desired) is 1500 mg. H (on hand) is 1300 mg. V (vehicle) is 2 mL. Put the values into the formula method.

$$\frac{1500\ mg}{1300\ mg}\times2\ mL$$

Step 2: Multiply the problem. Then divide 3000 by 1300 to figure out the amount. Round the answer to the nearest tenth.

$$\frac{1500\ mg}{1300\ mg}\times2\ mL = \frac{3000}{1300}$$

Answer: 2.3 mL

Liquid Medication Dose With Nonmatching Labels

Sometimes the stock medication's unit of measure does not directly match the order's unit of measure. For instance, the provider may want "ABC 500 mg" to be given. The stock vial indicates "1 g/mL." This might be confusing. The first step is to identify if there is a

Liquid Medication Dose With Nonmatching Labels: Proportion Method With Practice Problems

Problem: Order: ABC medication 1.5 g. Stock: ABC medication 1300 mg/2 mL. How much medication (in milliliters) should be given?

Solution for Problem

Step 1: Identify the two similar base unit labels. In this example, they are 1.5 g and 1300 mg. Essentially, a person could either convert the grams to milligrams or convert the milligrams to grams. This example shows how to convert from grams to milligrams (1.5 g = _____ mg). Set-up the problem and solve.

$$\frac{1.5 \text{ g}}{x \text{ mg}} = \frac{1 \text{ g}}{1000 \text{ mg}}$$

$$1.5 \times 1000 = 1500/1 = 1500 \text{ mg}$$

Answer: 1500 mg (If it helps, cross out the 1.5 g and write in 1500 mg.)

Step 2: Put the stock information into a fraction. The location of the numbers does not matter. Make sure to add the labels.

Stock

$$\frac{1300 \text{ mg}}{2 \text{ mL}}$$

Step 3: Put the order information on the other side. Make sure the labels are in the exact same location.

Stock   Order

$$\frac{1300 \text{ mg}}{2 \text{ mL}} = \frac{1500 \text{ mg}}{x \text{ mL}}$$

Step 4: Now solve for the unknown.

Using a calculator: Multiply in the diagonal direction of the two numbers (2 × 1500), then divide by the number in the other direction (1300). Round your answer to the nearest tenth.

Stock   Order

$$\frac{1300 \text{ mg}}{2 \text{ mL}} = \frac{1500 \text{ mg}}{x \text{ mL}}$$

$$2 \times 1500 = 3000/1300 = 2.3 \text{ mL}$$

To solve without a calculator: Multiply diagonally, and solve for x. Round your answer to the nearest tenth.

$$1300x = 1500 \times 2$$

$$1300x = 3000$$

$$\frac{1300x}{1300} = \frac{3000}{1300}$$

$$x = 2.3 \text{ mL}$$

Answer: 2.3 mL

Practice Problems

Directions: Solve the following problems. Round your answers to the nearest tenth.

1. Order: ABC 2500 mg
   Stock: ABC 2.8 g/2 mL
   How many milliliters will you give?
2. Order: ABC 1800 mg
   Stock: ABC 2 g/mL
   How many milliliters will you give?
3. Order: ABC 1.2 g
   Stock: ABC 2500 mg/2 mL
   How many milliliters will you give?
4. Order: ABC 450 mg
   Stock: ABC 1.2 g/2 mL
   How many milliliters will you give?
5. Order: ABC 420 mg
   Stock: ABC 1 g/2 mL
   How many milliliters will you give?
6. Order: ABC 750 mg
   Stock: ABC 1.2 g/2 mL
   How many milliliters will you give?
7. Order: ABC 650 mg
   Stock: ABC 1.8 g/3 mL
   How many milliliters will you give?
8. Order: ABC 400 mg
   Stock: ABC 3 g/2 mL
   How many milliliters will you give?

shared base unit between the order and the stock medication. In this example, they share the same base unit—gram. The second step is to change one of the shared unit labels (e.g., mg and gram) so it matches the other label. Remember that two of the labels need to match before you can solve the problem. Once the labels match, then the problem can be solved like the problems in the prior section.

Solutions

In the ambulatory care environment, many anesthetics used for minor surgeries come in a solution. For instance, a provider asks you to get the strongest Xylocaine vial in the cabinet. You see a 1% and a 2% vial. What does this mean?

When the manufacturer made the medication, the "recipe" called for powdered drug to be mixed with a liquid:

- A 1% solution means 1000 mg of powdered drug is mixed in 100 mL of liquid.
- A 2% solution means 2000 mg of powdered drug is mixed in 100 mL of liquid.

(The 100 mL of liquid always remains regardless of the number in front of the percentage sign.) Going back to the provider's request, you would give the provider the 2% vial, as it is the strongest solution (or contains the most powdered drug).

Solution Dose. If a medical assistant needs to calculate a dose of medication using a stock solution vial, the process is similar to that used for the prior problems. The initial step would require the medical assistant to change the percent into a fraction. Using a 5% solution as an example, the fraction would be 5000 mg/100 mL. The remaining steps would be the same as the previous problems.

Solution Dose: Proportion Method With Practice Problems

Problem: Order: ABC medication 20 mg. Stock: ABC medication 2% solution. How much medication (in milliliters) should be given?

Solution for Problem

Step 1: Change the 2% into a fraction. Tip: Take the number before the percentage sign. Add three zeros and "mg" after it. Then put it over 100 mL.

$$2\% = \frac{2000 \text{ mg}}{100 \text{ mL}}$$

Step 2: Use the fraction created in step 1 as the stock medication.

Stock
$$\frac{2000 \text{ mg}}{100 \text{ mL}}$$

Step 3: Put the order information on the other side. Make sure the labels are in the exact same location.

Stock   Order
$$\frac{2000 \text{ mg}}{100 \text{ mL}} = \frac{20 \text{ mg}}{x \text{ mL}}$$

Step 4: Now solve for the unknown.

Using a calculator: Multiply in the diagonal direction of the two numbers (100×20), then divide by the number in the other direction (2000). Round your answer to the nearest tenth.

Stock   Order
$$\frac{2000 \text{ mg}}{100 \text{ mL}} \diagup \frac{20 \text{ mg}}{x \text{ mL}}$$

$$100 \times 20 = 2000/2000 = 1 \text{ mL}$$

To solve without a calculator: Multiply diagonally, and solve for x. Round your answer to the nearest tenth.

$$2000x = 100 \times 20$$
$$2000x = 2000$$
$$\frac{2000x}{2000} = \frac{2000}{2000}$$
$$x = 1 \text{ mL}$$

Answer: 1 mL

Practice Problems

Directions: Solve the following problems. Round your answers to the nearest tenth.

1. ABC 60 mg. Stock: ABC 4% solution. How many milliliter(s) will you give?
2. ABC 80 mg. Stock: ABC 10% solution. How many milliliter(s) will you give?
3. ABC 30 mg. Stock: ABC 4% solution. How many milliliter(s) will you give?
4. ABC 70 mg. Stock: ABC 5% solution. How many milliliter(s) will you give?
5. ABC 120 mg. Stock: ABC 11% solution. How many milliliter(s) will you give?
6. ABC 50 mg. Stock: ABC 6% solution. How many milliliter(s) will you give?

Pediatric Dose

As with all medication calculations, it is important to be accurate for the safety of the patient. It is recommended that two people calculate a dose just to be sure of the accuracy.

Medication dosages for children are typically based on the children's weights. For this type of problem, the medical assistant needs the child's weight, the drug order, and the information on the stock medication label. For instance, a child's weight is 33 pounds (lbs), the drug order is ABC medication 0.1 mg/kg, and the stock medication label states "ABC medication 1 mg/mL." Notice the child's weight is in pounds and the order is 0.1 mg per every kilogram of weight. The unit of measure for weight is different, one being pounds and the other kilograms.

- Step 1: Convert the patient's weight to kilograms. This goes back to converting between the household and metric systems that was discussed earlier in the chapter.
- Step 2: Calculate the number of milligrams of medication the child needs. Imagine this scenario: A person tells you, you can have two chocolate bars for each kilogram you weigh. How would you figure it out? A simple way is to multiply the number of kilograms you weigh by 2 ($68 \times 2 = 136$ bars). You can use this same method to calculate the medication order—multiply the kilograms by the order.

- The final step is to calculate the liquid medication dose or the number of milliliters you will give. An example of this step was shown in a prior section of this chapter.

The following box shows the solution for solving this type of problem (see Procedure 14.1, p. 356). You can modify the steps and use the formula method if you like.

READING SYRINGES

For the safety of patients, it is important that medical assistants are accurate when measuring medications in syringes. Syringes have calibrations printed on the barrel. These markings are used when measuring the medication prior to administration. The calibration markings include longer or darker lines and shorter lines. The first step in reading a syringe is to identify the amount of each calibration line. With many types of syringes, a person should count the number of lines for 1 mL or for 0.1 mL, depending on the syringe.

Fig. 14.7 shows a 3-mL syringe, the most commonly used syringe in ambulatory care. The maximum amount that the syringe can hold is indicated at the bottom of the syringe. To identify what each line is worth, count the lines for 1 mL. For this syringe, there are 10 lines for 1 mL, which means each line is equal to 0.1 mL. Medication

Pediatric Dose: Proportion Method With Practice Problems

Problem: Patient's weight: 33 lb. Order: ABC medication 0.1 mg/kg. Stock: ABC medication 1 mg/mL. How much medication (in milliliters) should be given?

Solution for Problem

Tip on solving the problem: There are three main steps to this problem. When you complete a step, round two places beyond your answer. For instance, if your answer is to be in tenths, then during the problem, round to the thousandth (three places after the decimal). This will ensure accuracy in the answer.

Step 1: Convert the patient's weight into kilograms. This can be done several ways. Use your favorite method or follow the example and solve for the unknown.

Problem: 33 lb = _____ kg

$$\frac{33\,\text{lb}}{x\,\text{kg}} \,\diagdown\!\!\diagup\, \frac{2.2\,\text{lb}}{1\,\text{kg}}$$

Problem   Equivalent

Using a calculator: Multiply in the diagonal direction of the two numbers (33×1), then divide by the number in the other direction (2.2). Round your answer to the nearest thousandth (if needed).

To solve without a calculator: Multiply diagonally, and solve for x. Round your answer to the nearest thousandth (if needed).

$$33 \times 1 = 2.2x$$
$$33 = 2.2x$$
$$\frac{33}{2.2} = \frac{2.2x}{2.2}$$
$$15 = x$$

Updated weight: 15 kg

Step 2: Calculate the number of milligrams of medication needed. Again, there are several ways to do this. The easiest is to multiply the weight by the order (15 kg × 0.1 mg), or you can set it up like the example and solve it. Because this is in the middle of the problem, round to the nearest thousandth (if needed).

Order   Weight

$$\frac{0.1\,\text{mg}}{1\,\text{kg}} \,\diagdown\!\!\diagup\, \frac{x\,\text{mg}}{15\,\text{kg}}$$

$$0.1 \times 15 = \underline{1.5}/1 = \underline{1.5\,\text{mg}}$$

Updated order: ABC medication 1.5 mg

Step 3: Calculate the liquid medication dose. Put the stock information into a fraction. Put the order information on the other side. Make sure the labels are in the exact same location.

Stock   Order

$$\frac{1\,\text{mg}}{1\,\text{mL}} \,\diagdown\!\!\diagup\, \frac{1.5\,\text{mg}}{x\,\text{mL}}$$

Using a calculator: Multiply in the diagonal direction of the two numbers (1.5×1), then divide by the number in the other direction (1). Round your answer to the nearest thousandth (if needed).

To solve without a calculator: Multiply diagonally, and solve for x. Round your answer to the nearest thousandth (if needed).

$$1x = 1 \times 1.5$$
$$1x = 1.5$$
$$\frac{1x}{1} = \frac{1.5}{1}$$
$$x = 1.5\,\text{mL}$$

Answer: 1.5 mL

Practice Problems

Directions: Round to the nearest thousandth while solving, then round your answer to the nearest tenth.

1. Patient's weight: 40 lb
   Order: ABC medication 0.3 mg/kg
   Stock: ABC medication 2 mg/mL
   How many milliliters will you give?

2. Patient's weight: 58 lb
   Order: ABC medication 0.8 mg/kg
   Stock: ABC medication 60 mg/2 mL
   How many milliliters will you give?

3. Patient's weight: 145 lb
   Order: ABC medication 2 mg/kg
   Stock: ABC medication 80 mg/mL
   How many milliliters will you give?

4. Patient's weight: 31 lb
   Order: ABC medication 0.3 mg/kg
   Stock: ABC medication 2 mg/mL
   How many milliliters will you give?

5. Patient's weight: 60 lb
   Order: ABC medication 0.8 mg/kg
   Stock: ABC medication 50 mg/2 mL
   How many milliliters will you give?

6. Patient's weight: 86 lb
   Order: ABC medication 1.5 mg/kg
   Stock: ABC medication 80 mg/2 mL
   How many milliliters will you give?

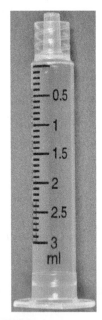

FIGURE 14.7 A 3-mL syringe.

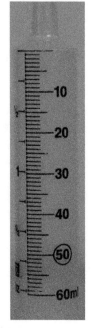

FIGURE 14.9 A 60-mL syringe.

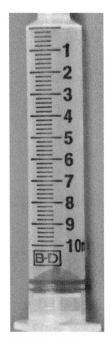

FIGURE 14.8 A 10-mL syringe.

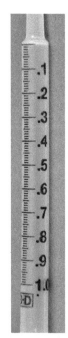

FIGURE 14.10 A 1-mL syringe.

amounts to the nearest tenth (one place after the decimal point) can be measured using this syringe.

Fig. 14.8 shows a 10-mL syringe. The calibration markings on this syringe are the same as on most 5-, 6-, 10- and 12-mL syringes. For this syringe, there are 5 lines for 1 mL, which means each line is equal to 0.2 mL. Syringes with this type of calibration can only measure medication ordered in even numbers (i.e. 1.2 mL, 2 mL, 3.6 mL).

Fig. 14.9 shows a 60-mL syringe. The calibration markings are different with this type of syringe. Unlike prior syringes, the numbers labeled are in increments of 5 (5, 10, 15, etc.). Each line is equal to 1 mL. Syringes with this type of calibration can only measure whole

number amounts (5, 9, 11, etc.). This type of syringe may be used in ambulatory care for irrigation.

Fig. 14.10 shows a 1-mL syringe. The numbers on this syringe are tenths (.1, .2, and so on). For this syringe, there are 10 lines for 0.1 mL, which means each line is equal to 0.01 mL. Syringes with this type of calibration can measure to the hundredth place (e.g., 0.08, 0.09, 0.15). The most common use of these syringes is for tuberculin (TB) skin tests.

If a medication order indicates that 0.14 mL is to be given, the medical assistant should find the calibration marking for 0.1. A trick is to think of 0.1 as 0.10. The next small line would be 0.11, then

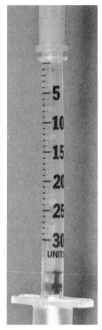

FIGURE 14.11 U-100 insulin syringe.

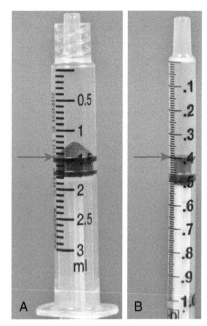

FIGURE 14.12 (A) The rubber stopper is pointed. **(B)** The rubber stopper is flat.

0.12, and so on. If a medication order indicates that 0.04 mL is to be given, the medical assistant should find the large line at the top of the syringe. This would be 0 and the next little line would be considered 0.01, followed by 0.02, and so on.

Fig. 14.11 shows an insulin syringe. Insulin is measured in units. The calibration markings are similar to the 60-mL syringe. The numbers labeled are in increments of 5 (5, 10, 15, etc.). Each line is equal to 1 unit. Syringes with this type of calibration can only measure whole number amounts (5, 9, 11, etc.). This type of syringe may be used in ambulatory care for U-100 insulin administration.

When using syringes, the rubber stopper on the plunger indicates the amount in the syringe. Some rubber stoppers are pointed (Fig. 14.12A) and others are flat (Fig. 14.12B). The top of the rubber stopper that touches the barrel is used for measuring. That part of the rubber stopper should be right on the correct calibration mark. The red arrow indicates this location on both rubber stoppers.

CLOSING COMMENTS

Patient Coaching

In some cases, the medical assistant needs to teach patients and parents how to read oral medical syringes. These syringes are used to draw up and administer oral medications, usually to young children. When coaching a patient or parent on using an oral syringe to measure medications, it is important for the medical assistant to refer to the provider's order. If the order states 1 teaspoon, the medical assistant should coach the person that this is the same as 5 mL. Prior to finishing the coaching session, the medical assistant should have the patient or parent draw up (with air) the dose ordered to determine if the person understands the procedure.

Legal and Ethical Issues

Not all states allow medical assistants to calculate medication dosages. It is important for the medical assistant to review the state's scope of practice laws. Some agencies may also have policies and procedures regarding calculating medication dosages. The medical assistant must follow both the state's scope of practice laws and the agency's policies and procedures.

Professional Behaviors

If a medical assistant needs to calculate a medication dosage, it is important to have another qualified staff person recheck the calculations. If a medical assistant forgets how to calculate a medical dosage or has questions regarding the procedure, the medical assistant must talk with the provider for clarification.

SUMMARY OF SCENARIO

Mark is enjoying working with Gabe. Mark was able to review the different types of commonly used math problems in ambulatory care. Besides working on calculations, Mark and Gabe reviewed syringes. The department carried 1-mL and 3-mL syringes for medication administration, 5-mL and 10-mL syringes for medication mixing procedures, and 60-mL syringes for wound irrigation procedures.

A small box of insulin syringes was also available in the department, should a patient need insulin administration directions. It took Mark a couple of days to get comfortable measuring medications using the various syringes. Being accurate when measuring medications is critical to the patient's safety.

SUMMARY OF LEARNING OBJECTIVES

1. **Summarize the important parts of a drug label.**
   The label shows the following information: brand name, generic name, strength, total amount or total volume, manufacturer, directions and storage, expiration date, lot number, and the National Drug Code. When preparing medications, the name, strength, and expiration date are important.

2. **Discuss math basics, including writing numbers in healthcare and rounding numbers.**
   Important healthcare rules when writing numbers include the following:
   - Follow the number with the correct abbreviation for the unit of measure. Leave a space between the number and the abbreviation. Do not use a period with the abbreviations.
   - Write a fraction of a dose as a decimal.
   - If the dose is less than 1, place a zero to the left of the decimal point.
   - Do not place a decimal point and a zero after a whole number.

   When rounding, remember the following:
   - 4 or below: drop the number(s) to the right of the place value
   - 5 or above: add 1 to the rounded place value and drop the number(s) to the right of the place value.

3. **Define basic units of measure in the household system and the metric system, and convert between measurement systems.**
   See the Household and Metric Problems box and the Metric Problems box for examples of solving household and metric problems.

4. **Convert between Fahrenheit and Celsius temperatures.**
   See the Temperature Conversion box for an example of converting between Fahrenheit and Celsius temperatures.

5. **Perform pharmacology calculations, such as quantity needed for a specific time period, number of tablets per dose, liquid medication doses, and pediatric doses.**
   See the following boxes for examples of solving these problems: Quantity Needed for a Specific Time Period, Number of Tablets per Dose, Liquid Medication Dose with Matching Labels, Liquid Medication Dose with Nonmatching Labels, Solution Dose, and Pediatric Dose.

6. **Read the calibration markings on various types of syringes.**
   When reading syringes, the first step is to identify how much each calibration line is worth.
   - If there are 10 lines per 1 mL, each line is equal to 0.1 mL.
   - If there are 5 lines per 1 mL, each line is equal to 0.2 mL.
   - If there are 10 lines per 0.1 mL, each line is equal to 0.01 mL.
   - Insulin syringes calibration lines are usually measured in 1-unit increments.

PROCEDURE 14.1   Calculate Medication Dosages

Task: Calculate dosages for oral medication, injectable medication, and children.

Orders:
Order 1: Dr. Martin orders ABC medication 135 mg. Stock bottle reads: 45 mg scored tablets
Order 2: Dr. Martin orders ABC medication 650 mg. Stock bottle reads: 1300 mg scored tablets
Order 3: Dr. Martin orders XYZ medication 430 mg IM. Stock vial reads: 1000 mg/2 mL
Order 4: Dr. Martin orders XYZ medication 680 mg IM. Stock vial reads: 1200 mg/mL
Order 5: Dr. Martin orders MNO medication 3 mg/kg IM. Child weighs 53 pounds. Stock vial reads: 125 mg/mL
Order 6: Dr. Martin orders MNO medication 5 mg/kg IM. Child weighs 71 pounds. Stock vial reads: 225 mg/mL

EQUIPMENT and SUPPLIES

- Provider's order
- Paper and pencil
- Calculator (optional per instructor)

PROCEDURE STEPS

1. Using Order 1, calculate the number of tablets to give the patient. Label your answer.
   PURPOSE: It is important to label your answer to avoid any mistakes in the dosage.

2. Using Order 2, calculate the number of tablets to give the patient. Label your answer.

3. Using Order 3, calculate the amount in milliliters to give the patient. Round your answer to the nearest tenth. Label your answer.
   PURPOSE: Most injections are measured in tenths of a milliliter.

4. Using Order 4, calculate the amount in milliliters to give the patient. Round your answer to the nearest tenth. Label your answer.

5. Using Order 5, calculate the amount in milliliters to give the patient. Round your answer to the nearest tenth. Label your answer.
   NOTE: When working through the problem, round your answer two places beyond your answer. In this situation, round your answers as you work to the thousandth place (or three places after the decimal point).

6. Using Order 6, calculate the amount in milliliters to give the patient. Round your answer to the nearest tenth. Label your answer.

7. Double-check your answers to ensure the correct dose will be given.
   PURPOSE: When calculating medications, it is important to recheck the work to ensure your answer is correct.

ADMINISTERING MEDICATIONS

15

SCENARIO

Gabe Garcia, CMA (AAMA), has worked for Walden-Martin Family Medical (WMFM) Clinic for 3 years. He was hired right after he completed his medical assistant program. He is currently Mark Allen's mentor for his practicum. Mark has been working with Gabe for 1 week. During the week, Gabe worked with Mark reviewing math for medications and prescriptions.

Mark's goal for his second week of practicum is to give medications. He has watched Gabe give injections to both children and adults. Mark is nervous, but excited at the same time. He is looking forward to improving his injection skills during practicum.

While studying this chapter, think about the following questions:

- What are the nine rights of medication administration? Why are they important?
- What forms and routes of medications are commonly used in the ambulatory care setting?
- How are oral medications given in the ambulatory care setting?
- How should a medical assistant uncap and recap needles? How should needles be switched?
- How are parenteral medications prepared?

- Why is tuberculin testing done? What is the procedure for tuberculin testing? What is two-step testing?
- What are administration techniques for intradermal, subcutaneous, and intramuscular injections?
- How does a medical assistant locate the sites for intradermal, subcutaneous, and intramuscular injections?
- How does a medical assistant administer intradermal, subcutaneous, and intramuscular injections?

LEARNING OBJECTIVES

1. Verify and discuss the rights of medication administration.
2. Discuss the various forms of medication.
3. Administer oral medications.
4. Describe other routes of medications, including sublingual, buccal, transdermal, inhalation, topical, irrigation, and parenteral.
5. Discuss types and parts of needles and syringes.
6. Prepare parenteral medications.
7. Prepare and administer intradermal injections.
8. Prepare and administer subcutaneous injections.
9. Prepare and administer intramuscular injections.
10. Describe the medical assistant's role in monitoring intravenous therapy.

VOCABULARY

aspirate (AS pi rayt) To withdraw fluid using suction.

diluent (DIL yoo ent) A liquid substance that dilutes or lessens the strength of a solution or mixture.

form Physical characteristics of a medication (e.g., tablet, suspension).

local Affecting the area where applied.

precipitate (pri SIP i tayt) Solid particles that settle out of a liquid.

reconstituted (ree KON sti toot ed) A dried substance (powder) that has been restored to a fluid form, so it can be injected.

route The means by which a drug enters the body.

systemic Affecting the entire body.

viscosity (vis KOS i tee) Resistance to flow; the thicker the liquid, the higher the viscosity.

Chapter 13 discussed the basics of pharmacology, and Chapter 14 discussed pharmacology-related math problems. You will use these skills when administering medications. This chapter discusses administration safety techniques, along with medication forms and routes. The techniques of preparing and administering medications will be the primary focus.

It is important to remember that medications can cause serious harm to patients. It is critical to pay attention to the details when you prepare and administer medications. Preventing errors and providing superior patient care are goals each time medication is given. Administering medication is an important responsibility for healthcare professionals.

State laws vary regarding whether or not medical assistants may administer medications. In some situations, the state law allows medical assistants to administer medications, but the facility's policies do not. It is important for medical assistants to know their state's laws and the facility's policies on medication administration.

NINE RIGHTS OF MEDICATION ADMINISTRATION

Throughout this chapter, administration procedures for various routes will be given. Before learning how to give medications, it is important to understand medication safety rights. Over the years the guidelines have grown to include additional steps to address patient education and the right to refuse the medication.

Each time you prepare and give medication, it is important that you follow the nine rights of medication administration. These rights are designed to help you look at the details and avoid making errors during the procedure (Fig. 15.1).

Right Medication

A prescription (or an order) from a provider is required before a medication can be given. As discussed in a prior chapter, orders can be written or verbal. For all verbal orders, make sure to write down the order and read it back to the provider. This helps to ensure the accuracy of the order. The order needs to include several factors, including the medication's name and **form**.

With the order in hand, the medical assistant must prepare the medication. This requires finding the correct medication. Use drug reference information if you are not familiar with the medication listed on the order. Sometimes the provider will give a brand name, but the stock medication will indicate only a generic name. Make sure you have the correct medication, which includes the correct **form** (e.g., tablet, suppository, suspension).

You will need to check the medication order against the label three times during the preparation process to ensure that you have the correct name and form of medication. You check the label:

- When you get the medication from the storage area (e.g., cabinet, freezer, or refrigerator)
- Before preparing the medication
- Before you return the medication to the storage area

It is important that you do an activity between each check. For instance, after you do the first check, assemble the supplies you need to prepare the medication. Then do the second check. As you clean up your area, you do the third check. Too often we reach for something based on the color, size, or location of the object. We may look at the label and think we see what we want to see. Checking the label three times, with activities between, helps to ensure that you have the right medication.

Right Dose

The dose of medication is on the order. The provider may have written the order in two different ways, even though the amount is the same. For example, both of these orders give the patient 1000 mg:

- Acetaminophen 500 mg, 2 tabs po × 1 dose
- Acetaminophen 1000 mg po × 1 dose

The first order shows the tablet strength (e.g., 500 mg) and the number of tablets (e.g., 2) to give. If the stock medication comes in 500-mg tablets, the medical assistant has no calculations to do. The second order just shows the number of milligrams to give (e.g., 1000 mg). The medical assistant would need to calculate how many tablets to give. (This procedure was discussed in Chapter 14.)

Right Route

Besides checking the label for the name and form, it is also important to check the **route**. The route of the medication must match the provider's order. The route should be checked, along with the name and form, three times before the medication is given.

Right Time

Medications need to be given at the right time. For most medication orders, the time is part of the order. Some orders are STAT, whereas others are every month. Vaccines are a little different. Timing for vaccines may not be written on the provider's order, but the medical assistant should ensure that it is the correct time for a vaccine to be given. The medical assistant will need to review the patient's vaccination history and the person's age. Using immunization schedules or the immunization tables in electronic health records (EHRs), the medical assistant can determine what vaccines are due.

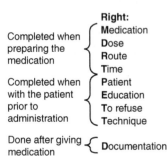

Right:
- Medication — Completed when preparing the medication
- Dose
- Route
- Time
- Patient — Completed when with the patient prior to administration
- Education
- To refuse
- Technique
- Documentation — Done after giving medication

Mnemonic: **M**aybe **D**ogs **R**eally **T**alk, **PET**s **T**ruly **D**o.

FIGURE 15.1 Mnemonic for the nine rights of medication administration.

Timing of Vaccines

Two main types of vaccines are available:
- *Live virus vaccines:* The microorganism is alive but *attenuated* (weakened) in the laboratory. Vaccine examples include MMR (measles, mumps, and rubella), varicella (chickenpox), zoster (shingles) (ZOSTAVAX), and yellow fever.
- *Inactivated vaccines:* The microorganism is dead. This type includes *toxoid vaccines* made from modified toxins of microorganisms (e.g., diphtheria and tetanus).

When vaccines are given, the immunization schedule must be followed. The immunization schedule indicates the person's age and the timing between doses. If a vaccination is administered too early or before the patient reaches a specific age, the patient will have to be revaccinated.

The provider will postpone vaccinations when patients have a moderate or severe acute illness. Specific vaccines are not given if a person has had a severe allergic reaction to a vaccine component, to latex, or to a prior dose. Patients may not receive a live virus vaccine if they meet the following conditions:

- Were vaccinated with another live virus vaccine less than 28 days earlier.
- Are pregnant or may become pregnant in the next month. The human papillomavirus (HPV) vaccine is also contraindicated with pregnancy.
- Are immunocompromised (e.g., cancer, leukemia, HIV/AIDS).
- Are receiving chemotherapy or high-dose steroid therapy.
- Recently received a blood transfusion, immune (gamma) globulin, or antiviral medication.

Consult the CDC website for information on vaccine schedules and catch-up schedules (https://www.cdc.gov/vaccines/index.html). The CDC also offers a free app that provides vaccine information.

Right Patient

Before administering the medication, it is important to correctly identify the patient. Ask the patient or parent/guardian to state his or her full name and date of birth. Some agencies require patients to spell their last names. Verify the information against the order and the patient's health record. All three must match. Any differences must be resolved before the medication is given.

In some agencies, patients are given identification bracelets that are scanned before medication is given. The medication is also scanned. An automatic entry is made in the EHR. This is a common practice in hospitals and is starting to be used in ambulatory care facilities. The identification process with bracelets still requires asking the patient's name and date of birth. The information is checked against the bracelet and the order.

CRITICAL THINKING APPLICATION 15.1

Gabe is introducing Mark to the facility's medication procedures. Gabe encourages Mark to have the patients give their complete name and date of birth. He also tells Mark it is a good idea to have the patients spell their last names. Why is spelling the last name an important safety check?

Right Education

Before administering the medication to the patient, the medical assistant must:

1. *Give the name of the medication and who ordered it.* For example, "Dr. Martin ordered acetaminophen for your fever."
2. *Explain the desired effect or action of the medication.* For example, "The acetaminophen will bring down your fever."

3. *Describe common side effects of the medication.* For example, "The acetaminophen may cause nausea, rash, and a headache."
4. Verify the patient's allergies.

If the patient is receiving a vaccination, the facility may require a questionnaire to be completed. The medical assistant may need to give a Vaccine Information Statement (VIS) prior to administering the vaccine. The VIS provides important information to the patient about the vaccine and common and uncommon side effects. If the patient cannot read, the medical assistant should review the VIS with the patient. VISs can be downloaded in about 40 different languages for patients who do not speak English.

Vaccine Information Statement (VIS)

The Vaccine Information Statement was created by the Centers for Disease Control and Prevention (CDC). A VIS provides information to the patient or to the guardian/parent on the benefits and risks of the vaccine. The National Childhood Vaccine Injury Act requires that all patients (or parents/guardians) get the appropriate VIS prior to every dose of vaccine administered, regardless of the age of the patient. The specific list of vaccines that require the VIS are listed on the CDC's website at https://www.cdc.gov/vaccines/hcp/vis/about/facts-vis.html.

The VIS can be displayed on a computer screen or as a laminated copy that the patient can read prior to administration of the vaccine. Copies of the VIS can be given to the patient or parent/guardian to take home. The provider must offer the information; however, the patient or parent/guardian has the right to decline to take the document.

Besides giving the patient or parent/guardian the VIS prior to the vaccination, the medical assistant must document the following in the patient's health record:

- The edition date of the VIS. This is found on the back of the document in the bottom right corner. Make sure to have the latest edition of the VIS.
- The date the VIS was provided and the date the vaccine was administered (usually the two are done on the same day).
- The office address, name, and title of the person who administered the vaccine.
- The vaccine's manufacturer and lot number.

From the Centers for Disease Control and Prevention (CDC): https://www.cdc.gov/hcp/vis/about/facts-vis.html. Accessed October 26, 2018.

CRITICAL THINKING APPLICATION 15.2

Part of the WMFM Clinic's policy is to explain to patients what was ordered and why they are getting it. Why is it important to tell patients the name of a medication or procedure and the reason it has been prescribed? How might this add to exceptional customer service?

Right to Refuse

The patient or the person legally responsible for the patient (e.g., parent, guardian) has a right to refuse any medication. If a patient refuses the medication, the medical assistant should respect the patient's wishes. Do not pressure the patient. Notify the provider that the ordered medication was refused, and specify the reason if it was shared. Document the refusal of the medication, and identify the provider who was informed. The provider will talk with the patient regarding other options.

Right Technique

When administering the medication, the medical assistant must give it in the right way. This may include an assessment before the medication is administered. Examples of right technique include the following:

- Obtain vital signs before giving a specific medication. For instance, digoxin must be withheld if an adult's pulse is under 60.
- Obtain information about the patient's pain level before giving an analgesic medication. The medical assistant can ask the patient to rate the pain using a 0–10 scale. Zero is no pain and 10 is the worst pain ever. Another pain assessment tool is the Wong-Baker FACES Pain Rating Scale (Fig. 15.2). The medical assistant should explain the scale to patients. Then patients can indicate how they feel. This scale works well for children.
- Some medications must be taken with food and others with a full glass of water. Medications that need to be taken on an empty stomach need to be taken 1 hour before meals or 2 hours after meals.

Information regarding the techniques to use when administering the medication can be found in drug reference information.

Right Documentation

After giving a medication, the medical assistant must document it in the patient's health record. If the medication is not documented, it will appear to others as though it were not given. The documentation will vary based on what the patient received. Some documentation is done in narrative form, whereas vaccines are documented on paper or in electronic vaccination forms. Elements that should be in the documentation include the following:

- Provider ordering the medication
- Assessment done (e.g., vital signs or pain level)
- Allergies
- Coaching/instructions given to patient (includes the edition date of the VIS for vaccine teaching)
- Name of medication (e.g., acetaminophen)
- Dose given (e.g., 650 mg)
- Route given (e.g., po)
- Lot number, expiration date, and manufacturer (usually only required for vaccines and controlled substances)
- How the patient tolerated the medication
- Additional information as needed (e.g., patient is resting on exam table)
- Signature if the note is handwritten (an electronic health record [EHR] uses automatic signatures for documentation entries)

FORMS OF MEDICATIONS

The form is the physical characteristics of the medication. Forms can be grouped into solids, semisolids, and liquids. Solid and semisolid medications are commonly prescribed and found in over-the-counter (OTC) products.

Solid Medication Forms

Examples of solid medication forms include the following:

- *Tablet:* Solid formed by compressed powdered medication; may be coated. Can come in various sizes and shapes (Fig. 15.3).
- *Chewable tablet:* Designed to be chewed prior to swallowing. Example: A chewable vitamin.
- *Caplet:* Coated, oval medication tablet.
- *Capsule:* Medication in a hard or soft gelatin shell.

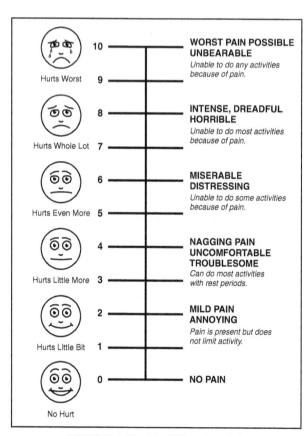

FIGURE 15.2 Wong-Baker FACES Pain Rating Scale.

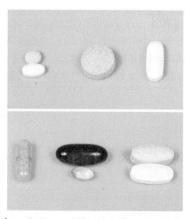

FIGURE 15.3 *Left to right:* Top row: Tablets, chewable, and caplet. Bottom row: Hard-shelled capsule, soft-shelled capsules, and scored caplets.

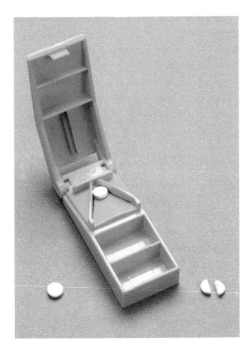

FIGURE 15.4 Pill cutter or splitter.

- *Scored tablet:* A notched tablet, which can be split into half with a pill cutter or splitter (Fig. 15.4).
- *Enteric coated tablets or capsules:* Coated to pass through the acidic environment of the stomach. Breaks down in the base environment of the intestines. These tablets should not be crushed, cut, or chewed because the protective property will be lost.
- *Buffered:* A solid medication containing the active medication and an antacid. The antacid neutralizes the stomach acid and thereby reduces stomach irritation. Example: Buffered aspirin.
- *Fast-dissolving tablet or film strip:* Also called *oral disintegrating tablets.* Solid form of medicine that is placed on the tongue (or by the cheek [buccal]) and breaks down rapidly in the presence of saliva. Examples: Fasprin and acetaminophen.
- *Extended release tablet or capsule:* Designed to break down over time. These tablets should not be crushed, cut, or chewed because doing so may cause an overdose. Many acronyms are used. Example: Calan SR.
- *Effervescent tablet:* Contains an acid substance and carbonate or bicarbonate. When placed in water, it releases carbon dioxide, creating a carbonated drink. Example: K-Lyte Effervescent Tablets.
- *Lozenge (troche):* Flat, round form containing active medication and a sweetened flavoring; dissolves on the tongue. Used for local treatment of the mouth and throat. Example: Cough drop.
- *Powder:* Nonpotent powdered medication that must be mixed with a liquid before it can be taken. Example: MiraLAX.

Some forms of medications can be crushed, whereas others cannot. Over the past few years, the U.S. Food and Drug Administration (FDA) has approved new drug delivery systems or drug forms. This has provided additional options to those who cannot swallow pills. It is common for patients or parents to have concerns about swallowing pills.

Examples of Acronyms for Slow-Release Tablets

CD — controlled delivery
CR — controlled release
DR — delayed release
ER — extended release
LA — long acting
SA — sustained action
SR — sustained release
TD — time delay
TR — time release
XL — extended release
XR — extended release

Crushing Medications

Children, older adults, and others may have problems swallowing solid medications. Crushing medications is sometimes an option. The medication should be placed in a small amount of food or liquid (e.g., pudding or jam). It is important to eat or drink all the food or liquid to get the entire dose of medication.

Solid medications typically have an unpleasant taste. It is important to share with parents that children sometimes shy away from foods with an unpleasant taste. For instance, if a parent mixes the medication with the milk in a bottle, the baby may not want to drink the milk. This can be a problem if the baby drinks only milk.

Medications that cannot be crushed include the following:

- Slow- or extended-release tablets: Crushing, chewing, or cutting the tablet can cause a person to get the dose faster than he or she should, resulting in an overdose.
- Enteric-coated tablets: Crushing, chewing, or cutting the tablet causes the protective nature of the coating to be lost. The person could have more stomach distress.

Semisolid Medication Forms

Examples of semisolid medication forms include the following:

- *Ointment* and *paste:* Semisolid, greasy drug preparations that are applied to the skin, rectum, or nasal mucosa. Pastes are thicker and less penetrating than ointments. Example: Nystatin Ointment.
- *Cream:* Semisolid drug preparation made of active medication, oil, and water. Example: Nystatin Cream.
- *Suppository* and *pessary:* Active medication mixed in an oil base (e.g., cocoa butter). Solid at room temperature but melts at body temperature. Suppositories are typically shaped like a small bullet and used in the rectum, urethra, or vagina. Pessaries are vaginal suppositories. Example: Dulcolax suppository.

Liquid Medication Forms

Liquid medications have various uses. They can be swallowed, rubbed on the skin, or instilled in the nose, eyes, or ears. Liquid medications are easily taken by children, older adults, and those with swallowing problems. With liquid medications, the active medication is mixed with water, alcohol, or both.

If the active medication dissolves in the liquid, the medication is a *solution*. The following are examples of solutions:

- *Tincture:* Very potent solution of alcohol or alcohol and water and the active medicine. Example: Iodine tincture.
- *Fluid extract:* Alcoholic plant source extractions; very concentrated and more potent than tinctures. Example: Belladonna fluid extract.
- *Spirit:* An alcoholic solution with substances that easily evaporate. Example: Aromatic ammonia spirit.
- *Elixir:* Clear sweetened liquid preparation that contains alcohol. Example: Digoxin elixir.
- *Syrup:* A sugar and water solution that contains flavoring and medicinal substance. Example: Cough syrup (some syrups contain alcohol).

If the active medication does not dissolve and becomes suspended in the liquid, it is called a *suspension*. Over time the suspended drug will settle to the bottom of the container. It is important to shake suspensions before pouring the medication. The following are examples of suspensions:

- *Emulsion:* A suspension of oil and water. Example: Ophthalmic cyclosporine.
- *Gel* and *magma:* Suspensions consisting of minerals and water. Gels are semisolids and contain finer particles than magmas. The minerals settle out with standing. Shake before using. Example: Milk of magnesia.
- *Liniment:* A suspension that is rubbed on the skin; used to reduce pain and stiffness. Example: Ben-Gay.
- *Lotion:* A water-based suspension that is applied to the skin. Example: Calamine lotion.
- *Aerosol:* A suspension of medication in a gas, usually used for respiratory or sinus conditions. Example: Albuterol metered-dose inhaler.

ROUTES OF MEDICATION

For drug administration, the route is how a drug enters the body. As discussed in the prior chapter, the dose of medication can differ based on the route. The following sections discuss common routes of medication. There are many other routes that are not commonly used in the ambulatory care environment.

Oral Route

Medications taken by the oral route (po) are those we take by mouth. Special administration techniques may be required for oral medications. These may include the following:

- Oral medications that coat the mouth or throat should not be immediately followed with water.
- Oral medications that require water for swallowing call for more than a sip. Some medications require a glass of water after taking the medication.
- A straw should be used for liquid medications that stain the teeth.
- Liquid medications should be measured only with a plastic medication cup or an oral medication syringe. Household measuring devices, such as spoons, are not accurate.

It is important to notify the provider if the patient is unable to take the medication due to nausea, vomiting, or problems swallowing. Do not attempt to see if the patient can swallow the pill. It is better to talk with the provider if the patient is concerned. Remember, some medications can be crushed safely, whereas others cannot. Procedure 15.1 on p. 383 describes the steps to follow when administering solid and liquid medications.

CRITICAL THINKING APPLICATION   15.3

Gabe and Mark are working with Charles Johnson, who has a temperature of 103.4° F. The provider orders acetaminophen 500 mg, 2 tabs po for the patient. Mr. Johnson tells Gabe and Mark that he cannot swallow pills. Can they give him liquid acetaminophen, or must they talk with the provider first about the situation?

Sublingual and Buccal Routes

Sublingual (SL) medications are placed under the tongue. *Buccal* medications are placed between the cheek and the gums. Both mucous membrane areas are rich in blood vessels. The medication is absorbed rapidly into the bloodstream. Special administration techniques may be required for SL and buccal medications. These may include the following:

- Do not eat or smoke prior to taking SL and buccal medications.
- Do not chew or swallow SL or buccal medications.
- Water can be taken prior to the medication to wet the mouth. No liquids can be taken until the medication has dissolved.
- Alternate cheeks used for buccal medication to avoid mucosal irritation.

Transdermal Route

Transdermal medications are placed on the skin and absorbed into the bloodstream. Transdermal medications are different from topical medications, which provide a **local** action. Transdermal medications provide a **systemic** action. The transdermal drug delivery system uses patches that adhere to the skin (Fig. 15.5). Medication in the patch is slowly absorbed through the skin. Depending on the medication, the patch may be worn for a part of a day to many days.

When replacing a patch or teaching a patient to use transdermal patches, follow these steps:

- Write the date and time on the new patch.
- Wear disposable gloves if changing a patch on another person.
- Remove the old patch. Fold the sticky sides together and discard. If the old patch is not removed, the person may be at risk for an overdose.
- Remove any residual medication from the skin using a tissue.
- Decide where to apply the new patch. Select a different location. Depending on the medication, it may be on the shoulder, back, upper arm, lower abdomen, or hip. Clean and dry the new site.
- Remove the protective liner on the patch. Do not use torn patches. Do not touch the sticky side of the patch.
- Place the patch's sticky side on the skin. Press down on the patch to ensure it adheres to the skin. Make sure the patch is smooth, without folds.

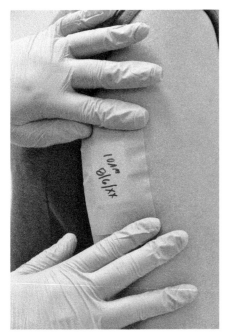

FIGURE 15.5 Transdermal patch.

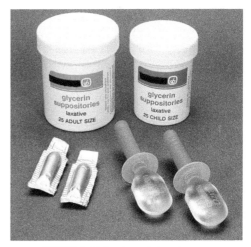

FIGURE 15.6 Rectal suppositories and enemas.

Inhalation Route

Medications for the nose, throat, and lungs can be inhaled. The small particles of medication are aerosolized in a fine mist. The medication is inhaled and reaches the mucous membrane or alveoli in the lungs, where it is absorbed. Metered-dose inhalers (MDIs) and nebulizers are common devices for inhaled drugs. (Chapter 25 discusses MDIs and nebulizers.)

Topical Route

Applying a drug to a mucous membrane or skin is considered use of the *topical route*. Absorption through the mucous membrane is usually faster than through the skin. Topical medications provide a local effect.

Many times, when a drug is ordered to be applied "topically," it means that it should be applied to the skin. Topical drugs may also be administered by other routes. The provider will indicate a more specific route, such as rectal, vaginal, ophthalmic, nasal, or optic, for these medications.

When the medical assistant applies a topical medication to a patient's skin, it is important to do the following:
- Wear gloves.
- Use a sterile applicator (tongue blade or swab) to remove medication from the container. To keep the container sterile, a new sterile applicator must be used each time.
- Rub creams gently into the skin, pat lotions onto the skin, and apply ointment using a sterile applicator.
- Liniments must be rubbed into the skin.
- For aerosol topical sprays, hold the bottle 3 to 6 inches from the skin and spray.

Vaginal Route

The vaginal route is used to insert suppositories, tablets, creams, and foams into the vagina. Typically, vaginal medications are used to treat local infections. Most medications can be inserted using the accompanying applicator. If no applicator is available, the patient should insert medications like suppositories using a finger. Usually, the medication must be inserted about 3 to 4 inches.

Vaginal instillation is most effective if the patient remains lying down after administration to prevent leakage. Many medications are intended to be used at bedtime. The patient may need to wear a pad to absorb drainage.

Rectal Route

Rectal medications are inserted into the rectum. Suppositories and enemas are the most common forms of rectal medications (Fig. 15.6). The medication is absorbed slowly and irregularly through the rectal mucous membrane. This route is useful when a patient cannot tolerate oral medications or if the patient is constipated. It is important for the medical assistant to remind patients to give both the enema and suppository time to work before using the bathroom.

Sometimes a medical assistant needs to teach a patient about inserting suppositories. It is helpful for the patient to know what supplies are needed and where the supplies can be purchased. Supplies required include the suppository, disposable gloves, and water-soluble jelly (K-Y Jelly). Encourage the patient to review the storage directions for the suppositories. The following tips are helpful for inserting a suppository:
- Remove the wrapping from the suppository.
- Lubricate the pointed part of the suppository with water-soluble jelly.
- Be in the Sims position (side-lying, with the knee drawn up toward the chest).
- Carefully insert the suppository pointed side first.
- For adults and older children: Use the gloved index finger to push the medication in. Both vaginal and rectal suppositories should be inserted about 3 to 4 inches. Have the person slowly breathe to help with the discomfort.
- For small children: Use the gloved little finger to insert the medication. Rectal suppositories should be advanced about 2 inches.

Nasal Route

Drugs given via the nasal route are breathed in through the nose. The medication is absorbed through the nasal mucous membrane. The medication can have local or systemic effects. If the medical assistant is administering the nasal medication, it is important to wear gloves. Patients should blow their nose prior to receiving the medication. They should sit in an upright position. The patient should sniff when the medication is given. Intranasal medications should be charted as "intranasal."

Ocular Route

Medication may be *instilled* (poured drop by drop) into the eye to treat an infection, soothe irritation, anesthetize the eye, or dilate the pupils before examination or treatment. Ophthalmic medications are available in different forms. Liquid drops usually are supplied in small squeeze bottles. The tip allows one drop at a time to be administered. Other bottles may have a dropper that is used to administer the medication. Eye ointments come in small metal or plastic tubes. The tip allows a small ribbon of ointment to be administered along the inner lower eyelid margin.

When instilling eye medications, avoid injuring the eye. Do not touch the eye with the tip or applicator. Always keep the tip or applicator sterile. If it gets contaminated, discard the container. See Chapter 16 for more information on eye medication instillation.

Otic Route

Ear conditions can cause pain and make hearing difficult. Medication may be instilled into the ear to treat infection or inflammation, or to soften cerumen. See Chapter 16 for more information on ear medication instillation.

Irrigation Route

As recommended by the FDA, irrigation is also a route of administration. *Irrigation* means to bathe or flush open wounds or body cavities. Irrigation can be used to remove foreign bodies or debris. It can also be used to bathe the area with medication. Wound, eye, and ear irrigations are commonly seen in ambulatory care settings. (Chapter 16 discusses eye and ear irrigations.)

Eye irrigation is done to remove foreign bodies or to flush irritants (e.g., chemicals) from the eye. Irrigation of the external auditory canal will do the following:

- Remove excessive or impacted cerumen
- Remove a foreign body (contraindicated if the item will absorb fluid [e.g., bean, pea, or corn kernel])
- Treat the inflamed ear with an antiseptic solution

Parenteral Route

The *parenteral route* involves administration by infusion, injection, or implantation. In the ambulatory care environment, injections and infusions are common. Vaccine administration in primary care settings (e.g., family practice and internal medicine) is a frequent duty of medical assistants. Types of injections performed by medical assistants include the following:

- *Intramuscular* (IM): Administration within a muscle
- *Subcutaneous* (subcut): Administration beneath the skin
- *Intradermal* (ID): Administration within the dermis

The rest of the chapter will focus on the parenteral route. The following topics are discussed: injection supplies, medication preparation, site location, and medication administration. The chapter concludes with a discussion on intravenous (IV) infusions and the role of the medical assistant. An intravenous infusion means fluid and medications are administered into a vein.

NEEDLES AND SYRINGES

Hypodermic Needles

A hypodermic needle attaches to a hypodermic syringe. Hypodermic needles come with syringes or are packaged separately. The entire needle needs to remain sterile for the injection. It is important for the medical assistant to know the parts of the needle (Fig. 15.7). The parts of a hypodermic needle include the following:

- *Hub*: Attaches or screws onto the syringe
- *Hilt*: Where the needle attaches
- *Bevel*: Slanted end of the shaft
- *Lumen*: Hollow space inside the needle; the size is indicated by the *gauge* number

Gauge and Length

Each needle has two measurements: the gauge (G) and the length. The lumen size is indicated by the gauge and is given a numeric value. The higher the gauge number, the smaller the lumen. The thickness of the needle wall increases along with the lumen size. This means that an 18 G needle makes a larger hole than a 25 G needle. The 18 G needle has a thicker wall than the 25 G needle. As the gauge

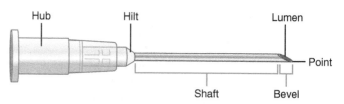

FIGURE 15.7 Parts of a hypodermic needle.

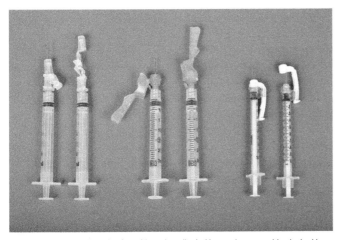

FIGURE 15.8 Protective sheaths and hinged needle shields must be activated by the healthcare professional. Each type of needle is shown before the injection and after the safety device has been activated.

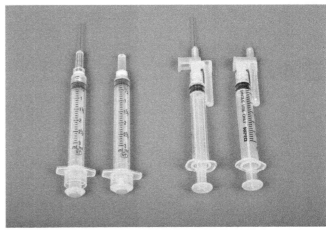

FIGURE 15.9 With retractable needles, the needle is retracted into the syringe or another chamber. Each type of needle is shown before the injection and after the needle has been retracted.

number increases, the needles bend more easily. Thicker-walled needles (smaller gauge numbers) are used for deeper injections. Thinner-walled needles (larger gauge numbers) are used for more superficial injections.

The medication's **viscosity** is also an important factor when selecting the gauge of the needle. A medication with a syrupy thickness (high viscosity) would be harder to push out of a needle compared with a medication as thin as water. Using a wider lumen needle (smaller gauge number) would be better for thicker medications. Using a finer lumen needle (a larger gauge number) would be more appropriate for watery medications.

The needle length refers to the length of the shaft. The needle length used is dependent on the type of injection given and the size of the patient. The length of the needle for an intradermal injection is smaller than that used for an intramuscular injection. The length of an intramuscular injection needle for a 300-pound person would be longer than that for a 100-pound person. Knowing the length and gauge required for an injection are important information for the medical assistant.

Safety Needles

Due to the Needlestick Safety and Prevention Act, safety needles are common in the ambulatory care setting. Safety needles are designed to reduce the risk of needlesticks after an injection. A *passive safety needle* is designed so that the needle is automatically covered after the injection. Passive safety needles are currently used with insulin pens (e.g., the BD AutoShield Duo pen needle). It is forecasted that in the next few years, more passive safety needles will be available. An *active safety needle* requires the healthcare professional to activate the safety device. These are most common for injections. Current active safety needles fall into two groups:

- *Protective sheaths* and *hinged needle shields*: The safety device is a sleeve over the syringe barrel or a hinged needle shield (Fig. 15.8). These devices are moved over the needle after the injection. Once in place, the needle cannot be uncovered. The risk of needlesticks decreases if the safety device is activated with the hand holding the syringe.

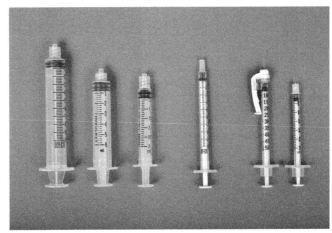

FIGURE 15.10 Syringes come in various sizes. Some come with the needles attached.

- *Retractable needles*: After the injection, the healthcare professional activates a device that retracts the needle either into the syringe or into another chamber (Fig. 15.9).

Hypodermic Syringes

Hypodermic syringes attach to needles and hold the medication for the injection. They come in many sizes (e.g., 1, 3, 5, 6, 10, and 12 mL), but usually the facility only stocks three or four sizes (Fig. 15.10). Fig. 15.11 shows the parts of the syringe. Syringes can have either a Luer-Lok tip or a slip tip (Fig. 15.12). Calibration marks are on the barrel of the syringe. It is important for the medical assistant to be able to read medication amounts in syringes.

Working With the Needle and Syringe

Syringes come packaged in different ways:

- A syringe can be packaged by itself. A needle must be added to the syringe when giving an injection.
- A syringe may be packaged with a needle. The unit must be assembled.

- A syringe and needle unit may come preassembled. Always tighten the needle on the syringe before using the unit.

The needle and syringe can be assembled with clean, ungloved hands.

When a syringe is packaged by itself, first open the syringe. When removing the syringe from the packaging, it is important not to touch the syringe tip to anything (Fig. 15.13A). The tip needs to

remain sterile because it attaches to the needle. The syringe should be held until the needle is attached. As you are holding the syringe, use your fingers to open the needle package (Fig. 15.13B). It is important to hold down the packaging flaps to prevent contaminating the needle. Attach the syringe to the needle, and lift the needle out of the package (Fig. 15.13C). The needle and syringe unit can be placed on the counter. The needle cover should remain on to protect the sterility of the needle.

When the needle and syringe are packaged together, yet not assembled, carefully open the packaging. Hold down the packaging flaps. Angle the contents so the syringe can be grasped without going over or touching the needle (Fig. 15.14A). Remove the syringe, then attach it to the needle (Fig. 15.14B). Remove the needle from the packaging. Once the syringe and needle are assembled, the unit can be placed on the counter.

When working with the plunger, only touch the section that remains outside of the syringe when the plunger is completely pushed

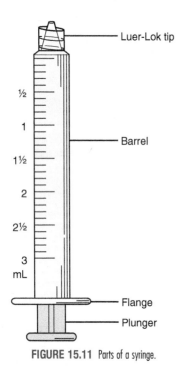

FIGURE 15.11 Parts of a syringe.

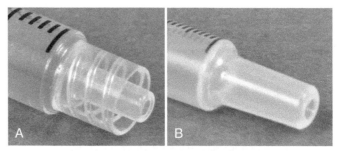

FIGURE 15.12 **(A)** Luer-Lok. **(B)** Slip tip.

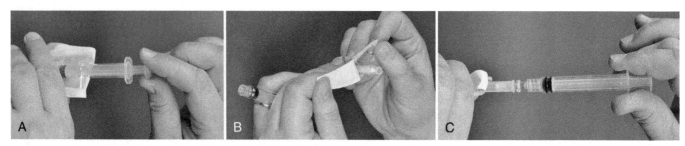

FIGURE 15.13 **(A)** When removing the syringe from the packaging, just touch the flange or barrel. **(B)** Place the syringe between your fingers with the tip face away from your fingers. Then open the needle package. **(C)** Hold down the packaging flaps to prevent contamination of the needle. Attach the syringe.

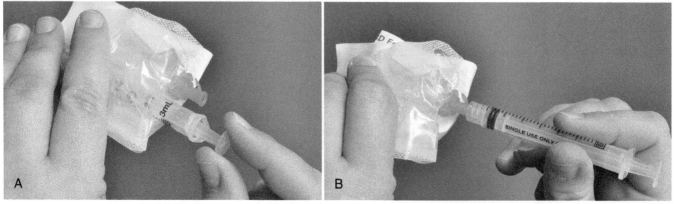

FIGURE 15.14 **(A)** Remove the syringe without touching the needle. **(B)** Continue to hold down the packaging flaps, and attach the needle to the syringe.

in (Fig. 15.15). Touching the plunger that goes inside the barrel could potentially contaminate the medication.

Uncapping and Recapping Needles

Never recap a needle that has been used on a patient. Needles can be recapped until they are used on a patient. As you prepare medication, you will need to uncap and recap the needle. It is important to maintain the sterility of the needle. If there is any doubt, consider the needle contaminated and replace it with a new one.

- *To uncap:* Hold the cover between the fingers and thumb of your nondominant hand. Hold the syringe with the fingers and thumb of your dominant hand. Pull your hands apart horizontally (side to side) in a smooth continuous motion (Fig. 15.16A).
- *To recap:* Use the one-handed scoop technique. Place the cover on a firm, flat surface. If the cover rolls, place a finger of your nondominant hand at the far end of the cover. This will keep the cover in place. Carefully insert the needle into the cover. If the needle touches the outside surface of the cover or any

other surface, it is contaminated and must be replaced. Scoop up the cover and secure the cover onto the needle (Fig. 15.16B).

Switching Needles

When switching needles, it is important not to give yourself a needlestick and to protect the sterility of the new needle. Several methods are used to switch needles. One method includes opening the new needle package. Hold the packaging flaps down with the index finger and thumb of your nondominant hand. With your dominant hand, place the syringe with the covered needle between the middle and ring fingers of your nondominant hand (Fig. 15.17A). Firmly grasp the covered needle in your palm. The syringe should be above the top of your hand. With your dominant hand, remove the syringe from the old needle and attach it to the new needle (Fig. 15.17B–C). Your nondominant hand should be holding both needles the entire time. Discard the old needle into the biohazard sharps container.

PREPARING PARENTERAL MEDICATION

As with all medication preparation, it is important to be in a well-lit room and to be free from distraction. The medical assistant must be focused on the procedure to reduce the risk of errors. For all parenteral medications:

- If the medication looks abnormal in color or clarity, discard it.
- Some medications will have **precipitate** at the bottom of the vial. If this is normal for that medication, make sure to mix

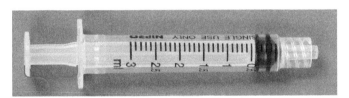
FIGURE 15.15 Touch only the part of the plunger that is outside of the barrel.

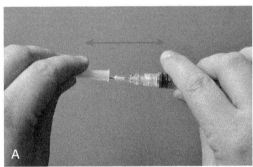
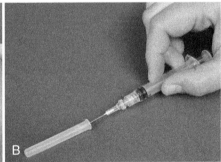
FIGURE 15.16 **(A)** Uncapping a needle. **(B)** One-handed scoop technique.

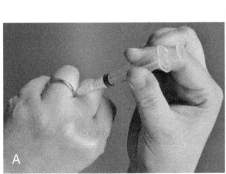
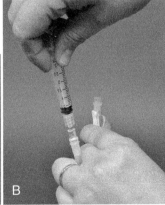
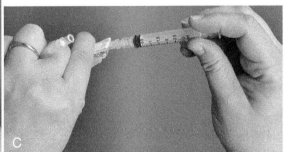
FIGURE 15.17 **(A)** Place the syringe unit between the fingers of your nondominant hand, and firmly grasp the covered needle. **(B)** Hold the old covered needle securely as you detach it from the syringe. **(C)** Attach the new needle while holding the old needle between your fingers.

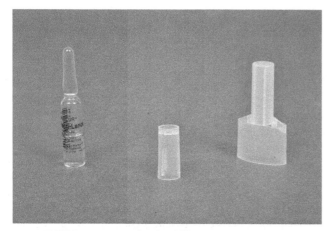

FIGURE 15.18 An ampule with two different ampule openers/breakers.

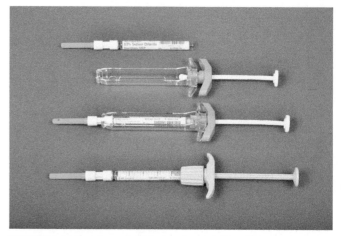

FIGURE 15.19 Top to bottom: Prefilled syringe, Carpuject holder, prefilled syringe in a Carpuject holder, and a prefilled syringe in a Tubex cartridge holder.

it prior to withdrawing medication. If the precipitate is abnormal, a chemical reaction may have occurred. The vial needs to be discarded.
- If the medication has expired, discard it.
- If the medication is no longer sterile, discard it.

Using an Ampule

Ampules contain a single dose of medication. They may contain more than the patient needs. The extra medication is wasted. Medications in ampules react to other substances and require the all-glass environment to remain stable. An ampule has a prescored neck, which is snapped off during the preparation process. An ampule opener or breaker is a safety device used to snap off the top of the ampule (Fig. 15.18). A filter needle on a syringe is used to **aspirate** the medication into the syringe. This needle has a small filter that catches glass particles before they enter the syringe barrel. The filter needle must be removed before the injection is given to the patient. Procedure 15.2 on p. 385 describes the steps required to prepare medication using an ampule.

Using a Prefilled Sterile Cartridge

A prefilled, sterile cartridge comes filled with a single dose of medication. It is not uncommon for the medication in the syringe to be more than what the provider ordered. The cartridge may come with or without a needle. A safety needle can be attached to the Luer-Lok on the prefilled cartridge. A reusable cartridge holder (e.g., Carpuject or Tubex) is needed to dispense the medication (Fig. 15.19). The medical assistant must assemble the cartridge and the reusable cartridge holder prior to administering the medication. Procedure 15.3 on p. 387 describes how to use a Carpuject holder and prepare the medication.

Specialty Syringe Units

Specialty syringe units are designed so that patients can administer their own medication. Different types of syringe units are available. Fig. 15.20 shows an insulin pen. The dose of insulin required can be set by the dial. The patient needs to change the needle with each dose. Insulin pens cannot be shared between patients.

The EpiPen and other epinephrine pens are automatic injector systems (Fig. 15.21). The pens are dosed for adults or children. People

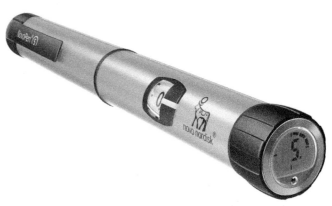

FIGURE 15.20 NovoPens use insulin cartridges. Patients change the cartridges and retain the pen.

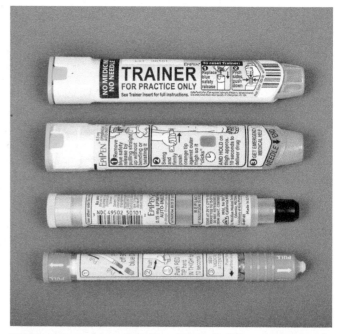

FIGURE 15.21 Top to bottom: EpiPen trainer, EpiPen for older children and adults, EpiPen Jr for children, and a generic epinephrine pen.

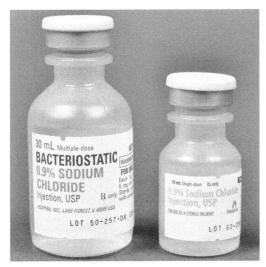

FIGURE 15.22 Multidose and single-dose vials.

Reconstituting Powdered Medication

As previously mentioned, vials can contain powdered medication. A powdered medication needs to be mixed with a **diluent**. Typically, sterile normal saline or sterile water is used as a diluent, although other medications may also be used (according to the provider's order and the manufacturer's directions). The most common powdered medications in primary care are live virus vaccines. These need to be **reconstituted** (see Procedure 15.5, p. 391).

If the vial is a multidose vial, it is important to write the expiration date on the label. The expiration dates for reconstituted medications will vary. See the manufacturer's insert for the length of time that the medication will remain stable after reconstitution. Besides the expiration date, include your initials and the fluid that was used to reconstitute the medication. These three pieces of information need to be on the multidose label.

There are four major steps in reconstituting powdered medication and withdrawing a dose of the medication (Fig. 15.23):

    Step 1: Remove air from the powdered medication vial and put air into the diluent vial.
    Step 2: Withdraw liquid from the diluent vial and add it to the powdered medication vial.
    Step 3: Mix the liquid with the powdered medication.
    Step 4: Add in air and withdraw the dose needed.

CRITICAL THINKING APPLICATION   **15.6**

Mark struggles to remember the steps to reconstitute powdered medication. What are the steps?

Mixing Insulins

Patients with diabetes may use insulin to help manage their disease. Taking insulin requires about four injections a day. Some patients may need two different insulins at the same time. Many premixed insulins are available for patients. However, for some individuals the premixed insulins are not an option, and they must mix the two insulins in one syringe. During this combination process, it is important that the vials do not become contaminated with another type of insulin. If by chance contamination occurs, it is better for the rapid-acting or short-acting insulin (Regular insulin) to be mixed in the intermediate-acting insulin vial (e.g., NPH insulin). This means that Regular insulin must be drawn up in the syringe first and then NPH is added (Fig. 15.24). Procedure 15.6 on p. 392 describes the steps for mixing two insulins in one syringe.

Depending on state laws and facility policies, administering insulin may be within the medical assistant's scope of practice. Understanding how to mix two insulins in the same syringe is important. Not all insulins can be mixed. Use drug reference information to ensure that the two insulins ordered can be mixed.

As discussed earlier in the chapter, insulin is measured in units. Special insulin syringes are available to measure small or large insulin dosages. Insulin is typically stored in the refrigerator and should be warmed to room temperature prior to administration. Cloudy insulins (e.g., NPH) are suspensions and need to be mixed before drawing up the insulin. Mix cloudy insulins by gently rolling the vial between

---

at risk for anaphylactic reactions (e.g., from food allergens, bee stings) should carry epinephrine pens to prevent a fatal reaction. Simulators can accompany some of the injector systems. These are useful when teaching patients how to give their own injections.

Using a Vial

A vial is a plastic or glass container with a rubber stopper that is covered by a cap. Vials contain powdered or liquid medications. Liquid medication is more common. The liquid can be a parenteral medication, sterile *normal saline* (0.9% sodium chloride), or sterile water. Vials come in single dose or multidose (Fig. 15.22). Single-dose or single-use vials are only good for a single patient and a single injection procedure. If the vial needs to be entered more than once for a single patient as part of a single procedure, then a new needle and syringe must be used. Discard the vial after the procedure. Single-dose vials do not contain any ingredients that would prohibit microorganism growth. Thus, they are only good for a single use.

Multidose vials contain many doses of medication. The label will clearly state that the vial is a multidose vial. These vials contain an antimicrobial preservative that prevents the growth of bacteria. The preservative does not help protect the fluid against viruses and other sources of contamination if safe injection practices are not followed. When multidose vials are opened (the cap is removed or the stopper is punctured), they are only good for 28 days (unless the manufacturer states otherwise). The new expiration date should be written on the label. If the manufacturer's expiration date comes sooner than the 28 days, then the earlier date must be used.

Each time the multidose vial is entered, the rubber stopper must be disinfected, and a sterile needle and syringe must be used. The vial is under pressure. You need to add air into the vial before you draw out the amount of liquid you need. The amount of air added should equal the amount of liquid you draw out. Always make sure you have the correct amount of medication in your syringe before you withdraw the needle. Never inject unneeded medication back into the vial once the needle has been removed. Procedure 15.4 on p. 389 describes how to prepare medication from a vial.

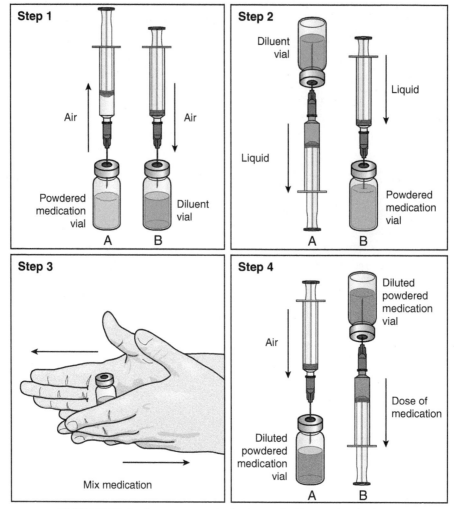

FIGURE 15.23 Steps for reconstituting powdered medication and withdrawing a dose of medication.

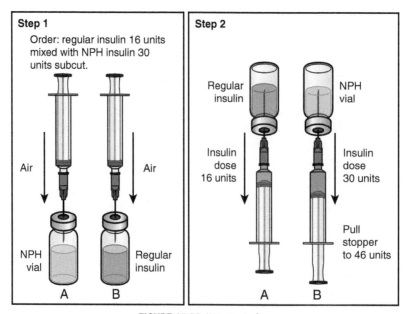

FIGURE 15.24 Mixing two insulins.

your hands. Clear insulin (e.g., Regular insulin) does not need to be mixed or rolled in your hand.

Patients receiving insulin must rotate their injection sites. This prevents tissue damage and absorption issues with the insulin. It might be helpful for patients to mark the site of the last injection with a spot bandage or a piece of tape. The easiest way to rotate sites is to give subsequent injections in a circular pattern around the first injection site in a specific location. The goal is to avoid using the same location again for another month.

CRITICAL THINKING APPLICATION   **15.7**
Mark struggles to remember the order for drawing up insulin. What might be a few good ways to remember the process of drawing up two insulins in the same syringe?

GIVING PARENTERAL MEDICATIONS

Some medications can be given by several routes. Other medications can only be given by injection. Parenteral medication administration has several advantages:

- It is useful when the patient has gastrointestinal distress or is unconscious.
- It offers good absorption compared with other routes, such as the oral route.
- The *onset* (time medication starts working) is more rapid than with other routes.
- Some types of parenteral medications have a longer *duration time* (time it works in the body).

Disadvantages of parenteral medication administration include the following:

- Pain with the injection
- Risk for infection due to the injection
- An unpredictable absorption rate for those with poor circulation (e.g., patients with peripheral artery disease, diabetes, obesity, or Raynaud disease)

When it comes to giving injections, over time you will gain confidence and it will become easy. Always do the following:

- Follow the nine rights of medication administration.
- Check the medication's label against the order three times.
- Know about the medication you are giving. (What is it, why is it being ordered, how is it given, and what are the common side effects?)
- Label all syringes with the name of the medication they contain.
- Follow medical asepsis and the Bloodborne Pathogens Standard established by the Occupational Safety and Health Administration (OSHA).
- Ensure that the needle is not directed at your hand holding the patient when giving an injection. Slight movement may cause a needlestick.

Following these guidelines will help you to perform injections safely and protect your patient from medication errors.

Guidelines for Parenteral Medications

Prepare and store medications in a separate area, away from the exam rooms. Medications can be prepared without the use of gloves. Ensure that all needles are tightly covered and placed on a tray when carrying them to the exam room. Never transport medication in your pockets. Bring only one patient's medication at a time to avoid confusion and error.

Follow these guidelines when selecting an injection site:

- Never give an injection near bones or blood vessels.
- Avoid scar tissue, a change in skin pigmentation or texture, or abnormal growth (e.g., mole or wart).
- Avoid abrasions, lesions, wounds, bruises, and edematous areas.
- Select a site that is large enough to hold the amount of medication injected.
- Avoid sites recently used (within the last month).

According to the Immunization Action Coalition (www.immunize.org), it is safe to give subcut and IM vaccines into a tattoo. However, it is not a good idea to inject into a newly tattooed area. If you must inject into a tattooed area, attempt to use a lighter pigmented area. All injections pose the risk of a reaction or an infection at the injection site. Dark pigments may mask a reaction or an infection.

Reducing Pain and Anxiety

To minimize pain with injections, insert subcut and IM needles swiftly. Inject the medication at the rate of 10 seconds per 1 mL to avoid unnecessary discomfort. Remove the needle quickly, using the same angle as used for entry.

Various techniques can be used to reduce a patient's pain and anxiety about injections:

- Giving a sugar-coated pacifier or sugar water (must be ordered by the provider), which helps to soothe children under age 1 year after injections.
- Applying a topical anesthetic skin refrigerant (e.g., Pain Ease), which works immediately (Fig. 15.25 and Fig. 15.26).
- Applying a topical anesthetic (e.g., EMLA cream) at the injection site, which works in about 30 to 40 minutes.
- Talking with the patient to distract him or her from the procedure.
- Having the patient move his or her toes or fingers on the extremity used when an IM injection is given. (Have a patient "play the piano" with his or her fingers when giving a deltoid injection.)

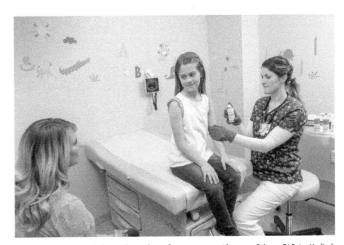

FIGURE 15.25 Topical anesthetic skin refrigerant spray. (Courtesy Gebauer-Tri-Point-Medical, Cleveland, Ohio.)

GEBAUER'S PAIN EASE®
MEDIUM STREAM SPRAY AND MIST SPRAY

CAUTION: Federal law restricts this device to sale by or on the order of a licensed healthcare practitioner.

Hold the can upright while spraying.

INDICATIONS FOR USE: Gebauer's Pain Ease Medium Stream Spray and Mist Spray are vapocoolants (skin refrigerants) intended for topical application to skin, intact mucous membranes (oral cavity, nasal passage ways and the lips) and minor open wounds. Pain Ease instantly controls pain associated with injections (venipuncture, IV starts, cosmetic procedures), minor surgical procedures (such as lancing boils, incisions, drainage of small abscesses and sutures) and the temporary relief of minor sports injuries (sprains, bruising, cuts and abrasions).

PRECAUTIONS:
1. Do not spray in the eyes.
2. Do not use this product on persons with poor circulation or insensitive skin.
3. When used to produce local freezing of tissues, adjacent skin areas should be protected by an application of petroleum.
4. The freezing and thawing process may be painful, and freezing may lower local resistance to infection and delay healing.
5. Over application of the product might cause frostbite and/or alter skin pigmentation.
6. Do not use on large areas of damaged skin, puncture wounds, animal bites or serious wounds.
7. Apply only to intact mucous membranes.
8. Do not use on genital mucous membranes.

ADVERSE REACTIONS: Freezing can occasionally alter skin pigmentation.

CONTRAINDICATIONS: Pain Ease is contraindicated in individuals with a history of hypersensitivity to 1,1,1,3,3-Pentafluoropropane and 1,1,1,2-Tetrafluoroethane. If skin irritation develops, discontinue use.

WARNINGS:
For external use only. Contents under pressure.
For use on minor open wounds only.
For use on intact mucous membranes only.
KEEP OUT OF THE REACH OF CHILDREN

INSTRUCTIONS: Press the actuator button firmly, allowing Pain Ease to spray from the can.

PRE-INJECTION & MINOR SURGICAL TOPICAL ANESTHESIA: Have all necessary equipment ready and prepare the procedure site per facility's protocol. Hold the can upright, 3 to 7 inches (8 to 18cm) from the procedure site, about a can's length away. Spray steadily 4 to 10 seconds or until the skin begins turning white, whichever comes first. Do not spray longer than 10 seconds. After spraying the site, immediately perform the procedure. The anesthetic effect of Pain Ease lasts about one minute. Reapply if necessary.
*Apply petrolatum to protect the adjacent area for minor surgical procedures.

TEMPORARY RELIEF OF MINOR SPORTS INJURIES:
The pain of bruises, contusions, swelling, minor sprains, cuts and abrasions may be controlled with Pain Ease. The amount of cooling depends on the dosage. Dosage varies with duration of application. The smallest dose needed to produce the desired effect should be used. The anesthetic effect of Pain Ease lasts about one minute. This time interval is usually sufficient to help reduce or relieve the initial trauma of the injury. Hold the can upright, 3 to 7 inches (8 to 18 cm) from the target area, about a can's length away. Spray steadily 4 to 10 seconds or until the skin begins turning white, whichever comes first. Do not spray longer than 10 seconds. Reapply if necessary.

CONTENTS: 1,1,1,3,3-Pentafluoropropane and 1,1,1,2-Tetrafluoroethane

STORAGE: Do not puncture or incinerate container. Do not expose to heat or store at temperatures above 50°C (120°F).

DISPOSAL: Dispose of in accordance with local and national regulations.

HOW SUPPLIED: Aerosol Can

Gebauer's Pain Ease® Medium Stream Spray
3.5 fl. oz. (103.5mL) - P/N 0386-0008-03
1.0 fl. oz. (30mL) - P/N 0386-0008-04

Gebauer's Pain Ease® Mist Spray
3.5 fl. oz. (103.5mL) - P/N 0386-0008-02
1.0 fl. oz. (30mL) - P/N 0386-0008-01

For more information about this product contact Gebauer Company.

Manufactured by:
Gebauer Company
Cleveland, OH 44128
1-800-321-9348
www.Gebauer.com
Products Made in the U.S.A
©2015 Gebauer Company, Rev 06/15

FIGURE 15.26 Package insert for Pain Ease, a vapocoolant (skin refrigerant). (Courtesy Gebauer-Tri-Point-Medical, Cleveland, Ohio.)

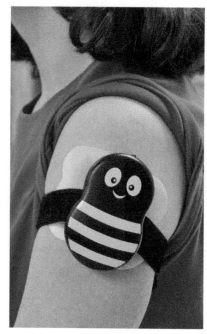

FIGURE 15.27 Buzzy helps reduce pain naturally by overwhelming the nerves with vibration and cold sensations.

- Using products that provide cold and vibration sensations (e.g., Buzzy), which overwhelm the nerves affected by the injection (Fig. 15.27).
- Administering the most painful injection last.

CRITICAL THINKING APPLICATION   15.8

Gabe talks with Mark about distractions to use when giving IM injections. He mentions having patients wiggle their toes or move their fingers when giving an injection on that extremity. He explains that he tells the patient about the movement prior to starting the injection. Gabe reminds the patient when he is aspirating, just prior to injecting the medication. What might be the benefit of reminding the patient when aspirating?

Special Situations

Even if the procedure was done correctly, sometimes things can go wrong. It is important for the medical assistant to know what to do in those situations.

If a needle breaks during an injection or if the needle separates from the syringe, pull out the needle, if it is visible. Discard the needle in the biohazard sharps container. If the needle breaks off and it is not visible, mark the spot with a pen and yell for help. If the injection was given in the arm, place a tourniquet above the spot to prevent the needle from moving in the body. Notify the provider immediately.

With intramuscular injections, sometimes the bone can be hit during the procedure. If this occurs, pull the needle out about ¼ inch, and give the medication.

With any medication, a patient can experience an anaphylactic reaction. *Anaphylaxis* is a severe allergic reaction that can be life-threatening. Having the patient wait 15 minutes after an injection allows you to monitor for unusual symptoms. If the patient is experiencing any unusual symptoms, it is important to tell the provider immediately. The first-line medication for anaphylaxis is epinephrine.

Signs and Symptoms of Anaphylaxis

- Anxiety, warm feeling, and flushing
- Shortness of breath, dyspnea (difficulty breathing), and wheezing
- Cough, throat tightening, and difficulty swallowing
- Pain, cramping, vomiting, and diarrhea
- Palpitations, dizziness, loss of consciousness, and shock

INTRADERMAL INJECTIONS

Intradermal (ID) injections are given just under the epidermis (Fig. 15.28). Because the drug is dispersed in an area where many nerves are present, it causes momentary burning or stinging. Small amounts of medication are injected.

Fig. 15.29 show sites recommended for intradermal injections. In ambulatory care, the following intradermal injections may be given:

- Mantoux tuberculin skin test (TST)
- Intradermal flu vaccine (e.g., Fluzone Intradermal)
- Allergy testing (discussed in Chapter 18)

Table 15.1 contains a summary of intradermal injection information.

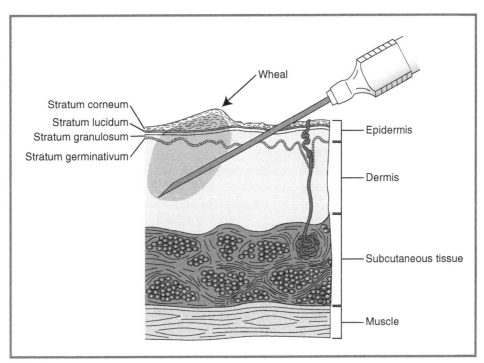

FIGURE 15.28 The intradermal (ID) injection is administered just under the epidermis.

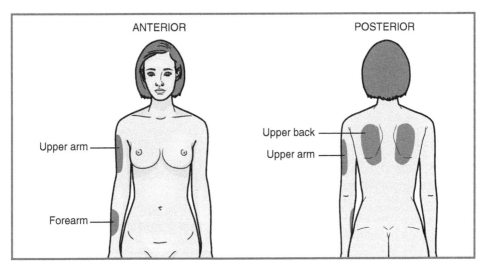

FIGURE 15.29 Sites recommended for intradermal injections.

Intradermal Flu Vaccine

Currently, the intradermal flu vaccine is the only intradermal vaccine. Fluzone Intradermal contains less antigen than the IM flu vaccines and is approved for use for adults age 18 to 64 years of age. Fluzone Intradermal uses a nontraditional ID site. The vaccine is given in the IM deltoid area, though it goes in the epidermis and not in the muscle like IM injections.

The vaccine comes in a prefilled microinjection syringe containing 0.1 mL of medication. The syringe contains a 30-G microneedle.

After preparing the site, hold the syringe between the thumb and middle finger of your dominant hand. With a quick, short motion, insert the needle at a 90-degree angle. Do not aspirate. Push the plunger and then remove the syringe. If the syringe comes with a needle shield, push firmly on the plunger to activate it.

Tuberculin Testing

Two types of tuberculin tests have been approved by the FDA: the skin test and the blood test. The Mantoux tuberculin skin test (TST) is used to determine whether a patient is infected with *Mycobacterium tuberculosis*. It is important for the medical assistant to be knowledgeable about and skilled at administering and reading the test.

The TST can be given to most patients, including infants, pregnant women, patients infected with the human immunodeficiency virus (HIV), and those vaccinated with bacillus Calmette-Guérin (BCG). Patients with a history of BCG vaccination may have a positive reaction to the TST. If a patient mentions a history of receiving BCG vaccine, it is important for the medical assistant to inform the provider before performing the skin test. The provider may opt to have the patient undergo the blood test instead.

The TST is contraindicated in patients who had the following:

- A severe reaction to a past TST (e.g., necrosis, ulcers, blisters, or anaphylaxis)
- A history of a positive TST result
- A live virus vaccine less than 4 to 6 weeks earlier (A TST and a live virus vaccine can be given on the same day, or the TST can be given 4 to 6 weeks after the vaccine.)

Tuberculin Skin Test Procedure and Reading

To perform the TST, tuberculin purified protein derivative (PPD) 0.1 mL is given ID into the inner surface of the forearm (see Procedure 15.7, p. 393). A tuberculin syringe and needle, with the bevel facing upward, is used to slowly inject the PPD, creating a wheal. A *wheal* is a tense, pale elevation of the skin. The wheal must measure 6 to 10 mm in diameter, or the test must be repeated.

The patient returns within 48 to 72 hours to have the test read. Reading before or after this time invalidates the results. When reading the test, palpate the site to check for a raised, hardened area, called an *induration*. If an induration is felt, measure the raised area across the forearm (perpendicular to the bone). The *erythema* (redness) is not measured. The diameter of the induration is read in millimeters (mm) and must be noted in the health record. The medical assistant can never state that the test result is positive or negative. The provider uses the test results and the patient history to determine if the patient has tuberculosis (TB). A TST reading between 5 and 15 mm can be positive for different populations. Table 15.2 describes the different populations.

TABLE 15.1	Summary of Intradermal Injections
Syringe used	1 mL (tuberculin syringe)
Needle size	¼ to ⅝ inch; 25–27 gauge
Angle of entry	5 to 15 degrees with bevel facing upward
Maximum volume	0.1 mL
Common sites	Forearm, upper arm, and back
Additional sites	Separate by at least 2 inches
Patient position	Sitting with arm extended
Administration	Pull skin taut at injection site

TABLE 15.2   Tuberculin Skin Reaction Categories

INDURATION ≥5 MM CONSIDERED POSITIVE IN PATIENTS WITH	INDURATION ≥10 MM CONSIDERED POSITIVE IN PATIENTS WITH	INDURATION ≥15 MM CONSIDERED POSITIVE IN PATIENTS WITH
• Human immunodeficiency virus (HIV) infection • Organ transplant • Immunosuppression • Recent contact with a person with tuberculosis (TB) • Fibrotic changes on a chest x-ray consistent with prior TB	• Recent immigrants (<5 years) from high-risk areas • Injection drug users • People living or working in high-risk areas (e.g., living in a group setting [jail, nursing home], employees in a clinical position with a high risk of TB exposure) • Children <4 years of age or children exposed to high-risk adults	• No known risk for TB

From Centers for Disease Control and Prevention (CDC): https://www.cdc.gov/tb/publications/factsheets/testing/skintesting.htm. Accessed October 5, 2018.

Incorrect Tuberculin Skin Test Readings

At times the TST reading may be incorrect. A false-positive reaction means the person reacted to the test even though no *M. tuberculosis* is present. Reasons for false-positive reactions with TST include the following:

- Lung infection with nontuberculous mycobacteria (NTM). This organism is found in the water and soil and is inhaled.
- Previous vaccination with bacillus Calmette-Guérin (BCG) vaccine. Many foreign-born patients from countries with a high risk of TB may have received BCG abroad. The BCG vaccine has been approved by the FDA, but it is used in very limited situations.
- Incorrect administration or reading of the TST.

A false-negative reaction means the person may not have reacted to the test. even though the patient is infected with *M. tuberculosis*. Reasons for false-negative results with TST include the following:

- Weakened immune system
- Exposure to TB infection within previous 8 to 10 weeks
- A very old TB infection
- Patient is younger than 6 months old
- Recently received a live virus vaccine (e.g., measles, yellow fever, chickenpox), or had a viral infection (e.g., influenza), or received corticosteroids or immunosuppressive medications (a false reaction may occur up to 5 to 6 weeks afterward)
- Incorrect administration or reading of TST

Two-Step Testing

In some patients who have had a TB infection, the body "forgets" to react to the TST. This can occur if the infection was many years before. The initial TST may be negative, and the person may have a false-negative reaction. Receiving a second TST can help the body "remember" the infection, thus causing a more accurate (positive) reading. This is called the *booster effect* or *booster phenomenon*. The second TST can be done 1 to 3 weeks after the initial test was read.

New residents in long-term care facilities (e.g., nursing homes) usually have a two-step TST done. Healthcare students and professionals also need to have a two-step TST. Once the two-step TST has been completed, they need yearly TSTs. If the time since the last TST exceeds 1 year, they may need to complete another two-step TST. Fig. 15.30 shows what occurs if the initial test result is positive or negative.

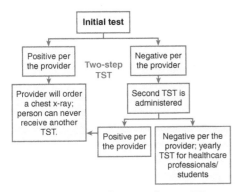

FIGURE 15.30 The process with two-step TST.

Tuberculin Blood Tests

The FDA has approved two tuberculin blood tests: the QuantiFERON-TB Gold In-Tube test (QFT-GIT) and the T-SPOT TB test (T-Spot). If a patient has had the BCG vaccine or is unable to return for the skin test reading, the blood test is preferred. The blood test replaces the skin test. A healthcare professional or student only needs one blood test initially, unlike the two-step skin test. After the initial test, a yearly skin or tuberculin blood tests is required.

After the medical assistant draws a patient's blood, it is sent to the laboratory for analysis. The error rate with a blood test is much lower than with the palpated, measured reading of the TST. The next step will depend on whether the TB blood test result is positive or negative:

- *Positive*: The person has been infected with TB. The provider will order additional tests to determine if the person has a latent TB infection or TB disease. (See Chapter 25 for more information on these two diseases.)
- *Negative*: It is unlikely the person has TB.

SUBCUTANEOUS INJECTIONS

Subcutaneous (subcut) injections involve placing medication into the subcutaneous layer, under the dermis (Fig. 15.31). The subcutaneous layer has fewer blood vessels than the muscles do. The medication absorbs slower in the subcutaneous layer compared with medications injected into the muscles. The patient may complain of discomfort or pain with a subcutaneous injection. Subcutaneous tissue contains pain receptors.

Common medications given via the subcutaneous route include several vaccines (e.g., measles-mumps-rubella [MMR], varicella, shingles [ZOSTAVAX], and polio), enoxaparin (Lovenox), heparin, and insulin.

Abbreviations for Subcutaneous Injections

There have been many abbreviations for subcutaneous injections over the years. Some may still be used in practice, although they are not recommended. The Institute for Safe Medication Practices (ISMP) discourages the use of SC, SQ, and subQ. Healthcare professionals should use *subcut* or *subcutaneously*. For more information, refer to the ISMP website at http://www.ismp.org/tools/errorproneabbreviations.pdf.

Administration Techniques

When a subcut injection is given, the angle depends on the needle length. If a ⅜-inch needle is used, then the medical assistant should

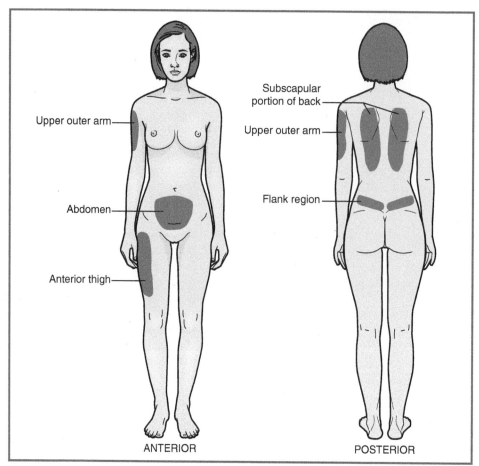

FIGURE 15.31 The subcutaneous (subcut) injection sites commonly used include the outer posterior aspect of the upper arm, the lower abdomen, and the anterior aspect of the thigh. The subscapular portion of the back and the flank region are other subcut sites.

use a 45-degree angle (Fig. 15.32). If a ½-inch needle is used, then a 90-degree angle should be applied. It is important to pinch up the tissue with the index finger and thumb of the nondominant hand. This ensures that the injection is given into the subcutaneous tissue. Table 15.3 contains a summary of subcutaneous injection information.

Aspiration

Aspiration is used to check if the needle is in a blood vessel. This is done once before the medication is given. (The aspiration technique will be discussed in detail in the Intramuscular Injections section, presented later in the chapter.) With subcut injections, the aspiration should be done if the medication manufacturer recommends it. It should also be done if it is part of the facility's policy.

Insulin is not aspirated. Subcut immunizations do not need to be aspirated, as recommended by the Centers for Disease Control and Prevention (CDC). Anticoagulants, such as enoxaparin and heparin, are administered in the abdomen. They are not aspirated, as specified by the manufacturers.

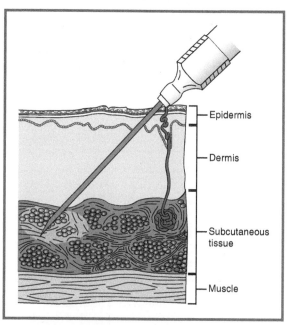

FIGURE 15.32 The subcutaneous (subcut) injection is administered in the subcutaneous layer. This method is used for small amounts of nonirritating medications in aqueous solution.

TABLE 15.3 Summary of Subcutaneous (Subcut) Injections

Syringe used	3 mL most common; 1 mL could be used
Needle size and angle of entry	25 gauge; ½ inch with a 90-degree angle of entry or ⅝ inch with a 45-degree angle of entry; the bevel position does not matter
Maximum volume	0.5–1.5 mL (0.5 mL in children)
Common sites	Lower abdomen, anterior thigh, and upper outer arm
Sites for vaccines	<1 year of age: anterior thigh >1 year of age: upper outer arm or anterior thigh
Additional sites	Separate sites by 1 inch
Patient position	Sitting
Administration technique	Pinch site; if 2 inches of tissue can be pinched, insert the needle at a 90-degree angle; if 1 inch of tissue can be pinched, insert the needle at a 45-degree angle; rotate sites

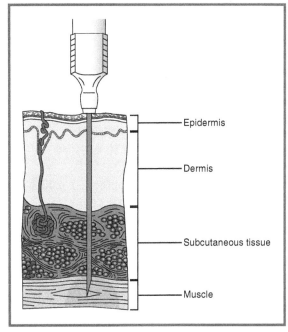

FIGURE 15.33 Anatomic illustration of the intramuscular (IM) injection. Note that the needle is inserted at a 90-degree angle, which deposits the medication into the large central part of the muscle.

Special Considerations When Giving Enoxaparin

When administering enoxaparin (Lovenox), follow these instructions:
- Make sure the drug is clear and colorless or pale yellow.
- Do not push any air or drug out of the syringe before giving the injection unless your healthcare provider tells you to. The air allows the medication to enter slower, reducing the risk of bruising.
- Using your finger and thumb, pinch a fold of skin 1 to 2 inches away from the umbilicus in the lower abdomen. Push the entire needle into the skin. Press down on the syringe plunger and inject the medication. Hold the pinched skin the entire time during the injection. Remove the needle. Do not rub or massage the site after the injection. Hold pressure to the site after the injection until the bleeding has stopped.

Subcutaneous Sites

Typically, three subcut sites are used in ambulatory care:
- *Abdominal site:* Have the patient remove the clothing in that area. Provide a drape sheet if needed to protect the patient's modesty. The site is located below the costal margins to the iliac crests. Stay 2 inches away from the umbilicus. It is important to stay away from the waistline and any scars. The patient may have more discomfort if the injection is given at the waistline due to the rubbing of clothing.
- *Outer posterior aspect of the upper arm:* Expose the arm. The outer posterior site extends from 3 inches above the elbow to about 3 fingerbreadths below the acromion process. It is important to stay away from the shoulder area.

- *Anterior aspect of the thigh:* Place one hand above the knee and the other hand below the greater trochanter. The site is the middle one-third of the thigh. The site extends from the front midline to the back midline, wrapping around the outer thigh. Usually only the middle one-third—from the front midline to the outer thigh—is used. Injections are not done on the back of the leg, because sitting would irritate the injection site.

Procedure 15.8 on p. 396 describes the steps to follow when giving a subcutaneous injection.

INTRAMUSCULAR INJECTIONS

Intramuscular injections involve placing medication into the muscle (Fig. 15.33). There are more blood vessels in the muscles; thus, absorption is faster than in the subcutaneous layer. For medications given by IM injection, *aqueous* (watery) medications should be given with a higher gauge needle than that used for oil-based medications. Table 15.4 contains a summary of intramuscular injection information. Common medications given via the intramuscular route include the following:
- Several vaccines; for example, hepatitis A and B; tetanus-diphtheria (Td), or with pertussis (Tdap); influenza; and meningococcal
- Antibiotics and medroxyprogesterone (Depo-Provera)

Administration Techniques

As with all injections, it is important to do the procedure safely. The medical assistant must identify the correct site and follow the guidelines for medical asepsis. When administering an IM injection,

TABLE 15.4   Summary of Intramuscular (IM) Injections

	DELTOID	VASTUS LATERALIS	VENTROGLUTEAL
Syrinige Used	3 mL		
Needle Length (Determined by the Patient's Size)	**1–11 yr**: ⅝–1 inch **Adults**: ⅝–1½ inch *By Weight:* **<130 lb**: ⅝ inch **130–152 lb**: 1 inch **Females 152–200 lb/males 152–260 lb**: 1–1½ inch **Females >200 lb/males >260 lb**: 1½ inch	**Birth–28 days**: ⅝ inch **1–12 mo**: 1 inch **1–18 yr**: 1–1¼ inch **18+ yr**: 1–1½ inch	**Birth–28 days**: ⅝ inch **1 mo–12 yr**: 1 inch **12+ yr**: 1–1½ inch
Needle Gauge (G) (Determined by the Medication)	22–25 G	**Children**: 22–25 G **Adults**: **oil-base**: 18–21 G; **aqueous**: 20–25 G	
Angle of Entry	90 degrees (bevel does not matter)		
Maximum Volume	1 mL for teens and adults	**Birth–1 yr**: 1 mL **1–11 yr**: 2 mL **12+ yr**: 3 mL	
Sites for Vaccines Per CDC	**1–3 yr**: Only if muscle mass is adequate **3+ yr**: Can be used	**Birth–1 yr**: Required **1–3 yr**: Preferred **3+ yr**: Can be used	
Additional Sites	Separate sites by 1 inch		
Patient /Position	Sitting	Sitting, supine	Side lying
Administration Technique	Stretch the skin over the injection site; use a 90-degree angle of entry		
Possible Complications	Necrosis, hematoma, ecchymosis (bruising), abscess, pain, and vascular and nerve injuries		

it is important to use a 90-degree angle for entry. The skin should be flattened or stretched over the site with the nondominant hand. Administration techniques for IM injections consist of the following:

- Being safe
- Minimizing pain
- Finding the correct site

The following sections address these three goals.

Aspiration

When giving an intramuscular injection, it is important to aspirate prior to injecting the medication. Once the needle is in the site, the medical assistant should pull back on the plunger for 5 seconds and check the barrel of the syringe. Lack of blood in the barrel means the needle is not in a blood vessel, so it is safe to inject the medication. If blood appears in the barrel, remove the needle, discard the syringe, and restart the procedure. Immunizations do not need to be aspirated, according to the CDC.

Air Lock Technique

When an IM injection is given, the air lock technique can be used. Remove the bubbles in the syringe, and measure the exact amount of medication needed. Once these steps have been done, add 0.2 to 0.5 mL of air into the syringe. This is the known as the *air lock technique*. When the IM injection is given, the medication is pushed in first, followed by the air. When the needle is withdrawn, the air creates a "lock," keeping the medication in the muscle. The air fills in the needle hole. The air lock prevents the irritating medication from tracking back up the tissues to the skin, creating pain for the patient.

Z-Track Technique

The Z-track technique is another injection method that can reduce pain and discomfort for the patient. Like the air lock technique, this method prevents the medication from tracking back through the subcutaneous tissue. The medication is sealed in the muscle, thus minimizing discomfort for the patient.

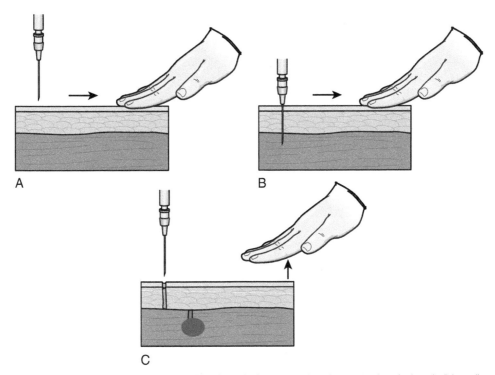

FIGURE 15.34 Z-track technique. **(A)** Displace and then cleanse the skin. **(B)** Inject the medication. **(C)** Release the skin and pull the needle out at the same time. The medication is locked in the muscle.

The **Z**-track technique should be used for irritating medications. The ventrogluteal site is the recommended site for injections of irritating medications. For the **Z**-track technique, the skin is pulled laterally with the medical assistant's nondominant hand. The site is cleansed, and the injection is given (Fig. 15.34A–B). As the needle is withdrawn, the skin is released (Fig. 15.34C).

Intramuscular Sites

Deltoid Site

The deltoid is a triangular-shaped muscle located near the shoulder and upper arm (Fig. 15.35). This muscle site is used to give a small volume of aqueous medications, such as vitamin B$_{12}$ and vaccines. The CDC recommends this site be used when vaccines are given to teens and adults. To find the site, expose the upper arm. Make sure the sleeve does not act as a tourniquet. If the sleeve is tight, have the patient slip the arm out of the shirt.

Palpate the acromion process. Place a finger on the acromion process and then 2 fingers below that. The top of the site is 1 to 2 inches (or 2 fingerbreadths) below the acromion process. The bottom of the site is at the anterior axillary fold (top of the axilla). The injection site should be somewhere between the top and the bottom of the site. Once the medical assistant finds the site, it is a good idea to have the patient lift his or her arm. The medical assistant can find the bulk (biggest part) of the deltoid muscle. The injection should be given into the bulk of the deltoid muscle.

Vastus Lateralis Site

The vastus lateralis site is used on patients from birth through adulthood. This site uses a thick, well-developed muscle. The CDC recommends this site until the deltoid muscle is the appropriate size

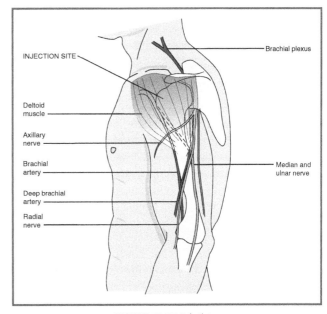

FIGURE 15.35 Deltoid site.

for vaccines (after the patient is 1 year or older). Have patients remove the clothing over the thigh. Remember to give patients a drape sheet to protect their modesty during the procedure.

To find the site, you will need to create a rectangle. Think about dividing the thigh into three sections. With adults, each of your hands will cover one-third of the thigh. Place one hand above the knee and the other hand below the greater trochanter (Fig. 15.36A). This creates the top and bottom borders of the rectangle (or the vastus lateralis site). The middle one-third is used for the injection

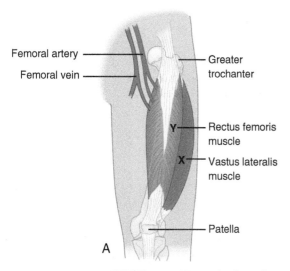

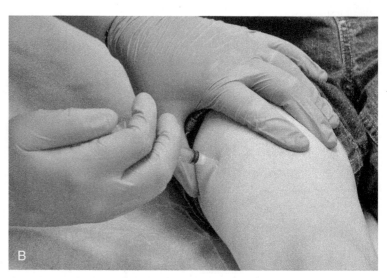

FIGURE 15.36 (A) Vastus lateralis site. The vastus lateralis muscle is typically used in ambulatory care. The rectus femoris muscle is used more by patients for intramuscular (IM) injections than by healthcare professionals. **(B)** The vastus lateralis is the recommended site for IM injections in infants and young children.

site. Next, find the midline of the thigh (remember, the midline creates equal right and left sides). That is the inner border of your rectangle. The final border is created by the midline of the outer thigh (i.e., it creates equal front and back sections of the thigh). Once the site is identified, the medical assistant should have the patient slightly lift the thigh. This allows the medical assistant to see if the injection site is in the bulk of the muscle, which is the goal (Fig. 15.36B). Procedure 15.9 on p. 398 describes the procedure for giving an intramuscular injection.

Ventrogluteal Site

The ventrogluteal site is an excellent site for oil-based medications and irritating medications. This site is being used more often, because the dorsogluteal site is no longer a recommended site for IM injections. To administer an injection in the ventrogluteal site, it is important to have patients remove clothing from this area. Offering a drape sheet to protect their modesty is important. For this injection, the patient needs to be in a side-lying position.

The most complex part of using the ventrogluteal site is to ensure that the correct hand is used to find the site. Remember to use the hand opposite the injection site. For instance, if the injection site is on the patient's left side, then use your right hand. Follow these steps to find the site:

- Place the palm of your hand on the patient's greater trochanter (Fig. 15.37).
- Your fingers need to point toward the patient's head, and your thumb to the patient's groin. (If your thumb is facing the patient's back side, you are using the wrong hand!)
- Place your index finger on the anterior superior iliac spine. If your fingers are short or if the patient is tall, point your index finger toward the anterior superior iliac spine.
- Move your middle finger back along the iliac crest toward the patient's buttock.

The positioning of your index and middle fingers forms a triangle. The injection point is at the center of the triangle. Remember, if you

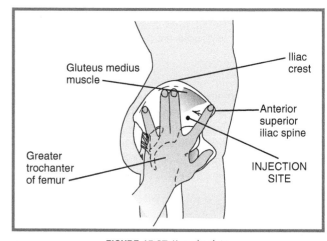

FIGURE 15.37 Ventrogluteal site.

are giving an irritating medication, use the **Z-track** method to reduce pain. Procedure 15.10 on p. 400 describes the steps of the Z-track technique.

Dorsogluteal Site

The dorsogluteal site was a common intramuscular (IM) site for irritating medications. However, the dorsogluteal site is near the sciatic nerve and large blood vessels. Over the years, many patients developed complications because of dorsogluteal injections. Agencies have had to defend lawsuits related to dorsogluteal injection complications.

Current evidence has demonstrated that dorsogluteal sites pose a high risk for injury. The current recommendation is that the dorsogluteal site should not be used. The ventrogluteal site is ideal for the medications that were always given in the dorsogluteal site. Many healthcare professions have moved away from administering medications at the dorsogluteal site since the recommendation became public.

MONITORING INTRAVENOUS THERAPY

Intravenous therapy is performed by nurses in ambulatory care facilities. IVs can be used to deliver medication and fluids. A needle inside a catheter is used to start the IV. The needle is removed, and the catheter is hooked up to the IV tubing that runs from the insertion site to the IV bag. The nurse must start the IV, adjust the flow, and monitor the patient during the procedure.

The medical assistant's role with IVs includes scheduling a patient for an IV infusion. It is important to schedule the IV infusion at the appropriate time. Sometimes the patient may need to come in for an IV medication that is scheduled every so many hours. It is important to keep the patient on schedule with the medication.

Sometimes the clinical medical assistant may assist the nurse with checking on the patient. The medical assistant should be aware of common problems that can arise with IVs. The nurse needs to be notified of any problems immediately. Common concerns with IV therapy include the following:

- Edema (swelling) or increasing pain at the IV insertion site
- Blood moving up the IV tubing
- An almost-empty bag of fluids
- A patient who is having difficulty breathing or who has increased audible wheezing

CLOSING COMMENTS

Patient Coaching

When administering medications, the medical assistant must be aware that several forms of liquid medications contain alcohol. This is a concern for patients who are recovering alcoholics or have other health issues, such as diabetes.

The medical assistant may need to teach patients about what types of medications contain alcohol. An Internet search can provide lists of medications with their alcohol content. Such online drug references also provide information on the ingredients.

If a patient mentions that he or she is a recovering alcoholic or addict, it is important for the medical assistant first to acknowledge the person's accomplishment. Then the medical assistant should communicate the information to the provider. This may make a difference in what medication the provider gives to the patient.

Legal and Ethical Issues

The medical assistant's scope of practice regarding injections differs across the nation. It is important for medical assistants to know their scope of practice in their state. Agencies may also have limitations on what medical assistants can do. For instance, if a scope of practice in the state allows medical assistants to give injections but the agency does not allow it, medical assistants must abide by the agency's policies and procedures.

Patient-Centered Care

For injections given to small children, the subcutaneous (subcut) and intramuscular (IM) sites in the thigh are in the same location. It is helpful to have the parent/guardian hold the child's upper body and hands (however, the medical assistant should anticipate that the adult may not hold securely). If another staff member is available, having him or her hold the lower extremities is helpful. Many times, children may need more than one injection. For this scenario, it is helpful to have two medical assistants each give an injection at the same time.

The medical assistant should hold the joint above the injection site with his or her nondominant hand. The child's lower leg can be carefully bent off the table and held between the side of the table and the medical assistant's body. If you use this technique, be careful not to hurt the child's leg. Injections for children need to be done using the one-hand technique, because the other hand is holding near the site.

Professional Behaviors

The medical assistant has an important role in administering medications. Paying attention to details is critical. If a medication error occurs, the medical assistant must act immediately to notify the provider. The provider will identify what steps need to be taken. The medical assistant needs to also complete an incident report. (Incident reports are discussed in Chapter 4 in the main text.) The supervisor needs to also be notified. In most cases the supervisor will ensure that the patient is not charged for the medication given in error. The supervisor may also need to complete a state or federal report on the medication error.

SUMMARY OF SCENARIO

Gabe and Mark continued to work together for the remaining weeks of practicum. Mark had the opportunity to give several TSTs. He was able to do subcut and IM injections also. Mark learned the importance of distracting patients during injections; they seemed to tolerate the injection much better.

One of the other medical assistants had a medication error. The medication was given to the wrong patient. This error really impressed on Mark the importance

of the nine rights of medication administration. He is adamant that he will never forget to follow each right each time he gives medications. He does not want to deal with a medication error.

SUMMARY OF LEARNING OBJECTIVES

1. **Verify and discuss the rights of medication administration.**

   Each time you prepare and give medication, it is important that you follow the nine rights of medication administration. These rights include the right medication, right dose, right route, right time, right patient, right education, right to refuse, right technique, and right documentation.

2. **Discuss the various forms of medication.**

   The form is the physical characteristics of the medication. Forms of medications include the following:

   - *Solid* medication forms: Examples include tablet, chewable tablet, caplet, capsule, scored tablet, and enteric-coated tablet.
   - *Semisolid* medication forms: Examples include ointment, paste, cream, suppository, and pessary.
   - *Liquid* medication forms: Examples include solutions and suspensions.
   - *Solution*: Examples include tincture, fluid extract, spirit, elixir, and syrup.
   - *Suspension*: Examples include emulsion, gel, magma, liniment, lotion, and aerosol.

3. **Administer oral medications.**

   Medications taken by the oral route (po) are medications we take by mouth. See Procedure 15.1 on p. 383 for the steps to administer solid and liquid medications.

4. **Describe other routes of medications, including sublingual, buccal, transdermal, inhalation, topical, irrigation, and parenteral.**

   Sublingual (SL) medications are placed under the tongue. *Buccal* medications are placed between the cheek and the gums. *Transdermal* medications are placed on the skin and absorbed into the bloodstream. Medications for the nose, throat, and lungs can be *inhaled*. Applying a drug to a mucous membrane or skin is considered use of the *topical* route. *Irrigation* means to bathe or flush open wounds or body cavities. The *parenteral* route involves administration by infusion, injection, or implantation.

5. **Discuss types and parts of needles and syringes.**

   The parts of a hypodermic needle include the following:

   - Hub: Attaches or screws onto the syringe
   - Hilt: Where the needle attaches
   - Bevel: Slanted end of the shaft
   - Lumen: Hollow space inside the needle.

   The parts of a hypodermic syringe are shown in Fig. 15.11 and include the Luer-Lok tip, barrel, flange, and plunger.

6. **Prepare parenteral medications.**

   This chapter described several procedures for preparing parenteral medications. See the following procedures for more information on preparing parenteral medications:

   - Procedure 15.2, p. 385: Prepare Medication From an Ampule
   - Procedure 15.3, p. 387: Prepare Medication Using a Prefilled Sterile Cartridge
   - Procedure 15.4, p. 389: Prepare Medication From a Vial
   - Procedure 15.5, p. 391: Reconstitute Powdered Medication
   - Procedure 15.6, p. 392: Mixing Two Insulins

7. **Prepare and administer intradermal injections.**

   Procedure 15.7 on p. 393 discusses how to administer an intradermal injection. A tuberculin skin test is one of the most common intradermal injections given by medical assistants. Table 15.1 provides a summary of intradermal injections.

8. **Prepare and administer subcutaneous injections.**

   Procedure 15.8 on p. 396 discusses how to administer a subcutaneous injection. Table 15.3 provides a summary of subcutaneous injections.

9. **Prepare and administer intramuscular injections.**

   Procedure 15.9 on p. 398 discusses how to administer an intramuscular injection, and Procedure 15.10 on p. 400 describes how to give an IM injection using the Z-track technique. Table 15.4 provides a summary of intramuscular injections.

10. **Describe the medical assistant's role in monitoring intravenous therapy.**

    Intravenous therapy is performed by nurses in ambulatory care facilities. The medical assistant's role includes scheduling a patient for an IV infusion. It is important to schedule the IV infusion at the appropriate time. Sometimes the clinical medical assistant may assist the nurse with checking on the patient. The nurse needs to be notified of any problems immediately.

| PROCEDURE 15.1 | Administer Oral Medications |

Tasks: Calculate the dose to give. Prepare a liquid and a solid medication, and administer medications to a patient. Document medication administration.

EQUIPMENT and SUPPLIES

- Provider's orders
- Patient health record
- Drug reference information
- Liquid medication and a solid medication
- Paper cup
- Plastic medication cup
- Marker
- Medication tray
- Glass of water

Orders: Diltiazem 240 mg po and Cephalexin Oral Suspension 375 mg po

PROCEDURAL STEPS

1. Using the drug reference information and the orders, review the information on the medications.
   PURPOSE: The medical assistant must know about the medication that is being given.

2. Using the orders and the labels in Fig. 1, calculate the amount of medication you need to give. Verify the right doses with the instructor. Verify if it is the right time for the order, if that applies.
   PURPOSE: The orders do not specify the number of tablets or the amount of liquid (mL) to give. The medical assistant must calculate both. It is important to check your answer with a peer in the workplace before preparing the medication. This is how to ensure that the right dose is being given.

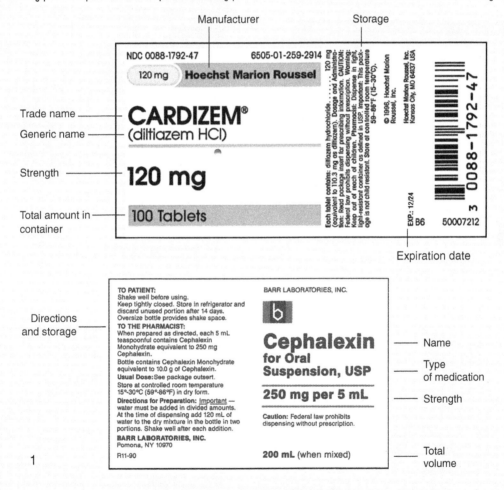

1

Continued

PROCEDURE 15.1   **Administer Oral Medications**—*continued*

3. Wash hands or use hand sanitizer. Select the right medications from the storage area. Check each medication label against the order. Check for the right name, form, and route. Check the expiration date to make sure the drug has not expired.

   PURPOSE: It is important to do the first check of the label when getting medications from the cabinet. Do not administer expired medications.

4. Assemble the supplies required to prepare the medications. Using the marker, write the medication name and dose on the appropriate cups (Fig. 2).

   PURPOSE: The paper cup will be used for the tablets, and the plastic cup will be used for the liquid. Make sure not to write over the measurement markings on the plastic cup. Labeling the cups is a safety measure. All medications prepared need to be labeled. Writing an assessment reminder on the cup is optional and can be helpful when the medical assistant needs to do an assessment (e.g., blood pressure) prior to administration.

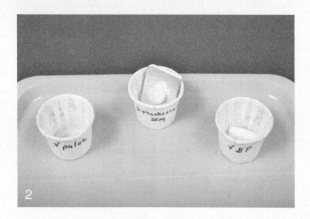

5. Perform the second medication check. Check each medication label against the order. Check for the right name, form, and route.

   PURPOSE: It is important to do the second check of the label before pouring the medications into the cups.

6. For the solid medication: Remove the cover of the container and hold it so the inside is facing up. Carefully pour the correct number of tablets into the cover. If you pour too many into the cover, pour the extra tablets back into the bottle. When you have the correct number of tablets in the cover, pour them from the cover into the paper cup. Place the cover on the container. Make sure not to contaminate the inside of the container or the cover.

   PURPOSE: The inside of the medication container and the cover are sterile. You can pour the tablets back and forth between these two sites until you have the correct number of tablets in the cover. Once you pour the tablets into the paper cup, they are no longer sterile. They cannot be put back into the sterile medication container. If using *unit dose* (individual packaged tablets [blister packs]), tear off the number of tablets needed, and place them in the paper cup. Do not open until you are with the patient. If the patient refuses the medication, the unopened unit dose medications can be returned to the original box.

7. For liquid medication:
   a. Place the plastic medication cup on a high, even surface. Uncover the bottle and place the cover on the counter, making sure the inside is facing up. Place your palm over the medication label. Position yourself so you are eye level with the medication cup (Fig. 3).

      PURPOSE: The cup needs to be on an even surface. Read the amount at eye level to ensure the accuracy of the measurement. Palming the label keeps the label clean as you pour the medication.

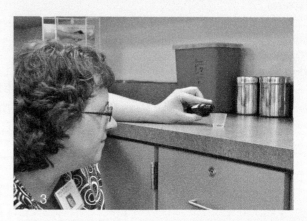

   b. Pour the medication into the cup until the lowest point of the meniscus is at the measurement needed (Fig. 4).

      PURPOSE: When liquid is poured into a container, it is higher at the edges than the middle. This is called the *meniscus*. The liquid must be measured at the lowest point of the meniscus.

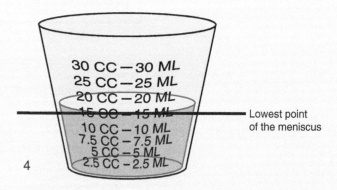

   c. If too much medication is poured into the cup, flush the extra down the sink. Replace the cover on the bottle without contaminating the inside of the cover or bottle.

      PURPOSE: Any extra medication in the cup cannot be poured back into the sterile medication bottle. The medication in the bottle and the inside cover need to remain sterile.

8. Place the medication cups on the medication tray. Clean up the area.

   PURPOSE: It is important for the medical assistant to clean up the work area.

PROCEDURE 15.1   Administer Oral Medications—*continued*

9. Perform the third medication check. Check each medication label against the order. Check for the right name, form, and route. Verify that the amount of medication in each cup is correct according to the order.
   PURPOSE: It is important to do the third check of the label before placing the medications back into the cabinet.

10. Prior to entering the exam room, knock on the door and wait a moment. Greet the patient. Identify yourself. Verify the patient's identity with full name and date of birth. Make sure the patient's information matches the order and the record. Explain what you are going to do.
    PURPOSE: It is important to identify the patient in two different ways to ensure that you have the correct patient. Explaining the procedure can make the patient feel more comfortable and reduces anxiety.

11. Provide the right education to the patient. Explain the medication ordered, the desired effect, and common side effects, and identify the provider who ordered it. Answer any questions the patient may have. Use language the patient can understand. Ask the patient if he or she has any allergies. If the patient refuses the medication, notify the provider.
    PURPOSE: The patient needs to be aware of what you are giving, the action, side effects, and who ordered it. It is also important to double-check the patient's allergies before administering the medication.

12. Perform the right technique. Do any assessments required prior to giving the medication. If the patient can have water with the medication, have water available.
    PURPOSE: Some medications require assessments prior to administration.

13. Allow the patient to take the medication in his or her hand or to use the cup. Stay with the patient until the medication has been taken.
    PURPOSE: The medical assistant needs to ensure that the medication is taken.

14. Document the procedure in the health record. Include assessments done; allergies; teaching or instructions provided; the name of the provider who ordered the medication; the medication's name, dose, and route; and how the patient tolerated the medication. For vaccines and controlled substances, add the lot number, the expiration date, and the manufacturer number.
    PURPOSE: The medications need to be documented to indicate that they were given.

Documentation Example:
10/30/20XX 0936 BP 162/92 left arm, sitting. NKA. Per Dr. Martin's order, administered Diltiazem 120 mg, 2 tabs po, and cephalexin suspension 250 mg/5 mL, 375 mg po. Medication action and side effects discussed with patient prior to administration. Pt had no questions and verbalized understanding. Pt tolerated the medications without problems._____
_____Gabe Garcia, CMA (AAMA)

Fig. 1 from Brown M, Mulholland JM: *Drug calculations: process and problems for clinical practice*, ed 9, St. Louis, 2012, Mosby.

PROCEDURE 15.2   Prepare Medication From an Ampule

Task: Prepare medication from an ampule.

EQUIPMENT and SUPPLIES

- Provider's order
- Ampule of medication
- Gauze or ampule breaker
- Alcohol wipes
- Filter needle and hypodermic safety needle
- 3-mL syringe
- Biohazard sharps container
- Waste container
- Drug reference information
- Marker

Order: 0.9% Sodium Chloride 0.7 mL IM

PROCEDURAL STEPS

1. Wash hands or use hand sanitizer. Using the drug reference information and the order, review the information on the medication if needed. Clarify any questions you have with the provider.
   PURPOSE: Hand sanitization is an important step for infection control. It is important to be knowledgeable about the medication you are giving.

2. Select the right medication from the storage area. Check the medication label against the order. Check for the right name, form, and route. Check the expiration date to make sure the drug has not expired. Verify the right dose and the right time.
   PURPOSE: It is important to do the first check of the label when getting medications from the cabinet. Do not administer expired medications.

Continued

PROCEDURE 15.2 **Prepare Medication From an Ampule**—*continued*

3. Assemble the supplies required for the procedure.
   <u>PURPOSE:</u> Remember to split up the three medication checks with activities between each check.

4. Perform the second medication check. Check the medication label against the order. Check for the right name, form, dose, and route.
   <u>PURPOSE:</u> It is important to do the second check of the label before proceeding with the procedure.

5. Attach the filter needle to the syringe. Using a marker, label the syringe with the medication name.
   <u>PURPOSE:</u> You will use the filter needle first during the procedure.

6. Gently tap the medication from the head of the ampule or hold the ampule securely, upright in your hand (Fig. 1). Quickly move your hand downward. After all the medication has drained into the body of the ampule, wipe the neck with an alcohol wipe.
   <u>PURPOSE:</u> Any medication left in the head will be lost after it is snapped off. Tapping or quickly bringing the ampule down will drain the medication into the body.

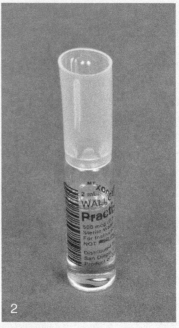

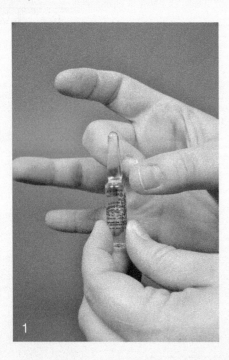

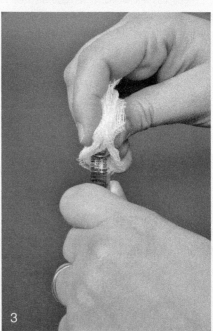

7. Place the ampule breaker over the head of the ampule (following the directions from the manufacturer), or wrap the neck with gauze (Figs. 2 and 3). Hold the body with your nondominant hand. With your dominant hand, firmly hold the head (or breaker) between your first two fingers and thumb. Quickly snap off the head of the ampule, making sure it breaks away from your body and others (Fig. 4).
   <u>PURPOSE:</u> It is important to protect your fingers from the broken glass.

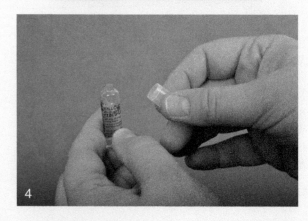

PROCEDURE 15.2   **Prepare Medication From an Ampule**—*continued*

8. Discard the breaker or gauze with the ampule head in a biohazard sharps container (Fig. 5).
   <u>PURPOSE:</u> It is important to discard the head immediately to protect yourself.

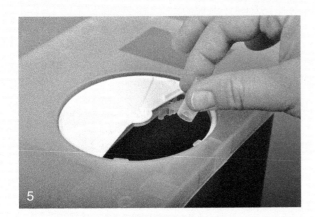

9. Place the ampule on a flat surface. Uncover the filter needle, and insert the needle into the ampule without contaminating the needle. Keeping the bevel in the medication, pull the plunger upward, aspirating the medication into the syringe. Tilt the ampule as you remove all the medication.
   <u>PURPOSE:</u> Keeping the bevel in the medication will prevent air from being aspirated into the syringe.

10. Recap the needle using the one-hand scoop technique. Perform the third medication check. Check the medication label against the order. Check for the right name, form, and route. Discard the ampule in the biohazard sharps container.

<u>PURPOSE:</u> It is important to do the third check of the label before seeing the patient.

11. Remove the filter needle, and attach a new needle without contaminating the unit. Discard the filter needle in the biohazard sharps container.
    <u>PURPOSE:</u> The filter needle needs to be removed before the injection is given.

12. Hold the syringe in a vertical position with the uncapped needle pointed upward. Tap the barrel carefully with the fingertips or a pen to move the air bubbles up to the top of the barrel. Once all the air bubbles are at the top, push the plunger slowly to the correct calibration marking for the ordered dose. Recap the needle.
    <u>PURPOSE:</u> The air needs to be at the top of the syringe before you measure the correct amount of medication.

13. Double-check the dose of medication measured against the order. Make sure no air bubbles are in the syringe.
    <u>PURPOSE:</u> Air bubbles take up space. If air bubbles are present, then the correct dose will not be given.

14. Maintain the sterility of the medication and the needle throughout the procedure.
    <u>PURPOSE:</u> The needle and medication need to be sterile for the injection.

15. Clean up the work area. Packaging and other waste should be discarded in the waste container.
    <u>PURPOSE:</u> It is professional to clean up after yourself. Never fill a biohazard sharps container with uncontaminated waste (e.g., packaging).

PROCEDURE 15.3   **Prepare Medication Using a Prefilled Sterile Cartridge**

Tasks: Prepare medication using a prefilled sterile cartridge. Discard a prefilled sterile cartridge with a reusable holder.

EQUIPMENT and SUPPLIES

- Provider's order
- Prefilled sterile cartridge
- Hypodermic safety needle (if needed)
- Carpuject cartridge holder
- Biohazard sharps container
- Waste container
- Drug reference information

Order: 0.9% Sodium Chloride 1.6 mL IM

PROCEDURAL STEPS

1. Wash hands or use hand sanitizer. Using the drug reference information and the order, review the information on the medication if needed. Clarify any questions you have with the provider.

<u>PURPOSE:</u> Hand sanitization is an important step for infection control. It is important to be knowledgeable about the medication you are giving.

2. Select the right medication from the storage area. Check the medication label against the order. Check for the right name, form, and route. Check the expiration date to make sure the drug has not expired. Verify the right dose and the right time.
   <u>PURPOSE:</u> It is important to do the first check of the label when getting the medication from the cabinet. Do not administer expired medications.

3. Assemble the supplies required for the procedure.
   <u>PURPOSE:</u> Remember to split up the three medication checks with activities between each check.

4. Perform the second medication check. Check the medication label against the order. Check for the right name, form, dose, and route.
   <u>PURPOSE:</u> It is important to do the second check of the label before proceeding with the procedure.

Continued

PROCEDURE 15.3 **Prepare Medication Using a Prefilled Sterile Cartridge**—*continued*

5. Break the seal. With one hand on the needle cover and the other on the barrel of the prefilled cartridge, move your hands together until you hear a pop. If needed, remove the cover on the cartridge and attach a covered needle.
   PURPOSE: This breaks the seal in the cartridge.
6. Hold the Carpuject holder so the opening (for the barrel) is facing up. Pull the plunger rod out until it clicks. Turn the blue lock until it clicks. This should increase the space between the blue lock and the flange (Fig. 1).
   PURPOSE: The Carpuject holder needs to be opened before the cartridge can be placed in it.

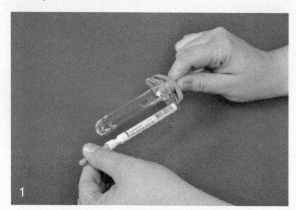

7. Insert the cartridge into the Carpuject holder (Fig. 2). To secure the cartridge, turn the blue lock on the Carpuject holder until it clicks. The space between the blue lock and the flange should decrease. Turn the white plunger rod until it screws onto the rubber stopper (Fig. 3).
   PURPOSE: The cartridge must be secured in the Carpuject holder.

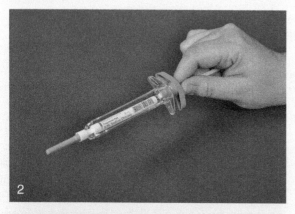

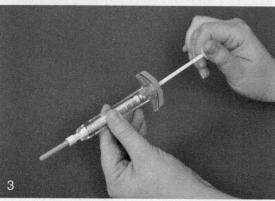

8. Remove the cover. Hold the syringe unit in a vertical position with the uncapped needle or tip pointed upward. Tap the barrel carefully with the fingertips or a pen to move the air bubbles up to the top of the barrel. Once all the air bubbles are at the top, push the plunger slowly to the correct calibration marking for the ordered dose.
   PURPOSE: The air needs to be at the top of the syringe before you measure the correct amount of medication.
9. Recap the needle using the one-hand scoop technique. Perform the third medication check. Check the medication label against the order. Check for the right name, form, and route.
   PURPOSE: It is important to do the third check of the label before seeing the patient.
10. Double-check the dose of medication measured against the order. Make sure no air bubbles are in the syringe.
    PURPOSE: Air bubbles take up space. If air bubbles are present, then the correct dose will not be given.
11. Maintain the sterility of the medication and the needle throughout the procedure.
    PURPOSE: The needle and medication need to be sterile for the injection.
12. After "giving" the injection, unscrew the plunger rod and pull out until it clicks. Turn the blue lock until it clicks. The space between the blue lock and the flange should increase in size.
    PURPOSE: The Carpuject holder needs to be opened to remove the used cartridge.
13. Carefully invert the Carpuject holder over a biohazard sharps container to discard the cartridge (Fig. 4). Hold the Carpuject holder firmly so it does not end up in the sharps container.
    PURPOSE: Only the cartridge should be discarded.

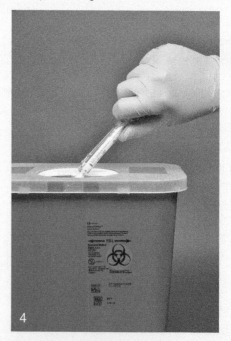

14. Disinfect the Carpuject holder. Clean up the work area. Waste should be put in the waste container.
    PURPOSE: Disinfection is an important step for infection control.

| PROCEDURE 15.4 | Prepare Medication From a Vial |

Task: Prepare medication from a vial.

EQUIPMENT and SUPPLIES

- Provider's order
- Vial of medication
- Alcohol wipes
- Hypodermic safety needle and 3-mL syringe or needle/syringe unit
- Biohazard sharps container
- Waste container
- Drug reference information
- Marker

Order: 0.9% Sodium Chloride 1.2 mL IM

PROCEDURAL STEPS

1. Wash hands or use hand sanitizer. Using the drug reference information and the order, review the information on the medication if needed. Clarify any questions you have with the provider.
   <u>PURPOSE:</u> Hand sanitization is an important step for infection control. It is important to be knowledgeable about the medication you are giving.

2. Select the right medication from the storage area. Check the medication label against the order. Check for the right name, form, and route. Check the expiration date to make sure the drug has not expired. Verify the right dose and the right time.
   <u>PURPOSE:</u> It is important to do the first check of the label when getting medications from the cabinet. Do not administer expired medications.

3. Assemble the supplies required for the procedure.
   <u>PURPOSE:</u> Remember to split up the three medication checks with activities between each check.

4. Perform the second medication check. Check the medication label against the order. Check for the right name, form, dose, and route.
   <u>PURPOSE:</u> It is important to do the second check of the label before proceeding with the procedure.

5. Open the syringe and needle. Tighten the preassembled syringe and needle unit (if needed), or attach the needle to the syringe. Using a marker, label the syringe with the medication name.
   <u>PURPOSE:</u> Labeling the medication is critical for medication safety.

6. Mix the medication by rolling it with your hands if needed (Fig. 1). Remove the cap on the vial (if present). Clean the rubber stopper with an alcohol wipe (Fig. 2). Let the stopper dry.
   <u>PURPOSE:</u> The rubber stopper must be disinfected each time you enter the vial with a needle.

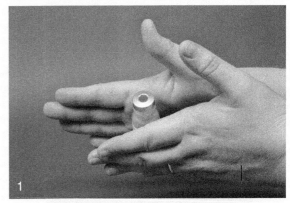

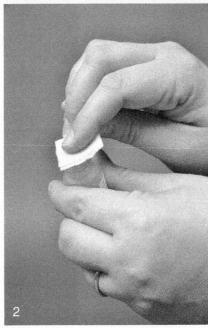

7. With the syringe in a vertical position, pull the syringe plunger down. Draw up an amount of air equal to the amount of medication ordered.
   <u>PURPOSE:</u> The vial is under pressure. When fluid is taken out, air must be added in. Not enough replaced air makes it difficult to withdraw the medication. Too much air causes the pressure to increase in the vial. The extra pressure causes the medication to be forced into the syringe without the plunger being pulled.

8. Hold the vial firmly against a flat surface. Insert the needle into the center of the dried rubber stopper. Inject the aspirated air above the fluid in the vial (Fig. 3).
   <u>PURPOSE:</u> Adding the air into the fluid will increase the bubbles.

Continued

PROCEDURE 15.4   **Prepare Medication From a Vial**—*continued*

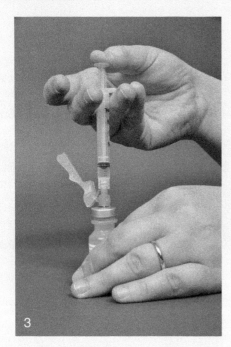

3

9. With the palm of your nondominant hand facing upward, grasp the vial between your middle and index fingers. Keeping the syringe unit in the vial, pick up and invert them. Use your thumb, ring, and little fingers of your nondominant hand to stabilize the syringe in the vial (Fig. 4).
   PURPOSE: It is important to stabilize the syringe, so the needle does not bend.

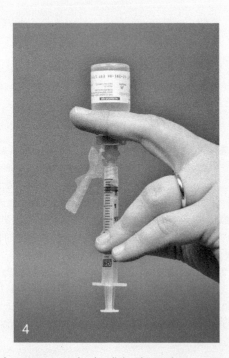

4

10. With the syringe at eye level, pull the plunger down using your dominant hand. Fill the syringe with more medication than what was ordered (Fig. 5).

PURPOSE: Air bubbles will need to be ejected back into the vial. The extra medication helps with this process.

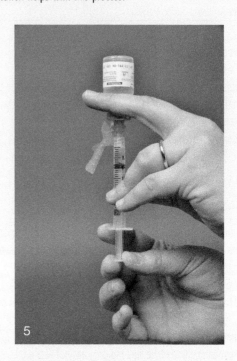

5

11. Continue to hold the vial/needle/syringe unit in a vertical position (with the needle pointing upward) with your nondominant hand. With your dominant hand, use either your fingers or a pen to tap the bubbles to the top of the barrel.
    PURPOSE: Bubbles rise to the top. With the syringe pointing straight up, the bubbles tend to move to the top of the barrel near the needle.

12. Once all the air bubbles are at the top, push the plunger slowly to the correct calibration marking for the ordered dose.
    PURPOSE: The air needs to be at the top of the syringe before you measure the correct amount of medication.

13. Double-check that no air bubbles are in the syringe and the right dose was measured. If everything is correct, remove the vial from the syringe/needle unit.
    PURPOSE: Air bubbles take up space. If air bubbles are present, then the correct dose will not be given.

14. Use the one-hand scoop technique to cover the needle. Perform the third medication check. Check each medication label against the order. Check for the right name, form, and route.
    PURPOSE: It is important to do the third check of the label before seeing the patient.

15. Maintain the sterility of the medication and the needle throughout the procedure.
    PURPOSE: The needle and medication need to be sterile for the injection.

16. Clean up the work area.
    PURPOSE: It is professional to clean up after yourself.

PROCEDURE 15.5   Reconstitute Powdered Medication

Tasks: Reconstitute powdered medication, and prepare the dose of medication.

EQUIPMENT and SUPPLIES

- Provider's order
- Vial of powdered medication
- Vial of diluent
- Alcohol wipes
- Two hypodermic syringes (a 3 mL and a larger syringe)
- Two hypodermic safety needles
- Biohazard sharps container
- Waste container
- Drug reference information
- Marker

Order: (Powdered medication name) 0.5 mL IM

PROCEDURAL STEPS

1. Wash hands or use hand sanitizer. Using the drug reference information and the order, review the information on the medication if needed. Clarify any questions you have with the provider.
   PURPOSE: Hand sanitization is an important step for infection control. It is important to be knowledgeable about the medication you are giving.

2. Select the right medication from the storage area. Check the medication label against the order. Check for the right name, form, and route. Check the expiration date to make sure the vials are not expired. Verify the right dose and the right time. Read the medication label to determine the correct diluent. Obtain the diluent, and check the name, route, and expiration date.
   PURPOSE: It is important to do the first check of the label when getting the medications from the cabinet. The label of the powdered medication will indicate the diluent to use. The diluent label must also be checked.

3. Assemble the supplies required for the procedure. If needed, calculate the dose of medication required.
   PURPOSE: Remember to split up the three medication checks with activities between each check.

4. Perform the second medication check. Check the medication labels against the order and directions for reconstituting the powder. Check for the right name, form, and route.
   PURPOSE: It is important to do the second check of the label before proceeding with the procedure.

5. Open and assemble the syringes and needles. Using a marker, label the 3-mL syringe with the medication name.
   PURPOSE: It is important to keep the needle sterile. If contamination occurs, discard the equipment, and start over.

6. Remove the caps on the vials. Clean the rubber stoppers with an alcohol wipe. Let the stoppers dry.
   PURPOSE: The rubber stopper must be disinfected each time you enter the vial with a needle.

7. With the powdered medication vial on a firm surface, insert the needle of the largest volume syringe unit. Make sure the tip stays out of the powder.

Pull back on the plunger, and withdraw air equal to the amount of diluent that must be added. Pull the needle/syringe out of the stopper.
PURPOSE: The vial is under pressure. When liquid is put in, the same volume of air must be removed to keep the pressure equal.

8. Using the syringe with the aspirated air (equal to the amount of diluent needed), insert the needle into the center of the dried rubber stopper of the diluent vial. Push the air into the vial, but do not force the air into the vial. Make sure the needle is not in the fluid.
   PURPOSE: Adding the air into the fluid will increase the bubbles. Forcing the air into the vial may cause the vial to have too much pressure.

9. With the palm of your nondominant hand facing upward, grasp the vial between your middle and index fingers. Keeping the syringe unit in the vial, pick up and invert them. Use your thumb, ring, and little fingers of your nondominant hand to stabilize the syringe in the vial. Pull down on the plunger until you have more diluent than what you need.
   PURPOSE: It is important to stabilize the syringe, so the needle does not bend.

10. Continue to hold the vial/needle/syringe unit in a vertical position (with the needle pointing upward) with your nondominant hand. With your dominant hand, use either your fingers or a pen to tap the bubbles to the top of the barrel.
    PURPOSE: Bubbles rise to the top. With the syringe pointing straight up, the bubbles tend to move to the top of the barrel near the needle.

11. Once all the air bubbles are at the top, push the plunger slowly to the correct calibration marking for the ordered dose. Keep the syringe at eye level.
    PURPOSE: The air needs to be at the top of the syringe before you measure the correct amount of medication.

12. Double-check that no air bubbles are in the syringe and the right dose was measured. If everything is correct, remove the vial from the syringe/needle unit.
    PURPOSE: Air bubbles take up space. If air bubbles are present, then the correct dose will not be given.

13. Using an alcohol wipe, clean the rubber stopper of the powdered medication vial. With the vial flat on a hard surface, insert the needle into the dried stopper. Push the diluent into the vial. If resistance is met, take your finger off the plunger, and allow air to fill in the syringe. Gradually work all the diluent into the vial. Withdraw the needle from the vial, and discard the needle and syringe in the biohazard sharps container.
    PURPOSE: Forcing the diluent into the vial may cause the vial to "explode" at the weakest point.

14. Gently mix the vial by rolling it in your palms. Mix the medication until all the powder has dissolved.
    PURPOSE: Powder needs to be totally dissolved so the correct dose is given.

15. Clean the rubber stopper of the powdered medication vial with an alcohol wipe. Let the stopper dry. With the second syringe in a vertical position,

Continued

PROCEDURE 15.5   Reconstitute Powdered Medication—*continued*

pull the syringe plunger down. Draw up an amount of air equal to the amount of medication ordered.

PURPOSE: Think of this step as starting over. Air needs to be inserted into the diluted powder vial to draw up the correct amount of medication.

16. Hold the vial firmly against a flat surface. Insert the needle into the center of the dried rubber stopper. Inject the aspirated air above the fluid in the vial.

PURPOSE: Adding the air into the fluid will increase the bubbles.

17. With the palm of your nondominant hand facing upward, grasp the vial between your middle and index fingers. Keeping the syringe unit in the vial, pick up and invert them. Use your thumb, ring, and little fingers of your nondominant hand to stabilize the syringe in the vial.

PURPOSE: It is important to stabilize the syringe, so the needle does not bend.

18. With the syringe at eye level, pull the plunger down using your dominant hand. Fill the syringe with more medication than what was ordered.

PURPOSE: Air bubbles will need to be ejected back into the vial. The extra medication helps with this process.

19. Continue to hold the vial/needle/syringe unit in a vertical position (with the needle pointing upward) with your nondominant hand. With your dominant hand, use either your fingers or a pen to tap the bubbles to the top of the barrel.

PURPOSE: Bubbles rise to the top. With the syringe pointing straight up, the bubbles tend to move to the top of the barrel near the needle.

20. Once all the air bubbles are at the top, push the plunger slowly to the correct calibration marking for the ordered dose.

PURPOSE: The air needs to be at the top of the syringe before you measure the correct amount of medication.

21. Double-check that no air bubbles are in the syringe and the right dose was measured. If everything is correct, remove the vial from the syringe/needle unit.

PURPOSE: Air bubbles take up space. If air bubbles are present, then the correct dose will not be given.

22. Use the one-hand scoop technique to cover the needle. Perform the third medication check. Check each medication label against the order. Check for the right name, form, and route.

PURPOSE: It is important to do the third check of the label before seeing the patient.

23. Maintain the sterility of the medication and the needle throughout the procedure.

PURPOSE: The needle and medication need to be sterile for the injection.

24. If the medication is in a multidose vial, label the vial with the expiration date, diluent added, and your initials. Clean up the work area. Put the packaging and other waste in the waste container. Discard the vial(s) in the biohazard waste container.

PURPOSE: It is professional to clean up after yourself.

PROCEDURE 15.6   Mixing Two Insulins

Task: Mixing two types of insulins in one syringe.

EQUIPMENT and SUPPLIES

- Provider's order
- Regular insulin vial
- NPH insulin vial
- Alcohol wipes
- Insulin needle and syringe unit
- Biohazard sharps container
- Waste container
- Drug reference information
- Marker

Order: Regular insulin 16 units mixed with NPH insulin 30 units subcut

PROCEDURAL STEPS

1. Wash hands or use hand sanitizer. Using the drug reference information and the order, review the information on the medication if needed. Clarify any questions you have with the provider.

PURPOSE: Hand sanitization is an important step for infection control. It is important to be knowledgeable about the medication you are giving.

2. Select the right medications from the storage area. Check the medication labels against the order. Check for the right name, form, and route. Check the expiration date to make sure the vials are not expired. Verify the right dose and the right time.

PURPOSE: It is important to do the first check of the label when getting the medications from the cabinet.

3. Assemble the supplies required for the procedure. If the insulin is cold, roll the vials in your hands to warm the medication.

PURPOSE: Remember to split up the three medication checks with activities between each check.

4. Perform the second medication check. Check the medication labels against the order. Check for the right name, form, and route.

PURPOSE: It is important to do the second check of the label before proceeding with the procedure.

PROCEDURE 15.6 Mixing Two Insulins—*continued*

5. Open and assemble the syringe and needle. Using a marker, label the syringe with the medication name. Mix the NPH insulin by rolling the vial in your hands. If present, remove the metal or plastic caps on the vials. Clean the rubber stoppers with an alcohol wipe. Let the stoppers dry.
   PURPOSE: The rubber stoppers must be disinfected each time you enter the vials with a needle.

6. With the syringe in a vertical position, pull the syringe plunger down. Draw up an amount of air equal to the amount of NPH insulin ordered. With the NPH vial on a firm surface, insert the needle in the rubber stopper. Inject the air into the NPH vial, keeping the needle tip out of the medication. Withdraw the needle from the stopper.
   PURPOSE: The vial is under pressure. Adding air is required before removing medication.

7. With the syringe in a vertical position, pull the syringe plunger down. Draw up an amount of air equal to the amount of Regular insulin ordered. With the Regular vial on a firm surface, insert the needle into the rubber stopper. Inject the air into the Regular vial, keeping the needle tip out of the medication.
   PURPOSE: The vial is under pressure. Adding air is required before removing medication.

8. With the palm of your nondominant hand facing upward, grasp the vial between your middle and index fingers. Keeping the syringe unit in the vial, pick up and invert them. Use your thumb, ring, and little fingers of your nondominant hand to stabilize the syringe in the vial. Pull down on the plunger until you have more Regular insulin than what you need.
   PURPOSE: It is important to stabilize the syringe, so the needle does not bend.

9. Continue to hold the vial/needle/syringe unit in a vertical position (with the needle pointing upward) with your nondominant hand. With your dominant hand, use either your fingers or a pen to tap the bubbles to the top of the barrel.
   PURPOSE: Bubbles rise to the top. With the syringe pointing straight up, the bubbles tend to move to the top of the barrel near the needle.

10. Once all the air bubbles are at the top, push the plunger slowly to the correct calibration marking for the ordered dose. Keep the syringe at eye level.
    PURPOSE: The air needs to be at the top of the syringe before you measure the correct amount of medication.

11. Double-check that no air bubbles are in the syringe and the right dose was measured. If everything is correct, remove the vial from the syringe/needle unit.
    PURPOSE: Air bubbles take up space. If air bubbles are present, then the correct dose will not be given.

12. Using an alcohol wipe, wipe the rubber stopper of the NPH vial. Calculate the total amount of insulin that needs to be given.
    PURPOSE: This total represents the calibration marking where the rubber stopper of the plunger needs to be pulled down to when withdrawing the NPH insulin.

13. With the NPH vial flat on a hard surface, insert the needle into the dried stopper. With the palm of your nondominant hand facing upward, grasp the vial between your middle and index fingers. Keeping the syringe unit in the vial, pick up and invert them. Use your thumb, ring, and little fingers of your nondominant hand to stabilize the syringe in the vial. Pull down on the plunger until the rubber stopper reaches the calibration mark required. Do not withdraw any extra NPH insulin.
    PURPOSE: If any additional NPH insulin is drawn up, the syringe must be discarded in the biohazard sharps container. No insulin can be injected into the NPH vial.

14. Double-check that no air bubbles are in the syringe and the right dose was measured. If everything is correct, remove the vial from the syringe/needle unit.
    PURPOSE: Air bubbles take up space. If air bubbles are present, discard the syringe and start over.

15. Use the one-hand scoop technique to cover the needle. Perform the third medication check. Check each medication label against the order. Check for the right name, form, and route.
    PURPOSE: It is important to do the third check of the label before seeing the patient.

16. Maintain the sterility of the medication and the needle throughout the procedure.
    PURPOSE: The needle and medication need to be sterile for the injection.

17. Clean up the work area. Put the packaging and other waste in the waste container. Place the insulin vials back in their storage location.
    PURPOSE: It is professional to clean up after yourself.

PROCEDURE 15.7 Administer an Intradermal Injection

Tasks: Prepare medication from a vial, administer an intradermal injection, read the tuberculin skin test, and document in the health record.

EQUIPMENT and SUPPLIES

- Provider's order
- Patient's health record
- Vial of medication

- Alcohol wipes
- 1-mL syringe with $\frac{1}{4}$- to $\frac{5}{8}$-inch, 25- to 27-gauge safety needle
- Bandage (if per facility's policy)
- Medication tray

Continued

PROCEDURE 15.7 | **Administer an Intradermal Injection**—*continued*

- Biohazard sharps container
- Waste container
- Drug reference information
- Gloves
- Marker and pen
- Millimeter ruler

Order: Tuberculin purified protein derivative (PPD) (5 tuberculin units) 0.1 mL ID

PROCEDURAL STEPS

1. Draw medication up from a vial (see Procedure 15.4).
2. Prior to entering the exam room, knock on the door and wait a moment. Greet the patient. Identify yourself. Verify the patient's identity with full name and date of birth. Make sure the patient's information matches the order and the record. Explain what you are going to do.
   PURPOSE: It is important to identify the patient in two different ways to ensure that you have the correct patient. Explaining the procedure can make the patient feel more comfortable and reduces anxiety.
3. Provide the right education to the patient. Explain the medication ordered, the desired effect, and common side effects; also identify the provider who ordered it. Answer any questions the patient may have. Use language the patient can understand. Ask the patient if he or she has any allergies. If the patient refuses the medication, notify the provider.
   PURPOSE: The patient needs to be aware of what you are giving, its action and side effects, and who ordered it. It is also important to double-check the patient's allergies before administering the medication.
4. Perform the right technique. Ask the patient the following questions:
   - Can you return in 48 to 72 hours for the reading?
   - Have you ever had BCG?
   - Have you ever had a TB skin test? If yes, did you have a reaction to it?
   PURPOSE: These questions are important to determine if the patient should get the test or if the medical assistant should talk with the provider.
5. Use hand sanitizer and put on gloves.
   PURPOSE: Hand sanitization is an important step for infection control.
6. Have the patient extend a forearm. With the palm facing upward, identify an appropriate site for an injection. The site should be 2 to 4 inches below the elbow. Loosen the cap on the needle, but still protect the needle from contamination. Open the alcohol wipes.
   PURPOSE: The site should be free from veins, scars, wounds, abrasions, and the like. If the person has a reaction, having the site away from the elbow does not limit its motion. Loosening the cap prior to starting allows you to remove the cap with one hand during the procedure.
7. Place your nondominant hand to the side of the site, pulling the skin taut (Fig. 1). Another option is to place your nondominant hand on the back of the patient's forearm, pulling the skin taut (Fig. 2).
   PURPOSE: The skin needs to be taut to insert the needle.

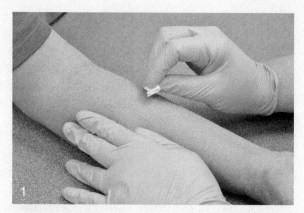

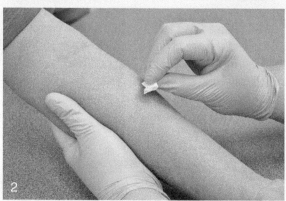

8. Cleanse the site with an alcohol wipe using a circular motion. Move from the center outward, using some friction to help clean the site. Create about a 2-inch circle at the site. Let the site dry while continuing to hold the area.
   PURPOSE: Cleaning from the inside to the outside prevents contamination of the cleaned area. Avoid waving over or blowing on the alcohol, which contaminates the site.
9. Pick up the syringe, and tip it to remove the cover. Grasp the syringe in your dominant hand, using your thumb and index finger. Make sure to have no fingers under the syringe. Ensure that the bevel is up.
   PURPOSE: The syringe needs to be lowered to the skin after it is inserted. Having fingers under the syringe changes the angle and can affect the administration.
10. At a 5- to 15-degree angle, slowly insert the needle until the bevel is covered with skin (Fig. 3). Carefully lower the syringe to the skin, and hold it steady with your dominant hand (Fig. 4).
    PURPOSE: If a greater angle is used or if more of the needle is inserted, the injection may be given deeper than it should be. Holding the syringe against the skin helps support it during the injection.

PROCEDURE 15.7 | Administer an Intradermal Injection—*continued*

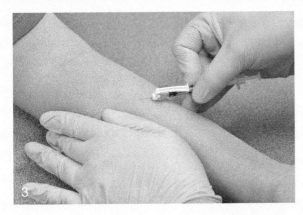

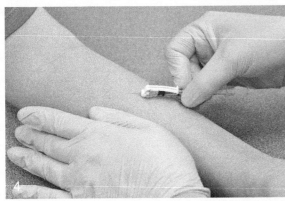

11. Carefully move your nondominant hand to the plunger. Slowly and steadily inject the medication by pressing on the plunger (Fig. 5). If a 6- to 10-mm wheal does not appear, repeat the test at least 2 inches from the site.
    PURPOSE: Any movement of the needle/syringe can dislodge the needle from the site.

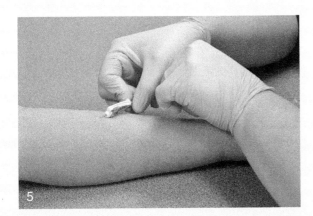

12. Double-check the barrel of the syringe to make sure all the medication was administered. Withdraw the needle. Activate the needle's safety device with one hand.
    PURPOSE: It is important to administer all the medication. Using more than one hand to activate the safety device increases the risk for needlestick injuries.

13. Discard the needle/syringe in a biohazard sharps container. Make sure to put the needle in first.
    PURPOSE: Safely discarding the needle/syringe will help prevent needlestick injuries.

14. Do not massage the area. According to the facility's policy, if the person is wearing a light-colored shirt with long sleeves, offer a bandage. Place the bandage on loosely to just absorb any blood from the site.
    PURPOSE: It is very important that the bandage not be put on snugly, because some of the medication could be lost at the site. If a bandage is used, it needs to be loosely applied. Some agencies will not allow the use of a bandage.

15. Observe the patient for any adverse reactions. Clean up the area. Discard the waste in the waste container. Sanitize your hands.
    PURPOSE: It is important to monitor the patient and clean up the work area.

16. Document the procedure in the health record. Include assessments done, allergies, teaching or instructions provided, the provider ordering the medication, the medication name, dose, route, and how the patient tolerated the medication. Also include the manufacturer, the lot number, and the expiration date of the vial.
    PURPOSE: Medications need to be documented to indicate they were given.

Scenario Update: The Patient Returns for the Reading

17. Check the health record to identify the location of the test. Greet the patient. Identify yourself. Verify the patient's identity with full name and date of birth. Make sure the patient's information matches the order and the record. Explain what you are going to do.
    PURPOSE: It is important to identify the patient in two different ways to ensure that you have the correct patient. Explaining the procedure can make the patient feel more comfortable and reduces anxiety.

18. Palpate the site for an induration. If an induration is felt, ask the patient if you can write on his or her arm. Using a ballpoint pen, draw a line toward the induration from the outer edge of the arm. Repeat on the other side (Fig. 6). Another option is to palpate the induration to find the edge and mark the edge with a pen. Repeat on the other side. Using a millimeter ruler, accurately measure the distance between the two points.
    PURPOSE: The ballpoint pen will stop at the edge of the induration. This provides you with two visible points to measure the size of the induration.

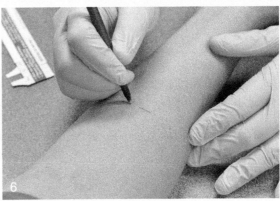

Continued

PROCEDURE 15.7   Administer an Intradermal Injection—*continued*

19. Document the reading in the patient's health record. Include the reason for the patient's visit, the test site, the size of the induration in millimeters, and the provider notified.
    PURPOSE: The medical assistant must document the size of the induration if one is present. If no induration is present, then document 0 mm. The provider will determine if the test is negative or positive.

Documentation Example: 1
11/1/20XX 0805 NKA. No prior history of TST. Per Dr. Martin's order, administered tuberculin purified protein derivative (PPD) 0.1 mL (5 tuberculin units) ID left forearm. (Vial: ABC Manufacturer, Lot#1345, Expires 10/20XX.) Pt tolerated test without a problem. Test side effects discussed with pt prior to administration. Pt instructed to return between 48 and 72 hours, and a follow-up appointment was made. Pt had no questions and verbalized understanding of instructions.
_____ Gabe Garcia, CMA (AAMA)

Documentation Example: 2
11/3/20XX 1005 Pt returned for TST reading. Left forearm induration measured 4 mm. Dr. Martin was notified._____ Gabe Garcia, CMA (AAMA)

PROCEDURE 15.8   Administer a Subcutaneous Injection

Tasks: Prepare medication from a vial, administer a subcutaneous injection, and document the medication administration in the health record.

Scenario: Dr. Martin ordered polio vaccine (IPV) 0.5 mL subcut for Johnny Parker (DOB 06/15/2010). (Vial information: ABC Manufacturer, Lot #1234, expires 1 year from today.)

EQUIPMENT and SUPPLIES

- Provider's order
- Patient's health record
- Vial of medication
- Alcohol wipes
- 3-mL syringe with ⅝-inch or ½-inch, 25-gauge needle
- Gauze
- Bandage
- Medication tray
- Biohazard sharps container
- Waste container
- Drug reference information
- VIS for polio vaccine (IPV) (optional)
- Gloves
- Marker

Order: Polio vaccine (IPV) 0.5 mL subcut

PROCEDURAL STEPS

1. Draw medication up from a vial (see Procedure 15.4).
2. (*Peer will play the parent.*) Prior to entering the exam room, knock on the door and wait a moment. Greet the parent/patient. Identify yourself. Verify the patient's identity with full name and date of birth. Make sure the patient's information matches the order and the record. Explain what you are going to do.
   PURPOSE: It is important to identify the patient in two different ways to ensure that you have the correct patient. Explaining the procedure can make the patient feel more comfortable and reduces anxiety.

3. Provide the right education to the parent/patient. Explain the medication ordered, the desired effect, and common side effects; also identify the provider who ordered it. Answer any questions the patient may have. Use language the patient can understand. Ask the patient if he or she has any allergies. If the patient refuses the medication, notify the provider.
   PURPOSE: The patient needs to be aware of what you are giving, its action and side effects, and who ordered it. It is also important to double-check the patient's allergies before administering the medication.
4. Use hand sanitizer and put on gloves.
   PURPOSE: Hand sanitization is an important step for infection control.
5. Loosen the cap on the needle, but still protect the needle from contamination. Open the alcohol wipes. Have gauze and a bandage available.
   PURPOSE: Loosening the cap prior to starting allows you to remove the cap with one hand during the procedure. You should never remove the cap with your teeth.
6. Find the injection site.
   PURPOSE: It is important to find the correct location for the injection.
7. Cleanse the site with an alcohol wipe using a circular motion (Fig. 1). Move from the center outward, using some friction to help clean the site. Create about a 2-inch circle at the site. Let the site dry.
   PURPOSE: Cleaning from the inside to the outside prevents contamination of the cleaned area. Avoid waving over or blowing on the alcohol, which contaminates the site.

PROCEDURE 15.8 | Administer a Subcutaneous Injection—*continued*

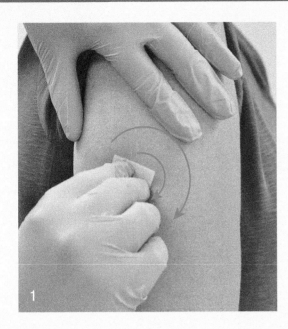

8. Perform the right technique. Place a gauze between the index and middle fingers of your nondominant hand. With that hand, use your index finger and thumb to pinch up at the cleansed area.
   PURPOSE: The site needs to be pinched for a subcut injection.
9. Pick up the syringe, and tip it to remove the cover. Hold the syringe between the thumb and index finger of your dominant hand (Fig. 2). Quickly and smoothly insert the needle into the site at a 45- or 90-degree angle, depending on the needle size. Insert the entire needle. Make sure the needle tip is not pointed toward your nondominant hand.
   PURPOSE: Ensuring that the tip is not pointed toward your hand will lessen the needlestick risk. Aspiration for subcut injections is based on the facility's policy and the recommendation from the manufacturer.

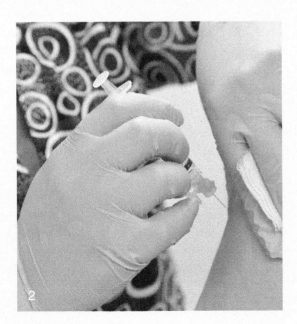

10. *One-hand option*: Continue to pinch the site. Securely grasp the syringe between the fingers of your dominant hand. With your dominant hand, aspirate if required, and then push the plunger to inject the medication. *Two-hand option*: Release the pinch and with the nondominant hand, aspirate if required, and then push the plunger to inject the medication.
    PURPOSE: Follow the facility's policy on whether to use the one- or two-hand option.
11. Inject the medication at a rate of 1 mL over 10 seconds. Ensure that all the medication has been injected before pulling out the needle at the same angle used for entry. Release the pinch if using the one-hand option.
    PURPOSE: Injecting the medication too slowly or too quickly can be uncomfortable for the patient.
12. Activate the needle's safety device with one hand while the other hand covers the site with gauze. Gently apply pressure at the site to stop any bleeding. Apply a bandage if the patient requests it.
    PURPOSE: Ask the patient if he or she would like a bandage if the site has stopped bleeding. Remember that some bandages may contain latex, which can be an allergen to some people. Some people may be allergic to the adhesive.
13. Discard the needle/syringe in a biohazard sharps container. Make sure the needle goes into the sharps container first.
    PURPOSE: Safely discarding the needle/syringe will help prevent needlestick injuries.
14. Observe the patient for any adverse reactions. Clean up the area. Discard the waste in the waste container. Sanitize your hands.
    PURPOSE: It is important to monitor the patient and to clean up the work area.
15. Document the procedure in the health record. Include assessments done; allergies; teaching or instructions provided; the name of the provider who ordered the medication; the medication's name, dose, and route; and how the patient tolerated the medication. Also include the manufacturer, the lot number, and the expiration date for the vaccines and controlled substances. Fig. 3 shows the documentation using an electronic health record.
    PURPOSE: Medications need to be documented to indicate they were given.

Continued

| PROCEDURE 15.8 | Administer a Subcutaneous Injection—*continued* |

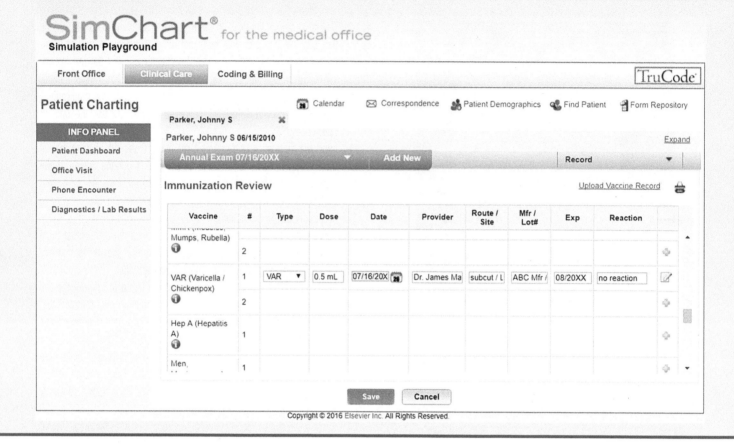

PROCEDURE 15.9 | Administer an Intramuscular Injection

Tasks: Prepare medication from a vial, administer an intramuscular injection, and document the medication administration in the health record.

Scenario: Dr. Martin ordered influenza vaccine (IIV) 0.5 mL IM for Erma Willis (DOB 12/09/1947). (Vial information: MN Manufacturer, Lot #7845, expires 1 year from today.)

EQUIPMENT and SUPPLIES

- Provider's order
- Patient's health record
- Vial of medication
- Alcohol wipes
- 3-mL syringe
- 22–25 gauge, 1–1½ -inch needle
- Gauze
- Bandage
- Medication tray
- Biohazard sharps container
- Waste container
- Drug reference information
- VIS for influenza vaccine (optional)

- Gloves
- Marker

Order: Influenza vaccine (IIV) 0.5 mL IM.

PROCEDURAL STEPS

1. Draw medication up from a vial (see Procedure 15.4).
2. Prior to entering the exam room, knock on the door and wait a moment. Greet the patient. Identify yourself. Verify the patient's identity with full name and date of birth. Make sure the patient's information matches the order and the record. Explain what you are going to do.
   <u>PURPOSE:</u> It is important to identify the patient in two different ways to ensure that you have the correct patient. Explaining the procedure can make the patient feel more comfortable and reduces anxiety.

PROCEDURE 15.9 **Administer an Intramuscular Injection**—*continued*

3. Provide the right education to the parent/patient. Explain the medication ordered, the desired effect, and common side effects; also identify the provider who ordered it. Answer any questions the patient may have. Use language the patient can understand. Ask the patient if he or she has any allergies. If the patient refuses the medication, notify the provider.
   PURPOSE: The patient needs to be aware of what you are giving, its action and side effects, and who ordered it. It is also important to double-check the patient's allergies before administering the medication.

4. Use hand sanitizer and put on gloves.
   PURPOSE: Hand sanitization is an important step for infection control.

5. Loosen the cap on the needle, but still protect the needle from contamination. Open the alcohol wipes. Have gauze and a bandage available.
   PURPOSE: Loosening the cap prior to starting allows you to remove the cap with one hand during the procedure. You should never remove the cap with your teeth.

6. Find the site using the landmarks.
   PURPOSE: It is important to find the correct location for the injection.

7. Cleanse the site with an alcohol wipe using a circular motion. Move from the center outward, using some friction to help clean the site. Create about a 2-inch circle at the site. Let the site dry.
   PURPOSE: Cleaning from the inside to the outside prevents contamination of the cleaned area. Avoid waving over or blowing on the alcohol, which contaminates the site.

8. Perform the right technique. Place a gauze between the index and middle fingers of your nondominant hand. With that hand, stretch or flatten the site. Hold the site.
   PURPOSE: The site needs to be flattened or stretched for an intramuscular injection.

9. Pick up the syringe, and tip it to remove the cover. Hold the syringe like a dart with your dominant hand (Fig. 1). Quickly and smoothly insert the needle into the site at a 90-degree angle. Insert the entire needle.
   PURPOSE: Inserting the needle quickly is important to minimize pain.

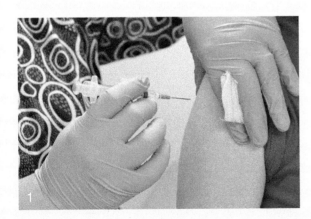

10. *One-hand option:* Continue to hold the site. Securely grasp the syringe between the fingers of your dominant hand. Place your thumb under the plunger edge, and push the plunger out farther to aspirate (Fig. 2).

Two-hand option: Move your nondominant hand to the plunger. Pull the plunger out farther to aspirate.
PURPOSE: It is important to aspirate before giving an IM injection. Follow the facility's policy on whether to use the one- or two-hand option.

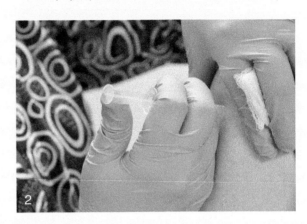

11. Aspirate for 5 seconds, and check the barrel for blood. If blood is seen, pull out the needle and discard it. Restart the procedure. If no blood is seen, inject the medication at a rate of about 10 seconds per milliliter. Ensure that all the medication has been injected before pulling out the needle at the same angle used for entry.
    PURPOSE: It is important not to give the injection if the needle is in the bloodstream.

12. Activate the needle's safety device with one hand while the other hand covers the site with gauze. Gently apply pressure at the site to stop any bleeding. Apply a bandage if the patient requests it.
    PURPOSE: Ask the patient if he or she would like a bandage if the site has stopped bleeding. Remember that some bandages may contain latex, which can be an allergen to some people. Some people may be allergic to the adhesive.

13. Discard the needle/syringe in a biohazard sharps container. Make sure to put the needle in first.
    PURPOSE: Safely discarding the needle/syringe will help prevent needlestick injuries.

14. Observe the patient for any adverse reactions. Clean up the area. Discard the waste in the waste container. Sanitize your hands.
    PURPOSE: It is important to monitor the patient and clean up the work area.

15. Document the procedure in the health record. Include assessments done; allergies; teaching or instructions provided; the name of the provider who ordered the medication; the medication's name, dose, and route; and how the patient tolerated the medication. Also include the manufacturer, the lot number, and the expiration date for the vaccines and controlled substances. Fig. 3 shows the documentation using an electronic health record.
    PURPOSE: Medications need to be documented to indicate they were given.

Continued

PROCEDURE 15.9 | Administer an Intramuscular Injection—*continued*

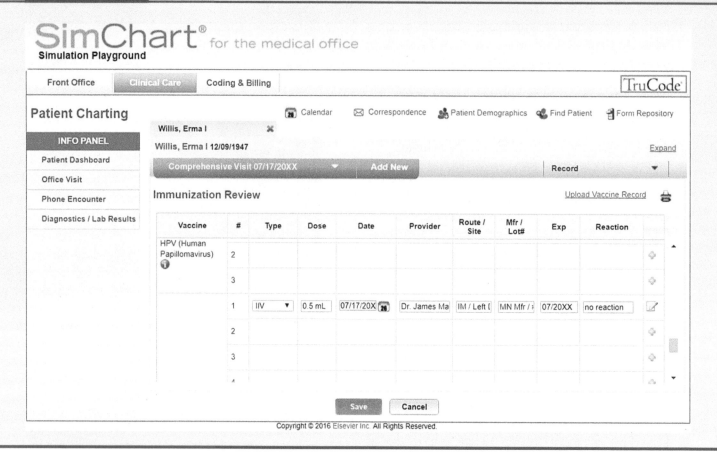

PROCEDURE 15.10 | **Administer an Intramuscular Injection Using the Z-Track Technique**

Tasks: Prepare medication from a vial, administer an intramuscular injection, and document the medication administration in the health record.

Scenario: Dr. Martin orders Iron Dextran 0.5 mL IM for Erma Willis (DOB 12/09/1947). (Vial information: FE Manufacturer, Lot #625, expires 1 year from today.)

EQUIPMENT and SUPPLIES

- Provider's order
- Patient's health record
- Vial of medication
- Alcohol wipes
- 3-mL syringe
- 22–25 gauge, 1–1½ -inch needle
- Gauze
- Bandage
- Medication tray
- Biohazard sharps container
- Waste container
- Drug reference information
- Gloves
- Marker

PROCEDURAL STEPS

1. Draw medication up from a vial (see Procedure 15.4).
2. Prior to entering the exam room, knock on the door and wait a moment. Greet the patient. Identify yourself. Verify the patient's identity with full name and date of birth. Make sure the patient's information matches the order and the record. Explain what you are going to do.
   PURPOSE: It is important to identify the patient in two different ways to ensure that you have the correct patient. Explaining the procedure can make the patient feel more comfortable and reduces anxiety.
3. Provide the right education to the parent/patient. Explain the medication ordered, the desired effect, and common side effects; also identify the provider who ordered it. Answer any questions the patient may have. Use language the patient can understand. Ask the patient if he or she has any allergies. If the patient refuses the medication, notify the provider.

PROCEDURE 15.10 | **Administer an Intramuscular Injection Using the Z-Track Technique—*continued***

PURPOSE: The patient needs to be aware of what you are giving, its action and side effects, and who ordered it. It is also important to double-check the patient's allergies before administering the medication.

4. Use hand sanitizer and put on gloves.
   PURPOSE: Hand sanitization is an important step for infection control.

5. Loosen the cap on the needle, but still protect the needle from contamination. Open the alcohol wipes. Have gauze and a bandage available.
   PURPOSE: Loosening the cap prior to starting allows you to remove the cap with one hand during the procedure. You should never remove the cap with your teeth.

6. Find the site using the landmarks.
   PURPOSE: It is important to find the correct site.

7. Perform the right technique. Place a gauze between the index and middle fingers of your nondominant hand. With that hand, displace the tissue.
   PURPOSE: The tissue needs to be displaced before you cleanse the site.

8. Cleanse the site with an alcohol wipe using a circular motion. Move from the center outward, using some friction to help clean the site. Create about a 2-inch circle at the site. Let the site dry while continuing to hold the area.
   PURPOSE: Cleaning from the inside to the outside prevents contamination of the cleaned area. Avoid waving over or blowing on the alcohol, which contaminates the site.

9. Pick up the syringe, and tip it to remove the cover. Hold the syringe like a dart with your dominant hand. Quickly and smoothly insert the needle into the site at a 90-degree angle. Insert the entire needle.
   PURPOSE: Inserting the needle quickly is important to minimize pain.

10. Continue to hold the site. Securely grasp the syringe between the fingers of your dominant hand. Place your thumb under the plunger edge, and push the plunger out farther to aspirate.
    PURPOSE: It is important to aspirate before giving an IM injection. Follow the facility's policy on whether to use the one- or two-hand option.

11. Aspirate for 5 seconds, and check the barrel for blood. If blood is seen, pull out the needle and discard it. Restart the procedure. If no blood is seen, inject the medication at a rate of about 10 seconds per milliliter.

Ensure that all the medication has been injected. Wait 10 seconds before withdrawing the needle and letting go with your nondominant hand.
PURPOSE: It is important not to give the injection if the needle is in the bloodstream. Waiting 10 seconds allows the medication to start absorbing.

12. Activate the needle's safety device with one hand while the other hand covers the site with gauze. Gently apply pressure at the site to stop any bleeding. Apply a bandage if the patient requests it.
    PURPOSE: Ask the patient if he or she would like a bandage if the site has stopped bleeding. Remember that some bandages may contain latex, which can be an allergen to some people. Some people may be allergic to the adhesive.

13. Discard the needle/syringe in a biohazard sharps container. Make sure to put the needle in first.
    PURPOSE: Safely discarding the needle/syringe will help prevent needlestick injuries.

14. Observe the patient for any adverse reactions. Clean up the area. Discard the waste in the waste container. Sanitize your hands.
    PURPOSE: It is important to monitor the patient and also clean up the work area.

15. Document the procedure in the health record. Include assessments done; allergies; teaching or instructions provided; the name of the provider who ordered the medication; the medication's name, dose, and route; and how the patient tolerated the medication. Also include the manufacturer, the lot number, and the expiration date for the vaccines and controlled substances.
    PURPOSE: Medications need to be documented to indicate they were given.

Documentation Example:
11/1/20XX 1420 NKA. Per Dr. Martin's order, administered Iron Dextran 0.5 mL IM in left ventrogluteal site using Z-track method. Pt stated she had pain initially but is feeling better. Side effects were discussed with pt prior to administration. Pt had no questions and verbalized understanding of instructions.
_____Gabe Garcia, CMA (AAMA)

16

OPHTHALMOLOGY AND OTOLARYNGOLOGY

Kim Tau, a certified medical assistant (CMA) through the American Association of Medical Assistants (AAMA), has worked at Walden-Martin Family Medical (WMFM) Clinic for several years. Kim has always enjoyed working with the ophthalmology and otolaryngology patients. Amy Ling was recently hired at WMFM, and Kim's supervisor asked her to help orient Amy to the practice. Amy recently graduated from a medical assistant program and is familiar with basic eye and ear procedures, but she has many questions about her responsibilities at the clinic. Amy will be responsible for performing initial Snellen and Ishihara

screening examinations on new patients and for assisting the ophthalmologist and the optician in the practice. She also must become proficient in conducting audiometry screening tests on pediatric patients, performing ear irrigations, and administering otic medications. Kim recognizes that it is important for Amy to be able to perform these skills with accuracy and confidence; however, she also must develop a sensitivity to the communication and education needs of patients with eye and ear disorders.

While studying this chapter, think about the following questions:

- What is the basic anatomy and physiology of the eye and of the ear?
- What are the major types of refractive errors?
- Which eye and ear disorders does Amy need to be familiar with on a routine basis?
- How is a Snellen test performed?
- What important steps should Amy follow when performing eye and ear irrigations and medication applications?
- How is an examination with an audiometer conducted?
- How should Kim prepare Amy to care for patients with sensory loss?

LEARNING OBJECTIVES

1. Explain the differences among an ophthalmologist, an optometrist, and an optician.
2. Identify the anatomic structures of the eye, and discuss the process of vision.
3. Identify the anatomic structures of the ear, and explain the functions of the external ear, middle ear, and inner ear.
4. Differentiate among the major types of refractive errors.
5. Summarize typical disorders of the eye and eyeball other than refractive errors.
6. Describe the conditions that can lead to hearing loss, including conductive and sensorineural impairments.
7. Define other major disorders of the ear, including otitis, impacted cerumen, and Ménière's disease.
8. Assist with the ophthalmology examination, and discuss what the acronym PERRLA stands for.
9. Assist with the otolaryngology examination, and discuss useful questions for gathering a history of ear problems.
10. Discuss distance visual acuity, and perform a visual acuity test using the Snellen chart.
11. Discuss visual acuity, and assess color acuity using the Ishihara test.
12. Assist with otolaryngology diagnostic procedures, and use an audiometer to accurately measure a patient's hearing acuity.
13. Assist with ophthalmology treatments, and explain the purposes of and the proper procedures for eye irrigation and the instillation of eye medication.
14. Assist with otolaryngology treatments, identify the purposes of ear irrigations and the instillation of ear medications, and demonstrate the proper procedures for both ear irrigation and instilling medicated eardrops.

VOCABULARY

accommodation Adjustment of the eye that allows a person to see various sizes of objects at different distances.

amblyopia (am blee OH pee ah) Dull or dim vision, with no apparent organic defect.

audible (AW di buhl) Capable of being heard.

audiologist (aw dee OL uh jist) Allied healthcare professional who specializes in the evaluation of hearing function, detection of hearing impairment, and determination of the anatomic site of impairment.

auditory cortex The region of the cerebral cortex that receives auditory data.

biconvex (bie KON veks) Having two outward curving surfaces, on a lens.

binocular (buh NOK yuh ler) Involving, relating, or seeing with both eyes.

dynamic (die NAM ik) **equilibrium** Relating to balance when moving at an angle or rotating.

equilibrium (ee kwi LIB ree uhm) A state of rest or balance due to the equal action of opposing forces.

evert (ih VURT) To turn the eyelid inside out; the provider typically does this to inspect the area for foreign bodies.

gonioscopy (goh nee AH skuh pee) Used to diagnose glaucoma and to inspect ocular movement.

hertz (hurts) The unit of measurement used in hearing examinations; a wave frequency equal to one cycle per second.

medulla oblongata (muh DUHL uh ob lawng GAH tah) The lowest part of the brain, continuous with the top of the spinal cord.

miotic (my OT ik) Any substance or medication that causes constriction of the pupil.

otosclerosis (oh tuh skleh ROH sis) The ossicles of the middle ear (malleolus, incus, and stapes) become fused and act as a single unit instead of individual bones.

ototoxic (oh tuh TOK sik) A medicine or substance capable of damaging cranial nerve VIII or the organs of hearing and balance.

photophobia (foh toh FOH bee ah) Extreme sensitivity to light.

psoriasis (suh RIE i sis) A usually chronic, recurrent skin disease marked by bright red patches covered with silvery scales.

seborrhea (seb uh REE ah) An excessive discharge of sebum from the sebaceous glands, forming greasy scales or crusty areas on the body.

sensorineural (sen suh ree NOOR uhl) Involving the sensory nerves, especially as they affect hearing.

serous (SEER uhs) A thin, watery serum-like drainage.

static (STAT ik) **equilibrium** Relating to balance when moving in a straight line.

suppurative (SUHP yuh ruh tiv) Characterized by the formation or discharge of pus.

thalamus (THAL uh muhs) The middle part of the brain through which sensory impulses pass to reach the cerebral cortex.

tinnitus (TIN it uhs) A noise sensation of ringing heard in one or both ears.

tonometer (toh NOM i ter) An instrument used to measure intraocular pressure.

vascular (VAS kyuh ler) Having (blood) vessels that conduct or circulate liquids (blood).

vertigo (VUR ti goh) Dizziness; abnormal sensations of movement when there is none.

A medical assistant is responsible for performing a wide variety of procedures in an ophthalmologic or otorhinolaryngologic practice. First, the medical assistant must be familiar with the normal anatomy and physiology of the eyes, ears, nose, and throat. With an understanding of how these specialty sensory organs function, the medical assistant can master the skills needed to become a valuable asset to providers who specialize in the treatment of eye and ear disorders.

Ophthalmology is the science of the eye and its disorders and diseases. A physician who specializes in the diagnosis and treatment of disorders and diseases of the eye is an *ophthalmologist*. An ophthalmologist is a licensed medical physician who can diagnose eye disorders, prescribe medication, conduct eye screenings, prescribe glasses or contact lenses, and perform optic surgery. An *optometrist* is not a medical doctor, but he or she is licensed and has earned a degree as a doctor of optometry (OD). An optometrist can perform eye examinations, diagnose vision problems and eye diseases, prescribe ophthalmic medications, and treat visual defects through corrective lenses and eye exercises. *Opticians* are trained to fill prescriptions written by ophthalmologists and optometrists for corrective lenses by grinding the lenses and dispensing eyewear.

Otorhinolaryngology is the medical specialty that deals with the ear, nose, and throat. It frequently is referred to as *otolaryngology* or even as a single specialty of otology or laryngology. Usually, the specialty otorhinolaryngology is referred to simply as *ear, nose, and throat* (ENT). An otolaryngologist is a licensed medical physician who is trained in the medical and surgical management and treatment of patients with diseases and disorders of the ear, nose, throat, and related structures of the head and neck.

ANATOMY OF THE EYE

The eye can be divided into the *ocular adnexa*, the structures that surround and support the function of the eyeball, and the structures of the eye itself.

Ocular Adnexa

Each of our paired eyes is encased in a protective, bony socket called the *orbit*. Our **binocular** vision sends two slightly different images to the brain that produce depth of vision. Within the orbit, a cushion of fatty tissue protects the eyeball. Only about one-sixth of the eye lies outside the orbit. The eyelid helps protect the eye from trauma. The eyebrows help keep irritants out of the eyes. The eyelashes line the margins of the eyelids and help trap foreign particles (Fig. 16.1).

The *conjunctiva* is a thin mucous membrane that lines the eyelid. It covers the outside of the eyeball except for the most central portion. The *cornea* covers the center of the eye. The mucus secreted from the conjunctiva helps keep the eye moist. The eye blinks about every 2 to 3 seconds. Blinking causes the *lacrimal gland*, located in the superior outer portion of the upper eyelid, to secrete tears. Tears move across the eyes, cleansing and moistening the surface of the eye. Tears drain into the lacrimal canals in the medial corner of the eye. The tears then drain into the nasal cavity through the *nasolacrimal*

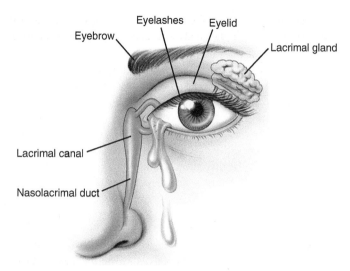

FIGURE 16.1 Ocular adnexa. (From Herlihy B, Maebius NK: *The human body in health and illness,* ed 4, Philadelphia, 2011, Saunders.)

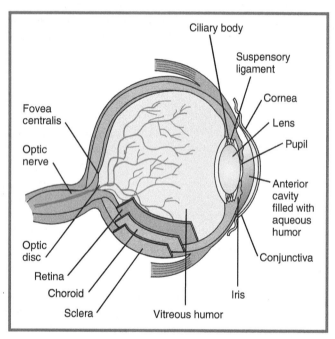

FIGURE 16.2 Anatomy of the eye.

duct. This is why when a person cries, the excess tears ultimately empty into the nose, producing a watery nasal discharge.

Eyeball

The eyeball consists of three layers. The outermost layer is made up of the white, opaque *sclera* (SKLAYR a) and the transparent cornea. The sclera is a tough, fibrous lining that protects the entire eyeball lying within the orbit. It is also known as the white of the eye. The transparent cornea covers the exposed one-sixth of the eyeball. The cornea acts like a window that allows light to enter the eye. The cornea also *refracts,* or bends the direction of light rays, after they enter the eye (Fig. 16.2).

The middle layer is made up of the *choroid,* the *iris,* and the *ciliary body.* The iris is the colored portion of the eye. It is doughnut shaped,

with an opening in the center called the *pupil.* The iris contains muscles that regulate the size of the pupil depending on the intensity of light. It becomes smaller in bright light and opens wider in dim light. The ciliary body contains both the ciliary muscle, which regulates the shape of the lens, and the ciliary processes, which secrete *aqueous humor.* The choroid is the posterior portion of the middle layer of the eye. It is the eye's **vascular** layer. It contains many blood vessels that supply nutrients to the outer layers of the *retina.* The choroid also has a brown pigment that absorbs excess light rays that could interfere with vision.

The inner layer of the eye includes the retina in the posterior portion and the lens in the anterior portion. The delicate tissue of the retina is composed of light-sensitive neurons called rods and cones. *Rods* are highly sensitive to light and can function in dim light. *Cones* function in bright light and detect color. Rods and cones convert light into nerve impulses. These impulses travel through the optic nerve to the brain, where they are converted into images.

The lens is a transparent, **biconvex** body that helps focus light after it passes through the cornea. The lens and the ciliary body divide the eye into two cavities. The posterior cavity, which is between the lens and the retina, contains the transparent, gel-like *vitreous humor.* The vitreous humor maintains the shape of the posterior eyeball. The anterior cavity, between the cornea and the lens, is filled with aqueous humor, which is continuously produced by the ciliary processes. Aqueous humor helps maintain normal pressure within the eye and provides nutrients to the lens and the cornea (see Fig. 16.2).

CRITICAL THINKING APPLICATION   16.1
To help Amy become familiar with the terminology used in ophthalmology, Kim asks her to describe the three layers of the eyeball. How would you respond?

PHYSIOLOGY OF THE EYE

Vision requires light and depends on the proper functioning of all parts of the eye (Table 16.1). A visual impulse begins with the passage of light through the cornea, where the light is refracted; it then passes through the aqueous humor and the pupil into the lens. The ciliary muscle adjusts the curvature of the lens to again refract the light rays so that they pass into the retina, triggering the photoreceptor cells of the rods and cones. At this point, the light energy is converted into an electrical impulse, which is sent through the optic nerve to the visual cortex of the occipital lobe of the brain; there, the light impulse is interpreted, and a picture is created.

ANATOMY OF THE EAR

The visible portion of the ear is only a small part of the actual organ of hearing. Most of the sensory structure lies hidden in the *temporal* bone of the skull. The ear is divided into the outer, middle, and inner ear (Fig. 16.3).

Outer (External) Ear

The outer ear consists of the *auricle,* or *pinna.* This is the fleshy part of the ear that can be seen on the side of the head. The next structure

TABLE 16.1 Functions of the Major Parts of the Eye

STRUCTURE	FUNCTION
Sclera	External protection
Cornea	Light refraction
Choroid	Blood supply
Iris	Light absorption and regulation of pupil width
Ciliary body	Secretion of vitreous fluid; changes the shape of the lens
Lens	Light refraction
Retinal layer	Light receptor that transforms optic signals into nerve impulses
Rods	Distinguish light from dark and perceive shape and movement
Cones	Color vision
Central fovea	Area of sharpest vision
Macula lutea	Center of the retina; contains the fovea centralis, the area of most highly acute vision
External ocular muscles	Move the eyeball
Optic nerve	One of a pair of nerves that transmit visual stimuli to (cranial nerve II) the brain
Lacrimal glands	Produce tears
Eyelid	Protects eye

Modified from Damjanov I: *Pathology for the health-related professions*, Philadelphia, 1996, Saunders.

is the external *auditory canal*, the tube that extends from the auricle into the *tympanic membrane* (eardrum).

The auricle collects sound waves and sends them into the auditory canal. The skin that lines the auditory canal contains numerous hair follicles and many nerve endings. Earwax, or *cerumen*, is secreted by modified sweat glands within the external auditory canal. Both the hair and the waxy cerumen help prevent foreign objects from reaching the eardrum. The canal has a slightly curved shape and is approximately 1 inch (2.5 cm) long.

Middle Ear

The middle ear is an air-filled cavity that contains three tiny bones called the *ossicles*: malleus, incus, and stapes. Tiny ligaments link these three tiny bones to form a bridge from the tympanic membrane to the inner ear. The ossicles transmit sound to the inner ear through the movement of the stapes. Within the middle ear is an opening for the *eustachian tube*. This is a connection between the ears and the throat. This connection helps equalize pressure within the middle ear. Without equalized pressure in the ear, hearing would not be possible.

The tympanic membrane is a thin, disc-shaped tissue that seals off the outer ear from the middle ear. Sound waves conducted through the external auditory canal hit the tympanic membrane and cause it to vibrate. The vibrations are picked up by the three ossicles and are changed from air-conducted sound waves to bone-conducted sound waves. The ossicles transmit the bone-conducted sound waves through the middle ear to the *oval window*. The oval window is a membrane that connects the middle ear and the inner ear. At the oval window, the sound waves move into the fluids of the inner ear. The fluid motion excites receptors, changing the bone-conducted sound into **sensorineural** impulses.

Inner Ear

Once sound is conducted to the oval window, it is transmitted to a structure called the *labyrinth*, or the inner ear. The inner ear is divided into the *cochlea* and the *semicircular canals*, which are joined by the *vestibule*. The semicircular canals and vestibule function to maintain **equilibrium**. The cochlea is responsible for the sense of hearing.

The *organ of Corti*, which contains the receptors for sound, is located within the cochlea. It is made up of hairlike sensory cells surrounded by sensory nerve fibers that form the cochlear branch of the eighth cranial nerve. Sound impulses cause the hairs to bend and rub against the nerve fibers, which initiate stimuli to travel through the cochlear nerve into the brain for sound interpretation.

The semicircular canals are responsible for evaluating the position of the head in relation to the pull of gravity. The three canals are positioned at right angles to one another, on different planes. When the head turns rapidly, these fluid-filled canals must rapidly adjust and send the information to the central nervous system (CNS). The CNS then interprets the information and initiates the desired response to maintain balance. The semicircular canals detect **dynamic equilibrium**. Within the vestibule, two saclike structures function to establish the body's **static equilibrium**. With repetitive or excessive stimulation to the equilibrium receptors, some people become nauseated and may vomit. This condition is known as *motion sensitivity* or *motion sickness*.

PHYSIOLOGY OF THE EAR

Hearing starts with the soundwaves reaching the tympanic membrane. Those sound waves cause the tympanic membrane to vibrate, which causes the ossicles to transmit the waves to the oval window. It is at the inner ear that the sensorineural impulses reach the cochlea.

The organ of Corti contains the receptors for sound and is located within the cochlea of the inner ear. Sound impulses cause the hairlike sensory cells of the cochlea to bend and rub against the nerve fibers. The movement initiates an auditory impulse, which travels through the cochlear nerve onto the eighth cranial nerve. The eighth cranial nerve transmits the auditory impulse to the **medulla oblongata**. The impulses then travel to the **thalamus** and on to the **auditory cortex** of the temporal lobe of the brain. The brain then interprets the auditory impulse into **audible** sound and speech patterns.

DISORDERS OF THE EYE

Refractive Errors

Four major types of refractive errors result when the eye is unable to focus light effectively on the retina. *Refraction* is the ability of the

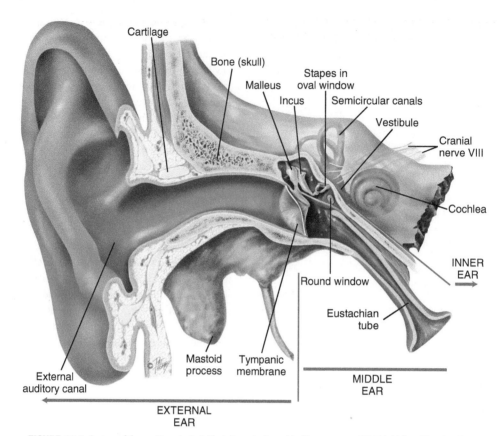

FIGURE 16.3 Anatomy of the ear. (From Jarvis C: *Physical examination and health assessment,* ed 7, Philadelphia, 2016, Saunders.)

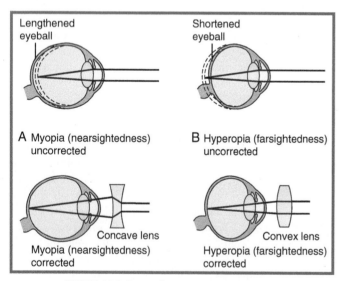

FIGURE 16.4 Errors in refraction. **(A)** Myopia. **(B)** Hyperopia.

lens of the eye to bend parallel light rays coming into the eye so that the rays are focused simultaneously on the retina. An *error of refraction* means that the light rays are not refracted or bent properly and consequently do not focus correctly on the retina. Defects in the shape of the eyeball can cause a refractive error. Most refractive errors can be corrected with corrective lenses, contacts, or surgery (Fig. 16.4).

Hyperopia (Farsightedness)

When light enters the eye and focuses behind the retina, a person has *hyperopia.* This disorder occurs when the eyeball is too short from the anterior to the posterior wall. An individual with hyperopia has difficulty seeing objects that are close, at reading or working level. A convex corrective lens helps the eye's internal lens place objects directly on the retina and creates a sharp, detailed image, or refractive surgery may be done to correct the shape of the lens.

Myopia (Nearsightedness)

Myopia occurs when light rays entering the eye focus in front of the retina, causing objects at a distance to appear blurry and dull. Objects viewed at reading or working level are seen clearly. In this disorder, the eyeball is elongated from the anterior to the posterior wall, and the image cannot be sharpened by the internal lens of the eye. A concave corrective lens is used to focus the light rays on the retina, or surgery can be done to change the shape of the cornea. However, the surgery is performed only on adults who have had a stable eye prescription for at least 1 year.

Presbyopia

As people age, the lens of the eye becomes less flexible, and the ciliary muscles weaken; consequently, changing the point of focus from distance to near becomes difficult. This is called *presbyopia.* The condition results in difficulty seeing at reading level. A combination corrective lens, known as a *bifocal lens* or a *progressive lens correction,* is used to focus both distal and proximal objects directly on the retina. Presbyopia actually starts at approximately age 10, but most people do not report an alteration in vision until their early 40s. Conductive keratoplasty is a laser surgical procedure used to treat presbyopia.

Astigmatism

Astigmatism occurs when light rays entering the eye are focused irregularly. This usually occurs because the cornea or the lens is not a smooth sphere, but rather has an irregular shape. Ophthalmologists describe the lens as being shaped like a football rather than a sphere, such as a basketball. This causes light rays to be unevenly or diffusely focused on the retina, resulting in blurred vision. It is like attempting to focus on objects seen through a wavy piece of window glass. Astigmatism can be corrected with glasses, contacts, or surgery. Surgical correction attempts to reshape the cornea into a more spherical or uniformly curved surface.

Signs and Symptoms of Refractive Errors

Refractive errors in vision can lead to squinting, frequent rubbing of the eyes, and headaches. The individual notices blurred vision, fading of words at reading level, or both. Some refractive errors are familial in nature.

Treatment of Refractive Errors

Eyeglasses and contact lenses are the traditional treatments for visual acuity problems caused by refractive errors. However, problems with the shape of the lens can be corrected surgically. Surgery is performed on an outpatient basis and requires only a short stay in the facility. Medical assistants employed in an outpatient eye surgery facility must be trained to fulfill this specialized role.

Surgical Correction of Refractive Errors

Most types of health insurance do not cover surgery for refractive corrections. On average, each eye costs $1500 to $3000. The following are some of the surgical procedures performed to correct refractive errors.

- *Photorefractive keratectomy (PRK):* The first surgical procedure developed to reshape the cornea with a laser. The same type of laser is used for PRK and LASIK. The major difference between the two types of surgery is the way the middle layer of the cornea is exposed before it is vaporized with the laser. In PRK, the top layer of the cornea (the epithelium) is scraped away to expose the stromal layer underneath. In LASIK, a flap is cut in the stromal layer.
- *Laser-assisted in situ keratomileusis (LASIK):* LASIK uses an excimer laser to reshape the central cornea to treat myopia, hyperopia, and astigmatism. A thin, hinged flap of cornea is created, the flap is lifted, and the exposed surface of the cornea is reshaped. After the corneal curvature has been corrected, the flap is replaced, and the area heals without stitches.
- *Laser-assisted epithelium keratomileusis (LASEK):* In LASEK surgery, the surface epithelial cells of the eye are softened with an alcohol solution, allowing the epithelial layer to be rolled back and the cornea to be exposed. A laser then is used to reshape the cornea and treat myopia, hyperopia, and astigmatism. The epithelial flap is returned to its original position, and a contact lens is placed

on the cornea as a bandage for several days to aid healing and reduce pain.
- *Conductive keratoplasty (CK):* CK uses heat created by a laser to reshape the cornea. Heat is applied to the cornea's outer edge to tighten and steepen the cornea. CK is used in patients older than 40 years of age who need correction for hyperopia, presbyopia, and myopia. The procedure causes little or no discomfort and improves vision almost instantly. The corneal changes are not permanent, and retreatment may be required.

CRITICAL THINKING APPLICATION 16.2

Amy is assisting Dr. Martin with visual acuity examinations. He asks her whether she understands the causes of refractive errors. Amy has difficulty explaining why refractive errors occur, so she tells Dr. Martin she will research the topic and get back to him. What have you learned about the different refractive disorders and why they occur?

Strabismus

Strabismus is failure of the eyes to track together, which means that both eyes do not look in the same direction at the same time. Adults can develop strabismus because of a condition or disease elsewhere in the body, such as diabetes mellitus, muscular dystrophy, or hypertension, or as the result of a head injury. In children, strabismus is caused by weakness in the muscles that control eye movement. If the condition appears in infancy or childhood, it is most commonly associated with **amblyopia**. Treatment involves having the child wear a patch over the unaffected eye so that the muscles of the "lazy" eye are strengthened or administering atropine eyedrops to the unaffected eye to medically decrease visual acuity in the "sound" eye, thereby forcing the amblyopic eye to compensate. It was once standard therapy that an eye patch would be worn up to 6 hours per day, but getting young children to comply with this treatment is very challenging. In children with moderate amblyopia, research shows that patching for 2 hours daily is as effective as patching for 6 hours daily, and daily atropine is as effective as daily patching. Children older than 7 years may still benefit from patching or atropine, particularly if they have not previously received treatment for amblyopia. Amblyopia recurs in 25% of children after patching is discontinued; however, slowly reducing the amount of time the patch is worn each day at the end of treatment reduces the risk of recurrence. The main symptom in all age groups is *diplopia* (double vision).

Nystagmus

A constant, involuntary movement of one or both eyes is called *nystagmus*. The eye can move in any direction, and the movement is accompanied by blurred vision. A child may be born with the problem (congenital nystagmus), or the condition may be acquired as a result of a brain tumor, an inner ear lesion, multiple sclerosis, or substance abuse. Nystagmus is caused by an abnormal function in the part of the brain that controls eye movements. Congenital nystagmus is more common than acquired nystagmus, is usually milder, does not worsen over time, and is not associated with any other disorder. A patient with signs and symptoms of nystagmus should initially have a neurologic evaluation to determine the cause of the disorder, with treatment based on those findings. However, congenital nystagmus has no cure. Affected individuals typically are not aware of the eye movements, but they may have a decrease in visual acuity that can be corrected with surgery or corrective lenses.

Infections of the Eye

Many acute disorders of the eye are seen in the ophthalmologist's office. These include the following:

- *Hordeolum* (sty): A localized, purulent infection of a sebaceous gland of the eyelid. The area is inflamed, swollen, and painful. The infection usually is caused by staphylococci, and it is treated with warm compresses and topical or systemic antibiotics.
- *Chalazion:* A small cyst that results from blockage of a meibomian gland (sebaceous gland) and lubricates the posterior margin of each eyelid. The cyst can become infected, inflamed, swollen, and painful. It may disappear spontaneously or may need to be removed surgically.
- *Keratitis*: Inflammation of the cornea that results in superficial ulcerations. It can be caused by the herpes simplex virus, bacteria, or fungi, or it may develop as a result of corneal trauma (e.g., intense light). Symptoms include inflammation, tearing, pain, and **photophobia**. The condition is treated with ophthalmic ointments, eyedrops, and use of an eye patch.
- *Conjunctivitis*: Inflammation of the conjunctiva caused by irritation, allergy, or bacterial infection. Bacterial conjunctivitis (pinkeye) is highly contagious and produces a purulent discharge. Symptoms include inflammation, swelling and itching of the sclera, photophobia, and tearing. Bacterial infections are treated with antibiotic ophthalmic preparations.
- *Blepharitis:* Inflammation of the glands and lash follicles along the margins of the eyelids that may be caused by staphylococcal infection, allergies, or irritation. Symptoms include itching and inflammation along the eyelash margins; the condition is treated with antibiotic ophthalmic ointment.

Disorders of the Eyeball

Corneal Abrasion

The cornea, the transparent outer covering of the eye, is prone to abrasion because of its location. Symptoms of corneal abrasion include pain, inflammation, tearing, and photophobia. The abrasion usually is caused by a foreign body in the eye or by direct trauma, such as from poorly fitting or dirty contact lenses. A corneal ulcer may form and become infected.

Diagnosis is based on the patient's signs and symptoms, but it can be confirmed with the instillation of fluorescein stain (Fig. 16.5). After instillation of the stain, the provider uses a cobalt blue filtered light to visualize the abrasions, which appear green (Fig. 16.6). If the abrasions are caused by a foreign body, it must be removed first; the eye then can be treated with antibiotic ophthalmic ointment to prevent infection. Although patching the affected eye has been recommended in the past, studies now show that patching does not reduce the patient's pain and may actually prolong healing time. Corneal abrasions are quite painful, so the patient may be prescribed topical nonsteroidal antiinflammatory ophthalmic drops, such as diclofenac (Voltaren) and ketorolac (Acular), in addition to oral analgesics. Most

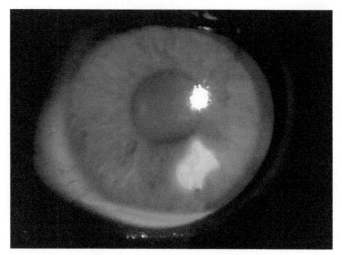

FIGURE 16.5 Corneal abrasion stained with fluorescein.

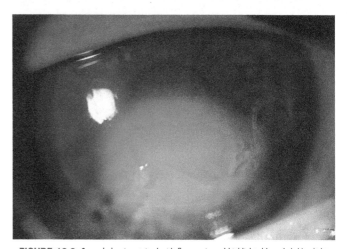

FIGURE 16.6 Corneal abrasion stained with fluorescein and highlighted by cobalt blue light.

corneal abrasions heal in 24 to 72 hours, but the patient should be aware that symptoms can worsen if the affected eye is exposed to bright light, if excessive blinking occurs, or if the patient rubs the injured surface of the cornea against the inside of the eyelid. Because the patient may develop a secondary infection from the corneal injury, topical antibiotics, including ciprofloxacin 0.3% (Ciloxan) ointment or drops and gentamicin 0.3% ointment or drops, may be prescribed. Patients with contact lenses may be prescribed oral antibiotics and should not wear their contacts until the abrasion has healed and the course of antibiotics has been completed.

Cataract

A cataract is a cloudy or opaque area in the normally clear lens of the eye that blocks the passage of light into the retina, causing impaired vision. This condition may result from injury to the eye, exposure to extreme heat or radiation, or inherited factors. However, most cataracts develop slowly and progressively as a result of the natural aging deterioration of the lens of the eye and typically occur after age 60. With advanced cataracts, the pupil of the eye appears white or gray (Fig. 16.7).

A cataract scatters the light as it passes through the lens, preventing a sharply defined image from reaching the retina resulting in blurred

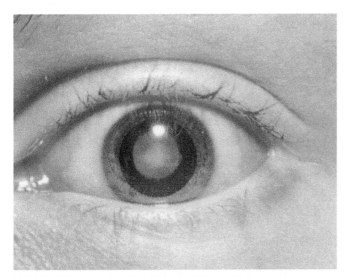

FIGURE 16.7 Cataract. (From Black JM, Hawks JH, Keene A: *Medical surgical nursing: clinical management for positive outcomes*, ed 8, Philadelphia, 2009, Saunders.)

and dimmed vision. The patient may need a brighter reading light or must hold objects closer to the eyes for better viewing. Continued clouding of the lens may cause diplopia. The patient also needs frequent changes of eyeglass prescriptions. Patients with cataracts report difficulty with *night vision* (nyctalopia), seeing halo images around lights, and increased sensitivity to glare. If left untreated, cataracts ultimately can lead to blindness.

When the patient's vision becomes distorted or appears to be deteriorating, the ophthalmologist performs a *slit lamp* procedure, in which he or she examines the structures at the front of the eye using a combination of a low-power microscope and a high-intensity light that shines into the eye as a slit beam.

The symptoms of early cataract may be improved with new eyeglasses, brighter lighting, and antiglare sunglasses. If these measures do not help, surgical removal of the lens is the only effective treatment. This is performed as an outpatient procedure in a clinic or hospital. After the eye has been anesthetized, the inner portions of the lens (the nucleus and the cortex) are removed. The provider may use an extracapsular extraction, in which the cataract is removed in one piece, or phacoemulsification, in which an ultrasonic probe is used to break up the cataract and the pieces are aspirated, before an artificial intraocular lens (IOL) is implanted. The incision may be closed with fine sutures, or it may be sutureless and self-sealing. The procedure usually takes 15 minutes, and the patient typically can leave the facility after 1 hour. Patients should be aware that they will not be able to drive until cleared by the ophthalmologist, and that they may need help at home until their vision is clear.

The patient is seen in the office the day after surgery and as frequently as needed for the next month. Vision gradually improves until it stabilizes, usually within 2 to 6 weeks; the patient then is fitted with new corrective lenses to match the improved vision.

Glaucoma

One of the most common and serious ocular disorders is a group of diseases known as *glaucoma*. Glaucoma is characterized by increased intraocular pressure (IOP), which damages the optic nerve and causes blindness if left untreated. It rarely occurs in people younger than

age 40 and usually is seen in individuals older than age 60. The cause is unknown, but a hereditary tendency toward development of the most common forms has been noted. Glaucoma is responsible for approximately 12% of all cases of blindness. After cataracts (which are typically age related and can be resolved surgically), glaucoma is the leading cause of blindness among African Americans. It is estimated that more than 3 million Americans have glaucoma, but only half of those know they have it.

The ciliary body constantly produces aqueous humor, which should circulate freely between the anterior and posterior chambers of the eye and eventually empty into the general circulation. A healthy eye is filled with fluid in an amount carefully regulated to maintain the shape of the eyeball. In chronic open-angle glaucoma, the channels that drain the fluid malfunction, and over time aqueous humor builds up, resulting in increased pressure, which affects the blood supply to the retina and the optic nerve. With acute closed-angle glaucoma, the opening of the drainage system narrows or closes completely, causing a sudden increase in IOP.

Patients can have chronic open-angle glaucoma for a long time before symptoms occur. Early detection through regular ophthalmic examinations that include IOP measurements is crucial to prevent permanent vision loss. The need to change eyeglass prescriptions frequently, loss of peripheral vision (often called "tunnel vision"), mild headaches, and impaired adaptation to the dark are some of the signs and symptoms that may be seen with chronic glaucoma. Acute closed-angle glaucoma has more obvious symptoms; the patient complains of severe pain, headaches, inflammation, photophobia, and seeing halos around lights. If left untreated, acute glaucoma can cause permanent blindness in a matter of days.

Screening for glaucoma is conducted during a complete eye examination. The ophthalmologist first uses a **tonometer** with a slit lamp to measure IOP. The air puff tonometer records the degree of indentation of the cornea from a puff of pressurized air without touching the eye. An applanation tonometer records the pressure needed to indent the cornea when the instrument is applied to the front surface of the eye. *Electronic tonometry* is the most recently developed technique. The ophthalmologist gently places the rounded tip of a tool that looks like a pen directly on the cornea, with results evident on a small computer panel. **Gonioscopy** also can be used to examine the aqueous fluid drainage system and to determine whether the glaucoma is the open- or closed-angle type. In addition, an ophthalmoscopic examination can identify cupping of the optic disc, which indicates atrophy of the optic nerve.

Diagnosis and immediate treatment for early stage, open-angle glaucoma can delay progression of the disease. Open-angle glaucoma can be relieved with **miotic** and beta-blocker eyedrops. The combinations of drugs used to treat glaucoma can vary considerably. Miotic medications increase the outflow of aqueous humor, and beta-blockers reduce the production of aqueous humor. It is imperative that the patient use prescribed eyedrops and take oral medications daily to prevent further damage to the optic nerve. Laser surgery may be performed to create an opening or to build a new channel for drainage of the aqueous humor. The goal of treatment in any type of glaucoma is to diagnose the disease early and to effectively treat its progression because any loss of sight that has occurred as the result of increased IOP cannot be regained. In closed-angle glaucoma, medications to lower IOP are prescribed so that surgery can be performed to create

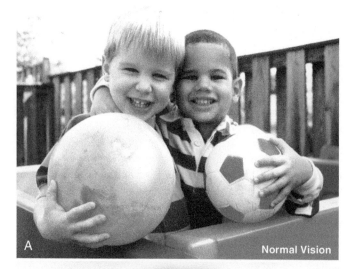

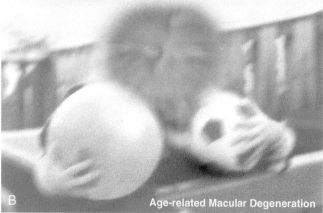

FIGURE 16.8 Visual field for a patient with macular degeneration. (From the National Eye Institute: Age-related macular degeneration: what you should know, National Institutes of Health, Bethesda, MD.)

a channel in which aqueous fluid can circulate. This is a medical emergency because the pressure must be relieved within a few hours or permanent vision damage occurs.

Macular Degeneration

The *macula lutea*, the part of the retina near the optic nerve, defines the center of the field of vision. Macular degeneration is progressive deterioration of the macula lutea, which causes loss of central vision; the patient can see only the edges of the visual field (Fig. 16.8). The condition affects more than 10 million Americans and is a leading cause of blindness in those older than 50.

Two types of macular degeneration can occur. The dry form accounts for most cases; it is painless and develops slowly, affecting sharp vision over time, so that reading and other activities that require fine, detailed vision become impossible. Wet macular degeneration causes 90% of all severe vision losses from the disease and has an acute onset and rapid progression. Dry macular degeneration is caused by the breakdown of light-sensitive cells in the region of the macula; the wet form is seen when new blood vessels behind the retina form and leak blood and fluid into the macula. The condition is age-related, but additional risk factors include cigarette smoking, obesity, family history, cardiovascular disease, elevated blood cholesterol levels, light

eye color, and excessive sun exposure. The disease has no known cure, but research indicates that antioxidants, including beta carotene and vitamins C and E with zinc and copper, may prevent the condition or may help treat the disease in people who have intermediate macular degeneration.

DISORDERS OF THE EAR

Hearing Loss

Two problems result in hearing loss: a conduction problem and a sensorineural impairment. Some individuals have both conditions.

Conductive hearing loss is caused by a problem originating in the external or middle ear that prevents sound vibrations from passing through the external auditory canal, limits the vibration of the tympanic membrane, or interferes with the passage of bone-conducted sound in the middle ear. Some common causative factors in conductive hearing loss include impacted cerumen; trauma to the tympanic membrane, especially with scar formation; hemorrhage or fluid in the middle ear; **otosclerosis**; and recurrent chronic ear infections. Patients with conductive hearing loss receive the greatest benefit from a hearing aid. If the hearing loss is caused by a malfunction or congenital abnormality of the ossicles, a surgical procedure can be performed to replace the damaged ossicles with manufactured models.

A sensorineural hearing loss results from an abnormality of the organ of Corti or of the auditory nerve. Viral infection (e.g., rubella, influenza, herpes) can result in hearing loss, as can head trauma or certain **ototoxic** medications. The first sign of ototoxic drug complications usually is **tinnitus**. This sometimes occurs with high doses of aspirin, certain antibiotics (erythromycin and vancomycin), and chemotherapeutic agents. A sensorineural hearing loss also can occur because of prolonged exposure to loud noise, such as repetitive noise in the workplace, or loud music, which damages the delicate cilia lining the organ of Corti.

Presbycusis, the hearing loss that affects older adults, is caused by a reduction in the number of receptor cells in the organ of Corti and also is classified as a sensorineural loss. Children can be born with a congenital hearing deficit or deafness because of an intrauterine infection, such as measles (rubella) (Fig. 16.9).

If the sensorineural hearing loss cannot be improved by hearing aids, an option is surgical insertion of cochlear implants. These are complex devices that use electrical impulses to stimulate the auditory nerve, which then carries the current to the brain to be interpreted as sound. Cochlear implants bypass damaged portions of the ear and directly stimulate the auditory nerve. These implants do not create normal hearing but provide increased sound for a person with profound or complete hearing loss.

Mixed hearing loss is a combination of conductive and sensory deafness. This type of loss can result from tumors, toxic levels of certain medications, hereditary factors, and stroke.

Otitis

There are two common types of otitis. The first affects the external ear canal and is called *otitis externa,* or swimmer's ear. Otitis externa may be caused by dermatologic conditions, such as **seborrhea** or **psoriasis**, trauma to the canal, or continuous use of earplugs or earphones. Swimmers frequently have otitis externa because water collects in the ears and mixes with cerumen to form an ideal culture

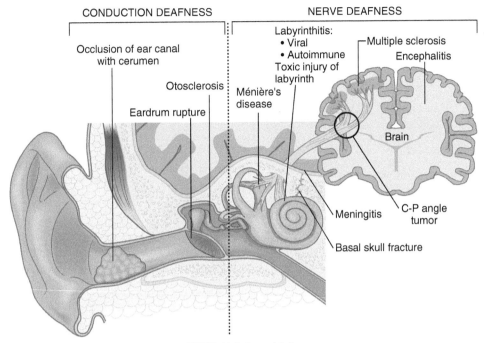

FIGURE 16.9 *Causes of deafness.*

medium for bacteria and fungus. Patients with otitis externa complain of severe pain and have inflammation and swelling of the external auditory canal, hearing loss, and possibly purulent (containing pus) or **serous** drainage. The inflammation is treated with antibiotic or steroid eardrops, and the canal must be kept clean and dry, or the condition can become chronic.

Otitis media is an inflammation of the normally air-filled middle ear that results in a collection of fluid behind the tympanic membrane. Otitis media can be serous or **suppurative**. Serous otitis media occurs because of a buildup of clear fluid in the middle ear; patients complain of a full feeling and some hearing loss. In suppurative otitis media, purulent fluid is present in the middle ear, and the patient has fever, pain, and hearing loss. Otitis media often is associated with an upper respiratory tract infection caused by a virus or an allergic reaction that results in swelling and inflammation of the sinuses and eustachian tubes. A child's eustachian tube is shorter, narrower, and more horizontal than that of an adult. The small size and decreased angle for drainage increases the chance that inflammation will block the tube and cause fluid to collect in the middle ear, which not only is uncomfortable but also interferes with the conduction hearing process (Fig. 16.10).

Risk Factors for Otitis Media

Factors That Cannot Be Controlled

- Sex (male)
- Age (infants and younger children [6 to 18 months])
- Premature birth
- Family history
- Siblings with infections
- Seasonal factors (most common during cold and flu season), seasonal allergies

- Underlying disease (cleft palate, Down syndrome, asthma, allergies)
- Ethnicity (Native American and Alaskan Inuit because of the shape of the eustachian tubes)
- Cochlear implants

Factors That Can Be Controlled

- Limit exposure to large-group child care settings.
- Do not expose the child to second-hand smoke.
- Hold the child upright during bottle feeding.
- Do not use pacifiers beyond 6 months, as this may increase the risk.
- Wash hands frequently to prevent the spread of colds and flu.
- Have the child immunized with the pneumococcal conjugate vaccine (Prevnar) and the flu vaccine.

An otoscopic examination reveals that the normally pearly gray tympanic membrane is inflamed (bright pink or red) and bulging (Fig. 16.11). Areas of fluid or pus may be visible through the membrane. A *tympanogram* may be done to determine the air pressure of the middle ear and the mobility of the tympanic membrane. During a tympanogram test, a small earphone is placed into the ear canal and the air pressure is gently changed. This test is helpful for showing whether an ear infection or fluid is present in the middle ear (Fig. 16.12). A tympanic membrane responding normally to an increase in air pressure will move, resulting in a peaked tympanogram. If fluid or pus in the middle ear is putting pressure on the tympanic membrane, the membrane moves only slightly or not at all, resulting in a slight peak or a flat tympanogram recording.

Treatment of otitis media may be a conservative "watch and wait" approach. However, if a fever and pronounced pain are present, the

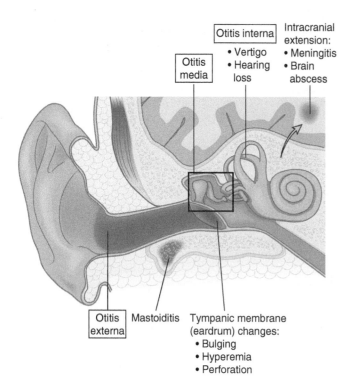

FIGURE 16.10 Inflammation and infection of the ear and surrounding tissues.

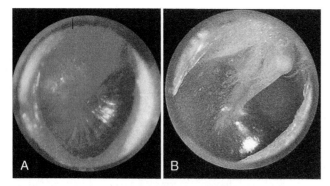

FIGURE 16.11 (A) Tympanic membrane with otitis media. **(B)** Normal tympanic membrane. (From LaFleur Brooks M: *Exploring medical language,* ed 9, St Louis, 2014, Mosby.)

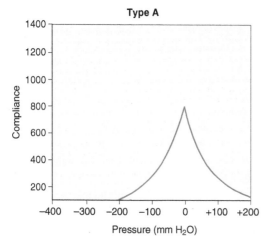

FIGURE 16.12 A normal tympanogram shows a peak at normal pressure (0). An ear with fluid produces a flat tympanogram.

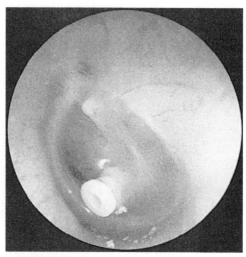

FIGURE 16.13 Tympanic membrane with a tympanostomy tube. (From Frazier MS, Drzymkowski JW: *Essentials of human diseases and conditions,* ed 5, St Louis, 2013, Saunders.)

individual may be given antibiotics and told to take over-the-counter analgesics such as acetaminophen or ibuprofen. If this condition becomes chronic, the provider may recommend a *myringotomy,* which is the creation of a surgical incision in the tympanic membrane to drain the fluid, followed by insertion of a tympanostomy tube to continually drain the middle ear of fluid. This may be necessary to prevent permanent hearing loss caused by damage to the ossicles (Fig. 16.13).

Recommendations for Treating Otitis Media

The development of drug-resistant strains of bacteria as a result of overprescribed antibiotics is a growing concern. The American Academy of Pediatrics recommends the following for the treatment of otitis media:

- Treatment with antibiotics should be delayed, giving the child's immune system a chance to fight the infection by itself. This delay should last 24 hours in children 6 to 24 months old and 72 hours for older children. Approximately 61% of children improve within 24 hours, regardless of whether they are treated. If the child's condition does not improve, an appropriate antibiotic can be prescribed.
- The child typically improves within 48 to 72 hours, but the parent should understand how important it is to complete the antibiotic medication as ordered to prevent the infection from recurring.
- The provider may decide to treat otitis media with a short course of antibiotics (i.e., 5 days) but at a higher dose. The drugs of choice include amoxicillin (Amoxil), azithromycin (Zithromax), and cefuroxime (Rocephin).
- Antibiotics will not help if otitis is caused by a virus. The child should be observed for possible complications, and analgesics should be administered for pain control. Viral otitis media typically resolves within 7 to 14 days.

Medical assistants play a key role in helping parents understand why antibiotic therapy may not be recommended. They also must educate parents about the importance of administering a prescribed antibiotic at the time ordered, using the correct dose, and completing the entire prescription.

Impacted Cerumen

Cerumen normally is a soft, yellowish, waxy substance that lubricates the external auditory canal.

Impacted cerumen that has been pushed up tightly against the eardrum is a common cause of conductive hearing loss because sound vibrations cannot pass through the cerumen to initiate movement of the tympanic membrane. Individuals with psoriasis, abnormally narrow ear canals, or an excessive amount of hair growing in the ear canals are more prone to this condition. Excessive secretion of cerumen can gradually cause hearing loss, tinnitus, a feeling of fullness, and *otalgia* (ear pain).

An otoscopic examination quickly reveals this problem. If impacted cerumen is found, it must be removed. This can be done by softening the wax with oily drops, such as carbamide peroxide (Debrox), and then irrigating the ear with warm water until the plug is removed. Because this condition can recur, the patient may need to schedule periodic examinations. If the patient is experiencing hearing loss because of the impaction, it is immediately remedied with removal of the cerumen.

Ménière's Disease

Ménière disease is a disorder of the inner ear. It is characterized by **vertigo**, tinnitus, progressive hearing loss, and sometimes a feeling of pressure or fullness in the ear. It usually only affects one ear. The cause of Ménière disease is not well understood. The inner ear of persons with this condition seems to have an abnormal amount of fluid (endolymph). What causes the excess fluid is not known. Research indicates the following possible causes: abnormal anatomy of the inner ear, genetic predisposition, possible autoimmune condition, head trauma, or migraines.

Ménière's disease causes swelling and edema in an endolymphatic sac of the semicircular canals, along with an overproduction or collection of excess endolymph. When an acute attack occurs, the patient may experience nausea, vomiting, and problems with balance. These attacks can last a few hours to several days, and they may increase in severity over time. Although the cause of this problem is unknown, Ménière's disease is a chronic, progressive condition that triggers episodes of recurring attacks of vertigo, tinnitus, a sensation of pressure in the affected ear, and advancing hearing loss.

During active periods of the disease, the patient is treated symptomatically with medications for nausea and vomiting. A salt-restricted diet, diuretics, and antihistamines may be prescribed to control edema in the labyrinth of the inner ear. Surgical destruction of the affected labyrinth is an option. Although this relieves symptoms, it may also result in permanent deafness if the cochlea is damaged.

Age-related macular degeneration (ARMD) and cataracts are the most common causes of blindness in older adults. Although there are several successful procedures to treat cataracts, currently there are no treatments to cure ARMD. Diabetic retinopathy is the most common cause of blindness, but it may also occur much earlier in life. Presbyopia is a visual disorder that usually accompanies aging and results in farsightedness.

Few babies are born with a hearing loss. The Universal Newborn Hearing Screening (UNHS) test is a means to detect deafness in infancy. Once an infant has been diagnosed, the parents can plan for future treatments and determine how to best handle the condition. Otitis media (OM) is the most frequently diagnosed childhood ear disease. In adults, hearing loss that may accompany the aging process is termed *presbycusis*.

THE MEDICAL ASSISTANT'S ROLE IN OPHTHALMOLOGY AND OTOLARYNGOLOGY PROCEDURES

Assisting With the Ophthalmology Examination

A complete examination of the eye is technical and requires expensive equipment and the expertise of an ophthalmologist or optometrist. However, a primary care provider performs some basic examinations and treatments of the eye. The ophthalmoscope is used to examine the interior of the eye. It projects a bright, narrow beam of light through the lens and illuminates the interior parts of the eye and retina. It is helpful for detecting disorders of the eyes and certain systemic disorders, such as capillary changes that occur with diabetes mellitus.

The eyelids are examined for edema, which may be the result of nephrosis, heart failure, allergy, or thyroid deficiency. *Blepharoptosis*, also called *ptosis*, is drooping of the upper eyelid that can be caused by a disorder of the third cranial nerve, muscular weakness as seen in muscular dystrophy, or myasthenia gravis.

The pupils of the eyes are normally round and equal. Normal pupils constrict rapidly in response to light. This is demonstrated by shining a bright, pinpoint light into one eye from the side of the patient's head. The pupil of an illuminated eye constricts, and the pupil of the other eye constricts equally. This test is called *light and accommodation* (L&A). An older patient's eyes do not accommodate as well as those of a younger person. Each eye is checked this way. The patient then is asked to look at the provider's finger as it is moved directly toward the patient's nose to check for eye coordination. If the pupils are equal and round, respond normally to light, and adjust and focus on objects at different distances in a reasonable length of time, the provider charts the acronym PERRLA (which stands for "pupils, equal, round, reactive to, light [and], accommodation").

Life Span Changes

In children, the most prevalent disorder of the eyes is conjunctivitis (commonly known as pinkeye), which accounts for a large number of pediatric visits. Because it is highly contagious, entire classrooms may be infected due to one student's infection. Most newborns receive erythromycin shortly after birth. This has significantly reduced the number of cases of ophthalmia neonatorum conjunctivitis, which is usually due to gonorrhea or a chlamydial infection.

PERRLA

P	Pupils
E	Equal
R	Round
R	Reactive to
L	Light (and)
A	**Accommodation**

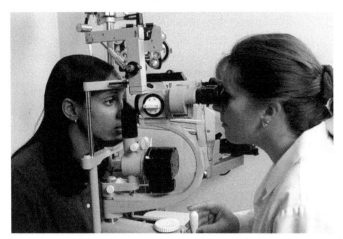

FIGURE 16.14 Slit lamp.

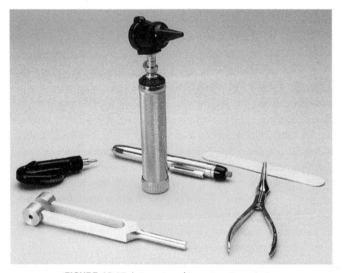

FIGURE 16.15 Instruments used in an otoscopic examination.

Special techniques used in the ophthalmologist's office include examinations performed with a slit lamp biomicroscope (Fig. 16.14). This device is used to view fine details in the anterior segments of the eye. It may be used to view a foreign body because it gives a well-illuminated and highly magnified view of the area. For this examination, the provider first orders administration of a *mydriatic* eyedrop to dilate the pupil and enhance visualization of eye structures.

A patient with *exophthalmia* (abnormal protrusion of the eye, possibly resulting from an overactive thyroid or a tumor behind the eyeball) is checked with an exophthalmometer. This instrument measures how far the eye protrudes beyond the edge of the eye socket and helps determine the level of tissue swelling and enlargement behind the eye.

Assisting With the Otolaryngology Examination

An ear examination involves viewing the external auditory canal with an otoscope covered by an ear speculum (Fig. 16.15). Disposable plastic speculum covers should be used each time to prevent disease transmission. A normal otoscopic examination reveals an external

auditory canal with a small amount of cerumen and a pearly gray and concave tympanic membrane. In addition to performing the otoscopic examination, the provider palpates the area around the pinna for abnormalities or sensations. A number of tests are used to assess hearing acuity, ranging from simple tuning fork tests to quantitative and qualitative audiometric testing. If a hearing loss is suspected, the next test usually is performed with a tuning fork.

Useful Questions for Gathering a History of Ear Problems

- Are you experiencing nausea, vomiting, dizziness, ear pain, fever, headache, upper respiratory infection, ringing of the ears, drainage, loss of balance, or hearing loss?
- What are the onset, duration, and frequency of symptoms?
- Have you taken any medication for the symptoms? If so, what medication? Has it helped?
- Do you have the problem in both ears?
- Are you experiencing pain? On a scale of 1 to 10, with 10 being the worst pain, how would you rate the pain? Is it localized or radiating, in one ear or both?
- Has anything you have tried relieved the symptoms?

Assisting With Ophthalmology Diagnostic Procedures
Distance Visual Acuity

Determining distance visual acuity frequently is part of a complete physical examination (see Procedure 16.1, p. 421). It is widely used in schools and industry and is the best single test available for vision screening. Many cases of myopia, astigmatism, and hyperopia have been detected with this routine test. The chart most commonly used is the Snellen alphabetical chart (Fig. 16.16A). This chart displays various letters of the alphabet, which the patient must identify in ever smaller font sizes. Patients with limited knowledge of the English alphabet can be tested with the **E** chart (Fig. 16.16B). In addition, a chart that uses pictures and symbols is available. This chart is used for young children or individuals who do not know the alphabet (Fig. 16.16C). To avoid patient confusion over the **E** chart or the symbol chart, the medical assistant should review the charts with patients first to make sure they know how to demonstrate the **E** visualized or the meaning of each picture or symbol. The symbol on the top line of the chart can be read at 200 feet by people with normal vision. In each of the succeeding rows, from the top down, the size of the symbols is reduced so that a person with normal vision can see them at distances of 100, 70, 50, 40, 30, and 20 feet, consecutively.

The patient must not be allowed to study the chart before taking the test. The room or hall should be long enough that the 20-foot distance can be marked off accurately and without interruptions from patient and staff traffic. The chart should be hung at the patient's eye level and illuminated with maximum light, without glare on the chart. Most adults do not need the standard Snellen chart explained, but if the **E** chart is used, an explanation must be given as to how the E's are to be read. The patient may point up or down or right or left toward the part of the letter that is open. If the **E** chart is to

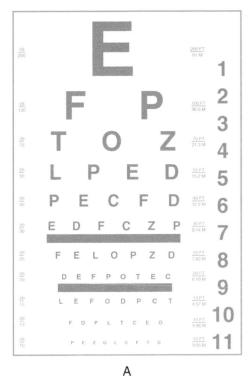

A

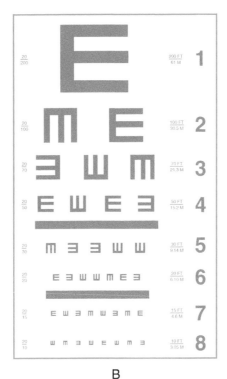

B

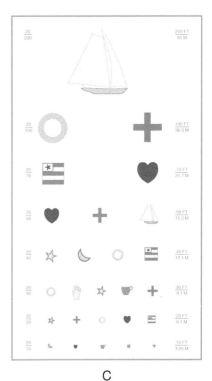

C

FIGURE 16.16 Different types of Snellen charts.

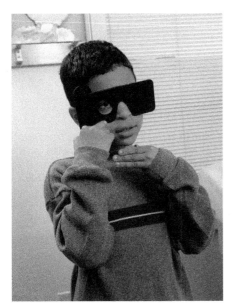

FIGURE 16.17 Visual acuity test with the E chart.

be used for a child, practice with an index card that has a large **E** drawn on it before the child is tested. Turn the card in different directions to simulate the position of the "fingers" of the **E** on the chart, and give the child the opportunity to demonstrate the direction of the **E** fingers by pointing his or her own fingers in the same direction (Fig. 16.17).

Because this is a gross screening of distance visual acuity, the eyes typically are tested with corrective lenses; the patient therefore should not remove glasses or contact lenses unless the provider requests it. Indicate in the patient's health record whether the assessment was

done with or without corrective lenses. Record the results of each eye separately and as fractions. The numerator (top number) is the distance of the patient from the chart (always 20 feet), and the denominator (bottom number) is the lowest line read satisfactorily by the patient. For example, if the patient reads the 20 line at 20 feet, the fraction 20/20 is recorded for that eye. *The last line the patient can read without squinting or straining and with no more than two mistakes is the line recorded in the patient's record for that eye.* The medical assistant should document the outcomes of the test, specifying the results for each eye and for both eyes. The Joint Commission no longer recommends the use of medical abbreviations for the eyes and ears because they are frequently confused or misinterpreted; therefore, the medical assistant must now document right eye, left eye, and both eyes.

Interpreting Snellen Results

- The patient always stands 20 feet from the chart.
- Each result is a record of how well the patient can see compared with normal vision.
- Example: A patient with a 20/40 reading can see that line correctly standing at 20 feet, but an individual with normal vision can see the same line correctly at 40 feet, so the patient's vision is not as acute as someone with normal vision.
- Example: A patient with a 20/15 reading can see that line accurately standing at 20 feet, but a person with normal vision must stand at 15 feet to have the same vision, meaning the patient's vision is better than someone with normal vision.

CRITICAL THINKING APPLICATION   16.3

Susie Anthony, a 19-year-old patient, is seen today for a general eye examination. The provider orders a routine Snellen test, and Kim administers it. Susie wears contacts. With her right eye, she reads without errors to the 20/25 line; however, she squints and makes three errors at the 20/20 line. With her left eye, Susie makes two mistakes at the 20/30 line; with both eyes, she reads the 20/25 without errors. How should Kim document this procedure?

Near Visual Acuity

Near visual acuity can be tested with the near vision acuity chart (Fig. 16.18). This test is given to screen for presbyopia or hyperopia. If the patient wears corrective lenses, they should be worn during the test. The size of the type on the card varies from newspaper headlines to print similar to that found in telephone books. The test should be given in a well-lit room, with the patient holding the card approximately 14 to 16 inches away. As with the Snellen examination, the near visual acuity test is given for each eye, starting with the right eye. The eye not being tested should be covered with an occluder but left open. The patient should be monitored for indications of difficulty, such as squinting or tearing. The patient reads the card, starting at the top, until reaching the smallest print that can be read. The medical assistant should document the number at which the patient had no more than two errors for each eye and also the two eyes together; whether corrective lenses were worn; and any signs of eyestrain.

Ishihara Color Vision Test

Defects in color vision are classified as congenital or acquired. Congenital defects are caused by an inherited color vision defect and are found most often in males. Acquired defects are caused by eye injury or disease. The Ishihara test is a simple, convenient, and accurate procedure that detects total color blindness, in addition to the red-green blindness prevalent in congenital blindness (see Procedure 16.2, p. 422). The test assesses the perception of primary colors and shades of colors.

The test booklet contains polychromatic plates made up of colored dots in numeric patterns. The numbers are one color, and the background dots are a different color. Patients with average visual acuity can read the number within the dot matrix without difficulty. Patients with color vision defects are unable to read the number, or they see a totally different number. A section of plates is included that contains colored line trails through a background of dots. These plates are designed to be used with children and adults who are unable to read numbers. In this situation, the patient uses a finger to follow the dotted trail through the picture.

The test should be administered in a quiet room that is well illuminated by sunlight, not by artificial lighting. If this cannot be done, the best situation possible is created by adjusting lights to resemble the effect of natural daylight. The test uses 14 color plates. The basic test consists of plates 1 through 11. Plates 12 through 14 are used if the patient appears to be having difficulty with red-green differentiations. The medical assistant records the number of plates read correctly. If the score is 10 or higher, the patient is within the

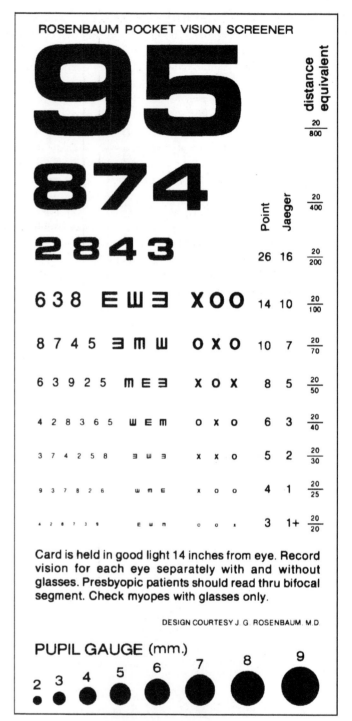

FIGURE 16.18 Near vision acuity chart.

average range. If the score is 7 or lower, the patient is suspected of having a color deficiency, and the ophthalmologist performs additional assessment tests using more precise color vision testing equipment.

Assisting With Otolaryngology Diagnostic Procedures

Tuning Fork Testing

Tuning fork tests measure hearing by air conduction and bone conduction. Remember that in bone conduction, the sound vibrates through the cranial bones to the inner ear. Tuning forks are available in different sizes, each with a different frequency. The most commonly used tuning fork is the 512 **hertz** (Hz), which means that it vibrates 512 cycles per second, the level of normal speech patterns. To activate the fork, the provider holds it by the stem and strikes the tines softly on the palm of the hand. Striking the tines too forcefully creates a tone that is too loud for diagnostic use. The two tests used to evaluate hearing are the Weber and Rinne tests. Both of these procedures are commonly used to evaluate conductive and sensory losses.

The Weber test is used if the patient reports that hearing is better in one ear than in the other. The vibrating fork is placed in the center of the top of the head, and the patient is asked in which ear the tone is louder, or if the tone is the same in both ears. Because the patient is hearing the tone by bone conduction through the head, a normal result is hearing the sound equally in both ears.

The Rinne test is designed to compare air conduction sound with bone conduction sound. In this test, the stem of the vibrating fork is placed on the patient's mastoid process, and the patient is instructed to raise a hand when the sound disappears. The fork is quickly inverted so that the vibrating tines are approximately 1 inch in front of the external ear canal. If hearing is normal, the patient should still hear a sound. In normal hearing, the sound is heard twice as long by air conduction as by bone conduction.

Audiometric Testing

An audiometric test may be done in an otology or a family practice and is performed by medical assistants who have received additional training. Audiometry measures the lowest intensity of sound an individual can hear (Fig. 16.19). The patient, frequently a child, is assisted in placing headphones over the ears.

Newer machines give the operator the choice of performing a traditional manual hearing test or an automated one. In the automatic mode, the patient is prompted through the earphones to press a hand button as soon as he or she hears a tone. The advantages of automated machines are that voice prompts are available in multiple languages and the test requires less time to complete. The medical assistant can watch the progress of the test on the audiometer's LCD screen. Whether the test is delivered manually or with an automated

model, each ear is tested by delivering a single frequency at a specific intensity, starting with low-frequency tones and going up to very high frequencies. The patient is asked to signal when he or she hears the sound. The results are printed on a graph, called an *audiogram,* or the medical assistant charts the results on a graph sheet (see Procedure 16.3, p. 423). An adult with normal hearing can hear tone frequencies below 25 decibels, and children with normal hearing can hear those below 15 decibels.

If initial screening indicates a hearing deficit, the provider may recommend an appointment with an **audiologist** for audiometric evaluation. The evaluation consists of a battery of tests that assesses the level of hearing impairment and provides valuable information as to how the patient may be helped. The first test evaluates speech comprehension and assesses the patient's ability to follow verbal instructions. Once this evaluation is complete, the patient is placed in a soundproof booth with earphones over the ears. From this point on, the audiologist speaks to the patient and conducts all testing through the earphones. The assessment includes testing the frequency, intensity, and audibility of sound. This process takes approximately 1 hour.

Assisting With Ophthalmology Treatments

Patients with ophthalmology conditions are prescribed a variety of medications. The following are some of the more common classifications of medications used for this specialty:

- *Topical antibiotic ointments*: Used to treat bacterial infections
- *Antiinflammatory agents*: Used to reduce inflammation
- *Antiinfectives*: Used to treat viral infections

Refer to Table 16.2 for information on the classification, including indications for use, desired effect, side effects, adverse reactions, and generic and trade names. Medical assistants should be familiar with medications that are prescribed to patients.

Eye Irrigation

The eye is irrigated to relieve inflammation, remove drainage, dilute chemicals, or wash away foreign bodies. Sterile technique and equipment must be used to prevent contamination (see Procedure

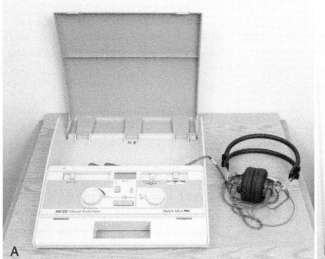
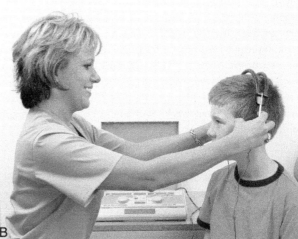

FIGURE 16.19 Audiometer with headset.

TABLE 16.2   Medication Classifications

Antivirals	**Indications for use:** Treat viral infections, including oral and genital herpes, influenza, and HIV. **Desired effects:** Inhibit the growth or reduce the spread of viral cells. **Side effects and adverse reactions:** Confusion, diarrhea, headache, kidney disease, urticaria, vomiting.	• **oseltamivir** (Tamiflu) • **acyclovir** (Zovirax)
Mydriatics	**Indications for use:** Ophthalmic procedures. **Desired effect:** Dilate the pupil, some cause paralysis of the ciliary muscle. **Side effects and adverse reactions:** Stinging, burning, dry mouth, urine retention.	• **atropine** (Isopto Atropine) • **cyclopentolate** (Cyclogyl, Pentolair)

16.4, p. 424). Follow the procedure as ordered, making sure the patient is comfortable. Record the treatment in the patient's health record immediately after it has been determined. Remember, if it is not recorded, it has not been done.

Foreign bodies in the eye are very irritating and may cause considerable pain. Most foreign bodies are superficial and can be removed easily. Occasionally, a foreign particle may be deeply embedded, requiring eye surgery. Notify the provider immediately if a patient comes into the office with something in his or her eye.

The first objective of the provider's examination is inspection. The patient is asked to look to either side and up and down so that the anterior surface of the eye can be inspected. For the provider to fully inspect under the upper lid, the patient must cooperate by looking downward while the provider **everts** the upper lid using a cotton-tipped applicator. While the lid is maintained in an everted position, any foreign materials may be rinsed away with sterile water or saline solution. If the provider's order is for you to remove the foreign body, do so with irrigation only. If this technique is unsuccessful, cover both of the patient's eyes with a gauze dressing, and notify your supervisor immediately. The eyes track each other, so to prevent movement in the affected eye, both eyes must be covered to prevent possible eye trauma.

Safety Alert

Never attempt to remove a foreign body from the cornea using a cotton-tipped applicator. Scratches to the cornea may result, causing scar formation and impaired vision.

CRITICAL THINKING APPLICATION   16.4

The provider tells Kim to irrigate the left eye of a 22-year-old patient to remove a foreign body. She is to irrigate the eye with sterile normal saline solution until clear. How should Kim document this procedure?

Instillation of Eye Medication

Medication may be instilled into the eye to treat an infection, soothe an eye irritation, anesthetize the eye, or dilate the pupils before examination or treatment (see Procedure 16.5, p. 426). Ophthalmic medications are available in several forms. Liquid drops usually are supplied in small squeeze bottles with tips that allow one drop at a time to be dispensed, or the bottle may contain a dropper with a small rubber attachment used to dispense the medication by drops. Eye ointments are dispensed in small metal or plastic tubes with an ophthalmic tip that allows them to be dispensed in a small ribbon of ointment directly into the bottom eyelid.

Safety Alert

Whatever the medication, the dispenser should never touch the eye while the prescribed amount of medication is administered. This can traumatize the eye and can contaminate the medication applicator. If the tip of the dispenser touches any surface, dispose of it in a biohazard waste container because it is contaminated.

Assisting With Otolaryngology Treatments

Ear Irrigation

Irrigation of the ear is done to remove excessive or impacted cerumen, to remove a foreign body, or to treat the inflamed ear with an antiseptic solution (see Procedure 16.6, p. 427). When the provider orders an ear irrigation, the medical assistant may perform the procedure if he or she has had the proper training and is competent in the technique. To prevent discomfort for the patient, it is important to administer the irrigating solution with the applicator tilted up, toward the top of the external canal, so that the solution is not directed at the tympanic membrane. Some discomforts the patient may experience during ear irrigation include vertigo, coughing, or a tickle in the back of the throat. Perform the procedure as prescribed, making sure the patient is comfortable. Always document the treatment and its results immediately after completion.

CRITICAL THINKING APPLICATION   16.5

Kim is instructed to perform a bilateral ear irrigation on a 68-year-old patient with impacted cerumen. Before the procedure, she uses an otoscope to check the auditory canal and sees a large amount of dark brown cerumen in the right ear, completely covering the tympanic membrane. The left ear has a moderate amount of golden-brown cerumen covering the bottom half of the tympanic membrane. After the procedure, both membranes are visible, and the patient tolerated the procedure without complaints. How should Kim document the procedure?

Instilling Otic Medications

Medication ordered for ear instillation is given to soften impacted cerumen, to relieve pain, or as an antibiotic drop for an infectious pathogen (see Procedure 16.7, p. 428). Patients with ear conditions may be in considerable pain and may have difficulty hearing, which makes health teaching a challenge. Wait until after the procedure has been completed and the patient is more comfortable to reinforce health behaviors.

CLOSING COMMENTS

Patient Coaching

Patients with vision or hearing impairment face serious challenges. For these patients, the medical assistant must use good listening skills, appropriate nonverbal methods, and touch to communicate empathy and understanding. Teaching may have to be adapted to meet the special needs of these patients. A person with a vision loss benefits from large-print forms and handouts, increased lighting, and verbal rather than written instructions to reinforce learning. For an individual with a hearing deficit, printed instructions, demonstrations of how to manage treatments, or even sign language interpretation should be available to ensure accurate communication. Including family members in the patient's treatment plan and offering referrals to appropriate community or professional resources may be very beneficial to a patient with sensory loss. Each patient must be assessed individually to determine the type of adaptation that he or she needs.

An important part of patient coaching for those administering eye medications at home is stressing the need to maintain the sterility of the medication. Patients and family members must be taught how to apply the medication while preventing trauma to the eye and contamination of the applicator. Patients administering ear treatments also must understand how to instill the medication.

Legal and Ethical Issues

The Americans with Disabilities Act (ADA) was passed in 1990, and amendments were added in 2008. The Americans with Disabilities Act Amendments (ADAA) prohibit discrimination based on disability. An individual with a disability is defined by the ADAA as a person who has a physical or mental impairment that substantially limits one or more major life activities, a person who has a history or record of such an impairment, or a person who is perceived by others as having such an impairment. Public facilities, including ambulatory care facilities and other healthcare buildings, must comply with ADAA requirements for physical accommodations. Public medical facilities must provide individuals with disabilities access to communication devices if they have a problem with vision, hearing, reading, or comprehension. Additional details can be found at http://www.ada.gov/nprm_adaaa/adaaa-nprm-qa.htm.

Patient-Centered Care

Diminished sight or hearing may render a patient seriously impaired. To prevent accidents and office injuries, always ask sight- or hearing-impaired patients whether they require assistance. When you escort the patient to an examination room, offer your arm and tell the patient the approximate distance you will be walking. If the patient is to have an examination that involves local anesthesia or eyedrops that dilate the pupil, be sure the patient has recovered, has sunglasses, and that someone is available to drive the patient home before allowing him or her to leave the facility. Never assume that the patient is capable of leaving alone. If the patient insists on leaving before the designated recovery time, inform the provider and record the time and circumstances surrounding the event in the patient's health record.

Professional Behaviors

Patients with vision and hearing problems require an extra level of professional courtesy and respectfulness. Imagine what it would be like if you could not see clearly or if you had difficulty understanding what your provider is saying to you. How would you like a family member who has sensory difficulties to be treated when he or she visits the provider? Focus on how you can adapt the facility's environment to accommodate the needs of these patients. Is there adequate lighting? Are patient education materials available that have been adapted for individuals with vision impairment? How can you most effectively and respectfully communicate with a patient who has a hearing loss? Many times, just the act of empathy—imagining yourself in the place of the patient—can help guide you to treat patients with the respect and courtesy they deserve.

SUMMARY OF SCENARIO

After observing Kim and asking many questions, Amy is beginning to understand her special responsibilities in the ophthalmology and otorhinolaryngology areas. She recognizes the need to be familiar with the anatomy and physiology of both the eye and the ear, in addition to the importance of being able to perform specialty-related skills, such as irrigations, medication instillations, and diagnostic procedures. Amy has become quite proficient at performing Snellen and Ishihara screening examinations and accurately documenting the results. Kim has taught her to use the audiometer and assisted her with the first few screenings, so she is now ready to do hearing tests on her own.

Although she learned about eye and ear medications in her medical assistant program, Amy found that instilling these medications in an actual patient is different from working on mannequins and classmates. Kim has reinforced the skills she learned in her program, continually emphasizing infection control procedures and reinforcing patient education information. Amy realizes that she needs to understand the pathologic conditions that can occur in the sensory organs so that she can assist the provider as needed and answer patients' questions.

After working with patients who have vision and hearing deficits, Amy understands the importance of adapting communication techniques to meet the needs of each patient. She has decided to take advantage of educational opportunities at the hospital and through her professional organization to continue to learn about this special area of practice.

SUMMARY OF LEARNING OBJECTIVES

1. **Explain the differences among an ophthalmologist, an optometrist, and an optician.**

   An *ophthalmologist* is a medical doctor who specializes in the diagnosis and treatment of the eye; an *optometrist* can examine and treat visual defects; an *optician* fills prescriptions for corrective lenses.

2. **Identify the anatomic structures of the eye, and discuss the process of vision.**

   The anatomy of the eye begins with the outer covering, the conjunctiva, and three layers of tissue: sclera, choroid, and retina. The retina is where light rays are converted into nervous energy for interpretation by the brain.

   Vision begins with the passage of light through the cornea, where it is refracted. The light rays then pass through the aqueous humor and pupil into the lens. The ciliary muscle adjusts the curvature of the lens to again refract the light rays so that they pass into the retina, triggering the photoreceptor cells of the rods and cones. Light energy is converted into an electrical impulse that is sent through the optic nerve to the brain, where interpretation occurs. Table 16.1 shows how vision requires light and depends on the proper functioning of all parts of the eye.

3. **Identify the anatomic structures of the ear, and explain the functions of the external ear, middle ear, and inner ear.**

   The anatomy of the ear begins with the outer ear, specifically the auricle. The next area is the middle ear where sound is transmitted via the ossicles to the inner ear. The inner ear is divided into the cochlea and the semicircular canals. Sound is then transmitted to the eighth cranial nerve and on to the brain.

   The external ear consists of the auricle, or pinna, and the external auditory canal, which transmits sound waves to the tympanic membrane. The middle ear is an air-filled cavity that contains the ossicles. The sound vibration passes through the tympanic membrane, causing the ossicles to vibrate. This bone-conducted vibration passes through the oval window into the inner ear. The organ of Corti, in the cochlea of the inner ear, converts sound waves into nervous energy, which is sent to the brain for interpretation. The semicircular canals in the inner ear maintain equilibrium.

4. **Differentiate among the major types of refractive errors.**

   Refractive errors include hyperopia, myopia, presbyopia, and astigmatism. All are caused by a problem with bending light so that it can be accurately focused on the retina. These conditions usually are caused by defects in the shape of the eyeball and can be corrected with glasses, contacts, or surgery.

5. **Summarize typical disorders of the eye and eyeball other than refractive errors.**

   Eye disorders can range from problems with eye movement, as in strabismus and nystagmus, to infections of the eye, including hordeolum, chalazions, keratitis, conjunctivitis, and blepharitis. Disorders of the eyeball include corneal abrasions, cataracts, glaucoma, and macular degeneration.

6. **Describe the conditions that can lead to hearing loss, including conductive and sensorineural impairments.**

   Conductive hearing loss is caused by a problem that originates in the external or middle ear and prevents sound vibrations from passing through the external auditory canal, limiting tympanic membrane vibrations or interfering with the passage of bone-conducted sound in the middle ear. A sensorineural hearing loss results from damage to the organ of Corti or the auditory nerve and prevents vibrations from being converted into nervous stimuli.

7. **Define other major disorders of the ear, including otitis, impacted cerumen, and Ménière's disease.**

   Otitis externa is an inflammation of the auditory canal, and otitis media is an inflammation of the normally air-filled middle ear, resulting in the collection of serous or suppurative fluid behind the tympanic membrane. Impacted cerumen is a common cause of conductive hearing loss. Ménière's disease is a chronic, progressive condition that affects the labyrinth and causes recurring attacks of vertigo, in addition to tinnitus, a sensation of pressure in the affected ear, and advancing hearing loss.

8. **Assist with the ophthalmology examination, and discuss what the acronym PERRLA stands for.**

   Diagnostic procedures for the eye begin with a visual examination of the eye with an ophthalmoscope. Next, the eyelids are examined for abnormalities, and the pupils are tested for PERRLA (pupils, equal, round, reactive to, light [and], accommodation). More advanced techniques include the use of a slit lamp to view the fine details of the eye and an exophthalmometer to measure the distance of the eyeball from the orbit. Distance visual acuity typically is assessed with a Snellen chart; near visual acuity is tested with a near vision acuity chart. A patient can be tested for a color vision defect with the Ishihara test.

9. **Assist with the otolaryngology examination, and discuss useful questions for gathering a history of ear problems.**

   An ear examination involves viewing the external auditory canal with an otoscope covered by an ear speculum. If hearing loss is suspected, the next test is usually performed with a tuning fork. Be sure to ask questions about symptoms (including onset, frequency, and duration), medications, if the problem is in both ears, and if pain is present.

10. **Discuss distance visual acuity, and perform a visual acuity test using the Snellen chart.**

    Procedure 16.1 on p. 421 explains the Snellen evaluation.

11. **Discuss visual acuity, and assess color acuity using the Ishihara test.**

    Procedure 16.2 on p. 422 outlines the color acuity examination.

12. **Assist with otolaryngology diagnostic procedures, and use an audiometer to accurately measure a patient's hearing acuity.**

    The ear exam begins with an otoscopic examination. It can include various tuning fork tests to detect conductive or sensorineural hearing deficits and more advanced audiometric testing. Procedure 16.3 on p. 423 explains the audiometry examination.

SUMMARY OF LEARNING OBJECTIVES—*continued*

13. **Assist with ophthalmology treatments, and explain the purposes of and the proper procedures for eye irrigation and the instillation of eye medication.**

    Eye irrigation relieves inflammation, removes drainage, dilutes chemicals, or washes away foreign bodies. Sterile technique and equipment must be used to prevent contamination. Medication may be instilled into the eye to treat an infection, soothe an eye irritation, anesthetize the eye, or dilate the pupils before examination or treatment. Procedure 16.4 on p. 424 describes the method for eye irrigation, and Procedure 16.5 on p. 426 explains how to administer eye medications.

14. **Assist with otolaryngology treatments, identify the purposes of ear irrigations and the instillation of ear medications, and demonstrate the proper procedures for both ear irrigation and instilling medicated eardrops.**

    Irrigation of the ear is performed to remove excess or impacted cerumen, to remove a foreign body, or to treat the inflamed ear with an antiseptic solution. Medication is instilled into the ear to soften impacted cerumen, relieve pain, or treat an infectious pathogen. Procedure 16.6 on p. 427 describes how to perform an ear irrigation. Procedure 16.7 on p. 428 explains how to administer otic drugs.

PROCEDURE 16.1 | Measuring Distance Visual Acuity

Task: Determine the patient's degree of visual clarity at a measured distance of 20 feet using the Snellen chart.

EQUIPMENT and SUPPLIES

- Patient's health record
- Provider's order
- Snellen eye chart
- Disposable eye occluder or an alcohol wipe to clean the occluder before use
- Pen or pencil and paper

PROCEDURAL STEPS

1. Wash hands or use hand sanitizer.
   <u>PURPOSE:</u> Hand sanitization is an important step for infection control.
2. Prepare the area. Make sure the room is well lit and that a distance marker is 20 feet from the chart.
3. Greet the patient. Identify yourself. Verify the patient's identity with full name and date of birth. Explain the procedure to be performed in a manner that the patient understands. Answer any questions the patient may have on the procedure. Instruct the patient not to squint during the test because this temporarily improves vision. The patient should not have an opportunity to study the chart before the test is given. If the patient wears corrective lenses, they should be worn during the test.
   <u>PURPOSE:</u> Explanations help gain the patient's cooperation and alleviate apprehension.
4. Assist the patient into a standing or sitting position at the 20-foot marker.
   <u>PURPOSE:</u> Twenty feet is the standard testing distance.
5. Check that the Snellen chart is positioned at the patient's eye level.
6. If the occluder is not disposable, disinfect it before the procedure starts. Then, instruct the patient to cover the left eye with the occluder and to keep both eyes open throughout the test to prevent squinting (Fig. 1).
   <u>PURPOSE:</u> Traditionally, the right eye is tested first.

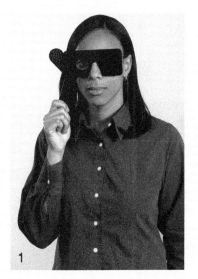

1

7. Stand beside the chart, and point to each row as the patient reads it aloud, starting with the 20/70 row (Fig. 2).
   <u>PURPOSE:</u> Starting with larger letters gives the patient confidence and allows for accommodation of vision.

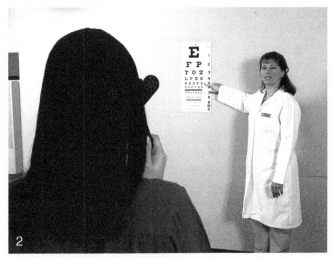

2

Continued

PROCEDURE 16.1 | **Measuring Distance Visual Acuity**—*continued*

8. Proceed down the rows of the chart until the smallest row the patient can read with a maximum of two errors is reached. If one or two letters are missed, the outcome is recorded with a minus sign and the number of errors (e.g., 20/40–2). If more than two errors are made, the previous line should be documented.

9. Record any of the patient's reactions while reading the chart.
   PURPOSE: Reactions such as squinting, leaning, tearing, or blinking may indicate that the patient is having difficulty with the test.

10. Repeat the procedure with the left eye, covering the right eye.

11. Repeat the procedure with both eyes uncovered.

12. Disinfect the occluder, if it is not disposable. Wash hands or use hand sanitizer.
    PURPOSE: To follow infection control procedures.

13. Document the procedure in the patient's record, including the date and time, visual acuity results, and any reactions by the patient. Also record whether corrective lenses were worn.
    PURPOSE: Procedures that are not recorded are considered not done.

Documentation Exercise:
The medical assistant conducted a Snellen exam on Carlene Anderson, who wears contacts. The results were right eye 20/60; left eye 20/30, but she missed one letter at the 20/30 line; both eyes 20/40. Carlene did not squint or strain during the exam.

Correct Documentation:
8/01/20XX 2:20 p.m. DVA completed c̄ Snellen chart. Right eye 20/60, left eye 20/30–1, both eyes 20/40 c̄ corrective lenses. No squinting noted.
_____Kim Tau, CMA, (AAMA)

PROCEDURE 16.2 | **Assess Color Acuity Using the Ishihara Test**

Task: Assess a patient's color acuity correctly, and record the results.

EQUIPMENT and SUPPLIES

- Patient's health record
- Provider's order
- Room with natural light if possible
- Ishihara color plate book
- Pen, pencil, and paper
- Watch with a second hand

PROCEDURAL STEPS

1. Assemble the equipment, and prepare the room for testing. The room should be quiet and illuminated with natural light.
   PURPOSE: Natural light is needed to test colors correctly.

2. Greet the patient. Identify yourself. Verify the patient's identity with full name and date of birth. Explain the procedure to be performed in a manner that the patient understands. Answer any questions the patient may have on the procedure. Use a practice card during the explanation, and make sure the patient understands that he or she has 3 seconds to identify each plate.
   PURPOSE: To make sure you have the right patient. Also, an informed patient is a cooperative patient. The first plate is a practice plate and is designed to be read correctly.

3. Hold up the first plate at a right angle to the patient's line of vision and 30 inches from the patient. Be sure both of the patient's eyes are kept open during the test (Fig. 1).

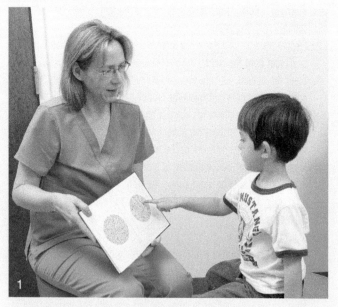

4. Ask the patient to tell you the number on the plate. Record the plate number and the patient's answer (Fig. 2).

PROCEDURE 16.2 **Assess Color Acuity Using the Ishihara Test**—*continued*

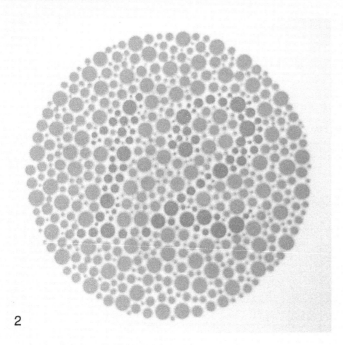

2

5. Continue this sequence until all 11 plates have been read. If the patient cannot identify the number on the plate, place an X in the record for that plate number. Your record should look like this:
   Plate 1 = pass, Plate 2 = pass, Plate 3 = X, Plate 4 = pass, and so on.
6. Include any unusual symptoms in your record, such as eye rubbing, squinting, or excessive blinking.
7. Place the book back in its cardboard sleeve, and return it to its storage space.
   PURPOSE: The Ishihara color plates must be stored in a closed position away from external light to protect the colors.
8. Document the procedure in the patient's health record, including the date and time, the testing results, and any patient symptoms shown during the test.
   PURPOSE: Procedures that are not recorded are considered not done.

PROCEDURE 16.3 **Measuring Hearing Acuity With an Audiometer**

Task: Perform audiometric testing of hearing acuity.

EQUIPMENT and SUPPLIES

- Patient's health record
- Provider's order
- Audiometer with adjustable headphones and graph paper
- Quiet area

PROCEDURAL STEPS

1. Wash hands or use hand sanitizer, assemble the equipment, and bring the patient into a quiet area.
   PURPOSE: The testing room should be free of distractions and noise, so the patient can concentrate completely on the hearing evaluation.
2. Greet the patient. Identify yourself. Verify the patient's identity with full name and date of birth. Explain the procedure to be performed in a manner that the patient understands. Answer any questions the patient may have on the procedure.
   PURPOSE: To make sure you have the right patient. Also, explanations help gain the patient's cooperation and ease apprehension.
3. Explain that the audiometer measures whether the patient can hear various sound wave frequencies through the headphones. Each ear is tested separately. When the patient hears a frequency, he or she should raise a hand or push the button to signal the medical assistant.
   PURPOSE: Patient education is needed for compliance with the examination.
4. Place the headphones over the patient's ears, making sure they are adjusted for comfort.
5. The audiometer tests each ear separately, starting at a low frequency. If the results are not automatically recorded by the machine, the medical assistant documents the patient's response to the frequencies on a graph or audiogram. Results for the left ear are marked with an X, and those for the right ear are marked with an O (see the following figure) (Fig. 1). More advanced machines automatically record the results. The medical assistant must have specialized training to conduct this test.

Continued

| PROCEDURE 16.3 | Measuring Hearing Acuity With an Audiometer—*continued* |

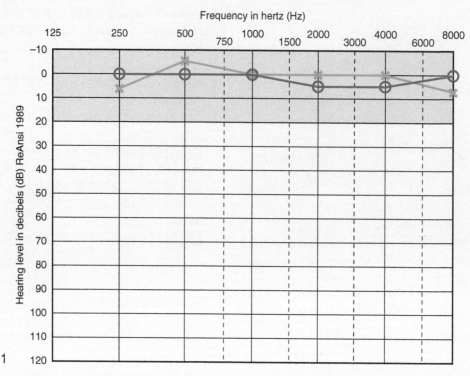

6. Frequencies are increased gradually to test the patient's ability to hear. Each response by the patient is documented.
7. After one ear has been tested, the other ear is then tested, and the results are documented.
8. The results are given to the provider for interpretation or downloaded into the patient's electronic health record for the provider to review.
9. The equipment is sanitized and disinfected according to the manufacturer's guidelines.
10. Wash hands or use hand sanitizer.

| PROCEDURE 16.4 | Irrigate a Patient's Eye |

Task: Irrigate a patient's eye, and document patient care.

EQUIPMENT and SUPPLIES

- Provider's order
- Patient health record
- Drug reference information
- Sterile ophthalmic irrigation solution and supplies
- Disposable waterproof pad and towels
- Basin
- Sterile gauze
- Gloves

PROCEDURAL STEPS

1. Wash hands or use hand sanitizer.
   PURPOSE: Hand sanitization is an important step for infection control.
2. Select the right medication (fluid) from the storage area. Check the medication label against the order. Check for the right name, form, and route.

Check the expiration date to make sure the fluid is not expired. Verify the right dose and the right time.
   PURPOSE: It is important to do the first check of the label when getting the medications from the cabinet. Do not administer expired medications or fluids.
3. Using the drug reference information and the order, review the information on the medication.
   PURPOSE: The medical assistant must know about the medication being given.
4. Perform the second medication check. Check the medication label against the order. Check for the right name, form, and route.
   PURPOSE: It is important to do the second check of the label before continuing with the procedure.
5. Assemble the supplies required for the procedure.
   PURPOSE: You need to have the supplies ready before going to the exam room.

PROCEDURE 16.4 **Irrigate a Patient's Eye**—*continued*

6. Perform the third medication check. Check each medication label against the order. Check for the right name, form, and route.
   PURPOSE: It is important to do the third check of the label before seeing the patient.

7. Prior to entering the exam room, knock on the door and give it a moment. Greet the patient. Identify yourself. Verify the patient's identity with full name and date of birth. Make sure the patient's information matches the order and the record. Explain what you are going to do.
   PURPOSE: It is important to identify the patient in two different ways to ensure that you have the correct patient. Explaining the procedure can make the patient feel more comfortable and reduces anxiety.

8. Provide the right education to the patient. Explain the procedure ordered, the name of the provider ordering the procedure, the desired effect, and common side effects. Answer any questions the patient may have. Use language the patient can understand. Ask the patient if he or she has any allergies. If the patient refuses the procedure, respectfully ask the patient the reason and notify the provider.
   PURPOSE: The patient needs to be aware of what you are giving, the action, side effects, and who ordered it. It is also important to double-check the patient's allergies before starting the procedure.

9. Using room temperature fluid, set up the equipment. If using an intravenous (IV) bag, prime or run fluid through the tubing. If using a prepackaged solution, remove the cover. If using a bulb syringe, pour the required fluid into a basin. Remember to palm the label. Draw the solution into the bulb syringe.
   PURPOSE: Having the fluid ready for the irrigation is important before you hold the eye open.

10. Assist the patient into a sitting or supine position. Have the patient remove glasses or contact lenses. Ask the patient to turn the head toward the side of the affected eye. Place the disposable waterproof pad over the patient's neck and shoulder. Place or have the patient hold the drainage basin next to the affected eye.
    PURPOSE: Protecting the unaffected eye from the solution is important so it does not also get contaminated. The basin will collect the irrigation fluid from the eye.

11. Put on gloves. Moisten a gauze pad with the irrigation fluid. Using the gauze, clean the eyelid from the inner to outer canthus (Fig. 1). Discard the gauze after each wipe.
    PURPOSE: Debris on the eyelid must be removed before the irrigation can be done.

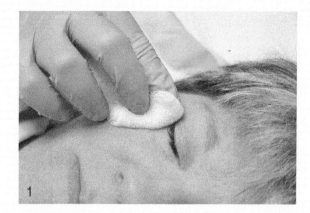

12. Perform the right technique. With your nondominant hand, separate and hold the eyelids using the index finger and thumb. With the dominant hand, hold the irrigation equipment on or near the bridge of the nose (Fig. 2).

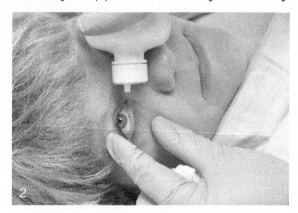

PURPOSE: Using the nose to help steady the irrigation will help to maintain a steady flow of fluid going into the eye.

13. Direct the solution toward the lower conjunctiva of the inner canthus. Allow a steady flow of solution to slowly flush the eye from the inner to the outer canthus. Do not touch the tip of the irrigation equipment to the eye.
    PURPOSE: Touching the eye with the irrigation equipment could lead to an eye injury.

14. Continue until the ordered amount of fluid has flushed the eye. Dry the eyelid with sterile gauze, moving from the inner to outer canthus.
    PURPOSE: It is important to follow the exact order of the provider.

15. Help the patient into a comfortable position. Clean up the area. Remove gloves, and wash hands or use hand sanitizer.
    PURPOSE: It is important that the patient is comfortable.

16. Document the procedure in the health record. Include allergies, teaching or instructions provided, the name of the provider ordering the irrigation, the fluid used for the irrigation, the amount used, the site, and how the patient tolerated the procedure.
    PURPOSE: The irrigation performed needs to be documented to indicate that it was done.

PROCEDURE 16.5   Instill an Eye Medication

Task: Instill an eyedrop or ointment, and document medication administration.

EQUIPMENT and SUPPLIES

- Provider's order
- Patient health record
- Drug reference information
- Sterile ophthalmic eyedrops or ointment
- Sterile gauze
- Gloves

PROCEDURAL STEPS

1. Wash hands or use hand sanitizer.
   PURPOSE: Hand sanitization is an important step for infection control.
2. Select the right medication from the storage area. Check the medication label against the order. Check for the right name, form, and route. Check the expiration date to make sure the drug is not expired. Verify the right dose and the right time.
   PURPOSE: It is important to do the first check of the label when getting the medications from the cabinet. Do not administer expired medications.
3. Using the drug reference information and the order, review the information on the medication.
   PURPOSE: The medical assistant must know about the medication being given.
4. Perform the second medication check. Check the medication label against the order. Check for the right name, form, and route.
   PURPOSE: It is important to do the second check of the label before continuing with the procedure.
5. Assemble the supplies required for the procedure.
   PURPOSE: You need to have the supplies ready before going to the exam room.
6. Perform the third medication check. Check each medication label against the order. Check for the right name, form, and route.
   PURPOSE: It is important to do the third check of the label before seeing the patient.
7. Prior to entering the exam room, knock on the door and wait a moment. Greet the patient. Identify yourself. Verify the patient's identity with full name and date of birth. Make sure the patient's information matches the order and the record. Explain what you are going to do.
   PURPOSE: It is important to identify the patient in two different ways to ensure that you have the correct patient. Explaining the procedure can make the patient feel more comfortable and reduces anxiety.
8. Provide the right education to the patient. Explain the medication ordered, identify the provider ordering the medication, describe the desired effect, and note the common side effects. Answer any questions the patient may have. Use language the patient can understand. Ask the patient if he or she has any allergies. If the patient refuses the medication, notify the provider.
   PURPOSE: The patient needs to be aware of what you are giving, the action, side effects, and who ordered it. It is also important to double-check the patient's allergies before administering the medication.

9. Assist the patient into a sitting or supine position. Ask the patient to tilt the head backward and look up.
   PURPOSE: These positions allow the medical assistant to instill the medication.
10. Put on gloves. If crusting or drainage is present on the eyelid, gently wash the area from the inner to outer canthus. Dry the area.
    PURPOSE: Gloves are used for infection control purposes. Washing and drying the eye prepares the area for the medication.
11. Perform the right technique. With your nondominant hand holding a sterile gauze, pull the lower conjunctival sac downward, creating a pocket for the medication (Fig. 1). Instruct the patient to look up.

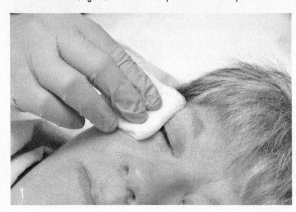

a. For the eyedrops: With your dominant hand, hold the bottle or the dropper ¾ inch away from the conjunctival sac. Drop the required number of drops into the eye (Fig. 2). If the drop misses the eye or the patient blinks, wipe the liquid on the skin and repeat the drop. Have the person keep the eye closed for 2 to 3 minutes after the administration of the drop. Have the person gently press against the inner corner of the eye and nose bone for 2 to 3 minutes.
   PURPOSE: Pressing in the corner after the drops keeps the medication from draining into the tear ducts and nose. This decreases the systemic effects of the medication.

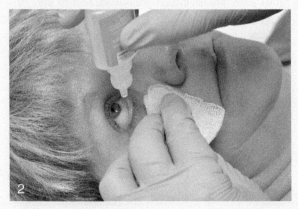

b. For eye ointment: With the dominant hand, hold the ointment container above the lower lid. Working from inner to outer canthus, apply a

PROCEDURE 16.5   Instill an Eye Medication—*continued*

small strip (about ½ inch of ointment along the inner lower lid margin) (Fig. 3). Have the patient close the eye for 1 to 2 minutes to allow the medication to be absorbed. Wipe any extra ointment from the eyelid.
PURPOSE: Rubbing the eyelid after administering the ointment helps to spread the medication over the eye.

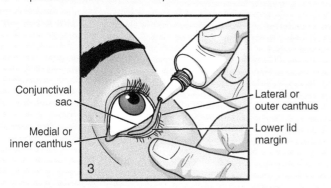

Conjunctival sac
Medial or inner canthus
Lateral or outer canthus
Lower lid margin
3

12. Help the patient into a comfortable position. Clean up the area. Remove gloves, and wash hands or use hand sanitizer.
PURPOSE: It is important that the patient is comfortable.
13. Document the procedure in the health record. Include allergies; teaching or instructions provided; the name of the provider ordering the medication; the medication name, dose, and route; and how the patient tolerated the medication.
PURPOSE: The medication needs to be documented to indicate it was given.

PROCEDURE 16.6   Irrigate a Patient's Ear

Task: Irrigate a patient's ear, and document patient care.

EQUIPMENT and SUPPLIES

- Provider's order
- Patient health record
- Ear wash basin
- Elephant ear wash system (or other ear wash system)
- Disposable waterproof pad and towels
- Thermometer (optional)
- Otoscope and disposable speculum (optional)
- Gauze
- Gloves
- Waste container

Order: Irrigate left ear with warm sterile water.

PROCEDURAL STEPS

1. Read order. Wash hands or use hand sanitizer.
PURPOSE: Hand sanitization is an important step for infection control.
2. Select the right medication (fluid) from the storage area. Check the medication label against the order. Check for the right name and route; check the expiration date.
PURPOSE: It is important to do the first check of the label when getting the medications from the cabinet.
3. Assemble the supplies required for the procedure. Perform the second medication check. Check the medication (fluid) name and route against the order.
PURPOSE: You need to have the supplies ready before going to the exam room.

4. Clean up the work area, and perform the third medication check. Check the medication (fluid) name and route against the order,
PURPOSE: It is important to do three checks before using the fluid.
5. Prior to entering the exam room, knock on the door and wait a moment. Greet the patient. Identify yourself. Verify the patient's identity with full name and date of birth. Make sure the patient's information matches the order and the record. Explain what you are going to do.
PURPOSE: It is important to identify the patient in two different ways to ensure that you have the correct patient. Explaining the procedure can make the patient feel more comfortable and reduces anxiety.
6. Provide the right education to the patient. Explain the procedure ordered, identify the provider ordering the procedure, describe the desired effect, and note the common side effects of ear irrigations. Answer any questions the patient may have. Use language the patient can understand. If the patient refuses the procedure, respectfully ask the patient the reason and notify the provider.
PURPOSE: The patient needs to be aware of what you are giving, the action, side effects of the procedure, and who ordered it.
7. Prepare the equipment. Warm the irrigating solution to body temperature (98.6°F [check with a thermometer]) or until it is lukewarm. Lukewarm is neither hot nor cold. Fill the spray bottle with water. Attach the disposal tip to the nozzle on the hose (Fig. 1). If another type of ear wash system is being used, prepare the equipment and the water.
PURPOSE: It is important to have the fluid ready for the irrigation before holding the ear.

Continued

PROCEDURE 16.6   Irrigate a Patient's Ear—*continued*

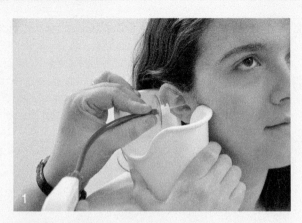

8. Assist the patient into a sitting position. Wrap a waterproof pad around the person's shoulder, protecting the clothing. Have a towel available for the patient if needed. Have the patient tilt his or her head toward the affected ear. Have the patient hold the ear wash basin under the affected ear.
   PURPOSE: It is important to protect the patient's clothing from the irrigating fluid.
9. Put on gloves. Using gauze, wipe any debris from the outer ear.
   PURPOSE: Debris on the outer ear must be removed before the irrigation can be done.
10. With your nondominant hand, gently pull the pinna up and back if the patient is older than age 3. For patients younger than 3, pull the pinna down and back. Insert the disposable tip gently into the ear. Do not insert too far because it could injure the canal.
   PURPOSE: Pulling the pinna helps to straighten the external auditory canal.
11. Keeping the tubing straight, spray the fluid in the ear canal. Aim the fluid toward the top of the ear canal.

PURPOSE: Aiming the fluid toward the top of the canal helps prevent injury to the tympanic membrane. It can also make the procedure more comfortable for the patient.
12. Continue irrigating until the solution is used, the maximum time has been reached, the desired result is achieved, or the patient has problems with the procedure. Empty the ear wash basin when it fills. Observe the fluid for any substances (i.e., cerumen).
   PURPOSE: The provider's order or the facility's procedures will indicate the amount of irrigation fluid to use or when to stop the irrigation.
13. Dry the outside of the ear with gauze. If agency procedure indicates, use an otoscope to observe the canal. Attach the speculum to the otoscope. Straighten the ear canal by pulling the appropriate direction on the pinna. Gently insert the otoscope. Observe the canal.
   PURPOSE: Observing the canal helps you check the results of the irrigation.
14. Place a clean, absorbent towel on the examination table. Have the patient rest quietly with the head turned to the irrigated side while you wait for the provider to return to check the affected ear.
   PURPOSE: Allows the fluid in the canal to drain out.
15. Clean up the work area. Remove your gloves, and dispose of them in the waste container. Wash hands or use hand sanitizer.
   PURPOSE: Hand sanitization is an important step for infection control.
16. Document the procedure in the health record. Include teaching or instructions provided, the name of the provider ordering the irrigation, the fluid used for the irrigation, the amount used, the site, and how the patient tolerated the procedure.
   PURPOSE: The irrigation performed needs to be documented to indicate that it was done.

PROCEDURE 16.7   Instill Eardrops

Task: Instill eardrops, and document medication administration.

EQUIPMENT and SUPPLIES

- Provider's order
- Patient health record
- Drug reference information
- Otic drops
- Gauze
- Gloves

PROCEDURAL STEPS

1. Wash hands or use hand sanitizer.
   PURPOSE: Hand sanitization is an important step for infection control.
2. Select the right medication from the storage area. Check the medication label against the order. Check for the right name, form, and route. Check

the expiration date to make sure the drug is not expired. Verify the right dose and the right time.
   PURPOSE: It is important to do the first check of the label when getting the medications from the cabinet. Do not administer expired medications.
3. Using the drug reference information and the order, review the information on the medication.
   PURPOSE: The medical assistant must know about the medication being given.
4. Perform the second medication check. Check the medication label against the order. Check for the right name, form, and route.
   PURPOSE: It is important to do the second check of the label before continuing with the procedure.

PROCEDURE 16.7   Instill Eardrops—*continued*

5. Assemble the supplies required for the procedure.
   PURPOSE: You need to have the supplies ready before going to the exam room.

6. Perform the third medication check. Check each medication label against the order. Check for the right name, form, and route.
   PURPOSE: It is important to do the third check of the label before seeing the patient.

7. Prior to entering the exam room, knock on the door and wait a moment. Greet the patient. Identify yourself. Verify the patient's identity with full name and date of birth. Make sure the patient's information matches the order and the record. Explain what you are going to do.
   PURPOSE: It is important to identify the patient in two different ways to ensure that you have the correct patient. Explaining the procedure can make the patient feel more comfortable and reduces anxiety.

8. Provide the right education to the patient. Explain the medication ordered, identify the provider ordering the medication, describe the desired effect, and note the common side effects. Answer any questions the patient may have. Use language the patient can understand. Ask the patient if he or she has any allergies. If the patient refuses the medication, respectfully ask the patient the reason and notify the provider.
   PURPOSE: The patient needs to be aware of what you are giving, the action, side effects, and who ordered it. It is also important to double-check the patient's allergies before administering the medication.

9. Assist the patient into a sitting position or in a side-lying position on the unaffected side.
   PURPOSE: These positions allow the medical assistant to instill the medication.

10. Warm the medication bottle with your hands if needed. The drops should be at room temperature. Shake the medication if needed. Put on gloves.
    PURPOSE: If the drops are too hot or too cold, the patient may experience nausea and vertigo. Gloves are used for infection control purposes.

11. Perform the right technique. Have the patient tilt his or her head so the affected ear is upward. If cerumen or drainage is blocking the canal, gently remove it with a cotton-tipped application.
    PURPOSE: The canal must be open to instill the drops.

12. With your nondominant hand, gently pull the pinna up and back if the patient is older than age 3. This straightens the external auditory canal. For patients younger than 3, pull the pinna down and back.
    PURPOSE: Straightening the canal allows the medication to flow down it.

13. Remove the cover of the bottle. Hold the dropper firmly in your dominant hand. Place the tip of the dropper about ½ inch above the ear canal (Fig. 1). Be sure not to contaminate the dropper by touching it to the patient. Carefully drop the required number of drops in the patient's ear. Replace the cover.
    PURPOSE: If the bottle tip gets contaminated, it needs to be discarded.

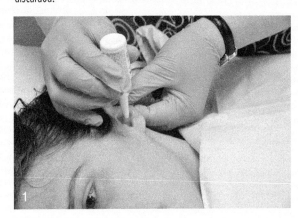

14. Have the patient keep the ear facing up for 3 to 5 minutes, depending on the medication (Fig. 2).
    PURPOSE: Allows the medication to move throughout the canal.

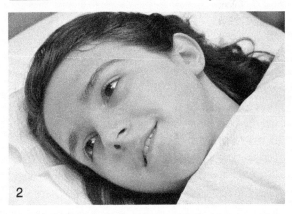

15. Help the patient into a comfortable position. Clean up the area. Remove and dispose of gloves in the waste container. Wash hands or use hand sanitizer.
    PURPOSE: It is important that the patient is comfortable.

16. Document the procedure in the health record. Include allergies; teaching or instructions provided; the name of the provider ordering the medication; the medication name, dose, and route; and how the patient tolerated the medication.
    PURPOSE: The medication needs to be documented to indicate it was given.

SCENARIO

Mai Vang is a medical assistant who has been working at the Walden Martin Family Medical (WMFM) Clinic for 2 years. She really wanted to work in a family practice clinic so that she could see patients of varying ages and medical conditions. Mai has noticed that skin conditions are a frequent reason for patient visits. When she was in high school, she visited her physician to get help for an acne breakout that would not go away. She remembers feeling self-conscious about the condition, so she tries to be especially sensitive to patients with skin diseases and disorders. There is a new patient on the schedule today, Casey Hernandez, and the scheduler indicates that the visit is to discuss possible treatments for acne. Mai understands that she needs to be familiar with common diseases and disorders that affect the skin, be ready to assist with dermatologic procedures, and be prepared to reinforce patient education about the treatment and prevention of dermatologic conditions.

While studying this chapter, think about the following questions:

- What are the basic anatomy and physiology of the integumentary system?
- What are common diseases and disorders that affect the integumentary system?
- How can Mai determine the difference between the levels of burn injuries?
- Why is it important that Mai understand the concepts of staging and grading of malignant tumors?
- What are the primary malignancies of the skin?
- What dermatologic procedures should Mai be prepared to assist with in a dermatology practice?

LEARNING OBJECTIVES

1. Describe the anatomic structures of the skin.
2. Discuss the physiology of the integumentary system.
3. Compare various skin lesions and give examples of each.
4. Describe typical integumentary system infections and infestations.
5. Differentiate among various inflammatory and autoimmune integumentary disorders.
6. Recognize burns and cold injuries to the skin.
7. Describe skin malignancies and their treatment and define the ABCDE rule for identifying a malignant melanoma.
8. Discuss how to assist with a dermatologic examination.
9. Explain dermatologic procedures performed in the ambulatory care setting.

VOCABULARY

basal Bottom layer.

benign A noncancerous condition; not malignant, harmless.

bilirubin A reddish pigment that results from the breakdown of red blood cells in the liver.

collagen (KAH lah jen) The most abundant structural protein found in skin and other connective tissues. It provides strength and cushioning to many parts of the body.

cryosurgery The technique of exposing tissue to extreme cold to produce a well-defined area of cell destruction.

elastin (ee LAS tin) A highly elastic protein in connective tissue that allows tissues to resume their shape after stretching or contracting. It is found abundantly in the dermis of the skin.

ecchymosis (ek i MOH sis) Discoloration of the skin caused by the escape of blood into the tissues from ruptured blood vessels; typically caused by bruising.

epithelial cells (ep i THEE lee al) Form cellular sheets that cover surfaces, both inside and outside the body. Epithelial cells are closely packed, take on different shapes, and strongly stick to each other.

excoriated (ik SKOHR ee ay ted) To strip off or remove the skin from an area.

glomerulonephritis (gloh mer yuh loh neh FRIE tis) Kidney disease affecting the capillaries of the nephron (glomeruli); characterized by albuminuria, edema, and hypertension.

hyperplasia (hahy per PLEY zhee uh) Enlargement due to an abnormal multiplication of cells.

jaundice A yellow discoloration of the skin and mucous membranes caused by deposits of bile.

leukoderma Lack of skin pigmentation, especially in patches.

VOCABULARY—*continued*

malignant A descriptive term for things or conditions that threaten life or well-being. Malignant is the opposite of benign.

melanocytes (meh LAN oh sites) Cells of the stratum germinativum that produce a brownish pigment called *melanin*. Melanin gives us our skin color.

opaque (oh PAYK) Not transparent, cloudy or murky.

pathogen A disease-causing organism.

petechiae (peh TEEK kee ah) Very small, round hemorrhage in the skin or mucous membrane.

pores Tiny openings in the surface of the skin that allow gases, liquids, or microscopic particles to pass.

strata Naturally or artificially formed layers of material, usually multiple layers.

synthesis (SIN theh sis) Formation of a chemical compound from simpler compounds or elements.

The skin is the largest organ of the human body. In an average-size adult, it covers a total area of about 20 square feet. Forming the outer boundary of the body, the skin performs several essential functions: it acts as a barrier to protect vital internal organs from infection and injury; it helps dissipate heat and regulate body temperature; and it synthesizes vitamin D when exposed to ultraviolet (UV) light. In addition, various sensory receptors present throughout the skin enable it to respond to such sensations as heat, cold, pain, and pressure.

The specialty of dermatology deals with the skin and its accessory structures: hair, nails, and sweat glands, and the subcutaneous tissue that lies beneath the skin. A physician who specializes in dermatology is called a *dermatologist*.

ANATOMY OF THE INTEGUMENTARY SYSTEM

The most important function of the skin (or integument) is protecting the body from disease. The skin provides a physical barrier that is our first line of defense against **pathogens.** It is the largest organ of the body, and, in addition to physically protecting the body, is also helps to:

- Regulate the body temperature
- Provide information about the environment through sensory activity
- Assist in the **synthesis** of vitamin D
- Eliminate waste products from the body

The skin functions together with accessory structures that include the hair; nails; *sebaceous* glands, or oil glands; and *sudoriferous* glands, or sweat glands. Any damage or injury to the skin has the potential to lessen its ability to carry out these functions, which can lead to disease.

Skin

The skin is considered a *cutaneous membrane,* made up of **epithelial cells,** that covers the entire body. The skin is composed of two layers: the *epidermis,* which forms the outermost layer, and the *dermis,* which forms the inner layer (Fig. 17.1). The dermis is attached to a layer of connective tissue called the *subcutaneous* layer, or hypodermis, which is mainly composed of fat or *adipose* tissue.

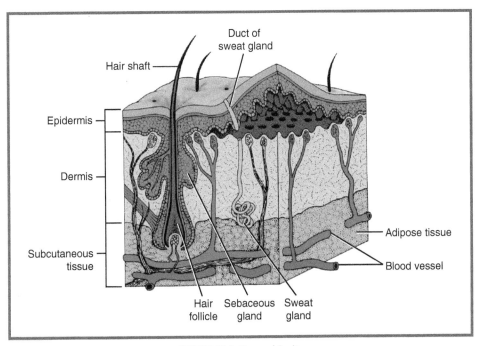

FIGURE 17.1 Diagram of the skin.

Epidermis

The epidermis is the top layer of the skin and is composed of several different **strata** of epithelial tissue. This type of tissue covers many of the external and internal surfaces of the body and has a microscopic scaly appearance.

The epidermis is *avascular*, which means it contains no blood vessels. New skin cells are formed in the **basal** layer of the epidermis, called the *stratum germinativum*. This layer is also where *melanin*, which is a pigment, is produced by **melanocytes**. When the skin is exposed to ultraviolet (UV) light, the melanocytes secrete more melanin. Birthmarks, age spots, and freckles result from clumps of melanin. Individuals have different skin colors because of varying numbers of melanocytes in the stratum germinativum of the skin.

New cells produced in the stratum germinativum move upward toward the top layer, or *stratum corneum*. During the transition from the basal layer to the upper layer, the cell's cytoplasm is replaced with *keratin*. Once this process is complete, the cells are called *keratinocytes*. Keratin is a hard protein material that enhances the skin by making it waterproof, abrasion resistant, and able to retain moisture in the body. These properties add to the protective nature of the skin.

A variety of microorganisms are normally found on the skin. These organisms are referred to as *normal flora*. Healthcare workers are taught to wash their hands or use hand sanitizer before and after each procedure. Good hand hygiene helps prevent the spread of microorganisms, reduces the likelihood of transferring possible pathogens, and decreases the risk of skin infections for our patients.

Dermal-Epidermal Junction

The *dermal-epidermal junction* is where the two layers of the skin meet. The top layer of the dermis contains *dermal papillae*, which are peglike projections that help fasten the dermis and epidermis together. This unique junction not only uses dermal papillae to create a bond, but it also uses a specialized gel that acts as a glue to keep the two layers of the skin connected.

If the dermal-epidermal junction is damaged by a burn, irritation, abrasion, or friction, a blister may occur. If the dermal-epidermal junction is destroyed, the skin will fall apart. If this happens in a small area, the body can heal the damage. If a large area of the junction is destroyed, it would result in an overwhelming infection that would be serious, possibly fatal.

CRITICAL THINKING APPLICATION   17.1

Yesterday Mai wore a new pair of shoes to work and developed a little blister on the heel of her right foot. What skin layers are affected by the formation of a blister? How should Mai properly care for her blister over the next few days?

Dermis

The *dermis* is the thick, underlying layer of the skin that is composed of vascular connective tissue arranged in two layers. The dermis gives the skin strength and stretch that the epidermis does not possess. The thin upper layer of the dermis is composed of fibers made from loose connective tissue, **collagen**, and some **elastin**. The lower, thicker layer of the dermis is composed of dense collagen. Collagen gives the skin toughness and elastin fibers help the skin stretch and have

flexibility. Distributed throughout the dermis are hair follicles, sweat glands, and old glands.

There are two types of sweat glands: *eccrine* and *apocrine*. Eccrine sweat glands are dispersed throughout the body and help maintain a constant body temperature by releasing sweat through **pores** in the skin. Apocrine sweat glands open into hair follicles and are concentrated in the axillae (armpits), scalp, face, and in the pigmented skin around the genitals. Apocrine sweat glands release a fatty sweat in response to stress. They enlarge and become more active at puberty.

The dermis contains many small blood vessels that supply the skin with nutrients and oxygen and take away waste product and carbon dioxide. Sensory receptors for the nervous system (pain, temperature, and pressure) are also located in the dermis.

Subcutaneous Tissue

The subcutaneous tissue is not a layer of the skin. It lies below the dermis and creates a connection between the skin and the structures that are below the skin, such as muscle or bone. Subcutaneous tissue is made up of loose connective tissue and adipose (fat) tissue. This tissue is not rigid but rather movable and pliable. The subcutaneous tissue can slip over underlying structures. Without subcutaneous tissue, our skin would tear with movement.

The subcutaneous tissue provides insulation for the body and serves as a calorie reserve in the adipose tissue. It also contains blood vessels, nerves, and the base of hair follicles. Subcutaneous tissue is distributed unevenly, and as the body ages it thins. This can make administering injections or drawing blood on elderly patients more challenging. Also the loss of subcutaneous tissue makes it more difficult for the elderly to regulate body temperature; they are hotter when temperatures rise and colder when temperatures drop. Aging skin can be very fragile and easily traumatized or damaged. The medical assistant must be very careful to avoid injuring the skin of elderly patients.

CRITICAL THINKING APPLICATION   17.2

Mai goes to the waiting area and calls back Casey Hernandez. She introduces herself and shows Casey back to the exam room. After vital signs are completed, Mai asks Casey the reason for her visit. Casey is looking down and is a bit shy as she talks. Mai notices that the palms of Casey's hands are sweaty. What types of glands produce sweat in the integumentary system? Where are they concentrated in the body?

PHYSIOLOGY OF THE INTEGUMENTARY SYSTEM

The five functions of the integumentary system are listed and discussed next:

- Protection
- Sensory organ activity
- Temperature regulation
- Excretion
- Synthesis of vitamin D

Protection

The skin protects the internal organs by providing a flexible, waterproof barrier to the outside environment. It is part of the first line of defense from microbial pathogens, toxic chemicals, and physical tears, cuts, and abrasions. The keratin in our skin cells protects us from excessive fluid loss and dehydration. Finally, the melanin in the epidermis of the skin protects the body from damaging UV light. Skin is so amazing!

Sensory Organ Activity

The skin has many sensory receptors scattered throughout the tissue. Sensory receptors can feel pain, pressure, heat, and cold. This allows us to respond to the environment and make appropriate changes to keep ourselves from harm.

Temperature Regulation

The skin is a very good thermoregulator. When we are cold, it constricts blood vessels close to the skin's surface. This preserves body heat and lessens the heat loss to the surrounding environment. When we are hot, it can produce sweat that evaporates and cools us off. Because of the extensive blood supply to the skin, the body can help regulate and maintain a consistent body temperature. This is all part of homeostasis.

Excretion

The body can regulate the amount of sweat produced and the chemical content of the sweat. When we sweat, we lose water, electrolytes, and small amounts of other waste products. The integumentary system can excrete substances through the skin to help maintain the necessary chemical balance in the body as a whole.

Synthesis of Vitamin D

The *synthesis* of vitamin D is a vital function of the body, and it all starts in the skin. When skin is exposed to the sun's ultraviolet rays, it manufactures a vitamin D precursor molecule. The molecule is carried to the liver and kidneys by way of the blood. The precursor molecule is then converted to the active form of vitamin D that the body can use. Research has uncovered many body functions affected by vitamin D, a few of which are:

- Proper absorption of calcium
- Maintaining normal calcium and phosphorus levels in the blood; calcium helps maintain strong bones, proper blood clotting, muscle function, and immunity
- Protection against osteoporosis, high blood pressure, and some forms of cancer
- Preventing consistently low vitamin D levels, which can put a person at a higher risk for developing multiple sclerosis, heart disease, osteoporosis, and depression

---

Life Span Changes

Children routinely appear at physician offices with skin disorders. Some of the most common are impetigo, acne, seborrheic dermatitis, cellulitis, and pediculosis. Although none of these are serious disorders, impetigo and pediculosis are highly contagious. Also seen are the different degrees of burns, usually accidental, but potentially life-threatening.

Older patients have a completely different set of diagnoses. The disorders categorized as those related to cornification, especially corns and calluses, are seen routinely in medical offices. These masses or thickenings of the skin are formed as a defensive response to constant friction, usually within shoes. Pressure sores (also called *bedsores* or *decubitus ulcers*) are seen most often in bedridden patients whose skin may already be atrophied and thin. Eczema, cellulitis, and fungal infections are also common complaints. The last category of skin disorders often seen in older adults is skin cancers. Although younger patients with skin cancers are often seen, older patients have had a longer time to be exposed to the sun and develop malignancies.

DISEASES AND DISORDERS OF THE INTEGUMENTARY SYSTEM

Diseases of the integumentary system are varied in appearance and cause. Fig. 17.2 shows examples of many common lesions of the skin. Many factors can cause skin diseases, such as bacterial, fungal, viral, and parasitic infections. Common signs and symptoms seen in patients with skin diseases and disorders include:

- Skin discoloration or redness
- Itching, weeping, or bleeding lesions
- Blisters, macules, papules (see Fig. 17.2 for examples)
- Scaly or flaky skin surface
- New or changing lesions

The underlying cause will vary and likely dictate the type of treatment needed.

A skin *lesion* is any visible, localized abnormality of skin tissue. It can be described as either primary or secondary. Primary lesions are early skin changes that have not yet undergone natural evolution or change caused by manipulation. Secondary lesions are the result of natural evolution or the manipulation of a primary lesion (see Fig. 17.2).

CRITICAL THINKING APPLICATION 17.3

Jean Burke, NP, comes into the exam room and greets Casey. Jean sits down, and she and Casey talk about the reason for Casey's visit, which is her acne, and what improvements Casey would like to see in her skin. Jean mentions that she had issues with acne as a teenager and assures Casey that they will develop a plan together. What type of lesions could Casey have with acne? Review Fig. 17.2 and share your thoughts with the class.

Skin Lesions

Skin lesions can be caused by a systemic problem, such as an allergic reaction to medication, or they may develop from a localized infection. When communicating with the provider and documenting in the patient's health record, always use correct medical terminology to describe skin lesions, such as, "The patient reports a widespread maculopapular rash across the anterior trunk" rather than "The patient has a red, raised rash on his stomach."

When you gather details from the patient about the characteristics of lesions, some elements you should consider include:

- Describe the color, elevation, and texture of the lesion.
- Does the patient have any pain or *pruritus* (itching)? If pruritus is present, is the area **excoriated** or inflamed?

PRIMARY LESIONS

SECONDARY LESIONS

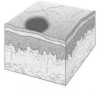

MACULE
Flat area of color change (no elevation or depression)

Example: Freckles

PAPULE
Solid elevation less than 0.5 cm in diameter

Example: Allergic eczema

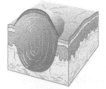

NODULE
Solid elevation 0.5 to 1 cm in diameter. Extends deeper into dermis than papule

Example: Mole

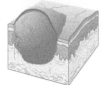

TUMOR
Solid mass—larger than 1 cm

Example: Squamous cell carcinoma

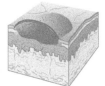

PLAQUE
Flat elevated surface found on skin or mucous membrane

Example: Thrush

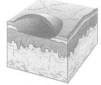

WHEAL
Type of plaque. Result is transient edema in dermis

Example: Intradermal skin test

VESICLE
Small blister—fluid within or under epidermis

Example: Herpesvirus infection

BULLA
Large blister (greater than 0.5 cm)

Example: Burn

PUSTULE
Vesicle filled with pus

Example: Acne

SCALES
Flakes of cornified skin layer

Example: Psoriasis

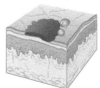

CRUST
Dried exudate on skin

Example: Impetigo

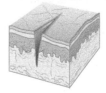

FISSURE
Cracks in skin

Example: Athlete's foot

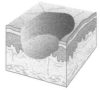

ULCER
Area of destruction of entire epidermis

Example: Decubitus (pressure sore)

SCAR
Excess collagen production after injury

Example: Surgical healing

ATROPHY
Loss of some portion of the skin

Example: Paralysis

FIGURE 17.2 Different types of skin lesions.

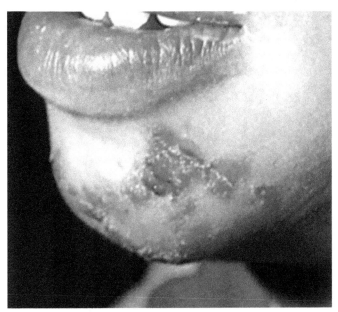

FIGURE 17.3 Impetigo. (From Marks J, Miller J: *Lookingbill and Marks' principles of dermatology*, ed 5, Philadelphia, 2014, Saunders.)

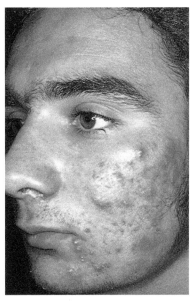

FIGURE 17.4 Acne. (From Paller A, Mancini A: *Hurwitz clinical pediatric dermatology: a textbook of skin disorders in childhood and adolescence*, ed 4, Philadelphia, 2011, Saunders.)

- Is any drainage present? If so, what are its characteristics?
- What is the exact anatomic location of the lesion? Have changes occurred over time?

Primary lesions are those that appear immediately. Macules, papules, plaques, nodules, cysts, wheals, and pustules all are primary lesions. *Secondary lesions* are the result of alterations in a primary lesion. Examples of secondary lesions include scales, crusts, fissures, erosions, ulcerations, and scars (see Fig. 17.2). For instance, vesicles (blisters) from a partial-thickness burn are primary lesions, but if the blisters break and ulcerations form, healing ends in a scar. Ulcerations and scars are secondary lesions.

Infections

Bacterial Infections

Impetigo. Impetigo is a common, superficial infection caused by *Streptococcus sp.* or *Staphylococcus aureus* that usually affects children. Initially impetigo looks like small vesicles on the face (especially around the nose and mouth) that quickly enlarge and rupture, excreting a honey-colored exudate. The exudate forms crusty lesions, and beneath the crust, the area is inflamed and moist (Fig. 17.3). Pruritus accompanies the infection, and scratching helps spread the lesions at the site. Impetigo is contagious, and bacteria are transmitted by direct contact with the drainage, whether at other sites or with other children through the sharing of toys and physical contact. Consistent hand washing is required to help break the chain of infection. It also is important to keep personal items that may be contaminated, such as washcloths, linens, and drinking glasses, away from other members of the family. If the areas of infection are limited, topical treatment with an antibiotic ointment may be effective. However, impetigo caused by streptococci may result in **glomerulonephritis**; more involved infections may require treatment with oral antibiotics.

Acne Vulgaris. Acne vulgaris is a skin condition that occurs when a hair follicle becomes plugged with oil and dead skin cells (Fig. 17.4). Acne is most common on the face, but it can occur on other sites of the body, such as the neck, chest, shoulders, and back. Acne is most common during adolescence, but it can occur at any age. Because acne can cause scarring, it is best treated as early as possible to minimize scars and emotional distress.

The main causes of acne include excess oil production, pores clogged with dead skin cells and oil, and bacterial infections. Once a pore is clogged, bacteria that are trapped in the pore multiply and cause inflammation. Risk factors for acne include age (adolescents are most prone due to hormonal changes), medications (corticosteroids, androgens, oral contraceptives, and lithium), stress, and diet (a diet that is high in dairy products and simple carbohydrates, such as refined sugars, processed foods, and sweets, can make acne worse). The signs and symptoms of acne can vary in severity. Common symptoms include:

- Whiteheads and blackheads
- Papules and pustules
- Large, solid, painful nodules
- Painful, pus-filled lumps beneath the skin's surface, known as *cystic acne*

There are many treatments used for acne, from simple over-the-counter (OTC) lotions to more extensive use of medications, antibiotics, and dermatologic procedures.

- Common medications include topical prescription-strength benzoyl peroxide, antibiotics, retinoids, and oral contraceptives.
- Common dermatologic procedures include light therapy, chemical peels, extraction of whiteheads and blackheads by a provider, and steroid injections.
- Common dietary changes recommended include reducing or eliminating dairy products, refined sugar, and simple carbohydrate foods. Examples include juice, soda, sweets, pasta, and bread.
- More extensive treatments include dermabrasion, laser resurfacing, and minor skin surgery to repair areas of damage or excessive scarring.

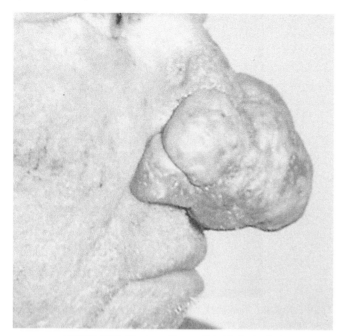

FIGURE 17.5 Rhinophyma. (Courtesy Michael O. Murphy, MD.)

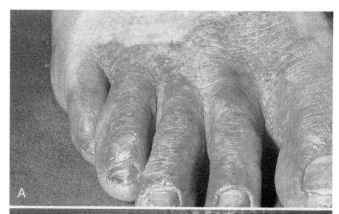

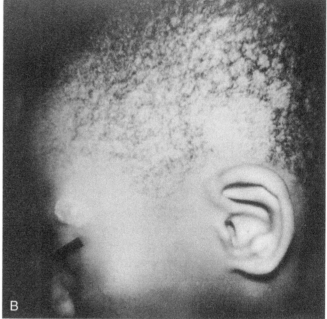

FIGURE 17.6 Fungal infections. **(A)** Tinea pedis. **(B)** Tinea corporis. (**A** from Gawkrodger D: *Dermatology*, ed 5, New York, 2012, Churchill Livingstone; **B** from Mahon CR et al: *Textbook of diagnostic microbiology*, ed 5, Philadelphia, 2015, Saunders.)

Acne often requires extended treatment and follow-up, depending on the severity of the condition.

Rosacea. Rosacea is a chronic disease seen most frequently in women between the ages of 30 and 60. It causes inflammation and pustule formation and begins as frequent flushing across the nose, forehead, cheeks, and chin.

As the condition progresses, capillaries of the face dilate and are visible across affected areas as small, red, edematous lines; these are accompanied by eye inflammation and photosensitivity. Over time, the face appears red, eye inflammation is more apparent, and painful nodules and pustules form. Men with rosacea may develop *rhinophyma*, a large, inflamed, bulbous nose caused by **hyperplasia** of sebaceous nasal tissue (Fig. 17.5). Individuals with rosacea eventually may develop an obvious thickening of the skin across the forehead, nose, cheeks, and chin.

The condition is treated with topical antibiotics and, as symptoms progress, with oral antibiotics, such as doxycycline (Oracea), which helps reduce the number of pimples and bumps on the face; however, it may not reduce the redness and flushing.

Furuncles and Carbuncles. A *furuncle*, or boil, is a localized staphylococcal infection that begins as inflammation of a hair follicle (folliculitis) or skin gland. The affected area is raised, inflamed, and painful and eventually may produce purulent drainage. A carbuncle is a collection of furuncles that have joined to form a large, infected area that may drain through multiple sites or form an abscess. Both infections are treated with oral antibiotics, frequent cleansing of the area, application of an antibiotic ointment and, in some cases, surgical incision and drainage of the purulent material.

Cellulitis. *Cellulitis* is an acute infection of the skin and subcutaneous tissue caused by staphylococci or streptococci. It begins from a small cut or as a result of a skin injury, or it develops at the site of a furuncle or an ulcer. The area surrounding the site becomes inflamed, edematous, and painful with red streaks along the lymph vessels that lead from the infection. The condition is treated with oral antibiotics. Warm compresses applied locally aid healing, and analgesics may be needed to relieve discomfort. It is important that patients with cellulitis are treated appropriately because a systemic infection can develop if the lymph glands become involved.

Fungal Infections (Dermatophytoses)

Fungal, or mycotic, infections, such as *tinea pedis* (athlete's foot) (Fig. 17.6A), *tinea cruris* (jock itch), and *tinea corporis* (ringworm) (Fig. 17.6B) are extremely common. These pathogens infect hair follicles or the nails, causing almost no inflammation in the underlying skin. The fungus invades the skin where it has been damaged or is consistently moist. All of these lesions are pruritic and are characterized by a distinct border with scaling areas that have a clear center. Secondary bacterial infections may occur with excoriation.

The provider typically diagnoses a fungal infection by noting the way the skin looks and the patient's complaints of pruritus. The skin may be scraped to obtain cells for examination under a microscope, and sometimes the provider may order a skin culture, in which a suspicious area is swabbed or scraped using sterile technique. The

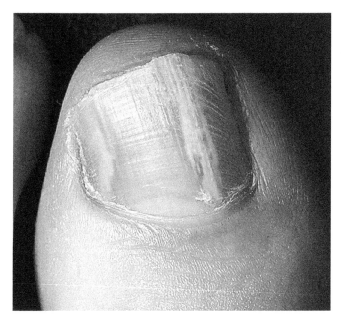

FIGURE 17.7 Tinea unguium. (From Habif TP: *Clinical dermatology*, ed 5, St Louis, 2010, Mosby.)

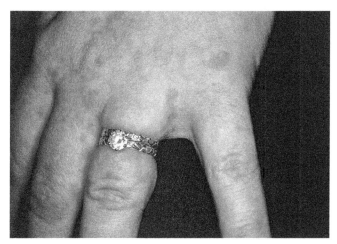

FIGURE 17.8 Scabies rash of the hand. (From James WD et al: *Andrews' diseases of the skin*, ed 11, Philadelphia, 2011, Saunders.)

sample is sent to the laboratory for analysis. Treatment consists of topical antifungal agents, such as clotrimazole (Lotrimin), ketoconazole (Nizoral), econazole, or nystatin (Mycostatin). Antibiotics may be necessary if a secondary infection occurs. Because mycotic infections thrive in dark, moist areas, the patient should be advised to keep the site clean and dry and to wear loose clothing if possible. All types of dermatophytoses can become chronic infections if not managed carefully.

Tinea unguium, or *onychomycosis* (Fig. 17.7), is a fungal infection of the toenails and fingernails. Unlike athlete's foot, which occurs on the skin's surface, nail fungus lives in the nail bed and the nail plate. The nail provides the fungus with an extremely well-protected place to live, which is why nail fungus may be especially difficult to treat. The primary sign of nail fungus is the appearance of the nail, which turns yellow, white, or **opaque**. The texture also changes, and the nail becomes thick and brittle. If the fungus has been present for a long time, the nail can become twisted or distorted. The most effective treatment for nail fungus is oral terbinafine hydrochloride (Lamisil) or itraconazole (Sporanox), which inhibit the production of fungal cells. However, the drug must be taken for 6 weeks to treat fungal infection of a fingernail and for 12 weeks for infection of a toenail; treatment carries the risk of liver complications.

Viral Infections

Warts. Warts, or verrucae, are caused by the human papillomavirus (HPV). Infection with HPV results in hyperplasia of the epidermis and a raised, cauliflower-like appearance. Verrucae can develop anywhere, but the most common sites are the fingers and the soles (plantar warts). Most warts resolve over time, but they can be treated with topical chemicals, excised surgically, vaporized with lasers, or removed with **cryosurgery**.

Herpes Simplex (Cold Sores). Cold sores, or fever blisters, are caused by herpes simplex virus type 1 (HSV-1). The initial infection may be asymptomatic or may cause painful ulcers along the gum lines of the mouth or on the lips. After the primary infection, the virus remains dormant in the trigeminal nerve and can be reactivated by exposure to the sun or to cold; by the presence of another infection, such as an upper respiratory infection; or when the patient is under stress. The patient reports a feeling of burning, tingling, or numbness before the eruption of vesicles. The blisters heal in 2 to 3 weeks, but the process may be speeded up by the use of topical antiviral drugs, such as acyclovir (Zovirax), docosanol (Abreva), or penciclovir cream (Denavir), or with oral antivirals, including famciclovir (Famvir), acyclovir, or valacyclovir (Valtrex). If started at the first indications of a cold sore, antiviral medications can limit the duration and severity of the outbreak.

Parasites

Parasitic infestations of the skin can occur at any age. They are spread in group settings, such as among families or in childcare groups, school classes, nursing homes, prisons, and dormitories. The two most common types of skin parasites seen are scabies (itch mites) and pediculosis (lice). Both parasites infect the skin and cause itching. Both parasites can be treated, and the infection resolved.

Scabies is caused by the itch mite *Sarcoptes scabiei.* This little mite burrows under the skin, causing intense itching (Fig. 17.8).

Pediculosis is caused by lice that populate three specific areas of the body (Fig. 17.9). A person can have head lice (*Pediculus capitis),* body lice *(Pediculus corporis),* or pubic lice, or crabs *(Pthirus pubis).* Lice crawl but cannot fly or hop.

Both itch mites and lice can move from person to person through close physical contact and through sharing of inanimate objects, or *fomites,* such as combs, brushes, clothes, and bedding.

The signs and symptoms of scabies and pediculosis are similar:
- Intense itching
- Tickling feeling as parasites move hair on the skin
- Lice: small red bumps on the skin and nits (eggs) on the body, facial, or pubic hair
- Scabies: little burrows or tunnels can be seen under the skin, frequently in areas of the skin that fold, such as between fingers and toes, around the waist, in the armpits, and on knees and elbows

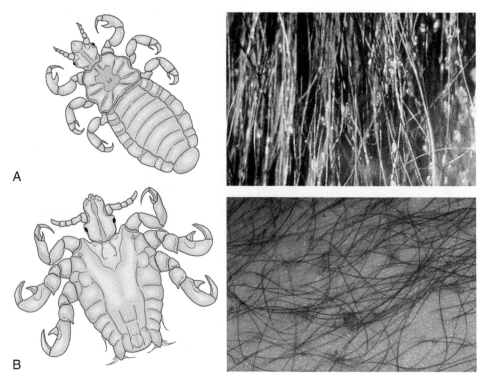

FIGURE 17.9 Types of lice. **(A)** *Pediculus humanus* capitis (head louse) and lice in the hair. **(B)** *Phthirus pubis* (pubic or crab louse) and pubic lice rash. (**A** from Lissauer T et al: *Illustrated textbook of paediatrics*, ed 4, London, 2012, Mosby; **B** from Long SS et al: *Principles and practice of pediatric infectious diseases*, ed 4, Philadelphia, 2012, Saunders.)

Diagnosis of lice infestation is often done with a magnifying lens to see the lice and nits on hair. A Wood light, which produces UV light, can also be used to detect the nits. They look pale blue. For scabies, physical examination involves looking for characteristic burrows under the skin. The provider may scrape the skin and examine it under the microscope to look for eggs. Prescription shampoo, body wash, and lotion can be used to kill the parasites on the head, hair, and body. The lice and mites are generally killed quickly, but the patient must follow all instructions to make sure eggs are also killed. There may be some itching after the parasites are killed, but that does not necessarily indicate a continued infection. Women who are pregnant and the parents of infants should consult their provider before applying antiparasitic products. They are strong chemicals that may cause complications for the very young and for pregnant women.

In addition to properly washing the hair and body, all clothing, bedding, personal items, furniture should also be cleaned with hot, soapy water. If all the eggs are not removed, reinfections can occur.

Inflammatory Skin Disorders

Seborrheic Dermatitis. Seborrheic dermatitis is one of the most common chronic inflammatory conditions of the sebaceous glands. It alters the amount and quality of the sebum, resulting in dry or moist, greasy-appearing scales and yellowish crusts on the scalp, eyebrows, eyelids, and sides of the nose, behind the ears, and in the middle of the chest. The condition has many different forms, including cradle cap in infants and dandruff in adults. Seborrheic dermatitis of the scalp can be treated with tar- or sulfur-based shampoos; inflammations of the skin usually are treated with topical corticosteroids, such as generic triamcinolone diacetate or betamethasone valerate,

or fluocinolone acetonide (Synalar). Seborrheic keratosis (age spots) is characterized by **benign**, slightly raised, tan to black lesions that occur with aging.

Contact Dermatitis. Contact dermatitis is an acute inflammatory response to a skin irritant or from exposure to a substance that causes an allergic reaction. An individual who is allergic to latex gloves or who has been exposed to poison ivy shows the signs and symptoms of contact dermatitis. The individual complains of redness (*erythema*), edema, pruritus, and vesicles. The patient should be encouraged to wash the affected area immediately after exposure to remove the irritant. Medical treatment includes application of a corticosteroid cream or the use of oral corticosteroid medications (e.g., prednisone, methylprednisolone [Medrol]) if the symptoms are severe.

Eczema (Atopic Dermatitis). Eczema, also known as *atopic dermatitis*, is a group of conditions that will make skin irritated, inflamed, red, and itchy. It is more common in children but can occur at any age. Eczema is a chronic condition that may become worse occasionally and then subside. Eczema is a group of conditions with an inherited tendency. It is often seen in combination with asthma or hay fever. Most children who develop eczema outgrow it by their 10th birthday. Some adults continue to have symptoms throughout their lifetime. The disease often can be controlled with proper treatment.

The cause of eczema is unknown, but it is more common in families with a history of allergies and asthma. Flare-ups can occur in response to specific substances, conditions, or triggers. Temperature, exposure to certain chemicals, fabric texture, pet dander, and stress are all examples of possible irritants. Some of the common signs and symptoms of eczema include; itchy skin; rash on the face, back of the knees, hands, wrists, or feet; and a dry, thickened, or scaly appearance of the skin that starts out pink or red but can turn brownish with time.

A pediatrician, dermatologist, or primary care provider will observe the rash and ask specific questions about the signs and symptoms. Sometimes the provider will perform allergy tests to try to pinpoint a specific trigger or irritant. Most frequently, observation and the patient history are sufficient to diagnose eczema. The treatment of eczema is focused on relieving itching and preventing scratching of the skin, which can lead to infection. Using a provider-recommended lotion or cream to keep the skin moist is the most common treatment. Applying topical treatments when the skin is damp (i.e., after a bath or shower) may help the skin to retain moisture. Cold compresses and 1% hydrocortisone cream are also common treatments.

If OTC remedies are not providing relief, creams and ointments that contain corticosteroids can be prescribed to lessen inflammation of the skin. Antibiotics may also be prescribed if an area becomes infected after vigorous itching. Additional treatments include antihistamines and UV light therapy. For patients with moderate to unresponsive eczema, cyclosporine or topical immunomodulators (TIMs) may be prescribed to help prevent flare-ups.

Autoimmune Skin Disorders

Psoriasis. Psoriasis is an autoimmune disease that affects the life cycle of skin cells. Psoriasis causes skin cells to build up rapidly on the surface of the skin. The extra skin cells form thick, silvery scales and itchy, dry, red patches that are sometimes painful. There may be times when symptoms get better, alternating with times when the psoriasis worsens.

Psoriasis is caused by a malfunction in the immune cells called T lymphocytes (T cells). T lymphocytes normally travel through the body looking for pathogens (bacteria and viruses) to destroy. But in people who have psoriasis, the T lymphocytes attack healthy skin cells. This T-cell overactivity causes the skin to produce too many new skin cells and the immune system to produce too many T cells.

It is unclear why the immune system of people with psoriasis acts this way. It can become a vicious circle of rapid skin cell production, which leads to the characteristic psoriasis plaques. Anyone can develop psoriasis, but risk factors include a family history of psoriasis, stress, a history of recurring streptococcal infections, obesity, and smoking. Signs and symptoms of psoriasis can vary, but plaques have a characteristic appearance that tends to be:

- Red patches of skin covered in silvery scales
- Dry, cracked skin that may bleed and small patches of scaly spots
- Itching, burning, and pain in and around plaques
- Thick, pitted, or ridged finger and toenails
- Swollen and stiff joints

Some people may only have a few spots of psoriasis; others may have large skin eruptions that may cover large areas of the body. Psoriasis may erupt, then get better, and continue this cycle for years.

Some of the most common forms of psoriasis are plaque, nail, scalp, and psoriatic arthritis, which also affects the joints (Fig. 17.10).

Discoid Lupus Erythematosus. Discoid lupus erythematosus is the most common form of chronic cutaneous lupus. It is a chronic autoimmune disease of the skin that presents as sores with inflammation and scarring favoring the face, ears, and scalp (sun-exposed areas)

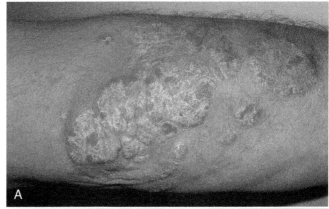
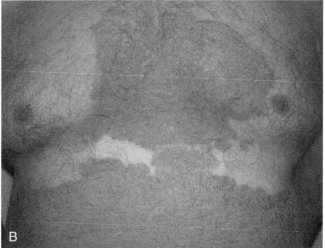

FIGURE 17.10 Psoriasis. (From Marks J, Miller J: *Lookingbill and Marks' principles of dermatology,* ed 5, Philadelphia, 2014, Saunders.)

and at times other body areas. The sores are usually coin-shaped red lesions with inflamed patches with a scaly or crusty appearance. These lesions can cause disfiguring scars. If the lesions are on the scalp there may be permanent hair loss after the lesions have healed.

Diagnosis is made with a physical examination with a complete history and laboratory evaluation. Patients with cutaneous lupus may not have any abnormal laboratory test results. A skin biopsy of a lesion may be done. Discoid lupus is very photosensitive, so prevention of sun exposure is very important. Treatments include the use of sunscreen and avoidance of sun exposure; corticosteroid creams or ointment may be used in conjunction with injections.

Burns

Burns are injuries to tissues that result from exposure to thermal, chemical, electrical, or radioactive agents. They are classified into four different degrees of severity, depending on the layers of the skin that are damaged. Burns that are second degree or higher should be further categorized according to the "rule of nines." The rule of nines regarding burns divides the body into percentages that are, for the most part, multiples of nine: the head and neck equal 9%, each upper limb 9%, each lower limb 18%, the front of the torso 18%, back of the torso 18%, and the genital area 1% (Fig. 17.11). Fig. 17.12 illustrates the different degrees of burns.

Because burns are injuries, the cause is trauma of some kind. Many risk factors could be included in this discussion, but particular caution should be exercised when participating in activities that involve fire, chemicals, or electrical hazards. Proper safety equipment should always be available and ready to use when burns are a possibility.

The categories of burns are:

- First-degree burn (superficial burn): A burn in which only the first layer of the skin, the epidermis, is damaged. It is characterized by redness (*erythema*), tenderness, and physical sensitivity (*hyperesthesia*), with no scar development.
- Second-degree burn (partial-thickness burn): A burn in which only the first and second layers of the skin (the epidermis and part of the dermis) are affected. If the burn extends to the papillary level, it is classified as a *superficial partial-thickness burn*. If it extends farther, to the reticular layer, it is classified as a *deep partial-thickness burn*. This type of burn is characterized by redness, blisters, and pain, with possible scar development.
- Third-degree burn (full-thickness burn): A burn that damages the epidermis, dermis, and subcutaneous tissue. Pain is not present because the nerve endings in the skin have been destroyed. The skin may appear deep red, pale gray, brown, or black. Scar formation is likely.
- Fourth-degree burn (deep full-thickness burn): Although not a universally accepted category, some burn specialists use this category to describe a rare burn that extends beyond the subcutaneous tissue into the muscle and bone.

Burns may not uniformly affect an injured area, so determining the depth of a burn and the extent of tissue damage is important. Burns are treated differently depending on the depth of damage. Treatment is based on the category of burn.

The American Burn Association defines a severe burn as a burn that affects 25% of the total body surface area or any burn involving the eyes, ears, face, hands, feet, or groin. With a severe burn, the patient may require additional testing, such as laboratory tests, x-rays, or other diagnostics. The treatment of burns listed in Table 17.1 is based on the category of burn.

Cold Injuries

Cold injuries usually are less severe than burns, but prolonged exposure to cold temperatures can result in infection, gangrene, amputation and, in severe cases, death. Frostbite is caused by exposure to subfreezing temperatures. Damage occurs at the level of the capillaries, which become permanently dilated and unable to regulate local blood flow. Signs and symptoms of superficial frostbite include burning, tingling, numbness, and a white or grayish color of the skin. With deep frostbite, blisters form and the area is hard, mottled, edematous, and blue or gray after thawing.

The extent of injury is determined by visual examination and the history of the exposure. Treatment consists of warming the area with immersion in warm water (100° F to 106° F [38° C to 41° C]). The affected site should never be rubbed because this increases cellular destruction. The person's vital signs should be monitored, and the provider's orders should be followed explicitly.

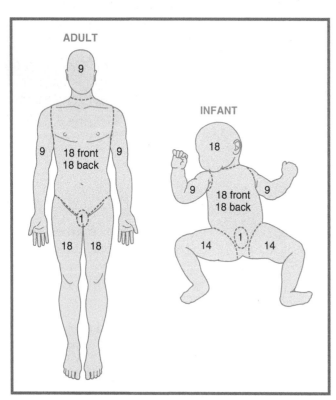

FIGURE 17.11 Rule of nines classification of burns.

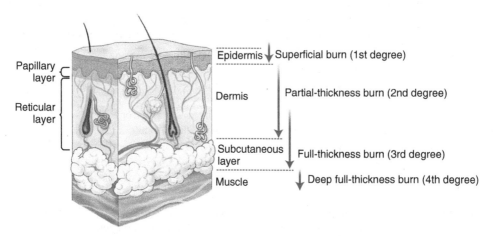

FIGURE 17.12 Burn category tissue involvement. (From Shiland B: *Mastering healthcare terminology*, ed 5, St. Louis, 2016, Elsevier.)

TABLE 17.1	Treatment of Burns		
	FIRST-DEGREE BURN	SECOND-DEGREE BURN	THIRD- AND FOURTH-DEGREE BURNS[a]
Treatment, nondrug	• Cool to cold water to immerse the affected area	Rinse burned skin with cool water until the pain stops, 10–30 minutes; additional cool compresses as needed • Do not break open blisters • Bandage the area if blisters are broken to prevent infection • Wrap area loosely; do not put pressure on the area • If the burn is on an arm or a leg, keep the area raised to reduce swelling	• Cover the affected area with sterile gauze or a clean cloth, depending on the size of the burn, until medical help arrives • Do not open blisters or remove clothing stuck to the burned area • Elevate body part if possible
Treatment, medications	• Analgesics for pain	• Analgesics for pain	• Pain medications consistent with pain needs; analgesics, opioids • Antibiotics
Surgical intervention	• None	• None	• Will often require skin grafts to close the wound and heal the affected area; plastic surgery and muscle/bone surgical restoration may be required; if bone and muscle are destroyed, amputation of affected areas may be necessary and prosthetics may be required
Other treatments	Topical OTC burn cream, aloe vera gel used to promote healing and limit scarring	Depending on the severity of the burn and tissue damage, the following services may be needed: • Physical therapy • Occupational therapy • Pain management • Counseling to deal with emotional issues during and after recovery	
Follow-up treatments	Seek medical attention if area looks infected or is not healing	Seek medical attention *immediately* if blistered area looks infected or is not healing	Ongoing depending on the extent of tissue damage

[a]This category of burn needs immediate and ongoing medical attention.

Carcinomas of the Skin

Skin cancer is the abnormal, **malignant** growth of skin cells. Skin that is exposed to the sun is at higher risk for developing skin cancer, but skin cancer can also occur on skin not ordinarily exposed to sunlight.

There are three major types of skin cancer:
• Basal cell carcinoma
• Squamous cell carcinoma
• Melanoma, often called *malignant melanoma*

Skin cancer starts with mutations that occur in the DNA of skin cells. The mutations cause the cells to grow out of control and form cancer cells. Skin cancer begins in the epidermis.

Skin cancer can happen in three different types of cells in the epidermis:
• *Squamous cells* lie just below the outer surface of the skin.
• *Basal cells* produce new skin cells and are located beneath the squamous cells.

• *Melanocytes* produce melanin, the pigment that gives skin its normal color. They are located in the lower part of the epidermis.

These cancers are thought to be caused by exposure to UV rays of the sun. UV rays can damage DNA in the skin's cells, which starts a mutation. However, not all cancers develop in areas of the body exposed to the sun; it is still unknown what other specific factors influence the start of a malignant mutation. Additional risk factors for skin cancer include fair skin with blond or red hair and light-colored eyes, and skin that freckles or sunburns easily; a history of sunburns that have blistered; moles that look irregular and are generally larger than normal moles; and a family history of skin cancer (if one parent or a sibling has had skin cancer, there may be an increased risk of the disease). Basal cell carcinoma most frequently appears on sun-exposed areas (Fig. 17.13) and may appear as:
• A pearly or waxy bump
• A flat, flesh-colored or brown scarlike lesion

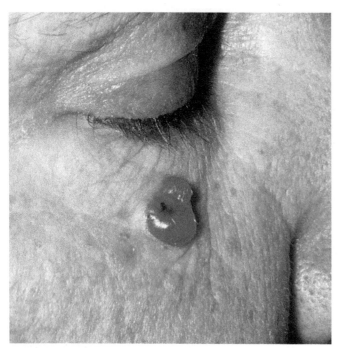

FIGURE 17.13 Basal cell carcinoma. (From James WD, et al: *Andrews' diseases of the skin*, ed 11, Philadelphia, 2011, Saunders.)

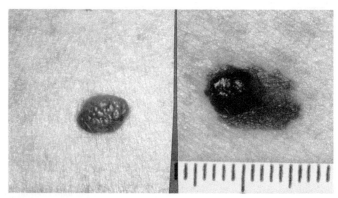

FIGURE 17.15 Pigmented skin lesions. *Left,* Benign pigmented nevus (mole). *Right,* Malignant melanoma. (Courtesy National Cancer Institute, Bethesda, MD.)

skin can develop melanoma on the palms of their hands or the soles of their feet, or even under fingernails or toenails. Melanoma may appear as:

- A large brownish spot with darker speckles
- A mole that changes in color, size, or feel or that bleeds
- A small lesion with an irregular border and portions that appear red, white, blue, or blue-black
- Dark lesions on the palms of the hands, soles of the feet, fingertips, or toes

To diagnose any type of skin cancer, the provider will do the following:

- Examine the skin and look for changes that are likely to be skin cancer.
- If abnormal areas of the skin are found, a skin biopsy will be performed. A biopsy will determine whether skin cancer is present and what type of cancer it is.
- Additional tests may be done to determine the extent or stage of the skin cancer. These tests might include:
  - Imaging tests to examine nearby lymph nodes for signs of cancer.
  - Removal of a nearby lymph node that will be tested for signs of cancer and staged; a skin cancer's stage helps determine which treatment options will be most effective.

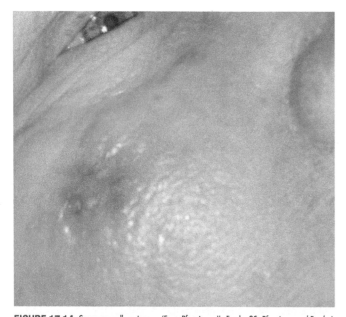

FIGURE 17.14 Squamous cell carcinoma. (From Pfenninger JL, Fowler GC: *Pfenninger and Fowler's procedures for primary care,* ed 3, Philadelphia, 2011, Saunders.)

Squamous cell carcinoma most frequently appears on sun-exposed areas (Fig. 17.14) and may appear as:

- A firm, red nodule
- A flat lesion with a scaly, crusted surface

Melanoma can develop anywhere on the body (Fig. 17.15). It can start in normal-looking skin or in an existing mole. Skin that has not been exposed to sunlight can still develop melanoma. Melanoma can affect people of any skin color. People with darker

Early Warning Signs of Malignant Melanoma

If a mole displays any of the following characteristics, a dermatologist should examine it immediately.

A	Asymmetry	One half of the mole does not match the other half.
B	Border	The edges of the mole are blurred or irregular.
C	Color	The mole is not the same color throughout and has shades of tan, brown, black, red, white, or blue.
D	Diameter	The mole is larger than 6 mm, about the size of a pencil eraser.
E	Elevation	A mole that once was flat against the skin now is raised and elevated.

CRITICAL THINKING APPLICATION 17.4

After Jean Burke and Casey go over the proposed treatment plan, Jean takes out a brochure on skin cancer. She shows the brochure to Casey and reminds her of how important her skin is. Even though Casey is young, precautions taken now could help prevent skin cancer in her future. List five preventive measures that she can take now in order to protect her skin from cancer. Share with the class.

Treatment for skin cancer varies greatly, depending on the type of skin cancer and its stage. Early detection and treatment are always the best options for any type of skin cancer, but that is not always possible.

Common treatments for basal cell and squamous cell carcinomas include:

- Mohs micrographic surgery
- Excisional surgery
- Topical medications and photodynamic therapy (PDT)
- Electrosurgery, cryosurgery, or laser surgery

Treatment for melanoma varies greatly, depending on the location and stage of the cancer. Treatment ranges from minor localized surgery to major surgery, radiation, and chemotherapy.

OTHER DISEASES AND DISORDERS OF THE INTEGUMENTARY SYSTEM

We have covered some of the more common diseases and disorders of the integumentary system, but there are many others. Table 17.2 lists additional diseases and disorders, along with a brief description.

ROLE OF THE MEDICAL ASSISTANT IN DERMATOLOGY

The integumentary system can reflect both internal and external reactions and disease processes. The skin holds information about the body's circulation and nutritional status and signs of systemic diseases. It also acts as a mirror, reflecting aging changes that occur in all organs of the body. For many people, self-esteem is linked to a youthful appearance, and dermatologic conditions may be very threatening to feelings of self-worth. As you prepare patients for a dermatologic examination, allow them to express their anxieties. The conditions that most frequently bring a patient to the dermatologist's office are cosmetic disfigurements caused by a skin disease, pain and pruritus, and interference with sensations or movements.

TABLE 17.2 Additional Diseases and Disorders of the Integumentary System

DISEASE/DISORDER	DESCRIPTION
Albinism	Complete lack of melanin production by existing melanocytes, resulting in pale skin, white hair, and pink iris of the eye
Callus	Common painless thickening of the stratum corneum at locations of external pressure or friction
Candidiasis	Yeast infection in moist, creased areas of the skin (armpits, inner thighs, underneath pendulous breasts) and mucous membranes; also called *moniliasis*
Decubitus ulcers	Also called *bedsore* or *pressure ulcer*. Injuries to the skin and underlying tissue from prolonged pressure to the skin. Most common on skin that covers bony areas of the body, such as heels, ankles, hips, tailbone, elbows, and shoulders.
Hyperhidrosis	Excessive perspiration. Possible causes include hyperthyroidism, menopause, hot temperatures, emotional situations, and infection.
Hypertrichosis	Also known as *hirsutism*. Abnormally hairy.
Kaposi sarcoma (KS)	A rare reddish-purple skin cancer. Seen frequently in patients with acquired immunodeficiency syndrome (AIDS) and other immunocompromised conditions. Causative agent is human herpes virus-8 (HHV8).
Scleroderma	An autoimmune disease. Local condition affects the skin. Systemic condition also affects internal organs. Demonstrates a chronic hardening and contraction of the skin and/or connective tissue. (See Chapter 18 for additional information on autoimmune diseases.)
Systemic lupus erythematosus (SLE)	An autoimmune disease. Can affect many systems or organs of the body, including skin, joints, kidneys, brain, lungs, and heart. (See Chapter 18 for additional information on autoimmune diseases.)
Urticaria	Also called *hives*. May be caused by an allergic reaction to specific foods or personal care products. Raised, round, red welts on the skin. Accompanied by intense itching.
Vitiligo	An autoimmune disease. Skin appears to have random areas with little or no pigment. Unknown etiology (Fig. 17.16)

Assisting With the Dermatologic Examination

During a dermatologic examination, the provider inspects the entire body, beginning with the scalp and continuing to the soles, including the genital area. Inspection of the skin is followed by detailed examination of suspicious areas through palpation, diascopy, and special tests. A *diascope* is a glass plate held firmly against the skin to permit observation of changes produced in underlying areas when pressure is applied. Inspection may include the use of a magnifying lens and a bright light to closely examine a suspicious lesion or growth. The dermatologist frequently asks the medical assistant to take photographs of moles and/or to document specific measurements and locations of suspicious lesions. These are placed in the health record for comparison when the patient returns for follow-up visits.

In the physical examination, concerns about the integumentary system include abnormal coloring, such as cyanosis, pallor, vitiligo, erythema, **leukoderma**, or excessive brown patches. **Jaundice** may indicate an increase in the level of **bilirubin** in the blood. Lesions, ulcers, and bruises may be the result of pathologic conditions. Localized red or purple discoloration may be caused by vascular neoplasms, birthmarks, or subcutaneous hemorrhages (**petechiae** and **ecchymosis**). Palpation helps confirm findings of the inspection. Therefore, inspection and palpation are interrelated in confirming the diagnosis of an integumentary system disorder. Palpated findings may include the skin's texture or elasticity or the presence of edema or a neoplasm.

Gowning and draping a patient for a skin examination depend on the area to be examined. Remember to expose the area adequately but also to protect the patient's privacy. Try to make the patient as comfortable as possible and offer support when it is needed.

Assisting With Diagnostic Procedures

Tissue Biopsy

Three methods are used to obtain a small piece of tissue for examination under a microscope. In an *excision biopsy,* such as removal of a mole, the entire lesion may be removed for analysis. A *punch biopsy* involves removal of a small section from a designated location in the lesion; the center usually is the optimum site. If the lesion is on the surface of the skin (e.g., a mole), this is done with a scalpel-like circular punch instrument (Fig. 17.17); in other cases, a large-gauge needle and syringe unit is used to aspirate cells and fluid from a suspicious area (e.g., a breast biopsy). A *shave biopsy* is performed with a scalpel or razor by cutting or shaving off the growth or lesion for a thin specimen of combined epidermis and upper dermis cells. This method is used to biopsy a possible squamous cell carcinoma lesion. The medical assistant may help the provider perform these biopsy procedures.

The medical assistant should follow these steps to assist with a tissue biopsy:

1. Assemble the necessary supplies for the procedure.
2. Prepare the patient with proper gowning, draping, and positioning and make sure the patient understands the procedure.
3. Confirm that the provider has obtained the patient's informed consent.

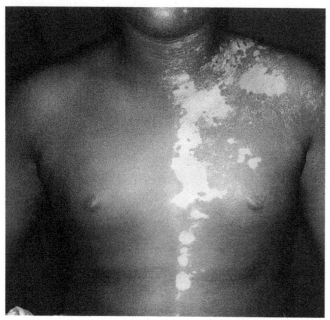

FIGURE 17.16 Vitiligo. (From Shiland B: *Mastering healthcare terminology,* ed 5, St. Louis, 2016, Elsevier.)

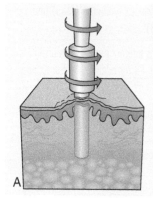 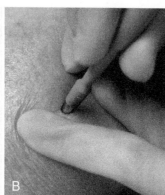 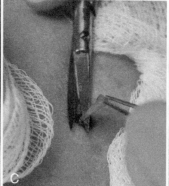 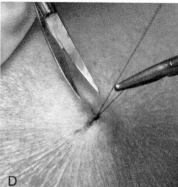

FIGURE 17.17 (A) Punch biopsy. **(B)** Punch biopsy instrument rotated into the skin. **(C)** Cutting the base of the specimen. **(D)** Closure of the biopsy wound with a simple epidermal stitch. (Modified from Bolognia J: *Dermatology,* ed 2, Edinburgh, 2008, Mosby.)

4. Prepare the site of the biopsy according to office protocol.

5. Assist the provider as needed, using appropriate personal protective equipment according to Standard Precautions.

6. Label the sample container and prepare it for transport to the testing laboratory. Remember to include laboratory request forms.

7. Clean the procedure area, properly dispose of all waste materials, and disinfect and sterilize equipment used in the procedure.

8. Sanitize your hands and document the procedure, including the patient education provided on biopsy site care.

Assisting With Treatments

Burns

The treatment of burns will vary, depending on the severity of the burn. Burns can be treated with medications, along with nonsurgical and surgical interventions. First-degree burns can be treated by immersing the affected area in cool to cold water and providing analgesics for pain. Topical OTC burn cream or aloe vera gel can be used to promote healing and limit scarring. Second-degree burns can be rinsed with cool water until the pain stops (10 to 30 minutes) and then additional cool compresses can be applied as needed. It is important to leave blisters intact. If a blister breaks open, the area should be bandaged to prevent infection. Elevating the limb can help to reduce the swelling. The same OTC creams suggested for first-degree burns can be used for second-degree burns. Both first- and second-degree burns can be treated at home, but the patient should seek medical attention if the area looks infected or is not healing. Third- and

fourth-degree burns need immediate and ongoing medical attention. The area should be covered with sterile gauze or a clean cloth until medical intervention is obtained. Clothing stuck to the burned area should not be removed, except by medical personnel. Pain medications may be prescribed, including analgesics or opioids. Antibiotics also will likely be prescribed. Third- and fourth-degree burns will often require skin grafts to close the wound. Treatment for these burns is an ongoing process.

Mohs Surgery

Mohs surgery is done to remove skin cancer lesions. The procedure involves repeated removal and microscopic examination of the layers of a lesion until no cancerous cells are seen (Fig. 17.18). As with any surgical procedure, sterile technique must be maintained.

Psoralen Plus Ultraviolet A (PUVA) Therapy

A psoralen topical medication plus ultraviolet A (PUVA) therapy is used to treat a number of different skin diseases and is commonly used for psoriasis. To treat small areas, the psoralen lotion or gel is applied to the affected area for 10 minutes before exposure to UVA.

Appearance Modification Procedures

Chemical Peel (Chemoexfoliation). Topical agents are used in chemical peels to minimize or remove minor skin features, such as acne scars, hyperpigmentation, and fine wrinkles. Agents used for chemical peels include tretinoin cream 0.05% to 0.1% concentration (Retin-A) and a number of different acidic preparations. During

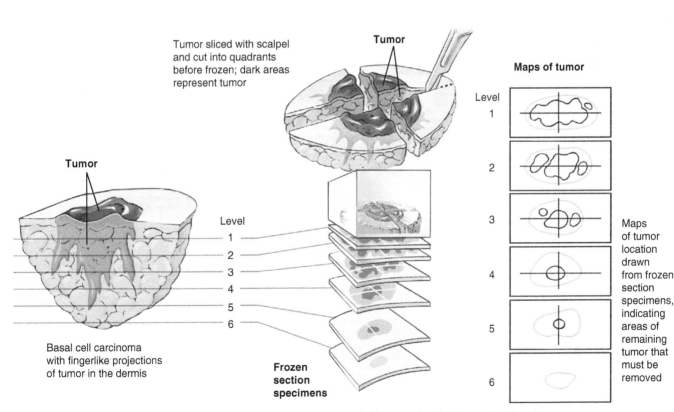

FIGURE 17.18 Mohs surgery. (From Shiland B: *Mastering healthcare terminology*, ed 5, St. Louis, 2016, Elsevier.)

application, care must be taken to prevent the solution from entering the eyes. The use of chemical exfoliating agents may cause the skin to appear inflamed and dry, with crusting and edema. The patient may complain of stinging and burning at the beginning of the treatment regimen. The patient should avoid sun exposure for the length of treatment and should use a sunscreen with a minimum SPF of 15 because photophobia (light sensitivity) is a typical side effect of treatment.

Dermabrasion. A dermabrader is a handheld device that mechanically evens the layers of dermal tissue. It is effective in the treatment of scars from acne vulgaris. Topical anesthetics (e.g., ethyl chloride) or locally injected anesthetics are used for the procedure. Besides the dermabrader, the dermatologist may use a variety of wire brushes, abrasive discs, or other devices to smooth scar tissue. Standard Precautions must be followed, including the use of face and eye guards, to prevent aerosol or splatter contamination from the site. The patient should be educated about wound care, signs of infection, and the presence of photophobia for 6 to 12 months after the procedure.

Laser Resurfacing (Photohermolysis). Laser therapy may be used for fine lines and wrinkles, pigmented areas, shallow scars, and tattoo removal. Typically, the patient is instructed to prepare the site 3 to 6 weeks before the procedure with tretinoin (Retin-A), alpha hydroxy solutions, or bleaches. Laser procedures are performed with the patient under local, regional, or general anesthesia. During the procedure, it is extremely important that the patient and all personnel wear the type of eye protection recommended by the laser manufacturer. After the procedure, cool packs are applied to help reduce swelling, and topical antibiotic ointment is used to prevent infection. The treated area appears inflamed and edematous and can take up to 2 weeks to heal; it can take as long as 6 months for the inflammation to fade.

Botox Injections. Botox is a strong neurotoxin (a substance toxic to nerves) produced by *Clostridium botulinum,* a bacterium that causes food poisoning. Two strains of the botulism bacterium are used in dermatologic procedures for appearance modification. Botox treatments involve injection of the substance around the eyes, mouth, and forehead. The toxin interferes with nervous stimulation, which temporarily paralyzes the muscles of the face that cause wrinkles to form. It also smoothes out the skin and makes it look younger and fresher. The effects are short term, so treatments must be repeated every 3 to 4 months, and some patients complain of an inability to show facial expression because of muscle paralysis.

CLOSING COMMENTS
Patient Coaching

When working with dermatology patients it is important to make them aware of the possible risks of skin cancer. The American Cancer Society has developed the acronym ABCDE to evaluate moles, birthmarks, or any skin changes. This is a great tool for patients. Any of these warning signs should be reported to the provider immediately. Early detection and self-examination are crucial to cancer survival.

- **A**symmetry: one area of the mole is changing
- **B**orders: moles are becoming irregular
- **C**olors: changes or uneven pigmentation
- **D**iameter: increasing size, more than 6 mm or one-fourth of an inch
- **E**levation: a mole that once was flat against the skin now is raised and elevated.

Legal and Ethical Issues

While working in dermatology, you will hear many patients express concern about skin disorders. Allow patients to express their concerns. Use therapeutic listening techniques but be careful when offering encouragement about the course and outcome of treatment. The improvement made with treatment of a skin disorder may be slow and gradual. Keep encouragement on a positive level. Help the patient recognize small improvements but remember that it is the provider's role to explain potential treatment outcomes. Making promises about outcomes could lead to a lawsuit.

Patient-Centered Care

The medical assistant must develop the ability to interact therapeutically with patients, families, co-workers, and other members of the healthcare team. When interacting with patients in a dermatology practice, the medical assistant needs to be especially sensitive to the patient's nonverbal behaviors and emotions. Many of the conditions seen in a dermatology practice affect how patients look and how they view themselves. Sensitivity to the importance of appearance, especially when skin conditions and/or treatments might alter a patient's appearance, is a crucial trait for healthcare professionals working in a dermatology practice.

SUMMARY OF SCENARIO

Casey is back at WMFM for her follow-up visit. In the past 2 months she has followed the treatment plan and is happy to show Mai and Jean Burke the improvements that have taken place. Her acne has improved greatly. She is pleased with the results and glad that she decided to visit WMFM about her skin issues. Casey also thanks Mai and Jean for being understanding on her first visit. How did Mai and Jean help Casey on her first visit? List three things that they did to help make Casey's experience positive.

SUMMARY OF LEARNING OBJECTIVES

1. **Describe the anatomic structures of the skin.**

   The skin is made up of three layers: the epidermis, which is the thin, uppermost layer; the dermis, the thicker layer beneath, which makes up approximately 90% of the skin mass; and the subcutaneous layer, which consists primarily of fatty or adipose tissue.

2. **Discuss the physiology of the integumentary system.**

   The five functions of the integumentary system are protection, sensory organ activity, temperature regulation, excretion, and synthesis of vitamin D.

3. **Compare various skin lesions and give examples of each.**

   Fig. 17.2 shows different types of skin lesions. The diagnosis of skin lesions is based on the color, elevation, and texture of the lesion; whether pruritus, excoriation, pain, or drainage is present; and whether the lesion is a primary or secondary growth.

4. **Describe typical integumentary system infections and infestations.**

   Integumentary system infections include bacterial infections, such as impetigo, acne vulgaris, furuncles, carbuncles, and cellulitis; fungal infections, including a variety of tinea growths; viral infections, which cause warts and herpes simplex; and scabies or lice infestations.

5. **Differentiate among various inflammatory and autoimmune integumentary disorders.**

   Inflammatory and autoimmune integumentary system disorders include a variety of seborrheic dermatitis inflammations, contact dermatitis, eczema, and the autoimmune disorders psoriasis, SLE, and scleroderma.

6. **Recognize burns and cold injuries to the skin.**

   Burns are classified as superficial, partial-thickness, or full-thickness, depending on the depth of the wound. The most important concern in the treatment of burns is the prevention of infection. Cold injuries usually are less severe than burns, but prolonged exposure can result in infection, gangrene, amputation, and death.

7. **Describe skin malignancies and their treatment and define the ABCDE rule for identifying a malignant melanoma.**

   Three cancerous lesions of the skin can occur: basal cell carcinoma, which is very slow growing and the most frequently seen form of skin cancer; squamous cell carcinoma, which grows rapidly and is more serious because it has a tendency to metastasize; and melanomas, which are pigmented lesions that are asymmetric, have irregular borders, and usually are larger than 6 mm. Treatment depends on the type of lesion, the level of invasion, and the location. The provider may surgically remove the tumor or may destroy it with cryosurgery, electrodesiccation, laser treatment, the application of chemotherapeutic agents, or Mohs surgery.

   The ABCDE rule includes examination of the site for any of the following: *a*symmetry, irregular *b*order, *c*hange in color, increase in *d*iameter, and *e*levation. If a mole displays any of these characteristics, a dermatologist should check it immediately.

8. **Discuss how to assist with a dermatologic examination.**

   During a dermatologic examination, the dermatologist frequently asks the medical assistant to take photographs of moles and/or to document specific measurements and locations of suspicious lesions.

9. **Explain dermatologic procedures performed in the ambulatory care setting.**

   Dermatologic procedures that can be performed in ambulatory care practices include allergy skin testing, which can be done with scratch, patch, or intradermal tests; drawing blood for a RAST test; treating allergies with immunotherapy; performing a biopsy or procedure to remove a cancerous area; and appearance modification procedures, including chemical peels, dermabrasion, laser resurfacing, and Botox injections.

ALLERGY AND INFECTIOUS DISEASE

Julia Shaw, CMA (AAMA), is a medical assistant working at Walden-Martin Family Medical (WMFM) Clinic. She is working with Dr. Angela Perez today. Julia enjoys the family practice setting and likes the variety of ages and conditions that she sees each day. Today, Dr. Perez and Julia will see a patient who is new to the clinic. The rest of their appointments are with existing patients. Each day is different. Each day is busy. Each day brings patients who need help and encouragement. Julia is a people person. Helping patients is Julia's passion.

While studying this chapter, think about the following questions:

- What are the structures related to the immune and lymphatic systems? What are the functions of the lymphatic and immune systems?
- What are the common pathologic conditions of the immune and lymphatic systems? What medical terms must you know to identify and explain these patient disorders?
- What diagnostic and treatment procedures typically are ordered for patients with immune and lymphatic disease?
- What are the medical assistant's primary responsibilities in working with patients with immune and lymphatic problems?
- What clinical skills are required in this specialty practice?

LEARNING OBJECTIVES

1. List the major organs and structures for the immune and lymphatic systems.
2. Describe the physiology of the immune and lymphatic systems. Also, discuss allergies and differentiate between active and passive immunity.
3. Identify the etiology, signs and symptoms, diagnostic procedures, and treatment of autoimmune diseases and disorders.
4. Identify the etiology, signs and symptoms, diagnostic procedures, and treatment of HIV/AIDS.
5. Identify the etiology, signs and symptoms, diagnostic procedures, and treatment of lymphoma.
6. Identify the etiology, signs and symptoms, diagnostic procedures, and treatment of multiple myeloma. Also, identify these factors for infectious diseases of the immune and lymphatic systems, such as viral hepatitis, sexually transmitted infections, and respiratory infections.
7. Describe the medical assistant's role in assisting with the examination and with diagnostic procedures associated with allergies and infectious diseases.
8. Describe treatments for allergies and respiratory infections.

VOCABULARY

antibody A protein substance produced in the blood or tissues in response to a specific antigen, that destroys or weakens the antigen. Part of the immune system.

antigen A substance that stimulates the production of an antibody when introduced into the body. Antigens include toxins, bacteria, viruses, and other foreign substances.

cytoplasm The cell substance that fills the area between the nucleus and the cell membrane. It contains the organelles of the cell.

debris (duh BREE) The remains of anything broken down or destroyed; ruins, rubble.

differentiate (dif uh REN shee ayt) To distinguish one thing from another. To make a distinction between items.

enzymes (EN ziemz) Special proteins that speed up a chemical reaction in the body.

homeostasis (hoh mee uh STAY sis) The internal environment of the body that is compatible with life. A steady state that is created by all the body systems working together to provide a consistent and unvarying internal environment.

inflammation (in fluh MAY shuhn) A pathology characterized by redness, swelling, pain, tenderness, heat, and disturbed function of an area of the body. Especially a reaction of tissues to injury.

intact (in TAKT) Complete or whole. Not altered; unbroken.

lymph (limf) A clear, yellowish fluid containing white blood cells in a liquid similar to plasma. The fluid comes from the tissues of the body and is moved through the lymphatic vessels and the bloodstream.

lymphocyte (LIM fuh site) A type of white blood cell that has a large, round nucleus that is surrounded by a thin layer of agranular cytoplasm.

macrophages (MACK roh fay jehs) Large white blood cells that live in the tissues. They engulf foreign particles, microorganisms, and cell debris.

microbiome (mIE kroh BIE ohm) The total collection of microorganisms, and their genetic material, present on or in the human body or a specific site in the human body.

microorganisms Any living organisms of microscopic size. Examples include bacteria, protozoa, fungi, parasites, and helminths. Some definitions include viruses, which are not alive.

monocyte (MON uh site) Agranulocyte that engulfs foreign particles, microorganisms, and cell debris.

pathogens (PATH uh jehns) Disease-causing organisms.

permeable (PUR mee ah buhl) A substance or structure that can be passed through, especially by liquids or gases.

Peyer patches (PAYH urh PACH ehz) Small masses of lymphatic tissue found mostly in the ileum of the small intestine. They are an important part of the immune system, because they monitor intestinal bacteria populations and prevent the growth of pathogenic bacteria in the intestines.

reflexes Movements or processes caused by a reflex response; a reflex is an automatic response that doesn't require thought.

replication The production of exact copies of a complex molecule, such as DNA.

stem cells Undifferentiated cells that can become specialized cells in the body.

vasoconstriction (vas oh kuhn STRIK shuhn) A contraction of muscles that causes narrowing of the inside tube of a vessel.

viability (vie a BIL ih tee) The ability to live.

When working with allergies and infectious diseases it is important to be familiar with the lymphatic and immune systems. They are two different systems; however, they cooperate and work together to maintain **homeostasis**. They also defend the body from foreign pathogens, which can cause infectious diseases. The cells, tissues, and organs of the lymphatic system and the immune system are almost the same. But the two systems help the body in very different ways. The lymphatic system can be described as mostly structural. It is the physical component of the two systems. The immune system can be described as mostly functional. The cells of the immune system work to keep the body safe from **pathogens**. These two systems together make up an amazingly complex and efficient means of maintaining the body's health.

The lymphatic system is responsible for a number of functions, with the help of the immune system. Lymphatic functions include cleansing the cellular environment, returning proteins and tissue fluids to the blood, providing a pathway for the absorption of fats into the bloodstream, and defending the body against disease.

Immunology is the healthcare specialty that deals with many immune- and lymphatic-related diseases and disorders. An *immunologist* is a specialist involved in the diagnosis, treatment, and prevention of disorders of the immune and lymphatic systems.

Other healthcare specialists who work with the diseases and disorders of the lymphatic and immune systems are cardiologists, otolaryngologists, allergists, rheumatologists, endocrinologists, pulmonologists, and nephrologists.

ANATOMY OF THE IMMUNE AND LYMPHATIC SYSTEMS

The immune and lymphatic systems are composed of many structures. **Lymph**, or interstitial fluid, flows through the lymphatic system (Fig. 18.1), which is composed of these structures:

- lymph vessels, lymph nodes, lymph glands, and lymphoid tissue
- lymph organs: the tonsils, adenoids, vermiform appendix, spleen, thymus gland, and **Peyer patches**

Two very important cells in the immune system, **monocytes** and **lymphocytes**, pass from the bloodstream through the blood capillary walls into the spaces between the cells in body tissue. When they pass into the lymph that surrounds cells, they perform their protective functions. Monocytes are in the blood, but once they are in the lymph, they are called **macrophages**. These cells destroy pathogens and collect **debris** from damaged cells. Lymphocytes are much more complicated. They are essential to the immune response, so they are discussed in a later section of this chapter.

Flow of Lymphatic Fluid

Lymph moves in one direction. This prevents pathogens from flowing through the entire body. The system filters out the **microorganisms** as the lymph passes through its various capillaries, vessels, and nodes.

Cells of the Immune System

The *immune system* is composed of organs, tissues, cells, and chemical messengers. The components of the immune system interact to protect the body from external invaders and from the body's own internally altered cells. The chemical messengers are *cytokines*. They are secreted by cells of the immune system that direct immune cellular interactions. Most of the cells involved in the lymphatic and immune systems are white blood cells (WBCs). A quick review of white blood cells may help in the discussion of the immune system.

Granular White Blood Cells

The three types of granular WBCs are *neutrophils*, *eosinophils*, and *basophils*. They are characterized by their heavily granulated **cytoplasm** and segmented nuclei. Neutrophils are aggressively *phagocytic*; that is, they engulf and destroy invading pathogens. Eosinophils are involved in allergies. Basophils play a part in inflammation.

Unlike red blood cells (RBCs), WBCs are found in both the bloodstream and the tissues. During **inflammation**, the blood carries neutrophils through blood vessels to the site of injury. Capillary walls become more **permeable**, and the granular cells squeeze through to the site of infection. Once at the site of infection or injury, the

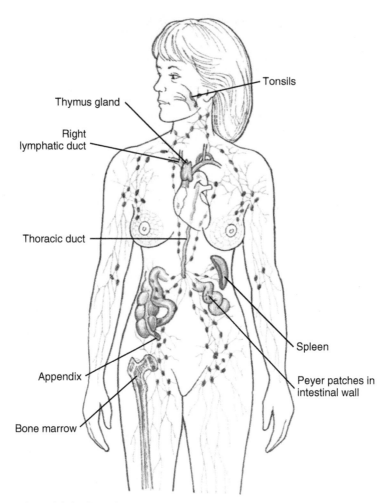

Thymus gland

Right
lymphatic duct

Thoracic duct

Appendix

Bone marrow

Tonsils

Spleen

Peyer patches in
intestinal wall

FIGURE 18.1 Organs of the lymphatic and immune systems. (From Shiland B: *Mastering healthcare terminology,* ed 5, St Louis, 2015, Elsevier.)

neutrophils engulf the invading microorganism. The collection of WBCs, dead WBCs, bacteria, and tissue cells creates *pus* at the site of infection.

CRITICAL THINKING APPLICATION   **18.1**

Julia needs to change a dressing on a patient's infected wound today. Robert Harrison has an abrasion that became infected. It is red and a little swollen, and there is pus at the margins of the wound.

What is pus? Write down a definition in your own words and be ready to share it with the class.

Agranular White Blood Cells

The two types of agranular leukocytes are *monocytes* and *lymphocytes.* They have a clear cytoplasm (no granules) and a solid nucleus. Monocytes are large and become *macrophages* when they enter tissues. Macrophages are also aggressively phagocytic cells that engulf pathogens and debris. Lymphocytes are small cells that have a big job! They are responsible for much of the work in specific immunity. Lymphocytes are further classified into T lymphocytes and B lymphocytes, depending on their function in the immune

response. B lymphocytes and T lymphocytes do not look different. But they function differently. B and T lymphocytes are also called *B cells* and *T cells.*

PHYSIOLOGY OF THE IMMUNE AND LYMPHATIC SYSTEMS

Immune System Levels of Defense

The best way to understand the immune system is to learn about the body's various levels of defense. The goal of foreign pathogens is to enter the body, reproduce, and damage healthy tissue. The immune system's primary function is to **differentiate** what is "self" from what is "foreign," and then destroy anything that is foreign. The immune system wants to stop pathogens from causing harm. Fig. 18.2 illustrates the levels of defense in the immune system. The two outside circles represent *nonspecific immunity* (also known as *innate immunity*) and its two levels of defense. The inner circle represents the various mechanisms of *specific immunity* (also known as *adaptive immunity*). These can be natural or acquired. Most pathogens can be contained by the first two lines of nonspecific defense. However, some pathogens get past nonspecific defenses. These pathogens are met with the third line of defense, or specific immunity.

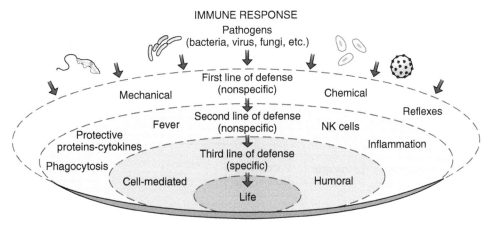

FIGURE 18.2 Immune system levels of defense. (From Shiland B: *Mastering healthcare terminology*, ed 5, St Louis, 2015, Elsevier.)

Nonspecific Immunity

The term *nonspecific immunity* refers to the many ways the body protects itself from pathogens without having to "recognize" them. The first line of defense in nonspecific immunity consists of the following methods of protection.

- *Physical:* Examples include **intact** skin and mucous membranes. These are physical barriers to pathogens. The skin protects the inside of the body from the outside environment. The sticky mucous membranes at many body openings trap pathogens.
- **Reflexes:** Examples include coughing, sneezing, vomiting, and diarrhea. These actions help get rid of pathogens by forcing them back out of the body.
- *Chemical:* Examples include tears, saliva, and perspiration. These have a slightly acidic pH, which discourages pathogens from entering the body. All these fluids also help wash the pathogens away. In addition, stomach acids and **enzymes** try to kill pathogens.

CRITICAL THINKING APPLICATION   **18.2**

What are the three methods of protection in the first line of defense? Write all three down and briefly describe each one in your own words. Share your answers with your classmates.

The second line of defense in nonspecific immunity goes to work if the pathogens make it past the first line of defense. The second line of defense uses cellular and chemical responses to destroy the pathogen. The following are the protective measures of the second line of defense.

- *Phagocytosis:* The process of cells engulfing and destroying invaders. Pathogens that make it past the first line of defense and enter the bloodstream may be consumed by neutrophils, monocytes, or macrophages.
- *Inflammation:* A protective response to irritation or injury. Signs and symptoms of inflammation include heat, swelling, redness, and pain. This process causes immediate **vasoconstriction**, followed by an increase in vascular permeability. These conditions provide a good environment for healing. If caused by a pathogen, the inflammation is called an *infection*.
- *Pyrexia:* The medical term for fever. When an infection is present, fever helps protect the infected area. Fever increases the action of

phagocytes and reduces the **viability** of certain pathogens. Most pathogens love normal body temperature, so when a fever is present the environment gets too hot and they cannot function as they should.

- *Protective proteins* are part of the second line of defense. These include *interferons*, which disrupt viral **replication** and limit a virus's ability to damage cells. *Complement* is a group of proteins made in the liver that is involved in blood clotting and blood antigen-antibody interactions. Complement proteins are inactive in the blood until they encounter bacteria. Meeting bacteria activates complement, enabling it to *lyse* (destroy) the organisms.
- *Natural killer* (NK) cells are the last cell type involved in the second line of defense. They are derived from **stem cells** in the bone marrow, concentrated in the liver and lungs, and involved in nonspecific immunity and inflammation. NK cells are also capable of destroying targeted cells, such as tumor cells and virus-infected cells. They are *not* phagocytic cells. This special kind of lymphocyte acts nonspecifically to kill cells that have been infected by certain viruses and cancer cells.

Fig. 18.3 presents an overview of nonspecific immunity.

CRITICAL THINKING APPLICATION   **18.3**

Review the second line of defense in nonspecific immunity. What are the five different chemical or cellular responses discussed in this text? Briefly describe each of the five protective measures. Can you name the characteristic signs and symptoms of inflammation? Write down your answers and share them with the class.

Specific Immunity

Specific immunity is different from nonspecific immunity in several ways.

- Specific immunity means that the immune response is generated against one specific **antigen**. The response will not be effective against any other antigens.
- Specific immunity counts on the immune cells to identify antigens and recognize them if they encounter them again. An antigen can be an infectious agent from outside the body (*exogenous*), or it can be a malignant or tumor cell inside the body (*endogenous*).

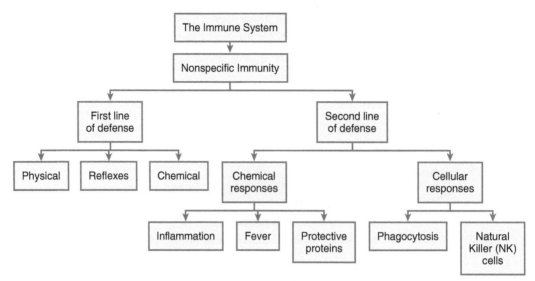

FIGURE 18.3 Nonspecific Immunity.

Both types of antigen are foreign, something that is not normal to the immune system.

- Specific immunity prepares a specific response (**antibody** production) to that unique antigen.
- Specific immunity intensifies with repeated challenges by the same antigen. When the body encounters a known antigen, it can respond more efficiently and react to the antigen quickly.
- Specific immunity may be either genetic or acquired. Genetic immunity is an inherited ability to resist certain diseases because of one's species, race, gender, or individual genetic makeup.

Antibodies belong to a group of proteins called *immunoglobulins* (Igs). There are five distinct classes of immunoglobulins: IgG, IgM, IgE, IgA, and IgD. Each class of immunoglobulin responds to different types of immune challenges, or antigens.

Specific immunity has two different methods of destroying pathogens: humoral immunity and cell-mediated immunity.

Humoral Immunity. *Humoral immunity*, also known as *antibody-mediated immunity*, involves the production of antibodies. B cells are formed from stem cells in the bone marrow. They then migrate to lymph organs (e.g., lymph nodes, spleen), where they multiply and live. B cells are the most important cell in humoral immunity, but T cells and macrophages are also involved in the process. When an antibody combines with an antigen, an antibody-antigen complex is formed.

Antibodies are protein molecules that specifically attach to antigens. They can neutralize toxins or destroy viruses directly. They can combine with larger antigens (e.g., bacteria) to form antibody-antigen complexes. These complexes signal neutrophils to come and destroy them. Neutrophils engulf the complexes and destroy the antigen.

Antibodies can protect the body in many ways. They circulate in the plasma and are present in secretions (i.e., tears, saliva, colostrum), ready to attach to unsuspecting antigens. However, there is one thing antibodies are unable to do – they cannot enter a cell. That can be a problem, because sometimes antigens go inside host cells. When that happens, antibodies cannot destroy the antigen. This is when cell-mediated immunity takes over.

Cell-Mediated Immunity. T cells are formed from stem cells in bone marrow. They then migrate to the thymus, where they mature and learn their role in the immune system. They are the most important cell in cell-mediated immunity. T cells do *not* produce antibodies, but they can help antibodies do their job. T cells are very effective against intracellular pathogens (antigens). When an antigen enters a cell, T cells help expose the antigen so that antibodies can destroy it. There are different types of T cells that have different roles in cell-mediated immunity.

Different Types of T Cells

Four main types of T cells work in specific immunity. Look at the following list and see how important T cells are to immunity in general.
1. *T helper cells* (T_H), also known as CD4+ T cells. They help in B-cell activation and activation of cytotoxic T cells.
2. *Cytotoxic T cells* (T_C), also known as CD8+ cells. They destroy virus-infected cells and tumor cells. They also can cause damage to or rejection of organ transplants. In addition, they can cause autoimmune diseases.
3. *Memory T cells* rapidly proliferate if an antigen is reexposed to the body.
4. *Regulatory T cells* (T_{reg}), also known as *suppressor T cells*. They help shut down the immune response when the antigen has been destroyed.

Cell-mediated immunity is particularly well suited to destroying viruses. Viruses must be inside a host cell to reproduce. Cytotoxic T cells destroy a virus once it gets inside a cell. Cell-mediated immunity helps stop the spread of viral infections within the body. Another job of cell-mediated immunity is to recognize and destroy cancer cells or tumor cells. Even though these cells are part of a person's body, they are not normal. They have changed and are now harming the body. Cell-mediated immunity recognizes malignant changes in

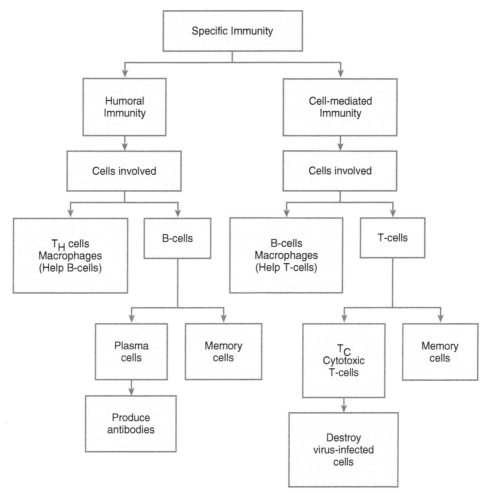

FIGURE 18.4 Specific Immunity.

cells. It works to destroy them before they cause disease (cancer) or tumors.

Fig. 18.4 presents an overview of specific immunity.

CRITICAL THINKING APPLICATION   18.4

T cells are very important cells in the immune system. List two ways T cells help protect the body from foreign antigens. Share your thoughts with the class.

ALLERGIES

The immune system is quite remarkable. When it works well, it keeps our bodies from harm. When it doesn't work properly, the immune system can harm the body. *Allergies* are an example of the immune system overreacting. Allergies are also known as hypersensitivity reactions.

Hypersensitivity Reactions

Hypersensitivity is defined as an immune response that causes tissue damage in the host. It is an excessive response to a stimulus or foreign agent. A hypersensitivity reaction does not occur the first time an antigen is encountered. It is when the person encounters the antigen for a second or subsequent exposure that the reaction develops.

An allergic reaction is a type I hypersensitivity reaction (Table 18.1). It is the body responding to an allergic trigger, called an *allergen*. Allergens are harmless environmental substances, but in an allergic reaction, the body overreacts to their presence.

When the body responds to an allergen, immune cells release *histamines, kinins,* and other inflammatory substances. This causes the characteristic allergy symptoms: runny nose, watery eyes, and possibly a rash or hives. Sometimes drugs called *antihistamines* are used to alleviate allergy symptoms.

If an allergic reaction is severe, it can cause a dangerous condition called *anaphylactic shock* (see Chapter 12). This can be a life-threatening condition. People who know they are highly allergic to a substance should carry an EpiPen with them to treat an anaphylactic reaction.

For specific emergency care during an anaphylactic reaction, see Chapter 12.

CRITICAL THINKING APPLICATION   18.5

What type of hypersensitivity is hemolytic disease of the newborn (HDN)?
What type of hypersensitivity is anaphylaxis?
What type of hypersensitivity is delayed hypersensitivity?

TABLE 18.1   Hypersensitivity Reactions

TYPE	REACTIONS	EXAMPLES
Type I — immediate hypersensitivity; also called an *allergic reaction*	Reactions may be local (runny nose, itching eyes). Reactions can also be systemic (swelling of the airway and tongue). Anaphylaxis is the systemic form of immediate hypersensitivity. It can be fatal.	Food allergies, insect venom allergies (bee and wasp stings), latex allergies
Type II	Antibodies to cell surface antigens are produced.	Hemolytic disease of the newborn (HDN), blood bank transfusion reactions
Type III	Antibody-antigen complexes are deposited in tissues of the body.	Organ damage with systemic lupus erythematosus (SLE), glomerulonephritis, rheumatic fever, rheumatoid arthritis
Type IV, also known as delayed hypersensitivity	Allergic reaction appears 24 to 48 hours after exposure to an antigen.	Poison ivy rash, tuberculosis (TB) skin tests, organ transplant rejection

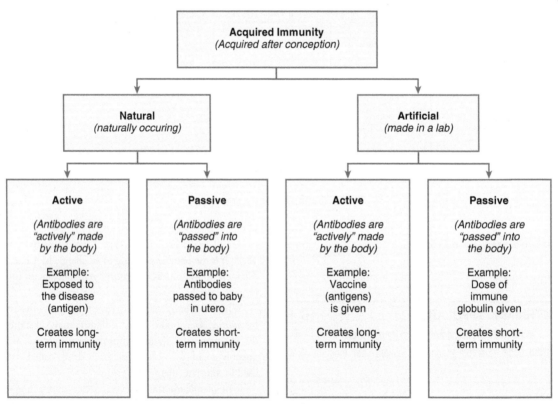

FIGURE 18.5 Acquired Immunity.

TYPES OF ACQUIRED IMMUNITY

Immunity is one way our body protects us from infectious diseases. Acquired immunity is classified as active or passive. *Active immunity* requires the body to respond to an antigen and produce antibodies for protection. *Passive immunity* does not require the body to do anything. In passive immunity, premade antibodies are given to a person. This occurs through transmission from the mother to the fetus or infant, or through an injection of immune globulin. The immune system is not required to make anything.

Active immunity and passive immunity are each categorized as natural immunity or artificial immunity. All four types of acquired immunity describe ways the body has acquired antibodies to specific diseases. Fig. 18.5 helps to explain acquired immunity.

CRITICAL THINKING APPLICATION   **18.6**

Rich and Jan Dallman have an appointment to see Dr. Perez today. They both want to get the shingles vaccine. Julia prepares their vaccinations and then sits down with Rich and Jan to go over the Vaccine Information Statement (VIS), which discusses the vaccine. What type of immunity is a vaccination, active or passive?

DISEASES AND DISORDERS OF THE IMMUNE AND LYMPHATIC SYSTEMS

Diseases of the lymphatic and immune systems are diverse and have many different causes but often have common signs and symptoms such as fatigue, joint pain, swollen joints, low-grade fever, skin changes, and weight loss. Many factors can be associated with lymphatic and immune system diseases, disorders, and infections. These diseases can involve the cells, tissues, and organs of the lymphatic system or the immune system.

Autoimmune Diseases and Disorders

Recall that the goal of the immune system is to protect the body from foreign pathogens and prevent infectious diseases. The immune system normally can distinguish *self* from *foreign*. However, in autoimmune diseases, something goes wrong in the immune system – it begins to attack healthy *self* cells.

According to the National Institutes of Health website MedlinePlus (*https://medlineplus.gov*), there are more than 80 different autoimmune diseases. The common factor among all autoimmune diseases is that a person's own immune system attacks healthy tissues. No matter what the symptoms are, the underlying cause of the disease is an immune system that is not working properly.

The cause of autoimmune diseases is a mystery. There are many theories about how the immune system becomes confused. The following is a brief list of suspected causes:

- A viral or bacterial infection that triggers the immune system to attack healthy cells
- Exposure over time to toxins (e.g., chemicals, pesticides, and food additives)
- A weakness in a person's immune system brought on by stress, past infections, and hormone fluctuations
- An imbalance in the intestinal **microbiome**
- Existing allergies (another type of immune system overreaction)

Many scientists think that a combination of all these possible causes influences a person's risk of developing an autoimmune disease. Autoimmune diseases are an area of intense scientific research, because more people are being diagnosed with autoimmune conditions. Risk factors for being diagnosed with an autoimmune disease include female gender, especially between the ages of 15 and 45, and African, Hispanic, or Native American race.

Common Autoimmune Diseases

- Rheumatoid arthritis
- Inflammatory bowel disease (IBD)
- Type 1 diabetes mellitus
- Psoriasis
- Myasthenia gravis
- Systemic lupus erythematosus (SLE)
- Multiple sclerosis (MS)
- Guillain-Barré syndrome
- Graves' disease
- Hashimoto's thyroiditis

Autoimmune diseases vary in their signs and symptoms, depending on the cells or tissues affected in the body. Some common signs and symptoms seem to affect a number of different autoimmune conditions. They include skin changes (discolorations, rashes, or lesions), joint pain, fatigue/malaise, low-grade fever, and general ill-feeling.

Commonly affected cells or tissues include joints, muscles, and skin, blood vessels and red blood cells, connective tissue, and endocrine glands (i.e., thyroid, pancreas).

To diagnose an autoimmune condition, the provider takes a complete history and performs a thorough physical examination. Laboratory and diagnostic testing procedures vary, depending on the patient's signs and symptoms. For most suspected autoimmune conditions, some or all of the following laboratory tests may be ordered.

- *Antinuclear antibody test* (ANA) – A blood test that looks for the presence of antibodies to the nucleus or the organelles of the nucleus. A serum sample is used for this type of test.
- *Autoantibody test* – A blood/serum test that looks for autoantibodies.
- *Complete blood cell count* (CBC) – A blood test. See Chapter 24 and Chapter 33 for more information. Some Clinical Laboratory Improvement Amendments (CLIA)-waived tests are available.
- *Comprehensive metabolic panel* (CMP) – A blood test. See Chapter 24 and Chapter 33 for more information. Some CLIA-waived tests are available.
- *C-reactive protein* (CRP) – A blood test that measures CRP. CRP is elevated in people with inflammation. Some CLIA-waived tests are available.
- *Erythrocyte sedimentation rate* (ESR) – A whole blood test. People with inflammation have elevated values. Some CLIA-waived tests are available.
- *Urinalysis* – See Chapter 31 for more information. Some CLIA-waived tests are available.

Imaging tests, such as joint and bone x-rays, magnetic resonance imaging (MRI), and ultrasound scans, in addition to tissue biopsies may be ordered. Information on each of these procedures can be found in Chapter 3.

Treatments will vary, depending on the signs and symptoms of the condition. However, common goals of treatment for most autoimmune conditions include diminishing the signs and symptoms of the condition and/or reducing their occurrence, controlling the autoimmune process, and maintaining the body's ability to fight disease and infections.

Treatments may include physical therapy, blood transfusions (if the condition affects blood cells), a modified diet (to reduce inflammation and boost the immune system with nutrient-dense foods), stress reduction, adequate sleep, regular exercise, and smoking cessation.

Medications may include nonsteroidal anti-inflammatory drugs (NSAIDs) (e.g., ibuprofen), corticosteroids, supplementation to replace substances lacking in the body (examples include thyroid hormones, insulin, vitamin B_{12}, and vitamin D), and immunosuppressive drugs to reduce the body's immune response (examples include prednisone, cyclosporine [Neoral], and adalimumab [Humira]).

Some alternative therapies that may bring symptom relief include yoga, massage therapy, and relaxation therapy. Special diets may also be used to help reduce inflammation or remove specific types of proteins from the diet (e.g., gluten-free diet, grain-free diet, elimination of sugar and natural/artificial sweeteners).

HIV/AIDS

Acquired immunodeficiency syndrome (AIDS) is a chronic condition caused by the human immunodeficiency virus (HIV). HIV attacks the immune system of its host and specifically damages the CD4$^+$ T lymphocytes (helper T cells). HIV impairs the immune system's ability to fight infectious agents that can cause disease.

Currently HIV/AIDS can be treated but not cured. And without proper and consistent treatment, it is a life-threatening disease. The treatment for HIV/AIDS that is available now slows the progression of the disease and allows a person to live a relatively normal life.

HIV is the causative agent of AIDS. HIV is a bloodborne virus that can be transmitted through sexual contact, through a sharps exposure (e.g., needlestick), or from mother to child during pregnancy or childbirth.

Risk factors for acquiring HIV include having unprotected sex, using intravenous drugs (especially if sharing needles), and having another sexually transmitted infection (STI). Being an uncircumcised man increases your risk of acquiring HIV if any of the other risk factors also exist.

A primary HIV infection occurs when a person is first exposed to the virus. Signs and symptoms of primary HIV include flu-like symptoms, swollen lymph nodes (especially in the neck), diarrhea, and weight loss.

After the initial infection with HIV, the virus becomes *latent* (shows no signs or symptoms). During this time, the person will test positive on an HIV blood test; however, he or she does not show signs or symptoms of the infection. HIV can remain latent for 18 months to 10 years. If an HIV-positive person is not treated with antiviral drugs, HIV will change from a latent infection to an active one, and progress to AIDS.

Signs and symptoms of AIDS include chronic and persistent diarrhea, recurring fevers, night sweats, profound fatigue, weight loss, skin rashes, continual white patches or lesions on the tongue or in the mouth, and repeated opportunistic infections.

Most individuals infected with HIV take about 12 weeks to produce anti-HIV antibodies. The diagnosis of HIV is made by testing a blood sample or a saliva sample for anti-HIV antibodies. Newer generation testing can also detect a protein made by the HIV virus shortly after infection, thus providing a quicker diagnosis. CLIA-waived kits are available for home use, but their results should be confirmed by laboratory tests. Confirmatory tests include the enzyme-linked immunosorbent assay (ELISA) and Western blot testing.

As mentioned, HIV/AIDS currently can be treated but not cured, and without proper and consistent treatment, it is a life-threatening disease. The goal of treatment is to slow the disease progression and allow the person to live a relatively normal life. A regimen of antiviral medications is available to control the virus. There are a number of different drug classes that can be used to control HIV. Most providers recommend using three drugs from at least two different drug classes. This helps to keep the virus from becoming resistant to a single drug. All HIV drugs block the virus from entering the CD4$^+$ T lymphocytes, but in different ways.

Lymphoma: Hodgkin's and Non-Hodgkin's

Lymphoma is a cancer of the lymphatic and immune systems. Lymphocytes, a type of white blood cell, mutate and reproduce rapidly in lymphoma. The overproduced, diseased lymphocytes crowd out healthy WBCs. This causes the patient to be more susceptible to infections.

There are two main types of lymphoma:
- Hodgkin's lymphoma: Also called *Hodgkin disease*. It is characterized by the presence of Reed-Sternberg cells in the blood. This type of cell is specific to Hodgkin's lymphoma.
- Non-Hodgkin's lymphoma: A collection of all other lymphatic cancers that are not Hodgkin's lymphoma; this is the more common of the two types.

The cause of lymphoma is not well understood or obvious in most cases. There isn't a direct link to any one event, chemical exposure, or genetic mutation that can predict the development of a lymphoma. However, some factors may increase a person's risk of developing this type of cancer.

Risk factors for developing Hodgkin's lymphoma include a family history of lymphoma, being 15 to 30 years old or over age 55, being male, and having had an Epstein-Barr (EBV) infection (infectious mononucleosis [mono]).

Risk factors for developing non-Hodgkin's lymphoma include being over age 60 years; being on immunosuppressive therapy or medications; and having had certain infections, such as EBV, HIV, or *Helicobacter pylori*, which causes stomach and intestinal ulcers.

Signs and symptoms of both Hodgkin's lymphoma and non-Hodgkin's lymphoma include painless swelling of lymph nodes (especially in the neck, armpits, or groin), fatigue, fever, chills, night sweats, and unexplained weight loss. Additional symptoms that are more common with non-Hodgkin's lymphoma are abdominal swelling and/or pain, trouble breathing, coughing, or chest pain.

For both types of lymphoma, the diagnostic process is the same. The provider will perform a physical exam specifically looking for enlarged and nontender lymph nodes, liver, and spleen. Blood and urine tests will be done to rule out other possible disease conditions and infections. Blood tests would likely include a CBC and differential and a CMP. Urinalysis also is likely. Imaging tests may include x-rays, computed tomography (CT), MRI, or positron emission tomography (PET) scans. Lymph node, tissue, and/or bone marrow biopsy may also be done. The provider can make an accurate diagnosis about the type of lymphoma present and the stage of the disease by using information obtained in a biopsy. Staging a cancer is important because it affects the treatment plan the provider will recommend.

Treatment depends on the type and stage of the lymphoma. Not all lymphomas are treated. For instance, some slowly progressing types of non-Hodgkin's lymphoma are monitored and may not be treated. Depending on the type and stage of the lymphoma, treatment may include chemotherapy, radiation therapy, and stem cell transplantation (bone marrow transplantation). A stem cell transplant is used to replace diseased bone marrow with healthy stem cells. Stem cells can then repopulate the bone marrow with healthy cells. Also, biologic drugs may be used to enhance the patient's immune system, helping it to destroy lymphoma cells.

Multiple Myeloma

Multiple myeloma is a cancer of the white blood cells called *plasma cells*. Plasma cells are a type of B lymphocyte that produce antibodies to help fight infection. In multiple myeloma, plasma cells reproduce so much that they crowd out healthy blood cells. The malignant plasma cells don't produce antibodies. Instead, they produce an abnormal protein (M protein) that can cause kidney damage.

This condition is called multiple myeloma because the tumors are found in many or multiple bones. If it occurs in only one bone or area, the tumor is referred to as a plasmacytoma.

The cause of multiple myeloma is unknown, or *idiopathic*. But for most people, multiple myeloma starts out as monoclonal gammopathy of undetermined significance (MGUS). People with MGUS also produce M protein but at such a low level it does not harm the body. Risk factors for developing multiple myeloma include being over the age of 60, male gender, blacks are more likely to develop multiple myeloma than whites, and a history of MGUS. This makes developing multiple myeloma more likely.

Signs and symptoms of multiple myeloma may be subtle at first. There may be no symptoms at all in the beginning. Noticeable signs and symptoms include bone pain, especially in the spine, chest, or hips; anemia; loss of kidney function; excessive thirst; nausea; loss of appetite; weight loss; constipation; fatigue; frequent infections; weakness or numbness in the legs; and mental confusion.

Tests that may be used to help diagnose multiple myeloma include blood tests, which may include a CBC and differential, tests for the presence of M protein, and a CMP (includes kidney and liver function tests); urinalysis (M proteins in the urine are called *Bence Jones proteins*); a bone marrow biopsy; and examination of cells. Imaging tests may include x-ray, MRI, CT, and PET scans. At diagnosis, multiple myeloma will be staged, and a treatment plan will be based on the staged diagnosis.

Treatment for asymptomatic multiple myeloma, MGUS, may not be needed. The provider will want to watch the condition and run periodic blood and urine tests to monitor signs of activity. Treatment for multiple myeloma includes targeted cancer therapy (designed to target specific weaknesses in myeloma cancer cells in order to kill the cells), biologic therapy, chemotherapy, radiation therapy, and possibly stem cell transplantation.

Infectious Diseases

Infectious diseases are those caused by organisms such as bacteria, viruses, fungi, or parasites. As healthcare professionals we know that many of our patients seek treatment for infectious diseases of all sorts. In the next several sections we will discuss common infectious diseases.

Viral Hepatitis

Hepatitis is an inflammation of the liver. Inflammation can damage the liver and cause impaired liver function. There are many causes for hepatitis in general, but this material will specifically cover hepatitis that has a viral cause. Viral hepatitis is an infectious disease that in most cases can be prevented. Viral hepatitis can be caused by five main viral strains: A, B, C, D, and E. Hepatitis A and hepatitis E are both transmitted primarily through fecal-oral contact. Hepatitis B, hepatitis C, and hepatitis D are transmitted as bloodborne pathogens. Table 18.2 provides detailed information on viral hepatitis.

Sexually Transmitted Infections

STIs can be seen in any individual who is sexually active. Signs and symptoms of STIs can be vague or nondescript. So anyone who is sexually active should be tested for STIs, especially if they have engaged in any high-risk behavior. Tables 18.3 and 18.4 give an overview of commonly encountered STIs. For additional information on STIs, please visit *https://www.cdc.gov/std/default.htm*.

Respiratory Infections
Strep Throat. Strep throat is a bacterial infection caused by *Streptococcus pyogenes*, also called *group A strep* (GAS). Strep throat is a common childhood infection, but it can affect patients of any age. Strep throat is highly contagious and can be spread from person to person by airborne droplets and by sharing food or beverages. If strep throat is not properly treated patients can develop serious complications, such as glomerulonephritis and rheumatic fever.

Signs and symptoms of strep throat include skin rash, nausea and vomiting, fever, headache, painful swallowing, sore throat, white spots at the back of the throat or on the tonsils, tiny red spots on the soft or hard palate on the roof of the mouth, swollen tonsils, and tender and enlarged lymph nodes under the jaw or in the neck.

If strep throat is suspected the patient should be tested to confirm the infection before being put on antibiotics. Some viral infections can exhibit similar signs and symptoms. Diagnosis includes the history and physical and a rapid streptococcus A antigen test (some CLIA-waived tests are available); if the rapid strep test is negative, an overnight throat culture should be performed. See Chapter 34 for the steps in a throat culture collection (Procedure 34.2, p. 884) and a rapid strep test (Procedure 34.3, p. 886).

Treatment for strep throat includes antibiotics. A person with strep throat should stay home until he or she has completed 24 hours of antibiotic therapy. Additional treatments include over-the-counter (OTC) analgesics to help relieve the pain and fever, such as acetaminophen. Extra rest and general supportive care are also recommended.
Influenza. Influenza is a viral respiratory infection that is referred to as the *flu*. Influenza affects a person's nose, throat, and lungs. For most healthy individuals the flu is an uncomfortable infection that resolves itself within a few weeks. But for the very young, the very old, or those with chronic medical conditions (asthma, diabetes, heart/liver/kidney disease, immunocompromised), influenza infections can cause very serious complications or even death.

Influenza is a contagious illness caused by an influenza virus that is spread by droplets from coughing, sneezing, or talking. It may also be transferred to a person by an inanimate object. Influenza viruses do not stay the same. They change and mutate so that antibodies you have produced to an influenza strain in the past may not be effective against the influenza virus that is presently causing people to become sick.

Signs and symptoms of influenza include fever, cough, sore throat, muscle aches, headaches, fatigue, and cough. For most people the flu is an infection that will last a few weeks but will resolve with no lingering effects. For the very young, very old, or chronically ill, complications are more likely, but anyone can develop complications to influenza. Complications include bronchitis, pneumonia, increased severity of asthma, heart conditions, and ear infections.

Diagnosis of influenza is made by conducting a history and physical examination, collecting a nasopharyngeal swab or nasal washing for rapid influenza diagnostic tests (some CLIA-waived tests are available).

Treatment for influenza includes bed rest, increased fluids, antiviral medications, and over-the-counter analgesics for muscle aches or

TABLE 18.2	Viral Hepatitis	
	HEPATITIS A (HAV) AND E (HEV)	**HEPATITIS B (HBV), C (HCV), AND D (HVD)**
Etiology and risk factors	Person-to-person transmission through fecal-oral contamination. Ingesting something that has been contaminated with the feces of an infected person. Ingesting contaminated food or water. Undercooked foods that are contaminated; examples include raw shellfish, vegetables, and fruits Sexual/intimate contact with an infected person.	Person-to-person transmission through activities that involve *percutaneous* (through the skin) or mucosal contact with infected blood or body fluids (semen, saliva). Sex with an infected partner. Injection drug use that involves sharing needles, syringes, or drug-preparation equipment. Birth to an infected mother. Needlesticks or sharp instrument exposure. Sharing personal items such as razors or toothbrushes with an infected person.
Signs and symptoms	Children younger than 6 years are frequently asymptomatic; older children and adults are frequently symptomatic. If symptoms occur, they can include fever, fatigue, loss of appetite, nausea, vomiting, abdominal pain, dark urine, jaundice, joint pain, and clay-colored feces.	Children younger than 5 years and newly infected immunosuppressed adults are frequently symptomatic. Among children older than 5 years, only about 30% to 50% are symptomatic.
Diagnostic procedures	A provider will perform a history and physical exam; if there is any indication of hepatitis, blood testing will most likely be done. For hepatitis A, B, C, and D, specific antibody testing is done to confirm the presence and type of hepatitis. There is no reliable antibody testing for hepatitis E; the history, physical exam, recent travel, and signs and symptoms are used to diagnose hepatitis E.	
Treatment	Lots of rest. Eat and drink tiny amounts at one time to cope with nausea. Do not drink alcohol, and consult the provider about any existing medications that may affect the liver; this includes OTC medications. For hepatitis A and E, treatment is generally supportive	*Hepatitis B or D — acute infection*: treatment is supportive. *Hepatitis B or D — chronic infection*: antiviral medications to prevent liver damage or liver cancer. *Hepatitis C — acute infection*: treated aggressively with antiviral medications to minimize the possibility of developing chronic hepatitis C. *Hepatitis C — chronic infection*: treated with antiviral medications to minimize the possibility of liver damage, cirrhosis, liver cancer, or organ failure.
Comments *With any type of viral hepatitis, serious complications can occur, including liver failure or death; liver failure requires liver transplantation.*	Hepatitis E is endemic in areas of Africa, the Middle East, Asia, and Mexico; if pregnant, consult the provider for travel recommendations.	Hepatitis D is only possible as a co-infection with hepatitis B; if a co-infection occurs, it can develop into a superinfection; a superinfection can cause liver failure and death. To prevent hepatitis D, vaccinate against hepatitis B.

Information summarized from the Centers for Disease Control and Prevention. *https://www.cdc.gov/hepatitis/index.htm.*

TABLE 18.3 Bacterial/Protozoal Sexually Transmitted Infections

FEATURE	CHLAMYDIA	GONORRHEA	SYPHILIS	TRICHOMONIASIS
Etiology	*Chlamydia trachomatis* (bacterium)	*Neisseria gonorrhoeae* (bacterium)	*Treponema pallidum* (spirochete bacteria)	*Trichomonas vaginalis* (protozoon)
Signs and symptoms – male	May be asymptomatic Dysuria Itching and thin, watery discharge from penis Testicular pain	Dysuria and urinary frequency Thick, cloudy, or bloody discharge from penis	Painless lesion (chancre) Serous discharge from chancre Lymphadenopathy	Asymptomatic Itching or irritation inside penis Burning after urination or ejaculation Some discharge from penis
Signs and symptoms – female	Asymptomatic Dysuria Urinary frequency Abdominal pain Increased vaginal discharge	Dysuria Urinary frequency Abdominal pain Increased vaginal discharge	Painless lesion (chancre) Serous discharge from chancre Lymphadenopathy	Asymptomatic Urinary frequency, urgency Dysuria Frothy, yellow-green vaginal discharge Pruritus
Diagnostic procedures	Testing a first-catch urine specimen (male) Collecting swab specimens from the endocervix or vagina (female) Nucleic acid amplification test (NAAT)	Urethral swab (male) Endocervical swab or vaginal swab (female) Urine specimen (both male and female) NAAT Gram stain for symptomatic males	Rapid plasma regain (RPR), Venereal Disease Research Laboratory (VDRL), fluorescent treponemal antibody absorption (FTA-ABS)	NAAT Wet mount preparation of the vaginal discharge examined under a microscope Culture of discharge Retest 3 months after treatment
Treatment, medications	Curable with antibiotic therapy; single dose of azithromycin or 1 week of doxycycline	Curable with antibiotic therapy; ceftriaxone, azithromycin, or doxycycline	Penicillin G; if patient is allergic to penicillin, doxycycline or tetracycline	Single dose of metronidazole or tinidazole; partner must be treated

TABLE 18.4 Viral Sexually Transmitted Infections

FEATURE	GENITAL HERPES	GENITAL WARTS	HIV/AIDS
Etiology	Herpes simplex virus-2 (HSV-2)	Human papillomavirus (HPV)	Human immunodeficiency virus (HIV)
Signs and symptoms – male	Painful genital vesicles and ulcers; erythema and pruritus; tingling or shooting pain 1–2 days before outbreak; cycle through episodes	Elevated papillomas on external genitalia; single or cluster of warts	Flulike symptoms, also referred to as *acute retroviral syndrome* (ARS) or *primary HIV infection*: Fever Swollen glands Sore throat Rash, muscle and joint aches and pains Headache
Signs and symptoms – female			
Diagnostic procedures		Examination and possible biopsy of warts	Enzyme-linked immunosorbent assay (ELISA); if positive, a Western blot test to confirm Saliva test Viral load test
Treatment, medications	No cure, but antiviral therapy during episodes shortens duration of lesions; acyclovir, famciclovir, valacyclovir	Topical medications; podofilox solution, imiquimod cream, cryosurgery, electrocautery	Antiretroviral (ART) medications: non-nucleoside reverse transcriptase inhibitors, nucleoside reverse transcriptase inhibitors, protease inhibitors, fusion inhibitors, integrase inhibitors

fever reducers to bring down a fever. Rest and supportive care are important to a full recovery.

Respiratory Syncytial Virus. Respiratory syncytial virus (RSV) produces upper respiratory "cold" symptoms in healthy older children and adults. RSV spreads by coughing or sneezing. For young children and adults with medical problems, it can cause pneumonia and severe breathing problems. For additional information about RSV, see Chapter 25.

Infectious Mononucleosis. *Infectious mononucleosis* is also known as mono, or the kissing disease. It is commonly acquired as a child or an adolescent. Most children do not show signs and symptoms, or they are very mild. People who acquire the disease in late childhood, adolescence, or young adulthood usually have signs and symptoms. It is generally a mild, self-limiting viral infection, but it can have serious complications, such as hepatosplenomegaly. Mono is passed from person to person via saliva – that's why it can be passed by kissing. It can also be passed by sneezing or coughing or by sharing eating or drinking utensils.

The most common cause of infectious mononucleosis is the Epstein-Barr virus, which is a type of herpes virus. Other viruses can also cause mono, but EBV is by far the most common. Most adults have antibodies to EBV by the end of their 20s. Once a person develops antibodies, he or she is considered immune and cannot have mono again. Although the disease is usually mild, some people can develop complications and may become very sick.

Risk factors for acquiring mono include contact with someone who has an active infection; for example, kissing, sharing food and drink, and sharing eating utensils or toothbrushes. EBV has an incubation period of 4 to 6 weeks for adolescents and young adults.

Signs and symptoms of infectious mononucleosis may include fatigue, fever, swollen lymph nodes in the neck and armpits, sore throat, swollen tonsils (may obstruct breathing or cause wheezing), headache, skin rash, swollen upper abdomen, and soft-swollen spleen. Signs and symptoms usually subside within 2 to 4 weeks. Fatigue and enlargement of the lymph nodes and spleen may last 4 to 6 weeks.

Complications of mono that may occur include an enlarged spleen and pain in the left upper abdomen (left untreated, the spleen could rupture), hepatitis, jaundice, anemia, and thrombocytopenia. Rarely, complications may include myocarditis, meningitis, encephalitis, and Guillain-Barré syndrome. Severe complications can occur in someone who is immune compromised, such as a person with HIV/AIDS or on immunosuppressive drugs.

Diagnostic procedures include the history and physical exam (to look for swollen lymph nodes, liver, and spleen; fever; and sore throat); blood tests, including a Monospot to detect antibodies to EBV; and a CBC and differential to look for an elevated WBC count and atypical lymphocytes in the blood (Fig. 18.6).

Treatment for mono is supportive care—it is a viral infection. Antibiotics are not necessary and are not useful for viral infections. Lots of rest, fluids (especially water), OTC pain- or fever-reducing medications (not aspirin), and a healthy diet are the best treatments for mono. Within 2 to 4 weeks the virus should run its course, and most people recover completely.

One more important treatment for mono is to limit activities while symptoms remain. Staying away from school or work, getting extra rest, and limiting physical activities and sports are

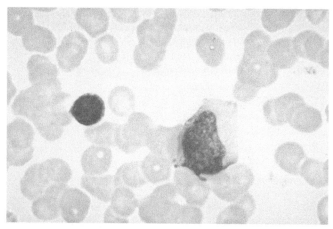

FIGURE 18.6 Atypical lymphocytes. (From Thibodeau GA, Patton KT: *Anatomy and physiology,* ed 7, St Louis, 2010, Mosby.)

recommended. The provider should give permission to resume a normal schedule.

Treating the complications of infectious mononucleosis may include these measures:

- Sometimes streptococcal throat infections can occur secondary to mono. Antibiotics should be used to treat streptococcal infections.
- If hepatosplenomegaly occurs, the person should seek medical attention. Sometimes corticosteroids are given to reduce the inflammation of the liver and spleen.

Life Span Changes

Childhood disorders of the lymphatic and immune systems include:
- hypersensitivities or allergies to foods, pollen, or pet dander
- childhood leukemias or lymphomas
- the development of autoimmune disease in late adolescence

Unlike children, adults and seniors will have a host of diagnoses from this chapter on their medical charts. Autoimmune diseases are most common in young adulthood to middle age. Cancers of these systems also appear in significant numbers. Non-Hodgkin's lymphoma and acute myelogenous leukemia (AML) account for thousands of hospitalizations every year. Multiple myeloma is most frequently diagnosed after age 60.

THE MEDICAL ASSISTANT'S ROLE IN ALLERGY AND INFECTIOUS DISEASE PROCEDURES

Assisting With the Examination

When working with patients who have infectious diseases it is important to protect yourself and other patients in the healthcare facility. If a patient has made an appointment to be seen for a cough or other respiratory issue, he or she may be asked to put on a mask when checking in for the appointment. This will help to protect the other patients in the reception area. Hand sanitizer is often available in the reception area so that patients can use it after they have sneezed, coughed or wiped their nose.

Many healthcare facilities will also have the medical assistant wear a mask when working with patients with a potentially infectious

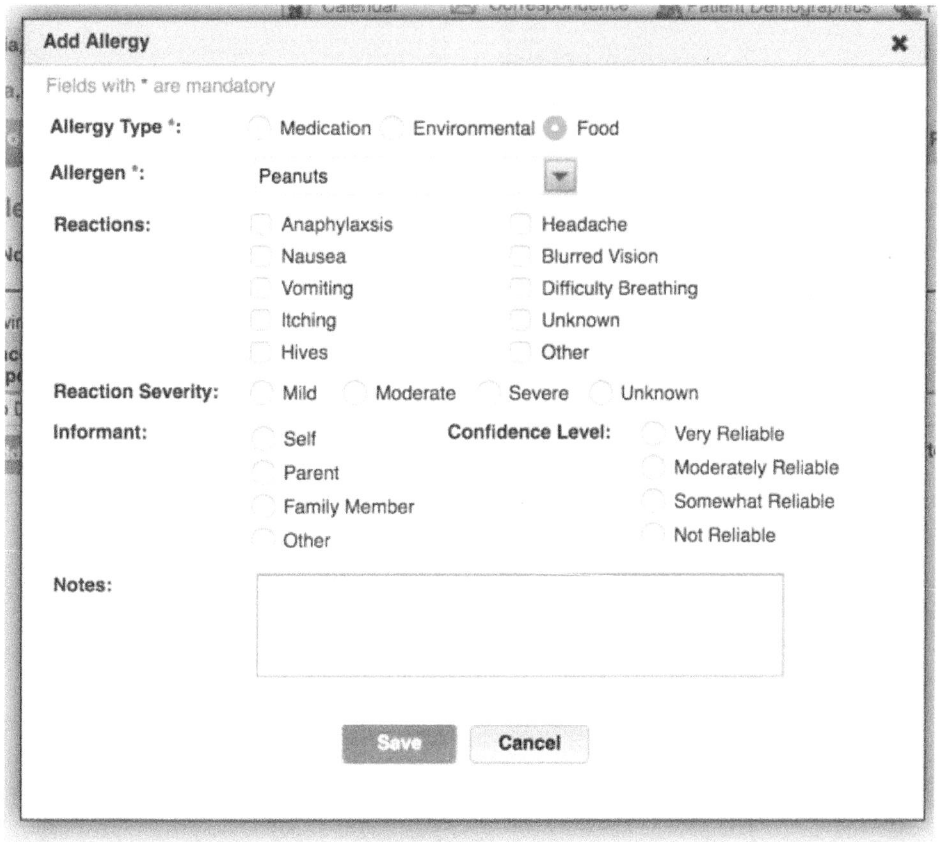

FIGURE 18.7 Allergy documentation in SimChart for the Medical Office.

disease, especially respiratory infections. A simple explanation that you are wearing the mask as a precaution will help to make the patient feel more comfortable with the situation.

Preparing a patient for an infectious disease examination includes having the patient disrobe appropriately, depending on which body system is involved. For allergy testing the patient usually must disrobe to the waist and the gown is open in the back.

An important part of any examination is taking a health history. When working with a patient who has a potential infectious disease the medical assistant should gather the history of the present illness (HPI) information and review the past medical history (PMH).

When working with a patient with potential allergies it is important to ask what the reaction to the allergen was. The reaction can indicate whether the patient has an allergy or a sensitivity. With a true allergy there is an immune system response that can affect many organs in the body (e.g., difficulty breathing or hives). Allergies can be severe or even life-threatening. With a *sensitivity* there is no immune system response, but there is an exaggeration of a normal side effect. This could range from digestive issues to neurologic issues. Fig. 18.7 is an example of how allergies would be documented in the electronic health record. Table 18.5 lists common allergens.

Assisting With Diagnostic Procedures
Skin Testing for Allergies
Skin testing to detect allergies requires percutaneous application or intradermal injection of a small amount of antigen (or groups of

TABLE 18.5 Common Medication, Environmental, and Food Allergens

MEDICATION	ENVIRONMENTAL	FOOD
Penicillin and related antibiotics	Dust mites	Eggs
Sulfonamides (antibiotics)	Pollen	Peanuts
Anticonvulsants	Pet dander	Tree nuts
Nonsteroidal anti-inflammatory drugs (NSAIDS)	Mold	Wheat
Chemotherapy drugs	Cigarette smoke	Shellfish

antigens) and later examination of the test sites for a visible reaction. The larger the localized skin reaction, the more profound the patient's allergic response to the tested allergen.

Percutaneous Test. A percutaneous, or scratch, test may be performed on the forearm, upper arm, or back. The back is favored in young children because of the large area of skin available. It also is easier to immobilize the child in this position. The skin surface is labeled or numbered in rows $1\frac{1}{2}$ to 2 inches apart, and a small amount of allergen is placed on the skin, which is then scratched or pricked to place the allergen just under the skin surface. Many

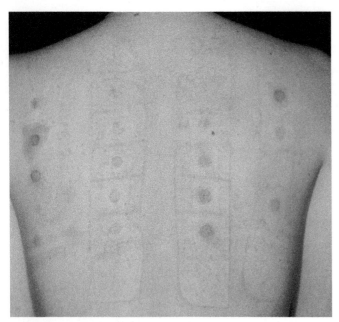

FIGURE 18.8 Results of allergy testing. (From Habif TP: *Clinical dermatology*, ed 5, St Louis, 2010, Mosby.)

> **Four Guidelines for Allergen Skin Testing**
>
> - The patient should stop taking all antihistamines or allergy medications 3 to 10 days before testing to prevent false-negative results.
> - Recommended sites for injection or application of the allergen are the anterior forearm, the upper arm, and the back.
> - Allergen sites must be specifically labeled and spaced approximately $1\frac{1}{2}$ to 2 inches apart.
> - If the patient shows signs of anaphylaxis, notify the provider immediately and prepare emergency supplies. Allergy testing should be performed only when the provider is on site.
> - Skin testing may cause a mild systemic allergic response, resulting in rhinitis, wheezing, and sneezing. The patient should contact the provider if a more severe reaction occurs.

allergists use a plastic device that is dipped into the designated allergens and lightly pressed into the skin so that the prick and allergen deposition occur at the same time. Seventy or more tests may be done at one time. It is essential to follow a pattern so that the site of each allergen can be easily identified. This type of allergy testing is used for allergic rhinitis, asthma, and detection of food allergies.

A reaction usually occurs within 10 to 30 minutes of exposure to the allergen. If the reaction is positive, a wheal (hive) forms at the site of the scratch (Fig. 18.8). Interpretation of the test result should always be based on a comparison of this reaction with that of the control, which is a scratch with a plain fluid free of any allergy-producing extract.

The interpretation, or reading, of the skin tests is performed by the provider or a trained technician. Reactions commonly are graded from 2 to 4. No precise definition of a reaction can be given, and the intensity of the response may vary among individuals. However, as a general rule, a 2 reaction implies a wheal that is definitely larger than that of the control. A larger wheal is interpreted as a 3, whereas the presence of pseudopods (fingerlike extensions around the periphery of the wheal) may be read as a 4. If a strong reaction occurs, the allergen extract should be carefully wiped off to prevent any further exposure. Frequently, large or significant reactions are accompanied by local itching. Patients should remain in the office for at least 30 minutes after completion of the test in case a delayed systemic allergic response occurs.

Patch Test. This test uses an allergen that is applied to a patch that is placed on the skin. Patch testing helps detect delayed allergic reactions associated with contact dermatitis. The patches are placed on the arms or back and must remain in place for 48 hours. The patient needs to avoid bathing and activities that cause heavy sweating. The patches are removed at a subsequent office visit. Skin irritation at the patch site indicates an allergy to that particular substance.

Intradermal (Intracutaneous) Test. The intradermal test is more sensitive than the percutaneous test and usually is used to diagnose allergies to penicillin and insect venom, such as from bee stings. Extracts are injected into the intradermal layer of the skin in doses of 0.1 to 0.2 mL. This method also is used for the tuberculin (purified protein derivative [PPD]) test and the Valley Fever coccidioidomycosis test. When intradermal injections are used for allergy testing, 10 to 15 allergens may be tested at one time on each arm. The reaction time is identical to that of the scratch test; however, the antigen is more dilute.

Radioallergosorbent Test. The radioallergosorbent test (RAST) measures the level of antibodies created when a sample of the patient's blood is mixed with allergens in the laboratory. The RAST is easier to perform than skin testing because it requires a single venipuncture. Although skin testing remains the preferred method of diagnosing hypersensitivity, the RAST may be indicated when the patient cannot stop antihistamine medications, when a skin disorder makes accurate interpretation of skin test results difficult, or when skin test results are negative but the patient's signs and symptoms support further investigation. RAST blood tests are primarily used to identify food allergies.

Testing for Respiratory Infections

When performing CLIA-waived tests for respiratory infections, it is important to wear the appropriate personal protective equipment (PPE) to protect yourself and your patients. If a patient has an active cough, he or she will likely be asked to wear a mask while in the reception area. This will need to be removed for the provider to do the examination. At that point the provider and the medical assistant will don face masks. In addition, a fluid-impermeable lab coat and disposable gloves should be used. Chapter 34 provides more information on performing the CLIA-waived tests.

Assisting With Treatments

Treatment of Allergies

The classic treatment of allergies is to encourage the patient to avoid known or suspected allergens. Unfortunately, this is not always possible, so the provider may prescribe antihistamine medications, such as levocetirizine (Xyzal), for relief of allergy symptoms. Over-the-counter antihistamines include Allegra, Zyrtec, and Claritin. Another option is the use of immunotherapy, a series of injections in which minute doses of known allergens are administered subcutaneously over time to desensitize the patient's immune system and ultimately develop a resistance to the immune response. This usually requires weekly or bimonthly injections over several years. Some patients are cured, whereas others have only a minor reduction in allergic symptoms. Immunotherapy is controversial because it is an expensive, invasive, and potentially dangerous treatment with unpredictable results. It is recommended only for patients with severe allergic symptoms that are not relieved by antihistamine medications.

If you are responsible for administering allergen injections, you must take great care to dispense the correct dose of each allergen; administer each subcutaneous injection in a separate site; accurately document the procedure and the exact location of each injection; record any local or systemic reactions; and observe the patient for at least 20 to 30 minutes after the injections to detect possible systemic allergic responses, including urticaria (hives), wheezing, or hypotension. If the patient shows any localized or systemic reactions, the provider should be notified.

Treatments for Respiratory Infections

Some infections, such as strep throat, will require the use of antibiotics for treatment. If the provider prescribes antibiotics, the medical assistant should make sure that the patient understands the importance of taking all of the medication and coming for any follow-up visits recommended by the provider.

If the infection is viral, the treatment will consist of using over-the-counter medication (acetaminophen [Tylenol]) for any fever and plenty of fluids to prevent dehydration. Patient education is the key to patient compliance and recovery.

It is also important to educate patients in proper hand hygiene when dealing with respiratory infections. Hand washing and the use of an alcohol-based hand sanitizer will help to prevent the spread of the infection. Covering a cough or sneeze will also help to prevent the spread of infection.

CLOSING COMMENTS

Patient Coaching

We know that proper hand hygiene plays a key role in preventing the spread of infectious diseases. Often our patients are not aware of how important it is. It is considered to be the most important element of infection control. Coaching our patients on the when and how of hand washing can help to keep everyone healthier. The CDC recommends washing your hands at the following times:
- Before, during, and after preparing food
- Before eating food
- Before and after caring for someone who is sick

- Before and after treating a cut or wound
- After using the toilet
- After changing diapers or cleaning up a child who has used the toilet
- After blowing your nose, coughing, or sneezing
- After touching an animal, animal feed, or animal waste
- After handling pet food or pet treats
- After touching garbage

Washing hands with soap and water is recommended, but if that is not available an alcohol-based hand sanitizer that is at least 60% alcohol can be used. When washing with soap and water, the hands should be scrubbed for at least 20 seconds. Be sure to lather the backs of your hands, between your fingers, and under your nails.

Legal and Ethical Issues

By law, diseases considered of great public health importance must be reported. Some diseases must be reported at the federal level, to the Centers for Disease Control and Prevention; others must be reported at the state level. Most states will have a "reportable diseases" list. Many of those diseases are also on the federal list.

It is important for medical assistants to know which diseases need to be reported for the state in which they are working. See Chapter 4 in the main text, Healthcare Laws, for more information on required reporting.

Patient-Centered Care

Part of providing care for patients with sexually transmitted infections is education on the prevention of those infections. This education must be presented in a nonjudgmental way. Abstinence, limiting the number of sex partners, and the use of male and female condoms and cervical diaphragms (for cervical gonorrhea, chlamydia, and trichomoniasis) are all ways to reduce the risk of contracting a sexually transmitted infection.

Professional Behaviors

When you have a strong work ethic, it becomes hard to stay home when you are sick. You may think, "I'm not that sick"; "We are shorthanded already"; "I don't want to put more work on my co-workers' shoulders," and so on. If you are sick, it is best for everyone for you to stay at home and get better. The quicker you get better, the quicker you will be back at work giving 100% again. It is also better for your co-workers and patients if you stay home, rather than risk spreading your illness to others. Many of your patients are at the healthcare facility because they are already ill. You risk exposing them to another illness if you go to work when you are sick. If you have a fever or have been vomiting, it is best to stay home.

SUMMARY OF SCENARIO

Julia has had a busy day with many different conditions being presented. She has helped with allergy testing and by working with Dr. Perez has a better understanding of what causes allergies and how allergies are diagnosed. Julia is discovering that the immune system is a complex system, and she plans on taking some continuing education courses to better understand it.

Julia has always understood the importance of preventing the spread of diseases, and she has had the opportunity today to educate patients. Proper hand hygiene can go a long way toward keeping people healthy.

SUMMARY OF LEARNING OBJECTIVES

1. **List the major organs and structures for the immune and lymphatic systems.**

   The lymphatic system is made up of lymph vessels, lymph nodes, lymph glands and lymphoid tissue. Lymph organs include the tonsils, adenoids, vermiform appendix, spleen, thymus gland, and Peyer patches.

   Within the immune system there are two very important cells, monocytes and lymphocytes. These cells move from the bloodstream into the lymph to perform their protective functions. The granular white blood cells play an important role in the immune system protection function.

2. **Describe the physiology of the immune and lymphatic systems. Also, discuss allergies and differentiate between active and passive immunity.**

   Nonspecific immunity uses physical methods of protection, along with reflexes and chemical methods, as the first line of defense. Phagocytosis, inflammation, pyrexia, protective proteins, and natural killer cells are all involved in the second line of defense.

   Specific immunity is another way that the body protects itself from infectious diseases. It is called specific immunity because the response is directed at one specific antigen. Specific immunity involves the development of antibodies. Humoral immunity and cell-mediated immunity are both parts of specific immunity.

   Allergies are also known as hypersensitivity reactions. A hypersensitivity reaction does not occur the first time an antigen is encountered. When the body responds to an allergen, immune cells release *histamines*, *kinins*, and other inflammatory substances. This causes the characteristic allergy symptoms: runny nose, watery eyes, and possibly a rash or hives. Sometimes drugs called *antihistamines* are used to alleviate allergy symptoms.

   Active immunity requires the body to produce antibodies in response to the presence of an antigen. Passive immunity does not require the body to do anything because the premade antibodies are given to the person.

3. **Identify the etiology, signs and symptoms, diagnostic procedures, and treatment of autoimmune diseases and disorders.**

   In autoimmune diseases and disorders, the body attacks healthy self-cells rather than foreign antigens. The cause of autoimmune diseases is unknown, but there are several suspected causes, including an infection that triggers the immune system to attack healthy cells, exposure over time to toxins, a weakness in a person's immune system, an imbalance in the intestinal microbiome, and/or existing allergies.

   Signs and symptoms vary, depending on the cells or tissues involved. The common signs and symptoms include skin changes, joint pain, fatigue/malaise, and a low-grade fever.

   A thorough history and physical examination, along with various blood tests, are used to help diagnose autoimmune diseases and disorders.

   Treatments vary, again depending on the cells or tissues involved, but could include physical therapy, blood transfusions, modified diet, stress reduction, NSAIDS, prescription corticosteroids, and immunosuppressive drugs.

4. **Identify the etiology, signs and symptoms, diagnostic procedures, and treatment of HIV/AIDS.**

   The human immunodeficiency virus is the virus that causes HIV/AIDS. It attacks the immune system and impairs its ability to fight infectious agents. AIDS is the last stage of the HIV infection.

   Signs and symptoms of AIDS include chronic and persistent diarrhea, recurring fevers, night sweats, profound fatigue, weight loss, skin rashes, continual white patches or lesions on the tongue or in the mouth, and repeated opportunistic infections.

   HIV can be diagnosed using a CLIA-waived test and then confirmed with ELISA or Western blot testing.

   There is no cure for HIV, but treatment includes a regimen of antiviral medication. Treatment should also include eating healthy, nutrient-rich food, getting adequate sleep, exercise, relaxation, and staying up to date on immunizations.

5. **Identify the etiology, signs and symptoms, diagnostic procedures, and treatment of lymphoma.**

   Hodgkin's and non-Hodgkin's are the two main types of lymphoma. The cause of lymphomas is not completely understood. Risk factors include a family history of lymphoma, being 15 to 30 years old or over age 55, being male, and having had an Epstein-Barr infection.

   Signs and symptoms include painless swelling of lymph nodes, fatigue, fever, chills, night sweats, and unexplained weight loss. With non-Hodgkin's lymphoma there could be abdominal swelling and/or pain, trouble breathing, coughing, or chest pain.

   A physical examination, along with blood and urine tests, will be done to diagnose Hodgkin's or non-Hodgkin's lymphoma. The provider may order imaging tests and a biopsy of lymph nodes, tissue, or bone marrow.

   Treatment depends on the type and stage of the lymphoma. Some types of non-Hodgkin's lymphoma may just be monitored. Hodgkin's lymphoma may be treated with chemotherapy, radiation therapy, or stem cell transplantation.

6. **Identify the etiology, signs and symptoms, diagnostic procedures, and treatment of multiple myeloma. Also, identify these factors for infectious diseases of the immune and lymphatic systems, such as viral hepatitis, sexually transmitted infections, and respiratory infections.**

   The cause of multiple myeloma is unknown. Risk factors include being over the age of 60, male gender, and a history of MGUS; blacks are more likely to develop multiple myeloma than whites.

   Signs and symptoms can be very subtle at first but when noticeable could include bone pain, especially in the spine, chest, or hips; anemia; loss of kidney function; excessive thirst; nausea; loss of appetite; weight loss; constipation; fatigue; frequent infections; weakness or numbness in the legs; and mental confusion.

   Blood tests, including a CBC and differential; tests for the presence of M protein; a comprehensive metabolic panel (CMP), which includes kidney and liver function tests, along with urinalysis; and bone marrow biopsy and examination of cells are used to help diagnose multiple myeloma. Imaging tests may include x-ray, MRI, CT, and PET scans. At diagnosis, multiple myeloma will be staged, and a treatment plan will be based on the staged diagnosis.

Often the provider will watch the condition and run periodic blood and urine tests to monitor asymptomatic multiple myeloma. Treatment for multiple myeloma includes targeted cancer therapy (designed to target specific weaknesses in myeloma cancer cells in order to kill the cells), biologic therapy, chemotherapy, radiation therapy, and possibly stem cell transplantation.

Infectious diseases are those caused by organisms such as bacteria, viruses, fungi, or parasites. Hepatitis is an inflammation of the liver. Sexually transmitted infections may be seen in any individual who is sexually active. Strep throat is a bacterial infection caused by *Streptococcus pyogenes*. Influenza is a viral respiratory infection that is referred to as the flu. Respiratory syncytial virus (RSV) produces upper respiratory "cold" symptoms. Infectious mononucleosis is a generally mild viral infection, but it can have serious complications.

7. **Describe the medical assistant's role in assisting with the examination and with diagnostic procedures associated with allergies and infectious diseases.**

The medical assistant must help where needed but also protect himself or herself by wearing a mask. Preparing a patient for an infectious disease examination includes having the patient disrobe appropriately, depending on which body system is involved. For allergy testing the patient usually must disrobe to the waist and the gown is open in the back.

Skin testing for allergies can be done with a percutaneous test, patch test, intradermal test, or a radioallergosorbent test. These tests can help to determine just what the patient is allergic to so that a treatment plan can be designed.

Diagnostic procedures for respiratory infections include many CLIA-waived tests.

8. **Describe treatments for allergies and respiratory infections.**

Treatments for allergies include encouraging patients to avoid the known or suspected allergen, but if that is not possible medications may be recommended. Another option is immunotherapy to desensitize the patient's immune system.

Treatments for respiratory infections could include the use of antibiotics for bacterial infections. For both bacterial and viral infections, the provider may recommend the use of over-the-counter medication for fever and plenty of fluids to prevent dehydration.

19

GASTROENTEROLOGY

SCENARIO

Keith Williams, CMA (AAMA), has been newly hired as a medical assistant at the Walden-Martin Family Medical (WMFM) Clinic. He just graduated from the local community college last semester, after returning to school to study for a second career. Now, at age 49, he has accepted a job at WMFM Clinic. He has been asked by his supervisor to assist the gastroenterology outreach team, which comes to WMFM Clinic twice a week.

Keith is excited about his new duties yet realizes that he needs to review the gastrointestinal (GI) system and related diseases. He decides to spend the next week reviewing the anatomy, physiology, and pathology related to the GI system, along with the diagnostic procedures and commonly ordered treatments.

While studying this chapter, think about the following questions:
- What terms relate to the gastrointestinal system?
- Where are the gastrointestinal system structures located?
- What are the functions of the gastrointestinal system?

- What are commonly diagnosed gastrointestinal diseases? What are their causes, signs and symptoms, diagnostic processes, and treatment?

LEARNING OBJECTIVES

1. Discuss the anatomy of the gastrointestinal system and the accessory organs. Also describe the sections of the small and large intestines, the functions of the liver, and life span changes associated with the gastrointestinal system.
2. Describe the four processes that occur in the gastrointestinal system and discuss the chemical digestion of carbohydrates, proteins, and fats.
3. Identify common signs, symptoms, and etiologies of gastrointestinal disorders and discuss disorders of the mouth, esophagus, and stomach.
4. Discuss disorders of the intestines.

5. Discuss disorders of the accessory organs and explain how hepatitis A, B, C, D, and E are transmitted.
6. Discuss cancers of the gastrointestinal system.
7. Describe the medical assistant's role in gastrointestinal procedures, list examples of screening questions, and describe the diagnostic tests and procedures for common gastrointestinal disorders.
8. Identify CLIA-waived tests associated with common gastrointestinal disorders.
9. Describe the treatments for common gastrointestinal disorders.

VOCABULARY

cholecystitis Inflammation of the gallbladder.

colostomy (koh LOS tuh mee) A surgical procedure in which the large intestine is brought though the abdominal wall, creating either a temporary or a permanent opening (stoma) to allow stool to pass out of the body.

dysphagia Difficulty swallowing.

emulsifies (ee MUL sih fyez) When a substance suspends tiny droplets of one liquid into a second liquid. By creating an emulsion, you can mix two liquids that usually do not mix well, such as oil and water.

endocrine A glandular secretion that is released into the blood or lymph directly (does not go through a duct).

enema Fluid introduced into the rectum for a therapeutic or diagnostic purpose.

epiglottis (ep i GLOT is) Lid-like structure over the glottis that prevents food and liquids from entering the trachea when swallowing occurs.

exocrine A glandular secretion released through a duct.

fissure A crack, cleft, or narrow opening.

fistula A permanent abnormal passageway between an abscess, organ, or cavity to the body surface or another organ resulting from a congenital disorder, disease, or injury.

hemolytic uremic syndrome Kidney disorder that can occur after a digestive infection with *E. coli*, shigella, or salmonella; red blood cells are destroyed and block the kidneys' filtering system, causing acute kidney failure.

intrinsic factor Secreted by the parietal cells of the stomach; necessary for the absorption of vitamin B_{12} to prevent pernicious anemia.

lumen The cavity, channel, or open space within a tube or tubular organ.

mucous membrane A mucus-producing membrane that lines tracts and structures of the body (e.g., GI tract, respiratory tract); also called *mucosa*.

occult Hidden or unseen.

peristalsis (payr i STAHL sis) Wave-like movement from alternate circulate contraction and relaxation of a tubular structure (e.g., intestine), which propels the content forward.

plaque Sticky substance made of mucus, food particles, and bacteria that builds up on the exposed part of the tooth.

polyp A growth or mass protruding from a mucous membrane (e.g., nose, bladder, intestine).

rebound pain Pain felt when the pressure on the abdomen is released.

resection Surgical removal of all or part of an organ.

rugae (ROO gah) Folds in the wall of an organ; when organ (e.g., stomach, bladder, uterus) fills or needs to expand, the rugae unfold.

sphincter (SFINGK ter) A circular muscle that either constricts and closes the opening or relaxes and allows substances to pass through the opening.

---

*G*astroenterology is the healthcare specialty that deals with most digestive diseases and disorders. A *gastroenterologist* is a specialist involved in the diagnosis, treatment, and prevention of disorders of the digestive organs and liver. A *proctologist* is a subspecialist who treats disorders of the rectum and anus. *Hepatology* is a subspecialty that deals with liver disorders. A *hepatologist* is a specialist who focuses only on the liver.

Gastrointestinal system disorders are common in the ambulatory care facility. Besides the gastroenterology department, patients with digestive concerns are seen in primary care, pediatrics, internal medicine, and urgent care settings.

ANATOMY OF THE GASTROINTESTINAL SYSTEM

The *gastrointestinal (GI) system* is also called the *digestive system*. It is made up of these structures:

* *Gastrointestinal tract*: Also called the *digestive tract* and the *alimentary canal*. It consists of a large, muscular tube that, with the help of hormones and enzymes, digests food. The GI tract starts at the mouth and extends to the anus. It includes the mouth, pharynx (throat), esophagus, stomach, small intestine, and large intestine.
* *Accessory organs*: The salivary glands, gallbladder, liver, and pancreas are considered the major accessory organs. These structures secrete fluids into the GI tract, aiding in digestion.

The following sections will discuss the GI tract structures and the accessory organs.

CRITICAL THINKING APPLICATION   19.1

As Keith starts to review the anatomy of the GI system, he tries to remember the major and accessory organs. List the major organs and accessory organs of the GI system.

Gastrointestinal Tract Structures

Mouth

The cheeks, lips, tongue, *hard palate*, and *soft palate* form the mouth (also called the *oral cavity* or *buccal cavity*). The roof of the mouth is created by the anterior hard palate and the posterior soft palate. The *uvula* is a fleshy structure that hangs above the throat, at the back of the soft palate. Adults have 32 permanent teeth that are set in the gums (also called *gingivae*). Saliva from the salivary glands helps to lubricate the food, making it easier to swallow. The salivary glands will be discussed later in the chapter.

Pharynx

When food or liquid is swallowed, it moves into the pharynx, or throat. The pharynx is divided into three sections:

* *Nasopharynx*: Located behind the nasal cavity.
* *Oropharynx*: Located behind the mouth and part of the respiratory and digestive systems.
* *Laryngopharynx*: Located between the **epiglottis** and the esophagus.

Esophagus

The esophagus connects the pharynx to the stomach (Fig. 19.1). This muscular tube runs behind the trachea and the heart. The esophagus is lined with a **mucous membrane** that secretes mucus, helping the mass of food, or *bolus*, pass into the stomach. Peristalsis, or the muscular contractions of the esophagus, helps to move the food into the stomach.

A **sphincter** is located at the top and bottom of the esophagus. When the *upper esophageal sphincter* (UES) constricts, it prevents air from entering the esophagus. The *lower esophageal sphincter* (LES), or the *cardiac sphincter*, is located between the esophagus and the stomach. When the LES constricts, it prevents the stomach contents from moving up the esophagus. When a person swallows, the LES relaxes, allowing the bolus to move into the stomach.

Stomach

The stomach serves as a reservoir for food. The stomach is divided into three sections:

* *Fundus*: Top of the stomach, sits just below the diaphragm
* *Body*: Main part of the stomach
* *Pylorus*: Bottom of the stomach, between the body and the small intestine

The stomach wall contains **rugae**, which when unfolded allow for greater expansion of the stomach size.

Tiny glands in the mucous membrane lining of the stomach produce digestive enzymes, **intrinsic factor**, hydrochloric acid, mucus, and bicarbonate, which make up the *gastric juice*. Gastric juice is continually being made, but the amounts vary. Certain things trigger more gastric juice to be made, including thoughts of eating, the smell of food, and the presence of food in the mouth and stomach. The smooth muscles in the stomach provide the churning and mixing action, which helps combine the gastric juice with the food ingested, creating a mixture called *chyme*. A continuous coating of mucus protects the stomach and the rest of the GI system from the acidic nature of chyme and the gastric juices.

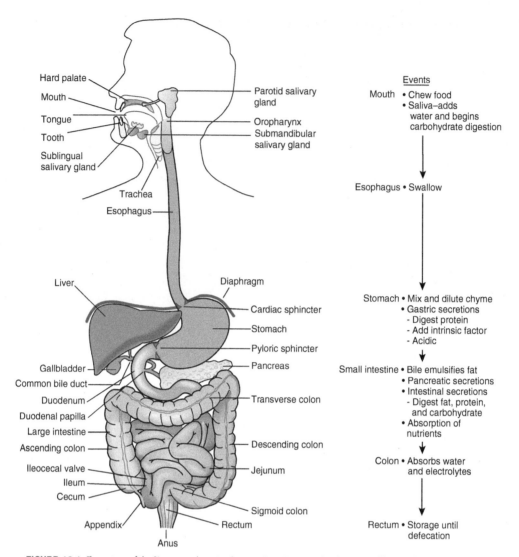

FIGURE 19.1 The anatomy of the GI system and associated events. (From VanMeter KC, Hubert RJ: *Gould's pathophysiology for the health professions*, ed 5, Philadelphia, 2015, Saunders.)

Besides being a food reservoir and secreting gastric juices, the stomach has additional roles, which include:

- Producing *gastrin*, a hormone that regulates the digestive functions
- Producing *ghrelin*, which increases the appetite
- Protecting the body by killing disease-causing bacteria in food
- Absorbing alcohol, some water, certain drugs, and some fatty acids

The *pyloric sphincter* is located between the pylorus and the small intestine and regulates the passage of food into the small intestine (see Fig. 19.1). When the pyloric sphincter relaxes, the chyme empties out of the stomach and into the small intestine.

CRITICAL THINKING APPLICATION   **19.2**

Keith tries to remember the roles of the stomach as he prepares for his day with the gastroenterologist. List the roles of the stomach.

Small Intestine

The small intestine has about a 1-inch **lumen** and is about 20 feet long. The small intestine loops around and fills most of the abdominal cavity. The small intestine is made up of three parts:

- *Duodenum*: Smallest part of the small intestine; connected to the stomach by the pyloric sphincter.
- *Jejunum*: Second largest part of the small intestine; connected to the duodenum and the ileum.
- *Ileum*: Largest part of the small intestine; connects to the jejunum and the large intestine. It joins the cecum at the ileocecal valve.

The lining of the small intestine has *plicae* (folds), which contain small projections called *villi*. The villi are covered by *microvilli* (epithelial cells that have a brush-like shape). The villi and microvilli increase the surface area of the small intestine and make absorption of nutrients more efficient. Each villus contains a *lacteal* (lymph vessel) that absorbs lipids (fats) and a blood capillary that absorbs glucose and amino acids.

Each of the three sections of the small intestine have important roles.

- *Duodenum*: Receives chyme from the stomach. Pancreatic enzymes, bile from the liver, and bicarbonate mix with the chyme. Pancreatic enzymes break down chyme. Bile helps break down and absorb fat. Bicarbonate neutralizes the acid from the stomach.
- *Jejunum*: Contains larger villi, thus absorption is the primary function of this section. Sugars, fatty acids, and amino acids are absorbed.
- *Ileum*: Limited absorption occurs in this section. Bile acids and vitamin B$_{12}$ are most often absorbed for reuse in the body.

Chyme from the stomach empties into the duodenum. **Peristalsis** moves the chyme through the duodenum, jejunum and the ileum. The *ileocecal* valve is found between the ileum (of the small intestine) and the cecum (of the large intestine). The ileocecal valve controls the passage of chyme into the cecum and prevents the backflow of chyme into the small intestine.

Large Intestine

The *large intestine* or *colon* has about a 3-inch lumen and is about 5 feet long. The large intestine is made up of these six sections:

- *Cecum*: A 2- to 3-inch pouch or tube-like structure in the lower right abdomen that is considered the first section of the large intestine. The main roles of the cecum include receiving chyme from the small intestine and absorbing fluids and salts. Mucus is also mixed with the chyme in the cecum. Attached to the cecum is the *vermiform appendix*. The function of the appendix is not known, though research suggests that it harbors "good bacteria," which will repopulate the intestines after an illness.
- *Ascending colon*: The second part of the large intestine, which extends vertically from the cecum to just below the liver (see Fig. 19.1).
- *Transverse colon*: Extends horizontally from the ascending colon to the descending colon.
- *Descending colon*: Extends vertically on the left side of the abdomen from the transverse colon to the sigmoid colon.
- *Sigmoid colon*: Forms an S-shaped curve; attaches to the descending colon and the rectum.
- *Rectum*: Stores the stool until defecation, or a bowel movement (BM), occurs and the stool is released through the anus.

The watery waste products move from the small intestine into the large intestine. The primary functions of the large intestine include:

- *Reabsorption of water and electrolytes*: The large intestine has no villi for nutrient absorption, but can reabsorb water and electrolytes (e.g., sodium and potassium). The longer stool is in the colon, the more water is absorbed. The quicker stool passes through the large intestine, the more water it contains.
- *Makes vitamin K*: The bacteria in the large intestine make vitamin K, which is used for blood coagulation, bone mineralization, and cardiovascular health.
- *Eliminates waste products from the body.*

CRITICAL THINKING APPLICATION   **19.3**

Keith is reviewing the anatomy of the GI tract. List the sections of the small and large intestines in order.

Bacteria in the Colon

The bacteria in the colon can help with the digestion of some materials. This digestive process can cause gas to be formed, and when it is released through the anus, it is called *flatus*. The bacteria in the colon produce vitamin K and biotin (vitamin B$_7$).

The majority of the colon bacteria are nonpathogenic. The bacteria colonized in the colon (also called *gut flora* or *microbiota*) are important for our maturation, immune system development, and metabolism. Cardiovascular disease, metabolic diseases (e.g., diabetes and obesity), and inflammatory bowel disease are some diseases that have been associated with changes in the intestinal bacteria. Antibiotic therapy can also change the delicate microbiota balance in the gut.

Usually the microbiota prevents *Clostridium difficile* colonization. With some antibiotic therapies, *C. difficile* may be allowed to grow, causing intestinal inflammation, diarrhea, and in some cases, death. *C. difficile* is spread by the fecal-oral route and is shed in the stool of infected patients. The *C. difficile* spores have a long survival life and are difficult to kill. They are not destroyed by alcohol-based hand sanitizers. *C. difficile* infections are treated with antibiotics, and the risk of reinfection is high.

Accessory Organs

Accessory organs have a role in digestive activities, though they are not part of the digestive tract. Accessory organs include the salivary glands, liver, gallbladder, and the pancreas. Each of these accessory organs will be discussed in the following sections.

Salivary Glands

Three pairs of salivary glands are found in the mouth. The parotid glands are near the ear in the cheeks. The submandibular glands are on the floor of the mouth, and the sublingual glands are under the tongue. These glands produce and secrete saliva, which mixes with the food eaten. Saliva not only moistens the food, it aids in the breakdown and swallowing of food. Saliva contains salivary amylase, an enzyme, which will be discussed later in the chapter.

Liver

The liver is one of the largest organs in the body and is located just below the diaphragm, in the right hypochondriac and epigastric regions (see Fig. 19.1). The liver is divided into two major lobes and two smaller lobes.

The hepatic artery brings oxygenated blood to the liver. The hepatic portal vein brings blood from the digestive tract, which can contain nutrients, medications, alcohol, and toxic substances. These substances are filtered from the blood and are processed, stored, changed, detoxified, and returned to the blood or eliminated in the stool. Besides these roles, the liver has additional important functions:

- Produces plasma proteins (e.g., albumin and blood clotting factors)
- Breaks down old or damaged blood cells
- Breaks down proteins and fats and produces energy
- Produces up to a liter of bile a day

- Removes extra minerals (e.g., iron and copper), vitamins (B_{12}, A, D, and K), and glucose from the blood and stores them in the liver. The liver releases them into the blood when needed. (For instance, the liver stores extra glucose as *glycogen*. When the blood glucose level decreases, the liver breaks down the glycogen and releases the glucose into the blood.)
- Manufactures triglycerides and cholesterol

Bile

Bile is made and released by the liver. It is stored in the gallbladder until it is secreted into the duodenum. Bile breaks down fats into fatty acids.

Bile contains the following substances:
- *Bilirubin,* a breakdown product of red blood cells
- Bile acid (also called *bile salts*)
- Cholesterol
- Water
- Body salts (e.g., sodium, potassium) and metals (e.g., copper)

CRITICAL THINKING APPLICATION   19.4

Keith is amazed at all of the activities that occur in the liver. List at least four roles of the liver.

Gallbladder

The gallbladder (GB) is found in a small area on the underside of the liver (see Fig. 19.1). The gallbladder stores and concentrates bile. The bile is made by the liver and then flows through the common bile duct to smaller ducts before going into the gallbladder, where it is stored. When a person eats, the gallbladder contracts and squeezes the bile through the bile duct into the common bile duct, which empties into the duodenum. If gallbladder emptying is delayed (as in pregnancy), gallstone formation can occur.

Pancreas

The pancreas is a gland found behind the stomach and in front of the spine (see Fig. 19.1). It is about 6 to 10 inches long. The pancreas has two main roles:

- **Exocrine** *function*: About 95% of the pancreas is made up of exocrine tissue that produces digestive enzymes. These enzymes are released into the duodenum.
- **Endocrine** *function*: About 5% of the pancreas is made up of endocrine cells, called *islets of Langerhans,* which make hormones (e.g., insulin) that regulate blood sugar and pancreatic secretions. (See Chapter 23 for additional details.)

The pancreatic enzymes created in the exocrine tissue include trypsin, chymotrypsin, amylase, and lipase. When food enters the stomach, pancreatic enzymes and sodium bicarbonate are released into the main pancreatic duct. This duct joins the common bile duct to form the ampulla of Vater (also called the *hepatopancreatic duct* or *ampulla*), which is located at the duodenum.

Life Span Changes

At birth the baby's digestive system is not fully mature. The infant does not have teeth to help break down food. Salivary secretions (which start starch breakdown) are insufficient until about 6 months of age. Pancreatic amylase levels may not be sufficient until 12 to 18 months of age. Bile salts and lipase levels are not sufficient until 6 to 9 months of age.

During pregnancy, progesterone (a hormone) causes the smooth muscles to relax. This causes less peristalsis in the digestive system, thus slowing digestion. Gallbladder emptying may be delayed, leading to gallstone formation. Morning sickness, constipation, and heartburn can result from digestive system changes.

With age, the stomach cannot accommodate as much food because of decreased elasticity. The stomach empties slower. Aging does not affect the secretion of gastric juices, and the most nutrient absorption occurs in the small intestines. The lactase levels decrease with age, leading to lactose intolerance (milk products). Bacterial overgrowth (excessive growth of certain intestinal bacteria) is more common with age and leads to bloating, weight loss, and pain. Bacterial overgrowth can also lead to reduced absorption of certain nutrients (e.g., iron, calcium, and vitamin B_{12}). With aging, constipation is more common and can be caused by many factors, including:

- Slowing of fecal contents through the large intestine, allowing for more water absorption
- Increased use of drugs that can cause constipation
- Decreased physical activity and fluid intake

Age-related changes can be seen with the accessory organs. A decrease of salivary flow is not related to age, although common in older adults. It is related to diseases, medications, and head and neck radiation therapy (used for cancers). The pancreas decreases in weight as some tissue is replaced with scar tissue, although these changes do not affect the organ's ability to produce digestive enzymes and sodium bicarbonate. With age, the liver gets smaller and blood flow decreases. Liver function test results are unchanged. Metabolism of many substances decreases, which affects drug metabolism; thus older adults may experience dose-related side effects. The production and flow of bile decreases with age, leading to more gallstones.

PHYSIOLOGY OF THE GASTROINTESTINAL SYSTEM

The role of the GI system is to provide nutrients to the cells of the body. Four processes occur in the GI system:

- *Ingestion:* The intake of food and liquids into the body
- *Digestion*: The breakdown of food into chemical substances
- *Absorption:* The passage of substances and liquids through the lining of the GI tract into the body fluids and tissues.
- *Excretion:* The elimination of indigestible materials and waste products of metabolism

The following sections will focus on digestion, absorption, and elimination processes in the body.

CRITICAL THINKING APPLICATION   19.5

Summarize the four processes that occur in the GI system.

Digestion

Once food is ingested, it must be digested for absorption to occur. Two digestive processes happen to break down food into chemical substances:

- *Mechanical digestion*: The breakdown of food into smaller particles. This process starts in the mouth as the food is being chewed. The smooth muscles in the stomach provide the churning and mixing action, which also aids in the breakdown of the food.
- *Chemical digestion*: The smaller particles of food are broken down into small molecules that can be absorbed.

Chemical Digestion

Chemical digestion starts in the mouth. During *mastication* (the process of chewing), saliva moistens the food. Saliva not only moistens the food; it aids in the breakdown and swallowing (*deglutition*) of food. Saliva contains an enzyme called *salivary amylase*, which starts to break down complex carbohydrates.

In the stomach, hydrochloric acid softens and breaks down proteins and other foods. The pH of hydrochloric acid also kills many pathogens (e.g., bacteria) that are consumed. Pepsin, an enzyme found in the gastric juices, breaks down proteins into polypeptides.

Hydrochloric acid, amino acids, or fatty acids in the stomach or duodenum stimulate the small intestine to secrete *cholecystokinin* (CCK), a hormone. CCK causes the gallbladder to contract and release bile into the duodenum through the common bile duct. Bile from the liver is also secreted in the duodenum and **emulsifies** fats. CCK also increases secretion of pancreatic juices, which contain the following enzymes:

- *Trypsin* and *chymotrypsin*: Break down proteins into amino acids
- *Amylase*: Breaks down carbohydrates into sugars
- *Lipase*: Breaks down fats into fatty acids and glycerol

Pancreatic juices also contain sodium bicarbonate, which helps to neutralize the acidity of the chyme in the duodenum.

In the small intestine, brush-border enzymes (sucrase, lactase, and maltase) are found in the microvilli. These enzymes help with the final breakdown of carbohydrates, including:

- *Sucrase*: Breaks down sucrose (or cane sugar) into glucose and fructose.
- *Lactase*: Breaks down lactose (found in milk) into galactose and glucose.
- *Maltase*: Breaks down maltose (from starches) into glucose.

CRITICAL THINKING APPLICATION   19.6

Summarize the chemical digestion of carbohydrates, proteins, and fats.

Absorption and Excretion

Once chemical digestion is complete, small nutrient molecules move from the small intestines into the bloodstream through the process of *absorption*. As mentioned earlier, the villi and microvilli in the small intestine increase the surface area, which makes absorption of nutrients more efficient. The lacteal in the villus absorbs lipids, and the capillary absorbs glucose and amino acids. Chemical digestion and nutrient absorption are completed by the time chyme leaves the small intestine.

As chyme moves through the large intestine, water and electrolytes are reabsorbed to prevent dehydration. The consistency of chyme changes to a soft-formed solid, called *feces,* which is excreted. The composition of feces is water, bacteria, undigested carbohydrates, fiber, and some protein and fat.

DISORDERS OF THE GASTROINTESTINAL SYSTEM

Many patients seen in ambulatory care facilities have GI system diseases. Common signs and symptoms include:

- Constipation, diarrhea, *hematochezia* (bloody stool), and *melena* (black, tarry stools)
- *Pyrosis* (heartburn), *dyspepsia* (indigestion), and *flatus* (gas)
- *Halitosis* (bad-smelling breath)
- Nausea, vomiting, and *hematemesis* (vomiting of blood)
- *Jaundice* (yellowing of the skin and whites of the eyes caused by elevated bilirubin levels)

Disorders of the Mouth

Orofacial Clefts

Orofacial clefts are one of the most common birth defects in the United States. Orofacial clefts include the following congenital disorders:

- *Cleft lip*: An opening in the upper lip caused by the lip tissues not completely joining before birth.
- *Cleft palate*: The tissue that makes up the palate (roof of the mouth) does not completely join before birth. The hard palate makes up the front section and the soft palate makes up the back section. Cleft palate can affect one or both palates.

Children can have a cleft lip, a cleft palate, or both (Fig. 19.2). Children with clefts can have problems with feeding, speaking, hearing, and ear infections.

In most cases the etiology is unknown, but researchers believe it involves genetics and environmental factors. Research studies have shown that women who smoke, have diabetes, or use certain

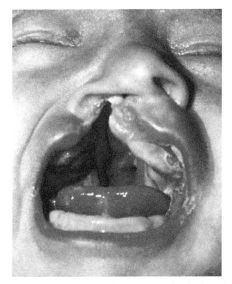

FIGURE 19.2 Cleft lip and cleft palate. (Zitelli BJ, Davis HW: *Atlas of pediatric physical diagnosis*, ed 4, St Louis, 2002, Mosby.)

medications (e.g., valproic acid) during pregnancy have an increased risk of having a baby with an orofacial cleft. The signs of an orofacial cleft are visible at birth. The child may have a split in the lip or the roof of the mouth. The cleft can affect one or both sides of the face.

The provider will identify the cleft right after birth. Sometimes the cleft is detected during a prenatal ultrasound. Treatment involves surgery to improve the child's ability to eat, speak, and hear. A team of specialists is involved with the treatment of the related complications.

Additional Disorders of the Mouth

Additional disorders of the mouth include:

* *Cavities*: Also called *tooth decay* or *dental caries*; **plaque** on the tooth creates the decay.
* *Gingivitis*: Early stages of periodontal disease; caused by plaque deposits on the tooth for a short amount of time. Gingivitis, an inflammatory disease of the gums, causes redness, swelling, and bleeding.
* *Herpetic stomatitis*: Inflammation of the mouth caused by the herpes simplex virus (also known as fever blister or a cold sore).
* *Leukoplakia*: A condition of white patches on the lips and buccal mucosa often associated with tobacco use.
* *Periodontal disease*: Infection and inflammation in the mouth that destroys the gums, periodontal ligaments, and bone that support the teeth.
* *Thrush*: A yeast infection of the mouth and tongue. Risk factors include older adults, infants, poor health, compromised immune system (e.g., HIV, AIDS, chemotherapy), and taking antibiotics.

Disorders of the Esophagus and Stomach

Gastroesophageal Reflux Disease

Gastroesophageal reflux (GER) occurs when the stomach contents back up into the esophagus, causing acid reflex or heartburn. Gastroesophageal reflux disease (GERD) is more serious and longer lasting than GER. GERD can occur in adults and infants. The presentation in infants is different from that in adults.

The cause of GERD is a weakened or an abnormal lower esophageal sphincter. The sphincter may relax when it should not, and stomach contents back up into the esophagus. The risk for GERD and GER in adults increases with pregnancy, being overweight, certain medications, and smoking. The most common symptom of GERD in adults is heartburn. Other common GERD symptoms in adults include bad breath, nausea, vomiting, chest pain, upper abdominal pain, respiratory problems, and erosion of the teeth.

A provider will do a history and physical examination. Treatment is based on the severity of the symptoms and can include lifestyle changes, medications, or surgery. Usually, patients are encouraged to reduce their intake of the foods and drinks that make the symptoms worse.

GERD in Infants

Infants can have GER and GERD. The cause of GER and GERD in infants is an immature (not fully developed) lower esophageal sphincter. The sphincter becomes weak or relaxed, and stomach contents back up into the esophagus.

The main symptoms of GERD in infants is spitting up more than normally. Additional symptoms include:

* Arching of the back during or right after feedings
* Colic, coughing, trouble breathing, wheezing, gagging, and projectile or forceful vomiting
* Poor feeding and refusal to feed
* Poor growth and weight gain, and malnutrition

Treatment for GERD focuses on feeding changes and medications. Rice cereal may be added to the milk. Holding the baby upright for 30 minutes after feeding and avoiding overfeeding the child may be encouraged. H_2 blockers or proton-pump inhibitors may be given to reduce acid production. Surgery may be recommended in severe cases. Most infant GERD resolves by 9 to 18 months of age.

Hiatal Hernia

A hiatal hernia occurs when a section of the upper stomach pushes through an opening of the diaphragm into the chest (Fig. 19.3).

The cause is unknown. The risk of hiatal hernias increases with age, obesity, and smoking. Often people over 50 years of age experience this condition. The signs and symptoms include chest pain, heartburn, and difficulty swallowing.

The provider will have a barium swallow x-ray and an esophago-gastroduodenoscopy (EGD) done to help diagnose the condition. The goal of treatment is to relieve symptoms and prevent complications. Treatment includes medications for acid reflux and surgery to repair the hernia. The person should avoid alcohol and use medications with care.

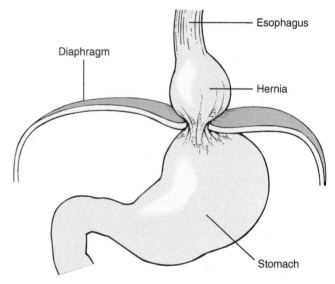

FIGURE 19.3 Hiatal hernia. (Frazier MS, Drzymkowski JW: *Essentials of human diseases and conditions*, ed 4, Philadelphia, 2008, Saunders.)

CRITICAL THINKING APPLICATION   **19.7**

What are the similarities and differences between GERD in adults and infants?

Peptic Ulcers

Peptic ulcers are also known as *duodenal, gastric,* and *stomach* ulcers. A peptic ulcer is a sore or breakdown in the lining of the stomach or duodenum. Gastric ulcers occur in the stomach, and duodenal ulcers occur in the first section of the small intestine.

The most common etiology for peptic ulcers is infection of the stomach by *Helicobacter pylori* (*H. pylori*). The risk for peptic ulcers may increase with drinking too much alcohol, regular use of aspirin or nonsteroidal anti-inflammatory drugs (NSAIDs) (e.g., ibuprofen and naproxen), using cigarettes and chewing tobacco, radiation treatments, and stress. Zollinger-Ellison syndrome can also cause peptic ulcers. Signs and symptoms include upper abdominal pain at night or when the stomach is empty (1 to 3 hours after a meal). Additional symptoms include: nausea, vomiting, melena, chest pain, fatigue, vomiting and hematemesis, and weight loss.

Besides a history and physical exam, the provider may order an upper endoscopy or an upper GI series to visibly examine the lining of the esophagus, stomach, and duodenum. Testing for *H. pylori* requires a biopsy of the stomach lining or a urea breath test. A stool occult blood test and a hemoglobin test may also be done. Treatment is based on the reasons for the ulcer. If *H. pylori* bacteria are present, the patient may need to take medication, such as antibiotics and an H₂ blocker (e.g., ranitidine [Zantac]) or a proton-pump inhibitor (PPI) (e.g., omeprazole [Prilosec], lansoprazole [Prevacid], or esomeprazole [Nexium]). Additional ulcer treatment may include a lining protectant, such as sucralfate.

Pyloric Stenosis

Pyloric stenosis is the narrowing of the pylorus, the muscular opening between the stomach and the small intestine. It occurs more often in males than females and in infants younger than 6 months.

The exact etiology is unknown, but there is a genetic link. Other risk factors include taking certain antibiotics, hyperacidity in the duodenum, and conditions such as type 1 diabetes mellitus. Vomiting is the most common sign. It can occur after feedings, may be projectile (forceful), and usually starts around 3 weeks of age. Other signs and symptoms include weight loss, constant hunger, dehydration, burping, abdominal pain, and a wave-like motion of the abdomen just before vomiting. Upon physical exam, the provider may feel an olive-sized mass in the upper abdomen.

The provider will order an ultrasound of the abdomen and barium x-ray to detect the stenosis and blood tests to identify electrolyte imbalances. Treatment depends on the severity of the stenosis and may include surgery to widen the pylorus (*pyloromyotomy*). If surgery cannot be done, an endoscope is inserted in the upper GI tract and a balloon is inflated to widen the pylorus. Medications or a feeding tube may also be used to relax the pylorus.

Additional Disorders of the Esophagus and Stomach

The following are additional disorders of the esophagus:

- *Achalasia*: The lower esophageal sphincter does not relax. Also, the esophageal peristalsis is reduced. Both factors delay the emptying of the food from the esophagus.
- *Barrett's esophagus*: Caused by GERD; the lining of the esophagus changes to resemble the lining of the intestines; this can lead to a potentially fatal condition called *esophageal adenocarcinoma.*

- *Esophageal atresia*: The esophagus ends in a blind pouch and does not connect to the stomach.
- *Esophageal varices*: Enlarged veins in the esophagus usually associated with severe liver disease; can leak or rupture, causing life-threatening bleeding.

Additional disorders of the stomach include:

- *Cyclic vomiting syndrome (CVS)*: Causes sudden, repeated episodes of severe nausea and vomiting. Vomiting episodes usually occur at the same time each day and last for about the same amount of time.
- *Dumping syndrome*: Rapid gastric emptying; occurs when foods (most commonly carbohydrates) empty too quickly into the duodenum. Can occur after bypass surgery or other types of bariatric surgeries for weight loss.
- *Gastritis*: Inflammation of the stomach lining; caused by bacteria, pain relievers, and alcohol.
- *Gastroparesis*: Stomach motility is slowed, causing delayed gastric emptying. Can be caused by certain medications (e.g., opioids, antidepressants, and antihypertensives).
- *Hypochlorhydria*: Deficiency in the hydrochloric acid in the stomach, which can lead to improper digestion, lack of nutrient absorption, infections, and other health issues.

Disorders of the Intestines

Acute Appendicitis

Appendicitis is an inflammation of the appendix. Commonly, it occurs between the ages of 10 and 30, though it can occur at any age.

The etiology is a blockage in the appendix, which can increase pressure, affect blood flow, and cause inflammation. If the blockage is not treated, the appendix can burst and cause *peritonitis* (inflammation of the peritoneum), a life-threatening condition. The pain usually begins near the umbilicus and then moves to the lower right side of the abdomen. **Rebound pain** can occur with peritonitis. Additional signs and symptoms include low fever, abdominal bloating, anorexia, nausea, vomiting, constipation, diarrhea, and inability to pass gas.

After the physical exam, blood and urine laboratory tests will be performed to rule out other conditions. A complete blood count (CBC) will show an elevated white blood cell count. Imaging tests (e.g., x-ray, computed tomography [CT] scan, ultrasound [US]) will be done to confirm appendicitis or rule out other conditions. Treatment consist of antibiotics and an appendectomy (surgical removal of the appendix). Laparoscopic surgery will result in a few small incisions. If a laparotomy is done, the incision may be 2 to 4 inches long. If the appendix bursts and an abscess forms, surgery may be delayed while the abscess is drained.

Celiac Disease

Celiac disease is a digestive and an immune disorder. When people with this disease eat foods with gluten, their immune system damages their small intestine. Gluten, a protein, is found in barley, rye, wheat, spelt, and triticale. It can also be found in other products, including vitamins and supplements, toothpastes, lip balm, and hair and skin products.

Celiac disease is a genetic, autoimmune disorder. The signs and symptoms of celiac disease can vary, depending on the age of the person. For example:

- *Young children*: Abdominal pain, vomiting, diarrhea, bloating, and constipation; irritability, emotional withdrawal, or very dependent behavior; failure to gain weight and grow; and obesity.
- *Teenagers*: Diarrhea, constipation, delayed puberty, hair loss, slowed growth, and short height.
- *Adults:* Diarrhea, constipation, fatigue, bone or joint pain, depression, anxiety, irritability, missed menstrual periods, anemia, and osteoporosis.

Celiac disease can also cause lactose intolerance, anemia, dermatitis herpetiformis (itchy, blistering skin condition), and canker sores in the mouth.

The provider will perform a history and physical exam. Blood tests and an intestinal biopsy may be ordered. Treatment consists of a gluten-free diet. Foods that are safe to eat include rice, oats, corn, quinoa, millet, and buckwheat.

Diverticulitis

Diverticula are small marble-sized pouches that form in the large intestine. The pouches protrude through the weakened walls of the large intestine. These pouches are common after age 40 and usually do not cause symptoms, unless they become inflamed or infected. When the diverticula become inflamed or infected, the condition is called *diverticulitis*.

When a diverticulum tears, inflammation and infection can occur. Risk factors include aging, obesity, smoking cigarettes, lack of exercise, low-fiber diets, and a high animal fat diet. Medications such as steroids, opioids, and NSAIDs can also increase the risk. Signs and symptoms of diverticulitis include constant lower left abdomen pain and tenderness, nausea, vomiting, diarrhea, constipation, and fever.

After a physical exam, the provider will order imaging and medical laboratory tests. Blood and urine tests are used to rule out infection, pregnancy, and liver disease. A CT scan can identify the inflamed pouches, thus confirming the diagnosis. Treatment depends on the symptoms. Antibiotics, over-the-counter (OTC) analgesics, and a liquid diet may be recommended. With severe attacks, intravenous (IV) antibiotics are given and drainage of abscesses, if present, is done. A primary bowel **resection** or a bowel resection with a **colostomy** may be done.

Foodborne Illnesses

Eating or drinking contaminated food can result in a foodborne illness. Typically, foodborne disorders are acute illnesses, which occur suddenly and last for a short time. Most people recover without treatments, though sometimes more serious complications can occur.

Many different types of bacteria, viruses, parasites, and chemicals can contaminate food, including:

- *Salmonella:* Found in raw or undercooked meat, poultry, and seafoods. It can also be found in dairy products, egg shells, and inside eggs.
- *Shigella*: Bacterium that spreads to others from one infected person who does not wash his or her hands after using the bathroom.
- *Escherichia coli (E. coli)*: Found in raw or undercooked hamburger, unpasteurized milk and fruit juices, and fresh produce.
- *Listeria monocytogenes*: Found in raw and undercooked meats, unpasteurized milk, deli meats, soft cheeses, and hot dogs.

- *Clostridium botulinum*: Found in improperly canned foods and smoked and salted fish.
- *Norovirus*: Found in foods prepared by infectious food handlers. Can cause inflammation of the intestines and stomach.
- *Hepatitis A*: A virus spread through food or drinks contaminated with a small amount of stool from an infected person.
- *Trichinella spiralis*: A roundworm parasite found in raw or undercooked pork or wild game.

Common signs and symptoms include vomiting, diarrhea, abdominal pain, chills, and fever. Symptoms may last for a few hours to a few days. Complications can lead to dehydration, **hemolytic uremic syndrome**, and other disorders, such as reactive arthritis and irritable bowel syndrome.

After a physical exam, the provider may order a stool culture and blood work. Treatment consists of replacing lost fluids and electrolytes. Over-the-counter antidiarrheal medications such as loperamide (Imodium) and bismuth subsalicylate (Pepto-Bismol, Kaopectate) can help decrease diarrhea in adults. These medications should not be used if the person has bloody diarrhea, which could be a sign of a parasitic or bacterial infection.

Hemorrhoids

Hemorrhoids are swollen and inflamed veins. *External hemorrhoids* are located around the anus, and *internal hemorrhoids* affect the lining of the anus and the lower rectum. About 50% of those over 50 years of age have hemorrhoids.

Hemorrhoids can be caused by straining during a bowel movement and by pregnancy, aging, chronic constipation, and diarrhea. The most common symptom of internal hemorrhoids is bright red bleeding, which usually goes away within a few days. Anal itching can occur with external hemorrhoids.

During the physical exam, the provider will check the anal area and perform a digital rectal exam. An anoscope, proctoscope, or sigmoidoscope may be used to examine the lower part of the large intestine and rectum. Home treatment includes a high-fiber diet, topical treatments (e.g., hydrocortisone, analgesic), sitz baths (soaking in a warm bath), cold packs, oral analgesics, and keep the area clean.

Hernia

A hernia is a common disorder that occurs when part of an internal organ (e.g., intestine) bulges through a weak area in the muscles. The hiatal hernia was already discussed in a prior section. Other types include:

- *Femoral hernia*: A bulge below the groin, in the upper thigh. More common in women.
- *Inguinal hernia*: Most common type of hernia. A bulge forms in the groin and may extend into the scrotum.
- *Umbilical hernia*: The muscle around the umbilicus does not close at birth and a bulge forms.

Inguinal Hernia. An inguinal hernia occurs when tissue (e.g., part of the intestine) protrudes through a weak spot in the abdominal muscles (Fig. 19.4). Sometimes people can gently push the hernia back into the abdomen, but other times the hernia may become trapped *(incarcerated),* and blood flow may be cut off to the tissue *(strangulation),* causing tissue death. This can be a life-threatening complication if it is not treated.

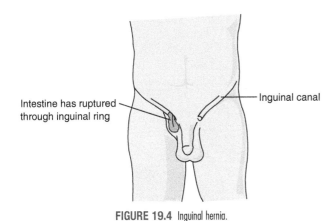

FIGURE 19.4 Inguinal hernia.

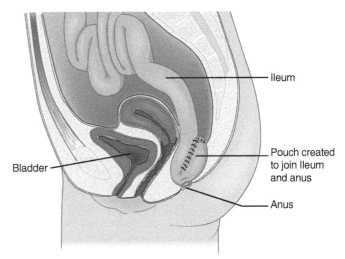

FIGURE 19.5 Ileal pouch–anal anastomosis (IPAA).

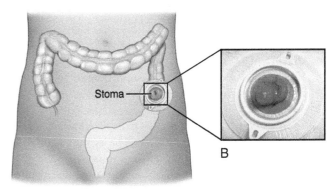

FIGURE 19.6 **(A)** Colostomy. **(B)** The inset shows the stoma. (Potter PA, Perry AG: *Fundamentals of nursing*, ed 7, St Louis, 2011, Mosby.)

For some inguinal hernias, the etiology is unknown. Other times straining, strenuous activities, pregnancy, or chronic coughing may cause it. Signs and symptoms include bulging on the side of the pubic bone, burning or aching at the bulge, and groin heaviness, pain, or pressure.

The provider will do a physical examination. The patient may be asked to stand and cough, which makes the inguinal hernia more prominent. A CT or magnetic resonance imaging (MRI) scan may be ordered if the hernia is not felt. For a small hernia that is asymptomatic, the provider may just wait and monitor it. Painful or enlarged hernias are treated with surgery (either an open hernia repair or a laparoscopic repair).

Inflammatory Bowel Disease

Inflammatory bowel disease (IBD) includes two chronic conditions that cause inflammation of the digestive tract:

- *Ulcerative colitis*: Usually starts in the rectum and spreads into the large intestine. Damaged areas are in patches along the intestine. The inflammation may affect many layers of the GI tract wall.
- *Crohn's disease*: Can affect any part of the GI tract, but most often affects the ileum. Damage appears in patches next to healthy tissue. The inflammation affects several layers of the GI tract walls.

The etiology of IBD is unknown, but it is the result of a defective immune system. IBD has a genetic component, and environmental triggers cause inflammation of the digestive tract. Common signs and symptoms of IBD include persistent diarrhea, abdominal pain, blood in the stool, weight loss, and fatigue.

After the medical history and physical exam, the provider will order imaging tests and endoscopy exams. Stool samples are tested to rule out other conditions. Treatment consists of corticosteroids, immunomodulators, and biologics. Severe IBD may require surgery to remove the damaged GI tract. Common surgical procedures include:

- *Colectomy*: Surgical removal of the colon
- *Proctocolectomy*: Surgical removal of the colon and rectum
- *Proctocolectomy with ileal pouch–anal anastomosis* (IPAA): Requires multiple surgeries; a proctocolectomy is done, but the anus and anal sphincter muscles remain. A pouch is created with the ileum when it is connected to the anus (Fig. 19.5).

- *Ileostomy*: The end of the ileum is brought to the surface of the abdomen through a *stoma* (hole created in the abdomen), allowing waste to drain from the body (Fig. 19.6B).

Intestinal Obstructions

Intestinal obstructions are also called *bowel obstructions*, *intestinal volvulus*, and *paralytic ileus*. The obstruction can be either partial or complete and prevents stool or food from moving through the intestine. A complete intestinal obstruction is a medical emergency.

The obstruction can be related to a mechanical cause, such as adhesions, hernias, and cancers, or to an ileus. An ileus can be caused by bacteria, viruses, electrolyte imbalances, abdominal surgery, a decreased blood supply to the intestines, and medications (e.g., narcotics). Signs and symptoms include severe abdominal pain, cramping, bloating, nausea, vomiting, swelling of the abdomen, loud bowel sounds, inability to pass *flatus* (gas), and constipation.

Tests to diagnose an intestinal obstruction can include an abdominal CT scan, an abdominal x-ray, a barium **enema**, and an upper GI and small bowel series. Treatment includes hospitalization and a *nasogastric tube* (a tube passed from the nose to the stomach), which is used to relieve abdominal contents and swelling. A bowel resection surgery may be required if the obstruction continues. A temporary or permanent colostomy may be done (Fig. 19.6A).

Irritable Bowel Syndrome

Irritable bowel syndrome (IBS) is a disorder of the large intestine, though it does not cause harm to the colon. IBS is a common disorder, affecting women twice as often as men. People younger than 45 often have IBS.

There is no known cause of IBS. The signs and symptoms include abdominal cramping, bloating, constipation, and diarrhea. Sometimes people go back and forth between diarrhea and constipation.

There is no specific test for IBS. The provider may do different diagnostic tests to rule out other diseases. Treatment for IBS includes dietary changes, stress management, medications, and probiotics.

Additional Disorders of the Intestines

The following list presents additional intestinal disorders.
- *Bowel incontinence*: Accidental passage of a stool; also called *accidental bowel leakage*.
- *Gastroenteritis*: Inflammation of the intestinal lining; caused by a virus, bacteria, or parasites. Viral gastroenteritis is a very common illness.
- *Hirschsprung's disease*: Congenital disorder caused by malformed intestinal nerves. Leads to severe constipation and intestinal obstructions.
- *Intestinal ischemia and infarction:* Occur when there is a partial or complete blockage in the arteries supplying the intestines. Can cause damage or death to the intestinal tissues.
- *Intestinal volvulus:* Occurs when the intestine twists around itself and the supporting mesentery, leading to an obstruction.
- *Intussusception:* Occurs when part of the intestine slides onto another portion of the intestine. It can cause an intestinal blockage. The blood supply may be constricted, leading to intestinal tissue death.
- *Small intestinal bacterial overgrowth* (SIBO): Caused when a large number of bacteria grow in the small intestine, which may use up important nutrients needed by the body, leading to malnourishment.

Disorders of the Accessory Organs

Cholelithiasis

Cholelithiasis (or gallstones) occur when the substances in the bile harden and form stones (Fig. 19.7). The stones can be small, like a piece of rice, or large, like a walnut. Cholesterol gallstones are the most common type and usually contain undissolved cholesterol. Pigment gallstones are darker black and occur when the bile contains too much bilirubin.

It is unclear why gallstones form, but it may be related to the bile containing too much cholesterol or bilirubin. They may also form if the gallbladder does not empty completely, causing the bile to become concentrated. Risk factors for gallstones include:
- Being: female, over 40 years of age, sedentary, and pregnant
- Eating: high-fat, high-cholesterol, or low-fiber diet
- Personal history: obesity, diabetes, liver, losing weight quickly, or taking estrogen-containing medications (e.g., oral contraceptives)
- Family history: gallstones

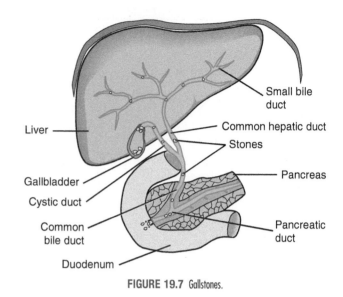

FIGURE 19.7 Gallstones.

If signs and symptoms are present, they may include pain in the upper back, right shoulder, upper right abdomen, or below the sternum; and nausea or vomiting. Many of these symptoms are similar to a heart attack, thus they can be scary for the patient.

After a physical exam, a hepatobiliary iminodiacetic acid (HIDA) scan, MRI, or endoscopic retrograde cholangiopancreatography (ERCP) may be done. Treatment is based on the intensity of the symptoms. A cholecystectomy (removal of the gallbladder) may be done. Gallstones can be removed during the ERCP. Patients who cannot undergo surgery may take medications to dissolve the gallstone, though it may take months or years to work.

CRITICAL THINKING APPLICATION   19.8

Keith is rooming a female patient who works as an office assistant. She has had upper back and right shoulder pain, nausea, and vomiting for 2 days. The patient states that she has lost 50 pounds in the past 3 months. She is on oral contraceptives and acetaminophen for pain as needed. After examining her, Dr. Martin wants her to have an MRI for possible gallstones. What risk factors does this patient have for gallstones? What signs and symptoms does she have that are related to gallstones?

Cirrhosis

Cirrhosis is a chronic liver disease. The liver cells are damaged and are replaced with scar tissue. The scar tissue reduces the liver's ability to function, and over time the liver fails.

Diseases such as alcoholic liver disease, nonalcoholic fatty liver disease, and chronic hepatitis B and C cause cirrhosis. The signs and symptoms of cirrhosis may not appear until the liver is significantly damaged. Cirrhosis can cause nosebleeds, abdominal swelling, hypertension, kidney failure, jaundice, severe itching, gallstones, varices in the stomach and esophagus, and increased sensitivity to medications. Cirrhosis, like other liver diseases, can cause *ascites*, a buildup of fluid in the space between the organs and the abdominal lining (Fig. 19.8).

Besides a medical history and physical exam, liver function tests, imaging tests, and a liver biopsy may be done. There is no cure for

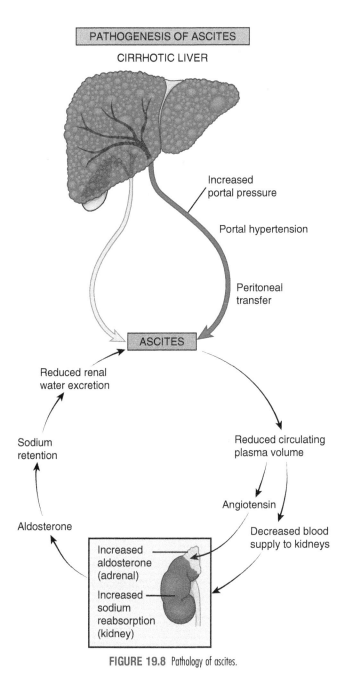

PATHOGENESIS OF ASCITES

CIRRHOTIC LIVER

Increased portal pressure

Portal hypertension

Peritoneal transfer

ASCITES

Reduced renal water excretion

Sodium retention

Aldosterone

Reduced circulating plasma volume

Angiotensin

Decreased blood supply to kidneys

Increased aldosterone (adrenal)

Increased sodium reabsorption (kidney)

FIGURE 19.8 Pathology of ascites.

cirrhosis. Treatment of the underlying disease causing the cirrhosis can help to slow liver destruction.

Hepatitis

Hepatitis is an inflammation of the liver. It can affect the functioning of the liver. Hepatitis is caused by alcohol use, toxins, certain medications and conditions, and viruses (Table 19.1). The signs and symptoms include fatigue, nausea, vomiting, anorexia, abdominal pain, clay-colored stools, dark urine, low-grade fever, joint pain, jaundice, and intense itching.

To diagnose hepatitis, the provider will order a blood test (e.g., hepatitis panel). A liver ultrasound and biopsy may also be done. The following sections will discuss specific information on several types of hepatitis.

CRITICAL THINKING APPLICATION 19.9

Summarize how hepatitis A, B, C, D, and E are transmitted. What prevention strategies can be taken to prevent the transmission of each type?

Jaundice in the Newborn

Jaundice in newborns can be life-threatening. *Jaundice* is a condition caused by high levels of bilirubin in the blood. *Bilirubin* is a yellow to orange pigment that results when heme (from red blood cells) is broken down.

The cause of jaundice in newborns is *hyperbilirubinemia* (excess bilirubin). During the first days of life, red blood cells are produced and broken down at a faster rate compared to adults. In infants the bilirubin can build up in the blood because the liver is not mature enough to get rid of it. Additional disorders that may cause jaundice in newborns include hemorrhage, infection, incompatibility between the mother's blood and the baby's blood, liver malfunction, red blood cell abnormality, and an enzyme deficiency. The risk for jaundice also increases with premature birth, significant bruising during birth, and breastfeeding. Signs and symptoms of jaundice include yellowish coloring to the skin and sclera, listlessness, poor feeding and weight gain, and high-pitched cries.

High levels of bilirubin can lead to severe complications in newborns. Acute bilirubin encephalopathy occurs when the bilirubin passes into the baby's brain. Signs and symptoms include listlessness,

TABLE 19.1	Types of Hepatitis		
VIRUS	**SPREAD THROUGH**	**TREATMENT**	**PREVENTION**
Hepatitis A virus (HAV)	Ingestion of contaminated food or drink (contaminated by infected fecal matter)	Rest and management of nausea	Hepatitis A vaccine
Hepatitis B virus (HBV)	Blood, semen, or other body fluids from an infected person	Rest, antiviral medication (adefovir, entecavir, lamivudine, telbivudine, and tenofovir), interferon, liver transplant	Hepatitis B vaccine
Hepatitis C virus (HCV)	Blood from an infected person	Rest and antiviral medication	None
Hepatitis D virus (HDV)	Blood or body fluids from an infected person	Supportive care	None
Hepatitis E (HEV)	Ingestion of contaminated food or drink (contaminated by infected fecal matter)	Bed rest and fluids	None

difficulty waking, high-pitched crying, fever, backward arching of the neck and back, poor sucking, and poor feeding. *Kernicterus* occurs if the acute encephalopathy causes permanent brain damage. Signs of kernicterus include involuntary and uncontrolled movements, a permanent upward gaze, and hearing loss.

The provider will do a physical exam and then order a blood test to measure the bilirubin level. Treatment may consist of these measures:

- *Phototherapy*: The infant is placed under a lamp that emits blue-green spectrum light, which changes the structure of the bilirubin molecule. The change allows the bilirubin to be excreted in the urine and stool. Light therapy can also be done using a light-emitting mattress or pad. The baby wears only a diaper and protective eye patches.
- *Intravenous immunoglobulin (IVIg)*: Used for blood incompatibility–related jaundice. The immunoglobulin reduces the levels of antibodies and may reduce the jaundice.
- *Exchange transfusion of blood*: Used for severe jaundice.

Nonalcoholic Fatty Liver Disease

Nonalcoholic fatty liver disease (NAFLD) causes a buildup of fat in the liver, unrelated to drinking alcohol.

The cause of NAFLD is unclear. The risks for NAFLD include obesity, prediabetes, type 2 diabetes, high cholesterol and triglycerides, and high blood pressure. Additional risks include rapid weight loss, gastric bypass surgery, bowel disease, and medications (e.g., calcium channel blockers and some chemotherapy drugs). Signs and symptoms include fatigue and upper right abdomen pain. If the person has liver damage, weakness, loss of appetite, nausea, jaundice, itching, leg and abdominal swelling, GI bleeding, and mental confusion may be experienced.

Often NAFLD is found during routine blood tests. The provider may order additional tests, including a CBC; prothrombin time; blood albumin level; ultrasound, MRI, and CT scans; and a liver biopsy. Treatment is focused on healthy choices, including losing weight, healthy eating, being physically active, and not drinking alcohol.

Pancreatitis

Pancreatitis is an inflammation of the pancreas. The digestive enzymes start to break down the pancreas. If treated, acute pancreatitis may last a few days, but chronic pancreatitis gets worse over time and permanent damage occurs.

Gallstones commonly cause acute pancreatitis, and patients may have severe upper abdominal pain radiating to the back, a rapid pulse, nausea, and vomiting. Heavy alcohol use, cystic fibrosis, some inherited and autoimmune diseases, and certain medications can lead to chronic pancreatitis. Signs and symptoms of chronic pancreatitis include nausea, vomiting, weight loss, and oily stools.

Besides a medical history and physical exam, lab and imaging tests are used to diagnose pancreatitis. Treatment includes hospitalization, IV fluids, analgesics, antibiotics, and nutritional support (e.g., low-fat diet, enteral feeding).

Additional Disorders of the Accessory Organs

The following conditions are liver disorders.

- *Primary biliary cirrhosis*: Chronic liver disease causing the bile ducts to be inflamed and damaged, leading to the buildup of bile in the liver.

- *Hemochromatosis*: Causes too much iron to build up in the body, especially in the liver, heart, and pancreas, which damages the organs.
- *Sialoliths*: The buildup of crystallized saliva deposits blocks the flow of saliva, causing pain and swelling; also called *salivary stones*.
- *Sialadenitis*: A bacterial infection of a salivary gland, usually related to blockage of the duct. Can cause a painful lump in the gland, severe pain, high fever, and a foul-tasting pus in the mouth.

Cancers of the Gastrointestinal System

Cancer can affect any part of the GI system. The cause of cancer is a mutation of the cells, which leads to a tumor. To diagnose the cancer, the provider will do a physical exam, endoscopy procedures, imaging tests, blood work, and a biopsy. Treatment consists of surgery, radiation therapy, and chemotherapy. Targeted therapy, which uses medications that attack only the cancer cells, can be used for some types of GI system cancers.

The risk factors, signs, and symptoms can vary between the different types of cancer. These will be discussed in the following sections.

Oral Cavity, Pharyngeal, and Laryngeal Cancers

Oral cavity, pharyngeal, and laryngeal cancers can form in any of the tissues in the mouth and throat. Men are more likely than women to have oral cavity or pharyngeal cancer.

Using alcohol and tobacco products (e.g., cigarettes, betel quid, and gutka) can increase the risk of these cancers. A personal history of oral or throat cancer, human papillomavirus (HPV) infection, or Epstein-Barr virus can also increase the risk. The signs and symptoms depend on the type of cancer:

- *Oral cancer*: White or red patches, bleeding, or a continuous sore in the mouth, loose teeth, pain with swallowing, earache, and lump in the neck
- *Throat cancer (pharyngeal and laryngeal cancers)*: Continuous sore throat, lump in the neck, ear pain, ringing in the ear, and problems swallowing

Stomach Cancer

About 65% of stomach cancer cases occur in adults over age 65. Diagnosing stomach cancer in its early stages can be difficult because the symptoms (e.g., indigestion and stomach discomfort) relate to other conditions.

Males have a greater risk of stomach cancer. A personal history of *H. pylori* infection or stomach inflammation is also a risk factor, along with a family history of stomach cancer. The risk of stomach cancer increases with cigarette smoking and consuming lots of smoked, pickled, or salted foods. Besides indigestion and stomach discomfort, other signs and symptoms include bloody stools, vomiting, weight loss, jaundice, and difficulty swallowing.

Pancreatic Cancer

Pancreatic cancer is difficult to diagnose in its early stages because the symptoms are vague and may go unnoticed. This type of cancer spreads quickly, and because the condition usually is diagnosed in the later stages of the disease, it can be difficult to treat.

Risk factors for pancreatic cancer include smoking, long-term diabetes mellitus, chronic pancreatitis, and certain hereditary disorders.

Signs and symptoms include jaundice, abdominal and back pain, weight loss, and fatigue.

Liver Cancer

Liver cancer can either be *primary* (the initial site) or *metastatic* (spread to the liver from the initial site elsewhere in the body). Primary liver cancer may be difficult to treat if it is diagnosed in an advanced stage.

Risk factors for primary liver cancer include a personal history of hepatitis B or C, cirrhosis, obesity, diabetes, hemochromatosis, and heavy alcohol use. Signs and symptoms include jaundice, right abdominal pain, and a lump in the right abdomen. The symptoms may not appear until the cancer is in an advanced stage.

Small Intestinal Cancer

Small intestinal cancer can also be called *duodenal, ileal,* and *jejunal cancer.* Adenocarcinoma is the most common form of small intestine cancer.

Risk factors for small intestine cancer include eating a high-fat diet or having a personal history of Crohn's disease, colonic polyps, or celiac disease. Signs and symptoms include abdominal pain, weight loss, bloody stools, and a lump in the abdomen.

Colorectal Cancer

Colorectal cancer is also called *colon cancer* and *rectal cancer.* Colorectal cancer affects both men and women. Screening is recommended to start at age 45 for those with an average risk.

Risk factors for colorectal cancer include being over 50 years of age, smoking tobacco, and eating a high-fat diet. A family history of colorectal cancer, ulcerative colitis, or Crohn's disease also increases the risk. Signs and symptoms include diarrhea, constipation, bloody stools, cramps, bloating, flatus (gas), nausea, vomiting, fatigue, or weight loss.

THE MEDICAL ASSISTANT'S ROLE IN GASTROINTESTINAL PROCEDURES

Many times, the medical assistant may get calls from patients or parents of patients who are experiencing gastrointestinal problems. It is important for the medical assistant to be able to screen these phone calls and gather information for the provider. Table 19.2 provides possible screening questions for common signs and symptoms (see Procedure 19.1, p. 487).

CRITICAL THINKING APPLICATION   19.10

List three screening questions for each of these symptoms a patient has: vomiting, abdominal pain, and diarrhea.

Assisting With the Examination

When a patient describes and points to the location of the pain, the medical assistant must know the underlying organs that may be involved. Record the abdominal quadrant or region in which the pain is located so that the provider can immediately assess this area when the examination begins. (See Chapter 3 for a discussion on the abdominopelvic quadrants and regions.)

The provider's inspection of the abdomen begins with noting any change in skin color, such as jaundice. *Striae* (silver stretch marks), *petechiae* (small, purple hemorrhagic spots), scars, and visible masses may be seen. The contour of the abdomen may be flat, rounded, or bulging in localized areas.

TABLE 19.2   Examples of Screening Questions for Common Complaints

SIGNS AND SYMPTOMS	EXAMPLES OF SCREENING QUESTIONS
Dysphagia	• Is there pain when you swallow? If so, what does the pain feel like? (For instance, is there burning pain?) • Does it feel like a blockage or something stuck in your throat?
Vomiting	• When did the vomiting start? How often does it occur? • What is the color of the vomit? • Is there anything that alleviates the vomiting? Is there anything that makes it worse?
Abdominal pain	• When did the pain start? • Where is the pain located? What does the pain feel like? (For instance, is it burning, cramping, sharp, or dull?) • Is the pain constant or is it intermittent? • How severe is the pain? (Use the 0–10 pain scale.) • Does anything relieve the pain? Does anything increase the pain?
Diarrhea	• How many stools do you have in a day? • Is there blood, pus, or mucus in the stool? • What color is the stool? • Is there anything that increases the diarrhea? Is there anything that decreases the diarrhea? • Do you have cramping with the diarrhea? Do you have a stool incontinence?
Constipation	• When did it start? When was your last stool? • Have you tried any over-the-counter medications? If so, did it help?

The provider uses palpation and percussion to evaluate the entire abdominal area. If the medical assistant is present for the examination, he or she should remove the drape from the area to be examined and should redrape the patient once this segment of the examination is completed. In addition, the provider may want the medical assistant to document findings as the examination progresses. If the provider wants to examine the anal area, have the patient turn onto his or her left side, and then assist the patient into the Sims position. As this is done, make sure the patient remains draped. After the patient is in the Sims position, adjust the drape on an angle so that it can be easily lifted for the final part of the examination.

A digital rectal exam (DRE) may be done to identify abnormalities in the rectum (see Chapter 26). The provider may use a proctoscope to examine the anal area. This allows for detection of hemorrhoids, **polyps**, **fissures**, **fistulas**, and abscesses.

Assisting With Diagnostic Procedures

There are many tests and procedures used to help diagnose gastrointestinal disorders. Table 19.3 describes common diagnostic procedures (Fig. 19.9). The medical assistant should be familiar with the description of these tests and the patient preparation required. Table 19.4 describes medical laboratory tests for gastrointestinal conditions.

Stool-Based Tests

There are several stool-based tests on the market used to screen for colorectal cancer. The fecal occult blood test (FOBT) checks a sample of stool for **occult** blood. Blood in the stools can be caused by hemorrhoids, diverticulosis, ulcers, colitis, and polyps. There are two main types of FOBT: the guaiac fecal occult blood test (gFOBT) and the fecal immunochemical test (FIT). Besides the FOBT, the multitargeted stool DNA test (MT-sDNA) may also be used. It detects

TABLE 19.3	Diagnostic Procedures for Gastrointestinal Conditions	
PROCEDURE	**DESCRIPTION**	**PATIENT PREPARATION**
Upper gastrointestinal (UGI) series (also called a barium swallow)	X-ray evaluation of the esophagus, stomach, and duodenum after the patient drinks barium sulfate. Used to diagnose swallowing issues, esophageal disorders, hiatal hernia, ulcers, tumors, and GERD. Also used to diagnose hiatal hernia, esophageal varices, strictures, and tumors.	May need to eat a low-fiber diet 2 or 3 days before the test. Food, liquids, and smoking restricted prior to the test. Must remove all jewelry. A consent form may be signed. The patient needs to drink the barium during the test. After the test, the patient may have white-colored stools for 24 to 72 hours. A mild laxative or enema may be given to help the barium pass.
Lower gastrointestinal (LGI) series, or barium enema	X-ray evaluation of large intestine after instillation of a barium sulfate enema. Used to diagnose colorectal cancer, inflammatory disease of the colon. It can detect polyps, diverticula, or obstructions.	Requires a clear liquid diet for 1 to 3 days before the test. The patient may need to take laxatives and/or enemas prior to the test. The intestine needs to be clear for the test. The medical assistant should screen for allergies. A consent form may need to be signed. An enema is given and may cause fullness, cramping, and general discomfort. The patient may need to change positions during the test. After the test, the patient may have white-colored stools for 24 to 72 hours. A mild laxative or enema may be given to help the barium pass.
Hepatobiliary (HIDA) scan (also known as cholescintigraphy and hepatobiliary scintigraphy)	Nuclear scan of the liver, gallbladder, and bile ducts. Used to diagnose **cholecystitis**, bile duct obstructions, and liver disorders; also used to evaluate liver transplants.	Food and fluid restrictions prior to the test. May need to sign a consent form. An IV radioactive tracer is given, which may cause a pressure or cold sensation. Sincalide, a drug, may be given to help the gallbladder contract and empty. After the test, the patient should drink plenty of fluids.
Endoscopic retrograde cholangiopancreatography (ERCP)	An endoscope is inserted into the mouth and passed through the stomach and duodenum, before it is inserted into the bile ducts. Used to treat stones, tumors, or narrowed areas of the ducts. Can obtain biopsies with this procedure.	Food and drink restrictions prior to the test. Must sign a consent form. Screen for an iodine allergy. An IV sedative may be given. Back of throat is sprayed with a local anesthetic to reduce gag reflex as tube is passed. Person may not have much memory of the test. The patient must avoid driving after the test. Bloating and gas may occur for 24 hours.
Ultrasound (US) – abdomen	High-frequency sound waves are used to produce a picture of the abdominal organs (e.g., liver, gallbladder, bile ducts, and pancreas). Used to diagnose liver disease, gallstones, pancreatic tumor, abscess, or inflammation.	May have food and fluid restrictions prior to the test.

TABLE 19.3 Diagnostic Procedures for Gastrointestinal Conditions—*continued*

PROCEDURE	DESCRIPTION	PATIENT PREPARATION
Flexible sigmoidoscopy	A sigmoidoscope is inserted into the rectum, sigmoid colon, and descending colon. Used to diagnose inflammatory diseases, ulcers, polyps, and cancer.	Usually clear liquids the day before the test. No red liquids allowed. Laxatives and/or enema(s) are used to clean the bowel. May have food and fluid restrictions prior to the test. During the test, air is instilled into the colon. The provider will examine the colon and may take biopsies.
Colonoscopy	An endoscope is inserted through the anus. Used to visualize the large intestine. Polyps can be removed during the procedure.	
Computed tomography (CT) colonography, or virtual colonoscopy	A small tube is inserted into the rectum. The lower colon is inflated with gas. CT images are taken of the colon and rectum.	
Upper gastrointestinal (UGI) endoscopy	Fiberoptic view of the esophagus and stomach. Used to diagnose GERD, ulcers, cancer, Barrett's esophagus, celiac disease, strictures, and blockages.	Food and fluid restrictions for 8 hours before the test. A consent form must be signed. An IV sedative is given. Back of the throat is sprayed with a local anesthetic to reduce gag reflex as tube is passed. The patient must avoid driving after the test.
Capsule endoscopy	Pill-sized video camera is swallowed, which allows examination of the small intestine. Used to detect bleeding, polyps, inflammatory bowel disease, ulcers, and tumors in the small intestine.	Food and drink restrictions for 12 hours before the procedure; screen for pacemaker, defibrillator, history of abdominal surgery or intestinal obstructions, and inflammatory bowel disease. Patient wears a small recording device that receives pictures from the camera. The capsule is excreted.

TABLE 19.4 Medical Laboratory Tests for Gastrointestinal Conditions

TEST	DESCRIPTION
Comprehensive metabolic panel	Includes glucose, electrolytes, liver function, and kidney function tests. Some CLIA-waived tests are available.
C-reactive protein (CRP)	The CRP increases with inflammation in the body. May be used as an inflammation marker test for IBD. Some CLIA-waived tests are available.
Fecal immunochemical test (FIT)	Also called the *immunochemical fecal occult blood test (iFOBT)*. Stool test that detects human hemoglobin from the large intestine.
Guaiac fecal occult blood test (gFOBT)	A test that detects occult blood in a stool smear; a CLIA-waived test
Helicobacter pylori testing	Includes blood test, breath test, and stool tests, all of which can be used to detect *H. pylori*. Some CLIA-waived tests are available.
Hepatitis virus panel	Series of blood tests used to detect current or past infection with hepatitis A, B, and C.
Liver function tests	Also called *hepatic function panel* and *liver panel*. Measures proteins, enzymes, and other substances. Examples of tests included in this panel include albumin, total protein, liver enzymes (alanine transaminase [ALT], aspartate transaminase [AST], alkaline phosphatase [ALP], and gamma-glutamyl transpeptidase [GGT]), bilirubin, and prothrombin time. Some CLIA-waived tests available.
Multitargeted stool DNA test (MT-sDNA)	Stool test that screens for DNA markers (cancer and precancerous cells) and the presence of occult hemoglobin.
Ova and parasite examination (O&P)	A microscopic exam that look for parasites and eggs (ova) in a stool specimen.
Stool culture	Also called *fecal culture*. A stool exam to test for the presence of pathogenic bacteria in the feces
Total bilirubin	A blood test or urine test used to measure the level of bilirubin. Some CLIA-waived tests available.

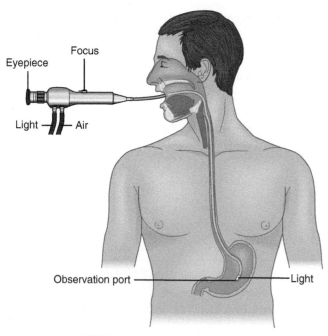

FIGURE 19.9 Upper gastrointestinal endoscopy.

abnormal DNA, along with the presence of occult hemoglobin in the stool. These three tests will be discussed in more depth in the following sections. Keep in mind the exact directions for the tests are in the kits and must be followed by the patient.

Guaiac Fecal Occult Blood Test. The guaiac fecal occult blood test is a stool test that looks for the presence of occult blood. This is a common test in the ambulatory care environment. The medical assistant needs to coach the patient on both the preparations for the gFOBT and how to collect the stool specimens (see Procedure 19.2, p. 487). Usually, the patient is asked to collect samples from two or three stools on consecutive days. Each Hemoccult card has two locations (A and B) for samples. One card should be used on each day.

When the Hemoccult cards are returned to the lab, it is recommended by the company to develop the test no sooner than 3 days after the stool sample was applied. If immediate testing is required, wait 3 to 5 minutes for the sample to penetrate the test paper. Open the back of the slide and apply two drops of the Hemoccult developer to the guaiac paper over each smear (see Procedure 19.3, p. 488). The medical assistant should read the results within 60 seconds. Any trace of blue on the specimen smear or near the edge is considered a positive test result for occult blood (Fig. 19.10). The medical assistant must also apply one drop of the developer between the positive and

Coaching for the Guaiac Fecal Occult Blood Test

To prepare for the test, the patient should avoid the following items for 3 days prior to the test and while collecting the sample(s):

- Aspirin and nonsteroidal anti-inflammatory drugs (NSAIDs) (e.g., ibuprofen and naproxen). *(If the patient is taking aspirin for a heart problem, the medical assistant should check with the provider to see if it needs to be stopped.)*
- More than 250 mg of vitamin C daily from supplements and foods (e.g., fruit and fruit juices)
- Red meats (e.g., pork, beef, and lamb)
- Horseradish, cantaloupe, raw turnips, broccoli, cauliflower, red radishes, and parsnips
- Antacids
- Antidiarrheal medications
- Iron supplements

(Note: The number of days to avoid these products can vary based on agencies.)

The patient may be asked to collect two or three samples on consecutive days. Keep the Hemoccult test cards in their envelopes (if given that way). Keep the cards at room temperature, away from heat, light, chemicals, children, and pets.

To collect the specimens:

- Prepare the cards by writing your name, age, and address on the front of each card, if they are not prelabeled by the provider.
- Before collecting the sample, write the date on the front of the card.
- Prepare to collect the stool, using one of these three ways:
  - Use a clean disposable container to collect the specimen.

- If given a flushable collection tissue with the Hemoccult card, unfold the tissue paper. Float it on the surface of the toilet water. The edges will stick to the side of the bowl, and your stool will fall on the tissue. Sometimes water will collect on the tissue; this is fine.
- If no collection tissue is provided, apply plastic wrap to the bowl.
- Remove the Hemoccult test card from the envelope and place it with the applicator stick in a dry location in the bathroom. Do not get them wet.
- Open the large flap on the front of the card. Sometimes there is a blue discoloration on the squares marked A and B, but this will not affect the test results.
- After collecting the stool, use the applicator stick and place a thin smear of stool in the square marked A.
- Do the same thing for the square marked B, but take a sample from another part of the stool. Wrap the applicator stick in toilet paper and discard in the wastebasket. Empty the stool in the toilet and flush.
- Close the flap on the Hemoccult test card and insert the front flap under the tab. Store the card in the envelope until you have completed collecting all the samples. Keep the card in a cool, dark place. Do not place it in a plastic bag or in the refrigerator.
- Wash your hands well with soap and water.
- Repeat these directions on day 2 and day 3.
- Return the Hemoccult cards to the provider or the laboratory. If you are to mail the cards back, allow the last Hemoccult card to dry overnight. Then place the cards in the special mailing pouch you received and seal. Return the cards immediately.

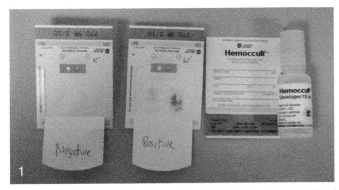

FIGURE 19.10 Negative and positive Hemoccult results. (From Roberts J, Hedges J: *Clinical procedures in emergency medicine,* ed 5, Philadelphia, 2010, Saunders.)

negative Performance Monitors areas, for quality control. The results must be read within 10 seconds. The Hemoccult card and the developer are functioning if a blue color appears in the positive Performance area and no blue appears in the negative Performance Monitors area.

Fecal Immunochemical Test. The fecal immunochemical test (FIT), also called the *immunochemical fecal occult blood test* (iFOBT), is a screening test for colon cancer. It only detects human hemoglobin from the large intestine (e.g., cecum, colon, or rectum). Hemoglobin from bleeding occurring from the mouth to the small intestine is generally degraded by the digestive and enzyme processes. Food and medications do not affect this test, so it tends to have fewer false positive results than the gFOBT.

InSure ONE

InSure ONE is an FIT that detects human hemoglobin in samples of toilet bowl water collected around the stool. The toilet bowl water is collected after the person brushes the stool surface to release any blood into the water.

The patient is given the test to take at home, with the following directions.

- Do not collect samples 3 days before or during, or 3 days after, the menstrual period; if the patient has bleeding hemorrhoids; or if there is visible blood in the urine.
- Store the collection kit at room temperature away from heat and direct sunlight.
- There are no preparations for the test.
- Label the card as indicated.
- Flush the toilet before starting. After having the bowel movement, put the used toilet paper in the wastebasket instead of the toilet.
- Follow the kit instructions. Use the brush from the kit to brush the surface of the stool for about 5 seconds Then dip the brush into the toilet water before touching the brush to the space indicated on the test card. Wrap the brush in toilet paper and discard it in the wastebasket.
- Seal the test card and return as directed to your provider or the laboratory.

Multitargeted Stool DNA Test. An example of a multitargeted stool DNA test (MT-sDNA) is the Cologuard, which tests stool for cancer and precancerous cells. Cologuard screens for DNA markers and the

presence of occult hemoglobin in stool. The patient is asked to obtain the sample at home and mail the test to the laboratory.

The patient is given the test to take at home with the following directions:

- Do not obtain the sample if you have diarrhea, obvious blood in the urine or stool (e.g., bleeding hemorrhoids, bleeding wounds on the hands, or menstruation).
- There is no preparation required for this test.
- Store the kit at room temperature, away from heat, direct sunlight, children, and pets.
- The kit contains a bracket, sample container, tube, bottle of preservative, shipping label, and sample labels.
- The bracket is placed in the toilet. The lid is removed from the stool sample container, and the container is placed into the bracket.
- When having the bowel movement, the person must avoid getting toilet paper and urine in the stool sample container.
- Following the test directions, the person must scrape the stool sample with the probe to get a small sample. In addition, the preservative must be poured onto the stool in the stool sample container.
- Both samples (probe tube and sample container) must be sealed tightly, labeled, packed in the special shipping box, and mailed to the lab within a day. The lab must get the sample within 3 days.

Colonoscopy

A colonoscopy is a procedure in which the provider uses a colonoscope to look in the rectum and colon. The visual inspection of the colon and rectum allows the provider to see irritation, swelling, ulcers, polyps, and potentially cancerous areas.

In the past, many providers did colonoscopies in the office setting, where it was important for the medical assistant to know how to set up and assist with the procedures. Today, anesthesia plays an important part in sedating patients for the procedure. This is one of the main reasons colonoscopies are now usually done in a hospital or ambulatory surgical center. The medical assistant's role is preparing patients for the procedure. Procedure 19.4 on p. 489 describes how a medical assistant should coach a patient on the procedure.

As with all procedures, the patient needs to be informed of any medication changes or when to not take medications. The provider will determine when the patient needs to stop taking any blood-thinning prescription and over-the-counter medications. If the patient is on diabetic, antihypertensive, or heart medications, the provider will determine how these should be handled. The medical assistant needs to communicate these instructions to the patient.

Assisting With Treatments

Patients with digestive disorders are prescribed a variety of medications. The following are some of the more common classifications of medications:

- *Antacids:* Used to treat gastric hyperacidity.
- *Antidiarrheal:* Used to treat diarrhea
- *Antiemetics:* Used to prevent and relieve nausea, vomiting, and motion sickness.
- *Laxatives:* Used to increase and hasten bowel evacuation.
- *Proton-pump inhibitors:* Used to treat GERD and ulcers.

Patient Coaching for a Colonoscopy

Dietary preparations:

- Two days before the procedure: Do not take fiber supplements or eat foods high in fiber (e.g., nuts, seeds, whole grains, and raw or cooked fruits and vegetables).
- One day before the procedure:
  - Do not eat solid foods, just drink clear liquids (e.g., broth, gelatin, coffee, tea, clear juice, popsicles, and sport drinks). Do not drink red liquids or eat red gelatin. Do not drink or eat dairy products or alcohol.
- On the day of the procedure:
  - Do not eat solid foods. Stop drinking clear liquids at least 2 hours before the procedure or as indicated by the provider.

Colon cleansing:

- Usually a split-dose preparation. The first dose of the preparation solution (e.g., GoLYTELY, Colyte) is taken the evening before the procedure. The second dose is taken the next morning and must be completed at least 2 hours before the procedure.
- How the patient will feel: Usually within 1 hour of starting the preparation solution, liquid stools can occur and continue until 2 hours after completing the solution. Chills, headache, cramping, weakness, nausea, vomiting and bloating can occur when taking the solution. Drinking the preparation slower can help reduce the severe vomiting and cramping.

Postprocedure instructions:

- Do not drive. Plan to have someone bring you home.

Refer to Table 19.5 for information on the medication classification, including indication for use, desired effect, side effects, adverse reactions, and generic and trade names. Medical assistants should be familiar with medications that are prescribed to patients.

CLOSING COMMENTS

Patient Coaching

After the medical assistant coaches a patient on a topic, it is important for the medical assistant to evaluate the patient's learning. The medical assistant should encourage the patient to "teach back" the preparation instructions or information so that he or she can evaluate whether the patient has an accurate understanding of the directions. Any errors or misunderstandings can be clarified. The patient should have a copy of directions or information to take home.

Legal and Ethical Issues

The medical assistant's responsibility is to assist the provider and act as the patient's advocate. All information discussed between the patient and the provider, and all testing procedures ordered and done, must remain confidential. Confidentiality and trust are very closely linked, and these two issues form the basis of a sound patient-provider relationship. The medical assistant is an important part of that relationship and can strengthen it through ethical, professional conduct.

TABLE 19.5 Medication Classifications

CLASSIFICATION	INFORMATION	GENERIC NAME (TRADE NAME)
Antacids	**Indications for use:** Treat gastric hyperacidity. **Desired effect:** Neutralizes stomach acid. **Side effects and adverse reactions:** GI distress, increased urination, metallic taste.	• **calcium carbonate** (Os-Cal 500, Rolaids, Tums)
Antidiarrheals	**Indications for use:** Used to control acute diarrhea and chronic diarrhea related to inflammatory bowel disease. **Desired effects:** Decreases the amount of fluids and electrolytes in the bowel and slows down the peristalsis. Some decrease intestinal inflammation. **Side effects and adverse reactions:** Constipation, fatigue, bloody stools, stomach pain or swelling, rash.	• **loperamide** (Imodium) • **bismuth subsalicylate** (Pepto-Bismol, Kaopectate, Bismusal)
Antiemetics	**Indications for use:** Prevent and relieve nausea and vomiting; manage motion sickness. **Desired effect:** Act on hypothalamic center in the brain to reduce or prevent nausea and vomiting. **Side effects and adverse reactions:** Dry mouth, sedation, drowsiness, diarrhea, blurred vision.	• **ondansetron** (Zofran, Zuplenz)
Laxatives	**Indications for use:** Increase and hasten bowel evacuation (defecation). **Desired effect:** Increase activity in the large intestine, promoting stools. **Side effects and adverse reactions:** Nausea, bloating, flatulence, cramping.	• **bisacodyl** (Dulcolax) • **psyllium** (Fiberall, Genfiber, Konsyl, Metamucil, V-Lax)
Proton-Pump Inhibitors	**Indications for use:** Treat gastroesophageal reflux disease (GERD) and ulcers. **Desired effect:** Decrease the amount of acid produced in the stomach. **Side effects and adverse reactions:** Confusion, drowsiness, arrhythmias, sweating, flushing.	• **omeprazole** (Prilosec) • **pantoprazole** (Protonix) • **esomeprazole** (Nexium)

Patient-Centered Care

When coaching patients about diagnostic procedures, it is important for the medical assistant to give the patient a list of supplies (e.g., laxatives, enemas) required for the preparation. Patients may even need directions on where to purchase the supplies. The medical assistant should encourage the patient to call if there are questions or concerns and to complete the preparation directions. If the patient is not completely prepared, the procedure may not be able to be done and may need to be rescheduled.

SUMMARY OF SCENARIO

Keith has learned a lot from the gastroenterology outreach team. He was able to shadow at the hospital to see several diagnostic procedures. Keith realizes that he will be continually learning with the team. He looks forward to learning more about gastrointestinal diseases, diagnostic procedures, and treatments. With everything he has seen to this point, he feels excited about his medical assistant career.

SUMMARY OF LEARNING OBJECTIVES

1. **Discuss the anatomy of the gastrointestinal system and the accessory organs. Also describe the sections of the small and large intestines, the functions of the liver, and life span changes associated with the gastrointestinal system.**
   - *Gastrointestinal tract*: It consists of a large, muscular tube that, with the help of hormones and enzymes, digests food. The GI tract includes the mouth, pharynx (throat), esophagus, stomach, small intestine, and large intestine.
   - *Accessory organs:* The salivary glands, gallbladder, liver, and pancreas are considered the major accessory organs. These structures secrete fluids into the GI tract, aiding in digestion.

   The small intestine is made up of three parts:
   - *Duodenum*: Smallest part of the small intestine; connected to the stomach by the pyloric sphincter.
   - *Jejunum*: Second largest part of the small intestine; connected to the duodenum and the ileum.
   - *Ileum*: Largest part of the small intestine; connects to the jejunum and the large intestine. It joins the cecum at the ileocecal valve.

   The large intestine is made up of six sections:
   - *Cecum*: A 2- to 3-inch pouch or tube-like structure in the lower right abdomen that is considered the first section of the large intestine. Attached to the cecum is the *vermiform appendix*.
   - *Ascending colon*: The second part of the large intestine, which extends vertically from the cecum to just below the liver.
   - *Transverse colon*: Extends horizontally from the ascending colon to the descending colon.
   - *Descending colon*: Extends vertically on the left side of the abdomen from the transverse colon to the sigmoid colon.
   - *Sigmoid colon*: Forms an S-shaped curve; attaches to the descending colon and the rectum.
   - *Rectum*: Stores the stool until defecation occurs and the stool is released through the anus.

   The liver:
   - The hepatic artery brings oxygenated blood to the liver. Substances are filtered from the blood and are processed, stored, changed, detoxified, and returned to the blood or eliminated in the stool. Produces plasma proteins (e.g., albumin and blood clotting factors).
   - Breaks down old or damaged blood cells
   - Breaks down proteins and fats and produces energy
   - Produces up to a liter of bile a day
   - Removes extra minerals (e.g., iron and copper), vitamins (B_{12}, A, D, and K), and glycose from the blood and stores them in the liver. The liver releases them into the blood when needed.
   - Manufactures triglycerides and cholesterol

   Refer to the unnumbered box in the text to discuss specific life span changes related to the gastrointestinal system. Changes in the GI system occur during the first years of life. During pregnancy, progesterone causes the smooth muscles to relax, which affects the digestive system. With age, the stomach empties slower. Aging does not affect nutrient absorption. Constipation is more common with aging.

2. **Describe the four processes that occur in the gastrointestinal system and discuss the chemical digestion of carbohydrates, proteins, and fats.**

   Four processes occur in the GI system:
   - *Ingestion*: The intake of food and liquids into the body
   - *Digestion*: The breakdown of food into chemical substances

Continued

- *Absorption*: The passage of substances and liquids through the lining of the GI tract into the body fluids and tissues
- *Excretion*: The elimination of indigestible materials and waste products of metabolism

The chemical digestion of carbohydrates, proteins, and fats:

- *Carbohydrates*: Saliva contains an enzyme called *salivary amylase*, which starts to break down complex carbohydrates. Pancreatic juices contain *amylase*, which breaks down carbohydrates into sugars. In the small intestine, brush-border enzymes (*sucrase*, *lactase*, and *maltase*) are found in the microvilli and help with the final breakdown of carbohydrates,
- *Proteins*: In the stomach, the hydrochloric acid softens and breaks down proteins and other foods. Pepsin, an enzyme found in the gastric juices, breaks down proteins into polypeptides. Pancreatic juices contain trypsin and chymotrypsin, which break down proteins into amino acids.
- Fats: Bile from the liver is also secreted in the duodenum and emulsifies fats. Pancreatic juices contain *lipase*, which breaks down fats into fatty acids and glycerol.

3. **Identify common signs, symptoms, and etiologies of gastrointestinal disorders and discuss disorders of the mouth, esophagus, and stomach.**

Common signs and symptoms include:

- Constipation, diarrhea, hematochezia, and melena
- Pyrosis, dyspepsia, and flatus
- Halitosis, nausea, vomiting, and hematemesis
- Jaundice

The etiologies of GI disorders vary; some examples include blockages, cell mutation, other disorders, genetics, and infections.

Disorders of the mouth include orofacial clefts (cleft lips and cleft palates), cavities, gingivitis, periodontal disease, and thrush. Refer to this chapter for more information on these disorders.

Disorders of the esophagus and stomach include gastroesophageal reflux disease, hiatal hernia, peptic ulcers, pyloric stenosis, cyclic vomiting syndrome, dumping syndrome, gastritis, gastroparesis, and hypochlorhydria. Refer to this chapter for more information on these disorders.

4. **Discuss disorders of the intestines.**

Disorders of the intestines include acute appendicitis, celiac disease, diverticulitis, foodborne illnesses, hemorrhoids, hernias (including inguinal hernias), inflammatory bowel disease, intestinal obstructions, irritable bowel syndrome, bowel incontinence, gastroenteritis, Hirschsprung's disease, intestinal ischemia and infarction, intestinal volvulus, intussusception, and small intestinal bacterial overgrowth. Refer to this chapter for more information on these disorders.

5. **Discuss disorders of the accessory organs and explain how hepatitis A, B, C, D, and E are transmitted.**

Disorders of the accessory organs include cholelithiasis, cirrhosis, hepatitis, jaundice in newborns, nonalcoholic fatty liver disease, pancreatitis, primary biliary cirrhosis, hemochromatosis, sialoliths, and sialadenitis. Refer to the chapter for more information on these disorders.

Hepatitis:

- *Hepatitis A virus*: Spread through ingestion of infected fecal matter. Typically, the virus is spread from contact with fecal-contaminated objects, food, or drinks.
- *Hepatitis B virus*: Spread through blood, semen, or other body fluids.
- *Hepatitis C virus*: Spread when the blood from an infected person enters the bloodstream of a noninfected person.
- *Hepatitis D virus*: Spread by infected blood and body fluids.
- *Hepatitis E virus*: Spread by water contaminated with fecal matter from an infected person.

6. **Discuss cancers of the gastrointestinal system.**

Cancers of the gastrointestinal system include cancers of the oral cavity, pharyngeal and laryngeal cancers, stomach cancer, pancreatic cancer, liver cancer, small intestinal cancer, and colorectal cancer. Refer to the chapter for more information on these cancers.

7. **Describe the medical assistant's role in gastrointestinal procedures, list examples of screening questions, and describe the diagnostic tests and procedures for common gastrointestinal disorders.**

When a patient describes and points to the location of the pain, the medical assistant must know the underlying organs that may be involved. Table 19.2 provides possible screening questions for common signs and symptoms.

Diagnostic tests include blood, urine, and stool tests. A comprehensive metabolic panel, CRP, hepatitis virus panel, *H. pylori* test, liver function tests, and total bilirubin were discussed. Examples of stool tests include fecal occult blood tests (e.g., gFOBT and FIT), multitargeted stool DNA test, O&P, and stool cultures. Table 19.3 discusses diagnostic procedures used for gastrointestinal conditions.

8. **Identify CLIA-waived tests associated with common gastrointestinal disorders.**

Refer to Table 19.4; CLIA-waived tests are available for:

- Comprehensive metabolic panel
- C-reactive protein (CRP)
- Guaiac fecal occult blood test (gFOBT)
- *Helicobacter pylori* testing
- Liver function tests
- Total bilirubin

9. **Describe the treatments for common gastrointestinal disorders.**

There are a variety of treatments for the various gastrointestinal diseases. The more common classifications of medications used for gastrointestinal disorders include antacids, antidiarrheal, antiemetics, laxatives, and proton-pump inhibitors. For specific treatments for the diseases discussed in this chapter, refer to those sections.

PROCEDURE 19.1	Use Critical Thinking When Performing Patient Screening

Tasks: Incorporate critical thinking skills when performing patient assessment. Document the patient's history and chief complaint.

Scenario 1: You work at Walden-Martin Family Medical (WMFM) Clinic. A patient calls and states that she or he has had nausea, vomiting, diarrhea, and abdominal pain for 3 days. You need to gather the patient's information before talking with the provider, per the facility's policy.

Scenario 2: You work at WMFM clinic. A patient calls and states that she or he has had vomiting and constipation for 4 days. You need to gather the patient's information before talking with the provider, per the facility's policy.

Directions: Role-play the scenario with a peer, who is the patient. Your instructor is the provider.

EQUIPMENT and SUPPLIES

- Phone log and pen
- Patient's health record
- Phone

PROCEDURAL STEPS

1. Answer the telephone by the third ring, speaking directly into the mouthpiece or headset. Speak distinctly, using a pleasant tone and expression, at a moderate rate, and with sufficient volume.
   PURPOSE: Answering promptly conveys interest in the caller. Proper positioning of the mouthpiece or headset allows for an audible tone.
2. Greet the caller, identify the facility and yourself, and offer to help the caller.
   PURPOSE: Giving the facility's name lets the patient knows she has reached the correct number, in addition to the name of the staff member to whom she is speaking.
3. Verify the identity of the caller and her date of birth; access the patient's record. Note the patient's phone number in case you are disconnected.
   PURPOSE: To have the patient's health record ready for reference about the health history and recent care.
4. Determine the caller's needs using therapeutic communication skills.
   PURPOSE: To gather comprehensive information about the caller's complaint and to communicate empathetically about the caller's needs.

5. Upon learning the patient's complaint, use critical thinking skills and ask appropriate questions to obtain information about the patient's condition for the provider. Identify the onset, frequency, and duration of the complaint. If related to pain, identify the exact location, quality (e.g., sharp, dull, stabbing), and rating (using a 0–10 pain scale). Identify significant history and factors that increase or decrease the complaint.
   PURPOSE: Gathering relevant information helps the provider form an opinion on the patient's care.
   Scenario update: You know the provider is available, and the patient is willing to be put on hold as you talk with the provider.
6. Discuss the patient's information with the provider. Present the information in an accurate, logical method.
   PURPOSE: Presenting the patient's information in a logical manner helps eliminate confusion and misunderstanding.
7. Upon returning to the phone, give the patient the information from the provider. Conclude the phone call.
8. Document the patient interaction, including the patient's medical history, the provider notified, and the information relayed to the patient.
   PURPOSE: Legally it is important to document all patient interactions.

PROCEDURE 19.2	Coach Patient on Health Maintenance: Guaiac Fecal Occult Blood Test

Tasks: Coach a patient on the guaiac fecal occult blood test (gFOBT), while considering the patient's developmental life stage. Document the coaching in the health record.

Background: When coaching patients, it is important to consider their developmental life stage. When working with older adults, it is important to communicate with dignity and respect. Use simpler language. Speak clearly and allow time for the patient to respond. It is important to find out what they know about the topic and respectfully correct any inaccuracies. Make sure to listen to their concerns and provide resources as needed.

Scenario: You work at WMFM Clinic. You are working with Dr. David Kahn, who asked you to coach Charles Johnson (date of birth [DOB] 03/03/1958) on the gFOBT. He is to receive 3 Hemoccult cards for stool smears.

Directions: Role-play the scenario with a peer, who is the patient. Your instructor is the provider.

Continued

PROCEDURE 19.2 | **Coach Patient on Health Maintenance: Guaiac Fecal Occult Blood Test**—*continued*

EQUIPMENT and SUPPLIES

- Hemoccult test kit (Hemoccult cards, applicator sticks, and if available flushable collection tissue)
- Patient instructions
- Patient's health record
- Pen

PROCEDURAL STEPS

1. Wash hands or use hand sanitizer.
   UNDERLINE PURPOSE: Hand sanitization is an important step for infection control.
2. Greet the patient. Identify yourself. Verify the patient's identity with full name and date of birth. Explain what you will be doing.
   PURPOSE: It is important to identify the patient in two different ways to ensure that you have the correct patient. Explaining the procedure can make the patient feel more comfortable and helps to reduce anxiety.
3. Use simpler language when talking. Speak clearly. Communicate with dignity and respect. Allow time for the patient to respond. Listen to the patient's concerns.
   PURPOSE: When working with older patients, it is important to treat them with respect and dignity. Listening is important.
4. Ask the patient if he has ever taken a guaiac fecal occult blood test. If so, ask him what he remembers about it.
   PURPOSE: It is important to find out what the patient already knows about the topic.
5. Discuss the purpose of the test and the supplies needed (e.g., Hemoccult cards, applicator kits, and, if available, flushable collection tissue). Show the supplies to the patient.

PURPOSE: It is important that the patient knows what supplies will be used.
6. Discuss how the patient needs to prepare for the tests and refer to the written instructions.
   PURPOSE: Referring to the written directions that will be sent home with the patient helps eliminate confusion.
7. Discuss how the patient should collect and return the Hemoccult cards. Use the written directions when coaching the patient. Write the patient's name, date of birth, and address on the Hemoccult cards if required by the agency.
   PURPOSE: The cards need to be labeled with the patient's information. Having the medical assistant label the cards ensures this step is completed.
8. Ask the patient to teach back the preparation and the collection to you. Clarify any misconceptions or inaccuracies. Answer any questions the patient may have.
   PURPOSE: Using the "teach back" method to evaluate the patient's understanding will help identify any misunderstandings the patient may have.
9. Document the coaching in the patient's health record. Include the provider's name, what was taught, and how the patient responded, and indicate the supplies and written directions sent home with the patient.
   PURPOSE: It is important to document the procedure in the health record to show it was done.
   08/14/20XX 1105 Per Dr. Kahn's order, instructed pt on the gFOBT test including the preparation and collection. Patient taught back the instructions accurately. Gave the patient the Hemoccult testing kit and the Hemoccult Patient Directions booklet. Patient will return the cards to the clinic later this week.
   _____Keith Williams, CMA (AAMA)

PROCEDURE 19.3 | **Develop a Hemoccult Card and Perform Quality Control**

Tasks: Develop a stool specimen using a Hemoccult card and perform a quality control test. Document the test results in the patient's health record.

Scenario: Charles Johnson (DOB 03/03/1958) returns his Hemoccult card(s). Dr. David Kahn is his provider. You need to develop (test) the sample.

EQUIPMENT and SUPPLIES

- Hemoccult card with stool smear applied
- Hemoccult developer
- Gloves
- Biohazard waste container
- Waste container
- Patient's health record
- Timer

PROCEDURAL STEPS

1. Wash hands or use hand sanitizer. Put on gloves.
   PURPOSE: Hand sanitization is an important step for infection control.

2. Identify when the specimen was applied and if testing can be done.
   PURPOSE: It is recommended by the company to wait 3 days from when the sample was applied. This allows for the degradation of fruit and vegetable peroxidases from the sample. If immediate testing is required, wait 3 to 5 minutes to allow the sample to penetrate the test paper.
3. Open the back of the card and apply two drops of the Hemoccult developer to the guaiac paper directly over each smear.
4. Within 60 seconds, read the result accurately.
   PURPOSE: Any trace of blue on or near the edge of the sample is considered positive for occult blood.

PROCEDURE 19.3 **Develop a Hemoccult Card and Perform Quality Control**—*continued*

5. Perform quality control on the card by applying one drop of the Hemoccult developer between the positive and negative Performance Monitors area.
PURPOSE: This quality control test will indicate if the card and developer are functional.
6. Within 10 seconds, accurately read the results.
PURPOSE: A blue color in the positive Performance Monitors area and no blue in the negative Performance Monitors area means the card and the developer are functional.
7. Discard the Hemoccult card in the biohazard bag. Clean up the area. Remove gloves and discard in the waste container.

PURPOSE: It is important to discard the Hemoccult card in the biohazard bag for infection control.
8. Wash hands or use hand sanitizer.
9. Document the test result and the provider notified in the patient's health record.
PURPOSE: It is important to document the procedure in the health record to show it was done.
08/18/20XX 1105 Hemoccult card × 3 developed. All results were negative. Dr. Kahn notified. _____ Keith Williams, CMA (AAMA)

PROCEDURE 19.4 **Coach Patient on Health Maintenance: Colonoscopy**

Tasks: Coach a patient on the colonoscopy preparation. Document the coaching in the health record.

Scenario: You work at WMFM Clinic. You are working with Dr. David Kahn, who has asked you to coach Charles Johnson (DOB 03/03/1958) on the colonoscopy preparation. Dr. Kahn wants Charles to take his antihypertensive medication the morning of the procedure, 1 hour after finishing the preparation solution.

The ambulatory surgical center requires that Charles does not drink anything 2 hours before the procedure. He needs to arrive 90 minutes before the procedure, which is scheduled at 11 a.m. He will be receiving IV sedation during the procedure and will need a driver to take him home.

Directions: Role-play the scenario with a peer, who is the patient. Your instructor is the provider.

EQUIPMENT and SUPPLIES

- Patient instructions
- Patient's health record

PROCEDURAL STEPS

1. Wash hands or use hand sanitizer.
PURPOSE: Hand sanitization is an important step for infection control.
2. Greet the patient. Identify yourself. Verify the patient's identity with full name and date of birth. Explain what you will be doing.
PURPOSE: It is important to identify the patient in two different ways to ensure that you have the correct patient. Explaining the procedure can make the patient feel more comfortable and helps to reduce anxiety.
3. Use simpler language when talking. Speak clearly. Communicate with dignity and respect. Allow time for the patient to respond. Listen to the patient's concerns.
PURPOSE: When working with older patients, it is important to treat them with respect and dignity. Listening is important.
4. Ask the patient if he has ever had a colonoscopy. If so, ask him what he remembers about it.
PURPOSE: It is important to find out what the patient already knows about the topic.

5. Discuss the purpose of the colonoscopy and the preparation involved. Refer to the written instructions that the patient will be taking home.
PURPOSE: Referring to the written directions that will be sent home with the patient helps eliminate confusion.
6. Ask the patient to teach back the preparation to you. Clarify any misconceptions or inaccuracies. Answer any questions the patient may have. Give the patient a phone number to call if he has questions.
PURPOSE: Using the "teach back" method to evaluate the patient's understanding will help identify any misunderstandings the patient may have.
7. Document the coaching in the patient's health record. Include the provider's name, what was taught, how the patient responded, and any written directions (including appointment information) sent home with the patient.
PURPOSE: It is important to document the procedure in the health record to show it was done.
08/14/20XX 1105 Per Dr. Kahn's order, instructed pt on the colonoscopy preparation. Patient taught back the instructions accurately. Gave the patient the Colonoscopy Patient Directions booklet. Pt was notified of appointment on 08/25/20XX at 11 AM at WMFM Surgical Center. _____
_____ Keith Williams, CMA (AAMA)

20

ORTHOPEDICS AND RHEUMATOLOGY

SCENARIO

Suzanne Peterson, CMA (AAMA), works with Dr. Kahn at the Walden-Martin Family Medical (WMFM) Clinic. Dr. Kahn hired Suzanne right out of school as a new graduate. She has seen a lot in her 20 years as a medical assistant (MA). Many aspects of her day have changed from when she first started as an MA, but one thing that has not changed is her love for helping patients.

Another busy day is scheduled, and Suzanne's first patient is Walter Biller. Walter is in his late 40s, is in good general health, is near his ideal weight, and has no chronic conditions. He saw Dr. Kahn a few weeks ago when he experienced worsening pain in his hands and knees. He had been planting in his garden and noticed that the next day that he had more pain and stiffness in his hands than usual. He also experienced pain in the muscle on the front of his forearm, just below the elbow. Bending down on his hands and knees in the garden was not as easy as it used to be. Dr. Kahn performed a physical exam and ordered lab tests. He asked Walter to make a follow-up appointment to go over the results. Today Walter is back at the clinic, and Suzanne is ready to room him for his appointment.

While studying this chapter, think about the following questions:
- What structures are in the musculoskeletal system? What is the function of the musculoskeletal system?
- What are the common pathologic conditions of the musculoskeletal system? What medical terms must you know to identify and explain these patient disorders?
- What diagnostic and treatment procedures typically are ordered for patients with musculoskeletal disease?
- What are the medical assistant's primary responsibilities in working with patients with musculoskeletal problems?
- What clinical skills are required in this specialty practice?

LEARNING OBJECTIVES

1. List the major structures of the musculoskeletal system and identify the anatomic location of the structures.
2. Describe the normal function and physiology of the musculoskeletal system.
3. Discuss the diseases and disorders related to the musculoskeletal system. Also:
   - Identify the common signs and symptoms of musculoskeletal conditions.
   - Identify the common etiology of musculoskeletal conditions.
- Describe diagnostic measures used for musculoskeletal conditions.
- Identify CLIA-waived tests associated with common musculoskeletal conditions.
- Describe treatment modalities used for musculoskeletal conditions.
4. Discuss the medical assistant's role in orthopedics and rheumatology procedures and describe topics to address when coaching a patient on cast care, hot and cold applications, and assistive devices.

VOCABULARY

analgesic (an ahl JEE zik) A drug that reduces or eliminates pain.
anticoagulant (an tee koe AG yoo lant) A substance (i.e., medication or chemical) that prevents clotting of blood.
anticonvulsant (an tee kuhn VUL sahnt) A drug used to prevent or treat seizures.
ATP (adenosine triphosphate) A high-energy molecule, found in every cell, that supplies large amounts of energy for various biochemical processes.
autoimmune An immune response against a person's own tissues, cells, or cell parts, as in autoimmune disease, leading to the deterioration of tissue.
biopsy (BIE op see) Removal of tissue or cells for examination by a pathologist.
cartilage (KAR tih lij) Flexible connective tissue that covers the ends of many bones at the joint.
compact bone Consists of tightly packed osteons; denser and heavier compared to spongy bone.
compartment syndrome A serious condition that involves increased pressure, usually in the muscles; it leads to compromised blood flow and muscle and nerve damage.
crepitation (krep i TAY shun) A dry, crackling sound or sensation.
electrodes Adhesive patches that conduct electricity from the body to machine wires (e.g., ECG and transcutaneous electrical nerve stimulation [TENS] unit).
fascia (FASH ee ah) A tough fibrous covering of the muscles.

hematopoiesis (hee mah toh poh EE sis) The formation of the blood cells and platelets.

immunosuppressant A drug used to suppress the immune system.

ligaments (LIH gah ments) Supportive connective tissue that connects bones at a joint.

modalities (moe DAL i tees) Therapeutic treatments for a disorder.

ossicles (OS i kahls) The three small bones of the middle ear (malleus, incus, and stapes) that transmit sound vibrations from the eardrum to the inner ear.

osteoblasts (OS tee oh blasts) Bone-forming cells.

osteoclasts (OS tee oh clasts) Bone cells that break down bone.

permeability (pur mee ah BIL i tee) A quality or characteristic of a material that allows another substance to pass through it.

photosensitivity (foe toe sen si TIV i tee) Increase in the reactivity of the skin to sunlight or ultraviolet radiation.

psoriasis (sah RIE ah sis) A usually chronic, recurrent skin disease marked by bright red patches covered with silvery scales.

red bone marrow Soft, gelatinous tissue that consists of blood stem cells that can become white or red blood cells or platelets. Found at the center of most bones.

remission The partial or complete disappearance of the clinical and subjective characteristics of a chronic or malignant disease.

spongy bone Lighter and less dense than compact bone; also called cancellous bone. Usually found at the ends of bones and contains red bone marrow.

stoma A temporary or permanent surgically created opening used for drainage (i.e., urine, stool).

synapse (SIN aps) A point of communication between two cells.

tendons (TEN duns) Connective tissue that attaches muscles to bone.

tripod position The standing position when using crutches; crutch tips are 4 to 6 inches to the side and front of each foot.

vasoconstriction (vay zoe kuhn STRIK shuhn) Contraction of the muscles that causes a narrowing of the inside tube of the blood vessel.

vertebrae (VUR teh bray) A series of small, irregular-shaped bones that form the spine. Each vertebra has several projections, joint surfaces, areas for muscle attachment, and a hole where the spinal cord passes.

yellow bone marrow Soft, gelatinous tissue that consists mostly of fat cells and a small amount of primitive blood cells.

Orthopedics is the healthcare specialty that deals with most musculoskeletal disorders. An *orthopedist* is a specialist involved in the diagnosis, treatment, and prevention of disorders of the musculoskeletal system.

Rheumatology is a specialty that deals with disorders of connective tissue, including bone and cartilage. Rheumatology also deals with many diseases that are classified as **autoimmune** disorders. The specialist is called a *rheumatologist*.

Musculoskeletal system disorders are common in the ambulatory care facility. Besides the orthopedic department, patients with musculoskeletal concerns are seen in primary care and urgent care settings. Medical assistants may need to coach patients on hot and cold **modalities**, cast care, and *assistive devices* (e.g., canes, walkers, crutches).

ANATOMY OF THE MUSCULOSKELETAL SYSTEM

The musculoskeletal system (MS) consists of bones, joints, muscles, and supportive connective tissues (**cartilage**, **tendons**, and **ligaments**). The musculoskeletal system is responsible for the following functions:

- Body movement
- Protection, support, and framework for the organ systems of the body
- Storage for important minerals such as calcium and phosphorus
- Continually forming new blood cells by the process of **hematopoiesis**, which occurs in the red bone marrow inside some bones. Red blood cells, white blood cells, and platelets are all made in the bone marrow.

Bones

The human skeleton is composed of more than 200 bones. Human bones appear in a variety of shapes and sizes that suit their function

in the body. Bones are divided into two categories – the axial skeleton and the appendicular skeleton (Fig. 20.1). The axial skeleton is composed of 80 bones, including these:

- *Skull*, which is made up of the cranium (which encloses and protects the brain), the facial bones, and the three **ossicles** in the middle ear cavity.
- *Rib cage*, which is made up of 12 pairs of ribs. Seven pairs of *true ribs* attach directly to the sternum (breastbone) and five pairs of *false ribs*. The first three pairs of false ribs attach to the sternum indirectly with cartilage. The last two pairs of false ribs are called *floating ribs*, because they are not attached in the front of the body.
- *Spinal* or *vertebral column*, which is divided into five regions – cervical, thoracic, lumbar, sacral, and coccygeal. The spinal column is composed of 26 **vertebrae**.
- *Hyoid bone*, which is at the base of the tongue.

The appendicular skeleton is composed of 126 bones and includes:

- *Scapula* (shoulder blade) and *clavicle* (collarbone); the *acromion process* is the lateral tip of the scapula and is used as a landmark when giving injections in the deltoid muscle.
- *Humerus* (upper arm bone), *radius* and *ulna* (lower arm bones), and the wrist bones (*carpals*, *metacarpals*, and *phalanges*).
- Pelvic girdle (hip bones), which includes the *ilium*, *ischium*, and *pubis*.
- *Femur* (thigh bone), *patella* (kneecap), *tibia* (shin bone), *fibula*, and ankle/feet bones (*tarsals*, *metatarsals*, and *phalanges*).

Bones generally are categorized by shape: long, short, flat, sesamoid, and irregular. A long bone is composed of a long shaft called the *diaphysis*, which is made of hard **compact bone** (Fig. 20.2). The hollow space inside the diaphysis is called the *medullary cavity* and contains **yellow bone marrow**. Each end of a long bone is called an *epiphysis* and is made up of **spongy bone**. *Epiphyseal plates* (growth

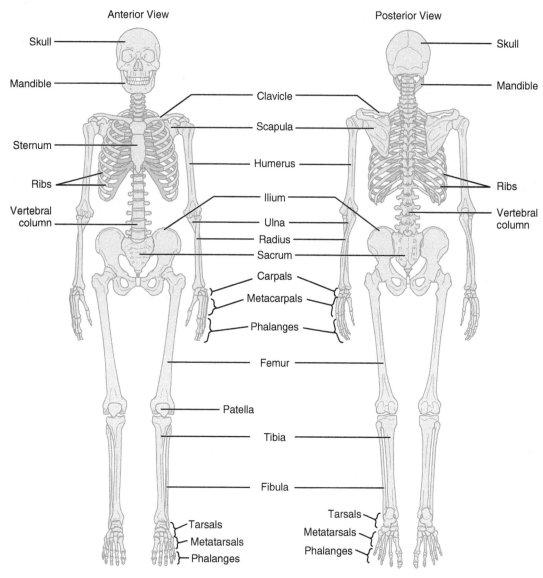

FIGURE 20.1 Axial skeletal bones *(outside columns)* and appendicular skeletal bones *(middle column)*.

plates) are at the end of the epiphysis, and this is where bone growth normally occurs. The epiphysis is covered with articular cartilage and is attached by ligaments to the epiphysis of another bone, forming a joint. Articular cartilage reduces the stress of weight bearing and the friction of movement. The thickness of the cartilage depends largely on the amount of stress placed on a particular joint.

Compact bone is made up of structural units called *osteons*, which are composed of osteocytes and calcified matrix. The nutrient foramina are small passageways that contain blood vessels that supply *osteocytes* (bone cells) with nutrients (see Fig. 20.2). Between the *periosteum* (outer covering of the bone) and the *endosteum* (inner lining), the **osteoblasts** and **osteoclasts** continuously remodel bones, making them strong, durable, and able to heal. Because bones have a good blood supply, they easily heal after trauma or a fracture. Spongy bone is less dense than compact bone and has a network of open spaces that contain **red bone marrow,** which produces blood cells.

CRITICAL THINKING APPLICATION   **20.1**

Suzanne was thinking about Walter as she prepared the exam room for his appointment. Walter's hands and knees were bothering him. The hands and knees are both part of the appendicular skeleton. She thought for a moment and quickly named the major structures in the appendicular and axial skeleton. Can you name them, too?

Joints

Bones are connected to each other at junctions known as joints *(articulations)*. The range through which a joint can extend and flex is called *range of motion* (ROM). Joints can be classified by their ROM and include:

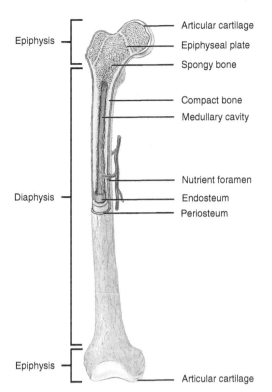

FIGURE 20.2 Long bone features. (From Applegate E: *The anatomy and physiology learning system,* ed 4, St Louis, 2011, Saunders.)

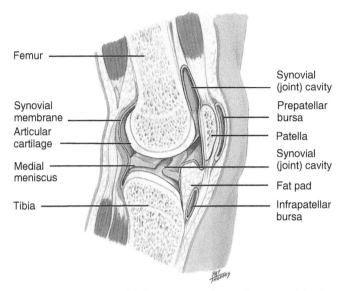

FIGURE 20.3 Sagittal section of the knee joint. (From Applegate E: *The anatomy and physiology learning system,* ed 4, St Louis, 2011, Saunders.)

- *Synarthroses*: Immovable (no ROM) joints held together by fibrous cartilaginous tissue. An example of this joint includes the suture lines of the skull.
- *Amphiarthroses*: Limited range of motion joints, which are joined together by cartilage that is slightly movable. Examples of these joints include the vertebrae and the pubic bones of the pelvic girdle.
- *Diarthroses* (or *synovial joints*): Full range of motion joints. Examples include the hinge joints in the knee and the ball-and-socket joint in the hip. The following section will provide more details on diarthrotic joints.

CRITICAL THINKING APPLICATION 20.2

As Dr. Kahn examines Walter's hands, he has Walter open and close his hands, wiggle his fingers, grip tightly around two of Dr. Kahn's fingers, and move his wrist. Throughout the whole exam, Dr. Kahn is watching Walter's hands and wrists. Dr. Kahn is looking at the ROM in Walter's hands. Describe in your own words what the acronym ROM means. List the three joint types (based on ROM) and give one example of each.

Diarthrotic Joints

Many of the diarthroses, or synovial joints, have *bursae,* sacs of fluid located between the bones of the joint and the tendons that hold the muscles in place. Bursae help cushion and support the joints when they move. Synovial joints also have joint capsules that enclose the ends of the bones (Fig. 20.3). A synovial membrane lines the joint capsules and secretes *synovial fluid* to lubricate the joint; joints also have cartilage that covers and protects the bone. The *meniscus*

consists of crescent-shaped cartilage in the knee joint that also cushions the joint. Ligaments are strong bands of white, fibrous connective tissue that connect one bone to another bone at the joints.

There are six classifications of *diarthroses* (or synovial joints). Each type has its own unique movement. These classifications include:

- *Ball-and-socket joint:* Allows free movement (rotation). Examples include the shoulder and hip joints.
- *Hinge joint:* Permits flexion and extension (Table 20.1). Examples include the elbow, knee, and finger joints.
- *Saddle joint:* Allows for flexion, extension, and other movement. An example is the thumb crossing over the palm of the hand.
- *Pivot joint:* Permits rotation. Pivot joints are found between the atlas and the axis (first and second cervical vertebrae).
- *Gliding joint:* Allows a bone to slide over another bone. This occurs in the wrist and between the vertebrae.
- *Condyloid joint:* Permits flexion, extension, and circular motion. An example would be the movement of the atlas.

Muscles

There are three types of muscles in the body:
1. *Skeletal muscles* are voluntary and *striated* (striped in appearance) and are attached to the bones of the skeleton by tendons (Fig. 20.4 and Fig. 20.5A). Special fibers in skeletal muscles allow them to shorten (contract) and lengthen (relax), which creates movement. Most skeletal muscle allows the body to move voluntarily at the joints.
2. *Smooth muscles* are involuntary and nonstriated (see Fig. 20.5B). They make up the walls of the hollow organs, blood vessels, and the respiratory system passageways. Smooth muscles move in a wavelike motion called *peristalsis,* which helps substances move through the organs easily and effectively.
3. *Cardiac muscles* are involuntary, striated muscles in the heart (see Fig. 20.5C). They contain *intercalated* disks (prominent dark bands) and interconnected fibers, which create an efficient and coordinated contraction of the heart.

Muscles, bones, and joints change with age.

TABLE 20.1 Types of Body Movement

MOVEMENT	DEFINITION OR EXAMPLE	MOVEMENT	DEFINITION OR EXAMPLE
Flexion	Reduces the angle of the joint and brings the two bones closer together.	Adduction	The opposite of abduction; moving the body part toward the midline of the body.
Extension	The opposite of flexion; increases the angle or distance between two bones or parts of the body.	Rotation	Moving a bone around its central axis; common in ball-and-socket joints.
Hyperextension	Extension 180 degrees (e.g., the neck is extended backward or the toes are pointed downward).	Circumduction	Circular movement of a limb; a combination of abduction, adduction, extension, and flexion.
Abduction	Moving the body part away from the midline or median plane of the body.	Dorsiflexion	Moving the instep of the foot up and dorsally, reducing the angle between the foot and the leg.

TABLE 20.1   Types of Body Movement—*continued*

MOVEMENT	DEFINITION OR EXAMPLE	MOVEMENT	DEFINITION OR EXAMPLE
Plantar flexion	A toe-down movement of the foot at the ankle; increases the angle of the joint.	Inversion	The opposite of eversion; turning the sole of the foot medially, or inward.
Eversion	Turning the sole of the foot laterally, or outward.	Pronation	Rotation of the forearm that turns the palm of the hand downward, or posteriorly.
		Supination	The opposite of pronation; rotation of the forearm that turns the palm of the hand upward, or anteriorly.

Life Span Changes

Common changes to the musculoskeletal system that occur with age:

- Bones lose calcium and other minerals, reducing bone mass or density and making them more brittle. This can lead to fractures.
- Loss of height from the compression and curving of the spinal column, which can cause a more stooped posture.
- Joints become stiffer and less flexible. Synovial fluid decreases and cartilage may wear away, causing degenerative changes. This can lead to inflammation, stiffness, pain, and deformities.
- Muscle mass decreases, resulting in a loss of strength and endurance.

PHYSIOLOGY OF THE MUSCULOSKELETAL SYSTEM

Muscle Cell in Action

Before a skeletal muscle can contract, it must be stimulated by an impulse that comes from the brain or spinal cord. The impulse moves away from the brain toward the muscle via a nerve cell, called a *motor neuron*. The point of contact between the nerve ending and the muscle fiber is called a *neuromuscular junction (NMJ)*, a type of **synapse**. At the synapse, there is a very small gap called a *synaptic cleft*. Chemical messengers called *neurotransmitters* are released by the motor neuron in response to a nerve impulse.

Neurotransmitters (e.g., acetylcholine [ACh]) must travel across the synaptic cleft to continue the stimulus and generate a muscle contraction. The released ACh triggers a change in the **permeability** of the individual muscle fiber. Then sodium ions flow into the fibers, causing calcium to be released from their storage area in the muscle fiber. When calcium is released, the thin actin fibers slide between the thick myosin fibers, causing the muscle to shorten, or *contract*. Muscles need calcium and energy in the form of **ATP (adenosine triphosphate)** to contract. The muscle will relax once the ACh is inactivated and the calcium ions are back in their storage areas of the muscle.

Types of Muscle Contractions

Even when we are not actively moving, our muscles are in a state of partial contraction called *muscle tone*. Nerve impulses help maintain muscle tone so that muscles are ready to act when needed. Muscle tone is an important factor in proper posture, too. The two types of muscle contractions that the body most frequently uses are:

- *Isotonic*: Muscle contraction that usually produces movement at a joint. The muscle usually shortens and thickens (bulges), and a task is done. Examples include walking, running, lifting weight, and twisting.
- *Isometric*: Muscle contraction usually does not produce movement. There is no change in muscle length, but there is an increase in muscle tension. Examples include pushing against an immovable object, pushing against a wall, and pushing the palms together – there is no movement, but there is an increase in muscle tension.

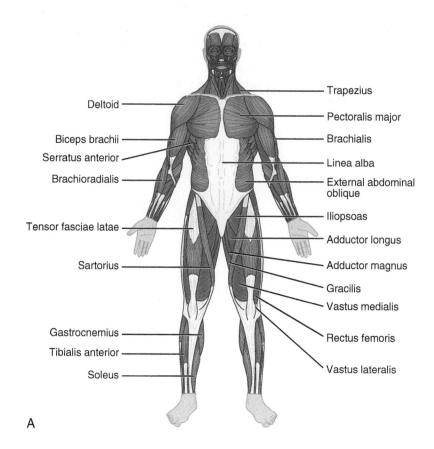

A

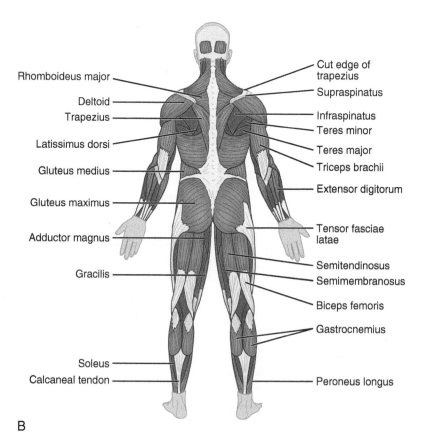

B

FIGURE 20.4 Muscles of the body. **(A)** Anterior view. **(B)** Posterior view.

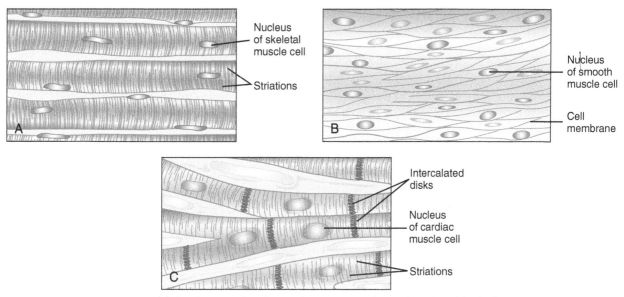

FIGURE 20.5 **(A)** Skeletal muscle. **(B)** Smooth muscle. **(C)** Cardiac muscle. (From Applegate E: *The anatomy and physiology learning system,* ed 4, St Louis, 2011, Saunders.)

CRITICAL THINKING APPLICATION 20.3

Walter tells Dr. Kahn about his love of gardening. He loves being outdoors and feeling the dirt on his hands. Dr. Kahn palpates the sore muscle on Walter's forearm and asks about the gardening activities that make the pain worse. Walter replies, "The activities that hurt the most are digging, pulling weeds, and pushing dirt in around the small plants." Which of these three actions are an isotonic contraction of the muscle, and which are isometric?

DISORDERS OF THE MUSCULOSKELETAL SYSTEM

The skeleton, muscles, and joints together work as a unit to move the body. Diseases of the musculoskeletal system often affect the ability to move with ease. Common signs and symptoms of musculoskeletal disorders include:

- Inflammation, pain, or swelling in the joints, muscles, or bones
- *Malaise* (generalized weakness or discomfort)
- *Myalgia* (muscle pain), *myositis* (inflammation of a muscle), and muscle tenderness
- Temporary loss of function or loss of normal mobility

The following sections describe in detail some of the more common diseases seen in the ambulatory care setting.

Skeletal Disorders

Fractures

A *fracture* is a broken bone. A simple fracture does not break through the skin, whereas a compound fracture does break through the skin. Table 20.2 describes types of fractures.

Fractures can occur from trauma, overuse, or diseases. A *pathologic fracture* or a *spontaneous fracture* results from an underlying disease, such as osteoporosis or cancer. Signs and symptoms of a fracture include pain, swelling, bruising, numbness or tingling, deformity, and difficulty using or inability to use the affected area. Bleeding at the site of the break will also occur with compound fractures.

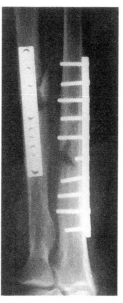

FIGURE 20.6 Orthopedic hardware from open reduction of fractures of the radius and ulna. (From Mettler MA: *Essentials of radiology,* ed 3, Philadelphia, 2004, Saunders.)

Most commonly, the provider will order an x-ray, but a bone scan, computed tomography (CT) scan, or magnetic resonance imaging (MRI) may also be used as a diagnostic test for some types of fractures. Depending on the type of fracture, treatment may include cast or splint immobilization, a brace, surgery, and **analgesics**. If bones are not aligned, surgery is required. During an open reduction and internal fixation (ORIF) surgery, the surgeon *reduces* (repositions and aligns) the bones and uses *internal fixators* (special metal devices [rods, screws, plates]) to hold the bones in place during the healing process (Fig. 20.6). Sometimes, external fixators and traction are used to hold the bones in place. Fractures may take several weeks to months to heal. Crutches or other assistive devices may be used for lower extremity fractures. Physical therapy may be ordered once the cast is removed.

TABLE 20.2   Types of Fractures

FRACTURE	DEFINITION	FRACTURE	DEFINITION
Closed, or simple	Broken bone is contained within intact skin.	Comminuted	Break is caused by severe, direct force, which creates a fracture with multiple fragments.
Open, or compound	Skin is broken above the fracture; open to the external environment, creating the potential for infection.	Impacted	Break is caused by strong forces that drive bone fragments firmly together.
Longitudinal	Fracture extends along the length of the bone.	Pathologic	Break results from weakening of the bones by disease, as in osteoporosis or sarcoma.
Transverse	Break is caused by direct force applied perpendicular to a bone; fracture runs across the bone.	Nondisplaced	Bone ends remain in alignment.
Oblique	Break is caused by a twisting force with an upward thrust; fracture ends are short and run at an oblique angle across the bone.	Displaced	Bone ends are moved out of alignment.
Greenstick	Break is caused by compression or angulation forces in the long bones of children under age 10; because of its softness, the bone is cracked on one side and intact on the other side.	Spiral	Break is caused by a twisting or rotary force, which results in long, sharp, pointed bone ends; suspicious as a child abuse injury.

TABLE 20.2 Types of Fractures—*continued*

FRACTURE	DEFINITION	FRACTURE	DEFINITION
Compression	Break is caused by forces that drive bones together; typically seen in the vertebrae.	Depression	Bone fragments of the skull are driven inward.
Avulsion	Break is caused by forceful contraction of a muscle against resistance, and a bone fragment tears at the site of muscle insertion.		

From Chester GA: *Modern medical assisting,* Philadelphia, 1999, Saunders.

CRITICAL THINKING APPLICATION   20.4

A patient comes into the clinic hopping on one foot and holding the other in the air. She says she thinks she broke her ankle when she stepped off the curb wrong and fell. What is the first thing Suzanne should do for this patient? What tests will Dr. Kahn most likely order? Why?

Osteomalacia and Rickets

Osteomalacia is the softening of bones due to the lack of vitamin D. Vitamin D helps the body absorb calcium. Calcium is needed for strong bones. Osteomalacia occurs in adults and children; in children, this disease is called *rickets*.

Osteomalacia and rickets are caused by a lack of vitamin D, which can be related to an absorption issue (e.g., after gastric bypass surgery) or a lack of dietary intake. Osteomalacia can also be related to kidney failure, liver disease, and certain medications (e.g., **anticonvulsants**). Signs and symptoms include bone fractures without related injuries, muscle weakness, and widespread bone pain, usually in the hips.

The provider will order blood tests to check the vitamin D level, along with creatinine, calcium, electrolyte, alkaline phosphatase, phosphate, and parathyroid hormone levels. Bone x-rays, a bone density test, and a bone **biopsy** may be done. Treatment involves oral supplements of vitamin D, calcium, and phosphorus. Sunlight for vitamin D production is also recommended.

Osteoporosis

Osteoporosis is a condition that causes bones to become brittle and weak. Healthy bone is constantly being broken down and remodeled. When a person has osteoporosis, bones are being broken down more quickly than new bone can be created. This leads to weak bones that are easily fractured, especially in the wrist, hip, and spine.

Peak bone mass is reached during a person's 20s. As people age, bone mass is lost faster than it can be produced, leading to osteoporosis. Increased risks for osteoporosis include menopause, family history, small body frame, white or Asian descent, hormonal imbalance, dietary deficiencies (low calcium intake), long-term corticosteroid use, celiac disease, kidney or liver disease, cancer, and some autoimmune conditions. A sedentary lifestyle, tobacco use, and excessive alcohol consumption are also risks for osteoporosis. Early osteoporosis is asymptomatic, but as the bones become weaker, back pain, height loss, stooped posture, and fractures can occur.

A bone density test is the only diagnostic tool for osteoporosis. This low-level x-ray determines the mineral content of the bone. Treatment for osteoporosis may include:

- Weight-bearing exercises to maintain bone density
- Modifying risk factors to prevent falls
- Appropriate calcium and vitamin D intake from food or supplements
- Medications: bisphosphonates and hormone replacement therapy (estrogen)

Osteoporosis is a chronic condition that can be managed, but it does progress with age.

CRITICAL THINKING APPLICATION   20.5

Mrs. Viola Carson, a 78-year-old patient, is being seen in the office today for follow-up after hip replacement surgery. Mrs. Carson fractured her hip from a simple fall at the grocery store. Why would the physician suspect she has osteoporosis? What treatment might be recommended to prevent further fractures in this patient?

Lordosis, Kyphosis, and Scoliosis

The spine has normal curves (Fig. 20.7). Abnormal curvatures of the spine deprive the body of important features related to spinal strength, balance, and posture. The three most common curvatures are:

- *Lordosis* (swayback): An exaggerated forward curve in the lumbar region, which makes the buttock appear larger.
- *Kyphosis* (hunchback): An exaggerated curve in the thoracic region.
- *Scoliosis*: An abnormal side-to-side (S or C) curvature that could be in both the thoracic and lumbar regions of the back.

Lordosis is caused by genetic and congenital conditions (e.g., muscular dystrophy, spondylolisthesis). Kyphosis can occur at any age, but more commonly occurs in adults as a result of degenerative diseases of the spine, fractures, and injury. Kyphosis can also be caused by Paget's disease, muscular dystrophy, scoliosis, and tumors.

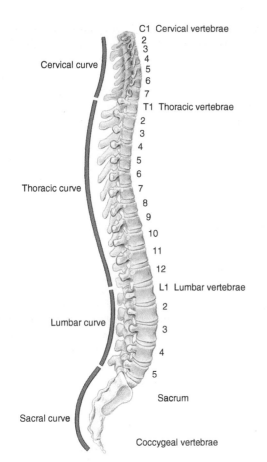

FIGURE 20.7 Normal curves of the spine. (From Applegate E: *The anatomy and physiology learning system*, ed 4, St Louis, 2011, Saunders.)

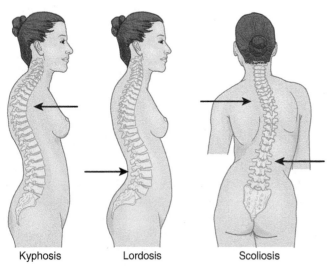

FIGURE 20.8 Spinal curve abnormalities.

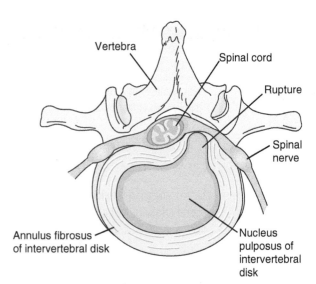

FIGURE 20.9 Herniation of a vertebral disk.

Many times, scoliosis occurs in children from age 10 to early teens, and the cause is unknown. Abnormalities in any of the spinal curves can cause pain and fatigue in the lower back and legs (Fig. 20.8).

The provider will perform a physical exam of the spine and a neurologic exam. A spinal x-ray, MRI, and CT scan are also used as diagnostic tools. The treatment depends on the severity of the curve and the patient's age and condition. Treatments include physical therapy, medications (analgesics, nonsteroidal anti-inflammatory drugs [NSAIDs], steroids, and muscle relaxants), spinal fusion surgery and, for scoliosis, a back brace and surgical placement of metal stabilizing rods.

Herniated Disk

The spine is made up of vertebrae. Soft disks filled with a jelly-like substance are between the vertebrae, to cushion and keep them in place. A herniated (slipped) disk occurs when it moves out of place. The disk can also rupture, causing the jelly-like center to leak out, irritating the local nerves (Fig. 20.9).

The disks can degenerate with age. Middle-aged and older men are more at risk for a herniated disk. Typically, herniation occurs with strenuous activities, but it can also occur with lifting heavy objects, obesity, repetitive movements involving the lower back, long periods of sitting or standing, inactivity, and smoking. Signs and symptoms of a lower back herniated disk include *sciatica* (pain and numbness from the hip down to the foot), back pain, and weakness. A herniated disk in the neck may cause pain and numbness from the shoulder down to the fingers. The pain usually starts slowly and gets worse with standing or sitting.

The provider will perform an examination checking reflexes and muscle strength. The provider may order diagnostic tests (e.g., myelogram and electromyography [EMG]) and imaging procedures (e.g., spine MRI, spine CT, and spine x-ray). Treatments usually include medications (e.g., NSAIDs, narcotics, and muscle relaxants), rest, physical therapy, and possibly surgery.

Plantar Fasciitis

The plantar **fascia** is a tough fibrous tissue that connects the toes to the heel on the bottom of the feet, creating the arch of the foot. Plantar fasciitis occurs when the plantar fascia becomes inflamed or swollen from being overstretched or overused. Plantar fasciitis is one of the most common foot issues.

People with flat feet or high arches are at risk for plantar fasciitis. Other risk factors include running long distances, obesity, wearing

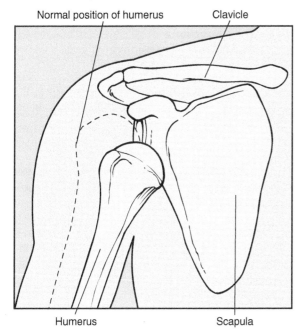

FIGURE 20.10 Dislocation (luxation) of the shoulder. (From Frazier MS, Drzymkowski JW: *Essentials of human diseases and conditions,* ed 3, Philadelphia, 2004, Saunders.)

shoes with poor arch support, and having a tight Achilles tendon. Signs and symptoms include foot pain immediately in the morning, after standing, sitting, or intense exercise, and when climbing stairs. The pain can be on the bottom of the foot or along the sole of the foot. Mild foot swelling, redness, or stiffness can also be seen.

The provider will do an examination. A foot x-ray may be ordered to rule out other issues. Treatment involves over-the-counter analgesics, heel and foot stretches, and good arch supports in shoes. Severe cases may require immobilization, custom-made shoe inserts, steroid injections in the heel, and surgery.

Joint Disorders

Dislocation and Subluxation

A *dislocation* (or *luxation*) occurs when a bone has been completely displaced from the joint (Fig. 20.10). A *subluxation* is a partial or incomplete dislocation of the joint. The most common site of joint dislocation in children is the elbow, whereas in the adult it is the shoulder. Other joints that can be dislocated include the ankle, knee, hip, jaw, toe, or finger.

The etiology of dislocations is related to sports and trauma (e.g., a blow or fall), which forces the joint out of position. The larger the joint, the greater the force needed for dislocation. Some people have a hereditary risk, because their ligaments are looser, and they are more prone to injury. Signs and symptoms include pain and swelling in the joint area and inability to move the extremity. Many times, a visual distortion in the joint area is seen. Once a joint is dislocated, there is a greater risk of dislocating it in the future.

A dislocated joint is an emergency and requires immobilization and application of a cold pack as first aid. Once the provider examines the joint, an x-ray may be ordered. Treatment depends on the severity of the injury and the joint involved. The joint needs to be manipulated back into position. Additional complications may require surgical

intervention. Once the joint is back into its normal position, the area may be immobilized in a splint or sling to heal. NSAIDs to reduce the inflammation and pain may be ordered.

CRITICAL THINKING APPLICATION   20.6

A patient comes into the office from her weekly softball game. After sliding into home plate, she immediately was unable to move her right arm, and she says that she has a lot of pain in her right shoulder. What steps should Suzanne take to help this patient?

Arthritis

Arthritis is a term that refers to any inflammatory joint condition. More than 54 million Americans have some form of arthritis. Arthritis is the leading cause of work disabilities in the United States. About 50% of arthritic cases are in those 65 years or older, though arthritis can occur at any age. According to the Arthritis Foundation, there are over 100 different types of arthritis. Surprisingly, diseases such as fibromyalgia and carpal tunnel syndrome are considered types of arthritis. Arthritis can be caused by autoimmunity, infection, injury, and genetic conditions. The following sections discuss common arthritic conditions, and Table 20.3 summarizes additional types of arthritis.

CRITICAL THINKING APPLICATION   20.7

Suzanne has been a runner for years, but recently she was diagnosed with bursitis in her knees. Explain how Suzanne's running may have contributed to this condition.

Carpal Tunnel Syndrome. Carpal tunnel syndrome results when the median nerve becomes compressed at the wrist. The carpal tunnel is a narrow passageway, located on the palm side of the wrist, that is surrounded by bones and ligaments. This tunnel protects the median nerve to the hand and the nine tendons that bend the fingers.

The etiology includes repetitive motions, trauma, injury to the wrist, and conditions such as thyroid disease and rheumatoid arthritis. Women are more likely to have carpal tunnel syndrome than men. Signs and symptoms start gradually, with tingling, burning, or numbness of the thumb and fingers, except for the little finger. Symptoms can come and go initially but can worsen and become more persistent with time. Without treatment, a person can lose grip strength and feeling in the fingertips.

The provider will examine the arm and wrist. X-rays and an electromyogram may be done. Treatments include limiting repetitive tasks, cold therapy, a wrist splint, NSAIDs, and corticosteroid injections. Surgery may be performed to relieve pressure on the median nerve.
Fibromyalgia. Fibromyalgia causes muscle pain, fatigue, and "tender points" on the legs, hips, back, arms, shoulders, and neck. It is estimated that 10 million people in the United States have fibromyalgia. Women develop fibromyalgia more often than men. Usually, the diagnosis occurs before age 50.

The etiology is unknown. Research indicates that trauma, infection, or injury may change how the central nervous system (CNS) responds to pain, leading to chronic pain. The signs and symptoms of fibromyalgia include widespread muscle pain, burning, aching,

TABLE 20.3   Types of Arthritis and Related Conditions

DISEASE	DESCRIPTION	ETIOLOGY; SIGNS AND SYMPTOMS	DIAGNOSTIC TESTS; TREATMENTS
Ankylosing spondylitis	Type of inflammatory arthritis affecting the back and spine, usually occurring between 17 and 35 years of age.	Heredity; low back pain and stiffness, especially in the night and morning	X-rays and blood test to check for HLA-B27 gene; medications (analgesics, NSAIDs, DMARDs, corticosteroids), and surgery
Bursitis	Inflammation of a bursa. Usually affects the hip, buttock, knees, calf, and shoulder.	Repetitive movements, injury, bad posture, side effect of certain medications, and metabolic conditions; pain, tenderness, and inflammation in joint area	Examination; rest, splint, hot and cold therapy, medications (NSAIDs, analgesics, and corticosteroid injection), and physical therapy
Chondromalacia patella	"Runner's knee," commonly seen in teens, young adults, women, and athletes	Activities that stress the knees; pain and tenderness in the front or side of the knee, grinding sensation with bending knee	Examination; rest, brace or elastic wrap, NSAIDs, strengthening exercises, and physical therapy
Chronic fatigue syndrome	Profound fatigue that lasts over 6 months regardless of bed rest	Unknown; generalized weakness, achy muscles and joints, low-grade fever, dizziness, problems sleeping	Examination; no treatment, focus is relief of symptoms
Developmental dysplasia of the hip	Dislocation of the hip joint; occurs in newborns	Unknown; uneven skinfold on the thigh or buttock, leg turns outward and is shorter	Examination, listening for a clicking sound when applying pressure, ultrasound, and x-ray; brace or harness, surgical intervention
Infectious arthritis	Septic arthritis; arthritis due to a joint infection	Bacteria (*Staphylococcus aureus*), viral, or fungal infections; pain, swelling in a joint, fever and chills	Examination, joint fluid analysis, and x-rays; antibiotics or antifungal medication, analgesic, NSAIDs
Systemic lupus erythematosus	Chronic autoimmune disease, affects joints, skin, kidneys, brain, and blood	Unknown; joint pain, rash, fatigue, **photosensitivity**, hair loss, sensitivity to light, memory problems, mouth sores, and low blood cell counts	Examination, blood tests (CBC, ANA, chemistry test), and urine test; medications (NSAIDs, corticosteroids, DMARDs, belimumab [Benlysta], and chemotherapy)
Paget's disease	Osteitis deformans, causes abnormal bone remodeling resulting in weakened, enlarged bones	Unknown; pain, enlarged and broken bones, damaged cartilage	Examination, blood tests, and x-rays; bisphosphonates to slow bone turnover and analgesics
Psoriatic arthritis	Chronic autoimmune disease that can occur with **psoriasis**	Unknown; joint pain and stiffness, fatigue, swelling of hands and feet, skin rashes, and eye problems	Examination, x-rays, and blood tests (C-reactive protein and rheumatoid factor [RF]); medications (NSAIDs, corticosteroids, and DMARDs), and light therapy
Raynaud's phenomenon	Causes vasoconstriction in the extremities	Unknown, episodes triggered by cold weather and emotional stress; skin color change (fingers, toes), coldness, numbness, and pain	Examination, blood tests (ANA, ESR); focused on preventing episodes, hypertensive medications to dilate blood vessels
Rheumatic fever	Inflammatory disease that can cause permanent heart damage	Group A streptococcus bacteria; joint pain, tenderness, and inflammation, fever, chest pain, and fatigue	Examination, blood test, ECG, and ECHO; medications (antibiotic, NSAIDs, and corticosteroids)
Tendinitis	Inflammation of a tendon	Repetitive movements, injury, bad posture, side effect of certain medications, and metabolic conditions; pain, tenderness, and inflammation in joint area	Examination; rest, splint, hot and cold therapy, NSAIDs, analgesics, corticosteroid injection, and physical therapy

ANA, Anti-nuclear antibody; *CBC,* complete blood count, *DMARDs,* disease-modifying antirheumatic drugs; *ECG,* electrocardiography; *ECHO,* echocardiography; *ESR,* erythrocyte sedimentation rate, sed rate; *NSAIDs,* nonsteroidal anti-inflammatory drugs.

stiffness, or soreness. Additional symptoms include fatigue, sleep disturbances, mood and concentration problems, anxiety, headache, abdominal pain, bloating, constipation, diarrhea, bladder spasms, dizziness, numbness or tingling in the hands and feet, and tender points around the body.

The provider will perform an examination and rule out other conditions. With no diagnostic tests for fibromyalgia, the provider may use these results:

- Widespread Pain Index (WPI) score, which evaluates 19 areas on the body for pain.
- Symptom Severity (SS) score, on which the patient scores specific fibromyalgia symptoms, including cognitive issues, fatigue, headache, and dizziness.

Treatments focus on minimizing the pain and fatigue experienced through the use of medications (e.g., pregabalin [Lyrica], duloxetine [Cymbalta], and milnacipran [Savella]), exercise, biofeedback, and acupuncture.

Gout. Gout (also called *gouty arthritis*) is a common form of arthritis. The great (big) toe is the most common site for gout, though it can affect the heel, ankle, knee, elbow, wrist, and fingers. Gout can be acute or chronic, and attacks can last longer as time progresses.

The etiology is a buildup of uric acid in the body (Fig. 20.11). Uric acid results from the breakdown of purines in foods (e.g., liver, dried peas and beans, and anchovies). The risk factors for gout include being male, a family history of gout, obesity, drinking alcohol, and eating too many purine-rich foods. Certain medications (e.g., diuretics, aspirin, niacin, and levodopa) may increase the risk of gout. The signs and symptoms of gout include swollen, red, warm, and stiff joints.

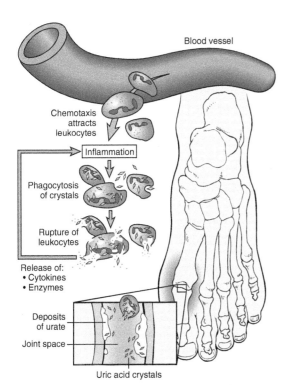

FIGURE 20.11 Gout is characterized by deposits of uric acid crystals in the connective tissue. The inflammation most often affects the joint of the big toe. (From Damjanov I: *Pathology for the health-related professions*, ed 4, St Louis, 2012, Saunders.)

To diagnose gout, the provider will do a physical examination and order an x-ray and lab tests. The provider may take a sample of fluid from the inflamed joint area to look for uric acid crystals. Pseudogout has a similar presentation, but it is caused by calcium phosphate. Treatment includes NSAIDs to reduce the pain and swelling. Corticosteroids (e.g., prednisone) can reduce the inflammation. Colchicine (Colcrys) should be taken within the first 12 hours of the attack. Full recovery may take up to 14 days. To treat gout or to prevent future attacks by reducing the uric acid level in the blood, the person may need to take allopurinol (Aloprim, Zyloprim), febuxostat (Uloric), probenecid (Probalan), or pegloticase (Krystexxa).

Juvenile Arthritis. Juvenile arthritis (JA) is a generic phrase for autoimmune, inflammatory, or rheumatic conditions that affect children under 16 years of age. Juvenile idiopathic arthritis (JIA) is the most common form of JA. Other types of JA are listed in Table 20.4.

There is no known cause of JA. For some types of JA, there may be a genetic predisposition for the condition. Signs and symptoms of JA depend on the specific condition. Most JA conditions cause pain, swelling, redness, and warmth in the joints. Some JA conditions may also cause issues with the eyes, muscles, digestive system, and the skin.

The provider will perform an examination and order lab work, though no specific blood test diagnoses JA. The goal of the treatment is to provide the child with the best quality of life; thus pain control and reducing inflammation are important. A combination of medications, physical therapy, and nutrition therapy may be used.

Lyme Disease. Lyme disease is the most common tickborne infectious disease in the United States. This bacterial infection is prevalent in Wisconsin, Minnesota, California, and between Virginia and Maine. Exposure to grassy and heavily wooded areas increases the risk for coming in contact with infected ticks.

Lyme disease is caused by *Borrelia burgdorferi* and *Borrelia mayonii* in the United States. Infected deer ticks and western black-legged ticks transmit the bacteria that cause Lyme disease. Early signs and symptoms of Lyme disease include flu-like symptoms (fever, chills, achiness, fatigue, swollen lymph nodes, and headache) and a rash (*erythema migrans*). The rash appears about 70% to 80% of the time, usually starting 3 to 30 days after the bite. The rash begins at the bite site and slowly expands over the skin, reaching up to 12 inches or more. The rash can appear as a bull's-eye or target. If left untreated, Lyme disease can cause arthritis, severe joint pain, meningitis, Bell's palsy, facial palsy (affecting both sides of the face), numbness and weakness in the extremities, heart palpitations (Lyme carditis), short-term memory issues, and eye inflammation.

TABLE 20.4	Types of Juvenile Arthritis
TYPE	**DESCRIPTION**
Juvenile dermatomyositis	Causes weakness and a rash on the eyelids and knuckles.
Juvenile systemic lupus erythematosus	Autoimmune disease that affects the kidneys, blood, skin, and joints.
Juvenile scleroderma	Causes skin to tighten and harden.
Kawasaki disease	Causes inflammation of blood vessels and heart damage.

After an examination, the provider will order an enzyme immunoassay (EIA) or immunofluorescence assay (IFA) blood test. If the results are positive or equivocal, further testing with IgM and/or IgG Western blot will be done. The lab test results are more reliable if a person has been infected for several weeks. Antibiotics, such as amoxicillin (Amoxil, Moxatag), cefuroxime (Ceftin), or doxycycline (Doryx, Oracea, Vibramycin), usually cure Lyme disease. Some people may have post-treatment Lyme disease syndrome, which will resolve in time.

Patient Education for Lyme Disease

- Minimize the risk for ticks in your yard by clearing tall grass, leaves, and brush.
- Treat clothing, boots, and camping gear with 0.5% permethrin.
- Use Environmental Protection Agency (EPA)–registered insect repellents. They contain DEET, picaridin, IR3535, Oil of Lemon Eucalyptus, para-menthane-diol (PMD), or 2-undecanone. You can also use the information found at the EPA website: https://www.epa.gov/insect-repellents/find-repellent-right-you.
- Wear pants tucked into socks and long-sleeved shirts when walking in wooded or grassy areas.
- Walk in the center of trails and avoid wooded and high-grass areas.
- Deer ticks are no bigger than the head of a pin. After you come indoors, check your entire body and your clothing, gear, and animals for ticks. Showering within 2 hours of potential exposure can reduce the chances of Lyme disease.
- If a person has a tick embedded, it needs to be removed. Wear gloves and use fine-tipped pointed tweezers. Get as close to the head as possible. Do not squeeze the abdomen, because it may inject secretions into the person's body. Slowly pull the head out. Do not twist. Do not burn it or use petroleum jelly or nail polish. Once the tick is removed, place it in a container of rubbing alcohol to kill it. Clean the site with antiseptic soap and water. Apply an antibiotic ointment. Monitor the site for infection or other complications.
- If you develop a rash or fever within several weeks of removing a tick, see your healthcare provider. Be sure to tell him or her about your recent tick bite and when the bite occurred.
- Do not assume you are immune. Lyme disease can occur in the same person more than once.

Centers for Disease Control and Prevention (CDC). https://www.cdc.gov/lyme/prev/index.html. Accessed June 6, 2018.

Osteoarthritis. Osteoarthritis (OA), also called *degenerative joint disease* (DJD), is the most common form of arthritis. OA can occur in any joint but most often affects the hands, hips, spine, and knees.

Osteoarthritis occurs when the cartilage at the end of the bones wears down, causing the bones to rub together, leading to permanent damage to the joint. Risk factors include genetics, being female, obesity, age, and injury to the joint. The signs and symptoms develop gradually and worsen over time. OA can cause pain, tenderness, stiffness, and swelling in joints, reducing the range of motion. Bone spurs may form around the affected joint.

The provider will examine the affected joints and check the range of motion. X-rays, MRI, joint fluid analysis, and blood tests may be ordered to check for joint damage and rule out other types of arthritis. Treatment is focused on slowing the progression by maintaining a healthy weight, and limiting pain with the use of analgesics, NSAIDs, and duloxetine (Cymbalta). Additional interventions include physical therapy, occupational therapy, and cortisone injections in the joint to relieve pain. Joint replacement surgery (*arthroplasty*) may also be done.

CRITICAL THINKING APPLICATION   20.8
An 80-year-old male patient with arthritis comes into the office complaining of severe pain in his knees, hips, and lower back. The pain makes it impossible for him to get up onto the examination table. What should Suzanne do? Is this patient required to get onto the examination table? Why or why not?

Rheumatoid Arthritis. Rheumatoid arthritis (RA) is an autoimmune and inflammatory disease. RA often starts in middle age and is common in older adults. A person can have the disease for a short time, or episodes may come and go. The severe form of RA is chronic.

With this autoimmune disease, the immune system attacks the healthy cells, causing inflammation in the joints, eyes, lungs, and mouth. Usually, it affects the wrist, finger, and knee joints. The lining of the joints becomes inflamed, causing damage to the joint tissue. Older adults and females are at most risk for RA, though women who breastfeed have a decreased risk. Other risk factors include genetics, cigarette use, and obesity. Signs and symptoms of RA include pain, achiness, stiffness, swelling, and tenderness in more than one joint. The person can experience weight loss, fever, weakness, and fatigue (Fig. 20.12).

Early stages of RA can be difficult to diagnose because the symptoms are similar to other joint diseases. During the examination, the provider will check the reflexes and muscle strength, and the joints for signs of inflammation (e.g., swelling, redness, and warmth). Imaging tests (x-rays, MRI, and ultrasound [US]) may be done, along with blood tests, including ESR, C-reactive protein (CRP), rheumatoid factor (RF), and anti–cyclin citrullinated peptide (anti-CCP) antibodies. There is no cure for RA, but recent research has shown that early use of disease-modifying antirheumatic drugs (DMARDs) can increase the chances of **remission**.

Muscular Disorders
Muscular Dystrophy
Muscular dystrophy (MD) is a collection of over 30 inherited diseases that cause muscle weakness and muscle loss. Some of these diseases affect children, whereas others appear in middle-aged adults. The most common form is Duchenne muscular dystrophy, which is usually diagnosed by the age of 3. About half of the people with MD have Duchenne muscular dystrophy. Boys are affected much more frequently than girls.

Muscular dystrophy may be congenital or caused by a genetic mutation that disrupts the body's ability to make muscle-protecting proteins. The signs, symptoms, onset, and affected muscle groups depend on the specific disease, though the main sign of MD is progressive muscle weakness. The signs and symptoms of Duchenne muscular dystrophy include frequent falls, trouble running and moving from lying to sitting position, muscle pain and stiffness, and learning disabilities.

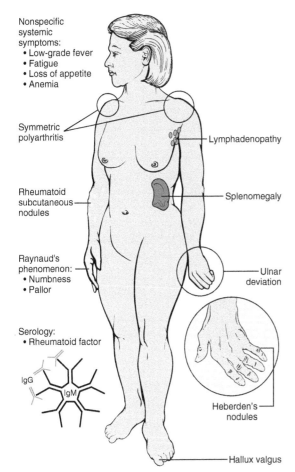

FIGURE 20.12 Signs and symptoms of rheumatoid arthritis. (From Damjanov I: *Pathology for the health-related professions*, ed 4, St Louis, 2012, Saunders.)

Labels on figure:

Nonspecific systemic symptoms:
• Low-grade fever
• Fatigue
• Loss of appetite
• Anemia

Symmetric polyarthritis

Rheumatoid subcutaneous nodules

Raynaud's phenomenon:
• Numbness
• Pallor

Serology:
• Rheumatoid factor

IgG

IgM

Lymphadenopathy

Splenomegaly

Ulnar deviation

Heberden's nodules

Hallux valgus

After the examination, the provider may order a creatine kinase (CK) blood test. Without trauma, high levels of CK suggest muscle disease, such as muscular dystrophy. Additional diagnostic tests include electromyography, genetic testing, and a muscle biopsy. There is no cure for muscular dystrophy. Treatments can help improve quality of life, help people to remain mobile for as long as possible, and reduce or prevent bone and spinal complications. Treatments include corticosteroids, heart medication, range of motion and stretching exercises, braces, and assistive devices (e.g., walkers, wheelchairs).

Myasthenia Gravis

Myasthenia gravis affects the voluntary muscles, causing weakness and fatigue with activity, which improves with rest. Myasthenia gravis is more common in men over 60 and women younger than 40 years of age.

The etiology is an autoimmune neuromuscular disease. The body produces antibodies that block the muscle cells from responding to neurotransmitters from nerve cells. Signs and symptoms include muscle weakness, leading to issues with breathing, chewing, swallowing, talking, climbing stairs, lifting objects, and maintaining a steady gaze. Additional symptoms include drooping eyelids, facial paralysis, fatigue, hoarseness, and double vision.

After a detailed neurologic examination, the provider will order imaging tests (CT or MRI), pulmonary function tests, and

electromyography (EMG). With myasthenia gravis, the person will have a positive result on an acetylcholine receptor antibody blood test. There is no cure for myasthenia gravis. The treatment is focused on increasing periods of remission. Lifestyle changes are encouraged, including resting, using eye patches, and avoiding stress and heat exposure, which can make symptoms worse. Medications such as neostigmine (Prostigmin) and pyridostigmine (Mestinon) can help with the neuromuscular communication process. **Immunosuppressants**, including prednisone, azathioprine (Azasan, Imuran), cyclosporine (Neoral, Sandimmune), and mycophenolate (CellCept, Myfortic), may also be used.

Sprains, Strains, and Spasms

A *sprain* is a traumatic injury to a ligament. A sprain can be graded to indicate the severity: grade I for a stretched ligament, grade II for a partial tear, and grade III for a complete tear of the ligament. Sprains of the ankle and wrist are the most common. A *strain* is a tear, partial tear, overuse, or overstretching of a muscle or tendon. A strain can occur suddenly or over time. Hamstring and back muscle strains are common.

Sprains occur when a person overextends or tears a ligament, when stressing a joint. Sprains can occur with sport injuries, falls, and walking on uneven surfaces. Acute strains occur with falling, jumping, and lifting heavy objects. Chronic strains occur with repetitive muscle movements, usually related to one's job or during a sport activity. Poor condition, fatigue, failing to do warm-up exercises, environmental conditions (e.g., ice), and poor equipment are risk factors for sprains and strains. Signs and symptoms of strains and sprains include pain, swelling, and difficulty moving the affected muscle. With sprains, a popping sound may be heard at the time of the injury and bruising may occur later. With strains, muscle spasms may be felt.

During the examination, the provider will check the affected area and the range of motion. X-rays and MRIs may be ordered to rule out other injuries. Treatment includes RICE (*r*est, *i*ce [cold applications], *c*ompression [elastic wraps], and *e*levation) to help minimize the swelling. NSAIDs and analgesics may be taken. With severe sprains and strains, a brace or splint may be used to immobilize the area. Surgery may be done to repair a torn ligament or ruptured muscle.

Restless Legs Syndrome

Restless legs syndrome (RLS) is also known as *restless legs syndrome/Willis-Ekborn disease* (RLS/WED). RLS causes a creeping, tingling, or burning sensation in the legs when the person is lying down or sitting. Moving the legs helps reduce the sensations for a short period of time. RLS can affect a person's quality of sleep. Most people with RLS can also have periodic limb movement disorder (PLMD), which causes the legs or arms to twitch or jerk uncontrollably in sleep. RLS can occur at any age and can worsen with age.

In many situations, there is no known cause for RLS. For some people, RLS is caused by a condition (e.g., pregnancy, anemia) or by a medication. Caffeine, alcohol, and tobacco can worsen the symptoms. Researchers believe that RLS may be related to a dopamine imbalance in the brain. There also may be a genetic cause, if the condition appears before age 40. Associated risk factors for RLS include peripheral neuropathy, iron deficiency, kidney failure, and spinal cord lesions. The signs and symptoms include abnormal sensations in the legs and feet that begin after rest (at night) and decrease with movement. The abnormal sensations can be described as itching, electric, aching, throbbing, pulling, crawling, or creeping. The symptoms may disappear for a while and then come back.

Besides an examination, the provider may order blood tests and a sleep study. Treatments include exercise and massage of the legs, stress reduction activities, and decreased caffeine and tobacco use. Medication therapy may include iron for anemia and medications to increase the dopamine in the brain, including ropinirole (Requip), pramipexole (Mirapex), and rotigotine (Neupro). Opioids and anticonvulsants, such as gabapentin (Neurontin, Horizant) and pregabalin (Lyrica), and clonazepam (Klonopin), may be used.

Additional Musculoskeletal System Diseases

There are many musculoskeletal diseases, including:

- *Adhesive capsulitis*: Also known as *frozen shoulder;* the movement in the shoulder is limited due to inflammation of the shoulder joint capsule.
- *Bunion*: An abnormal enlargement of the first metatarsophalangeal joint of the great toe, caused by inflammation of the synovial bursa. Over time, the enlargement can cause lateral displacement of the toe.
- *Collateral ligament injury*: The medial collateral ligament (MCL) runs along the inside of the knee, and the lateral collateral ligament (LCL) runs along the outside of the knee. When one or both ligaments are stretched or torn, the knee becomes unstable.
- *Contracture*: Occurs when the normal tissue is replaced with a nonstretchy fiber-like tissue and can affect the skin, muscles, ligaments, and tendons. The affected joint can have limited range of motion. Can be related to disorders (e.g., cerebral palsy, stroke), nerve damage, scarring, and reduced use of the joint.
- *Cruciate ligament injury*: The anterior cruciate ligament (ACL) is in the middle of the knee and works with the posterior cruciate ligament (PCL). When one or both ligaments are stretched or torn, the knee becomes unstable.
- *Cubital tunnel syndrome*: Pressure or stretching of the ulnar nerve causes numbness and tingling of the ring and small fingers, forearm pain, and hand weakness.
- *Hammertoe*: An abnormal bend in the middle joint of the second, third, or fourth toe.
- *Impingement syndrome*: Also called *swimmer's shoulder* and *pitcher's shoulder;* a group of symptoms, including impaired movement and progressive shoulder pain, caused by inflammation or injury to the rotator cuff and surrounding structures.
- *Lateral epicondylitis*: Also called *tennis elbow;* repeated use of the elbow causes small tears in the tendon, resulting in pain on the lateral side of the upper arm near the elbow.
- *Medial epicondylitis*: Also called *golfer's elbow* or *baseball elbow;* repeated use of the elbow causes small tears in the tendon, resulting in pain on the inside of the lower arm near the elbow.
- *Osteomyelitis*: A bacterial or fungal infection that comes from the bloodstream, surgery, or an injury. Signs and symptoms include chills, fever, and the infected area can be painful, warm, red, and swollen. Antibiotics and surgery if needed to remove dead bone tissue can be done to treat the infection.
- *Osteosarcoma*: Most common bone cancer in children. Usually found in large bones, although it can occur in any bone.

- *Polydactyly*: Often a genetic condition in which a person has more than five toes per foot or five fingers per hand. The extra digit is often poorly formed and is surgically removed.
- *Spina bifida occulta*: Mildest form; no spinal nerves are involved, but one or more vertebrae are malformed. No signs or symptoms may be present. The only indication may be an abnormal cluster of hair, a small dimple, or birthmark on the infant's back.
- *Spondylolisthesis*: A forward displacement of a vertebra over the one below it. Usually occurs in the lumbar or sacral area. Can be related to a birth defect or an acute trauma.
- *Syndactyly*: The digits (fingers and toes) are fused together or are webbed together. Most commonly seen with the second and third toes.
- *Talipes (clubfoot)*: Most common congenital disorder of the legs. One foot or both feet are turned inward and downward. The calf and foot may be slightly smaller. Treatment depends on the severity and can range from stretching, casting, braces, and surgery.
- *Torn meniscus*: The meniscus in the knee joint tears, causing pain, swelling, and locking of the knee.
- *Torticollis*: The neck muscles cause the head to turn or rotate to the side. The can be a genetic condition or can relate to a nervous or musculoskeletal problem.

THE MEDICAL ASSISTANT'S ROLE IN ORTHOPEDICS AND RHEUMATOLOGY PROCEDURES

Assisting With the Examination

When the medical assistant gathers a medical history on a patient with a musculoskeletal concern, it is important to ask about the symptoms, their onset, and what reduces or increases the symptoms, in addition to assessing the pain level. The medical assistant can ask the patient to rate the pain using a 0 to 10 scale. Zero is no pain, and 10 is the worst pain ever. Another pain assessment tool is the Wong-Baker FACES Pain Rating Scale, which is described in Chapter 15. The medical assistant should explain the scale to patients, and then patients can state how they feel. This scale works well for children. The healthcare facility may also require a functional assessment to be done, which gathers information on the patient's mobility and ability to do activities of daily living (ADLs) (e.g., toileting, bathing, grooming, and eating).

Assist the patient into a comfortable position by offering a pillow or folded blanket to support the painful or injured body part. For recent injuries, if ordered by providers, apply a cold application to the injured area. This procedure will be discussed later in the chapter.

Patients may have limited mobility because of pain. The medical assistant may need to help patients change into the examination gown. Make sure the patient is warm enough by offering an additional sheet or blanket. Explain clearly what is happening and what the patient can expect.

During the exam, the provider may use inspection, palpation, ROM testing, and muscle testing to examine the major skeletal muscles and joints. Many times, the unaffected side is examined first and compared to the affected side. The provider may compare the size, position, and strength of the extremities. Depending on the concern, the provider may also perform a gait analysis, which means the provider observes the patient walking. Gait abnormalities may be the cause or the result of different musculoskeletal conditions.

If the medical assistant is in the room for the exam, he or she may be responsible for taking notes, keeping the patient properly draped, and assisting by handing equipment to the provider. Always keep patient safety in mind, especially when the patient is transferring onto and off the exam table and changing positions.

Assisting With Diagnostic Procedures

The medical assistant assists with diagnostic procedures by scheduling and preparing patients for procedures. If tests require restrictions of food or fluids, the medical assistant should address the following points with the patient after talking with the provider:

- Can the patient have water prior to the test
- Which medications should the patient take prior to the test, or when can the patient resume the current medications

Table 20.5 describes common diagnostic procedures used for musculoskeletal conditions. The medical assistant may need to screen the patient for specific allergies, medications, and so on prior to scheduling the procedure. For some procedures, a signed consent

TABLE 20.5	Diagnostic Procedures for Musculoskeletal Conditions	
PROCEDURE	**DESCRIPTION**	**PATIENT PREPARATION**
Arthrogram	Provides visualization of the soft tissues in the joint (e.g., tendons, ligaments, cartilage). A series of x-rays are taken of a joint after a contrast medium (e.g., dye) is injected into the joint.	Screen for pregnancy, **anticoagulant** use, and for allergy to contrast medium (iodine) or other medications used. Sign a consent form. Patient may feel a sting when the medication is given. After the test, mild pain and swelling in the joint area may occur. Ice and analgesics are typically ordered.
Bone scan	Imaging test used to diagnose bone disease, tumor, or cancer. A small amount of radiotracer is injected into the vein and collects in the bones and organs. A camera slowly scans the body and takes pictures of the radiotracer that collects in the bones.	Screen for pregnancy. Patient should not take any medication with bismuth (e.g., Pepto-Bismol) for 4 days before the test. Have the patient remove all metal items (e.g., jewelry). A small amount of pain is felt when the needle is inserted. The scan is painless. Depending on the condition, an initial scan may be done as the radiotracer is injected and then in 3 to 4 hours after the radiotracer has collected in the bone.
Computed tomography (CT, CT scan)	Used to detect fractures, tumors, and other abnormalities. This imaging test takes cross-sectional pictures of the body. Contrast medium may be used.	Screen for pregnancy and for allergy to contrast medium (iodine). Patient should not eat or drink for 4–6 hours prior to the test if a contrast medium is used. Have the patient remove all metal items (e.g., jewelry) and put on a gown. When the contrast medium is given, the person may feel some burning and flushing and may have a metallic taste in the mouth.
Dual-energy x-ray absorptiometry (DEXA) scan	A bone density test used to measure the calcium and other minerals in the bone. Central DEXA requires the scanner to pass over the spine and hip. Peripheral DEXA measures the bone density in the wrist, fingers, legs, or heels.	Screen for pregnancy. Patient should not take calcium supplements for 24 hours before the test. Have the patient remove all metal items (e.g., jewelry). Test is painless. The test results are reported as a T-score (compares the bone density to that of a healthy woman) and Z-score (compares the bone density to other people of the same age, gender, and race).
Electromyography (EMG)	Checks the nerves and muscles. Thin needle electrodes are inserted through the skin into the muscle and picks up the electrical activity in the muscle.	Screen for anticoagulant use. No special preparation is required. The person may feel a little pain when the needles are inserted. The site may be tender or bruised for a few days after the test.
Myelogram	Uses fluoroscopy and contrast medium to evaluate the spinal cord and related structures.	Screen patient for pregnancy and allergy to iodine contrast medium. Anticoagulants should be stopped several days before the test. Patient may have food and liquid restrictions prior to the test. Patient will feel a brief sting when the medication is given. The table is moved into different positions as the images are taken.
Nerve conduction velocity (NCV)	Used with an EMG to test the speed of electrical signals through a nerve. Electrodes are placed on the skin. Each electrode gives off a mild electrical impulse that stimulates the nerve.	Screen the patient for a cardiac defibrillator or pacemaker. Patient should not wear lotion, perfume, or moisturizer. The impulse will feel like a small electric shock.

TABLE 20.6   Medical Laboratory Tests for Musculoskeletal Conditions

TERM	DEFINITION
C-reactive protein (CRP)	Blood test; some are CLIA-waived tests. CRP is produced by the liver and increases with inflammation. The CRP is a nonspecific indicator of inflammation.
Erythrocyte sedimentation rate (ESR)	CLIA-waived blood test. Measures how quickly the red blood cells (RBCs) in a blood sample settle to the bottom of the test tube. The quicker they settle, the more it indicates inflammation in the body. The ESR is a nonspecific indicator of inflammation.
Lyme disease blood antibodies	Blood or cerebrospinal fluid test; some are CLIA-waived tests. Also called Lyme Antibodies IgM/IgG by Western Blot. Test looks for antibodies to *Borrelia*, which causes Lyme disease.
Rheumatoid factor (RF) test	Blood test; some are CLIA-waived tests. Looks for RF present in the blood.

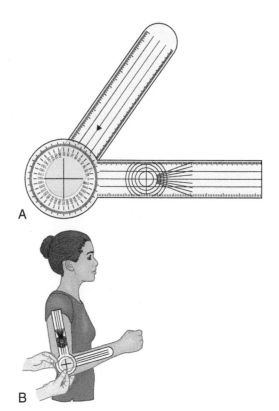

FIGURE 20.13 **(A)** Goniometer. **(B)** Correct position of the goniometer on the arm.

form is required. The patient should be notified of what he or she will experience during the procedure and any follow-up care required after the test. Table 20.6 lists common laboratory tests used for musculoskeletal conditions.

CRITICAL THINKING APPLICATION   **20.9**

As Dr. Kahn finishes his exam with Walter, he asks Suzanne to join them as they discuss Walter's test results. Dr. Kahn ordered an RF test, Lyme disease antibody test, ESR, and C-reactive protein (CRP) through the clinical laboratory. He also ordered a series of hand x-rays and knee x-rays. What information will each of the lab tests give Dr. Kahn? What will the x-rays of the hands and knees show him?

Range of Motion Measurement

Often orthopedic injuries severely affect the normal ROM of a joint. Measuring the ROM of specific joints is an objective measure of both the seriousness of an injury and the recovery progress. The joint may be evaluated with active and passive ROM. To determine the active ROM of a joint, the patient is asked to move the joint as far as possible. For evaluation of passive ROM, the provider moves the joint as far as possible.

A goniometer is the most common tool used to measure the ROM of a joint. Goniometers have calibration markings to indicate the measurement. A goniometer has two arms that are fixed together with a hinge joint at one end (Fig. 20.13A). Each of the arms is lined up with a bone on each side of the joint being tested (Fig. 20.13B). The degrees of motion are indicated on a scale on the hinged

center of the nondigital instrument or on the digital display of the digital goniometer. All ROMs are measured in degrees. Usually, pain, tenderness, or **crepitation** is also noted during the procedure.

CRITICAL THINKING APPLICATION   **20.10**

How can Suzanne best assist Dr. Kahn in testing upper extremity ROM in a new patient? What equipment should Suzanne have ready? What patient position would best facilitate this examination? Why?

Muscle Strength Evaluation

During the ROM evaluation, the provider also assesses each muscle group for strength. Normal muscle strength allows for complete voluntary ROM despite resistance. This resistance can be gravity, as when rising from a sitting to a standing position, or physical, as in pulling, pushing, or lifting an object. Muscle strength is bilaterally equal in normal conditions.

Hand grip strength can be measured with a dynamometer (Fig. 20.14). Digital and nondigital dynamometers are available. A dynamometer provides an objective measurement of hand grip strength. The patient holds the dynamometer in the hand being tested. Typically, the arm is at the side of the patient with the elbow bent at 90 degrees. Various arm and hand positions may be used for different assessments. If a dynamometer is not available, a blood pressure cuff can be used (Fig. 20.15).

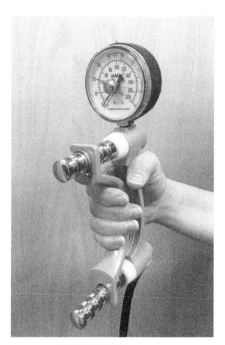

FIGURE 20.14 Dynamometer.

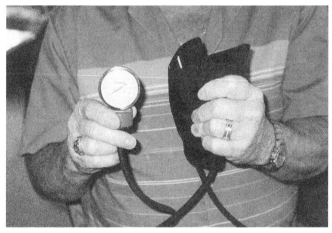

FIGURE 20.15 Assessing grip strength using a blood pressure cuff.

Using a Blood Pressure Cuff to Assess Grip Strength

1. Roll up an aneroid blood pressure cuff and have the patient hold it in one hand.
2. Inflate the cuff to 20 mm Hg of pressure and lock the valve.
3. Ask the patient to squeeze the cuff as tightly as possible.
4. Note the increase in pressure on the dial (a normal grip registers above 150 mm Hg).
5. Record the hand tested and the results of the test.
6. Repeat on the other hand.

Assisting With Treatments

Patients with orthopedic and rheumatology conditions are prescribed a variety of medications. The following are some of the more common classifications of medications for the orthopedic and rheumatology specialties:

- *Analgesics*: Relieve pain
- *Anticonvulsants*: Treat neuromuscular disorders and epilepsy
- *Antigout medications*: Treat gout
- *Anti-inflammatories*: Treat arthritis and other inflammatory disorders
- *Corticosteroids*: Treat chronic inflammatory diseases (e.g.,arthritis)
- *Muscle relaxants*: Treat painful musculoskeletal conditions (e.g., strains, sprains, and muscle injuries)
- *Osteoporosis agents*: Promote bone mineral density and reverse the progression of osteoporosis
- *Tumor necrosis factor (TNF) inhibitors:* Treat autoimmune disorders (e.g., rheumatoid arthritis)

Refer to Table 20.7 for information on the medication classification, including indications for use, desired effect, side effects, adverse reactions, and generic and trade names. Medical assistants should be familiar with medications that are prescribed to patients.

Casts and Splints

Splints and casts are applied to immobilize joints and bones after injury or surgery. A *splint* consists of a strip of rigid material that immobilizes an extremity. It provides partial protection while the site heals. The splint can be adjusted as the swelling changes. Ready-made splints and custom-designed splints are used in the ambulatory care environment. Ready-made splints usually have Velcro straps, which assist when taking off or putting on the splints. Custom-designed splints are used with elastic bandages. Casts provide additional protection to the injured area.

Casts are made from fiberglass or plaster. Fiberglass casts can be colorful, lightweight, durable, and porous. Fiberglass casts do not need to be removed during x-rays. Plaster casts are cheaper and easier to shape. The medical assistant can help the provider apply the cast and the custom-designed splints (see Procedure 20.1, p. 519). The medical assistant can remove casts (see Procedure 20.2, p. 521).

The medical assistant needs to provide cast care instructions to patients. It is important to teach patients about checking the **c**olor, **s**ensation, **m**otion, and **t**emperature (CSMT) of the casted extremity. Table 20.8 describes normal and abnormal CSMT findings. Any suspicious abnormal findings should be reported to the provider immediately.

Patient Education for Cast Care

- For a recent injury, elevate and ice the extremity to minimize swelling. Increased swelling can lead to **compartment syndrome**, damaging muscles, blood vessels, and nerves.
- Cover the cast with a plastic bag prior to bathing or showering. If the cast gets wet, use a hair dryer on a cool setting to dry a fiberglass cast. If the cast does not dry or if it becomes smelly or moldy, contact the provider.
- Avoid putting weight or pressure on the cast.
- Do not put anything inside the cast, including sharp objects, powder, or lotion.
- A metal file can be used to smooth down rough sections of a fiberglass cast.
- A sling can be used to help support a casted arm.

TABLE 20.7   Medication Classifications

CLASSIFICATION	INFORMATION	GENERIC NAME (TRADE NAME)
Analgesics	**Indications for use:** Relieve pain. **Desired effects:** Reduce the sensory function of the brain; block pain receptors. **Side effects and adverse reactions:** *Nonnarcotic:* GI distress, liver and kidney disorders, and tinnitus. *Narcotic:* hypotension, decreased respirations, agitation, blurred vision, confusion, constipation, sedation, restlessness.	***Nonnarcotic over-the-counter (OTCs):*** • **aspirin** (Ecotrin, Bayer Aspirin, Bufferin) • **acetaminophen** (Tylenol, Tempra) • **ibuprofen** (Advil, Motrin) ***Narcotic (opioids):*** • **oxycodone** (OxyContin) • **hydrocodone with acetaminophen** (Lortab, Norco, Vicodin) • **oxycodone with acetaminophen** (Percocet, Oxycet, Roxicet) • **tramadol** (Ultram, Conzip)
Anticonvulsants and Mood Stabilizer	**Indications for use:** Treat epilepsy, trigeminal neuralgia, mania and mixed episodes (mania and depression) with bipolar disorder **Desired effects:** Reduce the frequency and severity of seizures by reducing excessive stimulation of the brain. **Side effects and adverse reactions:** Sedation, vertigo, visual disturbances, GI disturbances, liver complications.	• **carbamazepine** (Tegretol, Equetro) • **lamotrigine** (Lamictal) • **topiramate** (Topamax) • **valproic acid** (Depakene, Depakote) • **gabapentin** (Neurontin, Horizant)
Antigout	**Indications for use:** Gout **Desired effects:** Reduce the uric acid in the body. **Side effects and adverse reactions:** GI distress, eye irritation, itching, rash, blood in urine.	• **allopurinol** (Zyloprim, Aloprim) • **febuxostat** (Uloric)
Anti-inflammatories	**Indications for use:** Treat arthritis and other inflammatory disorders (e.g., allergic rhinitis). **Desired effect:** Reduce inflammation. **Side effects and adverse reactions:** GI distress, GI bleeding, hepatitis, drowsiness, tinnitus, irregular heart rate, kidney disorders.	***Nonsteroidal anti-inflammatory drugs (NSAIDs):*** • **Ibuprofen** (Advil, Motrin, Midol) • **naproxen** (Naprosyn) • **meloxicam** (Mobic) ***Steroidal:*** • *See* Corticosteroids *(oral)*
Corticosteroids (oral)	**Indications for use:** Used to treat chronic inflammatory diseases (e.g., arthritis) and acute conditions (e.g., poison ivy, asthma). **Desired effects:** Reduce inflammation. **Side effects and adverse reactions:** Headache, mood changes, difficulty falling asleep or staying asleep, increased sweating, vision problems, depression, and weight gain.	• **prednisone** (Prednisone Intensol, Sterapred) • **prednisolone** (Flo-Pred, Orapred, Pediapred) • **methylprednisolone** (Medrol)
Muscle Relaxants	**Indications for use:** Painful musculoskeletal conditions (e.g., strains, sprains, muscle injuries) **Desired effect:** Decreases pain **Side effects and adverse reactions:** drowsiness, clumsiness, tachycardia, GI intolerance, difficulty breathing, fever, weakness, burning in the eyes, seizures	• **carisoprodol** (Soma) • **cyclobenzaprine** (Flexeril)
Osteoporosis agents	**Indications for use:** Promote bone mineral density and reverse progression of osteoporosis. **Desired effects:** Inhibit bone reabsorption and/or promote use of calcium. **Side effects and adverse reactions:** GI disorders, esophageal irritation.	• **alendronate** (Fosamax, Binosto) • **risedronate** (Actonel, Atelvia) • **ibandronate** (Boniva) • **raloxifene** (Evista)

TABLE 20.7   Medication Classifications—*continued*

CLASSIFICATION	INFORMATION	GENERIC NAME (TRADE NAME)
Tumor-necrosis factor (TNF) inhibitors	**Indications for use:** Autoimmune disorders (e.g., rheumatoid arthritis) **Desired effect:** Blocks the action of TNF, preventing inflammation. **Side effects and adverse reactions:** GI distress, weakness, seizures, bleeding	• **infliximab** (Remicade) • **etanercept** (Enbrel)

TABLE 20.8   CSMT Normal and Abnormal Findings

	NORMAL	ABNORMAL
Color	Color of extremity and nail beds should match the opposite extremity. Should be pink.	Pale or bluish skin.
Sensation	Normal sensation. Should be able to feel light touch on the fingers or toes.	Increased pain, burning, or stinging; "asleep" feeling or pins-and-needles sensation or numbness. Unable to feel light touch.
Motion	Movement of toes and fingers is normal. There should be no swelling.	Unable to move toes or fingers on the casted side. Swelling on injured side.
Temperature	Temperature matches the opposite extremity. Should be warm.	Cold or cooler than the opposite extremity.

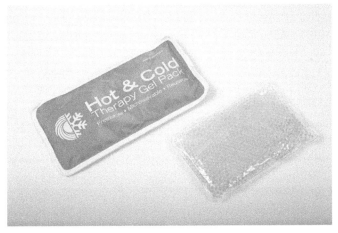

FIGURE 20.16 Many gel packs and bead packs are used for hot and cold therapy.

Cold and Hot Therapies

Cold and hot therapeutic modalities or treatments are used for orthopedic injuries and infections (Fig. 20.16). The applications can be dry or moist. Dry means no moisture is left on the skin; moist means moisture is left on the skin. Dry applications tend to pull moisture out of the skin. Moist applications tend to increase tissue elasticity and allow heat or cold to penetrate deeper into the tissues.

In some facilities, it is a common practice to provide a cold pack to a patient who comes in with a recent injury. When using hot or cold applications, the medical assistant should ask the patient if it feels too hot or too cold. The medical assistant should monitor the

area being treated. Some patients are at higher risk for tissue injury with hot or cold applications:

- Younger children because of their thinner skin
- Older adults due to their reduced sensitivity to pain
- People with impaired circulation (e.g., those with peripheral vascular diseases and diabetes mellitus)
- People with altered sensitivity (e.g., those who are confused or have neurologic disorders, including diabetic neuropathy and spinal cord damage)
- Those for whom the application is placed on an open wound, broken skin, or **stoma** (this tissue is more sensitive)
- Those for whom the application is placed on edematous or scarred areas (scars and edema reduce sensitivity)

Patient Education for Hot and Cold Applications

- Know what supplies are required and where they can be purchased.
- Use a protective covering between the skin and the application.
- Never fall asleep with an application on the skin.
- Never place an application over metal jewelry.
- Know the length of time for each application, the number of times a day ordered, and the number of days for treatment.
- Hot and cold therapy should be applied for 15 to 20 minutes. Additional time can harm the tissues.
- After the session, remove the application. Allow the skin to return to the normal temperature before applying again.
- Prolonged erythema or paleness, pain, swelling, and blisters should be reported to the provider.

Cold Therapy. Cold therapy is typically used for sprains, strains, fractures, joint injuries, shin splints, and other injuries. A cold application causes **vasoconstriction**, which reduces blood flow to the area. As a result, tissue metabolism decreases, less oxygen is used, and less waste accumulates. The nerve endings in the area become numb. The blood viscosity increases, which can cause clotting. Cold therapy helps to reduce pain and inflammation and prevents *edema* (swelling) in the area. Table 20.9 describes common types of cold applications. Procedure 20.3 on p. 522 describes how to apply a cold pack.

Heat Therapy. Heat therapy can be used to relieve:

- Acute pain (e.g., back and menstrual) and chronic pain (e.g., arthritis)
- Sinus congestion
- Infection (e.g., localized abscesses)

Heat therapy can help with muscle relaxation. It can produce local vasodilation, which increases circulation. The increased blood supply to a local area helps to absorb the extra fluid (from edema). Table 20.10 discusses the types of hot applications. Additional types of heat therapy will be discussed. Procedure 20.4 on p. 522 describes how to apply a hot pack.

Paraffin Bath Therapy. Paraffin provides deep heat therapy. The heat can reduce pain and tenderness. It has been found to maintain muscle strength and increase mobility. Paraffin therapy is a common treatment for arthritis and other conditions that cause pain and stiffness.

A paraffin bath uses melted paraffin and mineral oil warmed to about 125°F. The patient bathes a foot or hand in the bath. Once the extremity is coated, the patient should lift it out and let it dry for a few seconds (Fig. 20.17). This process is repeated until the patient has 10 to 12 layers of wax built up on the extremity. The foot or hand is wrapped in plastic and then in a towel to retain the moisture and heat. After 20 minutes, it is unwrapped and the wax is removed.

CRITICAL THINKING APPLICATION   **20.11**

Suzanne is helping a 56-year-old male patient with RA who is receiving a paraffin bath treatment for both hands. She did not check the temperature before having the patient put his hands in the bath, and when he puts his hands in, he immediately pulls them out and complains that it is too hot. How should Suzanne handle this situation? What should she say to the patient? What steps should she take to prevent this from occurring with another patient?

TABLE 20.9	Types of Cold Applications		
TYPE	**DRY OR MOIST**	**DESCRIPTION**	**USES**
Cold compress	Moist	Washcloth or other soft cloth is dampened with a cold solution (e.g., water) and applied to the skin.	Usually used on the face and forehead for discomfort and pain.
Chemical cold pack	Dry	Comes in a variety of sizes. Stored at room temperature. Contains inner areas of a dry chemical and water. When activated, the water and chemical mix creates coldness.	Used to reduce inflammation, prevent edema, reduce bleeding, and decrease pain. A towel or protective covering needs to be placed between the skin and the pack or bag. This protects the skin from a burn or from the cold.
Ice bag	Dry	A bag with cubes or pieces of ice.	
Gel pack	Dry	Aqueous gel that freezes. Reusable. Stored in freezer.	
Bead pack	Dry	Little beads of gel conform to the site even when frozen. Similar to a frozen bag of peas. Reusable. Stored in freezer.	

TABLE 20.10	Types of Hot Applications		
TYPE	**DRY OR MOIST**	**DESCRIPTION**	**USES**
Hot soak/whirlpool bath	Moist	Part of the body is submerged in warm water or a warm medicated solution. Should be warmed to 105°F–110°F.	Used to cleanse wounds. Helps to ease discomfort.
Hot compress	Moist	Washcloth or other soft cloth is dampened with a hot solution (e.g., water) and applied to the skin.	Can be used on many places on the body, including the face and eyes.
Heating pad	Dry	Electric pad that warms. Inspect for safety purposes.	Used for spasms and pain. Must be covered with a towel or protective covering.
Chemical hot pack	Dry	Comes in a variety of sizes. Stored at room temperature. Contains inner areas of a dry chemical and water. When activated, the water and chemical mix, creating heat for a period of time.	
Gel pack	Dry	Aqueous gel that can be microwaved. Reusable.	
Bead pack	Dry	Little beads of gel that can be microwaved. Reusable.	

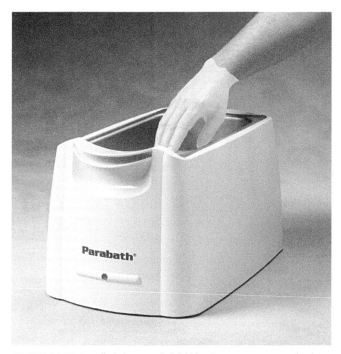

FIGURE 20.17 A paraffin bath is especially helpful for relieving pain in patients with arthritis.

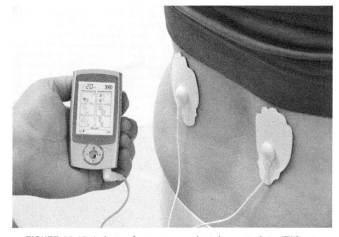

FIGURE 20.18 Application of a transcutaneous electrical nerve stimulation (TENS) unit.

Heat Lamp Therapy. Two commonly used heat lamp therapies include red light therapy and near infrared light therapy. Red light therapy is used to treat skin conditions. Near infrared light therapy penetrates deeper, killing pathogens, healing tissue, improving circulation, and relieving pain.

Ultrasound Therapy. Ultrasound therapy has been used for a long time to treat pain and promote healing. The ultrasound transducer head produces sound waves. Ultrasound gel is applied to the skin. As the transducer head is moved over the skin, the gel helps with the transmission of sound waves into the soft tissue. There are two main types of ultrasound therapy: thermal and mechanical. The main difference between these types is the speed at which the sound waves penetrate the soft tissue. Ultrasound therapy must be done by a trained therapist. This treatment is often provided in chiropractic, sports medicine, physical therapy, and occupational therapy facilities.

RICE Therapy

For orthopedic injuries, RICE is commonly ordered as a treatment for usually the first 48 to 72 hours. After 72 hours, moist heat is prescribed. RICE stands for rest, ice, compression, and elevation:

- **R**est: Reduce activities for a period of time. Crutches can help an injured leg/ankle rest.
- **I**ce: Apply a cold pack to the injured area for 15 to 20 minutes, 4 to 8 times daily. Always use a protective covering between the cold pack and the skin to prevent a cold injury or frostbite.
- **C**ompression: Use elastic wraps or splints to reduce swelling. It is important to monitor the CSMT of a wrapped extremity.
- **E**levation: Elevate the injured extremity higher than the level of the heart to help reduce swelling.

Exercise Therapy

Often patients are encouraged to exercise to maintain their strength and joint mobility. Patients recovering from surgery (e.g., orthopedic, cardiac) may need to see a physical therapist or an occupational therapist. These therapists work with patients to help them regain their mobility and strength. Isometric, isotonic, and range of motion exercises are encouraged to maintain strength, flexibility, and mobility.

Isometric contractions do not change the muscle length, but they do increase the muscle tension. Isometric exercises help to maintain a person's strength. Isotonic contractions cause movement at a joint. Isotonic exercises help restore movement after an injury and relieve stiffness and pain. ROM exercises help to maintain flexibility and joint mobility and reduce stiffness. *Active ROM exercises* are done by the patient, whereas *passive ROM exercises* are done by a caregiver or therapist. For patients who have had a stroke or other trauma that affects movement, daily ROM exercises are critical to prevent joints from freezing up. Frozen joints have limited to no movement.

Electrical Muscle Stimulation

A transcutaneous electrical nerve stimulation (TENS) unit is used for pain relief (Fig. 20.18). **Electrodes** are placed on the skin in specific locations. The adjustable low-voltage machine sends electrical current through disposable gel electrodes into the skin. The current stimulates specific nerves, producing a tingling or massaging sensation that reduces pain. TENS units have been used for passive exercise of muscles when a patient cannot exercise the extremity (e.g., due to injury or stroke). The electrical stimulation can prevent atrophy of normal muscles. TENS units are also used to treat the pain from muscle, joint, or other orthopedic conditions.

Assistive Devices

An *assistive device* is used to help a person perform a specific task, such as walking. Crutches, walkers, canes, and wheelchairs are considered assistive devices. Many times, these assistive devices can be purchased at pharmacies and medical supply stores. The medical assistant should know how to adjust the device to fit the patient. Medical assistants may also coach patients on the proper use of the assistive device. Improper use of assistive devices can lead to falls and injuries.

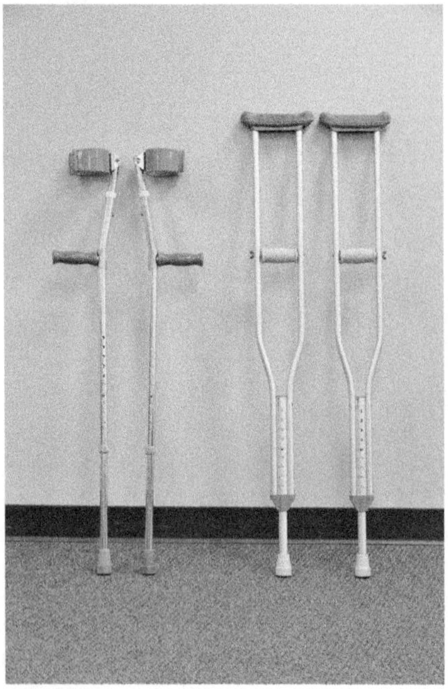

FIGURE 20.19 Forearm crutches *(left)* and axillary crutches *(right)*.

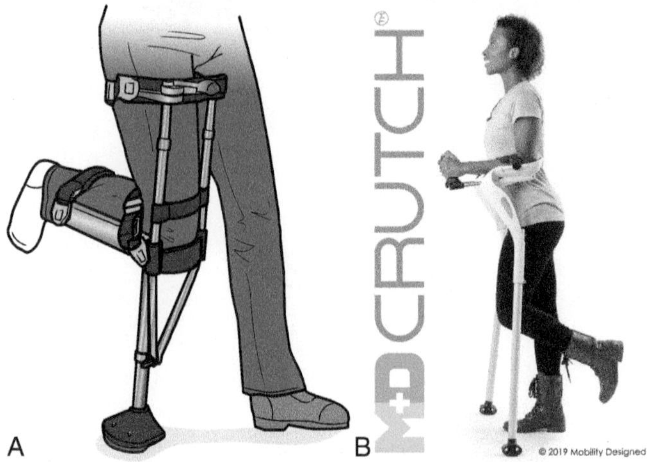

FIGURE 20.20 (A) Hands-free crutch. **(B)** M+D crutches by Mobility Designed, Inc. (Courtesy of Mobility Designed, Inc.)

CRITICAL THINKING APPLICATION 20.12

Suzanne has had to teach patients about assistive devices. She discusses ways to prevent falls and how to transfer between different positions. Why are both of these topics important to address?

Crutches. Crutches are used to help a person walk. Crutches can be made out of aluminum or wood and can be adjusted for the patient. The more common crutches include:

- *Axillary crutches*: Most common type; used when recovering from a foot, ankle, or leg injury or surgery (Fig. 20.19).
- *Forearm crutches*: Also called *Lofstrand* or *elbow crutches;* require more upper body strength. An open elbow cuff fits around the patient's forearm (see Fig. 20.19). These crutches help with proper posture and body mechanics.
- *Extension crutches*: Also called *Canadian crutches.* These combine the underarm crutch with an elbow cuff, which provides extra support for the patient.
- *Platform crutches*: Also called triceps crutches. They have padded armrests with handgrips. These crutches are used when patients cannot straighten their arms to hold the handgrip of the crutch.
- *Hands-free crutch*: Straps to the thigh and a platform supports the lower leg (Fig. 20.20A).
- *M+D crutches*: The hinged arm cradles the strap to the forearms, thus eliminating pressure in the axillae, wrists, and hands (Fig. 20.20B).

Axillary crutches need to be fitted correctly to allow for good body mechanics and to reduce the risk of injury. *Crutch palsy* can occur with poorly fitted crutches or if the patient rests on the top of the crutches while walking. The axillary nerves can be temporarily or permanently damaged. This can cause loss of hand strength and weakening of the wrist and forearm muscles. When you fit axillary crutches, the patient must be wearing shoes. Have the patient stand straight up. Fit the crutches so they are 1 to 1½ inches (about 2 finger-widths) below the armpit. The crutch should be about 4 to 6 inches to the side and front of each foot. Handgrips must be near the wrist and even with the top of the hip line. When the hands are on the handgrip, the elbow should be bent 15 to 30 degrees.

Providers will indicate the type of crutch, along with any limitations. Common limitations with crutches include:

- *Weight bearing as tolerated*: Patients can place more than half of their body weight on their "bad" or affected extremity if it is not painful.
- *Partial weight bearing*: The provider will indicate how much weight can be placed on the affected extremity.
- *Toe-touch weight bearing*: Patients can touch the ground with their toes on the affected side. The toe-touch helps with balance. No weight bearing is allowed on the affected extremity.
- *Non–weight bearing*: Patients cannot put weight on their affected extremity. This type of limitation would require the three-point crutch gait.

There are several *gaits,* or ways to walk, with crutches. The provider may also order the gait. The gait depends on whether the patient can put weight on the affected extremity. The following are common gaits.

- *Two-point crutch gait*: Mimics normal walking. The patient must be able to put some weight on both legs. From the **tripod position** (starting position) use this sequence: Move the right crutch with left foot forward and then move the left crutch with the right foot forward. There are two individual movements with this gait. Repeat this pattern (Fig. 20.21A).
- *Four-point crutch gait*: Must be able to put some weight on both legs. This gait is slower, but safer for those with generalized weakness. From the tripod position use this sequence: Move the right crutch forward, then the left foot forward, followed by the left crutch forward, and lastly bring the right foot forward. There are

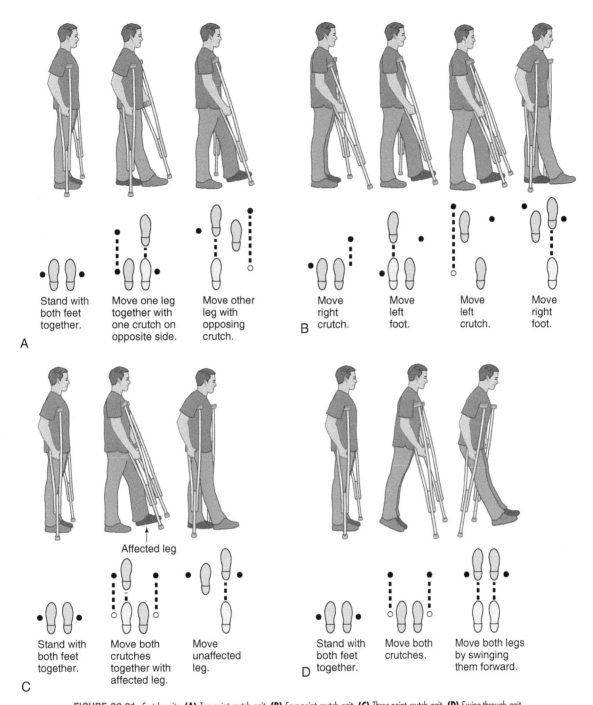

FIGURE 20.21 Crutch gaits. **(A)** Two-point crutch gait. **(B)** Four-point crutch gait. **(C)** Three-point crutch gait. **(D)** Swing-through gait.

four individual movements with this gait. Repeat this pattern (see Fig. 20.21B).

- *Three-point crutch gait:* Used when partial weight bearing or non–weight bearing is indicated. From the tripod position, use this sequence: Move both crutches and the affected leg forward, then move the "good" or unaffected leg forward. Repeat this pattern (see Fig. 20.21C and Procedure 20.5, p. 523).
  - *Swing to crutch gait:* Must be able to put some weight on both legs. From the tripod position, use this sequence: Move both crutches forward, then swing the body so the feet are *even with* the line of the crutches. Repeat this pattern.

- *Swing-through crutch gait:* Must be able to put some weight on both legs. From the tripod position, use this sequence: Move both crutches forward, then swing the body so the feet land *in front* of the line of the crutches. Repeat this pattern (see Fig. 20.21D).

Walkers. Some patients use walkers after surgery. Many older adults use walkers for help with balance and support. Walkers provide more support than canes. A walker's wide base helps stabilize the gait of the patient and can support up to 50% of the body weight. Walkers have a metal frame and can easily be adjusted to fit an individual. They are lightweight, and several types

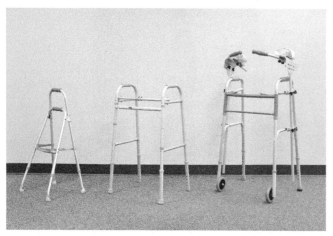

FIGURE 20.22 *Left to right:* Hemi walker, regular walker, and a two-wheel walker with a platform walker attachment. The platform attachment is designed for a patient who has limited strength and cannot grip the walker. An adjustable strap secures the patient's forearm onto the padded section of the attachment.

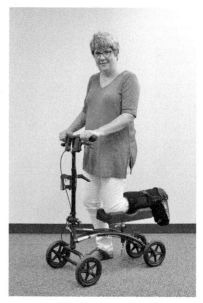

FIGURE 20.23 Knee walker.

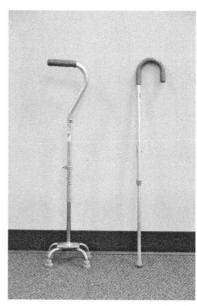

FIGURE 20.24 Four-tipped cane *(left)* and single-tipped cane *(right)*.

can fold flat for storage and travel. Several types of walkers are available:

- *Hemi walker*: Also called a one-hand walker. These walkers are used by patients who can only grasp the walker with one hand due to a stroke or arm/hand amputation (Fig. 20.22).
- *Standard walker*: A very common walker; it has four nonskid, rubber-tipped legs (see Fig. 20.22). A person needs to pick up the walker with every completed step. Sometimes tennis balls are inserted over the feet to help to move the walker easily across the floor.
- *Two-wheel walker*: Resembles the standard walker, but the front two legs have wheels. This type of walker is for those who need some help but not constant weight-bearing help (see Fig. 20.22).
- *Three-wheel walker* and *four-wheel walker*: Also called a *Rollator*. Each leg has a wheel, and many Rollators have brakes by the handles. Some models have a seat and a basket. These walkers are for people who do not need to lean on a walker for balance.
- *Knee walker*: A foot-propelled scooter that has platform to rest a knee and lower leg (Fig. 20.23). This is commonly used instead of axillary crutches for leg or foot conditions.

When you fit a walker, the patient must be wearing shoes. Have the patient step into the walker and relax the arms at the sides of the body. The top of the walker grip should be near the crease in the wrist and even with the top of the hip line. With the shoulders relaxed and the hands on the grips, the elbows should be bent 15 degrees. Procedure 20.6 on p. 525 discusses fitting a walker and coaching a patient to use a walker.

Canes. A cane can provide extra assistance for a person who has a minor balance or stability problem. There are two basic types of canes but several different grips or handles. The basic types of canes are:

- *Single-tipped cane*: Provides minimal assistance with walking (Fig. 20.24).
- *Four-tipped cane*: Also called a *quad cane*. It provides greater stability for patients than the single-tipped cane (see Fig. 20.24).

Tingling, numbness, or pain in the hand and fingers may indicate the handle is not appropriate for the person.

When you measure a cane, the patient must be wearing shoes and relax the arms at the sides of the body. The top of the cane should be near the crease in the wrist. With the shoulders relaxed and the hand on the cane, the elbow should be bent 15 degrees. Procedure 20.7 on p. 526 discusses measuring a cane and coaching a patient to use a cane.

Wheelchairs. Wheelchairs provide mobility for patients who cannot walk or who are able to walk only short distances. With a regular wheelchair, the patient uses arm muscles for mobility. Motorized wheelchairs are also available. The patient is referred to a medical equipment store, where the appropriate wheelchair is fitted to the individual. It is important to encourage the patient to always lock the wheels before transferring into and out of a wheelchair.

CLOSING COMMENTS

Patient Coaching

An informed patient is better prepared to continue with home care. Musculoskeletal conditions, particularly arthritis, can be so painful and debilitating that these patients may be easy prey for miracle drug promotions. It is important for you to recognize the need for patient education about the condition and to work diligently with the patient and family to encourage participation in effective care programs. When you work with the provider and the physical therapist in helping the patient, you become an important member of the healthcare team. This type of involvement leads to patient satisfaction and to personal satisfaction and a sense of achievement for the medical assistant.

Legal and Ethical Issues

Working with orthopedic patients may require assisting with assessments and performing procedures that directly involve the patient's recovery plan. Many of the procedures in this chapter are not the basic procedures you will be required to perform when you are first hired as a medical assistant. All of these techniques involve additional on-the-job training and practice. Before performing any of the described procedures, you should check with your local and state medical assistant organizations about the laws in your state. Whenever you perform the procedures and techniques described in this chapter, you are responsible for doing them correctly. The following steps are required before you perform any procedure on a patient:

- You must have a written order from the provider.
- You must follow the procedure precisely as it is ordered, without variation.
- Never advise the patient without permission.
- Make sure you know what instructions the provider gave the patient and reinforce them.
- If you have any concerns about a procedure, discuss them with the provider privately before proceeding.

- Do not perform a procedure if you are uncomfortable; get someone to help you.

Always remember – you are the assistant, and this is the provider's patient. The provider ultimately is responsible for every aspect of the patient's care. Always stay within the legal and ethical guidelines of the medical assisting profession in your state.

Patient-Centered Care

When patients are using assistive devices, falls can occur. The medical assistant should teach patients how to prevent falls when using assistive devices. These instructions should include:

- Wear shoes with rubber or nonskid soles.
- Remove items in the walkway that can cause falls (e.g., throw or loose rugs, cords, and clutter). Small indoor animals may also cause falls if they are near the person's feet.
- Make sure that floors are clean and dry.
- When attempting to sit, back up until the seat touches the back of the legs. With a free hand, grab the seat or armrest and lower yourself into the chair or onto the toilet.
- To stand, scoot forward in the chair and use the free hand to push up from the seat to stand up. Make sure to get your balance before moving.
- Consider adding handrails inside the tub and by the toilet.

Professional Behaviors

Musculoskeletal injuries and disorders are commonplace in the ambulatory care setting. Because of this, patients may ask for your advice on how to manage their health problems. Remember that as the medical assistant you should never diagnose or recommend treatment for a patient. That is the provider's responsibility. Responding professionally to inquiries and offering provider-approved educational materials and websites can be very helpful. Respectful and courteous behavior should be standard practice for a medical assistant when he or she interacts with patients and their families.

SUMMARY OF SCENARIO

Dr. Kahn, Suzanne, and Walter wrap up the appointment. Dr. Kahn has recommended that Walter garden for shorter stretches of time, use a knee cushion when weeding, and take acetaminophen when he needs pain relief. Degenerative joint disease is manageable, and with a few changes in Walter's gardening routine, the prognosis is good. As for the muscle strain that Walter

is feeling in his forearm, that, too, can be managed with muscle rest, ice, and acetaminophen.

Suzanne walks Walter out to the lobby. As she returns to the exam room, she reflects back on 20 years as a medical assistant and is so happy with the choice she made so many years ago.

SUMMARY OF LEARNING OBJECTIVES

1. **List the major structures of the musculoskeletal system and identify the anatomic location of the structures.**
   The musculoskeletal system (MS) consists of bones, joints, muscles, and supportive connective tissues (cartilage, tendons, and ligaments). The human skeleton is composed of more than 200 bones. Bones are divided into two categories – the axial skeleton and the appendicular skeleton. The axial skeletal is made up of the skull, rib cage, spinal column, and the hyoid bone. The appendicular skeleton is made up

   of the shoulders, arms, wrists, pelvic girdle–hip bones, legs, and ankle/feet bones.

2. **Describe the normal function and physiology of the musculoskeletal system.**
   The musculoskeletal system is responsible for the following functions:
   - Posture and body movement
   - Protection, support, and framework for the organ systems of the body

Continued

- Storage for important minerals, such as calcium and phosphorus
- Continually forming new blood cells by the process of hematopoiesis, which occurs in the red bone marrow inside some bones; red blood cells, white blood cells, and platelets are all made in the bone marrow
- Remodeling of the bones

3. **Discuss the diseases and disorders related to the musculoskeletal system. Also:**
   - *Identify the common signs and symptoms of musculoskeletal conditions.*
   Diseases of the musculoskeletal system often affect the ability to move with ease. Common signs and symptoms of musculoskeletal disorders include:
   - Inflammation, pain, or swelling in the joints, muscles, or bones
   - Malaise (generalized weakness or discomfort)
   - Myalgia (muscle pain), myositis (inflammation of a muscle), muscle tenderness
   - Temporary loss of function or loss of normal mobility
   - *Identify the etiologies of common musculoskeletal conditions.*
   Etiologies of musculoskeletal diseases include:
   - Trauma: Fractures, dislocations, subluxation, carpal tunnel syndrome, sprains, strains, and spasms
   - Vitamin and mineral deficiencies: Osteomalacia, rickets, and osteoporosis
   - Genetic and congenital: Lordosis and muscular dystrophy
   - Degeneration with age: Herniated disk and osteoarthritis
   - Unknown: Fibromyalgia, juvenile arthritis, and restless leg syndrome
   - Infection: Lyme disease
   - Autoimmune: Rheumatoid arthritis and myasthenia gravis
   - *Describe diagnostic measures used for the musculoskeletal conditions.*
   Diagnostic procedures used for musculoskeletal conditions include:
   - Arthrogram — x-rays with contrast medium to visualize the soft tissues of the joint
   - Bone scan — imaging test with radiotracer used to diagnose bone disease, tumor, or cancer
   - Computed tomography (CT, CT scan) — imaging test that takes cross-sectional pictures; used to detect fractures, tumors, and other abnormalities
   - Dual-energy x-ray absorptiometry (DEXA) scan — bone density test used for osteoporosis
   - Electromyography (EMG) — insertion of thin needle electrodes into the muscle to check the nerve and muscle responses
   - Myelogram — uses fluoroscopy and contrast medium to evaluate the spinal cord

- Nerve conduction velocity (NCV) — tests the speed of electrical signals through a nerve
- C-reactive protein (CRP) — blood test used as a nonspecific indicator of inflammation
- Erythrocyte sedimentation rate (ESR) — blood test used as a nonspecific indicator of inflammation
- Lyme disease blood antibodies — blood or cerebrospinal fluid test used to detect antibodies to *Borrelia* sp
- Rheumatoid factor (RF) test — blood test that looks for the RF
   - *Identify CLIA-waived tests associated with common musculoskeletal conditions.*
   CLIA-waived tests used for musculoskeletal diseases include the erythrocyte sedimentation rate (ESR), some Lyme disease blood antibodies, rheumatoid factor test, and C-reactive protein (CRP) test.
   - *Describe treatment modalities used for musculoskeletal conditions.*
   Treatment modalities used for musculoskeletal conditions include:
   - Medications: include analgesics, anticonvulsants, antigout drugs, anti-inflammatories, corticosteroids, muscle relaxants, osteoporosis agents, and tumor necrosis factor (TNF) inhibitors
   - Casts and splints: include plaster and fiberglass casts, ready-made splints, and custom-designed splints
   - Cold and hot therapies: include cold therapy (e.g., cold packs), hot therapy (e.g., hot packs), paraffin bath therapy, heat lamp therapy, and ultrasound therapy
   - RICE therapy: rest, ice, compression, and elevation
   - Exercise therapy: includes active and passive range of motion (ROM) exercises
   - Electrical muscle stimulation: used for pain relief
   - Assistive devices: include crutches, canes, walkers, and wheelchairs

4. **Discuss the medical assistant's role in orthopedics and rheumatology procedures and describe topics to address when coaching a patient on cast care, hot and cold applications, and assistive devices.**
   - For cast care, it is important to address how to minimize swelling initially. Other topics for cast care include protecting the cast from moisture, working with the rough sections of the cast, not putting weight on the cast, and not putting anything in the cast.
   - For hot and cold applications, patients need to know where to get the supplies, to always cover the application, and never to fall asleep with the application on. Patients also need the details of the treatment; for instance, the length to apply the application and how many times a day. They should also know when to contact the provider with concerns.
   - For assistive devices, patients need to know how to walk with the devices. They should be taught how walk up and down stairs and move between standing and sitting positions. Discussing safety tips and how to prevent falls is important.

| PROCEDURE 20.1 | Assist With Application of a Cast |

Tasks: To assist the provider in applying a fiberglass cast. Document the procedure in the patient's health record.

Scenario: You are working with Dr. David Kahn, and he needs to apply a fiberglass cast on the left lower leg of Johnny Parker (DOB 06/15/2010). You will assist the provider.

EQUIPMENT and SUPPLIES

- Patient's health record
- Rolls of fiberglass
- Basin for casting material
- Bandage
- Stockinette
- Gloves
- Sheet wadding and/or spongy padding
- Stand to support foot (lower extremity)
- Tape
- Scissors
- 2–3 Towels
- Water
- Cast care instructions (optional)

PROCEDURAL STEPS

1. Wash hands or use hand sanitizer. Assemble the necessary equipment.
   PURPOSE: Hand sanitization is an important step for infection control.

2. Assemble the necessary equipment

3. Greet the patient. Identify yourself. Verify the patient's identity with full name and date of birth. Explain the procedure to be performed in a manner that the patient understands. Answer any questions the patient may have about the procedure.
   PURPOSE: It is important to identify the patient in two different ways to ensure that you have the correct patient. Explaining the procedure can make the patient feel more comfortable and helps to reduce anxiety.

3. Seat the patient comfortably, as directed by the provider. If the cast is being applied to the lower extremity, the toes must be supported by a stand.
   PURPOSE: The amount of flexion of the ankle can be controlled by supporting the toes so that the patient can more easily maintain the desired position without fatigue.

4. Clean the area that the cast will cover. Note any objective signs and ask about subjective symptoms (chart them at the end of the procedure).
   PURPOSE: The condition of the area under the cast must be noted before the cast is applied so that it can be compared with the site when the cast is removed. Clean the area with a mild soap solution or as directed. Dry thoroughly.

5. Cut the stockinette to fit the area the cast will cover. Apply the stockinette smoothly to the area the cast will cover. Leave 1 or 2 inches of excess stockinette above and below the cast area to finish the cast (see the first of the following figures). Excess stockinette may be cut away where wrinkles form, such as at the front of the ankle (see the second of the following figures).

PURPOSE: The stockinette will help protect the skin. Stockinette must lie smoothly and cannot be too bulky or wrinkled because this may cause a pressure wound.

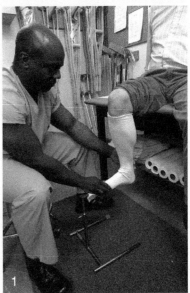

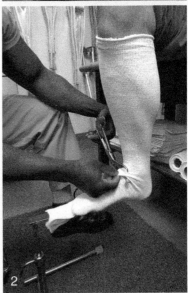

6. Apply sheet wadding along the length of the cast using a spiral bandage turn. Extra padding may be used over bony prominences, such as the bones of the elbow or ankle.
   PURPOSE: Padding the cast helps reduce pressure against bony prominences, which could cause skin breakdown.

7. Put on gloves. With lukewarm water in the basin, wet the fiberglass tape as directed by the provider (see the following figure).

Continued

PROCEDURE 20.1 | **Assist With Application of a Cast**—*continued*

PURPOSE: Immersing the roll of fiberglass tape in water begins the chemical reaction that will cause the cast to harden. The cast can be shaped while wet and will harden in the shape that is formed.

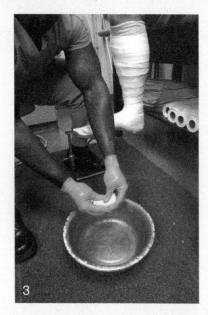

3

8. Assist as directed as the provider applies the inner layer of fiberglass tape. A length of 1 to 2 inches of stockinette is rolled over the inner layer of the cast to form a smooth edge when the outer layer is applied.
9. As directed by the provider, help to open and apply an outer layer of fiberglass tape (shown in the first of the following figures as blue).
10. Help shape the cast as directed. All contours must be smooth (see the second of the following figures).
    PURPOSE: If flat or dented areas develop on the cast, they may cause pressure on the skin below.

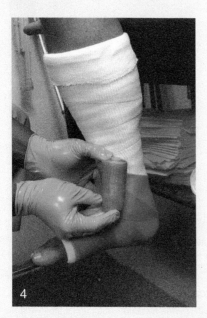

4

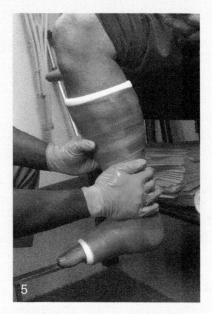

5

11. Discard the water and excess materials. Remove your gloves. Wash hands or use hand sanitizer.
12. Reassure the patient, review cast care verbally, and provide written instructions (optional).
13. Document the procedure in the patient's health record. Include the provider's name, the procedure, what was taught, and how the patient responded.
    PURPOSE: It is important to document the procedure in the health record to show it was done.

07/19/20XX 1005 Assisted Dr. Kahn with fiberglass cast application to left leg. Skin under cast dry and intact. Pt and mother given verbal and written cast care instructions. No questions. Instructed mother to call provider if there is numbness, tingling, swelling of toes, or blue discoloration. Reinforced the need for elevation and ice per Dr. Kahn's order. _____

_____ Suzanne Peterson, CMA (AAMA)

PROCEDURE 20.2 | Assist With Cast Removal

Tasks: To remove a cast. Document the procedure in the patient's health record.

Scenario: You are working with Dr. David Kahn, and he orders removal of the lower left leg cast on Johnny Parker (DOB 06/15/2010).

EQUIPMENT and SUPPLIES

- Patient's health record
- Cast cutter
- Cast spreader
- Large bandage scissors
- Basin of warm water
- Mild soap
- Towel
- Skin lotion

PROCEDURAL STEPS

1. Wash hands or use hand sanitizer. Assemble the necessary equipment.
   PURPOSE: Hand sanitization is an important step for infection control.
2. Greet the patient. Identify yourself. Verify the patient's identity with full name and date of birth. Explain the procedure to be performed in a manner that the patient understands. Answer any questions the patient may have about the procedure.
   PURPOSE: It is important to identify the patient in two different ways to ensure that you have the correct patient. Explaining the procedure can make the patient feel more comfortable and helps to reduce anxiety.
3. Provide adequate support for the limb throughout the procedure. Using the cast cutter, make a cut on the medial and lateral sides of the long axis of the cast (see the following figure).
   PURPOSE: To ensure the patient's comfort.

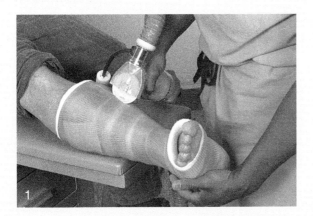

4. Use the cast spreader to pry apart the two halves using the cast spreader (see the following figure). Carefully remove the two parts of the cast. Use the large bandage scissors to cut away the stockinette and padding remaining.
   PURPOSE: A cast spreader is needed to pry apart the cast.

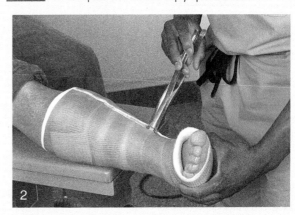

5. Gently wash the area that was covered by the cast with mild soap and warm water. Dry the area and apply a gentle skin lotion.
   PURPOSE: To ensure the patient's comfort.
6. Give the patient appropriate instructions about exercising and using the limb, as directed by the provider.
   PURPOSE: To enhance continued healing, restore lost strength, and prevent injury.
7. Clean up the area. Wash hands or use hand sanitizer.
8. Document the procedure in the patient's health record. Include the provider's name, the procedure, what was taught, and how the patient responded.
   PURPOSE: It is important to document the procedure in the health record to show it was done.

9/10/20XX 1205 Dr. Kahn ordered the left leg fiberglass cast to be removed. Cast removed, skin washed and dried. Lotion applied. Pt and mother instructed on appropriate exercises to do per the provider's order. Questions answered. Encouraged patient's mother to call with concerns. _____
_____ Suzanne Peterson, CMA (AAMA)

PROCEDURE 20.3 | Apply a Cold Pack

Tasks: Apply a cold pack (chemical, gel, or bead) to a body area to reduce pain and prevent further swelling per treatment plan. Document the procedure in the patient's health record.

Scenario: You are working with Dr. David Kahn. Johnny Parker (DOB 06/15/2010) arrives holding his arm and crying. Another medical assistant brings the patient and parent to the exam room. The medical assistant comes out and updates you on Johnny. His parent states that Johnny fell off his bike an hour ago and has since been complaining of pain in his right wrist. The department has a standing order to apply a cold pack to orthopedic injuries if the patient does not arrive with one in place. The medical assistant asks you to apply the cold pack as he completes the vital signs and medical history on Johnny.

EQUIPMENT and SUPPLIES

- Cold pack (chemical, gel, or bead)
- Towel or another type of protective covering for the cold pack
- Provider's order or standing order for orthopedic injuries
- Patient's health record

PROCEDURAL STEPS

1. Wash hands or use hand sanitizer.
   PURPOSE: Hand sanitization is an important step for infection control.
2. Read the standing order or the provider's order. Assemble the equipment. If using a chemical cold pack, activate the pack by squeezing it.
   PURPOSE: It is important to know the provider's order or the standing order before starting the procedure.
3. Greet the patient. Identify yourself. Verify the patient's identity with full name and date of birth. Explain the procedure to be performed in a manner that the patient understands. Answer any questions the patient may have about the procedure.
   PURPOSE: It is important to identify the patient in two different ways to ensure that you have the correct patient. Explaining the procedure can make the patient feel more comfortable and helps to reduce anxiety.
4. Cover the cold pack with a towel or protective covering.
   PURPOSE: The cold pack must never be put directly on the skin. Place a towel or protective covering between the cold pack and the skin to prevent injuries.
5. Assist the patient to position the cold pack over the injured area (see the following figure).
   PURPOSE: Some patients like to place the cold pack themselves on the injured area.

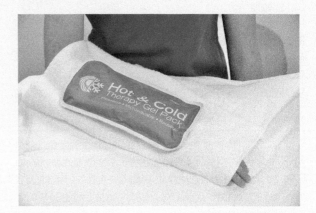

6. Coach patient on the use of a cold pack. Advise the patient to leave the cold pack in place for 15 to 20 minutes or until the area feels numb, whichever comes first. Wash hands or use hand sanitizer.
   PURPOSE: Cold applications are typically applied for 15 to 20 minutes or per the provider's order.
7. Document the procedure in the patient's health record. Include the provider's name, the order, what was taught, and how the patient responded.
   PURPOSE: It is important to document the procedure in the health record to show it was done.
   07/19/20XX 1505 Pt arrived holding right wrist and complaining of pain. Parent stated that he fell off his bike about 1 hour ago. Per Dr. Kahn's standing order, applied cold pack to pt's right wrist. Instructed pt and parent to keep the cold pack (covered with a towel) on the wrist for 15–20 minutes. Parent stated she would remove it at that time._____ Suzanne Peterson, CMA (AAMA)

PROCEDURE 20.4 | Apply a Hot Pack

Tasks: Apply a hot pack (chemical, gel, or bead) to the infected wound. Document the procedure in the patient's health record.

Scenario: Dr. Kahn orders a hot pack to be applied to the wound for 15 minutes and coaching the patient to continue the treatment at home four times a day for the next 3 days.

PROCEDURE 20.4 **Apply a Hot Pack**—*continued*

EQUIPMENT and SUPPLIES

- Hot pack (chemical, gel, or bead)
- Towel or another type of protective covering for the hot pack
- Provider's order
- Patient's health record

PROCEDURAL STEPS

1. Wash hands or use hand sanitizer.
   PURPOSE: Hand sanitization is an important step for infection control.
2. Read the provider's order. Assemble the equipment. If using a chemical hot pack, activate the pack by squeezing it. If pack needs to be warmed, follow the manufacturer's directions.
   PURPOSE: It is important to know the provider's order or the standing order before starting the procedure.
3. Greet the patient. Identify yourself. Verify the patient's identity with full name and date of birth. Explain the procedure to be performed in a manner that the patient understands. Answer any questions the patient may have about the procedure.
   PURPOSE: It is important to identify the patient in two different ways to ensure that you have the correct patient. Explaining the procedure can make the patient feel more comfortable and helps to reduce anxiety.
4. Cover the hot pack with a towel or protective covering.
   PURPOSE: The hot pack must never be put directly on the skin. Place a towel or protective covering between the hot pack and the skin to prevent injuries.

5. Assist the patient to position the hot pack over the covered wound.
   PURPOSE: Some patients like to place the hot pack themselves on the area.
6. Coach the patient on the use of a hot pack. Advise the patient to leave the hot pack in place for 15 minutes per the provider's order or until the area feels warm, whichever comes first. Wash hands or use hand sanitizer.
   PURPOSE: Hot applications are typically applied for 15 to 20 minutes or per the provider's order.
7. Document the procedure in the patient's health record. Include the provider's name, the order, what was taught, and how the patient responded.
   PURPOSE: It is important to document the procedure in the health record to show it was done.
   07/21/20XX 1505 Per Dr. Kahn's order, applied hot pack to pt's left lower arm. Instructed pt to keep the hot pack (covered with a towel) on the wound for 15 minutes. Instructed patient how to apply a hot pack at home. Instructed patient to apply a hot pack for 15 minutes, four times a day for the next 3 days. Pt's questions were answered. Pt was encouraged to call the department if he has additional questions or concerns. _____
   _____ Suzanne Peterson, CMA (AAMA)

PROCEDURE 20.5 **Coach a Patient in the Use of Axillary Crutches**

Tasks: Fit crutches to the patient. Coach the patient to use crutches properly, considering the patient's developmental life stage. Document your teaching in the patient's health record.

Scenario: You are working with Dr. David Kahn. He has ordered you to teach Daniel Miller (DOB 3/21/2012) how to use axillary crutches. Daniel broke his left leg, and his treatment plan requires that he not bear weight on the left leg for 6 weeks. Daniel's bedroom is on the second floor, so he has to learn how to use crutches on the stairs also.

EQUIPMENT and SUPPLIES

- Axillary crutches
- Handout on crutch walking (optional)
- Provider's order
- Patient's health record

PROCEDURAL STEPS

1. Wash hands or use hand sanitizer.
   PURPOSE: Hand sanitization is an important step for infection control.
2. Read the provider's order. Assemble the equipment.
   PURPOSE: It is important to know the provider's order before starting the procedure.

3. Greet the patient. Identify yourself. Verify the patient's identity with full name and date of birth. Explain the procedure to be performed in a manner that the patient understands. Answer any questions the patient may have about the procedure.
   PURPOSE: It is important to identify the patient in two different ways to ensure that you have the correct patient. Explaining the procedure can make the patient feel more comfortable and helps to reduce anxiety.
4. Ensure the patient is wearing shoes and ask the patient to stand up straight. Assist as needed. Fit the crutches to the patient so they are 1 to 1½ inches (about 2 finger-widths) below the armpit (see the following figure). The crutch should be about 4 to 6 inches to the side and front of each foot.

Continued

PROCEDURE 20.5 | **Coach a Patient in the Use of Axillary Crutches—*continued***

PURPOSE: Pressure in the axilla can cause crutch palsy. Adjust the length on the crutches as needed.

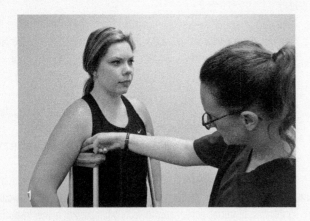

5. Adjust the handgrips so they are near the patient's wrist and even with the top of the hip line. This should allow for a 15- to 30-degree bend in the elbow when the patient's hands are on the handgrip.
   PURPOSE: This position allows for the most strength with the hands.
6. Coach the patient using strategies appropriate for the patient's developmental stage. Encourage discussion and questions. Use concrete terms when explaining the procedure. Show simple pictures.
   PURPOSE: Coaching a child requires strategies that are simple and concrete. Encourage the child to ask questions, which helps to clear up any misconceptions. See Chapter 7 for more information on communication and developmental life stage.
7. Using age-appropriate language, instruct the patient to keep the injured leg as relaxed as possible. The knee should be slightly bent, and the patient should look forward when walking. Instruct the patient not to bear weight on the axilla.
   PURPOSE: For a child, it is important to keep your language simple and to demonstrate what you are saying.
8. Have the patient start in the tripod position and then move the crutches about 12 inches in front of his or her body (or less for a child).
   PURPOSE: When doing the three-point crutch gait, placing the crutches in front of the body is the first step.
9. Have the patient put his weight on the crutches and move the body forward. Finish the step by having the patient swing the "good" or unaffected leg forward. Do not place weight on the "bad" or affected leg. Continue with these steps.
   PURPOSE: Placing weight on the affected extremity may harm the leg.
10. *To sit down:* Instruct the patient to do the following: Back up to the chair, toilet, or bed until the seat touches the back of the legs. Move the "bad"

or affected leg forward, balancing on the "good" or unaffected leg. Hold both crutches on the side with the "bad" or affected leg. Use the free hand to grab the seat or armrest. Slowly sit down.
   PURPOSE: Backing up until the seat touches the back of the legs is important to prevent falls.
11. *To stand up:* Instruct the patient to do the following: Move toward the front of the seat and move the "bad" or affected leg forward. Hold both crutches on the side with the "bad" or affected leg. Use the free hand to push up from the seat to stand up. Balance on the "good" or unaffected leg while placing a crutch in each hand. Balance is needed before moving.
   PURPOSE: If the person is unstable, the risk of falling is greater. Stand still until balance is achieved.
12. *To go up the stairs:* Instruct the patient to do the following: Step up with the "good" or unaffected leg first. Then bring the crutches up, one in each arm. Finally place weight on the "good" or unaffected leg and bring the "bad" or affected leg up.
   PURPOSE: It is important to go up the stairs, starting with the "good" or unaffected leg.
13. *To go down stairs:* Instruct the patient to do the following: With a crutch in each hand, place the crutches on the first step. Then move the "bad" or affected leg forward and down. Lastly, follow with the "good" or unaffected leg.
   PURPOSE: When going down stairs, the crutches and then the "bad" or affected leg come first.
14. Instruct the patient and family on ways to prevent falls. Wash hands or use hand sanitizer.
   PURPOSE: It is important to also educate the patient on how to prevent falls.
15. Document the patient education in the patient's health record. Include the provider's name, the order, what was taught, how the patient responded, how the patient did the demonstration, and any handouts provided.
   PURPOSE: It is important to document the patient education in the health record to show it was done.

07/21/20XX 1423 Per Dr. Kahn's order, pt fitted with crutches and taught with his mother on the 3-point crutch gait. They were told of the non-weight-bearing limitation on the left leg × 6 wks. Pt was able to correctly walk 20 feet using the 3-point gait. He was able to walk up and down the stairs safely with crutches. Pt was also taught to sit down and get up from a chair. Pt demonstrated the techniques correctly. Pt's mother was given the crutch booklet. All their questions were answered, and mother was given a follow-up number for additional questions. _____ Suzanne Peterson, CMA (AAMA)

PROCEDURE 20.6   Coach a Patient in the Use of a Walker

Tasks: Fit a standard walker to the patient. Coach patient to use a standard walker properly, considering the patient's communication barrier and developmental life stage. Document teaching in the patient's health record.

Scenario: You are working with Dr. David Kahn. He has ordered you to teach Jana Green (DOB 5/1/1936) how to use a standard walker. Jana needs the walker for extra stability. She has a hearing impairment. She can hear best with her right ear. She has no hearing in the left ear.

EQUIPMENT and SUPPLIES

- Standard walker
- Walker handout (optional)
- Provider's order
- Patient's health record

PROCEDURAL STEPS

1. Wash hands or use hand sanitizer.
   UNDERLINE PURPOSE: Hand sanitization is an important step for infection control.

2. Read the provider's order. Assemble the equipment.
   PURPOSE: It is important to know the provider's order before starting the procedure.

3. Greet the patient. Identify yourself. Verify the patient's identity with full name and date of birth. Explain the procedure to be performed in a manner that the patient understands. Answer any questions the patient may have about the procedure.
   PURPOSE: It is important to identify the patient in two different ways to ensure that you have the correct patient. Explaining the procedure can make the patient feel more comfortable and helps to reduce anxiety.

4. Face the person when speaking. Position yourself so your voice is directed toward the patient's good ear. Use a low-pitched voice and speak clearly, slowly, and distinctly. Speak naturally. Limit medical terminology as you speak.
   PURPOSE: It is important to speak naturally; do not shout. Listen to the patient and follow what he or she states works the best with the impairment. See Chapter 7 for more information on working with communication barriers.

5. Use simpler language when talking. Speak clearly. Communicate with dignity and respect. Allow time for the patient to respond. Listen to the patient's concerns.
   PURPOSE: When working with older patients, it is important to show respect and to value their dignity. Listening is important. See Chapter 7 for more information on communication and developmental life stage.

6. Ensure the patient is wearing shoes and ask the patient to step into the walker. The top of the walker grip should be even with the top of the hip line and near the crease in the wrist when the arms are at the side of the body. Adjust as needed. Keeping the shoulders relaxed and the hands on the grips will ensure the elbows are bent at a 15-degree angle (see the following figure).
   PURPOSE: For body mechanics, it is important to have the walker adjusted to fit the person. Using a walker that is too tall or too short can cause stress on the upper shoulders and back. A person should not lean over to walk because this increases the risk of falls.

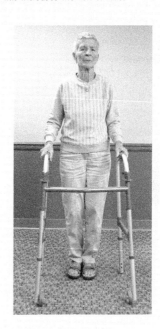

7. Have the patient place the walker one step ahead of his or her body. Instruct the patient to use the "bad" or affected leg to step into the walker. The patient should not touch the front bar with the leg. Have the patient step forward with his or her other leg to complete the step. The patient will continue with this pattern while holding up the head and looking forward.
   PURPOSE: Being too close to the front bar can affect the patient's stability.

8. *To sit down:* Instruct the patient to back up to the chair, toilet, or bed until the seat touches the back of the legs. The patient can then use one hand to grab the seat or armrest and slowly sit down.
   PURPOSE: Backing up until the seat touches the back of the legs is important to prevent falls.

9. *To stand up:* Instruct the patient to move toward the front of the seat. Have the walker in front of the person. Have the patient use one hand to push up from the seat to stand up and then place hands on the walker. Remind patients to make sure they have their balance before moving.
   PURPOSE: If the person is unstable, the risk of falling is greater. It is important to stand still until balance is achieved.

10. Instruct the patient on ways to prevent falls. The walker should never be used on stairs or an escalator. If the patient will be using a bag on the

Continued

PROCEDURE 20.6   Coach a Patient in the Use of a Walker—*continued*

front of the walker, instruct him or her to make sure not to overload it. Make sure to place all four legs of the walker on the ground before moving into the walker. Wash hands or use hand sanitizer.

PURPOSE: It is important to educate the patient on how to prevent falls. Too much weight in the front of the walker may cause it to tilt and the patient to fall.

11. Document the patient education in the patient's health record. Include the provider's name, the order, what was taught, how the patient responded, how the patient did the demonstration, and any handouts provided.

PURPOSE: It is important to document the patient education in the health record to show it was done.

07/21/20XX 1423 Per Dr. Kahn's order, patient was fitted with a walker and instructed how to use it. Pt was able to walk using the walker correctly. Pt was also able to sit and stand while using the walker. Pt demonstrated techniques correctly and safely. Coached patient on safety issues with the walker and how to reduce the risk of falls. Pt was able to verbalize four ways to prevent falls when using the walker. All the pt's questions were answered. Pt was given the walker booklet to take home. _____

_____ Suzanne Peterson, CMA (AAMA)

PROCEDURE 20.7   Coach a Patient in the Use of a Cane

Tasks: Fit a cane to a patient. Coach the patient to use a cane. Document teaching in the patient's health record.

Scenario: You are working with Dr. David Kahn. He has ordered you to teach Ella Rainwater (DOB 7/11/1959) how to use a cane. Ella has left side weakness.

EQUIPMENT and SUPPLIES

- Cane
- Handout on cane walking (optional)
- Provider's order
- Patient's health record

PROCEDURAL STEPS

1. Wash hands or use hand sanitizer.
   PURPOSE: Hand sanitization is an important step for infection control.
2. Read the provider's order. Assemble the equipment.
   PURPOSE: It is important to know the provider's order before starting the procedure.
3. Greet the patient. Identify yourself. Verify the patient's identity with full name and date of birth. Explain the procedure to be performed in a manner that the patient understands. Answer any questions the patient may have about the procedure.
   PURPOSE: It is important to identify the patient in two different ways to ensure that you have the correct patient. Explaining the procedure can make the patient feel more comfortable and helps to reduce anxiety.
4. Ensure the patient is wearing shoes. The top of the cane should be near the crease in the wrist when the arms are at the side of the body. Adjust as needed. With the patient's shoulders relaxed and hand on the cane, ensure the elbows are bent at a 15-degree angle.
   PURPOSE: For body mechanics, it is important to have the cane fitted correctly.
5. Instruct the patient to hold the cane on the "good" or unaffected side. The patient should take a step moving the "bad" or affected leg and the

cane forward at the same time and then step forward with the "good" leg. Instruct the patient to lean on the cane as needed.
   PURPOSE: The cane is held on the "good" or unaffected side so it can provide added support to the opposite leg.
6. *To sit down:* Instruct the patient to back up to the chair, toilet, or bed until the seat touches the back of the legs. The patient can then use a hand to grab the seat or armrest and slowly sit down.
   PURPOSE: Backing up until the seat touches the back of the legs is important to prevent falls.
7. *To stand up:* Instruct the patient to move toward the front of the seat and move the "bad" or affected leg forward. The patient can then use a hand to push up from the seat to stand up. Remind patients to make sure to get their balance before moving.
   PURPOSE: If the person is unstable, the risk of falling is greater. Instruct the patient to stand still until balance is achieved.
8. *To go up the stairs:* Instruct the patient to step up with the "good" or unaffected leg first while holding onto the rail. Then the patient should bring up the "bad" or affected leg to the same step. If there is no handrail, the cane and the "bad" leg should be placed on the stair at the same time.
   PURPOSE: It is important to go up the stairs, starting with the "good" or unaffected leg.
9. *To go down stairs:* Instruct the patient to hold onto the rail and move the "bad" or affected leg down first. Then the patient should place the "good" or unaffected leg on the same step as the "bad" leg. When there is no handrail, instruct the patient to place the cane on the lower step, then place the "bad" or affected leg, and lastly place the "good" or unaffected leg next to the "bad" or affected leg.

PROCEDURE 20.7 Coach a Patient in the Use of a Cane—*continued*

PURPOSE: When going down stairs, the cane and then the "bad" leg come down first, followed by the "good" leg.

10. Instruct the patient on ways to prevent falls. Wash hands or use hand sanitizer.

PURPOSE: It is important to also educate the patient on how to prevent falls.

11. Document the patient education in the patient's health record. Include the provider's name, the order, what was taught, how the patient responded, how the patient did the demonstration, and any handouts provided.

PURPOSE: It is important to document the patient education in the health record to show it was done.

07/25/20XX 1105 Per Dr. Kahn's order, pt was fitted with a cane and was instructed on walking with a cane, doing stairs, and sitting/standing. Pt was able to walk about 30 feet with a cane correctly. Pt was able to safely walk up and down and sit/stand while using the cane. Pt's questions were answered. Pt was given the "Using a Cane" booklet. _____ Suzanne Peterson, CMA (AAMA)

Nancy Gehir, CMA (AAMA), is a medical assistant at Walden-Martin Family Medical (WMFM) Clinic. She was hired at WMFM clinic shortly after passing her CMA exam. She has recently accepted a position to help the outreach providers. Outreach providers deliver specialty services that are not offered at WMFM Clinic.

Nancy will be assisting with the neurology providers, who come to the clinic weekly to see patients. Prior to starting with neurology, Nancy spent some time reviewing her anatomy textbook and researching common diseases. Today, she is helping Dr. Arzt and Tammy Tamar, nurse practitioner (NP).

While studying this chapter, think about the following questions:

- What structures are in the nervous system? What are the functions of the nervous system?
- What are the common pathologic conditions of the nervous system? What medical terms must you know to identify and explain these patient disorders?

- What diagnostic and treatment procedures typically are ordered for patients with neurological diseases?
- What are the medical assistant's primary responsibilities in working with patients with neurological conditions?

LEARNING OBJECTIVES

1. Summarize the anatomy of the nervous system and compare the structure and function of the nervous system across the life span.
2. Discuss the cells of the nervous system and describe polarization, depolarization, and repolarization.
3. Describe the autonomic nervous system, including the sympathetic and parasympathetic nervous systems.
4. Distinguish among common neurodegenerative diseases.
5. Discuss various functional disorders and describe the three types of seizures.
6. Compare and contrast encephalitis and meningitis.
7. Distinguish among neurological structural diseases.
8. Describe the types of strokes and related treatments.
9. Discuss the medical assistant's role in a neurological exam.
10. Summarize the medical assistant's role with a lumbar puncture procedure.
11. Summarize the patient coaching required for electroencephalography.

VOCABULARY

afferent (AF er uhnt) Pertaining to carrying toward a structure.

amygdala (ah MIG dah lah) A small mass of gray matter found in each temporal lobe of the cerebrum and involved with memories, emotions, and activating the fight-or-flight response; part of the limbic system.

analgesic (an ahl JEE zik) A drug that reduces or eliminates pain.

aneurysm (AN yeh rizm) An abnormal blood-filled sac formed from a localized dilation of the wall of a vein, artery, or heart.

aphasia (ah FAY zhah) Partial or complete loss of the ability to articulate ideas or understand written or spoken language.

axon (AK son) A long extension of a nerve fiber that conducts the impulse away from the nerve cell body.

autoimmune An immune response against a person's own tissues, cells, or cell parts, as in autoimmune disease, leading to the deterioration of tissue.

biomarkers Detectable cellular indicators used as a marker for a substance or disease process.

cataplexy (KAT ah PLEK see) A sudden loss of muscle strength and tone associated with an emotional stimulus.

choroid plexus (KOR oid PLEK sus) A network of capillaries found in the lateral ventricles and the third and fourth ventricles that secrete cerebrospinal fluid.

coma A state of deep, often prolonged unconsciousness, usually the result of a head injury, neurological disease, intoxication, or metabolic abnormalities.

concussion A type of brain injury resulting from a hit to the head or body that causes the brain to move rapidly back and forth.

efferent (EF er uhnt) Pertaining to carrying away from a structure.

evoked potential test A nerve response test that uses electrodes, which are placed on the scalp to measure brain reaction to a stimulus.

fissure (FISH er) A groove that divides an organ into lobes or parts.

fontanel (fon tah NEL) A soft membranous gap between the incompletely formed cranial bones of an infant; also called a *soft spot*.

foramen magnum (for AY men MAG num) A large opening in the base of the skull. It forms a passageway for the spinal cord.

Glasgow Coma Scale A scale used to measure the level of consciousness and severity of a head injury; the ability to open the eyes, verbal response, and motor response are evaluated and the score is determined based on the findings.

gray matter Nerve tissue that lacks the insulation that causes a white appearance to other nerves; thus, gray matter looks gray.

gyri (JIE rie) Folds or convolutions on the surface of the cerebral hemisphere, which increase the gray matter surface area. *Gyrus* (JIE rus) is the singular form.

hallucination (hah LOO si nae shun) A sensory experience (e.g., a smell, sound, sight, touch, or taste) involving something that is not present.

hematoma A localized collection of blood, usually clotted, caused by a break in a blood vessel wall.

hippocampus (hip oh KAM pus) A ridge in the floor of the lateral ventricle; composed of gray matter. Involved with the limbic system and with creating and filing new memories.

homeostasis (hoh mee oh STAY sis) The internal environment of the body that is compatible with life. A steady state that is created by all the body systems working together to provide a consistent and unvarying internal environment.

hydrocephalus (hi droe SEF ah luhs) An abnormal accumulation of cerebrospinal fluid that causes enlargement of the skull and compression of the brain.

limbic system Consists of several structures, including the amygdala, hippocampus, and hypothalamus; plays an important role in behavior, memories, and emotions.

meninges (meh NIN jeez) A protective covering around the brain and spinal cord.

myelin sheath (MIE uh lin sheeth) A protective insulation that covers the axons and helps with the transmission of nerve impulses.

neuralgia (noo RAL jah) Sharp, spasm-like pain in a nerve or along the course of one or more nerves.

neurotransmitter A chemical that helps a nerve cell communicate with another nerve cell or muscle.

paralysis A loss of muscle function and/or sensation causing the inability to move or use a body part.

pineal gland A small organ in the brain that secretes melatonin, a hormone that regulates the sleep/awake cycle.

shaken baby syndrome Condition resulting from internal head injuries that occur when a baby or young child is violently shaken.

sulci (SUL sie) Grooves or depressions on the surface of the brain between the gyri. *Sulcus* (SUL kus) is the singular form.

target tissue The destination, or intended tissue in the nervous impulse (e.g., a muscle).

tract A system of tissues (e.g., neuronal axons) and/or organs (e.g., intestines) that function together.

---

*N*eurology is the healthcare specialty that deals with the diseases and disorders of the nervous system. A *neurologist* is a specialist involved in the diagnosis, treatment, and prevention of nervous system diseases and disorders.

Besides the neurology department, patients with nervous system concerns can be seen in primary care and also urgent care departments. The medical assistant may help the provider with the examination and screening questions.

ANATOMY OF THE NERVOUS SYSTEM

The main structures of the nervous system include the brain, spinal cord, and nerves. Various other sense organs exist through the body, such as in the eyes. The nervous system is made up of nerve cells, or *neurons*. (Neurons are discussed in the Physiology of the Nervous System section.)

The nervous system is divided as follows:
- *Central nervous system* (CNS), which is composed of the brain and the spinal cord.
- *Peripheral nervous system* (PNS), which is made up of all the nervous tissue outside of the CNS, including the 12 pairs of cranial nerves and 31 pairs of spinal nerves. The PNS can be further divided into:
  - *Somatic nervous system*, which is voluntary. It collects information from and returns instructions to the skin, muscles, and joints.

- *Autonomic nervous system* (ANS), which is involuntary. It collects and returns information to involuntary structures (e.g., muscles, glands, organs).

Central Nervous System

Brain

The brain, enclosed in the skull, is one of the most complex organs of the body. It is divided into the cerebrum, cerebellum, diencephalon, and brainstem (Fig. 21.1).

Cerebrum. The cerebrum is the largest portion of the brain and is divided into two hemispheres by a deep **fissure**. The right hemisphere controls artistic functions, such as drawing, rhythm, and picture memory. The left hemisphere controls verbal functions, such as reading, writing, speaking, and mathematic calculations. The hemispheres are connected by the *corpus callosum*, a bundle of nerve tissue that facilitates communication between the two sides of the brain. If the corpus callosum only partially develops or is absent, the person is diagnosed with *corpus callosum agenesis*.

Most of the signals between the brain and body cross over. This means that the left cerebral hemisphere primarily controls the right side of the body. The right hemisphere primarily controls the left side of the body. For instance, if a person has a stroke affecting the right hemisphere, the symptoms will be seen on the left side of the body.

Each cerebral hemisphere is further divided into four sections, called *lobes*. These are the functions of the lobes:

Internal Structure of the Brain

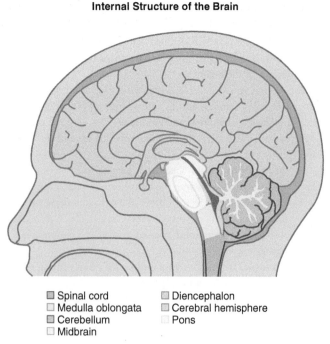

- Spinal cord
- Medulla oblongata
- Cerebellum
- Midbrain
- Diencephalon
- Cerebral hemisphere
- Pons

FIGURE 21.1 The structures of the brain.

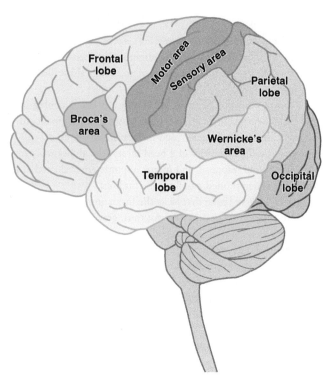

Frontal lobe

Motor area

Sensory area

Parietal lobe

Broca's area

Wernicke's area

Temporal lobe

Occipital lobe

FIGURE 21.2 The lobes of the cerebrum.

- *Frontal lobes*: Lie directly behind the forehead. These lobes are responsible for personality, intelligence, concentration, self-awareness, problem solving, short-term memory, planning, and judgment. In the back of the frontal lobe is a *motor area*, which controls the voluntary movements on the opposite side of the body. *Broca's area*, found on the left frontal lobe, is involved with speech (e.g., moving thoughts into words when speaking and writing) (Fig. 21.2). When damage occurs in Broca's area (e.g., stroke or head injury), **aphasia** can occur.
- *Parietal lobes*: Found behind the frontal lobes. These lobes are involved with reading and interpreting visual, auditory, motor, sensory, and memory signals, along with spatial and visual perceptions. The *sensory areas*, found near the motor area of the frontal lobe, receive information from the body regarding touch, pain, and temperature (see Fig. 21.2). Reading and math skills are also functions of the parietal lobe.
- *Occipital lobes*: Found at the back of the brain. These lobes handle images from the eyes and connect the information with stored image memories. Damage to or a lack of these lobes can cause blindness.
- *Temporal lobes*: Found in front of the occipital lobes on the right and left side of the brain. The top of each temporal lobe receives information from the ears, and the underside of the lobe forms and retrieves sound-related memories. *Wernicke's area*, found in the left temporal lobe, is important for language comprehension and speech (see Fig. 21.2). The temporal lobes are also responsible for processing memories and sensations of taste, touch, sight, and sounds. The **amygdala** is found in each temporal lobe and is involved with the **limbic system**.

The surfaces of the hemispheres are covered by **gray matter**, or *cerebral cortex*, a thin layer ranging from 1 to 4.5 mm in thickness. Most of the information processing in the brain takes place in the cerebral cortex. The folds (**gyri**) of the cerebral cortex add more surface area, thus increasing the gray matter and the amount of information that can be processed. **Sulci** (depressions) are also visible on the cerebral cortex.

Cerebellum. The cerebellum is located below the occipital lobe of the cerebrum. It is also covered by the cortex. The cerebellum gathers input from other parts of the brain and spinal cord to provide accurate timing for coordinated smooth movements. The cerebellum coordinates the equilibrium, or balance, posture, and muscle coordination. Damage to the cerebellum, as is caused by a stroke, can cause nausea, dizziness, and balance and coordination issues.

Diencephalon. The diencephalon is located just above the brainstem and is almost surrounded by the cerebral hemispheres. It serves as a relay station for sensory input neurons and other parts of the brain. It plays important roles in the functioning of the CNS, endocrine system, and the limbic system. The diencephalon is composed of the posterior pituitary gland and the **pineal gland**, which are part of the endocrine system. The diencephalon also includes two other parts:

- *Thalamus*: Processes information going to and from the body and the cerebrum.
- *Hypothalamus*: Controls body temperature, hunger, and thirst; also, part of the limbic system.

A **tract** of nerve cells connects the thalamus and hypothalamus to the **hippocampus**. The hippocampus works with memories, sending memories to cerebral hemispheres for storage (long-term memories) and then retrieving them when needed.

CRITICAL THINKING APPLICATION   **21.1**

Nancy roomed Elaine. While Nancy was taking her medical history, Elaine mentioned that she felt unsteady from time to time and lost her balance a few times. What part of the brain is involved in maintaining balance?

Brainstem. The brainstem connects the cerebral hemispheres to the spinal cord. It controls the flow of information from the body to the brain. The brainstem is composed of these structures:

- *Midbrain:* Connects the hemispheres of the cerebrum with the pons. It serves as a relay center for auditory, visual, and motor information. It also contains centers to regulate pupillary reflexes and eye movements.
- *Pons:* Serves as a bridge between the medulla oblongata and the cerebrum and helps to regulate respirations.
- *Medulla oblongata:* Lowest part of the brainstem. It contains vital centers of life (e.g., cardiac, respiratory, and vasomotor centers) that regulate the heart rate, respirations, and the diameter of blood vessels, which affect the blood pressure. Nonvital centers also are found in the medulla oblongata, including centers that regulate coughing, sneezing, hiccupping, vomiting, and swallowing. Some medications work to "quiet" these centers.

Spinal Cord

The spinal cord is a bundle of nervous tissue. It extends from the medulla oblongata to about the second lumbar vertebra (Fig. 21.3). The spinal cord passes through the **foramen magnum** in the skull and is protected by the vertebrae. It is covered by meninges. The spinal cord is composed of the cell bodies of motor neurons (gray matter), and the myelin-covered **axons** (*white matter*). Thirty-one pairs of spinal nerves extend from the spinal cord. Each nerve stimulates a specific organ or area of the body. The spinal cord carries messages between the spinal nerves and the brain. This can slow with age.

Life Span Changes in the Neurological System

Infants are born with an immature nervous system. Over the first few years of life, the process of myelination continues, causing an increase in the child's brain size. As the child matures, learning and thinking processes become more complex. During adulthood, the brain function is stable.

As a person ages, the nervous system changes. The brain and spinal cord lose nerve cells. Nerve cells break down in the brain and waste products accumulate, which can cause plaques and tangles to form. Nerve impulses become slower. This causes a slower reaction time, and tasks may take longer to perform. Reflexes can also be reduced. Slowing of thought, thinking, and memory is a normal part of aging.

Meninges

Meninges are a protective covering around the brain and spinal cord. They are composed of three membranes (Fig. 21.4):

- *Dura mater:* Outer layer of meninges; made up of a tough white fibrous connective tissue. The space below the dura mater is called the *subdural space,* which contains tiny blood vessels. Head trauma can cause these vessels to bleed, causing a subdural **hematoma.**
- *Arachnoid mater:* Middle layer of meninges; made up of a thin layer of threadlike strands resembling a cobweb. The space below the arachnoid is called the *subarachnoid space,* and it is filled with cerebrospinal fluid (CSF) and blood vessels.
- *Pia mater:* Innermost layer of meninges; a thin, highly vascular membrane that is tightly bound to the surface of the spinal cord and brain.

The ventricular system in the brain is made up of four connected *ventricles* (spaces or cavities). CSF originates in the **choroid plexus** in the ventricles. CSF is a clear fluid that resembles water, and it has three roles:

- Cushions the brain and spinal cord
- Removes waste products from cerebral metabolism
- Supplies nutrients to the nervous system tissues

CSF flows through the ventricles, exits into the cisterns at the base of the brain, and moves around the brain and spinal cord. Eventually, CSF is reabsorbed into the bloodstream. The balance between the CSF production and absorption is critical. Excessive amounts of CSF result in abnormal widening of the ventricles, which can put pressure on the brain tissue and lead to hydrocephalus.

Peripheral Nervous System

The peripheral nervous system is made up of the nerves that exit the brain or spinal cord. The peripheral nerves exiting the brain directly through the skull are called *cranial nerves.* Cranial nerves originate from the underside of the brain and relay information to and from the sensory organs and muscles of the face and neck (Table 21.1). Cranial nerves have either motor function, sensory function, or both.

The *spinal nerves* exit the spinal canal through spaces between the vertebrae. Spinal nerves closely mimic the organization of the vertebrae and provide stimulation to the rest of the body. If the nerve fibers from several spinal nerves form a network, it is called a *plexus.* Spinal nerves are named by their vertebrae location (e.g., cervical, thoracic) and by number. Spinal nerves carry information to and from the brain through the spinal cord. Sensory fibers in these nerves carry stimuli from the skin and internal organs to the CNS. Motor fibers carry messages from the CNS to skeletal muscles, causing them to contract.

Dermatomes are skin surface areas supplied by a single afferent spinal nerve. These areas are so specific, the body can be mapped by dermatomes (Fig. 21.5). Shingles, for example, appears on specific dermatomes based on which nerve the virus has infected.

CRITICAL THINKING APPLICATION   21.2

Using the mnemonic: "**O**n **O**ld **O**lympus **T**owering **T**op **A** **F**ine **V**ocal **G**erman **V**iewed **S**ome **H**ops" list the cranial nerves in order.

PHYSIOLOGY OF THE NERVOUS SYSTEM

The *nervous system* is a complex system that plays a major role in **homeostasis.** The nervous system works in partnership with the endocrine system to help the body respond to its internal and external environments. This effort is responsible for communication and control throughout the body. There are three main functions of the nervous system:

- Collecting information about the external and internal environments (sensing)
- Processing this information and making decisions about action (interpreting)
- Directing the body to put into action the decisions made (acting)

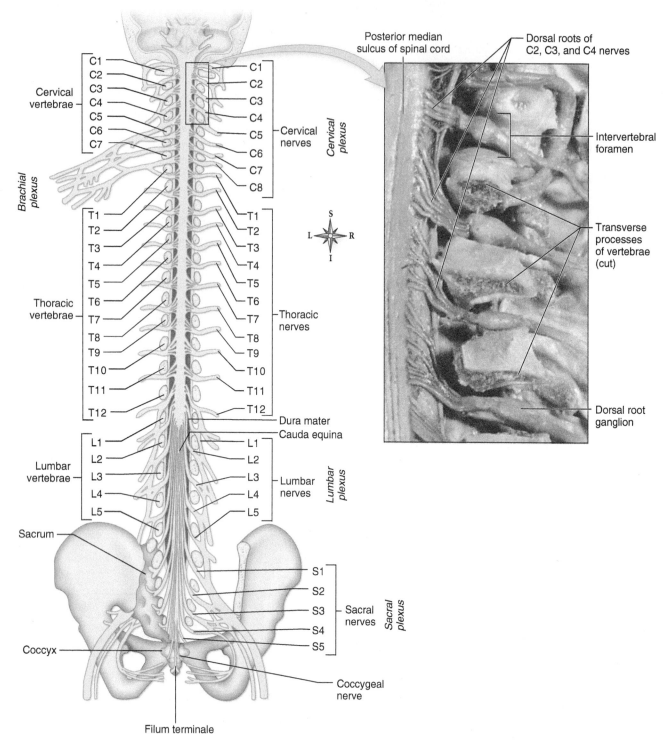

FIGURE 21.3 The spinal cord, showing the spinal nerves. (From Vidic B, Suarez FR: *Photographic atlas of the human body*, St Louis, 1984, Mosby.)

For example, the sensory function begins with a *stimulus* (e.g., the uncomfortable pinch of a tight shoe). That information travels to the brain, where it is *interpreted*. The return message is sent to *react to the stimulus* (e.g., remove the shoe).

To carry out its functions, the nervous system is divided into two main parts:

- *Peripheral nervous system*: Composed of the cranial and spinal nerves. The PNS consists of voluntary and involuntary nerves, which may be **afferent** (or sensory), carrying impulses to the brain and spinal cord, or **efferent** (or motor), carrying impulses from the brain and spinal cord to an organ, gland, or muscle.

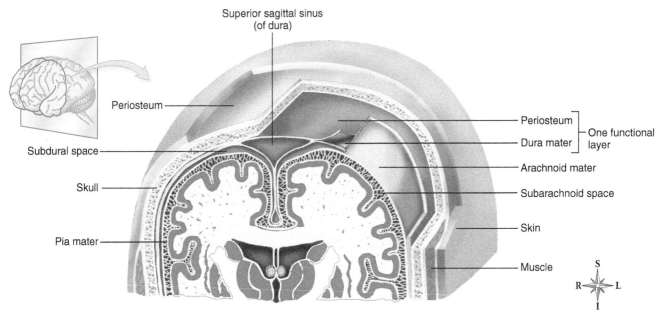

FIGURE 21.4 Protective coverings of the brain. (Modified from Patton K, Thibodeau G: *Anatomy and physiology,* ed 9, St. Louis, 2016, Mosby.)

TABLE 21.1	Cranial Nerves		
NUMBER	NAME	FUNCTION	HOW IT IS TESTED
I	Olfactory	*Sensory function:* Smell	Identify familiar odors, eyes are closed.
II	Optic	*Sensory function:* Vision	A visual acuity test may be given. A light may be shined in the eyes.
III	Oculomotor	*Sensory and motor functions:* Eye movement, pupil constriction and accommodation	The pupil is examined using a light. The patient may be asked to follow the light with his or her eyes, without moving the face.
IV	Trochlear	*Motor function:* Eye movement	Testing to see if the eyes can follow a moving light – as described for cranial nerve III.
V	Trigeminal	*Sensory and motor functions:* Muscles for chewing, general sensations from the anterior half of the head, including the face and meninges	The provider may feel the face in different locations and have the patient clench the teeth.
VI	Abducens	*Motor function:* Eye movement	Testing to see if the eyes can follow a moving light – as described for cranial nerve III.
VII	Facial	*Sensory and motor functions:* Muscles used for facial expressions; tearing, salivation, and taste	May be asked to identify common tastes, puff cheeks, smile, wrinkle forehead, and close eyes tightly.
VIII	Vestibulocochlear	*Sensory function:* Hearing and equilibrium	Assessed using a hearing acuity test.
IX	Glossopharyngeal	*Sensory and motor functions:* Swallowing and taste	Gag reflex is tested with a tongue blade.
X	Vagus	*Sensory and motor functions:* Breathing, speech, sweating, regulating heartbeat, stimulating muscles of the gastric region	Have patient say "ahh," swallow, and talk (voice quality assessed). Gag reflex is tested with a tongue blade.
XI	Spinal accessory	*Motor function:* Shoulder and head movements	Assessed by turning the head from side to side against mild resistance and shrugging the shoulders.
XII	Hypoglossal	*Motor function:* Tongue movements	Assessed by sticking out and moving the tongue from side to side.

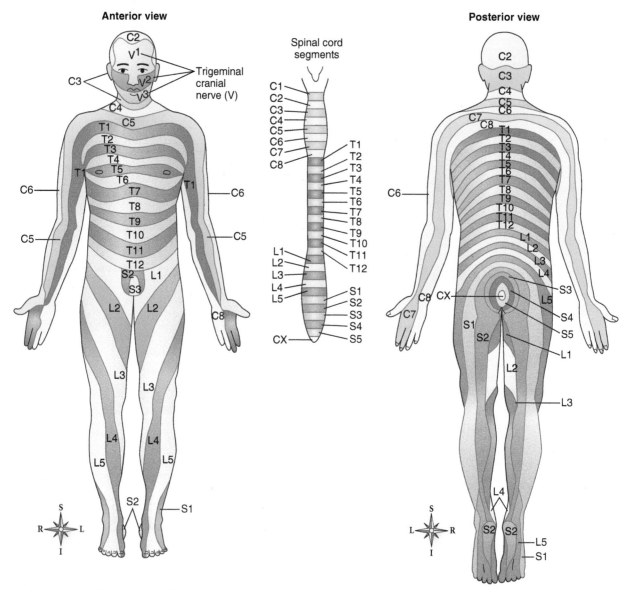

FIGURE 21.5 Map of the dermatomes. (From Patton K, Thibodeau G: *The human body in health & disease,* ed 7, St. Louis, 2018, Mosby.)

- *Central nervous system*: Composed of the brain and the spinal cord. It is the only site of nerve cells called *interneurons*, which connect sensory and motor neurons.

Cells of the Nervous System

The nervous system is made up of two types of cells:
- *Neurons*: Also called *parenchymal cells*, which carry out the work of the nervous system.
- *Neuroglia*: Also called *stromal cells* or *glia*. These cells provide a supportive function for the neurons.

Neurons

The nervous system is composed of nerve cells, or *neurons*. Neurons are composed of a cell body, dendrites, and an axon (Fig. 21.6). The *dendrites* are short projections off the cell body. They pick up the electrical impulses, say from other neurons, and send the signals along to the cell body. The impulse is then passed to the axon, which is a long extension off the cell body. Some axons can be over 3 feet

long. The axon transmits the impulse to other dendrites, glands, or muscles.

An *action potential* is a self-propagating wave of electrical impulse that travels along the surface of a neuron membrane. An action potential proceeds in the following steps:

1. A stimulus (e.g., pressure, temperature, sound wave) starts an impulse.
2. The resting nerve cell has a slightly positive charge (due to sodium ions) on the outside of the cell membrane, and a negative charge inside the cell. This state is called *polarization*.
3. When a section of the membrane is stimulated, the positively charged ions on the outside of the cell enter the nerve cell. This changes the outside charge to a negative charge. This state is called *depolarization*.
4. Almost immediately after the impulse passes, the positively charged ions move outside the nerve cells again. This returns the outside charge to a positive charge. This state is called *repolarization*.

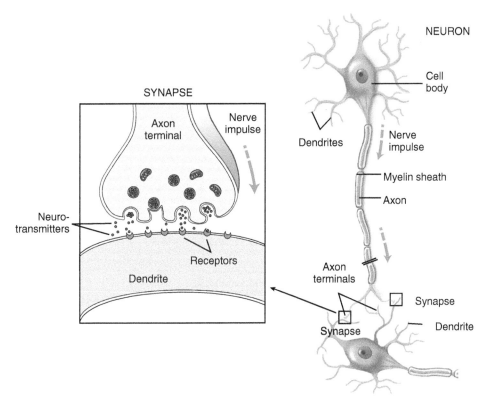

FIGURE 21.6 Neuron and synapse *(inset).* (From Shiland B: *Mastering healthcare terminology,* ed 5, St. Louis, 2016, Mosby.)

5. Once everything changes back, the cell is at rest again, and the cycle continues.

The transfer of the action potential begins as the electrical impulse travels down an axon. It becomes a chemical impulse while moving across the *synapse*, the gap between the neurons. The transfer of impulses from the end of one neuron to the dendrites of another is enhanced by chemical **neurotransmitters** found in the synapse. Examples of neurotransmitters include epinephrine, norepinephrine, dopamine, serotonins, endorphins, and enkephalins.

Neurotransmitters bind to specific receptor sites on the dendrites of the next neuron or the **target tissue**. Messages move throughout the entire nervous system in this manner. Impulses in the neuron are electrical; the impulses become chemical as a neurotransmitter is released at each synapse. The action potentials become electrical again as they are picked up by the next dendrites of another neuron or by the target tissue. Changes in the amount of available neurotransmitters can cause different conditions.

Neuroglia

Neuroglia cells care for and support neurons throughout the body. These specialized cells perform specific functions within the nervous system. There are several types of neuroglia, including:

- *Schwann cells:* Form the **myelin sheath**, which covers the axons of peripheral nerves.
- *Astrocytes:* Help form the *blood-brain barrier* (BBB), which closely regulates what substances enter the brain tissue. Oxygen, water, and glucose molecules easily pass into the brain. Many chemicals and drugs are prevented from moving into brain tissue.

- *Microglia:* Found in the CNS. If brain tissue is inflamed or damaged, microglia engulf and destroy microorganisms or debris.
- *Oligodendrocytes:* Found in the CNS; they myelinate the CNS axons and help hold nerve fibers together.

CRITICAL THINKING APPLICATION   21.3

What type of cell produces the myelin sheath that surrounds some nerve axons?

Autonomic Nervous System

The autonomic nervous system (ANS) consists of nerves that regulate involuntary function. The ANS is an automatic system that regulates body functions such as breathing, heart rate, sweating, circulation, and digestion. It also controls the actions of muscles in blood vessel walls, organs, and glands. The motor portion of this system is further divided into the sympathetic nervous system and the parasympathetic nervous system. These two opposing systems help maintain homeostasis throughout the body systems (Fig. 21.7).

Sympathetic Nervous System

The *sympathetic nervous system* can produce a "fight or flight" response. This is the part of the nervous system that helps the individual respond to perceived stress. It speeds up the heart rate, raises blood glucose levels, raises blood pressure, slows the digestive system, and widens the bronchioles, allowing more oxygen to enter the body quickly. It also stimulates the adrenal glands to increase their secretions.

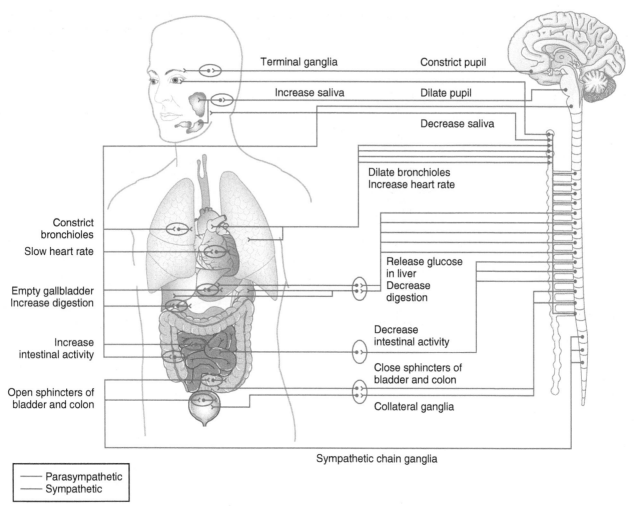

FIGURE 21.7 Structure and function of the autonomic nervous system. (From Applegate E: *The anatomy and physiology learning system,* ed 4, St. Louis, 2011, Saunders.)

Parasympathetic Nervous System

The *parasympathetic nervous system* does the opposite of the sympathetic nervous system. It slows the heart rate, lowers blood pressure, increases digestive functions, and reduces adrenal and sweat gland activity.

CRITICAL THINKING APPLICATION   **21.4**

It is important to know the differences between the sympathetic and parasympathetic nervous systems. List three characteristics of each and compare your list with a classmate. Do your lists agree?

DISORDERS OF THE NERVOUS SYSTEM

Common signs and symptoms of neurological disorders include:
- *Neuralgia* (nerve pain), *paresthesia* (feelings of prickling, burning, or numbness)
- *Spasms* (involuntary muscle contraction, such as stuttering and tics) and *tremors* (rhythmic, purposeless muscle movement)
- Recurrent headache, visual change, memory loss (*amnesia*), difficulty speaking or finding the right word
- Confusion, disorientation, or loss of consciousness

There are more than 600 neurological diseases. The conditions discussed are grouped as neurodegenerative diseases, functional disorders, infections, structural disorders, and vascular disorders.

Neurodegenerative Diseases

Neurodegenerative diseases affect a person's ability to move, talk, and breathe. These diseases can also affect a person's balance and heart function. The etiology may be genetic, related to a medical condition (e.g., tumor, stroke), or caused by a virus or toxin. With some diseases, the etiology is unknown.

Amyotrophic Lateral Sclerosis

Amyotrophic lateral sclerosis (ALS), or Lou Gehrig's disease, is a progressive neurological disorder that attacks the motor neurons in the brain and spinal cord. ALS usually affects adults between 40 and 60 years of age.

There is no known *etiology* (cause) for ALS, though there is a genetic component to the disease in up to 10% of the cases. Early signs and symptoms include mild muscle problems, including trouble walking, running, writing, swallowing (*dysphagia*), and speaking. The muscle weakness starts in the hands and feet and spreads throughout the body, leading to an inability to move the legs and arms. Eventually, the person has difficulty eating, speaking, and breathing. Some people experience memory issues and dementia.

The provider will do an examination which will show abnormal reflexes, weakness, twitching, and difficulty moving. Tests may be done to rule out other conditions, including blood tests, computed tomography (CT), magnetic resonance imaging (MRI), electromyography, and lumbar puncture. Breathing tests may be done to assess the lung muscles. There is no cure for ALS. Riluzole (Rilutek) may be prescribed to slow symptoms, and other medications may be given to help with the symptoms. Physical therapy, assistive devices (e.g., wheelchair, braces) may be used. A feeding tube may help with the nutritional status. Assistance with breathing may also be needed.

Dementia

Several disorders, such as a stroke or Alzheimer's disease (AD), cause dementia, though dementia is not a disease. It is a name for a group of symptoms that affect the brain. Symptoms of dementia include being unable to do normal activities of living (e.g., eating, dressing, grooming), solve problems, and control emotions. People with dementia need to have at least two or more problems with brain function (e.g., memory, language). Alzheimer's disease is the leading cause of dementia. Table 21.2 discusses other diseases causing dementia.

Alzheimer's Disease. AD is the most common cause of dementia. It damages and kills brain cells. Usually, AD begins after age 60, and the risk increases with age. The risk also increases if family members have AD.

Researchers feel that AD is caused by a combination of lifestyle, genetics, and environmental factors that affect the brain. Some research suggests a link between herpes simplex virus type 1 and AD. The causes are not fully understood. The signs and symptoms of AD begin slowly; initially, the person usually has difficulty remembering recent activities or the names of people he or she knows. AD affects

thinking, reasoning, making judgments and decisions, memory, performing familiar tasks, personality, and behavior. Over time, the symptoms worsen, affecting a person's ability to speak, read, write, or remember family members. Personality changes, aggression, and wandering away from home can occur.

The provider will do a medical history and physical. There is no specific test for AD. Neurological tests, CT, MRI, positron emission tomography (PET), psychiatric evaluation, and cognitive and neuropsychological tests may be done. Laboratory tests are done to rule out other conditions. A lumbar puncture may be done, and the cerebrospinal fluid may be examined for **biomarkers** that indicate AD. Current treatments may only keep symptoms from getting worse for a limited time; no cure is available. Medications that help treat cognitive symptoms include:

- Cholinesterase inhibitors: Boost the acetylcholine in the brain, which is depleted with AD. Common medications include donepezil (Aricept), rivastigmine (Exelon), and galantamine (Razadyne).
- Memantine (Namenda) is used for moderate to severe AD and may be used with cholinesterase inhibitors (donepezil and memantine [Namzaric]).

Huntington's Disease. Huntington's disease (HD), also called *Huntington's chorea*, is a progressive neurodegenerative disorder. There are two forms of HD:

- Early-onset HD: Begins during childhood or in the teen years; affects a small number of people.
- Adult-onset HD: Symptoms usually start in the 30s or 40s; most common form of HD.

Usually, people with HD die within 15 to 20 years.

HD is caused by a genetic defect. If the gene is inherited from one parent, the child has a 50% chance of getting the disease. As the gene is passed through families, the disease develops at an earlier age. Behavior issues are usually seen first and include behavioral

---

TABLE 21.2   Diseases Causing Dementia

DISEASE	DESCRIPTION AND ETIOLOGY	SIGNS AND SYMPTOMS	DIAGNOSTIC TESTS	TREATMENTS
Lewy body disease	Also called *dementia with Lewy bodies*; one of the more common causes of dementia. Lewy bodies (abnormal structures) build up in the brain.	Decreased alertness, hallucinations, muscle stiffness, confusion and loss of memory.	Physical and neurological examination, neuropsychological and mental status tests, imaging (CT, MRI), and blood tests.	No cure; treatments help with symptoms.
Frontotemporal dementia	Also called *Pick disease*. Rare condition that can start by age 20. Pick bodies and cells (abnormal proteins) are found in the damaged neurons.	Symptoms slowly get worse. Behavior changes, speech difficulty, and problems thinking occur.	Physical and neurological examination, imaging tests (MRI, CT), analysis of cerebrospinal fluid, electroencephalogram (EEG)	No specific treatment. Medications may be used to help with mood swings.
Vascular dementia	Second most common cause of dementia for people over 65. Caused from small strokes over time.	Difficulty performing tasks, language issues, misplacing items, sleep pattern changes, hallucinations, poor judgment, memory issues	Physical and neurological examination, imaging tests (CT, MRI), laboratory tests to rule out other conditions.	No treatment, goal is to control symptoms.

disturbances, hallucinations, moodiness, irritability, restlessness, psychosis, and paranoia. Abnormal movements can also occur and include facial grimacing, jerky movements, slow and uncontrolled movements, prancing gait. Dementia also occurs and affects the memory and speech.

The provider will do an examination and order additional tests, including psychological testing, head CT or MRI, and a PET scan of the brain. There is no cure for HD. The goal of the treatment is to slow the symptoms. Medications such as dopamine blockers help to reduce abnormal movements and behaviors, and amantadine may help to control extra movements.

Multiple Sclerosis

Multiple sclerosis (MS) is an **autoimmune** neurodegenerative disorder that affects the brain and spinal cord. The myelin sheath is damaged, leading to slowed or blocked messages to the brain. MS often occurs between the ages of 20 to 40 and affects women more than men. The disease can be mild, but some people may not be able to write, walk, or speak. There are four types of MS:

- *Clinically isolated syndrome (CIS)*: A person has an MS-like episode but does not meet the criteria for an MS diagnosis.
- *Relapsing-remitting MS (RRMS)*: Most common form; a person experiences relapses of the neurological symptoms, followed by periods of partial or complete remission (recovery).
- *Secondary progressive MS (SPMS)*: Follows the initial relapsing-remitting course; most people will eventually have worsening symptoms.
- *Primary progressive MS (PPMS)*: Symptoms worsen from the initial onset. The person does not experience early relapses or remissions.

The etiology is unknown, though it is an autoimmune disease. The immune system destroys the myelin sheath. Some risk factors include a family history, infection with the Epstein-Barr virus, and a history of thyroid disease, type 1 diabetes, or inflammatory bowel disease. Signs and symptoms include tingling, numbness, or weakness in the extremities, partial or complete loss of vision, double vision, slurred speech, fatigue, and lack of coordination.

The provider will perform an examination and evaluate the person's mental and language functions, along with movement and coordination. Vision and other senses will be evaluated. There are no blood tests to diagnose MS. The provider may order an MRI, cerebrospinal fluid analysis, and an **evoked potential test**. There is no cure for MS, though the goal of treatment is to slow the progression of the disease and speed up recovery time from attacks. Corticosteroid medications may be given to reduce nerve inflammation. Ocrelizumab (Ocrevus) may be used in some cases of MS.

Parkinson's Disease

Parkinson's disease (PD) is a progressive neurodegenerative disorder that affects movement. With PD, the dopamine-producing neurons in the brain gradually die. The dopamine levels decrease in the brain, leading to the symptoms. PD usually begins around age 60, and it is more common in men.

The cause of PD is unknown, but genetics and environmental triggers (e.g., exposure to certain toxins) can increase the risk of the disease. Signs and symptoms of PD include:

- Tremors and *pill-rolling tremors* (thumb and forefinger are rubbed back and forth)
- *Bradykinesia* (slow movement), shuffling gait, rigid muscles, impaired balance and posture, stooping, and writing changes
- Loss of automatic movements (e.g., blinking, smiling), *masked face* (facial appearance of depression or anger), and speech changes (e.g., slurring, soft voice)
- Loss of sense of smell, trouble sleeping, dizziness, constipation
- Excessive sweating or very little sweating, drooling

There are no specific tests for PD. The provider will do a neurological examination, and with the history of symptoms, the diagnosis can be made. Additional tests may be done to rule out other diseases. Medications can be used to manage the symptoms; some of these include:

- Carbidopa-levodopa (Sinemet): Used to increase the dopamine in the brain.
- Dopamine agonist: Used to mimic dopamine effect in the brain. Examples include pramipexole (Mirapex), ropinirole (Requip), and rotigotine (Neupro).
- MAO-B inhibitors: Prevent the breakdown of dopamine. Examples include safinamide (Xadago) and selegiline (Eldepryl, Zelapar).

Deep brain stimulation (DBS) may also be done. This treatment requires a generator to be implanted and the electrodes send impulses to the brain, which decrease the symptoms.

Other Neurodegenerative Diseases

Additional neurodegenerative diseases include the following:

- *Friedreich's ataxia*: An inherited disease that causes damage to the spinal cord and nerves. Signs and symptoms are seen as early as 5 years of age. The person can experience ataxia, difficulty walking, muscle weakness, scoliosis, heart palpitations, involuntary eye movements, and speech issues. There is no cure for this disease. Treatments may include assistive devices (e.g., wheelchair), braces, physical therapy, and surgery.
- *Tay-Sachs disease*: An inherited disease that progressively destroys the neurons in the brain and spinal cord. With the most common form, signs and symptoms are seen in infancy. The infant's motor skills (e.g., sitting, crawling, and rolling) are affected. As the disease progresses, the child can experience seizures, vision and hearing loss, intellectual disability, and **paralysis**.

CRITICAL THINKING APPLICATION   **21.5**

Nancy is trying to remember the different neurological diseases. Summarize the following neurodegenerative diseases discussed:
- Amyotrophic lateral sclerosis
- Alzheimer's disease
- Huntington's disease
- Multiple sclerosis
- Parkinson's disease

Functional Disorders

Headaches

Headaches are the most common form of pain experienced. Almost everyone has had a headache. There are different causes for headaches, including sinus issues (e.g., sinus headache) and stress. Many times, people try home treatments (e.g., rest, fluids, over-the-counter [OTC] **analgesics**), and these relieve the headache. People may be seen by providers if the headache is severe or recurring. The following sections will discuss commonly seen headaches.

Cluster Headaches. Cluster headaches occur in cyclical patterns or clusters. The person may awaken in the middle of the night with the headache on one side of the head. The cluster of headaches may last for weeks to months and then a remission period follows.

The etiology is unknown, but there may be an increase in the release of histamine or serotonin that causes the pain. The signs and symptoms include a severe, sudden, one-sided headache with tearing of the eyes, droopy eyelid, and stuffy nose. The onset commonly occurs 2 to 3 hours after falling asleep.

The provider will do a physical examination and may order an MRI to rule out other conditions. Often medications such as sumatriptan (Imitrex), dihydroergotamine (DHE), and analgesics may be ordered. Breathing in 100% pure oxygen may also help to reduce the headaches.

Migraine. Migraines are recurring headaches that can affect children through adults. The cause of migraines may include stress, anxiety, hormone changes, strong smells, and bright lights. Many times, migraines progress through four stages:

- *Prodrome* (1 to 2 days before): May cause mood changes, food cravings, neck stiffness, increase in thirst, and constipation.
- *Aura* (may occur before or during the migraine): May cause visual, sensory, motor, or verbal disturbances. Examples include hearing noises, difficulty speaking, vision loss, and jerking.
- *Attack* (may last up to 72 hours): May cause throbbing pain on one or both sides of the head; sensitivity to light, noise, and smells; nausea and vomiting, blurred vision, and lightheadedness.

- *Post-drome* (up to 24 hours after): May cause confusion, moodiness, dizziness, weakness, and sensitivity to noise and light.

The provider will do a physical and neurological examination. Treatment consists of rest, fluids and medications such as sumatriptan (Imitrex), dihydroergotamine (DHE), and analgesics.

Tension Headache. Tension headaches are the most common type of headaches. They occur when the neck and scalp muscles become tense.

Stress, depression, anxiety, and head injuries may cause tension headaches. Pain and muscle tightness in the head, scalp, or neck are usually seen.

Usually, the patient manages the pain with home treatments, such as OTC analgesics. Muscle relaxants and antidepressants may also be used.

Seizure Disorders

A *seizure* (or *convulsion*) is a sudden increase of electrical activity in one or more parts of the brain. Table 21.3 describes the three major groups of seizures. The seizures are classified based on how the abnormal brain activity begins.

Seizures can be caused by medications, high fevers, head injuries, diseases, and illegal drugs. The signs and symptoms of the different seizure classifications are listed on Table 21.3. Most seizures do not cause harm, but if they last longer than 5 minutes or if the person has repeated seizures without waking up between them, it is a medical emergency.

The provider will do a neurological exam and may order blood tests to check for conditions associated with seizures (e.g., infections). Additional tests may include neuropsychological tests, an electroencephalogram (EEG), CT, MRI, PET, and a single photon emission computed tomography (SPECT) scan. Depending on the type of seizure, antiseizure medication may be used.

TABLE 21.3	Seizure Classification				
NEW GROUPS (OLDER NAME)	**AFFECTS**	**TYPES – NEW CLASSIFICATION (OLDER NAME)**	**DESCRIPTION**		**SYMPTOMS**
Generalized onset (Generalized)	Both sides of the brain	*Tonic-clonic* (Grand mal)	Loses consciousness. Tonic phase (rigid muscles) comes first, followed by clonic phase (jerking rapidly). May be incontinent of stool and urine. Lasts 1–3 minutes; sleepy and confused after seizure.		Motor: sustained jerking (*clonic*), weak muscles (*atonic*), rigid muscles (*tonic*), brief twitching (myoclonus), and spasms Nonmotor: staring spells, twitching
		Absent (Petit mal)	Lapse of awareness of the environment; more common in children.		
Focal onset (Partial)	One area of the brain	*Focal aware* (Simple partial)	Awake and alert during seizure; lasts less than 2 minutes		Motor: clonic, atonic, tonic, myoclonus, spasms, automatic movements (e.g., lip-smacking, clapping, chewing) Nonmotor: changes in emotions, thinking, heart palpitations, goose bumps, lack of movement
		Focal impaired awareness (Complex partial)	Confused during seizure; lasts 1–2 minutes. Aura may occur.		
Unknown onset	Unknown		When seizure began is not known, or seizure was not witnessed		Motor: tonic-clonic, spasms Nonmotor: no movements, stares

From CDC, https://www.cdc.gov/epilepsy/communications/features/seizures.htm and Epilepsy Foundation, https://www.epilepsy.com/learn/types-seizures Accessed May 11, 2019.

CRITICAL THINKING APPLICATION   21.6
Nancy is attempting to remember the three classifications of seizures. What might be ways that she can remember them?

Epilepsy. Epilepsy is a disorder that causes recurring seizures. A person must have at least two unprovoked seizures before epilepsy is diagnosed. The type of seizure is classified either as generalized or focal. Epilepsy can affect anyone at any age, of any ethnic background, or of either gender. Children can outgrow epilepsy.

There are several causes of epilepsy, including genetics, brain injury, abnormal development, and illness. Many times, the cause is not known. Signs and symptoms vary based on the type of seizure and can include confusion, staring, uncontrolled jerking, and loss of consciousness (see Table 21.3). Status epilepticus, an emergency condition, occurs when a seizure lasts longer than 10 minutes or if the person has three or more seizures without regaining consciousness between them.

The provider will do a neurological examination and may order the tests listed in the Seizure section. Treatments include antiseizure medications, a ketogenic diet (eating foods high in fats and low in carbohydrates), vagus nerve stimulation, and deep brain stimulation (from a surgically implanted generator and electrodes). If medications fail to control the seizures, surgery can be done to remove the portion of the brain causing the seizures.

Other Functional Disorders
Additional functional disorders include the following:
- *Functional neurological disorder (FND)* (also called *conversion disorder* and *functional movement disorder*): A neurological disorder that affects the transmission of signals from the nervous system and the body. The cause is unknown. Symptoms include motor dysfunction (e.g., limb weakness, paralysis, spasms, problems walking), dysphagia, sensory dysfunction (e.g., numbness, loss of vision), syncope, and seizures.
- *Narcolepsy:* A chronic neurological disorder that affects the brain's ability to control the sleep-wake cycle, thus causing extreme daytime sleepiness, **cataplexy**, **hallucinations**, and sleep paralysis. Narcolepsy can be genetic and also an autoimmune disease.
- *Sciatica:* Occurs when the sciatic nerve can become compressed by a herniated disk, spinal stenosis, or a bone spur on the vertebrae. This condition causes burning or stabbing pain that radiates along the path of the sciatic nerve. The person can have pain and numbness in the lower back, hip, buttock, and leg on one side of the body.
- *Tourette Syndrome (TS):* A neurological disorder that causes tics and can be seen as early as 3 years of age. *Tics* are repetitive, involuntary movements and vocalizations. *Simple motor tics* involve a small number of muscle groups and cause sudden, brief, repetitive movements, such as eye blinking, facial grimacing, shoulder shrugging, and head jerking. *Complex motor tics* involve several muscle groups and several movements (e.g., grimacing, shrugging, and jerking). *Simple vocal tics* involve sounds made by moving air through the mouth or nose, causing barking, hissing, sniffing, grunting, or throat-clearing. *Complex vocal tics* may include repeating phrases, words, or sentences. People may repeat their own phrases, another person's words, or

obscene words. Tics can worsen with emotion (e.g., excitement and anxiety).

Infections
Encephalitis
Encephalitis is the inflammation of the brain. There are several types of encephalitis, including:
- *Japanese encephalitis:* Mosquito-transmitted viral infection that occurs in Asia and the western Pacific. Travelers can be vaccinated for prevention of this disease.
- *La Crosse encephalitis:* Mosquito-transmitted viral infection that occurs in the upper Midwestern, mid-Atlantic, and southeastern states.
- *Saint Louis encephalitis:* Mosquito-transmitted viral infection that occurs in the eastern and central states.

Encephalitis can be caused by a viral or bacterial infection. With a mild case, a person may have flu-like symptoms. With a severe case, a person may experience a severe headache, drowsiness, vomiting, confusion, seizures, and a sudden fever. Babies may constantly cry, not eat well, and have body stiffness and bulging **fontanels**.

After a physical and neurological examination, the provider may order a cerebrospinal fluid analysis, which requires a lumbar puncture. Blood laboratory tests and CT may also be done. Severe cases require hospitalization and intravenous (IV) medications to treat the infection and reduce the brain inflammation. Milder bacterial infections require oral antibiotics. Physical, speech, and occupational therapies may be required for some patients after other symptoms have resolved.

Meningitis
Meningitis is the inflammation of the meninges surrounding the brain and spinal cord. Viral meningitis, the most common form, is caused by a viral infection that affects the nose or mouth and travels to the brain. Bacterial meningitis, usually caused by pneumococcal or meningococcal infections, starts with a cold-like infection and can be deadly. The meningitis vaccine can help prevent certain types of bacterial infections that cause meningitis.

Meningitis can be caused by a viral, bacterial, or fungal infection. There is also a noninfectious meningitis and a cancer-related meningitis. The symptoms may include a sudden high fever, severe headache, stiff neck, nausea, and vomiting. Bacterial meningitis can cause hearing loss, brain damage, and a stroke.

After a physical and neurological examination, the provider will order blood tests (e.g., blood culture), imaging tests, and a lumbar puncture to test the cerebrospinal fluid. With bacterial meningitis, the patient usually receives IV antibiotics to treat the infection and corticosteroids to reduce the inflammation. With viral meningitis, bed rest, fluids, and OTC analgesics are usually prescribed. Antifungal medications will be given for a fungal meningitis. The underlying cause of the meningitis also needs to be treated.

Structural Disorders
Bell's Palsy
Bell's palsy is the most common cause of facial paralysis. The symptoms typically affect one side of the face, and the symptoms are at their worst about 48 hours after the onset.

Researchers believe that a viral infection causes the facial nerve inflammation. The risk of Bell's palsy increases with pregnancy, diabetes,

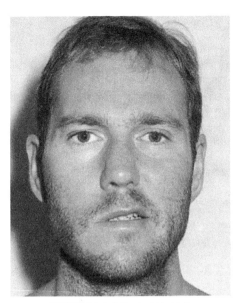

FIGURE 21.8 Bell's palsy (right-sided).

or with an upper respiratory viral infection. The signs and symptoms include facial twitching, weakness, and paralysis; drooping of the eyelid or corner of the mouth; dry eyes or excessive tearing; and drooling, dry mouth, and a diminished ability to taste (Fig. 21.8).

The provider will do a medical history and a physical examination. No other tests are usually ordered. Usually symptoms resolve within 2 weeks, but it may take 3 to 6 months to return to normal function. Some mild cases do not require treatment, whereas others may be treated with antiviral and corticosteroid medications. Protecting the eye from injury is important, thus eye drops for lubrication and a patch for protection may be used.

Guillain-Barré Syndrome

Guillain-Barré syndrome is a rare autoimmune disorder in which the immune system attacks the peripheral nervous system.

The etiology is unknown, but the disorder may be triggered by surgery, an infection, or vaccination. Weakness and tingling start in the legs and spread through the body, making the person almost paralyzed. The disease is life-threatening, and the person may require a respirator to breathe. It may take several weeks before the symptoms improve, and recovery can take up to a few years.

After the physical examination, the provider may order electromyography, nerve conduction studies, and a lumbar puncture. This disorder is difficult to diagnose. Treatment is aimed at relieving the symptoms and supporting breathing if needed.

Injuries

Traumatic Brain Injury. Traumatic brain injury (TBI) is an acquired brain injury. TBIs can occur as a result of falls, motor vehicle accidents, violence (e.g., **shaken baby syndrome**, gunshot wounds), sports injuries, and service in military combat zones. A **concussion** is a mild form of a TBI and is the most common type of sports injury. A *contusion* is bruising or swelling of the brain that occurs when small cerebral blood vessels bleed into brain tissue.

TBI can occur as a result of a violent jolt or blow to the head or body, or when something pierces the skull (e.g., bullet) and injures the brain tissue. Symptoms of TBI may not appear for weeks after the injury. TBI can be mild, moderate, severe, or life-threatening, depending on the brain damage.

- Mild TBI symptoms include headache, neck pain, nausea, ringing in the ear, dizziness, lightheadedness, blurred vision, tiredness, dazed feeling, mood changes, and trouble concentrating or remembering. Children experience irritability and changes in eating.
- Moderate or severe TBI symptoms are similar. The headache is constant and gets worse. The person may experience repeated vomiting, seizures, inability to awaken, dilation of one or both pupils, slurred speech, agitation, loss of coordination, and weakness in the extremities. Children may also be inconsolable and refuse to eat.

For severe injuries, emergency personnel will use the **Glasgow Coma Scale** to assess the patient. In the hospital, imaging tests (CT and MRI), along with intracranial pressure monitoring, will be done. In the ambulatory care facility, the provider will obtain information on the injury and perform a physical and neurological examination. A CT or MRI may be ordered to check for skull fractures. For mild TBIs, treatment consists of rest and OTC analgesics. For moderate to severe TBI, medications are given to reduce the brain swelling and prevent more damage. Surgery may be done to remove blood clots (*hematomas*), repair skull fractures, stop bleeding in the brain, and to relieve pressure (by removing a portion of the skull). Various rehabilitation specialists may be involved during the recovery phase.

Shaken Baby Syndrome

Shaken baby syndrome (SBS) is the leading cause of child abuse deaths. There are over 1300 cases a year in the United States, and about a quarter of the children die. SBS occurs when a child is violently shaken or when the head strikes against a hard surface (e.g., wall, counter, floor). Crying is the leading trigger for the violence that leads to SBS, and most babies are less than 6 months old when it occurs.

Signs and symptoms of SBS include lethargy, extreme irritability, bruises, rigidity, difficulty breathing, bulging fontanels, inability to focus the eyes or track movement, unequal pupil size, seizures, and poor feeding.

About 80% of the children who survive SBS have lifelong disabilities, including blindness, seizures, hearing loss, developmental delays (e.g., speech, learning, memory, attention), cerebral palsy, and severe mental retardation.

According the National Center on Shaken Baby Syndrome (*www.dontshake.org*), the Period of PURPLE Crying program is an evidence-based shaken baby syndrome prevention program that helps caregivers understand crying in infants and helps to prevent SBS. The letters in PURPLE describe important information for parents and caregivers.

- **P**eak of Crying: Crying may increase weekly until 2 months of age.
- **U**nexpected: The child may cry off and on, though the parent/caregiver may not know why.
- **R**esists Soothing: The child may not stop crying regardless of what the parent/caregiver does.
- **P**ain-like face: The child's facial appearance may indicate he or she is in pain, though it may not be the situation.
- **L**ong lasting: The child can cry more than 5 hours a day.
- **E**vening: Crying may increase in the late afternoon or evening.

Spinal Cord Injury. Spinal cord injuries occur when a blow, gunshot, or stabbing fractures or dislocates the vertebrae and the bone pieces cut into the cord or press on the nerves. Common causes include motor vehicle accidents, falls, acts of violence, alcohol, and diseases. Spinal cord injuries can be:

- *Complete*: No signals can be sent below the level of the injury and the person is paralyzed below the injury.
- *Incomplete*: Some signals can be sent below the injury, and thus the person has some movement and sensation below the injury.

The cause is an injury to the vertebrae. This is a medical emergency. Initially, the person may experience extreme back or neck pain, incontinence of bowel or bladder, difficulty breathing, and paralysis.

- *Quadriplegia* (or *tetraplegia*): The spinal cord injury affects the arms, hands, trunk, legs, and pelvic organs (e.g., bowel, bladder, and sexual functions).
- *Paraplegia*: The spinal cord injury affects some or all of the trunk, legs, and pelvic organs.

The emergency providers will perform a physical and neurological examination. Imaging studies (x-ray, myelogram, MRI, and CT) will be done. Treatments include surgery, traction, corticosteroids, and rehabilitation (e.g., physical and occupational therapies).

Peripheral Neuropathy

Peripheral neuropathy occurs as a result of damage to the peripheral nervous system. Over 100 types of peripheral neuropathy have been identified, each with its own symptoms. Diabetic neuropathy is one of the most common forms.

The cause may be inherited, acquired, or unknown (which is called *idiopathic*). Acquired peripheral neuropathy can be caused by:

- *Physical injury:* Related to trauma (accidents, sports-related activities, surgical procedures, and falls) or stress from repetitive activities.
- *Diseases:* Related to metabolic and endocrine disorders (e.g., diabetes mellitus), small vessel disease (e.g., vasculitis), autoimmune diseases (e.g., lupus, rheumatoid arthritis), kidney disorders, cancer, and infections (Lyme disease).
- *Exposure to toxins:* Includes medications, environmental and industrial toxins, and heavy alcohol consumption.

Signs and symptoms include tingling and numbness, paresthesia, weakness, increased sensitivity to stimuli, burning pain, muscle wasting, paralysis, and organ dysfunction. With diabetic neuropathy, pain and numbness are felt in both legs, with gradual progression up the legs. Eventually, the person may feel pain and numbness in the fingers, hands, and arms.

The provider will do physical and neurological examinations. Additional tests will be done, including nerve conduction velocity (NCV), electromyography (EMG), MRI, and nerve and skin biopsies. Treatment addresses the underlying causes and symptom management. Medications such as antidepressants, anticonvulsants, antiarrhythmics, narcotics, and nonsteroidal anti-inflammatory drugs (NSAIDs) may help ease the neuropathic pain.

CRITICAL THINKING APPLICATION   21.7
Nancy's last patient of the day has severe neuropathy in both her hands and feet. The patient stated she can't feel much with her hands. After rooming the patient, Nancy thought about her life if she could not feel much in her hands and feet. How might that affect a person's life? What complications might occur?

Shingles

Herpes zoster, also known as *shingles*, affects about 33% of all adults. Anyone who has had chickenpox can get shingles, including children. Typically, if a person gets shingles, it only occurs once, but there have been cases in which it has developed more than once. Vaccines are available to help prevent shingles.

Shingles is caused by the varicella zoster virus, the same virus that causes chickenpox. After a person has chickenpox, the virus remains inactive in the body. It can reactivate for unknown reasons and cause shingles. The beginning symptoms include tingling, pain, or itching on one side of the body or face, usually on the torso. This can occur 1 to 5 days before a rash with fluid-filled blisters develops (Fig. 21.9). The person is contagious to others who have not had chickenpox until the blisters scab over, in about 10 days. The rash clears up within 1 month. The person may also have fever, chills, headache, and nausea. Shingles can cause postherpetic **neuralgia**, vision loss, encephalitis, and facial paralysis.

The provider will do a history and physical examination to diagnose shingles. There is no cure, but antiviral medications may be ordered to help reduce complications and hasten recovery. Depending on the pain, the provider may also order anticonvulsants, antidepressants, or analgesics.

Spina Bifida

Spina bifida is a neural tube defect that occurs when the spinal column does not close during the first month of pregnancy. Spina bifida can cause damage to the nerves and spinal cord. Pregnant women are encouraged to take folic acid during pregnancy to reduce the risk of spina bifida.

The cause is unknown. There are four types of spina bifida:

- *Spina bifida occulta*: Mildest form; no spinal nerves are involved, but one or more vertebrae are malformed. No signs or symptoms may be present. The only indication may be an abnormal cluster of hair, a small dimple, or birthmark on the infant's back (Fig. 21.10).

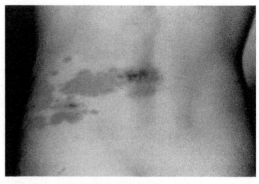

FIGURE 21.9 Herpes zoster (shingles).

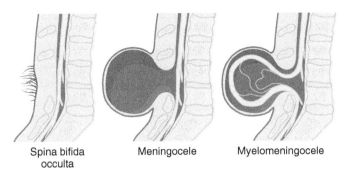

Spina bifida
occulta   Meningocele   Myelomeningocele

FIGURE 21.10 Types of Spina Bifida.

- *Closed neural tube defect*: Includes a malformation of the fat, bone, or meninges associated with the spinal cord. Symptoms range from no symptoms to incomplete paralysis with bowel and urinary dysfunction.
- *Meningocele*: The meninges protrude through an abnormal vertebral opening creating a sac. The sac is filled with fluid. Symptoms range from no symptoms to complete paralysis with bowel and bladder dysfunction.
- *Myelomeningocele*: The most serious type, because the spinal canal is open along several vertebrae. A sac containing fluid, part of the spinal cord, and nerves comes through the opening in the infant's back. This type can cause partial or complete paralysis below the opening. The child may have weakness or paralysis of the legs, bowel and bladder incontinence, lack of feeling in the legs, and an increase in cerebrospinal fluid (see Fig. 21.10).

During pregnancy, the mother can take a maternal serum alpha-fetoprotein (MSAFP) test. If abnormally high amounts of alpha-fetoprotein (AFP) are found, it suggests that the baby has a neural tube defect (e.g., spina bifida). The accuracy of the MSAFP test is not perfect. Even though abnormally high levels of AFP are found, the baby may be normal. With negative test results, there is a small risk of spina bifida. Amniocentesis can also be done, if the MSAFP test result comes back abnormal. Most of the time, ultrasound can detect the two most severe types of spina bifida during pregnancy. Prenatal surgery for spina bifida can occur around 26 weeks of pregnancy. The child may have fewer disabilities if the spinal cord is repaired at that time. Surgery can also occur after birth. Additional treatments focus on the complications that occur, including leg weakness, bowel or bladder problems, and **hydrocephalus**.

Shunt System

Hydrocephalus can be treated with surgical placement of a shunt system. The shunt system drains the extra CSF from the brain into another part of the body (e.g., abdomen), where it is absorbed into the bloodstream. The shunt system consists of a catheter that the CSF flows into, a regulation valve, and an outflow catheter, which drains the fluid into another part of the body. A shunt system needs to be replaced as the person ages or when it gets blocked. Increased intracranial pressure (ICP) is a sign that the shunt system is not functioning correctly. A person may experience a headache, nausea and vomiting, confusion, double vision, and decreased mental abilities with ICP.

Tumors

Benign (noncancerous) and *malignant* (cancerous) tumors can occur in the brain and spinal cord. Tumors can place pressure on the CNS, causing impaired function.

Tumors can be caused by genetic diseases (e.g., tuberous sclerosis), radiation exposure, or cancer-causing chemicals. Signs and symptoms depend on the tumor's location:

- Spinal cord tumors: Cause pain, numbness, and paralysis
- Brain tumors: Cause seizures, nausea and vomiting, poor vision or hearing, headaches, behavioral changes, changes in thinking, and balance and coordination problems

The provider will do a physical and neurological examination. Imaging tests (CT, MRI, and PET), laboratory tests, and a biopsy may be done. Treatment depends on the type of tumor. Surgery, radiation, chemotherapy, and corticosteroids may be prescribed.

Other Structural Disorders

Additional structural disorders include the following:

- *Cerebral palsy* (CP): A group of nonprogressive disorders caused by abnormal brain development or brain injury, resulting in muscle weakness or problems with using the muscles. CP can affect people's ability to move and maintain their posture and balance. Signs and symptoms usually appear during infancy or preschool years. The child can have abnormal reflexes, floppiness or rigidity of the extremities, abnormal posture, involuntary movements, and unsteady *gait* (manner or style of walking). CP is classified by the main type of movement disorder involved: *spasticity* (stiff muscles), *dyskinesia* (uncontrollable movements), and *ataxia* (poor balance and coordination).
- *Down Syndrome* (also called *Trisomy 21*): The most common chromosomal condition in the United States. It is a condition in which a person is born with an extra copy of chromosome 21. The complications from Down syndrome range and can include intellectual disabilities, dementia, heart disease, hearing and visual issues, thyroid disease, and musculoskeletal complications (e.g., poor muscle tone).

Vascular Disorders

Vascular disorders that affect the nervous system tend to affect the brain. These can include aneurysms and hemorrhages, which can lead to strokes.

Cerebrovascular Accident

A cerebrovascular accident (CVA), also called a *stroke*, is the fifth leading cause of death in the United States and a major cause of serious disability. Strokes can occur at any age, but they usually occur in older adults. A stroke is a medical emergency.

There are three types of strokes:

- *Ischemic stroke*: Occurs when the arterial blood flow to part of the brain is blocked. The brain cells start to die after a few minutes. This is the most common type of stroke. Two common types of ischemic strokes include:
  - *Thrombotic stroke*: A blood clot forms in an artery, blocking the blood to part of the brain.
  - *Embolic stroke*: A blood clot or other debris forms elsewhere in the body and moves into the brain arteries, blocking the blood flow.

TABLE 21.4   Cerebrovascular Accidents

RISK FACTORS	SIGNS AND SYMPTOMS
• Family history of stroke • Cardiovascular disease • Hypertension • High cholesterol • Diabetes • Cigarette smoking • Being overweight • Physical inactivity • Heavy or binge drinking • Use of illicit drugs (e.g., cocaine and methamphetamines)	• Confusion or mental changes • Speech difficulty (forming words, difficult to understand, or using words that do not make sense) • Numbness of the face, arm, or leg, usually on one side of the body • Problem seeing in one or both eyes • Trouble walking, lack of coordination or balance, or arm weakness • Sudden, severe headache • Facial drooping • *Hemiparesis* (weakness on one side of the body) and *hemiplegia* (one-sided paralysis)

- *Hemorrhagic stroke*: Occurs when an artery in the brain leaks or ruptures. The leaked blood puts pressure on the surrounding brain cells, causing damage. High blood pressure and **aneurysms** can cause hemorrhagic strokes. Two types of hemorrhagic strokes are:
  - *Intracerebral hemorrhage*: The most common type; it occurs when a cerebral aneurysm ruptures.
  - *Subarachnoid hemorrhage*: Bleeding occurs in the subarachnoid space, usually caused by small aneurysms.
- *Transient ischemic attack (TIA)*: Also called a "mini-stroke" because it lasts for only a few minutes. The blood supply to a part of the brain is briefly blocked. Symptoms are similar to stroke symptoms but do not last as long (e.g., 1 to 24 hours).

There are many risk factors (Table 21.4). The symptoms of a CVA relate to the part of the brain affected. The individual may not have all the symptoms.

The emergency department providers will perform a physical and neurological examination. Blood tests and imaging tests (CT, MRI, and cerebral angiogram) will indicate the type of stroke, which will then determine the treatment.

- Ischemic strokes are treated with clot-dissolving medications (e.g., a tissue plasminogen activator) that help the body break down the clot that is blocking the artery. The clot can also be removed by surgery if needed.
- Hemorrhagic strokes are treated with antihypertensives and surgical repair of the vessel. If the person is taking an anticoagulant or antiplatelet medication, medications to reverse the effects may be given.
- TIAs are treated with antihypertensive, anticoagulant, and antiplatelet medications. The goal is to prevent a future stroke.

Additional treatments address the life-changing complications of stroke. Physical, occupational, and speech therapies may be used to help with the disabilities.

CRITICAL THINKING APPLICATION   21.8

A patient had a stroke in the right side of her brain that affected her left arm and hand. What types of daily activities (e.g., bathing, grooming, eating) might she struggle with if she is left-hand dominant? What if she is right-hand dominant?

THE MEDICAL ASSISTANT'S ROLE IN NEUROLOGY PROCEDURES

Assisting With the Examination

As with other physical examinations, a careful history provides the provider with valuable clues in diagnosing neurological conditions. Such clues may include a record of seizures, *syncope* (faint), *diplopia* (double vision), incontinence, or any of the previously mentioned subjective symptoms. The patient's general health often complicates a neurological diagnosis.

As part of the medical history, a medical assistant may be asked by the provider to give and score a neurological status exam (if this is within the scope of practice for the state and agency). This exam tests the patient's cognitive functions and provides a baseline of neurological information for the provider (Fig. 21.11; also see Procedure 21.1, p. 552). Part of the exam also requires gathering information from the patient's caregiver.

The provider will do a neurological examination, also called a neuro exam, to evaluate the functioning of the patient's nervous system. During the examination, the provider may determine the effect of the symptoms on the patient's emotional status, intellectual performance, cognitive ability, and general behavior (see Procedure 21.2, p. 553). The patient's grooming and mannerisms are carefully observed, as is his or her ability to communicate effectively, including the appropriate use of speech, language, and writing skills. The exam may assess many different areas, including:

- *Mental status:* The patient's level of awareness is assessed. Is the person aware of person, place, and time? Providers may ask people to state their full name, where they are, and what the date is. If the person knows these three things, providers may document "Alert and oriented," "alert and oriented to person, place, and time," or "A&O×3." For neuro exams, it is always good to document what was asked and the patient's exact answer. The mental status is also assessed as the provider interacts with the patient. Is the patient's speech clear? Does the patient make sense when talking?
- *Functioning of the cranial nerves:* Table 21.1 describes how the nerves are assessed.
- *Motor function, balance, and coordination:* The patient may be asked to push and pull against the provider's hands as the provider checks all of the patient's extremities. The provider may have the patient walk or stand with his or her eyes closed to assess balance. The patient may be asked to walk normally or on a line on the floor. The provider may also have the patient touch his or her nose with the eyes closed.
- *Sensory function:* The provider may test the patient's ability to feel sensations by using sharp, dull, or light touch, as well as hot, cold, and vibrating items.
- *Reflexes (children and adults):* Using a reflex hammer, the provider will tap the extremities in different locations to check the reflexes

WALDEN–MARTIN
FAMILY MEDICAL CLINIC
1234 ANYSTREET | ANYTOWN, ANYSTATE 12345
PHONE 123-123-1234 | FAX 123-123-5678

Instructor: Becky Swisher

Neurological Status Exam

The Neurological Status Examination tests the individual's sense of cognitive functions and quickly allows the provider to screen for cognitive impairment and/or loss. In addition to testing language recall and motor skills, the NSE also allows you to test an individual's orientation to time, detail, and attention.

There are five sections. Each section of the test involves relating a series of questions or commands to a patient; the patient should receive one point for each correct answer. Conduct the test without interruptions in a well-lit, private exam room. Instruct the patient to listen carefully and to answer each question as accurately as possible. In the event that there is a caregiver accompanying the patient, ask the Caregiver Questions and record the responses (these are not part of the final score).

Read each question once and document the patient's response. Do not time the patient's answers or duration of the test overall; once completed, score the test immediately. To do so, add only the number of correct responses. The indivicual can receive a maximum score of 10 points; a score below 4 indicates cognitive impairment.

Patient Name: _____ Date of Birth: _____
Performed By: _____ Date: _____

Caregiver Questions (if available): (Yes, No, Not Aware)

Name of Caregiver: _____

	Yes	No	Not Aware
• Does the patient have difficulty remembering recent events or conversions?	☐	☐	☐
• Does the patient have difficulty performing activities of daily living (bath, driving, cooking, ets.)	☐	☐	☐
• Have you noticed changes to speech patterns?	☐	☐	☐

Patient Interview

Sequencing:

Read the following statement to the patient three consecutive times: **"Drive the red car to Washington Street".** Then ask the Patient to restate the sentence; you will ask the patient to recall the statement later in the test.

	Yes	No
The patient was able to repeat the exact statement to you	☐	☐

Total: _____

Time Orientation:

Ask the patient the following questions:

	Correct	Incorrect
• What is today's date?	☐	☐
• What season is it?	☐	☐
• What is the day of the week?	☐	☐

Total: _____

Drawing:

Give the individual a piece of paper and ask him/her to copy a design of the two intersecting shapes. Once point is awarded for correctly copying the shapes. All angles on both figures must be present, and the figures must have one overlapping angle.

	Correct	Incorrect
	☐	☐

Total: _____

Information:

Ask the patient the following questions:

	Correct	Incorrect
• Who is president of the United States?	☐	☐
• How may stars are on the American flag?	☐	☐

Total: _____

Recall:

Ask the patient to restate the sentence that you asked him/her at the beginning of the procedure. One point is given for repeating each of the following words.

	Correct	Incorrect
• Drive	☐	☐
• Red car	☐	☐
• Washington Street	☐	☐

Total: _____

Total Exam Score: _____

FIGURE 21.11 Neurological Status Exam Form.

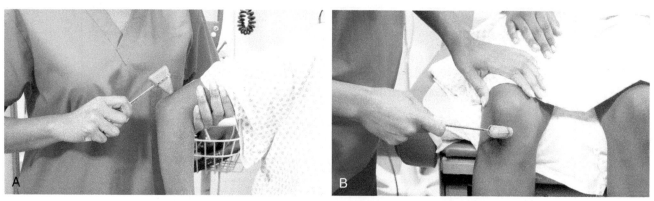

FIGURE 21.12 The provider checks **(A)** the triceps reflex and **(B)** the quadriceps reflex.

(Fig. 21.12). If the reflex is present and normal, a small movement of the extremity will occur.

- *Newborn and infant reflexes*: Different reflexes may be observed with these age groups. Examples include:
  - *Babinski reflex*: When the foot is stroked, the toes fan outward.
  - *Moro* or *startle reflex*: With sudden position changes or with loud noises, the infant moves the arms sideways with the palms up and the thumbs flexed, then pulls them toward the body.
  - *Palmar grasp*: When a finger is placed in the infant's palm, the fingers grasp it.

The medical assistant's role in the neuro exam differs among facilities. The medical assistant may need to set up for the exam. Some providers may have the medical assistant remain in the room and assist by handing supplies and helping the patient change positions. The medical assistant may also be asked to document the provider's findings during the exam.

Assisting With Diagnostic Procedures

The medical assistant assists with diagnostic procedures by scheduling and preparing patients for procedures. If tests require restrictions on food or fluids, the medical assistant should address the following points with the patient after talking with the provider:

- Can the patient have water prior to the test?
- Which medications should the patient take prior to the test, or when can the patient resume the current medications?

Table 21.5 describes common diagnostic procedures used for neurological conditions. The medical assistant may need to screen the patient for specific allergies, medications, and so on prior to the scheduling of the procedure. For some procedures, a signed consent form is required. The patient should be notified of what he or she will experience during the procedure and any follow-up care required after the test. The following sections will describe the lumbar puncture and the electroencephalography procedures in more detail.

Lumbar Puncture

A lumbar puncture (LP), also known as a spinal tap, is done to collect a small amount of CSF, to measure the pressure of the CSF, and to inject medication into the spinal cord structures. These medications may include spinal anesthetic for surgery, chemotherapy for

cancer treatment, and contrast dye (for x-ray procedures, such as myelography).

In ambulatory care, the most frequent reason for an LP is to obtain a sample of the CSF. The CSF is analyzed to help confirm or rule out many diseases, including meningitis, encephalitis, cancer, and dementia (Table 21.6).

In preparation for the procedure, the patient should be asked if he or she is taking a medication or herbal product that may increase the risk of bleeding (e.g., anticoagulant and antiplatelet medications, garlic, ginger, St. John's wort, and ginseng). The patient may be restricted from eating or drinking 3 or more hours prior to the procedure. The provider will explain the procedure to the patient, and a consent form is signed prior to the procedure.

The patient is placed in either a left side-lying position with the knees drawn up to the chest or in a sitting position leaning forward on a stable surface (see Procedure 21.3, p. 554). For an infant or young child, the medical assistant might need to hold the child in a side-lying position during the procedure.

The site is cleansed with an antiseptic, and a local anesthetic is injected to numb the area. The provider then inserts a hollow needle between the third and fourth or the fourth and fifth lumbar vertebrae and advances it into the subarachnoid space (Fig. 21.13). The CSF flows out of the needle into the sterile collection tubes. Usually 1 to 2 mL is collected in each tube, and multiple tubes may be collected. A total of about 10 to 15 mL is typically collected. The tubes need to be numbered in the order that they are collected. The needle is removed, and a bandage or small dressing is applied to the site.

After the procedure, the patient typically needs to lie down for about an hour and drink a lot of fluid. If more CSF is removed, the patient may need to lie down for a longer period of time. Prior to leaving the ambulatory care facility, the provider will check the insertion site and assess if the patient has any issues (e.g., problems moving the legs). The patient should not drive and will need to rest at home the remaining part of the day.

Lumbar punctures may cause:

- Post-lumbar puncture headaches, due to CSF leaking into nearby tissues. The patient may experience nausea, vomiting, and dizziness. Usually, the headaches resolve after lying down. These headaches may last for a week or more after the procedure.

TABLE 21.5   Diagnostic Procedures for Neurological Conditions

PROCEDURE	DESCRIPTION	PATIENT PREPARATION
Cerebral angiography	Used to see how the blood flows through the brain. A person must lie on the x-ray table without moving. The head is held still. A local anesthetic is given in the groin area, and a catheter is threaded through an artery in the groin until it reaches the neck. X-ray is used to help guide the process. A dye is injected and highlights the blood flow through the brain.	Screen for bleeding problems or taking anticoagulants, allergy to contrast dye, pregnancy, or kidney function problems. The patient may not eat or drink for 4 to 8 hours prior to the test. The patient may feel a brief discomfort during the anesthetic injection and the threading of the catheter. The contrast dye may cause a warming or burning feeling on the face and head.
Cerebral spinal fluid analysis	CSF is analyzed to determine any abnormalities. The specimen is gathered by a lumbar puncture (spinal tap) performed by a provider. An anesthetic will be given. A needle is inserted, and the fluid is collected. The CSF is then sent to the laboratory for testing.	Screen for bleeding problems or taking anticoagulants. A consent form must be signed. The patient may be put in an uncomfortable position during the test and will need to hold the position through the procedure. The patient may feel a sting when the anesthetic is injected.
Electromyography (EMG)	Used to test the health of nerves and muscles. A fine needle with an electrode is inserted into the muscle. The electrode picks up the electrical activity from the muscle during activity and at rest. The activity is recorded.	Screen if taking an anticoagulant. Patient should avoid using creams and lotions on the day of the test. The patient should have normal body temperature because a lowered temperature can affect the test. The patient may feel the insertion of the needles. After the test, the muscle may be tender. The patient may have bruising for a few days.
Nerve conduction velocity (NCV) test	Done with an EMG usually. Done to test the speed of electrical signals as they move through a nerve. Electrode patches are placed on the skin over nerves and give off a mild electrical impulse. The electrical activity is recorded by other electrodes.	Screen if the patient has a cardiac defibrillator or pacemaker. Patient should avoid any lotions, sunscreen, perfume, or moisturizer on the test day. The patient may feel the impulse and have some discomfort.
Nerve biopsy	The removal of a small piece of the nerve for examination. After applying an analgesic, the provider makes a small surgical incision and removes a piece of the nerve from either the ankle, forearm, or rib area.	There is no special preparation. The patient may feel the injection of the local anesthetic medication. The biopsy site will be sore for a few days after the test.

- Bleeding at the site or into the epidural space.
- Brainstem herniation.
- Back discomfort, tenderness, or pain in the lower back. Pain may radiate down the back of the legs.

The patient should notify the provider of any abnormalities, including numbness and tingling in the legs, draining or pain at the injection site, an increase in the number or intensity of headaches, and inability to urinate.

Electroencephalography

Electroencephalography (EEG) is used to record the brain wave activity of a patient. An EEG may be done to rule out or confirm seizure activity, AD, psychosis, and narcolepsy, a sleep disorder.

The medical assistant should coach the patient on the preparations for an EEG (see Procedure 21.4, p. 555). In preparation for the procedure, patients should wash their hair the evening before or the morning of the procedure. They should not use any conditioner or hair care products (e.g., gels, hairspray). Using hair care products can interfere with the electrodes adhering to the scalp. Providers may have patients hold (not take) certain medications before the test, if they may interfere with the EEG. Patients should avoid consuming any caffeine on the day of the test. If the EEG requires patients to sleep during the test, providers may encourage them to limit their sleep to 4 or 5 hours the night before.

During the procedure the patient will be relaxing in a bed or reclining chair. The technician will apply 16 to 25 electrodes to the scalp, either with a cap or paste. The wires from the electrodes bring the electrical impulses to the computer. The electrical activity in the brain is then recorded. The technician will record brain activity while the patient is at rest or asleep and with activities and stimuli (e.g., bright flashing light). The test takes between 45 minutes and 2 hours.

Once the test is done, the electrodes are removed and the paste is removed with warm water. If the patient was given a sedative, no

TABLE 21.6 Typical Laboratory Values for Cerebrospinal Fluid

	NORMAL CSF	ABNORMAL CSF AND RELATED CONDITIONS
Pressure ($mm\ H_2O$)	70–180	**Increased:** Increased intracranial pressure **Decreased:** Spinal cord tumor, fainting, diabetic coma, and shock
Appearance	Clear, colorless	**Cloudy:** Infection, elevated white blood cells or protein **Bloody or red:** Bleeding **Brown, orange, or yellow:** Increased protein or previous bleeding
Glucose (mg/dL)	50–80	**Increased:** Hyperglycemia (high blood glucose) **Decreased:** Hypoglycemia (low blood glucose), bacterial or fungal infection (e.g., bacterial meningitis), tuberculosis
Protein (mg/dL)	15–60	**Increased:** Blood in the CSF, diabetes, polyneuritis, injury, inflammation, infection, or tumor **Decreased:** Rapid CSF production
Blood Cells	0–5 White blood cells 0 Red blood cells	**Increase in white blood cells:** Meningitis, acute infection, tumor, abscess, stroke, multiple sclerosis **Increase in red blood cells:** Traumatic lumbar puncture, bleeding into the CSF

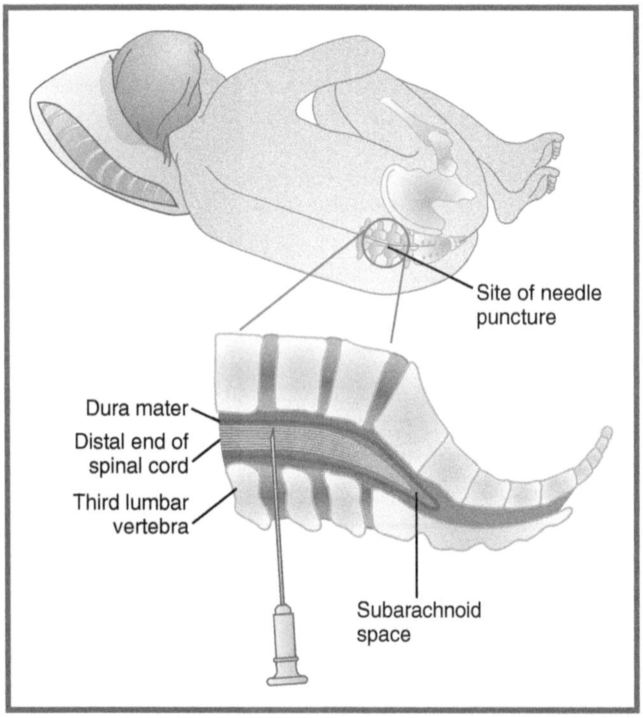

Site of needle puncture
Dura mater
Distal end of spinal cord
Third lumbar vertebra
Subarachnoid space

FIGURE 21.13 Lumbar puncture.

driving is allowed after the test. Mild skin irritation may occur for a few hours after the test. The patient should be informed of when to restart medications and when to anticipate the test results.

Assisting With Treatments

Patients with neurological disorders are prescribed a variety of medications. The following are some of the more common classifications of medications:

- *Analgesics*: Used to relieve pain
- *Anesthetics*: Used to produce local anesthesia or general anesthesia
- *Anti-Alzheimer*: Used to treat AD
- *Anticonvulsants*: Used to treat neuromuscular disorders and epilepsy
- *Antidepressants*: Used to treat depression, anxiety, and other neurological disorders
- *Antimigraines*: Used to treat migraine headaches
- *Corticosteroids*: Used to treat chronic inflammatory and some autoimmune diseases (e.g., multiple sclerosis)

Refer to Table 21.7 for information on the medication classification, including indication for use, desired effect, side effects, adverse reactions, and generic and trade names. Medical assistants should be familiar with medications that are prescribed to patients.

CLOSING COMMENTS

Patient Coaching

Often with neurological disorders, patients need to take medications daily or several times a day. With the symptoms of the disease, remembering can be difficult for some patients. The medical assistant may need to help patients figure out strategies to remember to take their medications. Some methods that can be used include:

- Placing medications near the kitchen table, if they need to be taken with food. (Always remember to keep medications out of the reach of children.)
- Get into a routine and always take the medications after doing a specific task (e.g., feeding the pet, brushing teeth, taking a shower).
- Using an alarm on a phone, clock, or app to remind about medication times.
- Have a family member call to check if the medication was taken.
- Cross out the day on the calendar after taking the medication.
- Use weekly pill boxes. Some pharmacies will help set up pill boxes; otherwise have a family member help set it up weekly if needed.

TABLE 21.7 Medication Classifications

CLASSIFICATION	INFORMATION	GENERIC NAME (TRADE NAME)
Analgesics	**Indications for use:** Relieve pain. **Desired effects:** Reduce the sensory function of the brain; block pain receptors. **Side effects and adverse reactions:** *Nonnarcotic:* GI distress, liver and kidney disorders, and tinnitus. *Narcotic:* hypotension, decreased respirations, agitation, blurred vision, confusion, constipation, sedation, restlessness.	*Nonnarcotic over-the-counter (OTCs):* • **aspirin** (Ecotrin, Bayer Aspirin, Bufferin) • **acetaminophen** (Tylenol, Tempra) (APAP) • **ibuprofen** (Advil, Motrin) *Narcotic (opioids):* • **oxycodone** (OxyContin) • **hydrocodone with acetaminophen** (Lortab, Norco, Vicodin) • **oxycodone with acetaminophen** (Percocet, Oxycet, Roxicet) • **tramadol** (Ultram, Conzip)
Anesthetics	**Indications for use:** Produce local anesthesia (no loss of consciousness) or general anesthesia (loss of consciousness). **Desired effects:** Produce insensibility to pain or the sensation of pain; block nerve impulses to the brain, resulting in unconsciousness. **Side effects and adverse reactions:** Hypotension, cardiopulmonary depression, sedation, nausea, vomiting, headaches.	*Local:* • **lidocaine** (Xylocaine) *General:* • **midazolam** (Versed)
Anti-Alzheimer	**Indications for use:** Alzheimer Disease **Desired effect:** Used to treat dementia be increasing naturally occurring substances in the brain. **Side effects and adverse reactions:** GI distress, frequent urination, muscle cramps, confusion, bradycardia, angina, bloody vomit or stools.	• **donepezil** (Aricept) • **memantine** (Namenda)
Anticonvulsants and Mood Stabilizer	**Indications for use:** Treat epilepsy, trigeminal neuralgia, mania and mixed episodes (mania and depression) with bipolar disorder **Desired effects:** Reduce the frequency and severity of seizures by reducing excessive stimulation of the brain. **Side effects and adverse reactions:** Sedation, vertigo, visual disturbances, GI disturbances, liver complications.	• **carbamazepine** (Tegretol, Equetro) • **lamotrigine** (Lamictal) • **topiramate** (Topamax) • **valproic acid** (Depakene, Depakote) • **gabapentin** (Neurontin, Horizant)
Antidepressants	**Indications for use:** Treat depression, anxiety, and other neurological disorders. **Desired effect:** Treat depression. **Side effects and adverse reactions:** Anorexia, anxiety, sexual dysfunction, fatigue, drowsiness, vertigo, weight gain, confusion, blurred vision.	*Selective serotonin reuptake inhibitors (SSRIs):* • **fluoxetine** (Prozac) • **citalopram** (Celexa) • **escitalopram** (Lexapro) • **sertraline** (Zoloft) *Serotonin and norepinephrine reuptake inhibitors (SNRIs):* • **venlafaxine** • **duloxetine** (Cymbalta) *Atypical antidepressants:* • **bupropion** (Wellbutrin, Zyban) *Serotonin modulators:* • **trazodone** (Oleptro) *Tricyclic antidepressants:* • **amitriptyline** *Monamine oxidase inhibitors (MAOIs):* • **phenelzine** (Nardil)

Continued

TABLE 21.7   Medication Classifications—*continued*

CLASSIFICATION	INFORMATION	GENERIC NAME (TRADE NAME)
Antimigraines	**Indications for use:** Treatment or prevention of migraine headaches. **Desired effect:** Alter circulation to the brain. **Side effects and adverse reactions:** Confusion, psychomotor slowing, difficulty concentrating, memory problems, rare but serious cardiac events.	• **sumatriptan** (Imitrex) • **zolmitriptan** (Zomig)
Corticosteroids (oral)	**Indications for use:** Used to treat chronic inflammatory diseases (e.g., arthritis) and acute conditions (e.g., poison ivy, asthma). **Desired effects:** Reduce inflammation. **Side effects and adverse reactions:** Headache, mood changes, difficulty falling asleep or staying asleep, increased sweating, vision problems, depression, and weight gain.	• **prednisone** (Prednisone Intensol, Sterapred) • **prednisolone** (Flo-Pred, Orapred, Pediapred) • **methylprednisolone** (Medrol)

The medical assistant should also provide the patient directions in writing about what to do if the medication was missed.

Legal and Ethical Issues

In neurology you will be faced with a variety of behaviors and personality changes that frequently are a part of neurological conditions. Often a patient is not aware of these changes and may act as though nothing is wrong. It is important for the medical assistant to remember to treat the patient with respect. All patient information, including pictures, audio recordings, and so on, are confidential. The medical assistant must also remember not to repeat information (gossip) to peers about the patient's actions and behaviors. Only staff immediately involved with the patient have a right to the information required for their care of the patient.

Patient-Centered Care

With many chronic neurological diseases, the patient may require a caregiver to assist with daily care (e.g., toileting, bathing, grooming), meal preparation, shopping, medical appointments, and so on. As the condition worsens, more burdens fall on the caregiver. In many situations the caregiver is the spouse or significant other of the patient; sometimes it may be an adult child. Providing 24/7 caregiving to a loved one is physically and emotionally stressful. With behavioral differences and with increasing dependency, relationship roles may change, and the stress can affect the caregiver's health. It is important for the caregiver to remember to take care of himself or herself.

The medical assistant needs to recognize the importance of the caregiver in the patient's life. The caregiver's concerns are important, just as are the patient's concerns. The medical assistant may need to provide the caregiver with emotional encouragement and resources for additional assistance, including in-home services, adult day care, support groups, and medical equipment.

Professional Behaviors

When working with patients with dementia, communicating with them can be challenging. The medical assistant should remember the following:
- Speak clearly and use short sentences.
- Make eye contact.
- Give them time to respond. Do not pressure them into giving a response.
- Allow them to speak for themselves.
- Keep the tone of your voice friendly and positive. Remain calm.
- Do not patronize or ridicule them.

SUMMARY OF SCENARIO

Nancy had a very busy day with the outreach neurological services providers. One of the most interesting parts of Nancy's day was talking with a patient's wife. The patient had had a stroke, and his wife shared with Nancy the different types of adaptive equipment available. Nancy learned that there were different types of walkers, shower chairs and tub benches, raised toilet seats with handles, dressing devices, grooming aids, kitchen utensils (e.g., rocker knives, cutting boards with suction cups), and specially shaped utensils. Many of the devices were designed to be used with one hand. Nancy was impressed with the variety of adaptive equipment available.

During the day, Nancy felt a little overwhelmed by the complexity of neuro tests and all the different types of test orders. She realizes that she needs to research more on neurological disorders and diagnostic tests before she assists the outreach providers next week. She enjoyed working with the patients and their caregivers and looks forward to getting to know them in the coming months.

SUMMARY OF LEARNING OBJECTIVES

1. **Summarize the anatomy of the nervous system and compare the structure and function of the nervous system across the life span.**

   The nervous system is composed of the central and peripheral nervous systems. The central nervous system is composed of the brain and spinal cord, which are covered by meninges. The cerebrum, cerebellum, diencephalon, and brainstem make up the brain. The peripheral nervous system is composed of the cranial nerves, which exit the brain, and the spinal nerves, which exit the spinal cord.

   The nervous system in infants is immature. Over childhood, the thinking and learning processes become more complex. During adulthood, the brain function is stable. As a person ages, the nervous system changes. Nerve impulses become slower, thus slowing down reaction time.

2. **Discuss the cells of the nervous system and describe polarization, depolarization, and repolarization.**

   The nervous system is composed of two types of cells: neurons and neuroglia. Neurons are made of a cell body, dendrites, and an axon. A stimulus starts an impulse. During polarization, the resting nerve cell has a slightly positive charge on the outside of the cell membrane and a negative charge inside the cell. When a section of the membrane is stimulated, the positively charged ions on the outside of the cell enter the nerve cell. This changes the outside charge to a negative charge. This state is called *depolarization*. Almost immediately after the impulse passes, the positively charged ions move outside the nerve cells again. This returns the outside charge to a positive charge. This state is called *repolarization*. Once everything changes back, the cell is at rest again, and the cycle continues.

3. **Describe the autonomic nervous system, including the sympathetic and parasympathetic nervous systems.**

   The autonomic nervous system consists of nerves that regulate involuntary function. The ANS is an automatic system that regulates body functions such as breathing, heart rate, sweating, circulation, and digestion. It also controls the actions of muscles in blood vessel walls, organs, and glands. The motor portion of this system is further divided into the sympathetic nervous system and the parasympathetic nervous system.

   The *sympathetic nervous system* can produce a "fight or flight" response. This is the part of the nervous system that helps the individual respond to perceived stress. It speeds up the heart rate, raises blood glucose levels, raises blood pressure, slows the digestive system, and widens the bronchioles, allowing more oxygen to enter the body quickly. The *parasympathetic nervous system* does the opposite of the sympathetic nervous system. It slows the heart rate, lowers blood pressure, increases digestive functions, and reduces adrenal and sweat gland activity.

4. **Distinguish among common neurodegenerative diseases.**

   Neurodegenerative diseases affect a person's ability to move, talk, and breathe. These diseases can also affect a person's balance and heart function. Neurodegenerative diseases include:

   - *Amyotrophic lateral sclerosis* (ALS), or Lou Gehrig's disease, a progressive neurological disorder that attacks the motor neurons in the brain and spinal cord.
   - *Alzheimer's disease* (AD), the most common reason for dementia. It damages and kills brain cells.
   - *Huntington's disease* (HD), also called *Huntington's chorea*, a progressive neurodegenerative disorder.
   - *Multiple sclerosis* (MS), an autoimmune neurodegenerative disorder that affects the brain and spinal cord.
   - *Parkinson's disease* (PD), a progressive neurodegenerative disorder that affects movement.

5. **Discuss various functional disorders and describe the three types of seizures.**

   Headaches are the most common form of pain experienced. Types of headaches include cluster headaches, migraines, and tension headaches.

   There are three classifications of seizures, including:

   - *Generalized onset.* Affects both sides of the brain. Includes tonic-clonic seizures, which cause loss of consciousness, and absent seizures, which cause lapses of awareness of the environment.
   - *Focal onset.* Affects one area of the brain. Includes focal aware seizures and focal impaired awareness seizures.
   - *Unknown onset.* Seizure that was not witnessed, or the beginning of the seizure was unknown.

6. **Compare and contrast encephalitis and meningitis.**

   Encephalitis is inflammation of the brain and can be caused by a viral or bacterial infection. With mild cases, a person may have flu-like symptoms. With severe cases, a person may experience a severe headache, drowsiness, vomiting, confusion, seizures, and a sudden fever.

   Meningitis is inflammation of the meninges surrounding the brain and spinal cord. Viral meningitis, the most common form, is caused by a viral infection of the nose or mouth that travels to the brain. Bacterial meningitis, usually caused by pneumococcal infections or meningococcal infections, starts with a cold-like infection but can be deadly.

7. **Distinguish among neurological structural diseases.**

   There are many types of neurological structural diseases, including:

   - *Bell's palsy.* The most common cause of facial paralysis. The symptoms typically only affect one side of the face, and the symptoms are at their worst about 48 hours after the onset.
   - *Guillain-Barré syndrome.* A rare autoimmune disorder in which the immune system attacks the peripheral nervous system.
   - *Traumatic brain injury* (TBI): An acquired brain injury that can occur as a result of falls, motor vehicle accidents, violence, sports injuries, and work in military combat zones.
   - *Spinal cord injuries.* Occur when a blow, gunshot, or stabbing fractures or dislocates the vertebrae and the bone pieces cut into the cord or press on the nerves.
   - *Peripheral neuropathy.* Occurs as a result of damage to the peripheral nervous system.

Continued

SUMMARY OF LEARNING OBJECTIVES—*continued*

- *Shingles (herpes zoster):* Caused by the varicella zoster virus, which also causes chickenpox.
- *Spina bifida:* A neural tube defect that occurs when the spinal column does not close during the first month of pregnancy.
- *Benign* and *malignant tumors:* Occur in the brain and spinal cord and can place pressure on the CNS, causing impaired function.

8. **Describe the types of strokes and related treatments.**
   There are three types of strokes:
   - *Ischemic stroke:* Occurs when the arterial blood flow to part of the brain is blocked. Two common types of ischemic strokes are thrombotic and embolic strokes. Ischemic strokes are treated with clot-dissolving medications.
   - *Hemorrhagic stroke:* Occurs when an artery in the brain leaks or ruptures. Two types of hemorrhagic strokes are intracerebral and subarachnoid strokes. Hemorrhagic strokes are treated with antihypertensives and surgical repair of the vessel.
   - *Transient ischemic attack (TIA):* Also called a "mini-stroke" because it lasts for only a few minutes. The blood supply to a part of the brain is briefly blocked. TIAs are treated with antihypertensive, anticoagulant, and antiplatelet medications.

9. **Discuss the medical assistant's role in a neurological exam.**
   The neurological exam may assess many different areas, including:
   - Mental status
   - Functioning of the cranial nerves
   - Motor function, balance, and coordination
   - Sensory function
   - Reflexes

10. **Summarize the medical assistant's role with a lumbar puncture procedure.**
    The medical assistant should provide the patient with the information needed to prepare for the procedure. During the procedure, the medical assistant needs to assist and, if required, hold the patient in the position required. Once the samples are obtained, the medical assistant must number the vials in the order they were obtained. The remaining activities include monitoring the patient after the procedure, preparing and sending the specimens to the medical laboratory, and cleaning the room.

11. **Summarize the patient coaching required for electroencephalography (EEG).**
    The medical assistant should provide the following coaching to a patient before an EEG:
    - Explain the purpose of an EEG. An EEG is done to check for changes in brain activity and can be helpful for diagnosing different disorders.
    - Explain how the patient should prepare for the test. The patient should avoid caffeine on the day of the test. Take daily medications unless the provider instructs to hold medications until after the test. Wash the hair the night before or the morning of the test, but do not use conditioners or any other hair care products. If the patient is to sleep during the EEG test, encourage the patient to stay up later the night before the test or to avoid sleeping.
    - Explain what the patient should expect during the test. Electrodes (patches with wires) will be attached to the head either with adhesive or by using a special cap.
    - Explain what the patient should expect after the test. The technician will remove the electrodes. If sedation was given, the patient will need a ride home, must rest for the remaining part of the day, and must not drive.
    - Let the patient know when to anticipate the results from the EEG. Also, give the patient the appointment information for the EEG, including the location and time.

PROCEDURE 21.1	Perform a Neurological Status Exam

Tasks: Administer and score the neurological status exam.

Scenario: Dr. Arzt ordered a neurological status exam form to be completed on Robert Caudill (date of birth [DOB] 10/31/1940). He is being accompanied by his caregiver. Role-play this scenario with two peers.

EQUIPMENT and SUPPLIES

- Patient's health record
- Order for the neurological status exam
- Neurological Status Exam Form (see Fig. 21.11) or SimChart for the Medical Office (SCMO).

PROCEDURAL STEPS

1. Wash hands or use hand sanitizer.
   PURPOSE: Hand sanitization is an important step for infection control.
2. **SCMO:** Click on the Form Repository and select the Neurological Status Exam on the INFO PANEL. Read the form.
   Paper form: Read the directions for the test.

PROCEDURE 21.1 Perform a Neurological Status Exam—*continued*

PURPOSE: To complete the test accurately, the directions need to be followed. Know the directions before completing the exam with the patient.

3. Greet the patient. Identify yourself. Verify the patient's identity with full name and date of birth. Explain the procedure to be performed in a manner that the patient understands. Answer any questions the patient may have about the procedure.
   PURPOSE: It is important to identify the patient in two different ways to ensure that you have the correct patient. Explaining the procedure can make the patient feel more comfortable and helps to reduce anxiety.

4. **SCMO:** Click on Patient Search. Select the patient and verify the DOB. Click Select and the patient's name and DOB will autofill into the form field. Key in the information for the performed by and the date fields.
   Paper form: Complete the following information on the exam form: patient name, date of birth, performed by and date.
   PURPOSE: The patient information needs to be completed on the form. Your name and the date also need to be completed.

5. Ask for the caregiver's name and clearly ask the caregiver related questions from the form. Accurately document the information obtained.
   PURPOSE: The caregiver's information is important for the completion of the exam.

6. Perform the patient interview, following the directions on the form. Clearly provide the patient with the directions and the questions. Accurately document the information obtained from the patient.
   PURPOSE: Accurately documenting the information is critical for the accuracy of the exam.

7. Accurately score the test as indicated by the directions.
   SCMO: Key the scores in the total fields. Save the form when completed.
   Paper form: Write the scores on the total line. Give the completed form to the provider.
   PURPOSE: The score is important for the provider for diagnostic purposes.

PROCEDURE 21.2 Assist With the Neurological Exam

Tasks: Set up for a neurological exam and prepare a patient for the procedure. Assist the provider and the patient during the neurological exam.

EQUIPMENT and SUPPLIES

- Patient's health record
- Patient gown
- Drape
- Otoscope
- Ophthalmoscope
- Percussion hammer
- Disposable pinwheel or other disposable sharp per provider
- Penlight
- Tuning fork
- Cotton ball
- Tongue depressor
- Small vials of warm, cold, sweet, and salty liquids
- Small vials of substances with distinct odors (e.g., spices, coffee, vanilla)
- Gloves
- Disinfecting wipes
- Biohazard sharps container
- Waste container

PROCEDURAL STEPS

1. Wash hands or use hand sanitizer.
   PURPOSE: Hand sanitization is an important step for infection control.

2. Assemble supplies and equipment in the exam room.
   PURPOSE: Having all the supplies and equipment for the procedure is important.

3. Greet the patient. Identify yourself. Verify the patient's identity with full name and date of birth. Explain the procedure to be performed in a manner that the patient understands. Answer any questions the patient may have about the procedure.
   PURPOSE: It is important to identify the patient in two different ways to ensure that you have the correct patient. Explaining the procedure can make the patient feel more comfortable and helps to reduce anxiety.

4. Instruct the patient to change into the gown. The opening should be in the back. Ask the patient if assistance is needed. If so, help. If not, leave the room and allow the patient time to change. When reentering the room, provide a courtesy knock on the door.
   PURPOSE: The patient needs to undress for the procedure. Patients require privacy to change.

5. During the examination, be prepared to assist the patient in changing positions as necessary. Have the necessary examination instruments ready for the provider at the appropriate time during the examination. Record all results from the examination as indicated by the provider.
   PURPOSE: Assisting the patient and provider helps to facilitate a thorough, accurate neurological examination

6. After the exam, put on gloves and clean the exam room. Discard sharps in the biohazard sharps container. Discard other waste in the appropriate waste containers. Disinfect equipment and surfaces (e.g., exam table). Remove gloves and discard.
   PURPOSE: Disinfecting equipment and surfaces is an important step for infection control.

7. Wash hands or use hand sanitizer.

PROCEDURE 21.3   Assist With a Lumbar Puncture

Tasks: Set up for a lumbar puncture and prepare a patient for the procedure. Assist the provider during the lumbar puncture procedure. Document the procedure in the patient's health record.

EQUIPMENT and SUPPLIES

- Patient's health record
- Patient gown
- Drape
- Local anesthetic vial
- Syringe and needle
- Alcohol wipes
- Sterile, disposable lumbar puncture kit with specimen tubes
- Mayo stand
- Permanent marker or printed patient labels
- Laboratory requisition and specimen transport bag
- Gloves
- Biohazard waste container
- Biohazard sharps container
- Waste container
- Consent form
- Lumbar puncture instructions (optional)

PROCEDURAL STEPS

1. Wash hands or use hand sanitizer.
   PURPOSE: Hand sanitization is an important step for infection control.
2. Assemble supplies and equipment in the treatment room.
   PURPOSE: Having all the supplies and equipment for the procedure is important.
3. Greet the patient. Identify yourself. Verify the patient's identity with full name and date of birth. Explain the procedure to be performed in a manner that the patient understands. Answer any questions the patient may have about the procedure. Encourage the patient to use the restroom before the procedure.
   PURPOSE: It is important to identify the patient in two different ways to ensure that you have the correct patient. Explaining the procedure can make the patient feel more comfortable and helps to reduce anxiety.
4. Check if the consent form was signed. If the consent was not signed, ask the patient if he or she has any questions. If there are no questions, explain the consent form and have the patient sign the form. If the patient has questions, let the provider know.
   PURPOSE: A signed consent form is needed for the procedure. If the patient has questions, the consent form cannot be signed. The provider should be notified so the questions can be answered.
5. Instruct the patient to change into the gown. The opening should be in the back. Ask the patient if assistance is needed. If so, help. If not, leave the room and allow the patient time to change. When reentering the room, provide a courtesy knock on the door.
   PURPOSE: The patient needs to be undressed for the procedure. Patients require privacy to change.

6. Assist the patient into a left side–lying position with the knees drawn up to the chest, or into a sitting position leaning forward on a stable surface. Support the patient's head with a pillow as necessary and provide a pillow for between the knees if needed.
   PURPOSE: To give the provider the easiest access to the lumbar region, while making the patient as comfortable as possible.
7. Prepare the skin preparation for the provider to use. Open the sterile disposable lumbar puncture kit on a Mayo stand. Without contaminating the supplies, add a sterile needle and sterile syringe to the sterile field.
   PURPOSE: To prevent contamination, the sterile kit should be opened as close to the start of the procedure as possible.
8. If needed, help the patient remain in the proper position. Use the drape to cover the patient. Give verbal encouragement to the patient during the procedure.
   PURPOSE: Encouraging the patient throughout the procedure helps to provide support to the patient.
9. Assist the provider as needed during the procedure. When the provider is ready for the anesthetic, wipe the top of the vial with alcohol. Show the label to the provider and then hold the vial upside down as the provider withdraws the medication needed.
   PURPOSE: To maintain sterile technique and expedite the procedure.
10. Attach the printed labels to the specimen tubes or, using the permanent marker, label the specimens #1, #2, #3, and so on in the order in which they are collected.
    PURPOSE: Different tests are done on different tubes. The accuracy of these tests depends on the tube on which they are performed.
11. Complete the laboratory requisition form and prepare the CSF specimens for transport to the laboratory.
    PURPOSE: To ensure that all the necessary tests are ordered correctly.
12. Put on gloves. Discard the needle/syringe in a biohazard sharps container. Make sure to put the needle in first. Clean up the area. Discard the waste in the appropriate waste container. Remove gloves and discard.
    PURPOSE: Sharps should be discarded as soon as possible after the procedure is over.
13. Wash hands or use hand sanitizer.
14. Monitor the patient and give liquids as directed by the provider. When the patient is ready to leave, instruct the patient to get dressed. Ask the patient if assistance is needed. If so, help. If not, leave the room and allow the patient time to change.
    PURPOSE: The patient needs to be watched after the procedure. The provider should be notified of any concerns or questions.
15. After the patient leaves, put on gloves and clean the room. Disinfect surfaces and discard waste. Remove gloves and discard.
    PURPOSE: Disinfecting surfaces is an important step for infection control.
16. Wash hands or use hand sanitizer.

PROCEDURE 21.3   Assist With a Lumbar Puncture—*continued*

17. Document the procedure in the patient's health record. Include the provider's name, the samples obtained, how the patient tolerated the procedure, and any instructions given.
    PURPOSE: A procedure is not complete until it has been documented accurately in the patient's health record.
    9/15/20XX 1402 Pt had no questions regarding procedure. Consent signed for the lumbar puncture, which was performed by Dr. Kahn. Four vials of 2 mL each of CSF were collected, labeled, and sent to the lab. Pt laid flat on exam table for 60 minutes after procedure. No drainage noted on dressing. Pt has no c/o discomfort. VS: P: 86 regular, strong; R: 20 regular, normal; BP 132/68 left arm, sitting. Patient was instructed to avoid strenuous activity for the rest of the day, to drink plenty of fluids, and to contact the provider if she gets a headache. The Lumbar Puncture instruction sheet was given to the patient. Pt had no questions._____Nancy Gehir, CMA (AAMA)

PROCEDURE 21.4   Coach a Patient for an Electroencephalogram

Tasks: Coach a patient on the preparation needed for an electroencephalogram. Document in the patient's health record.

Order: Provide EEG instructions.

EQUIPMENT and SUPPLIES

- Patient's health record
- Instruction sheet for electroencephalogram (optional)

PROCEDURAL STEPS

1. Wash hands or use hand sanitizer.
   PURPOSE: Hand sanitization is an important step for infection control.
2. Greet the patient. Identify yourself. Verify the patient's identity with full name and date of birth. Explain the procedure to be performed in a manner that the patient understands. Answer any questions the patient may have about the procedure.
   PURPOSE: It is important to identify the patient in two different ways to ensure that you have the correct patient. Explaining the procedure can make the patient feel more comfortable and helps to reduce anxiety.
3. Explain the purpose of an EEG. An EEG is done to check for changes in the brain activity and can be helpful when diagnosing different disorders.
   PURPOSE: The patient needs to understand why the EEG is being done.
4. Explain how the patient should prepare for the test. The patient should avoid caffeine on the day of the test. Take daily medications unless the provider indicates to hold medications until after the test. Wash hair the night before or the morning of the test, but do not use conditioners or any other hair care products. If the patient is to sleep during the EEG test, encourage the patient to stay up later the night before the test or to avoid sleeping.
   PURPOSE: Appropriate preparations are needed for quality test results.

5. Explain what the patient should expect during the test. Electrodes (patches with wires) will be attached to the head either with adhesive or by using a special cap. There will be little to no discomfort during the test. The technician may ask the patient questions during the test.
   PURPOSE: Explaining what to expect during the procedure will help reduce the patient's anxiety about the procedure.
6. Explain what the patient should expect after the test. The technician will remove the electrodes. If sedation was given, the patient will need a ride home, must rest for the remaining part of the day, and must not drive.
   PURPOSE: Letting the patient know any restrictions helps the patient plan for the procedure.
7. Let the patient know when to anticipate the results from the EEG. Also, give the patient the appointment information for the EEG, including the location and time.
   PURPOSE: Letting patients know when to expect test results helps to alleviate confusion and anxiety.
8. Document the teaching in the patient's health record. Include the provider's name and the information given, the type of instructions, appointment information, and any materials.
   PURPOSE: A procedure is not complete until it has been documented accurately in the patient's health record.
   9/12/20XX 1508 Per Dr. Kahn's order, EEG instructions were given to the pt. Pt's questions were answered. Appointment information and the EEG instruction document were given._____Nancy Gehir, CMA (AAMA)

22

BEHAVIORAL HEALTH

Mike Brewer, CMA (AAMA), is a medical assistant at Walden-Martin Family Medical (WMFM) Clinic. He has been with the clinic for 2 years. Mike currently assists outreach providers, who come to WMFM Clinic to provide services for patients. Recently, Mike has been working with the outreach behavioral health providers. During his medical assistant training, Mike learned about different behavioral health disorders, but never felt he wanted to go into that specialty. Over the past 2 years at WMFM Clinic, he has realized that no matter what position he holds, he works with patients who have behavioral health disorders, depression being the most common. He is looking forward to learning more about behavioral health disorders as he continues to help the outreach providers.

While studying this chapter, think about the following questions:
- What are the different healthcare professionals who work in behavioral health?
- What is the importance of the DSM-5 in behavioral health?
- What are early warning signs of behavioral health disorders?
- What are common mental health disorders, including signs, symptoms, diagnostic procedures, and treatments?
- What are common substance use disorders, including signs, symptoms, diagnostic procedures, and treatments?

LEARNING OBJECTIVES

1. Explore the differences between types of common behavioral health professionals.
2. Differentiate among common behavioral health disorders, including the etiology, signs, symptoms, diagnostic procedures, and treatments.
3. Discuss substance use disorders and other addictions. Also, list commonly used substances and describe a "standard" drink of alcohol.
4. Describe how a medical assistant should assist with a mental or behavioral health examination.
5. Explain the common diagnostic procedures for behavioral health disorders. Also, describe the common medication classifications used for behavioral health disorders.
6. Explain the legal issues and Health Insurance Portability and Accountability Act (HIPAA) applications associated with mental health disorders and substance use disorders.

VOCABULARY

affect The external emotional expression.

amnesia (am NEE zhah) Memory loss.

amygdala (ah MIG dah lah) A small mass of gray matter found in each temporal lobe of the cerebrum and involved with memories, emotions, and activating the fight-or-flight response; part of the limbic system.

delusion (de LOO zhun) Unshakable belief in something untrue; may be accompanied by hallucinations and/or paranoia.

depersonalization Alternative perception of the self; a person's own reality is lost. People feel they are not in control of their own actions or speech.

derealization Loss of sensation of the reality of one's surroundings.

euphoria (yoo FOR ee ah) An exaggerated sense of physical and mental well-being.

hallucination (hah loo si NAY shun) A sensory experience (e.g., a smell, sound, sight, touch, or taste) involving something that is not present.

mania (MAY nee ah) Abnormally elated mental state; the person may have feelings of euphoria, lack of inhibitions, sleeplessness, talkativeness, risk-taking behaviors, and irritability.

morbidity (more BID i tee) The rate of a disease in a population.

mortality (more TAL i tee) The relative frequency of deaths in a specific population.

orientation Awareness of one's environment, with reference to people, place, and time.

paranoia An unfounded or excessive suspicion of the motives of others.

psychotherapy (sie KOE ther ah pee) The treatment of behavioral health disorders through the use of psychological techniques, which encourage communication of conflicts and insights into the person's problems. The goals of this treatment include symptom relief, changes in behavior leading to improved social and vocational function, and personality growth.

psychotherapy notes Patient-provider details from private, group, or family therapy, including what the patient stated and the provider's analysis of the statements and situation.

Many times, healthcare students hear about mental health and quickly decide whether or not they are interested in that specialty. In today's healthcare environment, many healthcare professionals, including medical assistants, are involved with mental health and substance abuse issues, regardless of where they work. The number of people in the United States with a mental health or substance-use disorder has been increasing over the years. In 2016, about 44.7 million adults, or 18% of adults in the United States, had a mental illness, and more than 42,000 deaths were related to opioids.

According to the Centers for Disease Control and Prevention (CDC), *mental health* encompasses our psychological, emotional, and social welfare. Our mental health influences how we behave, feel, think, handle stress, interact with others, and make choices. Over the years, the field of mental health has changed and grown. *Psychiatry* is the healthcare specialty that studies the brain and its effects on the body. Today, the phrase "*behavioral health*" is used to refer to mental health, substance abuse, and associated physical disorders.

This chapter begins by describing behavioral health specialists and locations where patients are treated. Information on specific mental health, substance use disorder, and addiction disorders will follow. The chapter will conclude with information on behavioral health diagnostic procedures and treatments.

BEHAVIORAL HEALTH PROFESSIONALS

Psychotherapist is a general term for a healthcare professional who treats people with behavioral health conditions. This term is used for psychiatrists, psychologists, social workers, and so on. In behavioral health departments, there are people with many different credentials. Having a basic understanding of behavioral health professionals is important. The following are some of the more common behavioral health professionals:

- *Psychiatrist*: Trained as a medical doctor and has had 4 years of residency training in psychiatry, usually in a hospital setting. A psychiatrist assesses the mental and physical conditions related to psychological disorders. A psychiatrist treats patients with psychological disorders and can prescribe medications.
- *Psychologist*: Studied personality development, psychological problems, and how to diagnose mental and emotional disorders; must obtain a PhD or PsyD doctoral degree. Primarily focuses on providing **psychotherapy** and performing psychological testing. Most psychologists cannot prescribe medications.
- *Social worker*: Has a similar educational background as a psychologist but cannot provide psychological testing. The social worker provides psychotherapy. Depending on the state licensure, social workers may have different titles: Licensed Clinical Social Worker (LCSW), Licensed Independent Clinical Social Worker (LICSW), and Licensed Social Worker (LSW).

- *Cognitive behavioral therapist (CBT)*: Specializes in cognitive behavioral therapy and helping people change the way they think and behave in order to help manage their condition (e.g., depression, relationship issues).
- *Psychiatric nurse*: A registered nurse who has advanced training (e.g., master's or doctoral degree) in assessing and treating mental health issues.
- *Substance use (or addiction) therapist or counselor*: Has specialized training to treat patients with substance use disorders and other addictions.
- *Mental health therapist or counselor*: Trained to treat patients with mental health disorders (e.g., depression, anxiety).

In many states, most of these healthcare professionals need a license to practice. There are some exceptions. Some states allow unlicensed behavioral health professionals to provide treatment to patients, but their billing capacity is limited. State laws dictate the licensing and credential requirements for behavioral health professionals.

Patients with behavioral health conditions may be seen in community mental health clinics or in private practice clinics. When patients are a threat to themselves or others, they may be admitted to hospitals until their mental health conditions stabilize. Specialty inpatient settings for eating disorders and addictions are also available.

CRITICAL THINKING APPLICATION 22.1

Mike is asked by a patient to explain the difference between a psychiatrist and a psychologist. If you were asked this question, how would you respond?

DIAGNOSTIC AND STATISTICAL MANUAL OF MENTAL DISORDERS

The *Diagnostic and Statistical Manual of Mental Disorders* (DSM) is used by behavioral health professionals in the United States and other countries. The first DSM was published in 1952, and subsequent versions have been published since then; the latest is the DSM-5. The DSM provides descriptions, signs, symptoms, and other criteria for diagnosing behavioral health disorders. It provides a common language that is used in the behavioral health environment.

The DSM-5 contains the International Classification of Disease (ICD) codes required for insurance reimbursement and for monitoring **morbidity** and **mortality** statistics. In other words, the ICD codes allow researchers to gather information on how often the disorder occurs and how many deaths are attributed to the disease.

CRITICAL THINKING APPLICATION 22.2

Where have you seen or heard morbidity and mortality statistics? Explain your answer.

MENTAL HEALTH DISORDERS

Mental health disorders are conditions that cause changes in the mood, behavior, or thoughts of an individual. These disorders can affect how a person functions on a day-to-day basis, at work, school, and at home.

Biologic factors (e.g., genetics), life experiences, and a family history of mental health problems can contribute to mental health problems. It is important for a person to seek help immediately if signs of mental health disorders exist.

Behavioral Health Concerns Across a Life Span

Behavioral health problems are very common. Research has shown that 1 out of 7 children in the United States from ages 2 to 8 have been diagnosed with a mental, developmental, or behavioral disorder. Many times, the related factors included poverty, neighborhood concerns, parents with mental health issues, and childcare problems that affected the parent's job. Other studies have found that about half of all mental health disorders affect a person before the age of 14, and 75% of disorders begin before age 24. Less than 20% of children with a diagnosed mental health problem receive the treatment they need.

Behavioral health disorders in children cause changes in the way children learn, behave, or handle their emotions. This can cause problems getting through their days. Common disorders in childhood include anxiety, depression, oppositional defiant disorder, conduct disorder, ADHD, OCD, and PTSD. Substance abuse and suicides are occurring in growing numbers.

The National Alliance on Mental Illness (*www.nami.org*) states that about 1 in 5 adults experience a mental health disorder every year. About 20.2 million adults in the United States had a substance abuse disorder, and about 50% of these adults had a co-existing mental illness. With older adults, who have been diagnosed with heart disease, diabetes, and a stroke, research has shown that depression is more prevalent. Depression can complicate treatment and change a person's quality of life.

Early Warning Signs

- Withdrawing from others, isolating oneself
- Eating or sleeping too little or too much
- Having no or low amounts of energy
- Feeling helpless, hopeless, numb, or as if nothing matters
- Having unexplained pains and aches
- Smoking, drinking alcohol, or using drugs more than usual
- Feeling unusually forgetful, on edge, angry, worried, scared, confused, or upset
- Having persistent thoughts or memories "stuck" in your head
- Thinking of harming oneself or others
- Inability to function or do your daily activities
- Hearing voices or believing things that are not true

Anxiety Disorders

Having periodic anxiety about a problem or an important decision is normal. With an anxiety disorder, the anxious feeling is a constant companion and it gets worse with time. The anxiety interferes with daily living, for instance, school, work, and relationships.

The risk factors for anxiety disorders include shyness in childhood, being divorced or widowed, exposure to stressful life events, a family history of anxiety disorder, and a parental history of mental health disorder. The following sections will discuss the different types of anxiety disorders. Treatments will be discussed in further detail later in the chapter.

Generalized Anxiety Disorder

With generalized anxiety disorder (GAD), a person has many different worries. The person finds it difficult to control his or her anxiety. GAD is a common disorder that can affect a person at any age. GAD occurs more often in women than in men.

The cause of GAD is unknown, but genetics may be a factor. Stress also contributes to the development of GAD. The main symptom of GAD is excessive worrying for over 6 months about multiple issues without a clear reason. Other signs and symptoms of GAD include restlessness, easily fatiguability, irritability, difficulty concentrating, difficulty stopping or controlling the anxiety, muscle tension, and sleep problems.

There is no test to diagnose GAD. A physical exam and laboratory tests may be done to rule out other conditions. The provider will ask questions regarding the symptoms of GAD prior to making the diagnosis. The goal of treatment is to help the person feel and function better. Treatment includes psychotherapy or talk therapy. The most effective and common type of talk therapy is cognitive behavioral therapy (CBT). With CBT, a person learns to identify stressors, gain control of panic-causing thoughts, and manage stress, and also to relax. Medications such as antidepressants and sedative-hypnotics may be prescribed.

Obsessive-Compulsive and Related Disorders

Obsessive-compulsive disorder (OCD) causes a person to have frequent, upsetting thoughts (*obsessions*). Examples of obsessions include fear of germs or being hurt. Then, to control the thoughts, the person has an overwhelming urge to repeat certain behaviors (*compulsions*). Examples of compulsions include hand washing, counting, rechecking things (e.g., locked doors), or cleaning. The obsessions and compulsions affect the person's daily life.

The *etiology* (cause) of OCD is not completely understood, but it may relate to changes in brain function, genetics, and environmental factors. Risk factors include a family history of OCD, other mental health disorders (e.g., depression, substance use), and/or a traumatic event. Signs and symptoms of OCD include:

- Fear of touching items others touched.
- Items need to be in a certain position, organized, and orderly.
- Doubts about locking the door or turning off an appliance, causing continual rechecking.
- Avoidance of events that trigger the obsessions.
- Frequent hand washing, even to the point that the skin is raw.
- Silently repeating a prayer or phrase.

The symptoms start gradually and may increase in severity over time.

The provider will do a physical exam, laboratory tests (e.g., blood work, thyroid tests), and a psychological evaluation. Treatment consists of psychotherapy (e.g., cognitive behavioral therapy, exposure and response prevention) and antidepressants.

Hoarding Disorder. Hoarding disorder (HD) is the persistent difficulty of getting rid of personal possessions. People with HD feel they need to save items and are distressed at the thought of discarding them or having them touched or moved without their permission. Sometimes the thoughts center around "hurting the feelings" of the item if it is discarded. Others hold onto their possessions, because they may come in handy some day, or, if discarded, the memories attached to the object may be lost. As a result, people with HD have cluttered living areas that can become a significant public health burden and safety issue. It is estimated that up to 5% of the population has HD.

CRITICAL THINKING APPLICATION   **22.3**

List three safety issues related to hoarding and share them with your class.

Panic Disorder

Panic disorder causes recurrent unexpected *panic attacks*, or sudden feelings of terror without real dangers being present. A person experiencing a panic attack is very frightened and feels a loss of control.

The cause of panic disorders is unknown, but genetics, major stress, sensitivity to stress, and certain changes in brain function may play a factor. Signs and symptoms of panic attacks include a sense of impending doom, a rapid and pounding heart rate, sweating, trembling, chills and hot flashes, chest pain, abdominal cramping, nausea, dizziness, lightheadedness, and numbness. The signs and symptoms can mimic those of a heart attack, which can also increase the person's anxiety.

After a physical exam and laboratory tests to rule out other conditions, the provider will do a psychological evaluation. The DSM-5 criteria for panic disorder include:

- Having frequent, unexpected panic attacks
- One attack that is followed by 1 month or more of constant worry about having another attack
- The panic attack is not related to substance use, medications, or other medical or mental health conditions.

Treatment for panic disorder is similar to that for GAD; psychotherapy and medications can be helpful.

Phobia

A phobia is a type of anxiety disorder in which a person has a strong, irrational fear of something that causes little to no danger. There are many types of phobias (Table 22.1). Phobias typically start in childhood and continue into adulthood.

Phobias can be caused by negative experiences, genetics, changes in brain function, and the environment. Signs and symptoms of phobia can include panic, persistent and unreasonable fear, an increase in the heart rate, shortness of breath (SOB), trembling, and a strong desire to get away. A phobia can interfere with a person's daily life.

The provider will do a physical exam and gather a medical history. Often treatment includes psychotherapy, exposure therapy, and medication.

Social Anxiety Disorder

With social anxiety disorder, people have a persistent and irrational fear of social situations. People avoid situations in which they feel

TABLE 22.1 Examples of Phobias

TYPE	FEAR OF...
acrophobia	heights
agoraphobia	open spaces
algophobia	pain
aquaphobia	water
arachnophobia	spiders
aviophobia	flying
belonephobia	needles
brontophobia	thunder
cancerophobia	cancer
chionophobia	snow
claustrophobia	closed spaces
cyberphobia	computers
dentophobia	dentist or dental procedures
glossophobia	speaking in front of an audience
hemophobia	blood or injury
kleptophobia	stealing
nosophobia	disease
ochlophobia	crowds
spermaphobia, spermatophobia	germs

others will judge them. Some of the more common avoidances include attending social gatherings, eating and drinking in public, meeting new people, public speaking, and using public restrooms. This disorder affects a person's ability to go to school, function at work, and have relationships. The disorder may begin in a person's teenage years. Men and women are equally affected by this disorder.

The cause of social anxiety disorder may be related to overprotective parents or limited social opportunities. Other possible causes include genetics, learning behaviors early on in life, and an overactive **amygdala**, in the brain, which increases the fear response. Signs and symptoms of this disorder include blushing, an increased heart rate, trembling, sweating, nausea, dizziness, lightheadedness, SOB, and muscle tension. Elevated afternoon cortisol levels have also been reported.

After a physical exam and laboratory tests to rule out other conditions, the provider will do a psychological evaluation. The DSM-5 criteria for social anxiety disorder include:

- Persistent, intense anxiety or fear related to social situations in which one perceives others will be judgmental
- Avoidance of such social situations
- Excessive anxiety that interferes with daily life
- Fear or anxiety that is not related to substance use or a medical or mental health disorder

Treatment for social anxiety disorder includes psychotherapy and these medications:

- Antidepressants: Selective serotonin reuptake inhibitors (SSRIs): paroxetine (Paxil, Pexeva, Brisdelle), or sertraline (Zoloft)
- Antidepressants: Serotonin and norepinephrine reuptake inhibitor (SNRIs): venlafaxine
- Antianxiety medications, including benzodiazepines
- Beta blockers

Autism Spectrum Disorder

Autism spectrum disorder (ASD) is a developmental disorder with symptoms that appear by age 2. The child has difficulty interacting and communicating with others. The communication issues and behaviors, such as repetitive behaviors and limited interests, affect the person's ability to function at school and at home. There can be a wide range of symptoms and severity; thus it is known as a "spectrum" disorder. Prior diagnoses, such as Asperger's syndrome, are now included in ASD.

The exact cause of ASD is unknown, but research suggests that a person's genetics, with environmental influences, can affect development, leading to ASD. Risk factors for ASD include having a family member with ASD, older parents, certain genetic conditions, and a low birth weight. Signs and symptoms of autism spectrum disorder include:

- Social communication and interaction behavior issues: Little to no eye contact, not listening to others, failing to respond when being called, difficulty with holding a conversation, talks at length about a favorite topic without realizing others are not interested, body language does not match the verbal message, and having a singsong or flat, robot-like tone of voice.
- Restrictive and repetitive behaviors: Repeating certain behaviors or words, intense interest in certain topics (e.g., numbers, details, facts), getting upset with routine changes, and more or less sensitivity to light, noise, clothing, or temperature.

Often people with ASD have sleeping issues. They may be strong auditory and visual learners, who excel in art, music, science, or math. They may remember information for long periods of time and can learn information in detail.

The American Academy of Pediatrics recommends that children be screened for developmental delays during the 9-month, 18-month, and 24- or 30-month well-child visit. ASD screening tools are available. Children suspected of having ASD are referred for additional evaluation by a healthcare team specializing in diagnosing ASD. Treatment may consist of medication and behavioral, educational, and psychological therapies. These therapies focus on teaching the person life skills to live independently, including social, communication, and language skills.

Depression and Other Mood Disorders

Depression is the second leading mental health condition. The symptoms affect how a person acts, thinks, feels, and handles his or her daily life. Depression must be present for at least 2 weeks for a diagnosis to be given. Table 22.2 describes some types of depression. Depression can happen at any age.

The cause of depression is not known, but many factors may be involved, including changes in the brain and the functioning of neurotransmitters, hormone changes, and genetics. Risk factors

TABLE 22.2 Types of Depression	
TYPES	DESCRIPTION
Persistent depressive disorder	Also called *dysthymia*; depression that lasts for at least 2 years.
Postpartum depression	Occurs after giving birth. The person has feelings of extreme sadness, exhaustion, and anxiety. These feelings interfere with daily life and caring for the new baby.
Psychotic depression	Episodes of psychosis occur with severe depression. The person experiences **delusions** and **hallucinations**.
Seasonal affective disorder	Depression occurs during the winter months, when there is less sunlight. The depression usually lifts in the spring. During the winter, the person may experience increased sleepiness, weight gain, and social withdrawal.

include age (from teens to 30-year-olds), female, low self-esteem, stressful event, family history (of depression, bipolar disorder, alcoholism, or suicide), substance use, chronic medical or mental health illness, and certain medications. Signs and symptoms of depression include:

- Feeling sad, very tired, hopeless, irritable, anxious, or guilty
- Loss of interest in favorite activities (e.g., hobbies)
- Pain, headaches, cramps, digestive issues, anorexia, overeating
- Thoughts of death or suicide

The provider will do a physical exam, possibly laboratory tests (e.g., complete blood count, thyroid function tests), and radiology tests (Fig. 22.1). A psychiatric evaluation will also be completed to gather more information on the patient's symptoms, thoughts, feelings, and behaviors. Psychotherapy and medications are the most common treatments for depression. Common medications used for depression include:

- *Selective serotonin reuptake inhibitor (SSRI) antidepressants*: paroxetine (Paxil, Pexeva, Brisdelle), sertraline (Zoloft), escitalopram (Lexapro), fluoxetine (Prozac, Rapiflux), and vilazodone (Viibryd)
- *Serotonin and norepinephrine reuptake inhibitor (SNRI) antidepressants*: venlafaxine, duloxetine (Cymbalta), desvenlafaxine (Pristiq), and levomilnacipran (Fetzima)
- *Tricyclic antidepressants*: imipramine (Tofranil), amitriptyline, nortriptyline (Pamelor, Aventyl), doxepin, trimipramine (Surmontil), desipramine (Norpramin), and protriptyline (Vivactil)
- *Atypical antidepressants*: bupropion (Wellbutrin, Aplenzin, Forfivo XL), mirtazapine (Remeron), vortioxetine (Trintellix), trazodone (Oleptro), and nefazodone
- *Monoamine oxidase inhibitors (MAOIs)*: phenelzine (Nardil), isocarboxazid (Marplan), and tranylcypromine (Parnate).

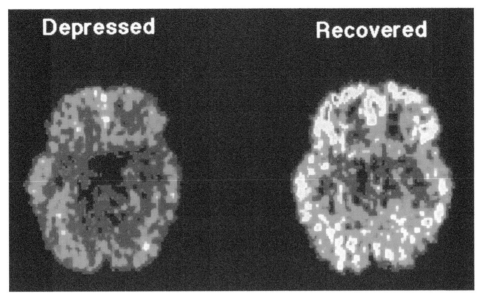

FIGURE 22.1 PET scans of an individual's brain when depressed *(left)* and after recovery through treatment with medication *(right)*. Several brain areas, particularly the prefrontal cortex *(at top)*, show diminished activity *(darker colors)* during depression. (From Fortinash KM: *Psychiatric mental health nursing*, ed 4, St Louis, 2008, Mosby.)

CRITICAL THINKING APPLICATION   22.4

Mike rooms Mrs. Johnson, who states she has not been sleeping well since her husband died 10 days ago. She states she has not been feeling hungry and is always tired. If you encountered a patient like Mrs. Johnson, how would you respond?

Bipolar Disorder

Bipolar disorder causes people to go from **mania** to depression. They cycle through highs and lows in their moods, with periods of normal moods. Bipolar disorder usually starts in the late teens to early adult years and lasts a lifetime.

The cause of bipolar disorder is unclear. There is a genetic link to the disorder, and abnormal brain structure and function may also be related. The signs and symptoms include:

- Mania and hypomania: **Euphoria** and energetic feelings, decreased need for sleep, distractibility, poor decision making, exaggerated sense of well-being
- Major depression episode: Insomnia or sleeping too much, fatigue, feelings of worthlessness, suicidal thoughts, feelings of no pleasure, and weight gain or loss

Moods affect relationships, school or job performance, and even cause suicide.

The provider will do a physical exam and a psychiatric assessment. Patients may be asked to chart their moods. Treatments include medications, lifelong treatments, psychotherapy, and support groups. Medications include:

- Anticonvulsants and mood stabilizers: valproic acid (Depakene, Depakote), carbamazepine (Tegretol, Equetro), and lamotrigine (Lamictal)
- Antidepressants and anxiolytics
- Antipsychotics: olanzapine (Zyprexa), risperidone (Risperdal), quetiapine (Seroquel), aripiprazole (Abilify), ziprasidone (Geodon), lurasidone (Latuda), and asenapine (Saphris)

Behavioral Disorders

Behavioral disorders in children involve a pattern of disruptive behaviors that cause issues at home, in school, and in social situations. According to the diagnostic criteria, the disruptive behaviors must have lasted at least 6 months. Behavioral disorders may involve defiant behavior, impulsiveness, hyperactivity, inattention, drug use, and criminal activity. Behavioral disorders include attention deficit hyperactivity disorder (ADHD), oppositional defiant disorder (ODD), and conduct disorder (CD). ODD and CD are also considered disruptive behavior disorders.

Disruptive behavior disorder involves uncooperative or hostile action patterns of behavior. The person may have temper tantrums, argue, demonstrate cruel and defiant behaviors, and fight with others. People with disruptive behavioral disorder have problems controlling their emotions and actions, leading to issues at school and home.

Attention Deficit Hyperactivity Disorder

ADHD is a chronic condition that affects children and can continue into adulthood. Often ADHD and ADD (attention deficit disorder) are used interchangeably, but the correct term is ADHD. Typically, symptoms begin before age 12, yet some have seen it in the toddler years. This disorder is more prevalent in males than in females.

The cause of ADHD is unknown, but possible factors include genetics, environmental factors (e.g., lead exposure), and developmental factors. Many conditions can co-exist with ADHD, including learning disabilities, anxiety, depression, bipolar disorder, and Tourette syndrome. Signs and symptoms include:

- Inattention: Fails to pay close attention, has problems staying focused, appears not to listen, has difficulty following directions, has trouble with organizational skills, and is easily distracted
- Hyperactivity and impulsivity: Fidgets, constantly moving, talking too much, difficulty waiting for his or her turn, and problems doing quiet activities.

Boys may be more hyperactive, whereas girls may be quietly inattentive. According to the diagnostic criteria, the symptoms can range from mild to severe and must last for at least 6 months, affecting school and home life. There are three subtypes of ADHD based on the symptoms: predominantly inattentive, predominantly hyperactive-impulsive, and combined (a mix of both).

There is no specific test for ADHD. The provider will do a physical exam, including vision and hearing, and ask questions of the parents and teachers. Treatments for ADHD include behavioral therapy to help manage the symptoms and provide coping skills. Medications can also be prescribed, including:

- Stimulants: methylphenidate (Ritalin LA, Concerta, Methylin) and amphetamine (Adzenys ER, Dyanavel XR, Evekeo). Stimulants provide a calming effect by increasing the dopamine in the brain, which helps with attention and motivation.
- Nonstimulants: atomoxetine (Strattera), guanfacine (Intuniv), and clonidine (Kapvay)

Conduct Disorder

With conduct disorder (CD), the person demonstrates disruptive and violent behaviors. The person hurts others and destroys property. Children with CD can have behavior problems that last into adulthood. Symptoms usually start during the preteen and teen years, though they can be seen in preschool. The disorder is more common in males.

There is no single cause for CD, but having a parent with a behavioral disorder; exposure to neglect, abuse, or violence; and having a high emotional reactivity can be risk factors. The signs and symptoms of CD include:

- Aggression toward animals and people: Includes bullying, threatening, starting fights, using weapons, forcing others into sexual activity, stealing from others, and physical cruelty to people or animals
- Destruction of property: For instance, setting fires
- Deceit or theft: Includes lying to get things, breaking in and stealing items, and shoplifting
- Serious violation of rules: Includes running away from home overnight at least twice, or once without returning for a long time, and truancy

There is no specific test for CD, so the provider will do a complete medical history. Treatment is based on the individual's need and addresses co-existing diseases. Common intervention programs include parent training, behavioral family therapy, and skills-based interventions, in addition to anger management and coping skills.

Oppositional Defiant Disorder

With oppositional defiant disorder (ODD), the child or teen demonstrates ongoing hostility to parents, friends, and teachers. ODD usually is diagnosed during preschool or childhood.

There is no single cause for ODD, but having a parent with a behavioral disorder; exposure to neglect, abuse, or violence; and having a high emotional reactivity can be risk factors. Depression and anxiety can co-exist with ODD. The signs and symptoms of ODD include ongoing hostility, defying rules, holding grudges, and rebel-like behaviors. These symptoms interfere with school and home life. Three types of ODD are:

- *Angry and irritable mood*: Annoyed by others easily, loses one's temper, and has rage outbursts
- *Argumentative and defiant behaviors*: Argues with those in authority, defies rules, purposely annoys others, and blames others
- *Vindictiveness*: Being cruel, nasty, vengeful, and mean

There is no specific test for ODD, so the provider will do a complete medical history. Treatment is based on the individual's need and addresses co-existing diseases. Common intervention programs include parent training, behavioral family therapy, and skills-based interventions, which teach the patient how to reduce behavior problems and learn how to appropriately interact with peers. Anger management and coping skills are also part of the intervention.

Dissociative Disorders

Dissociative disorders cause a person to involuntarily escape from reality. A person may have a disconnection between memories, thoughts, actions, identity, and surroundings. Dissociative disorder can cause a variety of conditions, such as **amnesia** and alternative identities. Table 22.3 describes types of dissociative disorders.

Dissociative disorders develop as a coping mechanism due to trauma (e.g., abuse, war, and natural disasters). A risk factor includes experiencing long-term sexual, physical, or emotional abuse during childhood. Signs and symptoms include amnesia, a sense of being detached from self, a distorted or unreal perception of others, an unclear sense of identity, significant stress and inability to cope, and mental health issues (e.g., depression, anxiety).

The provider will do a physical exam and a psychiatric evaluation. Treatment consists of psychotherapy and medications (e.g., antidepressants, antianxiety drugs, and antipsychotics).

TABLE 22.3	Types of Dissociative Disorders
TYPES	**DESCRIPTION**
Dissociative amnesia	Memory loss without an explained medical condition. No recollection of self, events, and familiar people. May involve confused wandering away from home (dissociative fugue). May last for hours to years.
Dissociative identity disorder	Formerly known as multiple personality disorder. People may feel two or more people "in their head" as if they have alternative identities. Each identity may have a name, history, and unique personality.
Depersonalization-derealization disorder	Episodic or long-term sense of detachment with **depersonalization** and **derealization**. People feel they are an outside observer of their thoughts, actions, and sensations. They also feel as if they are detached from their surroundings.

Eating Disorders

Eating disorders affect both genders, but the rate of eating disorders in females is 2.5 times greater than it is in males. Eating disorders typically appear during the teen years or young adulthood, but they can start earlier or later in life.

Eating disorders are real, treatable illnesses. They typically co-exist with other illnesses, including substance use, anxiety disorders, and depression. Eating disorders, especially anorexia, can be life-threatening without treatment.

Anorexia Nervosa

Anorexia nervosa causes people to lose more weight than is healthy. Individuals with this disorder have an intense fear of gaining weight (Fig. 22.2). Often it starts during the preteen to teen years. It is more prevalent in females.

The etiology is unknown. Genetics, hormones, and social attitudes may play a role in the development of anorexia nervosa. Risk factors for anorexia nervosa include:

- A history of anxiety disorder or eating problems as a child
- Worry about weight and shape of the body; negative self-image
- An exaggerated focus on rules and trying to be perfect

The provider will order extensive laboratory tests to look at thyroid, liver, and kidney function. An electrocardiogram and bone density test may also be ordered. Treatment focuses on helping these patients

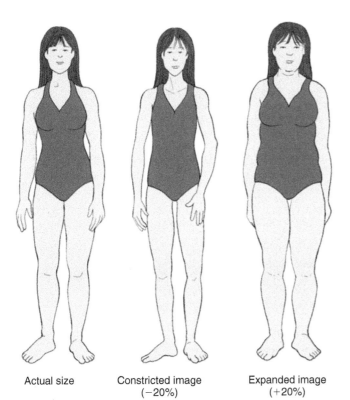

Actual size | **Constricted image (−20%)** | **Expanded image (+20%)**

FIGURE 22.2 The perception of body shape and size can be evaluated with the use of special computer drawing programs. These programs allow a subject to distort (increase or decrease) the width of an actual picture of a person's body by as much as 20%. Individuals with anorexia consistently adjusted their own body picture to a size 20% larger than its true form. This suggests that they have a major problem with the perception of self-image. (From Stuart GW, Laraia MT: *Principles and practice of psychiatric nursing,* ed 9, St Louis, 2009, Mosby.)

recognize they have an illness. Many types of treatments are available, including psychotherapy (e.g., cognitive behavioral therapy, group therapy, and family therapy) and support groups. Compliance with treatment is difficult, and it is common for the disease to return.

Symptoms of Anorexia Nervosa
• Underweight, intense fear of gaining weight
• Very distorted body image
• Severely limiting the amount of food eaten
• Exercising all the time
• Going to the bathroom right after meals, vomiting secretly after eating
• Refusing to eat around others
• Using diuretics, laxatives, or diet pills
• Blotchy or yellow dry skin covered with fine hair
• Confused, poor memory or judgment, slow thinking, depression
• Dry mouth
• Extreme sensitivity to cold
• Thinning of bones (osteoporosis)
• Wasting away of muscle
• Loss of body fat

Binge Eating Disorder

Binge eating disorder, also called compulsive overeating, is the most common eating disorder in the United States. It occurs when people regularly eat unusually large amounts of food in a short amount of time. They feel out of control, unable to manage what or how much they eat. A person may have binge eating disorder if this behavior occurs weekly for 3 months. It affects young women and middle-aged men.

The exact cause is unknown. Genetics, depression, stress, unhealthy dieting, and changes in brain chemicals may be factors in the condition. Signs and symptoms of binge eating disorder include:

- Eating very quickly and eating until uncomfortably full
- Eating when not hungry
- Eating huge amounts of food over a very short period of time
- Eating in secret
- Feeling disgusted, ashamed, or depressed about one's eating patterns
- Frequent dieting

A physical exam and a psychological evaluation will be done. Blood and urine tests (e.g., cholesterol, blood glucose) may be done to evaluate the consequences of binge eating. Treatment may consist of behavioral weight-loss programs and psychotherapy (e.g., cognitive behavioral therapy, interpersonal psychotherapy, and dialectical behavior therapy). Medications may also be used, including lisdexamfetamine (Vyvanse), topiramate (Topamax), and antidepressants.

Bulimia Nervosa

Bulimia nervosa, or bulimia, causes overeating that leads to purging and can be a life-threatening disorder. To prevent weight gain, self-induced vomiting, laxative use, weight-loss supplements, and enemas may be used. Bulimia may also occur with anorexia nervosa. More women than men have bulimia. It is more common in teens and young women.

The etiology is unknown. Genetics, hormones, and social attitudes may play a role in the development of bulimia. Symptoms that others see include:

- Excessive exercising
- Eating large amounts of food or buying large amounts of food that disappear right away
- Trips to the bathroom after meals
- Discarded boxes from laxatives, diet pills, and emetics to induce vomiting, or diuretics

The provider will do a physical exam and urine and blood tests. Treatment is usually on an outpatient basis unless the individual has a co-existing diagnosis. Support groups, counseling, and medications can be helpful.

Signs of Bulimia Nervosa

- Broken blood vessels in the eyes (this occurs from the strain of vomiting)
- Dry mouth, pouch-like look to the cheeks
- Rashes and pimples
- Small cuts and calluses on the tops of fingers (from inducing vomiting)
- Dehydration and electrolyte imbalance

CRITICAL THINKING APPLICATION 22.5
Describe the three types of eating disorders in your own words.

Personality Disorders

Personality disorders include a group of conditions that involve long-term patterns of unhealthy and inflexible thoughts and behaviors that affect relationships and work. Personality disorders cause people to have difficulty dealing with stresses and problems. Personality disorders are grouped by clusters (Table 22.4):

- Cluster A personality disorders: Cause odd, eccentric thinking and behaviors
- Cluster B personality disorders: Cause dramatic, overly emotional thinking and behaviors
- Cluster C personality disorders: Cause anxiety, fearful thinking and behaviors

The etiology of personality disorders is unknown, but childhood experiences and genetics may play a role in the disorders. The signs and symptoms can range from mild to severe and vary based on the type of disorder. People with a personality disorder may feel they do not have a problem and blame others for their problems.

The provider will do a physical exam and a psychiatric evaluation. Treatments involve psychotherapy and medications

TABLE 22.4 Types of Personality Disorders

CLUSTER	TYPES	DESCRIPTION
Cluster A personality disorders	Paranoid personality disorder	Unjustified beliefs that others are trying to do harm to him or her. Very suspicious, untrusting, angry, and hostile. May feel that the partner is unfaithful.
	Schizoid personality disorder	Avoidance of social activities and interacting with other people. The person may be seen as a loner and may not show emotion.
	Schizotypal personality disorder	Odd, peculiar, and unusual behaviors; flat or inappropriate emotional responses; belief in special powers, excessive social anxiety, and suspicious or paranoid thoughts.
Cluster B personality disorders	Antisocial personality disorder	No regard for others; persistent lying, and impulsive and aggressive behaviors
	Borderline personality disorder	Intense relationships, distorted self-image, impulsivity, and extreme emotions (e.g., intense fear of abandonment, anger, mood swings). Usually begins in early adulthood and may get better with age.
	Histrionic personality disorder	Seeks constant attention. Very dramatic, emotional, and opinionated.
	Narcissistic personality disorder	Inflated ego, an excessive need for attention, lacks empathy for others, has troubled relationships and a very fragile self-esteem.
Cluster C personality disorders	Avoidance personality disorder	Too sensitive to criticism; feels inadequate; avoids interpersonal contact or is extremely shy/withdrawn during social activities.
	Dependent personality disorder	Very clinging and dependent on another person. Fears being left alone. Lacks self-confidence.
	Obsessive-compulsive personality disorder	Preoccupied with rules, organization/orderliness, and details. Wants to control everything (e.g., tasks, situations, people, events).

(e.g., antidepressants, mood stabilizers, antipsychotic medications, and antianxiety medications).

Post-traumatic Stress Disorder

Post-traumatic stress disorder (PTSD) is a condition that occurs after experiencing or witnessing a traumatic or terrifying event. The symptoms of PTSD can vary over time and from person to person. Anyone can develop PTSD, from children, to war veterans, to people who have experienced the death of a loved one, physical or sexual assault, an accident, or a natural disaster. Women are more likely to have PTSD than men.

The cause of PTSD is experiencing a stressful, terrifying event. It is unknown why some get it and others do not. PTSD signs and symptoms include:

- *Intrusive memories*: Reliving the trauma (flashbacks); nightmares and recurrent distressful memories
- *Negative changes*: Negative thoughts, hopelessness, and difficulty maintaining close relationships
- *Changes in reactions*: Being easily frightened, self-destructive activities (drinking, drugs), trouble concentrating and sleeping, and aggressive behaviors
- *Avoidance*: Avoiding places, people and things that remind one of the situation; not talking about the event

The provider will do a physical exam and a psychological evaluation. Treatment is focused on regaining a sense of control. Psychotherapy, including cognitive therapy, eye movement desensitization and reprocessing (EMDR), and exposure therapy, may be prescribed. The following medications may also be prescribed for PTSD:

- Antidepressants (paroxetine [Paxil] and sertraline [Zoloft])
- Antianxiety medications
- Prazosin (Minipress) for nightmares

Schizophrenia

Schizophrenia causes disruptions in thought processes, perceptions, emotional responsiveness, and social interactions (Fig. 22.3). Schizophrenia is usually diagnosed in the late teen years to the early 30s. The symptoms tend to occur earlier for males than females. Schizophrenia is a debilitating disorder, and about half of those with it also have another mental or behavioral health disorder.

The cause of schizophrenia is unknown, but as with many other conditions, it is believed that a combination of brain chemistry, environmental factors, and genetics plays a role in the development of the disease. Signs and symptoms include delusions, hallucinations, disorganized thinking and speech, abnormal motor behavior, lack of response (no eye contact, lack of facial expression), and neglect of personal hygiene. Teens are more likely to withdraw and have insomnia.

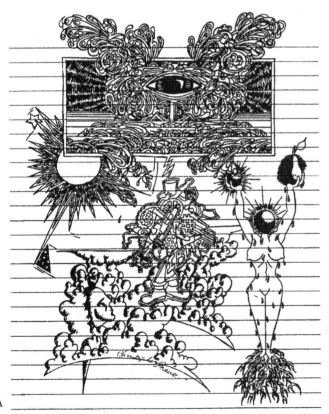

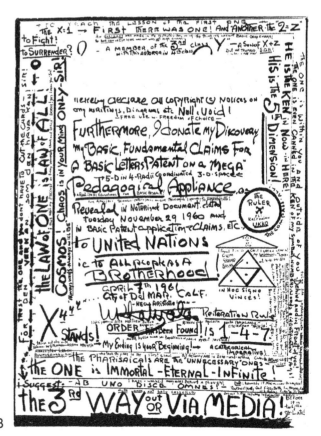

FIGURE 22.3 (A) Drawing by a delusional patient with schizophrenia. **(B)** This drawing by a patient with schizophrenia demonstrates thought disorder. (From Stuart GW, Laraia MT: *Principles and practice of psychiatric nursing*, ed 9, St Louis, 2009, Mosby.)

The provider will do a physical exam and may order an MRI or a CT scan to rule out other conditions. A psychiatric evaluation will be done. Treatment is lifelong and includes psychosocial therapy and antipsychotic medications. Hospitalization is required if the person experiences severe and/or life-threatening symptoms.

CRITICAL THINKING APPLICATION   22.6

Mike rooms Mr. James, who states he is seeing little green men coming out of the wall. If you encountered a patient like Mr. James, how would you respond?

Suicidal Behavior

Suicide is death caused by a self-inflicted injury with an intent to die as a result of the behavior. A *suicide attempt* is a nonfatal, self-directed, potentially harmful behavior with an intent to die as a result of the behavior. An injury may not be caused by the attempt. *Suicidal ideation* refers to thinking about, considering, or planning suicide.

In 2017, suicide was the tenth leading cause of death in the United States. More than 47,000 people committed suicide, or one person every 11 minutes. Suicide is the second leading cause of death between age 10 and 34, and the fourth leading cause of death between ages 35 and 54. The three most common methods of suicide are firearms, suffocation, and poisoning.

Certain factors increase the risk of suicide. Ninety percent of those who die by suicide have a mental disorder at the time, including depression, bipolar disorder, and schizophrenia. Additional risk factors include previous suicide attempts, a family history of suicide, substance use, incarceration, a low level of job satisfaction, and being the victim of bullying. Those who have the highest risk for suicide include men, people over age 45, Caucasians, American Indians, and Alaskan Natives. Veterans and other military personnel also have a higher risk of suicide. People with suicidal ideation are often overwhelmed with hopelessness and sadness. Warning signs of suicide include:

- Looking for a way to kill oneself
- Talking about killing oneself or wanting to die; feelings of hopelessness, feeling trapped or in unbearable pain; having no reason to live or being a burden on others
- Increased use of drugs or alcohol
- Socially withdrawn and isolated; agitation, feelings of rage, anxiousness, and behaving recklessly
- Sleeping too much or too little
- Extreme mood swings

If someone is showing some of these signs or symptoms, it is important to get help for him or her. The National Suicide Prevention Lifeline is 1-800-273-TALK (8255).

Protective factors help prevent suicidal thoughts and behaviors. The following are considered protective factors: effective clinical care for mental health conditions and for physical and substance use disorders; easy access to care; family and community support; support from ongoing medical and behavioral healthcare relationships; and skills in problem solving, conflict resolution, and nonviolent ways of handling disputes.

Treatment for suicide attempts includes treating any mental health disorders. Medications and psychotherapy (e.g., cognitive behavior therapy) may also be used.

SUBSTANCE USE DISORDERS AND OTHER ADDICTIONS

Substance Use Disorders

In the DSM-5, substance use disorder includes both substance use and substance dependence. Substance use disorder is measured from mild to severe. Each substance is addressed as a separate disorder; these substances include alcohol; cannabis; hallucinogens; opioids; inhalants; sedatives, hypnotics, and anxiolytics; tobacco; and stimulants. Caffeine is not included in the use disorder, though it may be in a future revision because there is sufficient evidence to support such a condition.

Substance use disorder occurs when a person uses alcohol or other substances (drugs) that lead to school, work, or home issues. Many people with substance use disorders also have other mental health conditions, including depression, anxiety, attention deficit disorder, and post-traumatic stress disorder. Table 22.5 describes commonly used drugs.

The exact cause of substance use disorders are unknown, but genetics, drug action, peer pressure, anxiety, depression, emotional distress, and stress can all be factors. Signs and symptoms include:

- Confusion, violence, hostility
- Making excuses to use drugs, lack of control over use, need for regular/daily use
- Continuing drug use even when work, family, and health are affected; missing work and school
- Secretive behaviors related to drugs
- Neglecting to eat or to care for one's appearance

To diagnose substance use, urine and blood drug tests (toxicology screens) are done. Treating substance use is not easy. Treatment starts by recognizing the problem. Substances may either be slowly withdrawn or stopped abruptly. Hospitalization or residential treatment programs address withdrawal symptoms and behaviors. Medications may be given for some withdrawal symptoms. Support groups are helpful.

Alcohol Use Disorder

Alcohol use disorder (AUD) is a chronic relapsing brain disease that includes a compulsion to use alcohol, loss of control over alcohol intake, and a negative emotional state when abstaining from alcohol. Many people are not aware of what a standard drink means. About 16 million people in the United States have AUD, including 623,000 children under age 18. AUD can range from mild to severe. AUD can include periods of alcohol intoxication and symptoms of withdrawal.

Psychological, genetic, and environmental factors can play a role in how alcohol affects one's body and behavior. Alcohol intoxication symptoms include inappropriate behavior, unstable moods, impaired judgment, slurred speech, impaired memory, poor coordination, and blackouts. Signs and symptoms of AUD include:

- Being unable to limit the amount of alcohol consumed
- Wanting to cut back on drinking or making unsuccessful attempts to do so
- Spending significant time obtaining alcohol, drinking, and recovering
- Having the effects of alcohol affect one's work, school, or home life
- Being unable to stop drinking even if it is causing problems in one's life

TABLE 22.5	Commonly Used Drugs			
DRUG	STREET NAMES	COMMON FORM/ WAYS TAKEN	POSSIBLE HEALTH EFFECTS	WITHDRAWAL SYMPTOMS
CNS depressants	*(Barbiturates, pentobarbital)* Barbs, Red Birds, Yellow Jackets	Pill, capsule, liquid/ swallowed, injected	Drowsiness, slurred speech, poor concentration, confusion, dizziness, problems with movement and memory, lowered blood pressure, slowed breathing.	Must be discussed with a health care provider; barbiturate withdrawal can cause a serious abstinence syndrome that may even include seizures.
	(Benzodiazepines) candy, downers, sleeping pills, tranks	Pill, capsule, liquid/ swallowed, snorted		
	(Sleep medications) Forget-me Pill, Mexican Valium, R2, Roche, Roofies, Roofinol, Rope, Rophies	Pill, capsule, liquid/ swallowed, snorted		
Cocaine	Blow, Bump, C, Candy, Charlie, Coke, Crack, Flake, Rock, Snow, Toot	White powder, whitish rock crystal/swallowed, snorted, smoked	Narrowed blood vessels; enlarged pupils; increased body temperature, heart rate, and blood pressure; headache; abdominal pain and nausea; euphoria; increased energy, alertness; insomnia, restlessness; anxiety; erratic and violent behavior, panic attacks, **paranoia**, psychosis; heart rhythm problems, heart attack; stroke, seizure, coma, loss of sense of smell, nosebleeds, nasal damage and trouble swallowing from snorting; infection and death of bowel tissue from decreased blood flow; poor nutrition and weight loss; lung damage from smoking.	Depression, tiredness, increased appetite, insomnia, vivid unpleasant dreams, slowed thinking and movement, restlessness.
Dimethyltryptamine	DMT, Dimitri	White or yellow crystalline powder/ smoked, injected	Intense visual hallucinations, depersonalization, auditory distortions, and an altered perception of time and body image, usually peaking in about 30 minutes when drunk as tea. Physical effects include hypertension, increased heart rate, agitation, seizures, dilated pupils.	Unknown
Gamma Hydroxybutyrate (GHB)	Home Boy, Liquid Ecstasy, Liquid X, Soap	Colorless, liquid, white powder/swallowed, often combined with alcohol and other beverages	Euphoria, drowsiness, nausea, vomiting, confusion, memory loss, unconsciousness, slowed heart rate and breathing, lower body temperature, seizures, coma, death.	Insomnia, anxiety, tremors, sweating, increased heart rate and blood pressure, psychotic thoughts.
Heroin	Brown Sugar, China White, Dope, H, Horse, Junk, Skag, Skunk, Smack, White Horse	White or brownish powder, or black sticky substance known as "black tar heroin"/ injected, smoked, snorted	Euphoria; dry mouth; itching; nausea; vomiting; analgesia; slowed breathing and heart rate. Collapsed veins; abscesses (swollen tissue with pus); infection of the lining and valves in the heart; constipation and stomach cramps; liver or kidney disease; pneumonia.	Restlessness, muscle and bone pain, insomnia, diarrhea, vomiting, cold flashes with goose bumps ("cold turkey").

Continued

TABLE 22.5	Commonly Used Drugs—*continued*			
DRUG	**STREET NAMES**	**COMMON FORM/ WAYS TAKEN**	**POSSIBLE HEALTH EFFECTS**	**WITHDRAWAL SYMPTOMS**
Ketamine	*(Anesthetic in veterinary practice)* Cat Valium, K, Special K, Vitamin K	Liquid, white powder/ injected, snorted, smoked, swallowed	Problems with attention, learning, and memory; dreamlike states, hallucinations; sedation; confusion; loss of memory; raised blood pressure; unconsciousness; dangerously slowed breathing; ulcers and pain in the bladder; kidney problems; stomach pain; depression; poor memory.	Unknown
Lysergic acid diethylamide (LSD)	Acid, Blotter, Blue Heaven, Cubes, Microdot, Yellow Sunshine	Tablet; capsule; clear liquid; small, decorated squares of absorbent paper that liquid has been added to/swallowed, absorbed through mouth tissues (paper squares)	Rapid emotional swings; distortion of a person's ability to recognize reality, think rationally, or communicate with others; raised blood pressure, heart rate, body temperature; dizziness; loss of appetite; tremors; enlarged pupils, frightening flashbacks (called *hallucinogen persisting perception disorder* [HPPD]); ongoing visual disturbances; disorganized thinking; paranoia; and mood swings.	Unknown
Marijuana	Blunt, Bud, Dope, Ganja, Grass, Green, Herb, Joint, Mary Jane, Pot, Reefer, Sinsemilla, Skunk, Smoke, Trees, Weed; Hashish: Boom, Gangster, Hash, Hemp	Greenish gray mixture of dried, shredded leaves, stems, seeds, and/or flowers; resin (hashish) or sticky, black liquid (hash oil)/smoked, eaten (mixed in food or brewed as tea)	Enhanced sensory perception and euphoria followed by drowsiness/ relaxation; slowed reaction time; problems with balance and coordination; increased heart rate and appetite; problems with learning and memory; anxiety; mental health problems; chronic cough; frequent respiratory infections.	Irritability, trouble sleeping, decreased appetite, anxiety
Mescaline	Buttons, Cactus, Mesc	Fresh or dried buttons, capsule/swallowed	Enhanced perception and feeling; hallucinations; euphoria; anxiety; increased body temperature, heart rate, blood pressure; sweating; problems with movement.	Unknown
Prescription opioids	Multiple names	Varies: tablet, capsule, liquid/swallowed, injected, snorted	Pain relief, drowsiness, nausea, constipation, euphoria, slowed breathing, death. Increased risk of overdose or addiction if misused.	Restlessness, muscle and bone pain, insomnia, diarrhea, vomiting, cold flashes with goose bumps ("cold turkey"), leg movements.

TABLE 22.5 Commonly Used Drugs—*continued*

DRUG	STREET NAMES	COMMON FORM/ WAYS TAKEN	POSSIBLE HEALTH EFFECTS	WITHDRAWAL SYMPTOMS
Phencyclidine (PCP, or "angel dust")	Angel Dust, Boat, Hog, Love Boat, Peace Pill	White or colored powder, tablet, or capsule; clear liquid/injected, snorted, swallowed, smoked	Delusions, hallucinations, paranoia, problems thinking, a sense of distance from one's environment, anxiety. *Low doses:* Slight increase in breathing rate; increased blood pressure and heart rate; shallow breathing; face redness and sweating; numbness of the hands or feet; problems with movement. *High doses:* Nausea; vomiting; flicking up and down of the eyes; drooling; loss of balance; dizziness; violence; seizures, coma, and death. Memory loss; problems with speech and thinking; loss of appetite; anxiety.	Headaches, increased appetite, sleepiness, depression
Psilocybin	Little Smoke, Magic Mushrooms, Purple Passion, Shrooms	Fresh or dried mushrooms with long, slender stems topped by caps with dark gills / swallowed	Hallucinations, altered perception of time, inability to tell fantasy from reality, panic, muscle relaxation or weakness, problems with movement, enlarged pupils, nausea, vomiting, drowsiness. Risk of flashbacks and memory problems.	Unknown
Rohypnol	*(Similar to Xanax and Valium)* Date rape drug, Mind Eraser, Mexican Valium, Roach	Tablet/swallowed	Drowsiness, sedation, sleep; amnesia, blackout; decreased anxiety; muscle relaxation, impaired reaction time and motor coordination; impaired mental functioning and judgment; confusion; aggression; excitability; slurred speech; headache; slowed breathing and heart rate.	Headache; muscle pain; extreme anxiety, tension, restlessness, confusion, irritability; numbness and tingling of hands or feet; hallucinations; delirium; convulsions; seizures; or shock.
Tobacco	Multiple brands	Cigarettes, cigars, bidis, hookahs, smokeless tobacco (snuff, spit tobacco, chew)/smoked, snorted, chewed, vaporized	Increased blood pressure, breathing, and heart rate. Greatly increased risk of cancer, especially lung cancer when smoked and oral cancers when chewed; chronic bronchitis; emphysema; heart disease; leukemia; cataracts; pneumonia.	Irritability, attention and sleep problems, depression, increased appetite.

From the National Institute of Drug Abuse. *https://www.drugabuse.gov/drugs-abuse.* Accessed June 12, 2018.

- Using alcohol in situations in which it is not safe (e.g., driving, boating, swimming)
- Feeling as if you need more alcohol to get the same effect
- Drinking to avoid withdrawal symptoms

The provider will do a physical exam, urine and blood tests, imaging tests, and a psychological evaluation. Treatment includes a medically managed detox and withdrawal in an inpatient setting.

Sedating medications may be required to help manage the withdrawal symptoms, which can last 2 to 7 days. Treatment also consists of psychological counseling, behavior change techniques, support groups, lifelong support, and medications, including:

- Naltrexone (ReVia [tablets] and Vivitrol [monthly injection]) blocks the "feel good" part of alcohol and reduces the urge to drink.

- Acamprosate (Campral) helps reduce the cravings.
- Disulfiram (Antabuse) helps prevent drinking by causing flushing, nausea, vomiting, and headaches if alcohol is consumed

---

Standard Drink

One "standard" drink is about 14 grams of pure alcohol. This can be found in:
- 12 fluid oz of regular beer (about 5% alcohol)
- 8–9 fluid oz of malt liquor (about 7% alcohol)
- 5 fluid oz of table wine (about 12% alcohol)
- 1.5 fluid oz of distilled spirits (gin, rum, tequila, vodka, and whiskey) (about 40% alcohol)

From the National Institute of Drug Abuse. *https://www.niaaa.nih.gov/alcohol-health/ overview-alcohol-consumption/what-standard-drink*. Accessed June 12, 2018.

Effects of Alcohol on the Body

- Changes moods and behavior; makes it harder to think clearly and move with coordination
- High blood pressure, stroke, *arrhythmias* (irregular heart beat), cardiomyopathy
- Liver inflammation, fatty liver, alcoholic hepatitis, fibrosis, and cirrhosis
- Pancreatitis
- Cancer of the mouth, esophagus, throat, liver, and breast
- Weakens the immune system

From the National Institute of Drug Abuse. *https://www.niaaa.nih.gov/alcohol-health/ alcohols-effects-body*. Accessed June 12, 2018.

Other Addictions

In the DSM-5, addictive disorders are addressed with substance use–related disorders. Research has shown similarities in the biology of addictions to that of substance use disorders. Comparing gambling disorder with substance use disorder shows that they share the following:

- An urge or craving state prior to using or gambling
- The activity reduces anxiety and results in a positive mood state ("a high")
- Co-existence of other types of substance use disorders. For instance, many with gambling addictions also have substance use disorder. Many with one type of substance use disorder also have another type.
- Similar abnormal functioning in the brain's cortex has been found in both.

There are several addictions recognized by the behavioral health professionals. The following are examples of addictions, though they are not all currently recognized as disorders in the ICD and DSM-5:

- *Exercise addiction*: This is a compulsive disorder that causes people to feel the uncontrollable need to exercise excessively; it can lead to illness or injury. This addiction can co-exist with anorexia nervosa or bulimia nervosa.

- *Gambling addiction*: With this disorder, people cannot control their gambling, and it affects their financial, social, recreational, familial, and occupational functioning. With gambling, dopamine is released in the brain (about 10 times the normal amount), causing a "feel good" sensation.
- *Gaming addiction*: With this serious disorder, a person excessively plays video games, which disturbs normal life activities, including school, work, and hygiene.
- *Internet addiction*: With this disorder, people have tremendous anxiety if they are forced to be without the internet (e.g., their phones, tablets, computers). They have excessive preoccupation or behaviors related to computer use and internet access. Excessive internet usage has been associated with other mental health and psychosocial conditions, including: social isolation, impaired social skills, ADHD, depression, and suicidal ideation.
- *Shopping addiction*: It is known by many names, including compulsive spending or compulsive buying disorder. The person has an intense preoccupation with buying and shopping and an uncontrollable urge to do these activities, even if negative consequences exist. It is estimated about 6% of the adults in the US have a shopping addiction.

In the future editions of the ICD and DSM, more addictions may be added. Currently, gambling is the only addictive disorder listed in the DSM-5.

THE MEDICAL ASSISTANT'S ROLE IN MENTAL AND BEHAVIORAL HEALTH PROCEDURES

Medical assistants working in behavioral health facilities may schedule appointments, work with patients' health records, handle telephone calls, assist with prescription refills, room patients and gather medical histories, perform phlebotomy, and obtain vital signs. When patients come for therapy appointments, usually the therapist gets the patients from the reception area. In many facilities, the medical assistants usually room the patients seeing the psychiatrist.

Assisting With the Examination

With patients diagnosed with eating disorders, many times the psychiatrist will want the patient to be weighed. When the medical assistant obtains the weight, it is important to have the patient empty his or her pockets and remove shoes and extra clothing. This will help to ensure the accuracy of the patient's weight, because the weight is an important sign in the treatment plan. Many healthcare facilities have patients with eating disorders get on the scale backwards, so they cannot see the weight (Fig. 22.4). They are not told what their weight is. If the person has an increase in his or her weight, that person may feel "fat," and it may not be helpful for the person's treatment. The provider will share the weight with the patient if he or she feels it is appropriate in the patient's treatment.

CRITICAL THINKING APPLICATION   **22.7**

Mike weighs Alexis White, who is being treated for anorexia. He has her step backwards on the scale and does not allow her to see the weight. She asks him repeatedly to tell her the weight. If you encountered a patient like Alexis, how would you handle the situation?

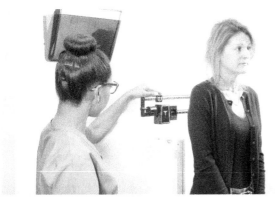

FIGURE 22.4 Weighing a patient backwards. The medical assistant should help, if needed, as the patient steps on and off the scale.

Assisting With Diagnostic Procedures

Some behavioral health facilities may have the medical assistant help with specimen collection and testing (e.g., venipuncture, urine drug test). Most of the diagnostic testing is done by psychologists, who perform psychological testing.

Mental Status Testing

Mental status testing (also called *neurocognitive testing*) assesses a person's ability to think. Providers are able to identify cognitive impairments. The testing involves the provider asking the patient a series of questions. Common tests include the Mini-Mental State Examination (MMSE), Folstein test, and the Montreal Cognitive Assessment. The provider's general observations are formed by assessing the following:

- *Physical appearance, behavior, and motor activity*: The provider checks the appropriateness of clothing, grooming, posture, facial expression, and eye contact. Does the stated age match the apparent physical appearance? Is the person friendly, withdrawn, shy, hostile, irritable, relaxed, or cooperative?
- *Mood and* **affect**: The provider asks the patient to give information on his or her emotional state or mood. The provider observes the patient's emotional state through body movements and facial expressions.

The provider assesses the cognitive functioning by examining the following:

- *Short- and long-term memory*: Questions relate to recent and past events. The person may be asked to remember something and in 5 minutes will need to recall what was remembered.
- *Attention span and concentration*: Can the person complete a thought and solve problems? The provider may ask the patient to count by fives or sevens.
- **Orientation**: Does the person know his or her name, age, and job? Does the person know the day, time, date, and season?
- *Language and communication skills*: Questions will examine the person's ability to form clear ideas. The patient may be asked to read or write a sentence.
- *Judgment and intelligence*: The person is given a scenario and is asked to solve it.

Types of Affect

The provider observes the person's affect or external expression of emotion. The provider uses the body language and the facial features to detect expressions of emotion. The following are types of affect:

- *Restricted* or *constricted affect*: A small reduction in the intensity of the affect
- *Blunted affect*: A severe reduction in the intensity of the affect; much less emotion is shown compared to the restricted affect
- *Flat affect*: A lack of emotional expression in both the face and the body language
- *Labile affect*: Rapidly changing emotions that are unrelated to external events
- *Inappropriate affect*: The emotional expressions are incongruent with the situation or the person's verbal message

Psychological Testing

There are many psychological tests used to help diagnose behavioral health disorders. Tests are available to examine:

- *Intellectual functioning*: There are a variety of tests available, including the *Wechsler Adult Intelligence Scale (WAIS)*, which measures the verbal intelligent quotient (IQ), performance IQ, and full-scale IQ. It is used for people 16 years of age or older. Other versions of the Wechsler can be used for younger children.
- *Academic achievement*: General tests along with specific tests for math, oral and written language, and reading are available. The *Boehm Test of Basic Concepts* is an example of a test in this category. It tests a child's understanding of basic positional concepts. Using pictures, the child must select the correct one when given cues such as "over," "least," and "left."
- *Psychological process*: There are a variety of tests that are available, based on the person's age. For instance, the *Bender Visual Motor Gestalt Test* is used to evaluate a person's visual-motor maturity. It is used to screen for developmental delays and can be used to assess for neurological issues and brain damage. This test is used for people age 5 years or older.
- *Adaptive behavior*: These tests are used to evaluate a person's learning difficulties, ADHD, or other impairments related to speech, language, hearing, and motor skills. The *Adaptive Behavior Assessment System* is an example.
- *Personality and attitudes*: There are a variety of tests available, including:
  - *Draw-a-Person (DAP) Test:* An analysis to measure nonverbal intelligence and to screen for behavioral or emotional disorders in children.
  - *Minnesota Multiphasic Personality Inventory (MMPI):* A widely used and researched personality assessment. It is used to diagnose behavioral health disorders, to screen for certain high-risk jobs, and as part of criminal defense and custody issues in legal cases.
  - *Thematic Apperception Test (TAT):* A test in which patients are asked to make up stories about the pictures on cards they are shown. This may provide information about a patient's thoughts, attitudes, and emotional responses.

Assisting With Treatments

Patients with behavioral health disorders are prescribed a variety of medications. The following are some of the more common classifications of medications for behavioral health disorders:

- *Antianxiety*: Used to reduce anxiety, produce calmness, and release muscle tension.
- *Anticonvulsants and mood stabilizers*: Used to treat mania and mixed episodes (mania and depression) with bipolar disorder.
- *Antidepressants*: Used to treat depression, anxiety, and other behavioral health disorders.
- *Antipsychotics*: Used to treat schizophrenia and bipolar disorder.
- *Sedative-hypnotics*: Used to treat insomnia.
- *Stimulants*: Used to treat ADHD.

Refer to Table 22.6 for information on the medication classification, including a drug's indication for use, desired effect, side effects, adverse reactions, and generic and trade names. Medical assistants should be familiar with medications that are prescribed to patients.

Psychotherapy

Psychotherapy is commonly referred to as "talk therapy." It is a general term used for a variety of treatment techniques that help a person identify and change troubling behaviors, thoughts, or emotions. Behavioral health therapists are trained in several types of psychotherapy. Based on the person and the disorder being treated, the therapist may use one or more types of psychotherapy.

- *Cognitive behavioral therapy (CBT)*: A scientifically proven treatment that produces changes in behavior by helping the person face fears, role-play situations, and learn problem-solving skills to cope with difficult issues. It is used for many behavioral health disorders including depression, anxiety disorders, substance use disorders, and eating disorders.

TABLE 22.6	Medication Classifications	
CLASSIFICATION	**INFORMATION**	**GENERIC NAME (TRADE NAME)**
Antianxiety	**Indications for use:** Produce calmness and release muscle tension; sedation. **Desired effects:** Reduce anxiety and tension. **Types:** SSRI, SNRIs, tricyclic antidepressants (see antidepressants), and benzodiazepines. **Side effects and adverse reactions:** Drowsiness, weakness, blurred vision, GI distress, hypersensitivity, jaundice, arrhythmias.	***Benzodiazepines:*** • **lorazepam** (Ativan) • **alprazolam** (Xanax) • **clonazepam** (Klonopin)
Anticonvulsants and Mood Stabilizer	**Indications for use:** Treat epilepsy, trigeminal neuralgia, mania and mixed episodes (mania and depression) with bipolar disorder **Desired effects:** Reduce the frequency and severity of seizures by reducing excessive stimulation of the brain. **Side effects and adverse reactions:** Sedation, vertigo, visual disturbances, GI disturbances, liver complications.	• **carbamazepine** (Tegretol, Equetro) • **lamotrigine** (Lamictal) • **topiramate** (Topamax) • **valproic acid** (Depakene, Depakote) • **gabapentin** (Neurontin, Horizant)
Antidepressants	**Indications for use:** Treat depression, anxiety, and other neurological disorders. **Desired effect:** Treat depression. **Side effects and adverse reactions:** Anorexia, anxiety, sexual dysfunction, fatigue, drowsiness, vertigo, weight gain, confusion, blurred vision.	***Selective serotonin reuptake inhibitors (SSRIs):*** • **fluoxetine** (Prozac) • **citalopram** (Celexa) • **escitalopram** (Lexapro) • **sertraline** (Zoloft) ***Serotonin and norepinephrine reuptake inhibitors (SNRIs):*** • **venlafaxine** • **duloxetine** (Cymbalta) ***Atypical antidepressants:*** • **bupropion** (Wellbutrin, Zyban) ***Serotonin modulators:*** • **trazodone** (Oleptro) ***Tricyclic antidepressants:*** • **amitriptyline** ***Monamine oxidase inhibitors (MAOIs):*** • **phenelzine** (Nardil)

TABLE 22.6 Medication Classifications—*continued*

CLASSIFICATION	INFORMATION	GENERIC NAME (TRADE NAME)
Antipsychotics	**Indications for use:** Treat the symptoms of schizophrenia and bipolar disorder. **Desired effect:** Alter chemical actions in the brain. **Side effects and adverse reactions:** GI distress, hypotension, electrocardiographic (ECG) changes, vertigo, sedation, headache, photosensitivity.	*Typical antipsychotics:* • **haloperidol** • **chlorpromazine** *Atypical antipsychotics:* • **olanzapine** (Zyprexa) • **lurasidone** (Latuda) • **aripiprazole** (Abilify) • **risperidone** (Risperdal) • **quetiapine**
Sedative-Hypnotics	**Indications for use:** Treat insomnia; obtain sedation (lower doses). **Desired effects:** Slowing activity in the brain to allow sleep. **Side effects and adverse reactions:** Daytime sedation, confusion, dry mouth, hypersensitivity.	• **eszopiclone** (Lunesta) • **temazepam** (Restoril) • **zolpidem** (Ambien, Edluar, Zolpimist)
Stimulants	**Indications for use:** Treat attention deficit/hyperactivity disorder (ADHD) and narcolepsy. **Desired effects:** Stimulate the brain and body; making the messages move faster between the brain and the body. The person becomes more alert and physically active. **Side effects and adverse reactions:** arrhythmias, aggression, memory loss, flushing, hypertension, restlessness, fainting.	• **atomoxetine** (Strattera) • **methylphenidate** (Concerta, Ritalin LA)

• *Dialectical behavioral therapy (DBT)*: This evidence-based CBT approach is used for individuals who are diagnosed with personality disorders, are suicidal, or engage in self-harm behaviors. DBT focuses behavioral change, problem solving, and regulation of emotions in a manner that is socially acceptable.

• *Exposure therapy*: A type of CBT that is used to help people process their traumatic experiences or feared situations. The person revisits and recounts the memories, which gradually helps the person emotionally process the experience or situation. The person may start by thinking about the object or situation, then progress to looking at pictures of it, then to getting near it, and then to touching it or experiencing it for short periods of time.

• *Eye movement desensitization and reprocessing (EMDR)*: Used to process and resolve traumatic memories (e.g., PTSD). During the therapy, the person concentrates on the memory while focusing on controlled stimuli (e.g., eye movements or sounds). The patient discusses any new thoughts that occur and continues until the memory is no longer distressing.

• *Interpersonal psychotherapy (IPT)*: Used to treat behavioral health disorders, such as eating disorders and major depression, by helping the person understand the relationship between symptoms and social interactions, thus improving social skills and functioning.

• *Play therapy*: Used for children who are experiencing behavioral, emotional, social, or relational disorders. Using play and the therapeutic relationship, the child is able to express feelings and thoughts.

• *Psychodynamic therapy*: Used to treat depression, addictions, social anxiety disorder, and eating disorders. It focuses on helping the patient recognize, express, and overcome negative feelings and repressed emotions, so that the person's interpersonal experiences and relationships improve.

CLOSING COMMENTS

Patient Coaching

In behavioral health, the medical assistant has an important role in coaching patients on their medications. Patients should be aware of:

• When and how to take the medication
• What to do if the medication is forgotten
• What side effects may occur
• When to contact the provider

Compliance can be an issue with medications in behavioral health. Patients who are experiencing issues may stop the medication. This may increase the signs and symptoms of the disorder. For some disorders, this can be a life-threatening complication. Sometimes hospitalization is required until medications can stabilize the situation.

Legal and Ethical Issues

Under HIPAA, **psychotherapy notes** are treated with higher levels of confidentiality than other health records. Psychotherapy notes need to be stored separately from the patient health record. They are not released with other health records and must be specifically indicated by the patient to be released.

If an electronic health record system is used, access to the psychotherapy notes must be limited to the behavioral health staff that require the notes for their job. Additional information from the visit is not held at a higher level of confidentiality and includes prescriptions, session times, types and frequency of treatments, and results of clinical tests.

Like HIPAA, many federal and state laws address the confidentiality of drug and substance abuse information. These laws require these patient health records to be held at a higher level of confidentiality.

Patient-Centered Care

In behavioral health, patient-centered care is important. Two principles of patient-centered care are emotional support and involvement of family. These two principles are addressed often in behavioral health. Behavioral health professionals need to develop a strong professional, therapeutic relationship with patients. This relationship provides the emotional support that helps patients feel accepted, so they share their concerns, thoughts, and feelings with behavioral health professionals.

Often families play an important part in the management and treatment of behavioral health. Some behavioral health disorders may come from issues related to family relationships. Other times, the family needs to provide emotional support to help assist the patient through treatment. Depending on the situation and the patient, family members may be brought into the therapy to ultimately help the patient through the situation or effectively manage the disorder.

Professional Behaviors

Medical assistants working outside the behavioral health department will often come in contact with patients who have behavioral health disorders. It is important for medical assistants to remain professional in their nonverbal and verbal communication. If patients make inappropriate or nonsensical statements, seem "off" in their affect, or demonstrate other unusual behaviors, the medical assistant should relay the information to the provider.

Inappropriate comments to the patient or about the patient to others is unprofessional and should not happen. Remember, all information about the patient is confidential.

SUMMARY OF SCENARIO

Mike learned a lot about the policies and procedures used by the behavioral health staff. At first, he was uncomfortable working with patients who were experiencing signs and symptoms of behavioral health disorders. To his surprise he found working with patients in behavioral health very interesting and rewarding. Having learned about these conditions in school, he was nervous, not knowing how he would deal with such situations. Mike was professional and felt he provided excellent patient-centered care. Mike realizes he still has a lot more to learn, because there are over 200 mental health disorders and many substance use disorders. He looks forward to spending more time with the behavioral health staff.

SUMMARY OF LEARNING OBJECTIVES

1. **Explore the differences between types of common behavioral health professionals.**

   Common behavioral health professionals include psychiatrists, psychologists, social workers, cognitive behavioral therapists (CBTs), psychiatric nurses, substance abuse (or addiction) therapists or counselors, and mental health therapists or counselors. In many states, most of these healthcare professionals need a license to practice, and they all have different degrees of training and specialties.

2. **Differentiate among common behavioral health disorders, including the etiology, signs, symptoms, diagnostic procedures, and treatments.**

   This chapter discussed anxiety disorders, including generalized anxiety disorder, OCD, panic disorder, phobias, and social anxiety disorder. Autism spectrum disorder, depression, behavioral disorder, dissociative disorder, eating disorders, personality disorders, post-traumatic stress disorder, schizophrenia, and suicidal behaviors were discussed. Substance use disorder, including drugs and alcohol, was discussed. Other addictions were also explained. Refer to each disorder for the specific etiology, signs, symptoms, diagnostic procedures, and treatments.

3. **Discuss substance use disorders and other addictions. Also, list commonly abused substances and describe a "standard" drink of alcohol.**

   In the DSM-5, substance use disorder includes both substance abuse and substance dependence. Substance use disorder is measured from mild to severe. Alcohol use disorder (AUD) is a chronic relapsing brain disease that includes a compulsion to use alcohol, loss of control over alcohol intake, and a negative emotional state when abstaining from alcohol. Other addictions include exercise, gambling, gaming, internet, and shopping. Currently, gambling is the only addictive disorder listed in the DSM-5. Commonly used substances, along with their street names, common forms, and ways to take the drug, in addition to possible health effects and withdrawal symptoms, were discussed. Common substances abused include CNS depressants, cocaine, DMT, GHB, heroin, ketamine, LSD, marijuana, mescaline, prescription opioids, phencyclidine, psilocybin, rohypnol, and tobacco.

   One "standard" drink is about 14 grams of pure alcohol. This can be found in:

   - 12 fluid oz of regular beer (about 5% alcohol)
   - 8–9 fluid oz of malt liquor (about 7% alcohol)
   - 5 fluid oz of table wine (about 12% alcohol)
   - 1.5 fluid oz of distilled spirits (gin, rum, tequila, vodka, and whiskey) (about 40% alcohol)

4. **Describe how a medical assistant should assist with a mental or behavioral health examination.**

   Medical assistants working in behavioral health facilities may schedule appointments, work with patients' health records, handle phone calls, assist with prescription refills, room patients and gather medical histories, perform phlebotomy, and obtain vital signs. When dealing with a patient diagnosed with an eating disorder, many healthcare facilities have the patient stand on the scale backwards, so that they cannot see their weight.

5. **Explain the common diagnostic procedures for mental and behavioral health disorders. Also, describe the common medication classifications used for behavioral health disorders.**

   Common diagnostic procedures for behavioral health disorders include:
   - Mental status testing (also called neurocognitive testing), which assesses a person's ability to think.
   - Psychological testing, which examines intellectual functioning, academic achievement, psychological process, adaptive behavior, personality, and attitudes.

   Patients with behavioral health disorders are prescribed a variety of medications. The following are some of the more common classifications of medications for behavioral health disorders:
   - *Antianxiety*: Used to reduce anxiety, produce calmness, and release muscle tension

   - *Anticonvulsants and mood stabilizers*: Used to treat mania and mixed episodes (mania and depression) with bipolar disorder
   - *Antidepressants*: Used to treat depression, anxiety, and other behavioral health disorders
   - *Antipsychotics*: Used to treat schizophrenia and bipolar disorder
   - *Sedative-hypnotics*: Used to treat insomnia
   - *Stimulants*: Used to treat ADHD

6. **Explain the legal issues and Health Insurance Portability and Accountability Act (HIPAA) applications associated with mental health disorders and substance use disorders.**

   Under HIPAA, psychotherapy notes are treated with higher levels of confidentiality than other health records. Psychotherapy notes need to be stored and released separately compared to regular health records. Only behavioral health staff that need the record should have access to it.

   Like HIPAA, many federal and state laws address the confidentiality of drug and substance abuse information. These laws require these patient health records to be held at a higher level of confidentiality.

23

ENDOCRINOLOGY

SCENARIO

Cecylia Cukier, CMA (AAMA), has worked at Walden-Martin Family Medical (WMFM) Clinic for 3 years. She enjoys working with the primary care providers. Working with the patients who have diabetes mellitus has been a special interest of hers since her medical assistant practicum in college. When a position was posted to work with the outreach endocrinology team, which came from a clinic 50 miles away, Cecylia applied for the position. She was accepted into the new position and now works 2 days a week with the endocrinology team, which sees WMFM Clinic patients. During the remaining 3 days, Cecylia continues to work with the primary care team.

Cecylia is excited to start working with the endocrinology team and patients. She has decided to review the anatomy, physiology, and pathology of the endocrine system in preparation for her new duties.

While studying this chapter, think about the following questions:
- What medical terminology relates to the endocrine system?
- What are the locations of the endocrine system structures?
- What are some of the common endocrine diseases?
- What are the differences between type 1 and type 2 diabetes mellitus?
- What complications may occur with diabetes mellitus?
- What diagnostic procedures are used for endocrine diseases?

LEARNING OBJECTIVES

1. Do the following related to the anatomy of the endocrine system:
   - Describe the anatomical location of the major organs of the endocrine system.
   - List the hormones secreted from the endocrine glands.
   - Describe life span changes related to the endocrine system.
2. Explain the physiology of the endocrine system.
3. Identify common disorders of the endocrine system and list common signs and symptoms of endocrine disorders.
4. Differentiate between type 1 and type 2 diabetes mellitus.
5. List signs and symptoms of hypoglycemia, hyperglycemia, and diabetic ketoacidosis, and describe the immediate care required for hypoglycemia and diabetic ketoacidosis.
6. Explain complications of diabetes and discuss gestational diabetes.
7. Discuss the medical assistant's role in endocrinology procedures, including assisting with the examination, diagnostic procedures, and treatments.

VOCABULARY

calcium A naturally occurring element that is necessary for many body functions, including strong bones and teeth, proper blood clotting, nerve conduction, and muscle contractions.

cataract Clouding of the lens, leading to decreased vision.

diabetic retinopathy (die ah BET ik reh tin OP ah thee) Diabetes mellitus damages the blood vessels in the retina, leading to loss of vision and eventual blindness.

diffuse To spread, scatter, disperse, or move.

electrolyte An inorganic compound, usually a salt. A major factor in controlling fluid balance within the body.

exocrine A glandular secretion released through a duct.

fatty acids Result when fats are broken down; used by the body for energy and tissue development.

glaucoma (glou KOE mah) Increase in the fluid pressure in the eye, can lead to blindness if not treated.

homeostasis (hoe mee oh STAY sis) The internal environment of the body that is compatible with life. A steady state that is created by all the body systems working together to provide a consistent and unvarying internal environment.

libido Sexual drive or instinct.

mediastinum (mee dee AH sti nuhm) The space in the thoracic cavity that lies between the lungs, containing the heart, trachea, and esophagus.

negative feedback An output or response that affects the input of a system.

nucleus A specialized organelle of a cell that is encased in a membrane and directs growth, metabolism, and reproduction of the cell.

organelle A structure within a cell that performs a specific function.

preeclampsia (pree ih KLAMP see ah) A form of toxemia during pregnancy, characterized by high blood pressure, fluid retention, and protein in the urine. May progress to eclampsia.

receptors Structures or sites on or in a cell that bind with substances such as hormones, antigens, or drugs.

target cell A cell selectively affected by a specific agent, such as a drug, hormone, or virus.

water deprivation test A test to measure the amount and concentration of urine produced when water is withheld from a patient for a period of time.

Endocrinology is the healthcare specialty that deals with endocrine disorders. These disorders relate to endocrine glands, hormones, and the hormonal effects on the body. An *endocrinologist* is a specialist involved in the diagnosis, treatment, and prevention of endocrine disorders.

Besides the endocrine department, patients with endocrine concerns are typically seen in primary care and urgent care departments. Medical assistants should have a strong understanding of the common endocrinology diseases, diagnostic tests, and treatments.

ANATOMY OF THE ENDOCRINE SYSTEM

The *endocrine system* is composed of ductless glands throughout the body. *Endocrine glands* release hormones directly into the bloodstream, and the blood transports them to **target cells**. The hormones act as messengers to the target cells, telling the cells to alter their functions to help maintain homeostasis in the body. Hormones function as the body's chemical messengers, transferring information from one group of cells to another. They control metabolism, growth, mood, sexual maturity, reproduction, and water and **electrolyte** balance. Hormone levels vary and can be affected by outside factors, such as illness and stress. Fig. 23.1 shows the location of the endocrine glands.

The nervous system and the endocrine system can work alone or together. Working jointly, as a *neuroendocrine system*, they perform communication functions and maintain homeostasis. The brain sends out signals to and continually receives feedback from the endocrine system. The nervous system communicates quickly through nerve impulses and delivers rapid responses to maintain homeostasis. The endocrine system communicates slowly through hormones, which maintain homeostasis for a longer period of time. The body needs both systems working together through communication to maintain homeostasis.

Hypothalamus

The *hypothalamus*, located in the middle of the brain, is the major connection for the neuroendocrine system. It plays an important role in controlling the endocrine system. When the hypothalamus detects rising levels of a target organ's hormones, it sends a signal to the pituitary gland to release or prevent the pituitary hormone production.

The hypothalamus is also responsible for the production of antidiuretic hormone (ADH) and oxytocin. These two hormones, though produced by the hypothalamus, are stored and secreted by the posterior lobe of the pituitary gland. They will be discussed in more detail in the next section.

Pituitary Gland

The *pituitary gland*, also known as the *hypophysis*, is a pea-sized gland that is connected to the hypothalamus by the *infundibulum*, a small

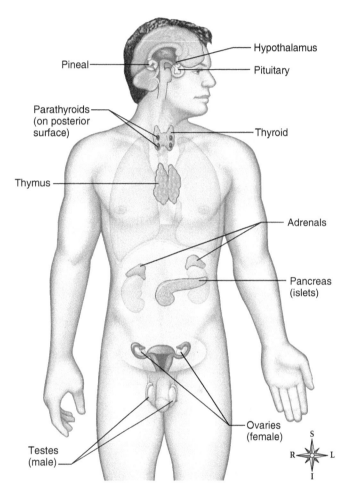

FIGURE 23.1 Location of the endocrine glands. (From Patton KT, Thibodeau GA: *Anatomy and physiology*, ed 9, St Louis, 2016, Mosby.)

stalk of tissue. The hormones from the pituitary control the other endocrine glands; thus the pituitary gland is called the "master gland." The pituitary gland is composed of two lobes that act as separate glands, the anterior lobe and the posterior lobe. Each lobe has its own functions.

Anterior Lobe of the Pituitary Gland

The anterior lobe, also known as the *adenohypophysis*, produces and secretes these hormones (Fig. 23.2):

- *Adrenocorticotropic hormone* (ACTH): Causes the adrenal cortex to produce and release steroids (e.g., cortisol).
- *Follicle-stimulating hormone* (FSH): Stimulates the development of ova (eggs) through ovulation in females and stimulates the seminiferous tubules to produce sperm in males.

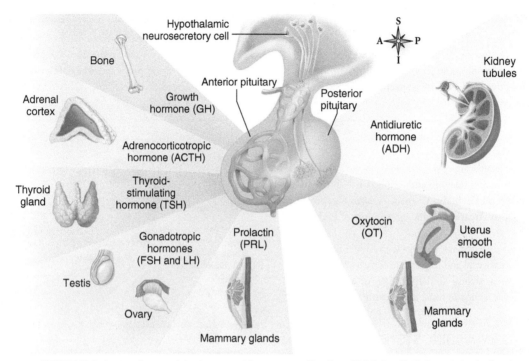

FIGURE 23.2 Anterior and posterior pituitary hormones and the target organs. (From Patton KT, Thibodeau GA: *The human body in health and disease,* ed 6, St Louis, 2014, Mosby.)

- *Growth hormone* (GH): Stimulates growth of the long bones and muscles in children and teens. Growth hormone is also involved with glucose metabolism in the body.
- *Luteinizing hormone* (LH): In females, it simulates the ovaries to produce estrogen, ova to mature, and the production of progesterone. LH also initiates ovulation and signals the corpus luteum to develop. In men, it stimulates interstitial cells in the testes to develop and secrete testosterone.
- *Prolactin (PRL)*: Stimulates breast tissue development and milk production toward the end of pregnancy and after childbirth.
- *Thyroid-stimulating hormone (TSH)*: Stimulates the thyroid gland to release T_3 and T_4. (More information about the thyroid will be presented later in the chapter.)

Posterior Lobe of the Pituitary Gland

The posterior lobe, also known as the *neurohypophysis*, is composed of nervous tissue. It does not produce hormones, but it stores hormones produced by the hypothalamus. The hormones are transported from the hypothalamus to the posterior lobe directly through the infundibulum. The posterior lobe stores the hormones until it gets a signal from the hypothalamus to release them into the bloodstream. The blood then carries the hormones to their target organ (see Fig. 23.2).

The two hormones released by the posterior lobe are:
- *Antidiuretic hormone* (ADH): Also called *vasopressin*. Stimulates contraction of the blood vessels, raising the blood pressure. It also stimulates the kidney tubules to reabsorb water, which concentrates the urine.
- *Oxytocin* (OT): Stimulates the uterine muscles to contract. OT also helps with releasing breast milk, by stimulating the contraction of the muscles surrounding the mammary ducts.

CRITICAL THINKING APPLICATION   23.1

Cecylia is struggling to remember the hormones from the posterior and anterior lobes of the pituitary gland. What might be some helpful ways to remember the hormones from this gland?

Thyroid Gland

The thyroid gland is a butterfly-shaped gland in the neck above the collarbone. The thyroid produces, stores, and secretes:
- *Triiodothyronine* (T_3): Regulates metabolism and increases the basal metabolic rate.
- *Thyroxine* (T_4): Regulates metabolism and increases the basal metabolic rate. It also supports the activities of growth hormone.
- *Calcitonin:* Helps lower blood **calcium** levels and helps to retain calcium in the bones.

When thyroid hormone levels decrease in the body, the hypothalamus secretes TSH-releasing hormone. This hormone "tells" the anterior lobe of the pituitary gland to produce TSH, which then stimulates the thyroid to produce hormones. Iodine from our diet is absorbed in the blood and carried to the thyroid gland. Iodine is required to produce T_3 and T_4.

Increasing the Basal Metabolic Rate

T_3 and T_4 hormones increase the basal metabolic rate, which:
- Causes an increase in the body temperature and pulse rate; also creates a stronger heartbeat
- Helps the brain mature in children and also promotes growth
- Improves concentration and faster reflexes
- Uses more energy (calories)

Parathyroid Glands

The parathyroid glands are four pea-sized glands located on the back side of the thyroid gland. They secrete *parathyroid hormone* (PTH), which helps regulate calcium and phosphorus levels in the body. When the blood calcium level decreases, PTH is secreted, causing calcium to be released from bone. The released calcium is absorbed in the blood, which increases the blood calcium levels.

A balance needs to be maintained. If too much PTH is secreted, *hyperparathyroidism* occurs, causing bones to lose calcium and the blood calcium level to rise. If too little PTH is secreted, *hypoparathyroidism* occurs. The blood calcium level decreases, and the blood phosphorus level increases.

Adrenal Glands

The adrenal glands are located on the top of each kidney. The outer part of the gland is the *adrenal cortex*, and the inner part is called the *adrenal medulla*.

Adrenal Cortex

The adrenal cortex produces cortical hormones, also called *steroids*. As a group, these three hormones are called *corticosteroids*. They include:

- *Mineralocorticoids*: Regulate the electrolytes in the body. *Aldosterone,* the most important mineralocorticoid, regulates the sodium and water balance in the body through the reabsorption of sodium and water in the kidneys. As the sodium is reabsorbed into the blood, hydrogen or potassium is excreted into the urine.
- *Glucocorticoids*: Regulate protein, fat, and carbohydrate metabolism. They also hasten the breakdown of proteins into amino acids, which are converted to glucose in the liver. This process increases the blood glucose level. Norepinephrine and epinephrine need glucocorticoids to constrict blood vessels, which increases the blood pressure. Lastly, glucocorticoids have anti-inflammatory properties. The main glucocorticoid secreted is *cortisol* (also called *hydrocortisone*). Cortisone and corticosterone are produced in lesser amounts. Stress can increase the amount of glucocorticoids secreted.
- *Gonadocorticoids*: Small amounts of male sex hormones (androgens) are secreted and responsible for some of the secondary sexual characteristics (e.g., pubic and axillary hair) in both males and females during puberty.

The hypothalamus and the anterior lobe of the pituitary gland (through the secretion of ACTH) regulate the corticosteroids secreted by the adrenal cortex.

CRITICAL THINKING APPLICATION   23.2

The actions of mineralocorticoids and glucocorticoids confuse Cecylia. Summarize the actions of these two corticosteroids.

Adrenal Medulla

The hypothalamus, with the help of the sympathetic nervous system, stimulates the adrenal medulla to secrete these nonsteroid hormones:

- *Epinephrine* (*adrenaline*): Secreted in response to physical or mental stress, providing the fight-or-flight response. It increases the heart rate and strength of the contractions, blood pressure, and blood glucose level. It also relaxes the smooth muscles in the bronchioles. These changes allow more glucose and oxygenated blood to get to the cells for the fight-or-flight response.
- *Norepinephrine* (*noradrenalin*): Also secreted in times of stress. It increases the blood glucose level, heart rate, and the force of the heart's contractions; in addition, it causes vasoconstriction, thus raising the blood pressure.

Pancreas

The *pancreas* is located inferior and posterior to the stomach. It has both endocrine and **exocrine** functions. As already discussed, an endocrine gland releases hormones into the blood, whereas an *exocrine gland* releases secretions through ducts. The pancreas releases digestive enzymes into the small intestine through pancreatic ducts.

The pancreas contains *pancreatic islets* or *islets of Langerhans*, which produce hormones. The pancreas produces several hormones, including:

- *Glucagon*: Secreted by the alpha islet cells. It raises the blood glucose level two different ways. It stimulates the stored glycogen in the liver to be converted into glucose. It also stimulates **fatty acids** and amino acids in the liver to be converted into glucose. The glucose is absorbed by the bloodstream, which increases the blood glucose level.
- *Insulin*: Secreted by the beta islet cells. It promotes the movement of fatty acids, amino acids, and glucose out of the blood and into the cells, which lowers the blood glucose level.
- *Somatostatin*: Secreted by the delta islet cells; it regulates the other pancreatic hormones and also inhibits the secretion of growth hormone.
- *Ghrelin* (GHRL): Secreted by the epsilon islet cells. Research has found that GHRL works in the brain to regulate body weight, glucose metabolism, and food intake. Multiple additional actions of ghrelin have been reported in research studies, including involvement with learning, memory, gut motility, gastric acid secretion, sleep/wake rhythm (*circadian rhythms*), reward-seeking behavior, and taste sensation.

Thymus Gland

The *thymus gland* is in the **mediastinum** behind the sternum (breastbone) and secretes thymosin and thymopoietin hormones. These hormones stimulate the production and maturity of T cells, a type of lymphocyte (white blood cells). T cells have an important role in immunity.

Gonads

The **gonads** are considered the primary sex organs. The male gonads are the testes, and the female gonads are the ovaries. Both types of gonads produce hormones. The testes secrete testosterone, which stimulates the development of male secondary sexual characteristics (e.g., voice changes, growth of facial and pubic hair). Testosterone also promotes sperm production and muscle development. The ovaries produce estrogen and progesterone. Estrogen stimulates the development of breasts and other female secondary sexual characteristics. Progesterone helps maintain a pregnancy. Both estrogen and progesterone are important in the menstrual cycle.

Pineal Gland

The *pineal gland* is located deep within the brain and secretes the hormone *melatonin*. Melatonin helps regulate waking and sleeping patterns and may affect seasonal reactions to the availability of sunlight.

PHYSIOLOGY OF THE ENDOCRINE SYSTEM

Mechanisms of Hormone Regulation

The goal of hormone regulation is to maintain **homeostasis**. Nervous system stimulation, endocrine control, and feedback systems regulate hormone secretion. The following examples demonstrate these three mechanisms.

- *Nervous system regulation*: During a stressful event, the adrenal medulla releases adrenaline (epinephrine) in response to stimulation from the sympathetic nervous system.
- *Endocrine control regulation*: TSH from the anterior pituitary stimulates the thyroid to secrete T_3 and T_4. (A hormone from one gland stimulates another gland to secrete a hormone.)
- *Feedback system regulation*: A **negative feedback** system example: If the calcium blood level falls below normal, the parathyroid glands are stimulated to release PTH. PTH increases blood calcium levels by stimulating the absorption of calcium from the intestines or by chemically breaking down bone to release stored calcium into the blood. The change in the blood calcium level is detected by the parathyroid gland, which then stops production of PTH. (An imbalance activates the endocrine gland, which then acts to correct the imbalance by stopping the hormone secretion process.)

Target Cells

Each hormone released into the bloodstream has specific target cells for action. The target cells have **receptors** that attract only certain hormones. The cell membrane only lets selected hormones pass into the cell and affect cellular action.

Hormone Action

There are two categories of hormones, nonsteroid hormones and steroid hormones. All hormones are messengers, but how they deliver their message is where they differ. Both types of hormones maintain homeostasis.

Nonsteroid hormones are made up of protein or amino acids. This type of hormone attaches to a target cell membrane. Another molecule takes the message from the nonsteroid hormone and carries it to the target cell **nucleus** or **organelle**, which then puts the message into action in the cell.

Steroid hormones are small *lipid-soluble* (fat-soluble) molecules that attach to a target cell membrane and then pass directly into the target cell. Once inside the target cell, steroid hormones travel to and enter the nucleus. They bind to a receptor site, which creates a hormone-receptor site complex. This complex communicates its message with DNA in the nucleus, and the DNA tells the cell how to put the hormone's message into action.

Prostaglandins

Prostaglandins (PGs), also known as *tissue hormones*, are substances found in many body tissues. PGs are produced in tissues and **diffuse** only a short distance to affect cells in their local area. They help regulate processes such as respiration, blood pressure, digestive system secretions, and reproductive functions. They are powerful molecules that are made locally and act locally.

DISORDERS OF THE ENDOCRINE SYSTEM

Many diseases affect the endocrine system. Most of the pathology of the endocrine system is the result of either *hyper-* (too much) or *hypo-* (too little) hormonal secretion. Table 23.1 defines terms related to signs and symptoms of endocrine conditions. The following sections describe in detail some of the more common diseases seen in the ambulatory care setting.

TABLE 23.1	Signs and Symptoms of Endocrine Conditions
MEDICAL TERM	**DEFINITION**
Exophthalmia	Noticeable protrusion of the eyeball
Glucosuria	Presence of glucose in the urine.
Goiter	Swelling of the neck and visible enlargement of the thyroid gland.
Hypocalcemia	A low blood calcium level
Hypoglycemia	A low blood glucose (sugar) level
Ketoacidosis	Presence of ketones in the blood that cause *metabolic acidosis* (a pH imbalance due to too much acid)
Ketonuria	Presence of ketones in the urine.
Polydipsia	Excessive thirst.
Polyphagia	Excessive eating.
Polyuria	Excessive urine volume

Pituitary Gland Diseases

Many hormones are secreted by the anterior and posterior pituitary glands. Table 23.2 describes pituitary gland disorders. Fig. 23.3 displays the signs of acromegaly and Figs. 23.4 and 23.5 show signs of growth hormone disorders. Diabetes insipidus is discussed in more detail in the next section.

Diabetes Insipidus

Diabetes insipidus (DI) is caused by a hyposecretion of ADH. The hypothalamus does not produce enough of the hormone, or the posterior pituitary does not release a sufficient amount of it.

There are several types of DI and the causes vary, including genetics, a tumor, trauma, or pituitary gland surgery. Diabetes insipidus can also occur if there is an inadequate response to ADH in the renal tubules in the nephrons, due to kidney disease or certain medications. The signs and symptoms usually have an acute onset and include:

- Polydipsia, polyuria, *nocturia* (frequent urination at night), and very dilute urine
- Trouble sleeping, fussiness, and irritability
- Fever, vomiting, diarrhea, and *hypotension* (low blood pressure)
- Delayed growth and weight loss in children

Complications may occur, such as hypernatremia (high blood sodium levels), severe dehydration, electrolyte imbalance, and low blood pressure.

The provider will do a physical exam and may order laboratory tests, including a urinalysis and blood tests. A **water deprivation test** and imaging tests can also be done. ID can be fatal if not adequately treated. Treatment focuses on the cause of the condition. Medications such as a synthetic ADH hormone (desmopressin [DDAVP]) and diuretics may be given.

CRITICAL THINKING APPLICATION   23.3

Cecylia is working with Landon, who was just diagnosed with diabetes insipidus. Landon's mother asks Cecylia how often he would need to take insulin. How would you address this question? Could you as a medical assistant correct the mother's misconception about diabetes insipidus?

TABLE 23.2 Pituitary Gland Disorders

GLAND	HORMONE	CONDITION	DESCRIPTION
Anterior pituitary	Growth hormone, hypersecretion	*Acromegaly*	Occurs after normal growth has finished (e.g., during adulthood). Usually caused by an adenoma of the pituitary gland. Leads to an enlargement of the extremities (hands and feet), jaw, nose, and forehead (see Fig. 23.3). Also causes an overgrowth of soft tissue. Treatment includes surgery and radiation to reduce the size of the pituitary gland.
		Gigantism	Occurs during childhood, leading to excessive growth (see Fig. 23.4). Treatment includes surgery and radiation to reduce the size of the pituitary gland.
	Growth hormone, hyposecretion	*Dwarfism*	Occurs during childhood, leading to smaller than normal body frame (see Fig. 23.5). Treated with injections of growth hormone during childhood.
	Prolactin, hypersecretion	*Prolactinoma*	Most common type of pituitary tumor. *Women:* Causes abnormal lactation and affects the menstrual cycle. *Men:* Causes impotence.
	Prolactin, hyposecretion	——	*Women:* Unable to maintain breast milk production.
	All hormones, hyposecretion	*Panhypopituitarism*	Destruction or deficiency of the entire anterior lobe. Most common in women. Causes hypotension, weight loss, weakness, and loss of libido.
Posterior pituitary	Antidiuretic hormone (ADH), hypersecretion	*Syndrome of inappropriate antidiuretic hormone (SIADH)*	Causes inability to produce and secrete diluted urine. Water retention, hyponatremia, and weight gain are seen.
	Antidiuretic hormone (ADH), hyposecretion	*Diabetes insipidus*	Causes the patient to excrete large quantities of diluted urine.

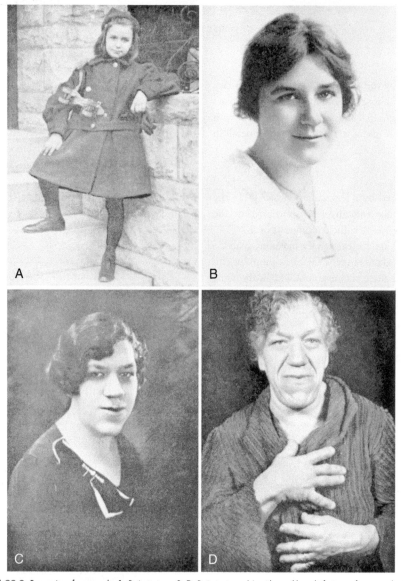

FIGURE 23.3 Progression of acromegaly. **A,** Patient at age 9. **B,** Patient at age 16, with possible early features of acromegaly. **C,** Patient at age 33, with well-established acromegaly. **D,** Patient at age 52, end-stage acromegaly. (From Clinical Pathological Conference, *Am J Med* 20:133, 1956.)

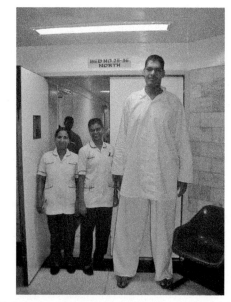

FIGURE 23.4 Gigantism. (From Sainani GS, Joshi VR, Sainani RG: *Manual of clinical & practical medicine,* New Delhi, 2010, Elsevier India.)

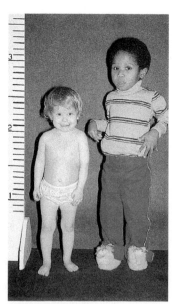

FIGURE 23.5 The normal 3½-year-old boy is in the 50th percentile for height. The short 3-year-old girl exhibits the characteristic "kewpie doll" appearance, suggesting a diagnosis of growth hormone deficiency (GHD). (From Zitelli BJ, Davis HW: *Atlas of pediatric physical diagnosis,* ed 5, St Louis, 2007, Mosby.)

Thyroid Gland Diseases

Thyroid diseases cause hypersecretion or hyposecretion of thyroid hormone. Table 23.3 describes thyroid diseases. Hyperthyroidism and hypothyroidism are described in depth in the following sections.

Hyperthyroidism

Hyperthyroidism occurs when too much thyroid hormone is produced. The most common cause of hyperthyroidism is Graves disease, and additional causes include thyroid nodules, pituitary disorders and tumors, and thyroiditis (see Table 23.3). Risk factors include a family history of thyroid disorders and having an existing autoimmune disease. Hyperthyroidism is more common in women, people with other thyroid conditions, and those over 60 years of age. Common signs and symptoms of hyperthyroidism include:

- Fatigue, muscle weakness, sensitivity to heat, and increased sweating
- More frequent bowel movements and weight loss, even with adequate food intake and an increased appetite
- Difficulty sleeping, restlessness, irritability, nervousness, and anxiety
- Rapid heart rate, irregular heart rate, and palpitations
- Goiter and exophthalmia (Figs. 23.6 and 23.7)
- Changes in menstrual cycle
- *Thyrotoxicosis* (thyroid storm), a life-threatening condition that causes elevated vital signs (e.g., temperature, pulse, respiration, and blood pressure).

After performing a physical exam, the provider may order thyroid function tests and a radioactive iodine uptake (RAIU) scan. Treatment includes radioactive iodine therapy to shrink the thyroid, antithyroid medication (e.g., methimazole [Tapazole]), and a thyroidectomy.

TABLE 23.3	Conditions That Cause Hyperthyroidism and Hypothyroidism	
CONDITION	**THYROID FUNCTION**	**DESCRIPTION**
Simple goiter	Hyperthyroidism or hypothyroidism	Simple enlargement of the thyroid gland, causing swelling in the neck. Usually not malignant. Can be caused by iodine deficiency, immune disorders, infections, medications, and other thyroid conditions. More common in people over 40, women, and those with a family history of goiters. Depending on the symptoms, may be treated with potassium iodide or thyroid hormone.
Thyroid nodule	Hyperthyroidism or hypothyroidism	A growth in the thyroid gland. Can be benign or malignant. More common in women. Causes neck enlargement, pain, hoarseness, and problems swallowing. Treatment may consist of monitoring, surgery, and thyroid hormone if hypothyroidism is occurring.
Thyroiditis	Hyperthyroidism or hypothyroidism	Inflammation of the thyroid. Several types of thyroiditis. Can be an autoimmune condition or caused by a virus, bacteria, or medication. For several types, the patient may start with hyperthyroidism symptoms and then have hypothyroidism symptoms. Treatment depends on the symptoms and type.
Thyroid carcinoma	Hyperthyroidism or hypothyroidism	The most common types of thyroid carcinoma are follicular and papillary. Both have high 5-year survival rates. Women are three times more at risk for thyroid cancer. Causes a hard, painless lump in the thyroid gland. May cause hoarseness and enlargement of the neck. Treatment depends on the type of cancer; may include surgery, chemotherapy, radiation, and thyroid hormone.
Graves disease	Hyperthyroidism	Autoimmune disease that results in hypersecretion of the thyroid hormone. Most common cause of hyperthyroidism. Causes heat intolerance, heart *palpitations* (pounding heart in chest), weight loss, and nervousness. Can cause Graves eye disease or Graves ophthalmopathy (e.g., bulging of the eyes [*exophthalmia*], double vision, light sensitivity, and irritation).
Cretinism	Hypothyroidism	Occurs during infancy and childhood. Leads to low metabolic rate, stunted growth and sexual development, and cognitive deficits. Treated with thyroid hormone.
Myxedema	Hypothyroidism	Occurs during adolescence and adulthood. Symptoms include menorrhagia; dry, scaly skin with no perspiration; weakness; fatigue; bloating; facial puffiness; cold intolerance; and cognition issues. Treated with thyroid hormone.
Hashimoto thyroiditis	Hypothyroidism	A chronic immune system disease that attacks the thyroid gland. Often occurs in middle-aged females. Occurs slowly, leading to difficulty thinking, dry skin, goiter, fatigue, hair loss, cold intolerance, mild weight gain, and irregular periods. Treatment may include thyroid medication.

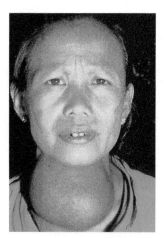

FIGURE 23.6 Goiter.

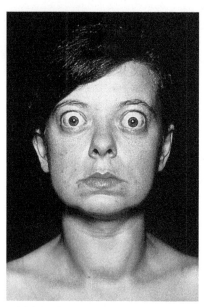

FIGURE 23.7 Exophthalmos in Graves' disease. (From Seidel HM et al: *Mosby's guide to physical examination*, ed 6, St Louis, 2006, Mosby.)

Hypothyroidism

Hypothyroidism occurs when too little thyroid hormone is produced. Hypothyroidism occurs after thyroidectomy and radiation therapy. Table 23.3 describes additional conditions that cause hypothyroidism. Risk factors for hypothyroidism include having a history of an autoimmune disease, a family history of hypothyroidism, or pregnancy in the past 6 months. Another risk factor is being a female over 60 years of age. The signs and symptoms relate to the metabolism slowing down and may include:

- Fatigue, muscle weakness, tenderness, aches, and stiffness
- Constipation and weight gain
- Dry skin, sensitivity to cold, and thinning hair
- Slowed heart rate, hoarseness, and depression
- Elevated blood cholesterol

After the provider performs the physical exam, thyroid function tests and a thyroid ultrasound may be done. Treatment requires taking lifelong synthetic thyroid hormone (e.g., levothyroxine [Levothroid, Synthroid]).

> **CRITICAL THINKING APPLICATION**   23.4
>
> Cecylia is working with a patient who has been diagnosed with hypothyroidism. What are the signs and symptoms of hypothyroidism? What treatments are usually prescribed?

Parathyroid Gland Diseases

Hyperparathyroidism

Hyperparathyroidism is a relatively common disorder. It occurs when one or more of the four parathyroid glands oversecrete parathyroid hormone (PTH) causing *hyperparathyroidism*. Hyperparathyroidism causes excessive bone resorption, and the calcium from the bones increases the blood calcium levels (*hypercalcemia*).

Primary hyperparathyroidism occurs as a result of an adenoma or a hyperplasia of one of the four glands, causing the increase in PTH secretion. Secondary hyperparathyroidism occurs with renal disease, which causes hypocalcemia and low vitamin D levels that trigger PTH secretion. The signs and symptoms are related to hypercalcemia and include:

- Muscle pain, atrophy, and weakness
- Gastrointestinal pain, nausea, vomiting, and anorexia
- Cardiac arrhythmias, renal calculi, bone tenderness, and fractures

After the physical exam, the provider may order blood tests (e.g., calcium, phosphorus) and imaging tests (e.g., x-ray studies, bone density test, radioimmunoassay studies). Treatment depends on the cause. Minimally invasive surgery may be done to remove a tumor or gland(s). When hyperplasia occurs, all but half of a gland can be removed. For secondary hyperparathyroidism, the underlying cause is treated. Medications may be prescribed to help increase calcium excretion by the kidneys.

> **CRITICAL THINKING APPLICATION**   23.5
>
> Cecylia is rooming Mr. Jones, who came with his wife, Sally. Over the past few months, he has been depressed, forgetful, and weak. At times he has experienced abdominal pain and joint pain. His primary care provider diagnosed him with hyperparathyroidism, and today he came in to see the specialist. Mr. Jones had never heard about the parathyroid gland, and he asks Cecylia about it. How would you explain the parathyroid gland to a patient?

Hypoparathyroidism

Hypoparathyroidism occurs when there is hyposecretion of parathyroid hormone. This reduction of PTH causes hypocalcemia to occur.

Hypoparathyroidism results from injury or damage to the parathyroid glands. Damage and destruction of the glands can result from cancer, radiation, and surgery (e.g., thyroidectomy). The signs and symptoms relate to the hypocalcemia. The patient may experience:

- Numbness and tingling, spasms, and twitching in the hands and feet
- Confusion and irritability
- *Tetany* (continuous muscle spasms), laryngospasm, arrhythmias, respiratory paralysis, and death

The provider will perform a physical exam and order blood tests (e.g., calcium, phosphate), an electrocardiogram, and imaging tests (e.g., radioimmunoassay studies). Lifelong treatment includes calcium and vitamin D supplements and a high-calcium diet.

Adrenal Gland Diseases

Adrenal gland diseases are described in Table 23.4. Addison disease and Cushing disease are described in more detail in the following sections.

Addison Disease

Addison disease is a malfunction of the adrenal cortex, leading to adrenal insufficiency (hyposecretion) of cortisol. Addison disease affects adults ages 30 to 50, though it can occur at any age. Addison disease can be acute or chronic. Acute Addison disease may be called *Addisonian crisis*, a condition marked by life-threatening symptoms. A crisis can be brought on by stressful situations, infections, minor illness, or surgery.

The causes of Addison disease include an autoimmune reaction, tuberculosis, and damage to or disease of the adrenal glands or pituitary gland. Acute Addison disease may have the following signs and symptoms:

- Pain in the lower back, abdomen, or legs
- Severe vomiting and diarrhea, dehydration, and low blood pressure
- Loss of consciousness
- High blood potassium (*hyperkalemia*) and low blood sodium (*hyponatremia*)

Signs and symptoms of chronic Addison disease may occur over weeks to months and include:

- Irritability, extreme fatigue, weight loss, lack of appetite, and a craving for salt
- Darkening of the skin and buccal membranes (*hyperpigmentation*) (Fig. 23.8)
- Hypotension, fainting, nausea, diarrhea, and vomiting
- Low blood sugar (*hypoglycemia*)
- Muscle pain, depression, and loss of body hair

After a physical exam, the provider may order blood tests (e.g., cortisol, sodium, potassium, and ACTH), imaging tests, and an ACTH stimulation test. The *ACTH stimulation test* measures the blood cortisol level before and after an injection of synthetic ACTH. If the adrenal gland is damaged, cortisol levels after ACTH stimulation will still be low or absent. Addisonian crisis treatment requires immediate administration of an intravenous saline and dextrose solution with corticosteroids. Other treatments involve corticosteroids to replace cortisol and aldosterone and dietary changes (e.g., a diet high in carbohydrates and protein; adequate sodium and fluids).

Cushing Disease

Cushing disease is a malfunction of the cortex of the adrenal gland, causing increased levels of cortisol. Cushing disease can be caused by a benign pituitary tumor, an adrenal adenoma (benign adrenal cortex tumor), a tumor that secretes ACTH, and taking long-term corticosteroids for another medical condition (e.g., organ transplantation, severe asthma, or rheumatoid arthritis). Signs and symptoms of Cushing disease include:

- High blood pressure; weight gain, especially in the abdomen, upper back, face (moon face), and between the shoulder blades (buffalo hump) (Fig. 23.9).
- Pink or purple stretch marks on the abdomen, thighs, breasts, and arms; fragile, thin skin that bruises easily
- Infections, slow-healing wounds, and acne
- Severe fatigue, muscle weakness, and headaches
- Depression, anxiety, irritability, loss of emotional control, and difficulty thinking clearly
- In children: slowed or impaired growth
- In women: thicker or more noticeable facial and body hair (*hirsutism* or *hypertrichosis*) (Fig. 23.10)
- In men: decreased **libido** and infertility

After obtaining a medical history and performing a physical exam, the provider may order blood, saliva, and urine tests to measure

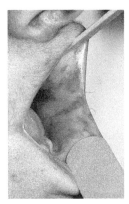

FIGURE 23.8 Hyperpigmentation caused by Addison disease. (From Thibodeau GA, Patton KT: *The human body in health and disease,* ed 5. St. Louis, 2010, Mosby.)

TABLE 23.4 Adrenal Gland Diseases

GLAND	HORMONE	CONDITION	DEFINITION
Adrenal cortex	Cortisol, hypersecretion	*Cushing disease*	Malfunction of the cortex, leading to many symptoms, including weight gain, decreased healing of wounds, depression, and impaired growth.
	Cortisol, hyposecretion	*Addison disease*	Malfunction of the cortex, leading to many symptoms, including low back pain, low blood pressure, and electrolyte imbalance.
Adrenal medulla	Epinephrine and norepinephrine, hypersecretion	*Pheochromocytoma*	Usually benign tumor that causes headache, palpitations, sweating, hyperglycemia, flushing, nausea, vomiting, and syncope. Condition can lead to hypertension (high blood pressure), arrhythmias, and heart failure.

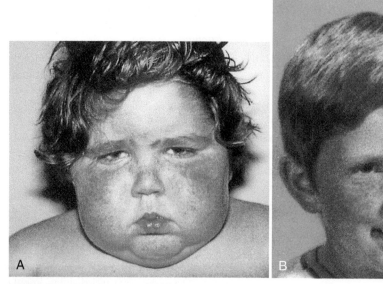

FIGURE 23.9 Cushing disease. **(A)** First diagnosed. **(B)** After 4 months of treatment. (From Shiland B: *Mastering healthcare terminology*, ed 5, St Louis, 2016, Elsevier.)

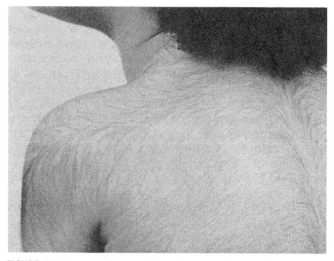

FIGURE 23.10 Hirsutism. (From *Mosby's medical, nursing, and allied health dictionary*, ed 8, St Louis, 2009, Mosby.)

TABLE 23.5	Pancreatic Diseases
CONDITION	**DESCRIPTION**
Type 1 diabetes mellitus	Condition resulting from a total lack of insulin production. Requires insulin injections.
Latent autoimmune diabetes in adults (LADA)	Slowly developing condition that causes the pancreas to stop producing insulin. Sometimes this condition is called type 1.5 diabetes. Requires insulin injections as the condition advances.
Type 2 diabetes mellitus	Condition resulting from deficient insulin production. Insulin is produced, but the body does not respond to it.
Prediabetes	Condition in which the blood glucose level is higher than normal, but not high enough for a diagnosis of type 2 diabetes.
Gestational diabetes	Insulin resistance acquired during pregnancy.
Hyperinsulinism	Hypersecretion of insulin; seen in some newborns of diabetic mothers. Causes severe hypoglycemia.
Islet cell carcinoma	Also called *pancreatic cancer*; fourth leading cause of cancer death in the US. Treated with a Whipple procedure (pancreatoduodenectomy).

cortisol levels; an ACTH stimulation test; and imaging tests. Treatment is focused on the cause of the disorder and may include medications to control cortisol levels, radiation therapy to shrink the tumor, or surgery to remove the tumor.

Pancreatic Diseases

Pancreatic diseases are described in Table 23.5. *Diabetes mellitus* (DM) is the most common pancreatic disease. DM is a group of metabolic disorders characterized by an inadequate production of insulin, a resistance to insulin, or a combination of both. The following sections discuss type 1, type 2, and gestational diabetes.

Type 1 and Type 2 Diabetes Mellitus

DM is a chronic condition in which the body cannot regulate the blood glucose levels. Table 23.6 describes type 1 and type 2 DM.

The exact cause of DM is unknown (see Table 23.6). Hyperglycemia signs and symptoms include polydipsia, polyuria, polyphagia, weight loss, fatigue, blurred vision, frequent infections, and slow-healing wounds.

The following diagnostic results suggest diabetes:

• Glycated hemoglobin (A_{1C}) test, 6.5% or greater on two separate samples

TABLE 23.6   Type 1 and Type 2 Diabetes Mellitus

	TYPE 1 DIABETES MELLITUS	TYPE 2 DIABETES MELLITUS
Onset	Occurs at any age, though it is often diagnosed between childhood and the young adult years.	More common in older adults, but with the rise in obesity, children and younger adults are also diagnosed with it.
Insulin Use	The pancreas produces very little or no insulin.	Insulin resistance occurs, or the pancreas does not make enough insulin to meet the body's needs, leading to hyperglycemia.
Etiology	Exact cause is unknown; may include environmental factors, genetics, and viruses. The immune system destroys the beta islet cells of the pancreas.	Exact cause is unknown; some factors could be genetics and environmental factors (e.g., obesity and lack of exercise).
Risk Factors	Family history of type 1 DM, genetics, age (peaks between ages 4 to 7 and then again between ages 10 to 14). Possible viral or environmental exposure.	Obesity, extra fat carried in the abdominal area, inactivity, family history of type 2 DM, race (greater risk if Native American, Asian American, Hispanic, or black), greater risk if over 45 years of age, or with a history of prediabetes, gestational diabetes, or polycystic ovarian syndrome.
Signs and Symptoms	Onset occurs rapidly; signs and symptoms relate to *hyperglycemia* (elevated blood sugar or glucose), especially with children. Adults may present with DKA.	Onset is usually gradual; no signs or symptoms may be experienced. If present, they relate to hyperglycemia.
Treatment	Insulin injections, regular exercise, frequent blood glucose monitoring, and dietary changes, including carbohydrate, fat, and protein counting.	Healthy eating, regular exercise, lose weight if obese, medications (e.g., antihyperglycemics, insulin), and glucose monitoring. Bariatric surgery if body mass index (BMI) is 35 or greater.

- Fasting blood sugar test, 126 mg/dL or greater on two separate samples
- Oral glucose tolerance test, greater than 200 mg/dL for the 2-hour level
- Random blood sugar test, no matter when the person ate last, with a value of 200 mg/dL or greater and diabetes symptoms

CRITICAL THINKING APPLICATION   23.6

Summarize the difference between type 1 and type 2 diabetes mellitus.

Diabetic Ketoacidosis. Hyperglycemia occurs when the blood glucose level is elevated or above the normal limit. With a fasting blood glucose test, the normal level is 70 to 99 mg/dL. Diabetic ketoacidosis (DKA) is a life-threatening hyperglycemic condition that is more commonly seen with type 1 diabetes. DKA occurs when there is not enough insulin in the body, which helps the blood glucose move to the cells. Because the cells need energy, the body starts rapidly breaking down fats, which leads to a buildup of ketones in the blood and urine, causing ketoacidosis.

Sometimes children not yet diagnosed with DM present with DKA, but more times undiagnosed adults will present with DKA. Eating too many carbohydrates without enough insulin, an infection or injury, missing insulin injections, and surgery are reasons for hyperglycemia to occur. Signs and symptoms of DKA include:

- Decreased alertness and headache
- Nausea, vomiting, abdominal pain, and dry mouth
- Muscle aches or stiffness, dry skin, and flushed face
- Frequent urination or thirst lasting for 1 or more days
- Fruity-smelling breath

To diagnose DKA, blood glucose and ketone levels are tested. A urine ketone test and a basic metabolic panel (which includes electrolytes [e.g., sodium and potassium levels]) may be done. The goals of treatment are to correct the hyperglycemic level, replace lost fluids, and correct any electrolyte imbalances. Treatment usually consists of insulin, intravenous (IV) fluids, and frequent glucose and electrolyte monitoring. Sometimes, DKA treatment can be done in an ambulatory care facility, and other times patients will be transported to the local emergency department for care.

It is important for the medical assistant to remember that blood glucose levels increase with infection, injury, and surgery, regardless of the number of carbohydrates eaten. Usually during an illness, people with type 1 DM have a special diabetic management plan to follow, which may include extra insulin and increased blood glucose monitoring.

Hypoglycemia. *Hypoglycemia* means low blood glucose (below 70 mg/dL). Hypoglycemia is commonly seen with DM but can be seen with other conditions too.

Hypoglycemia in DM usually occurs related to a medication side effect. A person takes too much insulin or oral medication for the amount of carbohydrates consumed, thus dropping the blood glucose level. Signs and symptoms of early hypoglycemia include:

- Irregular heart rhythm
- Pale skin, sweating, shakiness, and fatigue
- Irritability, hunger, and tingling sensation around the mouth
- Crying out while sleeping

As hypoglycemia worsens (the blood glucose level drops more), signs and symptoms include: visual disturbances, blurred vision, confusion, clumsy movements, seizures, abnormal behavior (e.g., incoherent speech, slurring words, inability to complete routine tasks), and loss of consciousness. The behavior may be similar to being intoxicated.

Immediate treatment is required and involves increasing the blood glucose level. If people are alert and can swallow, they should follow the 15/15 rule. For an unconscious adult patient, glucagon 1 mL should be given subcutaneously or IM to treat hypoglycemia. This dose should be repeated in 15 minutes if the patient is unconscious. Children younger than 6 years of age should get glucagon 0.5 mL. The blood glucose should be monitored, and once the person is alert and able to swallow, additional food should be given.

15/15 Rule

The 15/15 rule is used to treat hypoglycemia. After the person tests the glucose level and determines it is low, he or she should eat 15 grams of fast-acting carbohydrate. The person should wait 15 minutes for the glucose to get into the blood and then retest the blood glucose level. This cycle should be followed until the blood glucose level returns to the normal level. At that time, the person should eat a small, balanced snack that contains both a protein and a carbohydrate if the next meal is more than 2 hours away.

Examples of 15 grams of fast-acting carbohydrate include:

- 3 glucose tablets
- 4 ounces or ½ cup of fruit juice or regular soda (not diet soda)
- 6 to 7 hard candies
- 1 tablespoon of sugar

Complications With Diabetes Mellitus. According to the CDC (*www.cdc.gov*), during the last twenty years the number of people with DM has tripled. During that same time span, the top complications of DM, heart attack, and stroke have decreased because of the advances in DM education and care. The complications of diabetes mellitus develop over time. Two factors increase the risk of complications: the longer a person has DM and the more uncontrolled the blood glucose.

Diabetes affects the entire body. The following list provides a snapshot of possible complications of diabetes mellitus:

- *Cardiovascular disease*: People with DM have twice the risk of having a heart attack and stroke compared to people without diabetes mellitus. Diabetes increases the risk for coronary artery disease with *angina* (chest pain) and *atherosclerosis* (narrowing of the arteries).
- *Blindness and eye conditions*: **Diabetic retinopathy**, **glaucoma**, and **cataracts** can lead to vision loss. Early prevention and screening can prevent blindness with diabetic retinopathy. It is recommended that people with diabetes have their eyes checked every 4 to 6 months.
- *Neuropathy*: One of the most common complications of DM is nerve damage affecting the gastrointestinal (GI) system, reproductive system, cardiovascular system, and the extremities. Capillaries help nourish the nerves in the body, but hyperglycemia can damage the capillary walls, thus also causing nerve damage. Damage to the nerves in the GI system can cause nausea, vomiting, constipation, or diarrhea. Men can have erectile dysfunction. A person with neuropathy can experience burning, tingling, pain, and numbness in the fingers and toes, which gradually moves up the

extremities. If left untreated, a loss of feeling in the extremities may occur, which can affect functioning.

- *Poor healing of wounds*: Diabetes also makes a person more susceptible to bacterial and fungal skin infections. With the lack of feeling in the extremities, the person is more at risk for foot sores, blisters, and cuts. Left untreated, they can become infected, which increases the blood glucose levels. This affects the healing process, which may lead to amputations to stop the spread of infection.
- *Kidney disease*: Hyperglycemia also damages the tiny blood vessels (glomeruli) in the kidney, leading to chronic kidney disease (CKD). Untreated CKD leads to kidney failure, which requires dialysis or a kidney transplant.
- *Dementia*: Type 2 diabetes increases a person's risk of dementia-related disorders (e.g., Alzheimer's disease).
- *Depression*: Is common in patients with type 1 and type 2 DM.
- *Periodontal disease*: Gum infections and tooth loss can occur, which also increases hyperglycemia. It is recommended that patients with diabetes have dental cleanings and exams twice a year.

CRITICAL THINKING APPLICATION   23.7

Cecylia is rooming Susie Westwood, who has had type 2 DM for 4 years. Cecylia asks Susie when she last had her eyes checked and had a dental exam. Susie could not remember and asked Cecylia why that was important. How would you answer Susie?

Gestational Diabetes

Gestational diabetes develops during pregnancy. The hyperglycemia can affect the health of the pregnancy and the baby. Usually after the pregnancy, gestational diabetes resolves, though there is a greater risk for type 2 DM.

The exact cause is unknown, though hormones produced by the placenta impair the action of insulin, leading to hyperglycemia. Risk factors include being older than 25, having a family history of type 2 DM, a personal history of prediabetes, being overweight, and race (greater risk if Native American, Asian American, Hispanic, or black). There are no signs or symptoms of gestational diabetes.

A routine oral glucose tolerance test is usually done during weeks 24 to 28 of pregnancy.

Treatment for gestational diabetes includes eating a healthy diet, monitoring blood glucose levels, regular exercise, insulin injections, and closer follow-up for both the patient and baby.

Complications With Gestational Diabetes. Complications of gestational diabetes can include issues with the baby and the mother. For the baby, complications include:

- *Excessive growth in utero*: The extra glucose in the mother's blood passes into the baby's bloodstream, causing the baby's pancreas to make extra insulin. This causes extra weight to be added to the baby, thus increasing the likelihood the child may be delivered by a C-section.
- *Death*: If the mother does not get treated for gestational diabetes, the risk of death for the baby during pregnancy or after birth increases.
- *Hypoglycemia shortly after birth*: With the extra insulin production in utero, the baby may be at risk for hypoglycemia shortly after birth.
- *Risk of developing obesity and type 2 DM later in life*

For the mother, complications include **preeclampsia** and C-section delivery. She is at a greater risk for gestational diabetes with future pregnancies and having type 2 DM later in life.

THE MEDICAL ASSISTANT'S ROLE IN ENDOCRINOLOGY PROCEDURES

Assisting With the Examination

When the medical assistant is rooming a patient, it is important to accurately measure the vital signs and obtain the medical history. Encouraging the patient to voice any concerns or issues is vital. The medical assistant may be required to ask specific screening questions. Peripheral neuropathy screening questions for patients with DM may include:

- Do you have tingling, burning, numbness, cramps, or sharp pains in your hands and feet?
- Do you have a reduced ability to feel temperatures or pain in your hands and feet?
- Are your hands or feet more sensitive to touch?
- Do your hands or feet feel weaker?
- Do you have any problems with loss of balance or coordination?
- Do you have any sores, blisters, or any concerns with your feet?

When completing the medication section of the medical history, the medical assistant must verify the medication name, dose amount, and the number of doses taken each day. Sometimes the information in the health record is different from what the patient is really doing. Having accurate information in the health record helps the provider evaluate the complete picture of the patient's health.

During the physical exam, the provider often needs to examine the patient's feet for any abnormalities. The medical assistant should assist the patient as needed to remove shoes and socks. For infection control purposes, the patient's bare feet should never touch the floor. The medical assistant should place a piece of paper towel or some other barrier between the patient's feet and the floor.

Peripheral Neuropathy Screening

Many providers have medical assistants perform peripheral neuropathy screening by doing the monofilament foot exam. This is commonly done for diabetic patients but needs to be done for any patient experiencing peripheral neuropathy symptoms. Procedure 23.1 on p. 596 describes the monofilament foot exam procedure.

Assisting With Diagnostic Procedures

Tables 23.7 to 23.10 provide information about common diagnostic procedures and medical laboratory tests done for endocrine conditions. The medical assistant may be responsible for coaching patients on diagnostic procedures done in other departments. As with other diagnostic procedures, the medical assistant should coach the patient regarding:

- Patient preparation (e.g., dietary restrictions and medications to hold)
- Location and time of the test
- What to expect during the procedure
- Any follow-up required after the procedure

Assisting With Treatments

Patients with endocrine conditions are prescribed a variety of medications. The following are some of the more common classifications of medications:

- *Antihyperglycemics*: Used to manage diabetes mellitus
- *Hormone replacement*: Used to maintain adequate hormone levels
  - *Estrogen*: Used for menopause
  - *Estrogen and progestin*: Used for menopause
  - *Insulin*: Used to treat type 1 and type 2 diabetes mellitus
  - *Thyroid hormone*: Used for hypothyroidism
  - *Vasopressin*: Used for diabetes insipidus

Refer to Table 23.11, Medication Classifications, for information on drug classification, including indication for use, desired effect, side effects, adverse reactions, and generic and trade names. Medical assistants should be familiar with medications that are prescribed to patients.

TABLE 23.7 Diagnostic Procedures for Endocrine Conditions

PROCEDURE	DESCRIPTION	PATIENT PREPARATION
Thyroid ultrasound	Ultrasound of the thyroid gland. Used to check for nodules and other abnormalities in the gland.	Patient is asked to remove jewelry and clothing around the neck. The sonographer will apply warm gel to the neck and gently press a transducer along the neck.
Thyroid scan	Uses a radioactive iodine tracer to examine the thyroid gland. The patient swallows a pill with the radioactive iodine. The scan is done 4 to 6 hours later as the iodine collects in the thyroid. Often done with the radioactive iodine uptake test.	Screen the patient for allergies (e.g., iodine, shellfish), diarrhea, and history of CT scans using iodine in the past 2 weeks. The patient must remove jewelry, dentures, and other metal products. During the scan, the patient must remain still.
Radioactive iodine uptake (RAIU) scan	Uses a radioactive iodine tracer to measure the uptake of iodine in the thyroid. As with the thyroid scan, the patient swallows the iodine pill. A scan is done 4 to 6 hours after the pill is taken and then again 24 hours later. Often done with the thyroid scan.	Screen the patient for allergies (e.g., iodine, shellfish), diarrhea, and a history of CT scans using iodine in the past 2 weeks. The patient must remove jewelry, dentures, and other metal products. During the scan, the patient must remain still.

TABLE 23.8   Medical Laboratory Tests for Endocrine Conditions

TEST	DESCRIPTION
A_{1C}	Also called HbA_{1C} and Hemoglobin A_{1C} test. Measures the average blood glucose level over the past 3 months (see Table 23.9). Some CLIA-waived tests available.
Blood calcium test	Measures the calcium level in the blood. *Total calcium test* measures the calcium attached to specific proteins in the blood. *Ionized calcium test* measures the calcium unattached to proteins in the blood.
Fasting blood glucose (FBG) test	Measures the glucose level in the blood after fasting (see Table 23.10). Some CLIA-waived tests available.
Urine glucose test	Measures the amount of glucose in the urine sample. Some CLIA-waived tests available.
Hormone tests	Measures the amount of hormone in the blood. For example, TSH test, FSH test, growth hormone test, ADH hormone test, and so on.
Urine ketone test	Measures the amount of ketones in the urine sample. Some CLIA-waived tests available.
Oral glucose tolerance test (OGTT)	Blood test to measure the body's response to a concentrated glucose solution. Patient fasts for 8 to 12 hours and then drinks 75 or 100 grams of glucose. Blood may be drawn and tested prior to the drink and then every 30 to 60 minutes for up to 2 to 3 hours after taking the glucose (see Table 23.10).
Random blood glucose test	Measures the glucose level in the blood without fasting. A *glucometer* (a handheld instrument) may be used at home or in the ambulatory care environment. Some CLIA-waived tests available.
Thyroid antibody test	Measures the thyroid antibodies in the blood. Used to diagnose autoimmune thyroid disorders.
Thyroid function tests (TFTs)	Measures the levels of TSH, T_3, and T_4 in the blood. Used to evaluate the thyroid function. Some CLIA-waived tests available.

TABLE 23.9   Relationship Between A_{1c} and Average Blood Glucose Levels

A_{1C} (%)	AVERAGE BLOOD GLUCOSE (mg/dL)	LEVELS
4	65	*Normal:* <5.7%
5	97	*Prediabetes:* 5.7%–6.4%
6	126	*Type 2 diabetes:* ≥6.5%
7	154	
8	183	
9	212	
10	240	
11	269	
12	298	
13	326	

From the American Diabetes Association. https://professional.diabetes.org/sites/professional.diabetes.org/files/media/average_glucose_flyer.pdf Accessed on May 9, 2019.

In the ambulatory care facility, when a patient is prescribed insulin for the first time, the medical assistant may need to do some coaching, if the patient is not seeing a diabetic educator immediately. If it is within the scope of practice for the medical assistant, the following topics should be addressed with the patient:

- How to draw up and give an insulin injection (discussed in Chapter 15)
- Signs and symptoms of hyperglycemia and hypoglycemia
- Immediate treatments for hyperglycemia and hypoglycemia
- How to use a glucometer to monitor blood glucose levels (discussed in Chapter 33)
- When to contact the provider or seek additional care
- Storage of supplies and how to discard used needles

Insulin

Insulin is used to treat type 1 and in some cases type 2 diabetes mellitus. Most commonly insulin is injected subcutaneously several times a day. Table 23.12 describes the different types of insulins. The *onset* is the length of time before the insulin begins to work. The *peak* is the period when the insulin is most effective. The *duration* is the length of time the insulin exerts an effect on the body.

Many people take two types of insulin a day. Premixed insulins available in the United States include:

- *Premixed – Intermediate- and rapid-acting:* 70% insulin lispro protamine, 25% insulin lispro (Humalog Mix 75/25, Humalog Mix 50/50); 70% NPH human insulin, 30% human insulin (Humalog 70/30); and 70% insulin aspart protamine, 30% insulin aspart (NovoLog Mix 70/30)

TABLE 23.10   Test Results for Diabetes

TEST	NORMAL LEVEL	INDICATES PREDIABETES	INDICATES DIABETES
A$_{1C}$	<5.7%	5.7%–6.4%	>6.5%
Oral glucose tolerance test (OGTT) – not pregnant	Fasting: 60–100 mg/dL 1 hr: <200 mg/dL 2 hr: <140 mg/dL	2 hr: 140–200 mg/dL	>200 mg/dL
Random blood glucose test	<125 mg/dL	—	>200 mg/dL
Fasting blood glucose (FBG) test	70–99 mg/dL	100–125 mg/dL	>126 mg/dL

TABLE 23.11   Medication Classifications

CLASSIFICATION	INFORMATION	GENERIC NAME (TRADE NAME)
antihyperglycemics (non-insulin)	**Indications for use:** Manage diabetes mellitus. **Desired effect:** Reduce blood glucose level. **Side effects and adverse reactions:** GI irritation, fatigue, hypoglycemia, vertigo; possible hypersensitivity reaction	*Oral (Type 2):* • **rosiglitazone** (Avandia) • **sitagliptin (**Januvia) • **glipizide** (Glucotrol) • **glyburide** (DiaBeta, Glynase) • **metformin** (Glucophage, Fortamet, Glumetza) *Injectable (Type 2):* • **exenatide** (Byetta) • **dulaglutide** (Trulicity) *Injectable (used with other Type 1 or 2 medications):* • **pramlintide** (SymlinPen 60)
Hormone Replacement - *Estrogen*	**Indications for use:** Maintain adequate hormone levels. **Desired effects:** Replace hormones or compensate for hormone deficiency. **Side effects and adverse reactions:** Hot flashes, decreased sex drive, nausea, vomiting.	• **estrogen** (Estrace, Ortho-est, Premarin)
Hormone Replacement - *Estrogen and progestin*	**Indications for use:** Maintain adequate hormone levels. **Desired effects:** Replace hormones or compensate for hormone deficiency. **Side effects and adverse reactions:** Double vision, depression, unusual bleeding, acne, swelling of the hands and feet, nervousness, brown or black skin patches	• **estrogen and progestin** (Premphase, Prempro)
Hormone Replacement - *Insulin*	**Indications for use:** Type 1 and Type 2 diabetes mellitus **Desired effects:** Lower the blood glucose level. **Side effects and adverse reactions:** Shortness of breath, blurred vision, tachycardia, sweating, weakness, muscle cramps, arrhythmias, and other hypoglycemic symptoms	*Rapid-acting Insulin:* • **insulin aspart** (NovoLog, Novolog Mix 70/30, Fiasp) • **insulin glulisine** (Apidra) • **insulin lispro** (Humalog, Admelog) *Short-acting Insulin:* • **regular insulin** (Humulin R, Novolin R) *Intermediate-acting Insulin:* • **NPH human insulin** (Humulin N, Novolin N) *Long-acting Insulins:* • **insulin degludec** (Tresiba) • **insulin detemir** (Levemir) • **insulin glargine** (Basaglar, Lantus) *Ultra Long-acting Insulin:* • **insulin glargine U-300** (Toujeo)

Continued

TABLE 23.11	Medication Classifications—*continued*	
CLASSIFICATION	**INFORMATION**	**GENERIC NAME (TRADE NAME)**
Hormone Replacement - *Thyroid hormone*	**Indications for use:** Maintain adequate hormone levels. **Desired effects:** Replace hormones or compensate for hormone deficiency. **Side effects and adverse reactions:** Weight loss, tremor, headache, chest pain, arrhythmias	• **levothyroxine** (Synthroid, Levothroid, Levoxyl)
Hormone Replacement - *Vasopressin*	**Indications for use:** Maintain adequate hormone levels. **Desired effects:** Replace hormones or compensate for hormone deficiency. **Side effects and adverse reactions:** Restlessness, seizures, hallucinations, slowed reflexes, tiredness	• **desmopressin** (DDAVP)

TABLE 23.12	Types of Insulin				
TYPE	**GENERIC NAME (BRAND NAME)**	**ONSET**	**PEAK**	**DURATION**	**FORM/ADMINISTRATION**
Rapid-acting	insulin glulisine (Apidra), insulin lispro (Humalog, Admelog), insulin aspart (NovoLog, Fiasp)	About 15 min	About 1 hr	2 – 4 hr	Clear liquid/Take 5–15 min before meal
Rapid-acting inhaled	(Afrezza)	About 15 min	About 1 hr	2.5 – 3 hr	White powder/Take at start of meal
Short-acting	regular human insulin (Humulin R, Novolin R)	About 30 min	2–3 hr	3–6 hr	Clear/Take 30–45 min before meal
Intermediate-acting	NPH human insulin (Humulin N, Novolin N)	2–4 hr	6–8 hr	12–18 hr	Cloudy/Take 30 min before meal
Long-acting	insulin glargine (Basaglar, Lantus), insulin detemir (Levemir), insulin degludec (Tresiba)	2–4 hr	Does not apply	Up to 24 hr +	Clear/Does not need to be taken with meal
Ultra long-acting	insulin glargine U-300 (Toujeo)	6 hr	Does not apply	Up to 36 hr	Clear/Does not need to be taken with meal

From FDA, https://www.fda.gov/consumers/free-publications-women/insulin and American Diabetes Association, http://www.diabetes.org/living-with-diabetes/treatment-and-care/medication/insulin/insulin-basics.html Accessed on May 9, 2019.

- *Premixed – Intermediate- and short-acting*: 70% NPH, 30% regular insulin (Novolin 70/30, Humulin 70/30)
- *Premixed – Long- and rapid-acting*: 70% insulin degludec, 30% insulin aspart (Ryzodeg 70/30)

Insulin can be given in the following ways:

- *Syringe and vial*: Insulin is drawn up in the syringe, and then the injection is given. Adaptive equipment is available to help patients see the calibration lines on the syringe.
- *Insulin pump*: This is a computerized device that administers insulin through a needle-tipped catheter attached to tubing and the medication container. The needle can be inserted in several locations, including the abdomen, outer thigh, back of the arm, hip, and buttock. The pump is programmed to deliver a *basal rate*, or the continuous infusion of a small dose of insulin over a 24-hour period. The person can also set the pump to deliver extra insulin

to cover the carbohydrate being consumed. This method more closely resembles the body's normal surge of insulin and is designed to maintain blood glucose levels consistently within normal limits.

- *Injector pen*: An injection device that is preloaded with insulin cartridges for easy use (Fig. 23.11). Insulin pens are disposable or refillable and easily portable and therefore can be used by patients with diabetes when they are away from home.
- *Inhaler*: A cartridge containing the insulin is loaded in the inhaler. The person breathes in the insulin.

CRITICAL THINKING APPLICATION   23.8

Explain why it is important for patients who take insulin to be aware of the onset, peak, and duration of the insulin.

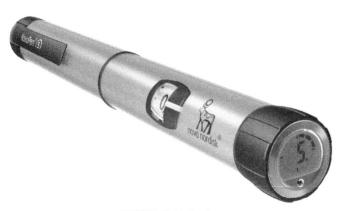

FIGURE 23.11 NovoPen.

Insulin Strengths. U-100 is the most common insulin strength in the United States. U-100 means that 100 units of insulin are dissolved or suspended in each milliliter (mL) of fluid. Additional insulin strengths are more concentrated.

- Insulin glargine U-300 (Toujeo) contains 300 units of insulin in each mL of fluid or three times the amount of insulin compared to U-100 insulin.
- Human R U-500 contains 500 units of insulin in each mL of fluid or five times the amount of insulin compared to U-100 insulin.

More concentrated forms of insulin require additional patient education and special equipment (e.g., syringes or pens) to prevent insulin overdoses.

Storage of Insulin. Most insulin manufacturers recommend that insulin should be stored in the refrigerator. Because injecting cold insulin is uncomfortable, usually the vial being used is stored at room temperature. An insulin vial stored at room temperature will last for about 1 month. It is important to keep insulin away from extreme heat or cold (e.g., freezer, direct sunlight, or in the glove compartment of a vehicle).

Afrezza, the inhaled insulin, should be stored in the refrigerator in the original closed container. Before using, the cartridge should warm at room temperature for 10 minutes. At room temperature, unopened medication packs are good for 10 days. Once the pack is opened, the cartridges are good for 3 days. The inhaler can be used for up to 15 days before it must be discarded.

CLOSING COMMENTS

Patient Coaching

The medical assistant can coach the patient on proper foot care. It is important for patients to examine and care for their feet daily. The following points should be reinforced with patients who have neuropathy:

- Check your shoes for damaged areas or stones before putting them on. Wear good-fitting shoes at all times to protect your feet.
- Check your feet when taking off your shoes. Look at all sides of the feet and between the toes. Check for redness, blisters, swelling, sores, and so forth.
- Keep your nails trimmed to a proper length.
- Wash your feet every day with lukewarm water and soap. Dry well with a soft towel. Use lotion, lanolin, or oil on dry skin,

but do not put it between the toes because this could cause an infection.
- Seek medical care immediately for foot sores.
- Avoid putting pressure for long periods of time on areas with nerve damage.
- Use an elbow instead of the toes or hands to check bathwater temperature.

Legal and Ethical Issues

Pathophysiology of the endocrine system can have far-reaching effects on the body's ability to function. Patient education interventions should be documented completely to establish legal proof of the information shared with the patient. Never just assume that the patient understands the disease process and treatment recommendations. The following suggestions can help ensure the patient's welfare and promote risk management.

- Advise patients that a MedicAlert bracelet with their diagnosis and medication information is an important safeguard.
- Patients must take medication as prescribed, following the directions for dosage, route of administration, and storage; they also must be alert for possible side effects.
- Patients newly diagnosed with diabetes should not drive until glycemic control has stabilized. These patients also should be warned about possible visual impairment from the disease.
- Remember that you are always representing your profession and employer and respond to each situation accordingly.
- Ask for assistance or further information if you feel unprepared to perform a procedure or to give accurate information.

Patient-Centered Care

Part of patient-centered care involves providing patients and families with information, education, and emotional support. When working with patients with endocrinology disorders, especially diabetes mellitus, the medical assistant has an important role in connecting patients with additional resources. These can include local support groups, medication discount programs, and websites, including:

- American Diabetes Association: *www.diabetes.org*
- Centers for Disease Control and Prevention: *www.cdc.gov*
- National Institutes of Health: Genetic and Rare Diseases Information Center: *rarediseases.info.nih.gov*
- US National Library of Medicine: MedlinePlus: *medlineplus. gov*

Professional Behaviors

An important part of becoming a professional medical assistant is a commitment to lifelong learning. This chapter focused on the details of diabetes mellitus because it is the most common endocrine system disease and also one of the most serious. Regardless of where you work as a medical assistant, you will end up caring for patients with diabetes and interacting with their families on some level. Diabetes researchers are constantly discovering more information about the disease: how it is diagnosed, the best treatment methods, and the pathophysiology of possible complications. You must commit to continual learning about diabetes so that you are best prepared to care for patients with this life-threatening disorder.

SUMMARY OF SCENARIO

Cecylia enjoyed working with the endocrinology team and patients. She was able to observe the diabetic nurse educator work with a newly diagnosed patient. The amount of information that newly diagnosed diabetic patients need to learn to manage their disease is incredible. All of the information was not given to the patient during the first visit. The nurse educator explained that over the coming weeks, the patient would get the information. During the first visit, the patient needed to learn how to administer insulin, test blood glucose levels, and learn about hypoglycemia and hyperglycemia. These topics were most critical at this stage.

Cecylia was also able to observe the diabetic nurse educator work with a patient who was learning about an insulin pump. The patient was preparing to switch from insulin injections to an insulin pump. The nurse explained to Cecylia that patients are better controlled on insulin pumps, but it is not a delivery method for everyone.

Later in the day, Cecylia observed the dietitian working with a patient with type 2 DM. The patient stated he enjoyed his beer, snack foods, and his sweets and really did not want to give them up. Cecylia was impressed by how the dietitian worked with the patient, so that eventually, the patient was willing to cut back on some of his "not so healthy" habits. Cecylia's experiences just reinforced her belief that she had made the right decision in volunteering to work with the endocrinology team.

SUMMARY OF LEARNING OBJECTIVES

1. **Do the following related to the anatomy of the endocrine system:**
   - *Describe the anatomical location of the major organs of the endocrine system.*

     The endocrine system is composed of ductless glands throughout the body. The hypothalamus, located in the middle of the brain, is the major connection between the nervous and endocrine systems and controls the endocrine system. When it detects rising levels of a target organ's hormones, it sends a signal to the pituitary gland to release or prevent pituitary hormone production.

     The pituitary gland is connected to the hypothalamus and is composed of two lobes that act as separate glands, the anterior lobe and the posterior lobe. The thyroid gland is a butterfly-shaped gland in the neck above the collarbone. The parathyroid glands are four pea-sized glands located on the thyroid gland. The adrenal glands are located on the top of each kidney. The outer part of the gland is the adrenal cortex; the inner part is called the *adrenal medulla*. The pancreas is located inferior and posterior to the stomach. The thymus gland is in the mediastinum behind the sternum (breastbone) and secretes thymosin and thymopoietin hormones. The male gonads are the testes, and the female gonads are the ovaries.
   - *List the hormones secreted from the endocrine glands.*
     - *Anterior lobe of the pituitary gland:* Adrenocorticotropic hormone, follicle-stimulating hormone, growth hormone, luteinizing hormone, prolactin, and thyroid-stimulating hormone.
     - *Posterior lobe of the pituitary gland:* Antidiuretic hormone and oxytocin
     - *Thyroid gland:* Triiodothyronine, thyroxine, and calcitonin
     - *Parathyroid glands:* Parathyroid hormone
     - *Adrenal cortex:* Mineralocorticoids, glucocorticoids, and gonadocorticoids
     - *Adrenal medulla:* Epinephrine and norepinephrine
     - *Pancreas:* Glucagon, insulin, somatostatin, and ghrelin
     - *Thymus gland:* Thymosin
     - *Gonads:* Testosterone, estrogen, and progesterone
     - *Pineal gland:* Melatonin

   - *Describe life span changes related to the endocrine system.*

     Changes in hormone levels vary with age. The hormones that decrease with age include estrogen, testosterone, growth hormone, and melatonin. Cortisol, insulin, and thyroid hormone usually remain unchanged or slightly decrease with age. Norepinephrine, epinephrine, parathyroid hormone, follicle-stimulating hormone, and luteinizing hormone may increase with age.

2. **Explain the physiology of the endocrine system.**

   The goal of hormone regulation is to maintain homeostasis. Nervous system stimulation, endocrine control, and feedback systems regulate hormone secretion. Each hormone released into the bloodstream has specific target cells for action. The target cells have receptors that attract only certain hormones. The cell membrane only lets selected hormones pass into the cell and affect cellular action.

   There are two categories of hormones, nonsteroid hormones and steroid hormones. Nonsteroid hormones attach to a target cell membrane. Another molecule takes the message from the nonsteroid hormone and carries it to the target cell nucleus or organelle, which then puts the message into action in the cell. Steroid hormones are attached to a target cell membrane, then pass directly into the target cell, and bind to receptor sites. This complex communicates its message with DNA in the nucleus, and the DNA tells the cell how to put the hormone's message into action.

   Prostaglandins are produced in tissues and diffuse only a short distance to affect cells in their local area. They help regulate processes such as respiration, blood pressure, digestive system secretions, and reproductive functions.

3. **Identify common disorders of the endocrine system and list common signs and symptoms of endocrine disorders.**

   Common disorders of the endocrine system include:
   - *Posterior lobe of the pituitary gland:* Diabetes insipidus
   - *Thyroid gland:* Hypothyroidism and hyperthyroidism
   - *Parathyroid glands:* Hypoparathyroidism and hyperparathyroidism
   - *Adrenal glands:* Addison disease and Cushing disease
   - *Pancreas:* Type 1 and type 2 diabetes mellitus and gestational diabetes

Some of the signs and symptoms of endocrine disorders include:

- Exophthalmia and goiter
- Glucosuria, hypocalcemia, hypoglycemia, ketoacidosis, and ketonuria
- Polydipsia and polyphagia

4. Differentiate between type 1 and type 2 diabetes mellitus.

Type 1 DM can occur at any age, though it is often diagnosed between childhood and the young adult years. The exact cause of type 1 DM is unknown. Usually the cause is autoimmune-related; other causes may include genetics, viruses, and environmental factors. The signs and symptoms occur rapidly. Children usually have hyperglycemia-related signs and symptoms. Treatment consists of insulin injections, regular exercise, frequent blood glucose monitoring, and dietary changes, including carbohydrate, fat, and protein counting.

Type 2 DM is more common in older adults, but with the rise in obesity, more children and younger adults are being diagnosed with it. The exact cause is unknown; some factors could be genetics and environmental factors (e.g., obesity and lack of exercise). The onset is usually gradual, with no signs or symptoms experienced. If signs and symptoms are present, they relate to hyperglycemia. Treatment consists of healthy eating, regular exercise, losing weight if obese, medications (e.g., antihyperglycemics, insulin), and glucose monitoring.

5. List signs and symptoms of hypoglycemia, hyperglycemia, and diabetic ketoacidosis and describe the immediate care required for hypoglycemia and diabetic ketoacidosis.

Signs and symptoms of early hypoglycemia include an irregular heart rhythm, pale skin, sweating, shakiness, fatigue, irritability, hunger, a tingling sensation around the mouth, and crying out while sleeping. Hyperglycemia signs and symptoms include polydipsia, polyuria, polyphagia, weight loss, fatigue, blurred vision, frequent infections, and slow-healing wounds. Signs and symptoms of DKA include decreased alertness, headache, dry mouth and skin, flushed face, nausea, vomiting, abdominal pain, muscle aches or stiffness, frequent urination or thirst lasting for 1 or more days, and fruity-smelling breath.

Hypoglycemia means low blood glucose. If the person is alert and can swallow, the 15/15 rule should be followed to treat hypoglycemia. After the person tests the glucose level and determines it is low, he or she should eat 15 grams of fast-acting carbohydrate. The person should wait 15 minutes for the glucose to get into the blood and then retest the blood glucose level. This cycle should be followed until the blood glucose level returns to the normal level. At that time, the person should eat a small, balanced snack that contains both a protein and a carbohydrate if the next meal is more than 1 hour away.

For an unconscious adult patient, glucagon 1 mL should be given subcutaneously or IM to treat hypoglycemia. This dose should be repeated in 15 minutes if the patient is unconscious. Children younger than 6 years of age get 0.5 mL of glucagon. The blood glucose should be monitored, and once the person is alert and able to swallow, additional food should be given.

The goals of treatment for DKA are to correct the hyperglycemic level, replace lost fluids, and correct any electrolyte imbalances. Treatment usually consists of insulin, intravenous fluids, and frequent glucose and electrolyte monitoring.

6. Explain complications of diabetes and discuss gestational diabetes.

Two factors increase the risk of complications: the longer a person has DM, and the more uncontrolled the blood glucose. Diabetes affects the entire body. The following provides a snapshot of possible complications of diabetes mellitus:

- Cardiovascular disease and kidney disease
- Blindness and eye conditions
- Neuropathy
- Poor healing of wounds
- Dementia and depression
- Periodontal disease

Gestational diabetes develops during pregnancy, and the hyperglycemia can affect the health of the mother and the baby. The exact cause is unknown. A routine oral glucose tolerance test is usually done during weeks 24 to 28 of pregnancy; treatment varies but involves eating a healthy diet, monitoring blood glucose levels, regular exercise, insulin injections, and closer follow-up for the patient and baby.

7. Discuss the medical assistant's role in endocrinology procedures, including assisting with the examination, diagnostic procedures, and treatments.

During an endocrinology examination, a medical assistant may be required to ask specific screening questions. When completing the medication section of the medical history, the medical assistant must verify the medication name, dose amount, and number of doses taken daily. During the physical exam, the medical assistant should assist the patient as needed to remove shoes and socks. Many providers have medical assistants perform peripheral neuropathy screening by doing a monofilament foot exam.

Insulin can be given in the following ways: syringe and vial, insulin pump, injector pen, and inhaler. Special care should be taken when storing insulin, because most insulin manufacturers recommend that insulin should be stored in the refrigerator.

Some diagnostic procedures for endocrine conditions include:

- *Thyroid ultrasound*: Ultrasound of the thyroid gland. Used to check for nodules and other abnormalities in the gland.
- *Thyroid scan* and the *radioactive iodine uptake test*: A radioactive iodine tracer is used to examine the thyroid gland. The patient swallows a pill with the radioactive iodine. A scan is done 4 to 6 hours after the pill is taken and then again 24 hours later. This scan often is done with the thyroid scan.

Some medical laboratory tests for endocrine conditions include:

- A1c, also called the HbA1c and Hemoglobin A1c test
- Fasting blood glucose
- Urine glucose test
- Urine ketone test
- Random blood glucose test
- Thyroid function tests

PROCEDURE 23.1   Perform a Monofilament Foot Exam

Tasks: Perform a monofilament foot exam to screen for peripheral neuropathy. Give health maintenance coaching by providing foot care instructions. Document test results in the patient's health record.

EQUIPMENT and SUPPLIES

- 10 g monofilament tool
- Gloves
- Paper towel
- Provider's order or standing order
- Patient's health record

PROCEDURAL STEPS

1. Wash hands or use hand sanitizer.
   <u>PURPOSE</u>: Hand sanitization is an important step for infection control.

2. Read the provider's order. Assemble the equipment.
   <u>PURPOSE</u>: It is important to know the provider's order before starting the procedure.

3. Greet the patient. Identify yourself. Verify the patient's identity with full name and date of birth. Explain the procedure to be performed in a manner that the patient understands. Answer any questions the patient may have about the procedure.
   <u>PURPOSE</u>: It is important to identify the patient in two different ways to ensure that you have the correct patient. Explaining the procedure can make the patient feel more comfortable and helps to reduce anxiety.

4. Ask the patient to remove socks and shoes and rest the feet on the paper towel. The paper towel should be placed under the person's feet either on the floor or on the exam table step.
   <u>PURPOSE</u>: This prepares the patient for the test.

5. Using your hand, demonstrate that the monofilament is flexible and not sharp. Also demonstrate the monofilament on the patient's hand. Put gloves on.
   <u>PURPOSE</u>: This alleviates the patient's anxiety. Demonstrating on the patient's hand allows the patient to know how it feels.

6. Instruct the patient to close his or her eyes. Tell the patient to say "yes" when he or she feels the monofilament on the foot.
   <u>PURPOSE</u>: The patient's eyes must be closed for this test to be accurate.

7. Start with the great toe and place the monofilament perpendicular to the skin. Press the monofilament until it bends, hold for 1 second, and release (see the following figure). Pause to give the patient an opportunity to confirm it was felt. A confirmation is a positive or normal response. The test result is abnormal if the patient cannot feel in one area.
   <u>PURPOSE</u>: It is important to hold the monofilament for 1 second for accurate results.

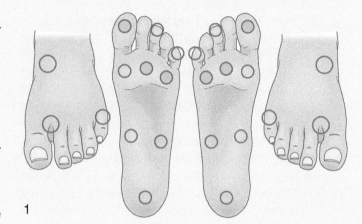

1

8. Do not cue the patient if no confirmation is given. Just move to the next location. Randomly test 9 to 12 locations on the anterior and posterior side of each foot or as the provider indicates (see Fig. 1). If a patient does not feel the site, check it three times randomly. Make sure to space out testing times (e.g., the time between each check).
   <u>PURPOSE</u>: If the test is done in a rhythmic way, the patient may confirm the feeling without really feeling the test.

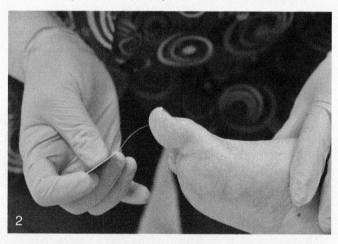

2

9. Discard supplies in the waste container. Remove gloves and wash hands.
   <u>PURPOSE</u>: Washing hands is important for infection control.

PROCEDURE 23.1 | **Perform a Monofilament Foot Exam**—*continued*

10. Coach the patient on proper foot care to prevent sores. Include when to check the feet, what to look for, and how to care for the feet daily. Suspicious areas need to be watched carefully and reported to the provider if they do not return to normal.
    PURPOSE: Careful monitoring can help prevent serious foot sores.

11. Document the test results in the patient's health record. Include the provider's name, the order, and the results of the test. For the test, the first number indicates the total number of sites felt and the last number indicates the total times done. Indicate all sites where the patient did not feel the test. If the provider indicates specific areas to test, documentation should reflect these areas. Include any teaching done.
    PURPOSE: It is important to document the patient education in the health record to show it was done.

07/19/20XX 1625 Per Dr. Kahn's order, performed a monofilament exam on both feet. Right foot 9/12 and left foot 12/12. Right posterior great toe 0/3. Pt coached on foot care. Stressed daily foot care and inspections. Pt listed the foot care he needs to do daily. He indicated what and where on his feet he needs to examine daily. All his questions were answered. The "Feet Guide for Neuropathy" brochure was given to the patient. _____

_____ Cecylia Cukier, CMA (AAMA)

24

CARDIOLOGY

SCENARIO

Rebecca White is a certified medical assistant (CMA) at Walden-Martin Family Medical (WMFM) Clinic. She was hired 8 months ago. She works with several family practice providers at the clinic. Many of the patients she works with have cardiovascular diseases. High blood pressure, or hypertension, seems to be the most common cardiovascular disease seen in her patients.

During her first few months at the clinic, Rebecca spent a lot of time learning about cardiovascular diseases, diagnostic procedures, and treatments. She found out that learning about the cardiovascular system takes time, but she is proud of how much she has learned over the months.

Rebecca's supervisor approached her and asked her to mentor a medical assistant student, Lizzy, for her practicum experience. Rebecca is excited about the opportunity, but she is a bit nervous to teach someone else about her job.

While studying this chapter, think about the following questions:
- What medical terminology relates to the cardiovascular system?
- What is the location of each of the cardiovascular system structures?
- What is the process of the conduction system?
- What factors impact blood pressure?
- What are some of the more common cardiovascular diseases?
- What diagnostic procedures are used for cardiovascular disorders?

LEARNING OBJECTIVES

1. Describe the anatomy of the cardiovascular system.
2. Explain the pulmonary and systemic circulations.
3. Describe coronary circulation, hepatic portal circulation, and fetal circulation.
4. Explain the components in blood, and discuss blood types.
5. Describe life span changes related to the cardiovascular system.
6. Describe the conduction system of the heart, including the three states of a cardiac cell.
7. Describe factors that influence blood pressure.
8. List common signs and symptoms of cardiovascular disorders.
9. Identify disorders of the cardiovascular system, list risk factors for heart disease, and describe the types of shock.
10. Discuss the medical assistant's role in assisting with the cardiology examination.
11. Describe diagnostic procedures, including angiography, cardiac catheterization, Doppler ultrasound, and echocardiography.
12. Describe cardiovascular treatments, including a pacemaker and an implantable cardioverter-defibrillator.

VOCABULARY

arteriosclerosis A disease in which the arterial walls become thickened and lose their elasticity.

atheroma (ath uh ROH mah) A waxy lesion, made up of cholesterol, fat, calcium, cells, and other substances, that builds up on the inner wall of an artery.

bilirubin (bil i ROO bin) A reddish pigment that results from the breakdown of red blood cells in the liver.

cardiac defibrillator An external or implantable device that provides an electric shock to the heart to restore a normal sinus rhythm.

constrict To contract or shrink.

deoxygenated Oxygen deficient; oxygen was removed.

ectopic pregnancy A pregnancy in which the fertilized egg implants outside the uterus (e.g., fallopian tubes).

electrocardiography The recording of electrical impulses of the heart as wave deflections on an instrument called an *electrocardiograph*. The record, or recording, is called an *electrocardiogram*.

embolus (EM boh lus) An air bubble, blood clot, or foreign body that travels through the bloodstream and blocks a blood vessel.

filamentous (fil ah MEN tuhs) Composed of or containing filaments or strands of a substance.

glucose A simple sugar that is absorbed by the intestines and found in the blood. Used by cells for energy, and the extra is stored in the liver as glycogen.

incompetent valves Valves do not close completely and allow blood to leak backward into the prior chamber; also called "leaky valves."

infarction (in FARK shuhn) Tissue death.

insufficiency Also called regurgitation or incompetence; the valve does not close completely, and blood leaks backward across the valve into the prior chamber.

orthostatic (postural) hypotension A temporary fall in blood pressure that occurs when a person rapidly changes from a recumbent position to a standing position.

pitting edema Excessive fluid in the intercellular spaces in the tissue; when external pressure (e.g., socks, finger pressure) is relieved, a depression is seen in the tissue.

polycythemia (pol ee sie THEE mee ah) A condition caused by an abnormally large number of red blood cells (RBCs) in the blood.

purpura Hemorrhage into the tissue.

solvent A liquid that is able to dissolve other substances.

stem cells Undifferentiated cells that can become specialized cells in the body.

stenosis (sten OH sis) Occurs when the heart valve flaps are stiff or fused together, thus narrowing the valve.

thrombus (THRAHM bus) A blood clot that blocks the flow of blood.

valvulitis Inflammatory condition of a valve that results in valve stenosis and obstructed blood flow; caused most commonly by rheumatic fever, bacterial endocarditis, or syphilis.

Cardiology is the healthcare specialty that deals with cardiovascular disorders. A *cardiologist* is a specialist involved in the diagnosis, treatment, and prevention of disorders of the cardiovascular system.

Cardiology-related tests are common in the ambulatory care setting. Patients with cardiovascular diseases are seen in primary care, urgent care, and specialty departments. Patients seen for other conditions may also have cardiovascular disease. Medical assistants may need to coach patients on cardiovascular procedures. Having a strong understanding of the cardiovascular system and common diseases is important for medical assistants.

ANATOMY OF THE CARDIOVASCULAR SYSTEM

The *cardiovascular system* is also called the *circulatory system*. The cardiovascular system brings oxygen (O_2), nutrients, water, and other substances (e.g., salts and hormones) to the body's cells. It also carries waste products (e.g., metabolic waste and carbon dioxide [CO_2]) away from the cells to be excreted.

The cardiovascular system is a closed system that includes the following:

- Blood vessels, consisting of arteries, arterioles, capillaries, venules, and veins that act as pipes to carry the blood around the body
- A heart, which pumps the blood
- Blood, which contains the nutrients for the cells and the waste products to be excreted

Cellular injury and death of the cells will occur if the system malfunctions and critical substances are withheld from the cells.

Blood Vessels

Blood vessels create a "pipeline" for blood to move out to the body and back to the heart. Blood vessels differ in their role, structure, and size.

- *Arteries*: Strong, stretchy, thick-walled vessels that carry blood from the heart. They are made to withstand the pressure of the blood being pumped out from the heart. Arteries are involved with maintaining blood pressure (Fig. 24.1).
- *Arterioles*: Smaller arteries that move blood to the capillaries and are also involved with maintaining blood pressure.
- *Capillaries*: Thin-walled vessels that allow for exchange of oxygen, nutrients, waste products, and other substances between the blood and cells. The diameter of the capillaries is so tiny that only one blood cell can pass through at a time.

- *Venules*: Vessels that collect blood from capillaries and begin the return journey to the heart.
- *Veins*: Vessels that collect blood from the venules and return blood to the heart. Medium to large veins have valves, which help keep blood moving in one direction. The skeletal muscle contractions help move the blood toward the heart. Vessel walls are thinner and less rigid than arteries. Veins hold about 70% of the blood supply at any one time.

The Heart

The heart, the size of a fist, is a complex muscular organ that pumps blood around the body. It is located in the mediastinum of the thoracic cavity, slightly left of the midline. The *apex* (pointed tip) of the heart rests just above the diaphragm. The area of the chest wall anterior to the heart and lower thorax is referred to as the *precordium*.

Heart Chambers

The heart has two sets of chambers. The two upper chambers are called *atria* and are smaller chambers with thinner walls. The right atrium receives blood from the body, and the left atrium receives blood from the lungs. The two larger lower chambers with thick muscular walls are called the right and left *ventricles* (Fig. 24.2). They pump blood to the body and the lungs.

The *septum* is the thick muscular wall that divides the heart into a right and left section. The *interatrial septum* separates the left and right atria, and the *interventricular septum* divides the right and left ventricles.

The heart wall is composed of three layers:

- *Endocardium*: The inner thin endothelial layer that lines the chambers and valves.
- *Myocardium*: The middle and thickest layer of the heart, composed of cardiac muscles.
- *Epicardium* or *visceral pericardium*: The outer layer that covers the heart. A space separates the epicardium from the *parietal pericardium*, which loosely covers the heart like a sac. The two layers of pericardium are serous membranes. As the heart beats, the two layers rub against each other, and the moisture between the layers decreases the amount of friction.

Heart Valves

The heart has valves between the chambers and the arteries. The valves allow the blood to flow in one direction. Valves are

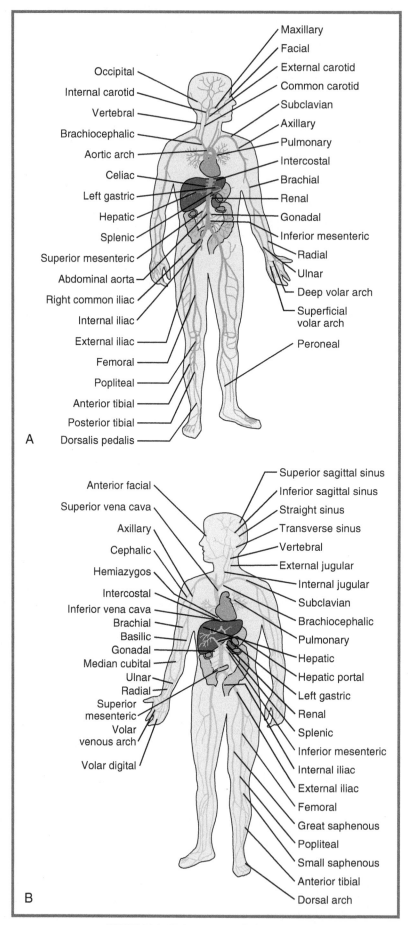

FIGURE 24.1 (A) Systemic arteries. **(B)** Systemic veins.

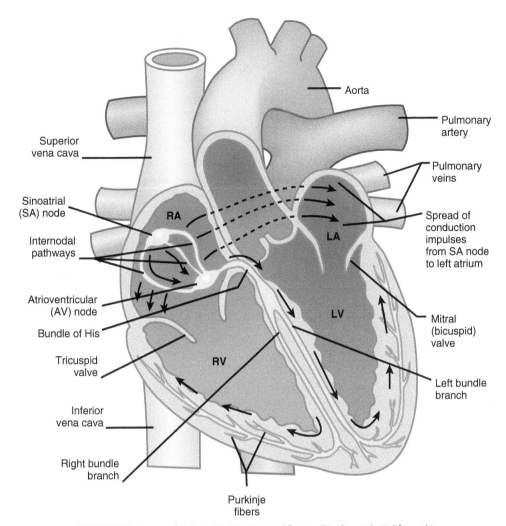

FIGURE 24.2 Structures of the heart (RA: right atrium; LA: left atrium; RV: right ventricle; LV: left ventricle).

competent if they open and close properly, letting through or holding back an expected amount of blood. The heart has two sets of valves: atrioventricular (AV) valves and semilunar (SL) valves.

An AV valve is found between each atrium and ventricle and when opened allows blood to flow into the ventricle. When closed, it prevents the backflow of blood into the atrium. The AV valves open and close with the help of the papillary muscles, which are attached to the valve by the *chordae tendineae*, tendon-like cords. The AV valves are located as follows:

- *Bicuspid* or *mitral valve*: Found between the left atrium and ventricle and made up of two cusps or flaps (see Fig. 24.2)
- *Tricuspid valve*: Found between the right atrium and ventricle and made up of three cusps.

The SL valves are found between the ventricles and the arteries leading out of the heart. The SL valves allow blood to flow out of the heart and prevent the backflow of blood into the ventricles. The valves are created by flaps from the pulmonary artery and aorta. The SL valves are located as follows:

- *Pulmonary valve*: Between the right ventricle and the pulmonary artery
- *Aortic valve*: Between the left ventricle and the aorta

CRITICAL THINKING APPLICATION   24.1

Lizzy, the medical assistant student, asks Rebecca how she can remember the chambers and valves of the heart. What is a way to remember the chambers and the names of the valves in the heart? (Be creative.)

Heartbeat

A provider listens to the heart sounds with a stethoscope. The normal sound is a *lub dup*. The *lub* sound occurs from the AV valves closing as the ventricles contract. This is a lower pitch, longer sound, which is followed by a pause. The *dup* sound occurs from the closing of the SL valves. With **incompetent valves**, the provider might hear additional abnormal noises.

A complete heartbeat or *cardiac cycle* can be divided into the diastole and systole phases. During the *diastole* phase, the heart is at rest and the atria fill with blood. The *systole* phase occurs when the heart is contracting.

Blood Flow

The body has several types of blood flow pathways or circulations. The heart, being a double pump, sends blood in two different directions, resulting in two major circulatory pathways:

• *Pulmonary circulation*: **Deoxygenated** blood is pumped from the right side of the heart to the lungs, gas is exchanged, and oxygenated blood returns to the heart.
• *Systemic circulation*: Oxygenated blood is pumped from the left side of the heart and moves through the body. Oxygen, nutrients, and other substances are brought to the cells while the blood picks up waste products. The deoxygenated blood returns to the heart.

Since the pulmonary circulation and the systemic circulation are closely tied, they will be discussed together. The coronary circulation (blood flow through the heart tissues) and fetal circulation (blood flow of an unborn baby) will also be examined.

Pulmonary and Systemic Circulations

Pulmonary circulation begins as the blood returns from the body. The superior vena cava and the inferior vena cava bring deoxygenated blood from the body to the right atrium. As the atria contract, the blood from the right atrium passes the tricuspid valve and empties into the right ventricle. When the ventricles contract, the blood in the right ventricle is pushed out past the pulmonary valve and enters the pulmonary artery trunk. The pulmonary artery trunk splits into the right and left pulmonary arteries. From there, the blood moves into the arterioles and then into the pulmonary capillaries in the lungs. The gas exchange occurs. Carbon dioxide leaves the blood and enters the lungs to be expelled. Oxygen enters the blood from the lungs. The oxygenated blood leaves the pulmonary capillaries and enters the pulmonary veins. The right and left pulmonary veins bring the blood back to the left atrium. This is the start of systemic circulation.

When the atria are full of blood, they contract. The oxygenated blood in the left atrium moves past the bicuspid or mitral valve and empties into the left ventricle. When the ventricles contract, the blood in the left ventricle moves out of the heart, passing the aortic valve, and empties into the aorta. From here, the blood will move through the body before it returns to the heart. Blood from the head, neck, and upper extremities empties into the superior vena cava before returning to the right atrium. Blood from the lower body empties into the inferior vena cava before returning to the right atrium.

CRITICAL THINKING APPLICATION   24.2

Rebecca is helping Lizzy review the blood flow through the body. She asks Lizzy to explain the blood flow through the pulmonary and systemic circulations, starting with the blood returning from the body. How should Lizzy answer her?

Coronary Circulation

The heart has its own blood vessels that support the tissues. The right and left coronary arteries are the first branches off the ascending aorta (Fig. 24.3). The coronary arteries bring nutrients and oxygen to the heart tissue. The blood moves from the arteries to the capillaries in the myocardium. From there, the blood moves into the coronary veins. The coronary veins remove the waste products from the heart tissue. Blood from the coronary veins drains into the coronary sinus, which opens into the right atrium.

Coronary arteries have the important role of maintaining the myocardium. If a branch of the coronary artery becomes blocked, a person will experience a heart attack. The tissue supplied by the blocked artery will be deprived of oxygen and nutrients.

Hepatic Portal Circulation

In most cases, veins leaving an abdominal organ empty blood into the inferior vena cava as it heads to the heart. Veins from the spleen, gallbladder, pancreas, stomach, and intestines take an alternative route. Veins from these organs dump the blood into the hepatic portal vein, which takes the blood to the liver. In the liver, the blood moves through capillaries as it is filtered. Eventually, the blood drains into the hepatic veins before emptying into the inferior vena cava.

The liver has a special role in filtering the blood and metabolizes or breaks down substances. The hepatic portal system has many advantages:

• The **glucose** absorbed can be filtered and stored in the liver as glycogen. It will later be added back to the blood when the glucose levels are low.
• Toxic substances like alcohol or medications can be partially filtered before moving to the rest of the body.

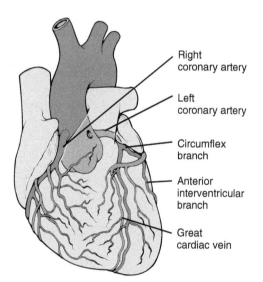
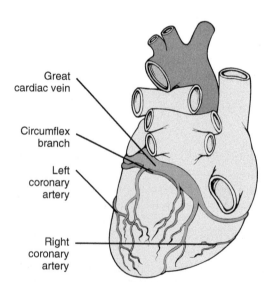

FIGURE 24.3 Coronary arteries. (From Frazier MS, et al: *Essentials of human diseases and conditions*, ed 5, St. Louis, 2013, Saunders.)

Fetal Circulation

Prior to birth, the baby is called a *fetus*. Fetal circulation differs from what we have discussed so far in this chapter. Before birth, the baby's lungs, gastrointestinal tract, and kidneys are not functioning like they will after birth. Toward the end of pregnancy, babies "practice" breathing, as they breathe in the amniotic fluid. No gas exchange occurs. Babies also urinate, but the waste products in their blood are being removed by their mothers' blood. Nutrients are being passed through the blood from the mother.

During the early weeks of pregnancy, the placenta (reproductive organ) begins to grow. It attaches to the mother's uterus and connects to the growing baby via the umbilical cord. The umbilical cord contains two umbilical arteries and one umbilical vein. The arteries carry the fetal blood to the placenta. The umbilical vein carries oxygen and nutrient-rich blood to the baby. The waste, oxygen, and nutrient exchange occurs in the placenta. There is a very thin wall separating the fetal blood from the mother's blood. There is no mixing of the two different blood supplies, though substances can pass between the separating wall. Oxygen and nutrients move from the mother's bloodstream to the fetal blood. Waste products (i.e., carbon dioxide) move from the fetal blood to the mother's blood.

Other structures that are unique to the growing baby in utero include the following:

- *Ductus venosus*: Shifts the majority of the blood from the umbilical vein and empties it into the inferior vena cava (Fig. 24.4). This structure helps the blood bypass the immature liver. After birth, with the lack of blood flow from the umbilical vein, the ductus venosus constricts. Within 1 to 3 months from birth, it is permanently sealed.
- *Foramen ovale*: A small flaplike opening in the interatrial septum that allows blood to move from the right atrium to the left atrium (see Fig. 24.4). This allows most of the blood to bypass the immature lungs. After birth, the flap opening is forced closed with the pressure of the blood pumping in the heart. During infancy, the flap should seal permanently.
- *Ductus arteriosus*: A short vessel that connects the pulmonary artery with the aorta. About 90% of the blood in the pulmonary artery is redirected to the aorta, bypassing the immature lungs. Usually it closes at birth or shortly after.

At birth, when a baby takes his or her first breath and the umbilical cord is cut, these special structures are no longer needed. With the first breath, more pressure is caused in the cardiovascular system. This helps with the closure of the foramen ovale. With the cutting of the umbilical cord, the remaining structures (ductus venosus, ductus arteriosus, and umbilical vessels) collapse.

Life Span Changes

An unborn child receives oxygen and nutrients from the mother's blood through the placenta. As described earlier in this chapter, the ductus venosus, ductus arteriosus, foramen ovale, and the umbilical vessels are special structures that help with fetal circulation. After birth, these structures are no longer necessary.

As a child grows and matures, the heart rate decreases. The systemic vascular resistance increases with age. This means that the resistance for blood flow increases and thus the blood pressure increases with age.

During pregnancy, the mother's cardiovascular system undergoes changes:

- Cardiac output (amount of blood pushed out of the heart in 1 minute) increases.
- Extracellular fluid volume increases, thus the blood volume is more.
- Total peripheral resistance decreases, thus decreasing the blood pressure.
- Blood flow to various organs increases.
- As the pregnancy progresses into the third trimester, the blood pressure increases.

As a person ages, the heart and blood vessels undergo changes. Heart changes that occur include the following:

- SA node loses some cells, thus the heart rate can be slower.
- The left ventricle may increase in size, thus decreasing the amount of blood that it can hold.
- Normal ECG changes can occur with age.
- Valves can become thicker and stiffer, causing a heart murmur.

Arterial walls become stiffer, thus increasing the blood pressure. *Baroreceptors* in the carotid arteries and aorta detect changes in blood pressure and help maintain a fairly constant blood pressure with position changes. With age, the baroreceptors become less sensitive, making older people more at risk for orthostatic hypotension when changing positions.

Blood

Blood is made up of two components:

- *Liquid portion*: Called plasma and makes up about 55% of the total blood volume.
- *Formed elements*: Includes red blood cells (RBCs), white blood cells (WBCs), and platelets. The formed elements are suspended (freely float) in the plasma and make up about 45% of the total blood volume.

A milliliter of blood has approximately 4.2 million to 6 million RBCs, 4500 to 11,000 WBCs, and 150,000 to 450,000 platelets. The average 150-pound (68 kg) person has approximately 5 liters of blood circulating throughout the body. The following sections will discuss plasma, platelets, WBCs, and RBCs in more detail.

Plasma

Plasma is the liquid portion of whole blood. Plasma contains 90% water. Water is the **solvent** for all the dissolved substances that travel in the plasma. Plasma also contains the following:

- Plasma proteins: Made in the liver and include the following:
  - *Albumin*: It is the most abundant protein in plasma, and it attracts water. It normally stays in the blood vessel; thus, it helps to maintain the blood volume.
  - *Globulins*: Antibodies are a type of globulin; they protect against infections.
  - *Clotting factors*: Include fibrinogen and prothrombin, which are important in the blood clotting or coagulation process.
  - *Complement*: A group of enzymes that assist antibodies protect the body.
- Inorganic substances and electrolytes (sodium, calcium, potassium, chloride, magnesium, bicarbonate)

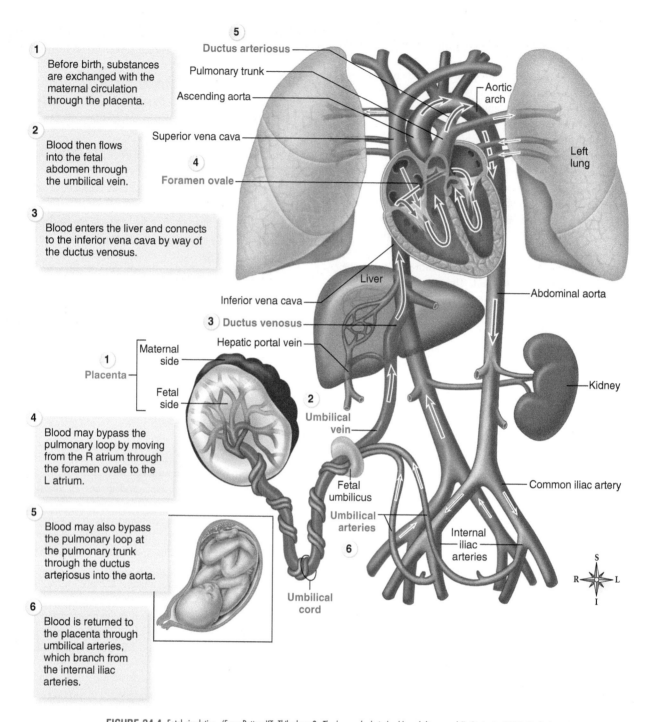

1 Before birth, substances are exchanged with the maternal circulation through the placenta.

2 Blood then flows into the fetal abdomen through the umbilical vein.

3 Blood enters the liver and connects to the inferior vena cava by way of the ductus venosus.

4 Blood may bypass the pulmonary loop by moving from the R atrium through the foramen ovale to the L atrium.

5 Blood may also bypass the pulmonary loop at the pulmonary trunk through the ductus arteriosus into the aorta.

6 Blood is returned to the placenta through umbilical arteries, which branch from the internal iliac arteries.

FIGURE 24.4 Fetal circulation. (From Patton KT, Thibodeau G: *The human body in health and disease*, ed 7, St. Louis, 2018, Mosby.)

- Organic substances (amino acids, glucose, fats, cholesterol, hormones)
- Waste products (urea, uric acid, ammonia, creatinine)

Organic and inorganic substances are needed for metabolism and cellular function, repair, and reproduction. Cellular metabolism waste products are dissolved in the plasma and are transported to the liver, kidneys, and lungs for excretion.

Plasma has a very narrow pH range (7.35 to 7.45), which is necessary to make sure that red blood cells can transport the optimal level of oxygen in the blood. The range also allows needed chemical reactions in the body to continue to work. Most chemical reactions in the body are pH-dependent. Without a stable blood pH, homeostasis is unlikely to be maintained.

Thrombocytes

Thrombocytes, also called platelets, have an irregular round or oval shape. They are formed in the bone marrow from **stem cells**. They are just a small piece or fragment of a much larger cell called a megakaryocyte that is in the bone marrow. Platelets aid in *coagulation*, the process of changing a liquid to a solid. When an injury to a blood vessel occurs,

TABLE 24.1	Types of White Blood Cells	
TYPE	DESCRIPTION	ROLE
Granulocytes		
Neutrophils	Also called segs, polys, or polymorphonucleocytes (PMNs); most abundant WBC	Phagocytic (protect by engulfing and destroying foreign substances); clean up the infection site and aid in the healing process
Eosinophils	Also called eos; make up about 1% of the WBCs	Increase in number when the body is defending against allergens and parasites
Basophils	Also called basos; make up 1% or less of the WBCs in the circulation	Respond to allergic reaction by releasing histamine, which causes an inflammatory response; also release heparin (an anticoagulant)
Agranulocytes		
Monocytes	Also called monos; contain a single, large nucleus; largest phagocytic WBC; transform into macrophages when in lymphatic tissue	Very aggressive phagocytic cells that can destroy pathogens, malignant cells, and tumor cells in the body
Lymphocytes	Also called lymphs; two types: B cells and T cells	Involved in the immune response and destroy pathogens; B cells produce antibodies; T cells attack foreign substances and assist B cells

platelets rush to the area and *agglutinate*, or clump together. This stops or slows the bleeding, thus controlling the blood flow (*hemostasis*).

Leukocytes

Leukocytes, also called white blood cells (WBCs), protect the body from invading pathogens. The two main types of WBCs are granulocytes and agranulocytes (Table 24.1).

Named for their appearance, granulocytes have granules within the cytoplasm, and they also have a segmented or multilobed nucleus. There are three types of granulocytes: neutrophils, eosinophils, and basophils. Each has its own role in immunity.

Agranulocytes lack granules in the cytoplasm, and they have one nucleus. Granulocytes originate in the bone marrow and mature after entering the lymphatic system. There are two types of agranulocytes: monocytes and lymphocytes.

Erythrocytes

Erythrocytes, or red blood cells (RBCs), have the important function of transporting O_2 and CO_2 throughout the body. Hemoglobin, a molecule on the RBC, is capable of binding, transporting, and releasing oxygen and carbon dioxide. Hemoglobin is made up of protein and iron.

RBC production is stimulated by *erythropoietin*, a hormone produced in the kidneys. The formation of RBCs takes place in red bone marrow. Stem cells produce immature RBCs that contain a nucleus. As an RBC matures, it loses its nucleus and is released into the bloodstream. RBCs are *biconcave* (curved inward on both sides), which allows for more surface area for the hemoglobin, thus allowing more O_2 and CO_2 to be carried. The shape also allows more flexibility as the RBC moves through the tiny capillaries.

Red blood cells have a life span of approximately 120 days. When an RBC is no longer useful, it is broken down into iron and **bilirubin** in the spleen. The iron is stored mainly in the liver and is recycled into new RBCs. The bilirubin is further broken down into bile, which is excreted by the liver.

Blood Types. Two major classification systems are used with blood types, the ABO system and the Rh system. Using the ABO system, each person has either an A, B, ABO, or O blood type. With the Rh system, a person is either Rh-positive or Rh-negative. For example, a person may have O-negative blood. Using the ABO system, the person has type O blood and is Rh-negative. These two systems will be explained in more detail in the following sections.

With the ABO system, each blood type is unique based on the specific antigens present or absent on the surface of the RBCs and specific antibodies circulating in the plasma (Table 24.2). Remember, antigens are foreign substances to the body, and the immune system makes specific antibodies to fight off specific antigens. When a person receives a blood transfusion, the blood given must be compatible with the person's blood. If an antibody is present in the recipient's blood, the corresponding antigen cannot be in the donor's blood. For example, type O blood contains both A and B antibodies, thus blood with A or B antigens cannot be given. The only type of blood that is compatible with type O is type O. Another example is a person with type AB blood, which contains no antibodies. These people can receive all four blood types because they have no antibodies to attack the donor blood. Type AB blood is considered the *universal recipient*, because it does not contain any antibodies. Type O is considered the *universal donor*, because it does not contain any antigens and everyone can receive O blood.

With the Rh system, there is a collection of 47 antigens that act together as a group and are referred to as the Rh antigen or Rh factor. When the Rh antigen is present, the person is said to be Rh-positive. About 85% of the population in the United States is Rh-positive, and 15% are Rh-negative.

Rh antibodies are different from ABO antibodies. Rh antibodies are not preformed (present before antigen exposure) like ABO

TABLE 24.2	Blood Types			
TYPE	ANTIGENS PRESENT	ANTIBODIES PRESENT	CAN GIVE BLOOD TO	CAN RECEIVE BLOOD FROM
ABO System				
A	A antigen	B antibodies	A, AB	A, O
B	B antigen	A antibodies	B, AB	B, O
AB	A and B antigens	None	AB	AB, A, B, O
O	None	A and B antibodies	O, A, B, AB	O
Rh System				
Negative	Rh not present		Negative and positive	Negative
Positive	Rh present		Positive	Positive and negative

antibodies. The first time a person is exposed to the Rh antigen, the immune system produces antibodies. This process is called *sensitization.* Nothing is noticeable during the first exposure, though subsequent exposures to the Rh antigen will cause *lysis* (destruction) of RBCs.

Blood typing is the process of determining a person's blood type. If the person receives the wrong type of blood, a transfusion reaction can occur, which may be a serious, life-threatening situation. For instance, if a person with type A blood is transfused with type B blood, the anti-B antibodies in the recipient's blood will attack the B antigens in the donor's blood, causing *agglutination* (blood clumping) or *lysis* (blood cell rupture).

Erythroblastosis Fetalis

The Rh factor is an important consideration during pregnancy for Rh-negative mothers due to erythroblastosis fetalis (also called hemolytic disease of the newborn [HDN]). In this disorder, an Rh-negative mother who is carrying an Rh-positive fetus will develop antibodies to the Rh-positive blood if fetal blood exposure occurs. If another pregnancy occurs with an Rh-positive fetus, the mother's immune system produces antibodies that cross the placenta and destroy the fetal red blood cells.

To prevent this disorder, it is standard practice for the pregnant mother's blood to be tested *(typed)* early in pregnancy, if the blood type is unknown. Mothers with Rh-negative blood receive an injection of RhoGAM around week 26 to 28 of pregnancy. After the baby is born, the cord blood is tested. If the baby has Rh-positive blood, the mother receives another injection of RhoGAM within 72 hours of delivery.

MICRhoGram (a smaller dose of RhoGAM) should be given to Rh-negative women 72 hours after a threatened or actual termination of pregnancy (spontaneous [miscarriage] or induced) through week 12 of the pregnancy. For threatened or actual exposure to Rh-positive blood (e.g., through an invasive procedure, trauma, **ectopic pregnancy**, or pregnancy termination), Rh-negative women should receive RhoGAM within 72 hours. RhoGAM and MICRhoGAM are Rh_o (D) human immune globulin, a blood product, which prevents Rh immunization by binding to Rh-positive cells that sneak into the bloodstream, making them invisible to the mother's immune system.

PHYSIOLOGY OF THE CARDIOVASCULAR SYSTEM

To explore the physiology of the cardiovascular system, the action of the heart, blood vessels, and the blood components will be examined. The following sections discuss the conduction system, factors that impact blood pressure, and coagulation.

Conduction System

To understand the conduction system, it is first necessary to learn the cardiac muscle characteristics and the three states they must undergo for each impulse. Following this discussion, the conduction system and the blood volume will be examined.

Cardiac Muscle

There are two kinds of cardiac cells, electrical or conduction system cells and myocardial cells. The electrical cells are found in the conduction system. They have three unique characteristics:

- *Automaticity*: The cells create and discharge the electrical impulse.
- *Excitability*: The cells respond to the electrical impulse.
- *Conductivity*: The cells transmit electrical impulses to other cells.

The myocardial cells are found in the myocardium. They can shorten and lengthen their fibers for contraction (called *contractility*). The fibers made from the myocardial cells can contract for prolonged periods of time without fatigue and use less adenosine triphosphate (ATP) than other muscles. These features are beneficial for the heart.

Cardiac muscle fibers are electrically linked, forming one unit. A myocardial cell forms a strong, electrical connection to the next cells through special junctions called intercalated disks. The intercalated disks are responsible for the cell-to-cell communication that is required for coordinated muscle contract. The intercalated disks help the muscle fibers form one unit that contracts all at once instead of a little at a time. The "one-unit" approach is important, as the atrial chambers need to contract together and then the ventricles contract at about the same time.

Conduction System Structures

As previously stated, the electrical cells make up the conduction system of the heart. These cells are found throughout the myocardium. They can respond to and transmit electronic impulses to neighboring cells. The conduction system is composed of five structures (see Fig. 24.2):

- *Sinoatrial* (SA) *node:* Located in the posterior, superior wall of the right atrium, the SA node is called the "pacemaker of the heart." This is because the electrical cells in the SA node generate the impulse that starts the heartbeat. When the SA node discharges the impulse, it travels in many directions through the heart muscle. The impulse also moves quickly across special bands of tissue called *internodal tracts.* The *Bachmann bundle,* a specialized internodal tract, takes the impulse to the left atrium. Other internodal tracts take the impulse quickly to the atrioventricular (AV) node. The impulse moving through the atrial chambers triggers the chambers to contract.
- *Atrioventricular* (AV) *node:* The AV node is located at the base of the interatrial septum. When the impulse reaches the AV node, it moves very slowly through the node.
- *Bundle of His* (also called the *atrioventricular* [AV] *bundle):* The bundle of His is located in the upper interventricular septum. When the impulse leaves the AV node, it moves to the bundle of His.
- *Right and left bundle branches:* The bundle branches are located in the lower interventricular septum. After the impulse passes through the bundle of His, it enters the right and left bundle branches. The right bundle branch brings the impulse to the right ventricle. The left bundle branch brings the impulse to the left ventricle.
- *Purkinje fibers:* The bundle branches split into many Purkinje fibers. Purkinje fibers transmit the impulse quickly and efficiently to the ventricular myocardial cells. This causes the ventricular chambers to contract.

CRITICAL THINKING APPLICATION 24.3

Rebecca is helping Lizzy review the conduction system of the heart. To see what Lizzy can remember, Rebecca has her write down the five conduction system structures. What should Lizzy write down? What might be a creative way to remember these structures in order?

States of Cardiac Cell

The cardiac cells cycle through three states or steps in the same sequence for each impulse:

1. *Polarized state:* Before the impulse hits the cells, they are in a polarized state. There is no electrical activity during the polarized state. Think of this as the "waiting" stage.
2. *Depolarized state:* When the impulse hits the cells, the cells' charges change. This is due to the movement of the ions (e.g., sodium, potassium, and calcium) across the cells' membrane. The change of the cells' charges allows the impulse to move through the cell causing *action potential,* also called depolarization. Electrical activity can be recorded on an electrocardiogram (ECG) when the cells are in the depolarized state. ECGs are discussed in Chapter 11.
3. *Repolarized state:* After the impulse passes over the cells, the ions move back to their original location. This causes the cells' charge to change. This recovery phase is called the repolarized state. Electrical activity (less than the depolarized state) can be recorded on an ECG during the repolarized state.

CRITICAL THINKING APPLICATION 24.4

Lizzy struggles with remembering what occurs with polarization, depolarization, and repolarization. Rebecca encourages her to keep the definitions simple, maybe using one to two words to summarize what is occurring. How might Lizzy define each of these words?

When discussing the three states and the chambers impacted, the chamber (atrial, ventricular) comes before the state (e.g., atrial polarization, ventricular depolarization). This terminology will be used as we examine the blood flow and the conduction system together.

Conduction System and Blood Flow

The conduction system is the electrical system in the heart. As already mentioned, it is recorded on the ECG. Electrical impulses from the conduction system cause the chambers of the heart to contract. This contraction is a mechanical action, and, as a result, blood moves through the heart. The mechanical action can be seen with echocardiography, which will be described later in this chapter.

Table 24.3 summarizes an impulse's path through the conduction system and the resulting mechanical action with the blood flow movement. Notice that the atrial chamber state is always one step ahead of the ventricular chambers.

Conduction System and the Nervous System

Cardiac muscle is different from other muscles in the body. The heart is controlled by the autonomic nervous system and the heart's own conduction system. When the heart rate needs to change to meet the demands of the body, the autonomic nervous system automatically kicks in.

Blood Pressure

About one in every three American adults has high blood pressure. This means that many of the patients seen in an ambulatory care center may be diagnosed with high blood pressure, or *hypertension.* More information on hypertension will be provided later in the chapter. By contrast, low blood pressure, or *hypotension,* can be life-threatening in some cases.

The pressure of the blood is highest in the arteries and lowest in the veins. Thus, we measure arterial blood pressure. ***Blood pressure*** **(BP)** can be defined as the resulting *force* of blood against the walls of the arteries. Two measurements are taken during the *cardiac cycle* (a complete heartbeat):

- ***Systole*** or the contractive phase: systolic pressure is measured when the heart is contracting and pumping out the blood.
- ***Diastole*** or the relaxation phase: diastolic pressure is measured when the heart is resting between contractions.

You will learn more about the procedure to take blood pressures in Chapter 5. This section addresses the factors that can influence blood pressure.

Blood Volume

Blood volume, or the amount of circulating blood, has a direct influence on blood pressure. The greater the blood volume, the more force it makes on the arterial walls. If the blood volume is low, less force or pressure will be on the arterial walls. Think of a garden hose attached to a faucet. If you turn on the faucet to the maximum level, there

TABLE 24.3	Impulse Pathway Through the Conduction System With the Triggered Mechanical Actions				
IMPULSE MOVING THROUGH CONDUCTION SYSTEM	**ATRIAL CARDIAC CELLS' STATE**	**VENTRICULAR CARDIAC CELLS' STATE**	**MECHANICAL ACTION TRIGGERED BY IMPULSE**		
			RIGHT SIDE OF HEART	**LEFT SIDE OF HEART**	
SA node (pacemaker) generates the impulse, which travels to the AV node	Atrial depolarization	Ventricular polarization	Right atrium contracts; blood passes the tricuspid valves and empties into the right ventricle	Left atrium contracts; blood passes the bicuspid valves and empties into the left ventricle	
Impulse moves slowly through AV node			Allows the atrial chambers to finish contracting		
Impulse leaves the AV node and moves to the bundle of His, to the right and left bundle branches, and to the Purkinje fibers	Atrial repolarization	Ventricular depolarization	Right ventricle contracts; blood passes the pulmonary valve before emptying into the pulmonary artery as it heads to the lungs	Left ventricle contracts; blood passes the aortic valve before emptying into the aorta as it goes to the body	
(The impulse is now done.)	Atrial polarization	Ventricular repolarization (then moves into ventricular polarization)	Right atrium fills with deoxygenated blood from the body via the inferior vena cava and the superior vena cava	Left atrium fills with oxygenated blood from the lungs via the pulmonary vein	

will be a lot of water pressure in the hose. If you turn on the faucet to get a trickle, then there is very little water pressure in the hose.

Let's briefly examine the factors that increase and decrease blood volume. The blood volume can be raised by the following:

- Blood, plasma, and fluid (intravenous [IV]) transfusions
- Increased sodium intake (because water follows sodium, more water will be drawn into the bloodstream due to the elevated sodium levels)

Fluid volume can decrease due to *hemorrhage* (bleeding), dehydration, and diuretic medications. Diuretics help pull water and sodium from the blood, thus lowering blood volume.

Strength of Ventricular Contractions

The left ventricle pumps blood to the body. The greater the force of the contraction, the more blood is pumped into the arteries. This increases the blood pressure. If the left ventricular contraction is weak, less blood is pumped out of the heart and thus the blood pressure is lower. Digoxin is a medication that decreases the heart rate and strengthens the contractions of the heart.

With heart disease, tests are done to check how the left ventricle is functioning. The *stroke volume* is the amount of blood that is pushed out of the left ventricle compared with the total volume of blood that filled the ventricle. It is a measure of the ejection fraction of the cardiac output. As heart disease occurs, the stroke volume can decrease.

Resistance to Blood Flow

Any factor that increases the resistance for blood to flow through the arteries will increase the blood pressure. Factors that increase resistance

include the size of the *lumen* (inner opening) of the arteries, the elasticity of the arterial walls, and the *viscosity* (thickness) of the blood.

The *peripheral resistance* of blood vessels refers to the size of the lumen and the amount of blood flowing through it. The smaller the vessel's lumen, the greater the resistance to blood flow, thus increasing blood pressure. Several dynamics lead to decreased lumen size, including the following:

- *Plaque* (waxy substance) builds up in the arteries and hardens over time. This buildup narrows the arteries and causes higher blood pressure.
- Smoking.
- Constriction of smooth muscles causing vasoconstriction. Several medications, including benazepril, lisinopril, and losartan, relax smooth muscles, thus decreasing blood pressure.

Another factor that increases blood flow resistance is the loss of vessel elasticity. The inner layer of an artery contains elastic-like fibers that allow the vessel to expand and contract. Arteries dilate as the blood is pumped out of the heart and narrow between heartbeats to help maintain blood pressure. Increasing age and plaque buildup decrease the elasticity of the vessels. To understand the effect of plaque on the vessels, think of dried glue on a balloon. The dried glue prevents that section of the balloon from expanding. The plaque is like the dried glue. It prevents the walls from expanding.

Lastly, the viscosity of blood influences the resistance of blood flow. As the viscosity of the blood increases, so does the resistance, and the blood pressure rises. The thickness of blood increases when more blood cells are present (e.g., **polycythemia**, blood transfusion).

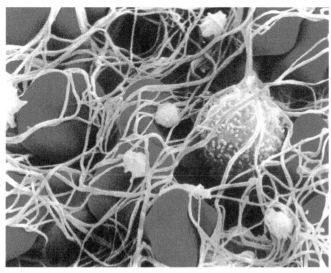

FIGURE 24.5 Fibrin clot. (Reprinted with permission of CNRI/Photo Researchers, Inc.)

In summary, blood pressure can be influenced by blood volume, the strength of ventricular contractions, and the resistance of blood flow. Resistance can be increased by the following:

- Narrowed lumen (e.g., due to plaque, smoking, and vasoconstriction)
- Loss of vessel elasticity due to aging and plaque
- Increased viscosity of the blood

CRITICAL THINKING APPLICATION   **24.5**

With many of their patients having high blood pressure, Rebecca wants to make sure Lizzy understands the factors that impact blood pressure. She asks Lizzy to summarize factors that increase blood pressure. How might Lizzy respond?

Coagulation and Hemostasis

The process involved in forming a blood clot is complicated, with many specific chemical reactions and clotting factors involved. What follows is a simplified version of this process.

First, a damaged vessel will **constrict** to slow the flow of blood through the vessel. In response to the injury, platelets become sticky and clump together (*aggregation*). Platelets then stick to the area of injury (*adhesion*). Because of platelet aggregation and adhesion, a *platelet plug* is formed over the injury and platelets release clotting factors, which aid in the process of coagulation. The injured blood vessel tissue also activates clotting factors in the blood plasma. The interaction between the clotting factors works to form *fibrin*, a white, **filamentous**, tough protein strand that creates a netlike structure (Fig. 24.5). The fibrin net traps red blood cells and more platelets to form a **thrombus**. This process is called *blood clotting* or *coagulation*. When the body stops the flow of blood through coagulation, the process is called *hemostasis*.

DISORDERS OF THE CARDIOVASCULAR SYSTEM

Many patients seen in the ambulatory care facility have cardiovascular diseases. Common signs and symptoms include the following:

- *Angina* (chest pain), *bradycardia* (heartbeat >60 beats per minute [bpm]), *tachycardia* (heartbeat <100 bpm), and *palpitation* (unusually fast, strong, or irregular heartbeat)
- *Cyanosis* (bluish discoloration of the skin, lips, and nail beds), *pallor* (paleness of the skin), *dyspnea* (difficulty breathing), *orthopnea* (dyspnea with lying flat, relieved when sitting up), and *shortness of breath* (SOB) (breathlessness)
- *Diaphoresis* (profuse sweating), *edema* (swelling), and *syncope* (fainting)

The following sections describe in detail some of the cardiovascular and blood-related diseases.

Cardiovascular-Related Disorders

Arrhythmias

An *arrhythmia* or *dysrhythmia* means the heart rate or rhythm is abnormal. The rhythm may be irregular, or tachycardia or bradycardia may be occurring. The most common arrhythmia is *atrial fibrillation*, which means the rate is fast and the rhythm is irregular.

Arrhythmias are caused by an issue with the heart's conduction system, including an extra beat, and the impulse is blocked, slowed, or takes a different pathway through the heart. Arrhythmias can be caused by diseases (e.g., heart failure), stress, substances (e.g., medications, caffeine), and electrolyte imbalances. Arrhythmias may be intermittent or constant.

Signs and symptoms of arrhythmias include the following:

- Fast or slow heart rate
- Irregular, skipping, or uneven heartbeats
- Lightheadedness, dizziness, SOB
- Pallor, angina, sweating

The provider will listen to the heart with a stethoscope. An ECG is usually the first test done. Heart monitoring devices (e.g., the Holter monitor and an event monitor) provide ECG monitoring over days to weeks. Other tests ordered may include echocardiography, coronary angiography, and an *electrophysiology study* (EPS), an in-depth study of the heart's electrical system. Treatment depends on the severity of the arrhythmia. Treatments may include defibrillation or cardioversion, which shocks the heart into a normal rhythm, or an implantable pacemaker to help establish a normal rate and rhythm. Antiarrhythmic medications, cardiac ablation, and an implantable **cardiac defibrillator** may also be used.

Atherosclerosis-Related Diseases

Atherosclerosis is a condition in which plaque or **atheromas** build up and narrow the artery. The plaque can prevent the arteries from properly constricting and dilating. At times, small cracks in the vessel wall can occur, causing a **thrombus** to form over the atheroma, and partially or completely occluding the vessel. If a section of the thrombus breaks away and travels in the bloodstream, this is an **embolus** (Fig. 24.6). Several diseases can result from plaque buildup. See Table 24.4 for atherosclerosis-related diseases.

The cause of atherosclerosis is unknown. Studies have shown that it can develop in childhood and gets worse with age. Risk factors for atherosclerosis include smoking, an unhealthy diet, lack of physical activity, high blood pressure, unhealthy cholesterol levels, and uncontrolled diabetes mellitus.

Diagnostic procedures include blood tests to check the cholesterol, glucose, and protein levels. Additional tests include an ECG,

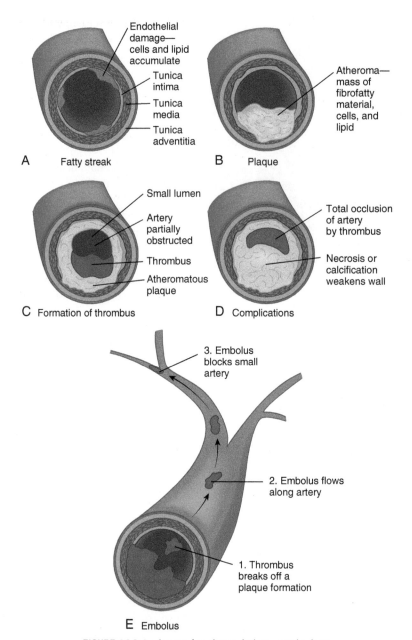

FIGURE 24.6 Development of an atheroma, leading to arterial occlusion.

TABLE 24.4	Atherosclerosis-Related Diseases	
DISEASE	**DESCRIPTION**	**SIGNS AND SYMPTOMS**
Carotid artery disease	Plaque builds up in the carotid arteries and may lead to a stroke.	Sudden weakness or paralysis (inability to move), numbness, confusion, problems speaking or seeing, dizziness, and other symptoms of a stroke
Coronary heart disease (CHD) or coronary artery disease (CAD)	Plaque builds up in the coronary arteries. Can lead to angina (chest pain) or myocardial infarction (heart attack). Also known as ischemic heart disease.	Angina; pain in the shoulder, arm, neck, jaw, or back; indigestion, shortness of breath, arrhythmias
Coronary microvascular disease (MVD)	Plaque builds up in the tiny coronary arteries damaging the vessel walls.	Angina, shortness of breath, fatigue, lack of energy, sleep problems
Peripheral artery disease (PAD)	Plaque builds up in the large arteries of the legs, arms, and pelvis.	Numbness, pain, and life-threatening infections
Chronic kidney disease	Plaque builds up in the renal arteries and can cause kidney damage.	Tiredness, loss of appetite, nausea, swelling of hands or feet, numbness, changes in amount of urine

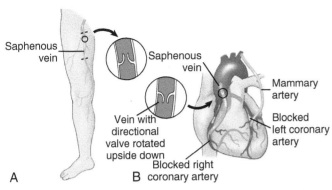

FIGURE 24.7 Coronary artery bypass graft (CABG). **(A)** A section of vein is harvested from the right leg and is anastomosed to a coronary artery to bypass an occlusion of the right coronary artery. **(B)** Bypass of the left coronary artery with a mammary artery. (From Shiland B: *Medical terminology and anatomy for ICD-10 coding*, ed 2, St. Louis, 2016, Mosby.)

echocardiography, chest x-ray, CT scan, angiography, and stress test. The goals of treatment are to lower the risk of blood clot formation, prevent diseases, and widen the affected arteries. Heart-healthy lifestyle changes will be encouraged. This involves exercise, a healthy diet, building stress-coping and management skills, maintaining a healthy weight, and smoking cessation. Medications that lower cholesterol levels may be used. Percutaneous coronary intervention, coronary artery bypass grafting (CABG), or a carotid endarterectomy may also be performed (Fig. 24.7).

CRITICAL THINKING APPLICATION   24.6

Lizzy is working with Ken Thomas, a patient. He asks her about plaque in the arteries and what can happen if a person has a lot of plaque. How might Lizzy answer Ken's questions?

Cardiomyopathy

With cardiomyopathy, the heart muscle becomes abnormal. It may become thin and weakened, enlarged and thick, or rigid. As the disease worsens, the heart becomes less efficient at pumping blood and maintaining a normal electrical rhythm. Cardiomyopathy can lead to arrhythmias, heart failure, edema, and heart valve problems.

There are many types of cardiomyopathy; some develop due to other diseases, and others are inherited. Some people may never have symptoms, whereas others do not experience symptoms during the early stages of the disease. As the condition worsens, a person may experience: shortness of breath, especially after activity; swelling of the legs, feet, ankles, abdomen, and neck veins; and fatigue.

The provider obtains a history and performs a physical exam. Abnormal heart sounds and lung sounds might be heard with a stethoscope. A heart murmur may be present. Crackling in the lungs may indicate fluid in the lungs. Swelling can also be seen, as mentioned in the prior section. A chest x-ray, an ECG, echocardiography, and a stress test may be ordered. Further procedures may include a cardiac catheterization, coronary angiography, or myocardial biopsy.

Treatments depend on the severity of the condition. Treatments may include healthy lifestyle changes and medications (antiarrhythmics,

anticoagulants, diuretics, and beta-blockers). Surgery to treat the heart area, a heart transplant, and a pacemaker may also be included.

Congenital Heart Defects

There are numerous congenital heart defects. Table 24.5 describes common defects. Depending on the type and severity of the defect, the newborn baby may require immediate surgery.

The cause of these congenital defects may be genetic, chromosomal, or unknown. The signs and symptoms of the defect will depend on its type and severity. For some, there are no symptoms, and the person may not realize the condition exists until adulthood. Other defects may cause the baby to have the following conditions:

- *Cyanosis* (blue-tinted nails or lips), increased respiration rate, breathing difficulties
- Difficulty feeding, tiredness with feeding, weight loss
- Abnormal heart murmur
- Sweating with feeding or crying

Some of the defects may be identified during the pregnancy. Fetal echocardiography can be used on unborn babies to detect cardiac abnormalities. After birth, echocardiography, pulse oximetry, ECG, and chest x-rays may be performed to help diagnose the defect. Treatment for congenital heart defects depends on the type and severity of the defect. Some holes may close on their own, whereas others may require surgery to patch them. Some defects will be monitored, but no treatment will be required. Life-threatening defects will require emergency surgery after birth and follow-up through childhood.

Congestive Heart Failure

Congestive heart failure (CHF), also called heart failure, occurs when the heart does not efficiently pump blood. Blood backs up behind the failing pump (side of the heart). *Systolic heart failure* occurs when the heart muscle cannot pump the blood out of the heart. *Diastolic heart failure* occurs when the chamber muscle is stiff and does not completely fill up with blood. Heart failure can impact one or both sides of the heart. Types of heart failure include the following:

- *Right-sided heart failure*: Fluid may back up into the body, causing swelling in the legs, feet, and abdomen
- *Left-sided heart failure*: Fluid may back up into the lungs, causing shortness of breath and abnormal lung sounds
- *Cor pulmonale*: Right-sided heart failure caused by high blood pressure in the right ventricle and pulmonary arteries

Coronary artery disease (CAD) and high blood pressure are the most common causes of heart failure. Other causes include congenital problems, heart attack, faulty valves, arrhythmias, infections, and other diseases (e.g., thyroid problems). Symptoms can develop slowly or suddenly, depending on the cause. Symptoms can differ based on the side of the heart that is failing. Common symptoms include the following:

- Cough and shortness of breath with reclining or activity
- Fatigue, faintness, weakness, and loss of appetite
- Fast or irregular pulse, and palpitations
- **Pitting edema** (swelling) in feet and legs, swollen liver and abdomen; weight gain (Fig. 24.8)

During the physical exam, the provider will listen for abnormal heart and lung sounds and check for edema. Echocardiography, imaging tests, and blood tests may be ordered. Treatment includes monitoring weight; limiting dietary cholesterol, salts, and fluids; and

TABLE 24.5	Congenital Heart Defects
DEFECT	**DESCRIPTION**
Atrial septal defect (ASD)	A hole in the interatrial septum allows oxygen-rich blood from the left atrium to flow into the right atrium. May not have many symptoms. Hole may close on its own or with surgery.
Atrioventricular septal defect	Holes are between the right and left chambers, and the valves are malformed. Surgery is required to patch holes.
Coarctation of the aorta	Narrowing of the aorta resulting in blood back-flowing into the left ventricle, high blood pressure, and weakened pulses in the legs. Surgery or balloon angioplasty can correct the condition.
Dextro-transposition of the great arteries	The pulmonary artery and the aorta are switched. Oxygen-rich blood is pumped back to the lungs, and the deoxygenated blood is pumped back to the body. Requires emergency surgery.
Hypoplastic left heart syndrome	Structures on the left side of the heart are not correctly developed. Treated with medications and surgery to improve blood flow.
Patent foramen ovale (PFO)	Foramen ovale does not close during infancy. It remains open or patent. May not have any symptoms and may not require treatment.
Patent ductus arteriosus (PDA)	Ductus arteriosus does not close soon after birth, causing too much blood to move into the pulmonary circulation. A heart murmur may be the only sign.
Pulmonary atresia	Pulmonary valve does not form, and blood cannot flow to the lungs. Requires immediate surgery after birth to improve blood flow to the lungs.
Tetralogy of Fallot (TOF)	Consists of four major conditions: ventricular septal defect, pulmonary stenosis, defective aortic valve, and ventricular hypertrophy. Requires immediate surgery.
Ventricular septal defect (VSD)	Septal wall is not fully developed between the ventricles, causing a hole. Blood tends to flow from the left ventricle into the right ventricle, stressing the pulmonary system.

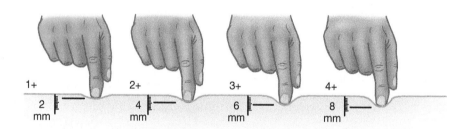

FIGURE 24.8 Providers measure pitting edema from 1+ to 4+. (From Ball J, et al: *Seidel's guide to physical examination*, St. Louis, 2019, Mosby.)

medications (e.g., diuretics, antihypertensives, and digoxin). Surgery, a pacemaker, an implantable defibrillator, or a heart transplant may also be needed.

Deep Vein Thrombosis

Deep vein thrombosis (DVT) or thrombophlebitis occurs when a **thrombus** forms in a vein deep in the body, usually in the legs. DVTs can occur at any age, but they most commonly occur in people over the age of 60. An embolus can occur from a DVT, which can lead to life-threatening conditions including a pulmonary embolism (PE), cerebrovascular accident (*stroke*), or myocardial **infarction** (heart attack).

Blood clots can form when the vein's inner lining and valves are damaged from surgery, injuries, inflammation, or from an immune response. Blood clots can also occur when the blood flow is slow or if the blood has an increase in viscosity. Estrogen, birth control pills, and inherited conditions can cause an increased risk for clotting. Signs and symptoms include leg pain, swelling, warmth, and redness (Fig. 24.9).

The provider will do a history and physical exam. An ultrasound may be ordered as well as blood tests (e.g., D-dimer blood test, antithrombin levels, and complete blood count [CBC]). Treatment includes anticoagulant medications, compression stockings, and possible surgery to remove the clot.

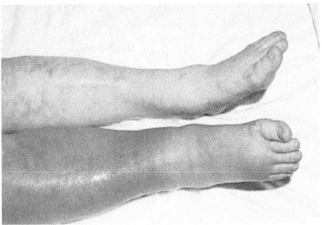

FIGURE 24.9 Deep vein thrombosis (DVT). (From Lewis SM: *Medical-surgical nursing: assessment and management of clinical problems*, ed 8, St. Louis, 2011, Mosby.)

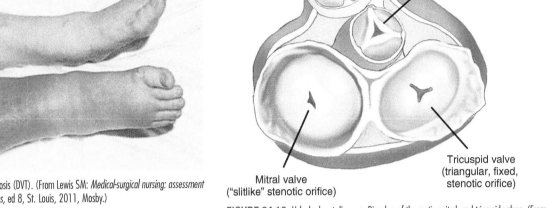

FIGURE 24.10 Valvular heart diseases. Disorders of the aortic, mitral, and tricuspid valves. (From Shiland B: *Medical terminology and anatomy for ICD-10 coding*, ed 2, St. Louis, 2016, Mosby.)

CRITICAL THINKING APPLICATION 24.7

Lizzy is preparing for a national exam. She is struggling to remember the difference between an embolus and a thrombus. What is a creative way to remember the differences between the two terms?

Heart Valve Diseases

There are many types of valvular disease. Two types of heart valve disease can occur to each of the valves, including **stenosis** and **insufficiency** (also called regurgitation or incompetence). When naming the disease, the valve is followed by stenosis or insufficiency (e.g., tricuspid stenosis, tricuspid insufficiency). With stenosis, the heart may need to work harder to push blood through the smaller opening. With insufficiency, the valve does not close completely, and blood leaks backward across the valve into the prior chamber (Fig. 24.10). The following sections will discuss more common valvular diseases.

Aortic Insufficiency. With aortic insufficiency, the aortic valve does not close tightly. The blood backs up into the left ventricle. This is more common in males between age 30 and 60.

Many conditions cause this disease, including high blood pressure, syphilis, congenital problem, and endocarditis. Signs and symptoms may not be present or be slow to develop. They include a bounding pulse, angina, fainting, fatigue, palpitations, SOB, and swelling of the feet.

Besides the physical exam, a person may have aortic angiography, echocardiography, left heart catheterization, magnetic resonance imaging (MRI), and transthoracic echocardiography done to diagnose the condition. The treatment goal is to reduce blood pressure through medications. The patient may need surgery to replace the valve.

Mitral Valve Prolapse. Mitral valve prolapse occurs when one or both cusps of the mitral valve protrude back into the left atrium during ventricular systole.

This condition is congenital or genetic. The patient may experience palpitations, SOB, cough, fatigue, dizziness, anxiety, migraines, and chest discomfort.

The provider will do a physical exam and additional tests will be ordered, including echocardiography, Doppler ultrasound, chest x-ray,

and an ECG. Treatment consists of medications (beta-blockers, diuretics, vasodilators) and surgery to repair or replace the valve.

Rheumatic Fever. Rheumatic fever is an inflammatory reaction that affects the heart valves (**valvulitis**) and causes swelling and scarring of the valves. Permanent damage of the valves leads to rheumatic heart disease.

Antibodies made by the body to attack the streptococcal infection start attacking the body tissues (joints and heart valves), causing inflammation, swelling, and scarring. It usually occurs 2 to 4 weeks after a strep throat infection. The patient may have a fever, joint pain, stomach pain, weakness, SOB, nodules (small bumps) under the skin by the elbows and knees, and rash on the chest, abdomen, or back.

Following the physical exam, the provider may order blood tests, chest x-rays, and an ECG. Treatment consists of antibiotics for the infection and, if needed, surgery to repair the valve.

Hypertension

Hypertension, or high blood pressure, occurs when the force of the blood pushing against the artery wall is elevated. Table 24.6 lists the stages of blood pressure. There are three types of hypertension:

- *Primary hypertension* (or *essential hypertension*): The most common type with no identifiable cause; develops with age.
- *Secondary hypertension*: High blood pressure is caused by another disease condition or medication. If the disease is treated or the medication is removed, the high blood pressure resolves.
- *Malignant hypertension*: Very high blood pressure that causes organ damage.

Hypertension can be caused by genetics, environmental factors (e.g., high sodium diet, obesity, smoking), kidney disease, and changes in the elasticity of the blood vessel walls. High blood pressure has no symptoms. The only sign is a high blood pressure reading. Hypertension can cause serious problems including stroke, heart attack, heart failure, and kidney failure.

Blood pressure is measured and recorded as two numbers (systolic pressure over diastolic pressure). Treatment involves a low-salt or heart-healthy diet, maintaining a healthy weight, stopping smoking, exercise, limiting alcohol intake, and developing healthy strategies to

TABLE 24.6   Blood Pressure Stages for Adults

CATEGORY	SYSTOLIC	AND/OR	DIASTOLIC
Normal blood pressure	Less than 120 mm Hg		Less than 80 mm Hg
Elevated	120–129 mm Hg	And	Less than 80 mm Hg
Hypertension stage 1	130–139 mm Hg	Or	80–89 mm Hg
Hypertension stage 2	At least 140 mm Hg	Or	At least 90 mm Hg
Hypertensive crisis	More than 180 mm Hg	And/or	More than 120 mm Hg

mm Hg (millimeters of mercury).

TABLE 24.7   Risk Factors for Heart Disease

FACTORS THAT *CANNOT* BE CHANGED	FACTORS THAT *CAN* BE CHANGED
• Age: Risk increases with age • Gender: Males have higher risk; after menopause, females have almost the same risk as males • Genetics: Family history increases risk • Race: African Americans, Mexican Americans, Native Americans, and Hawaiians have a greater risk	• Smoking • High cholesterol • High blood pressure • Uncontrolled diabetes • Lack of exercise • Obesity • Stress • Alcohol

cope with stress. Medications may also be used, including diuretics, angiotensin II receptor blockers (ARBs), angiotensin-converting enzyme (ACE) inhibitors, calcium channel blockers (CCBs), and alpha-blockers.

Myocardial Infarction

Myocardial infarction (MI), also called a heart attack, affects more than 1 million people in the United States a year, and about half of them die as a result. With an MI, the blood flow is limited or blocked, and the heart muscle cells die due to the lack of oxygen.

An MI can be caused by a blood clot or plaque buildup in the coronary arteries. Table 24.7 discusses the risk factors for heart disease. The most common warning symptoms of MIs include the following:

- *Angina pectoris* (chest pain): May also be described as mild or severe heaviness, squeezing, pressure, or heartburn; pain may be constant or intermittent
- Upper body discomfort or pain in one or both arms, shoulders, neck, jaw, upper part of the abdomen
- Shortness of breath with activity or rest
- Cold sweat, tiredness without a reason, nausea and vomiting, dizziness, lightheadedness, arrhythmias, palpitations

- Women may have sharp, burning chest pain, back pain; two-thirds have no symptoms

Diagnostic tests for an MI include an ECG and blood tests (i.e., troponin, creatine kinase [CK], creatine kinase–MB [CK-MB], and serum myoglobin tests). CK-MB is an enzyme found in the heart muscle cell. Within hours of a heart attack, the CK-MB level increases in the blood. It peaks within 12 to 24 hours and returns to normal by 48 to 72 hours. The blood tests may be repeated over time to look for changes. Angiocardiography may be done to study the coronary blood flow and to identify blockages. Immediate treatment involves chewing an aspirin, taking nitroglycerin, and oxygen therapy. Thrombolytic medications may be given to help the body dissolve blood clots. Percutaneous coronary intervention may be done to open the coronary artery.

CRITICAL THINKING APPLICATION   24.8

Rebecca reviews the chest pain protocol with Lizzy. It states that patients with chest pain need to chew an aspirin. Nitroglycerin and oxygen must also be administered to the patient. Rebecca asks Lizzy why aspirin, nitroglycerin, and oxygen are important if a person is experiencing chest pain. How might Lizzy answer this question?

Postural Orthostatic Tachycardia Syndrome

Postural orthostatic tachycardia syndrome (POTS) is estimated to affect 1 million to 3 million Americans and can occur at any age, though it commonly affects females between 15 and 50 years of age. POTS is considered a dysautonomia, an abnormal condition of the autonomic nervous system (ANS). The ANS does not control the blood pressure or heart rate when standing up.

Many times, the underlying cause of a person's POTS is unknown. Diseases that cause or are associated with POTS include autoimmune diseases, diabetes, infections (e.g., mononucleosis, Epstein-Barr virus, Lyme disease), multiple sclerosis, trauma, and vitamin deficiencies. The signs and symptoms can vary but may include *hypovolemia* (low blood volume), tachycardia, and **orthostatic (postural) hypotension**. Other symptoms include the following:

- Fatigue, exercise intolerance, nausea, headaches, and poor concentration
- Lightheadedness, blurred vision, *syncope* (fainting), heart palpitations, chest pain, and shortness of breath
- Cold or painful extremities (fingers and toes)
- Fainting with blood draws (phlebotomy) or deep breathing

With some the symptoms are mild and do not interfere with daily activity. Others experience significant symptoms that interfere with eating, moving, bathing, and working. About 25% of patients with POTS are disabled and cannot work.

Diagnostic testing for POTS includes orthostatic vital signs and the tilt table test, which is used to assess the patient during position changes. Treatment varies and may include medications to regulate the heart rate and blood pressure. Drinking plenty of fluids (2 to 3 L per day); eating a high-salt, low-carbohydrate diet; exercise; and compression stockings may also be encouraged as part of the treatment.

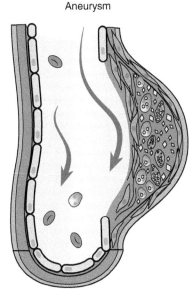

Aneurysm

FIGURE 24.11 Aneurysm caused by weakening of the vessel wall. (From Damjanov I: *Pathology for the health-related professions*, ed 4, St. Louis, 2012, Saunders.)

Shock

Shock occurs when there is not enough blood and oxygen getting to the organs and tissues. It causes very low blood pressure. Shock usually happens with a serious injury and can be life-threatening.

There are several types of shock:

- *Anaphylactic*: Severe allergic reaction; caused by exposure to an allergen (e.g., insect bites/stings, food allergy, drug allergy).
- *Cardiogenic*: The damaged heart cannot pump blood effectively; caused by a heart attack, arrhythmias, pulmonary embolism, or congestive heart failure.
- *Hypovolemic*: Excessive loss of blood or body fluids from internal or external hemorrhage (bleeding); severe dehydration, burns, vomiting, or diarrhea.
- *Neurogenic*: Peripheral vessels dilate due to a neurologic injury or disorder (e.g., spinal cord injury).
- *Septic*: Overwhelming infection; caused by bacteria, fungi, and rarely viruses.

Signs and symptoms of shock include a weak rapid pulse and rapid shallow respirations; changes in the level of consciousness (e.g., confusion, lack of alertness, loss of consciousness); dizziness, lightheadedness, or faintness; sweaty, pale skin; cool hands and feet; bluish lips and fingernails; and decreased or no urine output.

Shock is diagnosed based on the history, exam, and vital signs of the patient. If time allows, additional testing may be done to identify the cause. The goals of medical treatment include increasing the cardiac output and blood pressure with medications and IV blood and fluids. Additional treatments address the cause of the shock.

Varicose Veins

Varicose veins are swollen, twisted veins seen under the skin, usually in the legs or rectum (hemorrhoids). This is a common disorder.

The cause is the one-way valves in the veins, which keeps blood flowing toward the heart. If the valves become weakened or damaged, the blood backs up or pools, leading to swollen or varicose veins. Risk factors include family history of varicose veins, prolong standing, heavy lifting, multiple pregnancies, and an increase in age. Signs and symptoms include dark purple or blue twisty veins; swelling; and feelings of heaviness, fullness, aching, pain, fatigue, or cramping.

The provider will examine the legs and feet (or other areas involved) during the physical exam. An ultrasound may be ordered to check the functioning of the vein valves. Treatment includes wearing compression stockings, exercising, losing weight, avoiding standing for long periods of time, and elevating legs. There are many other treatments for varicose veins:

- *Sclerotherapy:* Involves an injection of a substance that closes the vein and within a few weeks the varicose vein should fade.
- *Foam sclerotherapy:* Used for large veins and involves injecting a foam substance in the vein to close it.
- *Laser surgery:* Involves using a laser to close off small veins.
- *High ligation and vein stripping:* Involve tying off the vein and removing the vein through small incisions.

Additional Cardiovascular System Diseases

There are many cardiovascular diseases. The following provides a brief description of some of them:

- *Aneurysm*: Bulging of the arterial wall that can burst, causing bleeding and possible death of the blood vessel wall (Fig. 24.11). Most commonly seen aneurysms occur in the aorta (aortic aneurysm). A brain aneurysm that ruptures causes a stroke.
- *Cardiac tamponade*: Blood or fluid build up in the pericardial sac, causing pressure on the heart.
- *Endocarditis*: Also called infective endocarditis (IE). The inner lining of the heart is inflamed. Bacterial endocarditis is most common and can damage the valves.
- *Esophageal varices*: Enlarged veins in the esophagus that can rupture. Found in people with cirrhosis of the liver.
- *Metabolic syndrome*: A group of factors that increase a person's risk for heart disease, diabetes, and stroke. Having three of the five risk factors leads to the diagnosis: large waistline, high triglyceride level, low high-density lipoprotein (HDL) cholesterol level, high blood pressure, and high fasting blood sugar.
- *Pericarditis*: Inflammation of the pericardium.

- *Raynaud disease*: Rare blood vessel disorder, affecting the toes and fingers. With cold temperatures or stress, the blood vessels narrow, and blood cannot get to the surface of the skin. The toes and fingers affected turn white or blue (Fig. 24.12). When the blood flow returns, the skin is red and painful.

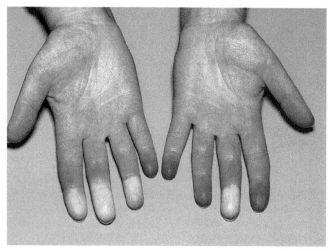

FIGURE 24.12 Raynaud disease. (From Hallett J, et al: *Comprehensive vascular and endovascular surgery*, ed 2, Philadelphia, 2009, Mosby.)

Blood-Related Disorders

Anemia

Anemia is a common blood disorder and occurs when the blood does not have enough healthy red blood cells (RBCs) or enough hemoglobin, which carries oxygen to the rest of the body. The cause of anemia depends on the type (Table 24.8). Usually, the body does not make enough RBCs, the destruction rate of RBCs is greater than the production rate, or the person is bleeding too quickly for the body to replace the RBCs. Signs and symptoms include weakness, fatigue, pale skin, arrhythmias, SOB, dizziness, lightheadedness, cold hands and feet, headache, and chest pain.

A physical exam and a CBC will be done. Additional tests may be done to rule out or confirm the type of anemia. Treatment is based on the type of anemia.

Hemophilia

Hemophilia is a genetic bleeding disorder that can lead to spontaneous bleeding. The mutation impacts the X chromosome. With men having one X chromosome, if it contains the mutation, that male will have hemophilia. If a female has two X chromosomes with the mutation, then she would have hemophilia, which happens rarely. If a female has only one X chromosome with the mutation, she will be a carrier of hemophilia. There are two types of hemophilia:

TABLE 24.8	Types of Anemias		
TYPE	**DESCRIPTION**	**ETIOLOGY**	**TREATMENT**
Aplastic anemia	Rare, life-threatening condition; the body does not produce enough RBCs	Caused by infections, certain medications, exposure to toxic chemicals, and autoimmune disorders	Blood transfusions, stem cell transplant, immunosuppressant medications, and bone marrow stimulants
Hemolytic anemia	Early destruction of RBCs occurs; bone marrow is not making enough RBCs to replace the destroyed RBCs	Autoimmune disorder, genetic RBC defect, infection, blood clots	Blood transfusions and treat the cause
Iron deficiency anemia	Most common form; not enough iron to make RBCs	Heavy menstrual periods, intestinal disease (e.g., Crohn disease, cancer), use of aspirin, ibuprofen, or arthritis medication, ulcers; not enough dietary iron	Iron supplements or iron medications
Sickle cell anemia	Inherited disorder that causes the RBCs to form a sickle (crescent) shape, get stuck in the blood vessels and break apart	Caused by a defected form of hemoglobin (hemoglobin S)	Manage and control the symptoms to prevent crises; folic acid supplements; blood transfusions, pain medications and fluids during crisis
Thalassemia	Inherited condition causing an abnormal form or inadequate amount of hemoglobin	Genetic condition	Blood transfusions and folate supplements
Vitamin B_{12}–deficiency anemia	A low RBC count due to a lack of vitamin B_{12}	Lack of dietary B_{12}, chronic alcoholism, Crohn disease, bariatric surgery, antacids	Depends on the cause; vitamin B_{12} supplements or monthly injections of vitamin B_{12}
Pernicious anemia	A type of vitamin B_{12}–deficiency anemia	Body destroys the cells that make intrinsic factor, which absorbs dietary vitamin B_{12} in the intestine	Monthly injections of vitamin B_{12}

- *Hemophilia A or classic hemophilia:* Caused by a lack or decrease of clotting factor VIII.
- *Hemophilia B or Christmas disease:* Caused by a lack or decrease of clotting factor IX.

About 20,000 males in the United States live with the disorder.

Hemophilia is caused by a mutation on a gene that provides information to make clotting factor proteins needed for making a blood clot. Signs and symptoms include bleeding within the joints, skin, mouth, nose, and gums. Blood can be in the urine or stool. Bleeding can occur after surgery or injury. Complications include chronic joint disease and pain, seizures, paralysis, and possible death.

If hemophilia runs in the family, the provider will test the male newborn. Blood clotting tests are performed and, if abnormal, clotting factor tests (factor assays) will be done. Treatment consists of infusing commercially prepared factor concentrates as a prophylaxis (prevention) or when bleeding occurs.

Idiopathic Thrombocytopenic Purpura

Idiopathic thrombocytopenic **purpura** (ITP) is also called immune thrombocytopenia and immune thrombocytopenic purpura. ITP is a rare autoimmune disease that results in the destruction of platelets.

The immune system produces antibodies that destroy platelets, thus causing ITP. In children, ITP sometimes occurs after a viral infection. In adults, ITP is a chronic disease that can occur after a viral infection, pregnancy, or *Helicobacter pylori*. The signs and symptoms include abnormally heavy menses, petechial rash (a rash with pinpoint red spots), easy bruising, nosebleeds, or bleeding.

After the physical exam, the provider will order a blood test to check the patient's platelet levels. A biopsy or bone marrow aspiration may also be done. Treatment for adults consists of steroids and immunosuppressant medications, high-dose gamma globulin infusions, drugs to stimulate the bone marrow, and a splenectomy.

Leukemia

Leukemia is cancer of the white blood cells. The bone marrow produces abnormal white blood cells. There are different types of leukemia (Table 24.9).

A specific type of WBCs is elevated, depending on the type of leukemia. The cause of leukemia varies according to the type. Some types advance quickly (e.g., acute), whereas chronic leukemia progresses slowly. The signs and symptoms depend on the type of leukemia.

After the examination, a blood test will be ordered. A bone marrow biopsy may also be done. Treatment for acute leukemia is more aggressive and consists of chemotherapy, radiation, and in some cases a splenectomy. With chronic leukemia, as the disease worsens, the patient may receive chemotherapy and radiation. Biologic therapy can also be used for leukemia. It boosts the body's natural ability to fight cancer. Targeted therapy may also be used, which uses substances that fight cancer cells, yet do not harm normal cells.

THE MEDICAL ASSISTANT'S ROLE IN CARDIOLOGY PROCEDURES

Assisting With the Examination

The cardiovascular examination begins with the medical assistant measuring the patient's height and weight, temperature, radial pulses, respirations, and blood pressure in both arms. Most cardiologists also want a complete list of the vitamins as well as the herbal, prescription, and over-the-counter (OTC) medications the patient is taking, including the strength and frequency of use for each.

A large part of the provider's examination focuses on subjective symptoms. The physical examination covers the chest, heart, and vascular systems. The patient's general appearance will be observed, as well as color of the skin, symmetry, temperature of the extremities, and breathing patterns. The veins in the neck may be examined for *distension* (enlargement). Using a stethoscope, the provider will listen to the lungs, for abnormal sounds that may indicate *congestion* (fluid in the lungs), and to the heart. A *murmur* (fluttering sound) is an abnormal heart sound. The provider may also use a doppler to check the pulses (Fig. 24.13). A *bruit* (blowing or swishing sound) can be heard over a carotid artery, aorta, or an organ and is caused by the blood flowing through a narrow artery.

TABLE 24.9	Type of Leukemia		
TYPE	DESCRIPTION	SIGNS AND SYMPTOMS	
Acute lymphocytic leukemia (ALL)	Also called acute lymphoblastic leukemia; most common cause of cancer in children. With ALL, there are too many lymphocytes (lymphoblasts).	Weakness, fever, bleeding, shortness of breath, and weight loss; bone, stomach, or rib pain; painless lumps in the underarm, neck, and stomach.	
Acute myeloid leukemia (AML)	Also called acute myelogenous leukemia; most common type of acute leukemia in adults. With AML, there are too many myeloblasts.	Fever, shortness of breath, bleeding, bruising, tiredness, weight loss.	
Chronic lymphocytic leukemia (CLL)	Second most common type of leukemia in adults. Occurs during middle age. With CLL, there are too many lymphocytes.	May not have symptoms. If present, may have painless swelling in the lymph nodes in the neck, stomach, groin, or underarm; fatigue, rib pain, fever, infection, and weight loss.	
Chronic myeloid leukemia (CML)	Also called chronic granulocytic or chronic myelogenous leukemia. With CML, there are too many granulocytes. A gene mutation called the Philadelphia chromosome is often seen.	May not have symptoms. If present, may have fatigue, fever, rib pain, night sweats, and weight loss.	

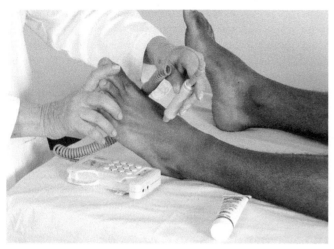

FIGURE 24.13 Using a Doppler to check the pulse. (From Jarvis C: *Physical examination and health assessment*, ed 7, St. Louis, 2016, Saunders.)

Assisting With Diagnostic Procedures

The medical assistant can support the provider by doing some diagnostic tests in the exam room. Obtaining the blood pressure in both arms and performing orthostatic vital signs are common procedures (see Procedure 24.1, p. 625). The medical assistant can also perform **electrocardiography** and Holter monitor testing, which are discussed in Chapter 11. Besides these procedures, assisting with scheduling and preparing patients for procedures outside of the department also fall into the medical assistant's scope of practice.

Tables 24.10 and 24.11 provide information on additional diagnostic procedures and tests. The medical assistant may need to screen the patient for specific allergies, medications, and so on prior to the scheduling of the procedure. For some procedures, a signed consent form is required. The patient should be notified of what he or she will experience during the procedure and any follow-up care required after the test.

TABLE 24.10	**Diagnostic Procedures for Cardiovascular Conditions**	
PROCEDURE	**DESCRIPTION**	**PATIENT PREPARATION**
Carotid ultrasound	Ultrasound of the carotid arteries on each side of the neck. Used to check for narrowed or blocked carotid arteries that can increase the risk of stroke.	Patient is asked to remove jewelry and clothing around the neck. The sonographer will apply warm gel to the neck and gently press a transducer along the neck.
Electrocardiography	Ten electrodes are placed on the chest and extremities. A tracing of the heart rhythm is obtained while the patient rests on the exam table.	Patient is asked to remove jewelry and clothing above the waist. No discomfort is felt during the quick test.
Exercise stress test	Electrodes are placed on the body and monitor the heart rhythm while the person exercises on a treadmill or exercise bicycle. The blood pressure is also monitored during the test.	The patient should dress for exercise. Food, drink, and nicotine are restricted 3 or more hours before the test, and no caffeine is allowed for 24 hours prior to the test. A consent form needs to be completed. Patient should let the provider know if any chest discomfort or pain, dizziness, palpitations, or shortness of breath occur during the test.
Holter monitor	Electrodes are placed on the body and record the heart rhythm for usually 24 hours. The patient also keeps a diary of activities during the test.	Patient is asked to remove jewelry and clothing above the waist. Electrodes are applied to the chest. The patient receives information on how to complete the journal and use the monitor for the study.
Nuclear stress test	Nuclear imaging test that shows blood flow into the heart at rest and with activity. Many names for the test, which reflect the substance given (e.g., sestamibi stress test).	Caffeine is restricted 24 hours before test. The patient should dress for exercise (if treadmill will be used). During the test, a radioactive substance (e.g., thallium or sestamibi) is given IV. A camera takes pictures while patient is at rest and then with activity or with medication that simulates activity by increasing the heart rate.
Nuclear ventriculography	A nuclear medicine test; a small amount of tracer (radioactive substance) is injected. X-ray video (fluoroscopy) shows the heart in motion and can measure the amount of blood pumped with each heartbeat (ejection fraction). Test is known by many names, including radionuclide angiogram (RNA), cardiac blood pooling scan, nuclear heart scan, multiple-gated acquisition (MUGA) scan, and radionuclide ventriculography.	Screen patient for allergies, pacemaker, breast-feeding, and pregnancy. A consent form needs to be signed. Tobacco, caffeine, food, and fluids may be restricted for 3 to 4 hours. During the procedure, an IV line is inserted, and the tracer is injected. A gamma camera takes continuous pictures of the heart. After the test, the patient must drink plenty of fluids for 2 days.

TABLE 24.11   Medical Laboratory Tests for Cardiovascular Conditions

TEST	DESCRIPTION
CLIA-waived tests	Done to diagnose and monitor disease: • *Cholesterol testing:* for heart disease. • *Prothrombin testing:* for anticoagulant therapy and heart disease.
Cardiac enzymes test	Blood test that measures the number of cardiac enzymes characteristically released during a heart attack (myocardial infarction); determines the amount of lactate dehydrogenase (LDH) and creatine phosphokinase (CPK) in the blood.
Lipid profile	Blood test to measure the lipids (cholesterol and triglycerides) in the circulating blood.

Angiography

Angiography is used to study blood vessels and to detect occlusions, aneurysms, and structural defects. The procedure uses x-rays, computed tomography (CT), or magnetic resonance imaging (MRI) with contrast medium. The contrast medium makes the blood vessel become visible on the x-ray images.

For regular angiography, the patient may be NPO (nothing by mouth) midnight before the procedure. During the procedure, an intravenous (IV) line may be inserted and sedative given to help relax the patient. The heart and blood pressure may be monitored during the procedure. After the area (e.g., groin) is shaved and cleansed, a small incision is made. A catheter is threaded into the blood vessel (e.g., femoral or carotid arteries) and advanced to the area that will be studied. Radiopaque contrast medium is injected to make the blood vessel appear on the x-ray. The patient may experience a burning or warming sensation in the location where the medium is given. A series of x-rays are taken. Some treatments can be done during the angiography. After the procedure, the patient is monitored as the medication wears off. The incision is monitored for bleeding. The patient needs to drink plenty of fluids to flush the dye from the body.

There are several types of angiography, including the following:
- *Arteriography:* A type of angiography that involves the study of arteries.
- *Cerebral angiography:* Used to detect blood clots, aneurysms, and other vascular conditions in the brain.
- *Coronary angiography:* A series of x-rays are taken of the heart. The catheter can also monitor the blood pressure in the heart. Coronary angiography is part of a group of procedures known as cardiac catheterization, which will be discussed in a following section.
- *Pulmonary angiography:* This test is used to evaluate the pulmonary artery for blood circulation conditions (e.g., pulmonary embolism).

A computed tomography angiography (CTA) and a magnetic resonance angiography (MRA) differ from a regular angiography. They are noninvasive and do not require recovery time, though no treatments can be done during the procedure. To prepare, caffeinated beverages may be restricted 12 hours before the test, and the patient may not eat for 4 hours before the test. The patient can drive before and after the test. A patient may receive a beta-blocker to slow the heartbeat or nitroglycerin to dilate the coronary arteries, making the images clearer. During the procedure, the contrast medium is given intravenously. Electrodes are placed on the patient's chest to monitor the heart during the procedure. After the test, the patient can resume normal activities, though it is important to increase the fluids consumed in order to flush the contrast medium from the body.

Cardiac Catheterization

Cardiac catheterization is a procedure to diagnose and treat certain heart diseases. The patient preparation is similar to that for an angiography, though the patient may be restricted from eating and drinking for a longer period of time.

During the cardiac catheterization, a regular coronary angiography is done. The catheter is inserted in an artery in the groin and threaded to the heart (Fig. 24.14). The contrast medium is injected, and narrowed or blocked arteries can be observed. The provider can also measure pressure, blood flow, and oxygen amounts in the chambers and large arteries. Blood samples and biopsies can be collected.

Based on what is found during the catheterization, the provider may also treat the condition. These treatments may include the following:
- *Repair of congenital heart defects*
- *Angioplasty:* A treatment to open narrowed blood vessels by expanding a small balloon at the site, which widens the vessel; a stent (small metal coil) may be inserted to help keep the vessel opened (Fig. 24.15)
- *Replacement or repair of a heart valve*
- *Balloon valvuloplasty:* A treatment to open narrowed heart valves, using a catheter with a balloon
- *Ablation:* A treatment for arrhythmias that involves using a catheter with heat (radiofrequency energy or laser) or cold (nitrous oxide) to destroy abnormal tissue causing the arrhythmias

Doppler Ultrasound

The Doppler ultrasound exam provides information on the blood flow in the arms and legs. This test is used to help diagnose **arteriosclerosis**, arterial occlusion (from blood clots), peripheral artery disease, aneurysms, arterial stenosis, and venous insufficiency. There is no special preparation for this test. The patient needs to remove clothing on the extremity being tested.

During the test, the sonographer applies gel to the extremity and places a handheld transducer on the patient. The transducer directs ultrasound waves (high-frequency sound waves) over the vein or artery being checked, and the waves bounce off the circulating RBCs. This test helps to estimate the blood flow through the vein or artery.

A simple handheld Doppler can often be used in the exam room to check the pulses in the extremities. An absent pulse means there is no blood flow through the artery, which is a medical emergency. With training, a medical assistant can use a handheld Doppler to check the pulses.

Echocardiography

An echocardiogram is a sonographic test that uses sound waves to create pictures of the heart structures. It shows the heart beating and the heart valves and other structures in motion.

Most people have a transthoracic echocardiogram (TTE). There is no special preparation for this test. The patient must remove any clothing and jewelry from the waist up and lie on the exam table in a supine position. A trained echocardiogram sonographer spreads warmed gel over the patient's chest and then moves a transducer slowly over the chest (Fig. 24.16). The transducer releases high-frequency sound waves and picks up the waves. The waves are transmitted as electrical impulses that are converted by the echocardiography machine into moving pictures. During the process, the sonographer can take still pictures of the heart's structures.

A transesophageal echocardiogram (TEE) is done less often, and it requires the patient to not eat or drink for several hours before the test. The patient may be given a sedative for the procedure. The patient's throat is numbed before the provider guides a probe (a long flexible tube) with a small ultrasound transducer down the throat and to the stomach. The TEE can get clearer echocardiographic images of the heart than the TTE can.

Assisting With Treatments

Patients with cardiovascular disorders are prescribed a variety of medications. The following are some of the more common classifications of medications:

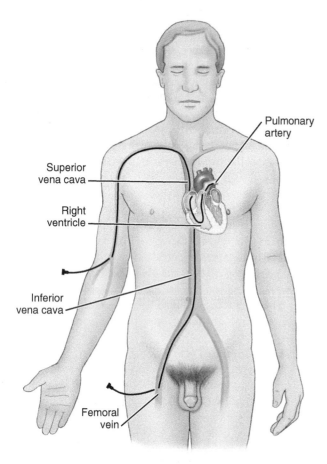

FIGURE 24.14 Cardiac catheterization. The catheter is inserted in the femoral or brachial vein and then is advanced through the right atrium and ventricle, into the pulmonary artery. (From Shiland B: *Medical terminology and anatomy for ICD-10 coding,* ed 2, St. Louis, 2016, Mosby.)

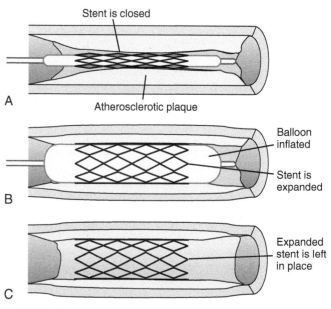

FIGURE 24.15 Angioplasty with stent placement. (From LaFleur Brooks M: *Exploring medical language,* ed 9, St. Louis, 2014, Mosby.)

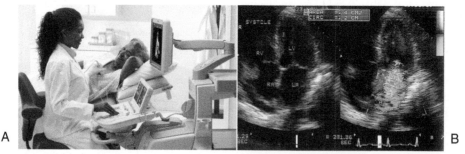

FIGURE 24.16 Person undergoing echocardiography (ECHO). (From Frank ED, Long BW, Smith BJ: *Merrill's atlas of radiographic positions and radiologic procedures,* ed 12, St. Louis, 2012, Mosby.)

- *Antiarrhythmics:* Used to treat arrhythmias
- *Anticoagulants:* Used to prevent blood clots from forming
- *Antihypertensives:* Used to lower and control the blood pressure; several categories include the following:
  - *Beta-blockers:* Reduce the heart rate, the workload, and the output of the heart.
  - *Angiotensin-converting enzyme* (ACE) *inhibitors:* Decrease angiotensin production, which causes blood vessels to dilate
  - *Angiotensin II receptor antagonists:* Block the effects of angiotensin and blood vessels dilate
  - *Calcium channel blockers:* Prevent calcium from entering the heart and arteries' smooth muscles; decrease contraction force, dilate blood vessels, and reduce heart rate
  - *Alpha blockers:* Dilate arteries
- *Antiplatelets:* Post treatment of stroke, heart attack, or angina
- *Cholesterol lowering agents:* Reduce low-density lipoprotein (LDL) and triglycerides; increase high-density lipoprotein (HDL)
- *Diuretics:* Increase urinary output and lower the blood pressure
- *Hematopoietics:* Treat anemia in patients undergoing chemotherapy
- *Hemostatics:* Control acute or chronic blood-clotting disorder; promote formation of absorbable, artificial clot

Refer to Table 24.12, Medication Classification, for information on the classification, including indications for use, desired effect, side effects, adverse reactions, and generic and trade names. Medical assistants should be familiar with medications that are prescribed to patients.

Pacemakers and Implantable Cardioverter-Defibrillators

A pacemaker uses low-energy electrical pulses to assist the heart when arrhythmias, tachycardia, or bradycardia occurs. There are two types of pacemakers:

- *Temporary pacemaker:* Used in an emergency until the permanent pacemaker can be placed. Also used for temporary conditions (e.g., heart attack and medication overdose).
- *Permanent pacemaker:* Surgically inserted into the chest or abdomen (Fig. 24.17). Patients can use technology (e.g., smart phones) to transmit their pacemaker data to their provider.

An implantable cardioverter-defibrillator (ICD) is similar to a pacemaker in that it uses low-energy electrical pulses to treat arrhythmias. However, ICDs differ from pacemakers because they can also use high-energy pulses when a life-threatening arrhythmia occurs.

TABLE 24.12	Medication Classifications	
CLASSIFICATION	**INFORMATION**	**GENERIC NAME (TRADE NAME)**
Antiarrhythmic	**Indications for use:** Arrhythmias. **Desired effects:** helps the heart work better, controls heart rate. **Side effects and adverse reactions:** arrhythmias, weight gain, difficulty breathing, swelling of hands and feet.	• **amiodarone** (Cordarone, Pacerone) • **procainamide** • **flecainide** (Tambocor) • **digoxin** (Lanoxin, Digitek, Cardoxin)
Anticoagulants	**Indication for use:** Prevent blood clots from forming. **Desired effects:** Decrease blood-clotting ability. **Side effects and adverse reactions:** Increased bleeding; blood irregularities; hypersensitivity	• **heparin** • **enoxaparin** (Lovenox) • **dabigatran** (Pradaxa) • **warfarin** (Coumadin, Jantoven) • **rivaroxaban** (Xarelto)
Antihypertensives	**Indications for use:** Reduce and control blood pressure. **Desired effects:** Lowers blood pressure **Side effects and adverse reactions:** Headache, vertigo, GI disturbances, rash, hypotension, nonproductive cough	*Beta-blockers:* • **propranolol** (Inderal) • **atenolol** (Tenormin) *Angiotensin-converting enzyme (ACE) inhibitors:* • **quinapril** (Accupril) • **benazepril** (Lotensin) • **lisinopril** • **metoprolol** (Lopressor) • **carvedilol** (Coreg) *Angiotensin II receptor antagonists:* • **losartan** (Cozaar) • **valsartan** (Diovan) *Calcium channel blockers:* • **diltiazem** (Cardizem, Cartia, Tiazac) • **amlodipine** (Norvasc) *Alpha blockers:* • **doxazosin** (Cardura)

Continued

TABLE 24.12   Medication Classifications—*continued*

CLASSIFICATION	INFORMATION	GENERIC NAME (TRADE NAME)
Antiplatelets	**Indications for use:** Post treatment of stroke, heart attack or angina. **Desired effect:** Inhibit the function of platelets (the formation of clots). **Side effects and adverse reactions:** GI distress, bleeding, weakness or numbness	• **clopidogrel** (Plavix)
Cholesterol lowering agents	**Indications for use:** Reduce low-density lipoprotein (LDL) and triglycerides; increase high-density lipoprotein (HDL). **Desired effects:** Prevents absorption of cholesterol in the intestine. **Side effects and adverse reactions:** GI discomfort, muscle pain and weakness, liver complications, hypersensitivity, cataracts, myopathy.	• **ezetimibe** (Vytorin, Zetia) • **atorvastatin** (Lipitor) • **rosuvastatin** (Crestor) • **simvastatin** (Zocor)
Diuretics	**Indications for use:** Increase urinary output; lower blood pressure. **Desired effects:** Inhibit reabsorption of sodium and chloride in the kidneys; promote excretion of excess fluid in the body. **Side effects and adverse reactions:** Dehydration, muscle weakness, fatigue, electrolyte imbalance.	• **triamterene** (Dyrenium) • **furosemide** (Lasix) • **hydrochlorothiazide** (HCTZ) (Microzide, Oretic)
Hematopoietics	**Indication for use:** Treat anemia in patients undergoing chemotherapy. **Desired effect:** Promote blood cell production. **Side effects and adverse reactions:** Headache, arthralgia, nausea, hypertension, diarrhea.	• **pegfilgrastim** (Neulasta)
Hemostatics	**Indications for use:** Control acute or chronic blood-clotting disorder; promote formation of absorbable, artificial clot. **Desired effects:** Control bleeding; act as a blood coagulant (clots blood). **Side effects and adverse reactions:** Hypersensitivity reactions, transient flushing, dizziness; newborn hyperbilirubinemia.	• **phytonadione** (Vitamin K)

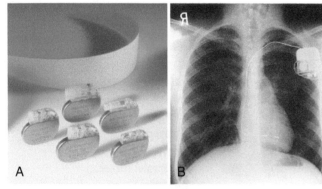

FIGURE 24.17 (A) Pacemakers. **(B)** Chest x-ray of a patient with a permanent implanted pacemaker. (From Frank ED, Long BW, Smith BJ: *Merrill's atlas of radiographic positions and radiologic procedures,* ed 12, St. Louis, 2012, Mosby.)

Patients with a pacemaker or ICD need to have the device checked on a routine basis. The batteries usually last 5 to 7 years, and a replacement requires a surgical procedure. When using a pacemaker or ICD, the person needs to stay away from magnets and strong electrical fields. This would include devices such as iPods, cell phones, microwaves, MRIs, power-generating equipment, and some metal detectors for screening. They should carry identification that indicates they have a pacemaker or an ICD.

CLOSING COMMENTS

Patient Coaching

Heart disease and stroke account for more than one-third of all deaths in the United States. Genetics, predisposition, and lifestyle factors, such as smoking, lack of exercise, and poor diet, play significant roles in the development of heart disease. Successful management of cardiovascular disease requires major lifestyle changes for most patients. The medical assistant can help by providing encouragement and support and by using community resources to help the patient find assistance with these changes.

Sources for information include the American Heart Association (www.heart.org), Nutrition.gov (www.nutrition.gov), United States Department of Agriculture (USDA) ChooseMyPlate.gov (www.chosemyplate.gov), local workshops and conferences, and reputable Internet sites.

Because many patients learn best through visual aids, providing them with pictures, brochures, and pamphlets is an effective means of helping them in this learning process. Always document education interventions so that the provider or medical assistant can clarify or expand upon the information on a return visit.

Legal and Ethical Issues

Diagnostic procedures can have a marked effect on the patient's treatment. When entrusted with performing testing procedures, the medical assistant assumes responsibility for the test's accuracy and for performing the test precisely. This is an important role because the results submitted could strongly influence the plan of treatment.

Patient-Centered Care

Two important aspects of patient-centered care are information and education. Many of the more common cardiovascular diseases require patients to be on medication for treatment. It is important that patients know the following:

- Name of the medication
- Reason for the medication
- Side effects/adverse reactions to report to the provider

When a patient is put on a new medication, providing information on the medication is important. The medical assistant should review the information with the patient. Also, giving the patient a handout to take home and a phone number to call if questions arise promotes patient-centered care.

Professional Behaviors

Critical thinking is a crucial part of professional behavior. The ability to question patients logically and comprehensively about possible cardiac signs and symptoms can greatly contribute to high-quality care. The provider relies on the medical assistant for initial information about the patient. Given the seriousness of cardiac conditions, the medical assistant must use his or her knowledge about the topic to gather and analyze the patient's comments so that the provider is better prepared to make an accurate diagnosis and develop an effective treatment plan.

SUMMARY OF SCENARIO

As the weeks followed, Lizzy became more independent in the practicum. She was very excited to interview for a medical assistant position in a cardiology department in a nearby city. During her last day with Rebecca, they celebrated her completion of the practicum. Lizzy shared that she was offered the medical assistant position, which she accepted.

In the weeks that followed Lizzy's last day, Rebecca thought about all the information she shared with Lizzy. She realized that she too had learned a lot from the practicum experience and found that she really enjoyed mentoring students. Rebecca plans to talk with her supervisor about future opportunities to mentor students in the department.

SUMMARY OF LEARNING OBJECTIVES

1. **Describe the anatomy of the cardiovascular system.**
   The cardiovascular system is a closed system that includes the following:
   - Blood vessels, consisting of arteries, arterioles, capillaries, venules, and veins that act as pipes to carry the blood around the body
   - A heart, which pumps the blood
   - Blood, which contains the nutrients for the cells and the waste products to be excreted

   The heart, which is the size of a fist, is a complex muscular organ that pumps blood around the body. It is located in the mediastinum of the thoracic cavity, slightly left of the midline. The *apex* (pointed tip) of the heart rests just above the diaphragm. The heart has two sets of chambers, the atria and ventricles. The septum divides the heart into a right and left section. The heart wall is composed of three layers: the endocardium, the myocardium, and the epicardium.

2. **Explain the pulmonary and systemic circulations.**
   Pulmonary circulation begins as the blood returns from the body. The superior vena cava and the inferior vena cava bring deoxygenated blood from the body to the right atrium. The blood passes the tricuspid valve and empties into the right ventricle. When the ventricles contract, the blood in the right ventricle is pushed out past the pulmonary valve and enters the pulmonary artery trunk, which splits into the

   right and left pulmonary arteries. In the lungs, gas exchange occurs and oxygenated blood returns to the lungs by the right and left pulmonary veins.

   Then the systemic circulation starts. The oxygenated blood in the left atrium moves past the bicuspid or mitral valve and empties into the left ventricle, before passing the aortic valve and emptying into the aorta. From here, the blood will move through the body before it returns to the heart. Blood from the head, neck, and upper extremities empties into the superior vena cava before returning to the right atrium. Blood from the lower body empties into the inferior vena cava before returning to the right atrium.

3. **Describe coronary circulation, hepatic portal circulation, and fetal circulation.**
   The coronary veins remove waste products from the heart tissue, and the coronary arteries bring nutrients and oxygen to the heart tissue. The liver has a special role in filtering the blood and metabolizes or breaks down substances.

   The umbilical cord contains two umbilical arteries and one umbilical vein. The arteries carry the fetal blood to the placenta. The umbilical vein carries oxygen and nutrient-rich blood to the baby. The waste, oxygen, and nutrient exchange occurs in the placenta. Other structures that are unique to the growing baby include the following:

Continued

- *Ductus venosus*: Shifts the majority of the blood from the umbilical vein and empties it into the inferior vena cava, thus bypassing the immature liver
- *Foramen ovale*: A small flaplike opening in the interatrial septum that allows blood to move from the right atrium to the left atrium, thus bypassing the immature lungs
- *Ductus arteriosus*: A short vessel that connects the pulmonary artery with the aorta, and most of the blood is redirected from the pulmonary artery to the aorta, thus bypassing the immature lungs

4. **Explain the components in blood, and discuss blood types.**
   Blood is made up of two components:
   - *Liquid portion*: Plasma is the liquid portion of whole blood; it also contains plasma proteins (e.g., albumin, globulins, clotting factors, and complement), inorganic substances, electrolytes, organic substances, and waste products
   - *Formed elements*: Includes red blood cells (RBCs), white blood cells (WBCs), and platelets

   The two major classification systems for blood typing are the ABO system and the Rh system. With the ABO system, each person has the A, B, ABO, or O blood type. With the Rh system, a person is either Rh-positive or Rh-negative.

5. **Describe life span changes related to the cardiovascular system.**
   As a child grows and matures, the heart rate decreases. The systemic vascular resistance increases with age. This means that the resistance for blood flow increases, and thus the blood pressure increases with age. As a person ages, the heart and blood vessels undergo changes. Heart changes that occur include a loss of some SA node cells and an increase in the left ventricle size. Normal ECG changes can occur with age. Valves can become thicker and stiffer, causing a heart murmur. Arterial walls become stiffer, thus increasing the blood pressure.

6. **Describe the conduction system of the heart, including the three states of a cardiac cell.**
   The electrical cells in the SA node generate the impulse that starts the heartbeat. When the SA node discharges the impulse, it travels in many directions through the heart muscle. The Bachmann bundle, a specialized internodal tract, takes the impulse to the left atrium. Other internodal tracts take the impulse quickly to the atrioventricular (AV) node. In the AV node, the impulse moves very slowly and then it moves to the bundle of His. After the impulse passes through the bundle of His, it enters the right and left bundle branches. The right bundle branch brings the impulse to the right ventricle. The left bundle branch brings the impulse to the left ventricle. The bundle branches split into many Purkinje fibers.
   The cardiac cells cycle through three states or steps in the same sequence for each impulse:
   - *Polarized state*: Before the impulse hits the cells, they are in a polarized or "waiting" state.
   - *Depolarized state*: When the impulse hits the cells, the cells' charges change. The change of the cells' charges allows the impulse to move through the cell, causing *action potential*, also called depolarization.
   - *Repolarized state*: After the impulse passes over the cell, the ions move back to their original location. This causes the cell's charge to change. This recovery phase is called the repolarized state.

7. **Describe factors that influence blood pressure.**
   - *Blood volume*: The amount of circulating blood has a direct influence on blood pressure. The greater the blood volume, the more force it makes on the arterial walls. If the blood volume is low, less force or pressure will be on the arterial walls.
   - *Strength of ventricular contractions*: The greater the force of the contraction, the more blood is pumped into the arteries. This increases the blood pressure. If the left ventricular contraction is weak, less blood is pumped out of the heart and thus the blood pressure is lower.
   - *Resistance to blood flow*: Any factor that increases the resistance for blood to flow through the arteries will increase the blood pressure. Factors that increase resistance include the size of the lumen of the arteries, the elasticity of the arterial walls, and the viscosity of the blood.

8. **List common signs and symptoms of cardiovascular disorders.**
   Common signs and symptoms include angina, bradycardia, tachycardia, palpitation, cyanosis, pallor, dyspnea, orthopnea, shortness of breath, diaphoresis, edema, and syncope.

9. **Identify disorders of the cardiovascular system, list risk factors for heart disease, and describe the types of shock.**
   This chapter discussed the following diseases:
   - *Cardiovascular disorders*: arrhythmias, atherosclerosis-related diseases (carotid artery disease, coronary heart disease, coronary microvascular disease, peripheral artery disease, and chronic kidney disease), cardiomyopathy, congenital heart defects (atrial septal defect, atrioventricular septal defect, coarctation of the aorta, dextro-transposition of the great arteries, patent foramen ovale, patent ductus arteriosus, pulmonary atresia, tetralogy of Fallot, and ventricular septal defect), congestive heart failure (right-sided heart failure, left-sided heart failure, and cor pulmonale), deep vein thrombosis, heart valve disease (stenosis and insufficiency can impact all valves; examples of diseases include aortic insufficiency, mitral valve prolapses, and rheumatic fever), hypertension (primary hypertension, secondary hypertension, and malignant hypertension), myocardial infarction, postural orthostatic tachycardia syndrome, shock, and varicose veins
   - *Blood disorders*: Anemia (aplastic anemia, hemolytic anemia, iron deficiency anemia, sickle cell anemia, thalassemia, vitamin B_{12} deficiency anemia, and pernicious anemia), hemophilia, idiopathic thrombocytopenic purpura, and leukemia (acute lymphocytic leukemia, acute myeloid leukemia, chronic lymphocytic leukemia, and chronic myeloid leukemia)

   Risk factors for heart disease that cannot be changed include age, gender, genetics, and race. Risk factors that can be changed are smoking, high cholesterol, high blood pressure, uncontrolled diabetes, lack of exercise, obesity, stress, and alcohol.

There are several types of shock:

- *Anaphylactic*: Severe allergic reaction; caused by exposure to an allergen.
- *Cardiogenic*: The damaged heart cannot pump blood effectively.
- *Hypovolemic*: Excessive loss of blood or body fluids from internal or external hemorrhage.
- *Neurogenic*: Peripheral vessels dilate due to a neurologic injury or disorder.
- *Septic*: Overwhelming infection.

10. **Discuss the medical assistant's role in assisting with the cardiology examination.**

   The cardiovascular examination begins with the medical assistant measuring the patient's height and weight, temperature, radial pulses, respirations, and blood pressure in both arms. A large part of the provider's examination focuses on subjective symptoms.

11. **Describe cardiovascular diagnostic procedures, including angiography, cardiac catheterization, Doppler ultrasound, and echocardiography.**

   - *Angiography*: A study of the blood vessels. The procedure uses x-rays, computed tomography (CT), or magnetic resonance imaging (MRI) with contrast medium. The contrast medium makes the blood vessel become visible on the x-ray images. The invasive procedure includes a catheter being inserted and guided to the location being examined.

The noninvasive procedure involves a CT or MRI with contrast medium.

   - *Cardiac catheterization*: An angiography procedure is done. Based on the patient's diagnosis, treatment for certain heart diseases can be done during the catheterization.
   - *Doppler ultrasound*: Provides information on the blood flow in the arms and legs. During the test, the sonographer applies gel to the extremity and places a handheld transducer on the patient. The transducer directs ultrasound waves (high-frequency sound waves) over the vein or artery being checked, and the waves bounce off the circulating RBCs. This test helps to estimate the blood flow through the vein or artery.
   - *Echocardiogram*: A sonographic test that uses sound waves to create pictures of the heart structures. It shows the heart beating and the heart valves and other structures in motion.

12. **Describe cardiovascular treatments, including a pacemaker and an implantable cardioverter-defibrillator.**

   A pacemaker uses low-energy electrical pulses to assist the heart when arrythmias, tachycardia, or bradycardia occurs. There are two types of pacemakers: a temporary pacemaker and a permanent pacemaker. An implantable cardioverter-defibrillator (ICD) is similar to a pacemaker in that it uses low-energy electrical pulses to treat arrhythmias. However, ICDs differ from pacemakers because they can also use high-energy pulses when a life-threatening arrhythmia occurs.

PROCEDURE 24.1   Measuring Orthostatic Vital Signs

Task: Obtain orthostatic vital signs. Document results in the patient's health record.

EQUIPMENT and SUPPLIES

- Sphygmomanometer and stethoscope or digital blood pressure monitor
- Watch

Scenario: Dr. Walden ordered orthostatic vital signs to be completed on Erma Willis (date of birth [DOB] 12/09/1947). She has had episodes of dizziness and lightheadedness with standing up. Role-play this scenario with a peer.

PROCEDURAL STEPS

1. Wash hands or use hand sanitizer.
   PURPOSE: Hand sanitization is an important step for infection control.
2. Greet the patient. Identify yourself. Verify the patient's identity with full name and date of birth. Explain the procedure to be performed in a manner that the patient understands. Answer any questions the patient may have about the procedure.
   PURPOSE: It is important to identify the patient in two different ways to ensure that you have the correct patient. Explaining the procedure can make the patient feel more comfortable and reduces anxiety.

3. Assist the patient onto the exam table, and have patient lie down for 5 minutes.
   PURPOSE: For this procedure, the patient needs to rest on the exam table for 5 minutes.
4. After 5 minutes, accurately obtain the patient's blood pressure and pulse rate. Keep the cuff on the patient. Write down the vital signs, and indicate the patient's position and time.
   PURPOSE: It is necessary to establish a baseline resting blood pressure and pulse.
5. Assist the patient into a standing position, and note the time. Ask the patient if he or she has any lightheadedness or dizziness. Continue to check with the patient throughout the procedure.
   PURPOSE: Lightheadedness or dizziness are considered abnormal during the procedure. They should be noted and reported to the provider.
6. After 1 minute of standing, accurately obtain the patient's blood pressure and pulse rate. Write down the vital signs, and indicate the patient's position and time.
   PURPOSE: Changes in the vital signs after 1 minute of standing can indicate orthostatic hypotension.

Continued

PROCEDURE 24.1   **Measuring Orthostatic Vital Signs**—*continued*

7. After 3 minutes of standing, accurately obtain the patient's blood pressure and pulse rate. Write down the vital signs, and indicate the patient's position and time.
   <u>PURPOSE</u>: Between the first and the last set of vital signs, a drop in blood pressure ≥ 20 mm Hg or a drop in the diastolic BP ≥ 10 mm Hg can indicate orthostatic hypotension.

8. Assist the patient to the chair or exam table, if he or she is not dizzy. If the patient is dizzy, have the patient lie on the exam table.
   <u>PURPOSE</u>: The patient could fall if he or she is sitting on the exam table and has an episode of dizziness or lightheadedness.

9. Wash hands or use hand sanitizer.

10. Accurately document the vital signs in the patient's health record. Include the name of the provider ordering the test, the patient's position, and the length of time in the position. Specify the arm used to check the blood pressure.
   <u>PURPOSE</u>: For the procedure to be considered done, it must be documented.

06/23/20XX 1420 Per Dr. Walden's order, orthostatic vital signs obtained. After resting on the exam table for 5 minutes: BP 142/76, right arm, laying; P 78, regular, strong. After 1 minute of standing: BP 134/70, right arm, standing; P 86, regular, strong. After 3 minutes of standing: BP 128/62, right arm, standing; P 94, regular, strong. No complaints of lightheadedness or dizziness. Patient lying on the exam table resting. _____
_____ Rebecca White, CMA (AAMA)

25

PULMONOLOGY

Renee Thomas, a certified medical assistant (CMA) through the American Association of Medical Assistants (AAMA), was hired 6 months ago. She assists the specialists who hold outreach clinics at Walden-Martin Family Medical (WMFM) Clinic. On Tuesdays the pulmonologist from a local larger city comes for a pulmonary outreach clinic. The pulmonologist brings his own equipment and one medical assistant, John.

Renee's job is to help the pulmonology medicine team because she knows the WMFM Clinic and the local community resources. Renee studied the anatomy and physiology of the respiratory system during her medical assistant training. She learned about common diseases, but she found that she has a lot more to learn. Besides obtaining patients' vital signs and medical histories, Renee does a pulse oximetry measurement on most of her patients. She has observed John performing a spirometry test, which she will learn to do in the future.

In her work with the pulmonologist and John, Renee sees patients with many interesting respiratory diseases. She continues to learn from her work with the specialist and the patients.

While studying this chapter, think about the following questions:
- What structures are in the upper and lower tracts of the respiratory system? What occurs during the ventilation process?
- What are the common pathologic conditions of the pulmonary system?
- What medical terms must Renee know to identify and explain these patient disorders?
- What diagnostic and treatment procedures typically are ordered for patients with pulmonary disease?
- What are the medical assistant's primary responsibilities in working with patients with pulmonary problems?
- What clinical skills are required in this specialty practice?

LEARNING OBJECTIVES

1. Describe the organs of the respiratory system, including their function and anatomical location, and compare the structure and function of the respiratory system across the life span.
2. Discuss the physiology of the respiratory system, and explain the process of ventilation.
3. Discuss common chronic and acute respiratory system disorders, including signs, symptoms, etiology, diagnostic procedures, and treatments. In addition, discuss the hazards of using tobacco products, including cigarettes, smokeless tobacco, and e-cigarettes (vaping).
4. Discuss the medical assistant's role in pulmonary procedures, including assisting with examination and diagnostic procedures such as measuring the peak flow rate and performing spirometry.
5. Describe pulmonary treatments, including metered-dose inhalers, nebulizer treatments, and oxygen therapy.

VOCABULARY

accessory muscles Muscles in the neck, abdomen, and back that assist in breathing.

analgesic (an ahl JEE zik) A drug that reduces or eliminates pain.

antipyretic (an tee pie RET ik) A drug that is used to reduce a fever.

bronchodilator A drug that relaxes smooth muscle contractions in the bronchioles to improve lung ventilation.

corticosteroids (kor ti koe STER oids) A group of steroid hormones produced in the body or given as a medication. Some have metabolic functions, and others reduce tissue inflammation. Glucocorticoids and mineralocorticoids are two types.

decongestant A drug that is used for nasal congestion.

diaphragm (DIE uh fram) A broad, dome-shaped muscle used for breathing. It separates the thoracic and abdominopelvic cavities.

expiration Exhaling; movement of waste gases from the alveoli into the atmosphere.

inspiration Inhaling; movement of O_2 from the atmosphere into the alveoli.

intercostal (in tur KOS tul) muscles Muscles located between the ribs that help with quiet respiration.

paranasal sinuses (pair uh NAY zul SIE nus suhs) Hollow, air-filled cavities in the skull and facial bones. They lighten the weight of the skull and increase the tone, or resonance, of speech.

pharyngitis Inflammation or infection of the pharynx, usually causing the symptoms of a sore throat.

productive cough A cough that produces phlegm or mucus.

pulmonary hypertension High blood pressure that affects the pulmonary system (pulmonary arteries and the right side of the heart).

respiratory arrest Stoppage of breathing.

sputum Mucous secretion coughed up from the lungs and expectorated through the mouth.

surfactant (sur FACK tunt) A mixture of protein and fats that lines the alveoli and prevents the tissues from sticking together and collapsing during exhalation.

thoracentesis (thor ah sen TEE sis) Aspiration of a fluid from the pleural cavity.

Pulmonology is the healthcare specialty that deals with respiratory disorders. A *pulmonologist* is a specialist involved in the diagnosis, treatment, and prevention of disorders of the respiratory system.

Pulmonary procedures and treatments are common in the ambulatory care area. Besides the pulmonary department, patients with respiratory concerns are typically seen in primary care and urgent care departments. Medical assistants measure peak flow rates, perform spirometry, and assist with pulmonary treatments. Nebulizer treatments and oxygen therapy are the most frequent pulmonary treatments in ambulatory care.

ANATOMY OF THE RESPIRATORY SYSTEM

The respiratory system is divided into the upper respiratory tract and the lower respiratory tract. The upper respiratory tract structures are considered passageways for the air, whereas the lower respiratory tract structures are involved in gas exchange.

Upper Respiratory Tract

The upper respiratory tract is composed of structures from the nose to the larynx. These organs are located outside the chest cavity. The main functions of the upper respiratory tract include warming and cleaning the inspired air, serving as a passageway for air, and providing the sense of smell.

Air can enter through the mouth or the two nares (nostrils) in the nose. The nasal septum separates the nares. The air then moves into the nasal cavity. The surface capillaries, mucous membrane, and cilia (small hairs) found in the nasal cavity clean, warm, and moisten the air. The cilia continually move in a wavelike motion to push mucus and debris out of the respiratory tract. Receptors for smell are in the nasal cavity. The nasal cavity is connected to four pairs of **paranasal sinuses** called maxillary, frontal, sphenoid, and ethmoid.

Air continues to travel into the pharynx (throat) (Fig. 25.1), which is divided into three sections:

- *Nasopharynx*: Located behind the nasal cavity. The eustachian tube connects the middle ear to the nasopharynx and equalizes the pressure in the ear with the air pressure outside the body.
- *Oropharynx*: Located behind the mouth and part of the respiratory and digestive systems.
- *Laryngopharynx*: Located between the epiglottis and the esophagus. The *epiglottis*, a flap of cartilage at the larynx opening, closes off the trachea when food is swallowed. As air passes back out through the opening, the *larynx* (vocal cords) vibrates to produce speech. The vocal cords are paired bands of cartilaginous tissue.

Lower Respiratory Tract

The lower respiratory tract consists of the trachea, bronchial tubes, and lungs (see Fig. 25.1). These structures are also lined with mucous membranes and cilia. The *trachea* (windpipe) lies in the space between the lungs, called the *mediastinum*. Air travels from the larynx through the trachea, and then the trachea branches into the right and left bronchi. The right bronchus is wider than the left bronchus.

The bronchi divide into smaller branches, called *bronchioles*. These bronchioles end in microscopic ducts capped by air sacs, called *alveoli*. Each thin-walled alveolus is in contact with a blood capillary. This contact between the two structures allows the exchange of gases. It is at this point that oxygen (O_2) from the inspired air moves across the one-cell membrane into the blood cells. Carbon dioxide (CO_2) moves in the other direction, from the blood into the air to be expired. Each alveolus is coated with a substance called **surfactant,** which keeps it from collapsing. Without surfactant, the alveoli stick together during exhalation and deflate. Inhalation becomes more difficult, and less O_2 is able to move into the bloodstream. This condition is life-threatening. Babies born before 37 to 39 weeks of gestation are at risk for not having enough surfactant.

The bronchial tree and alveoli are the major structures in the right and left lungs. The lungs are soft and spongy because of the air sacs that make up most of their mass. They hang in the right and left sides of the chest, separated by the pericardial sac, which contains the heart. Each lung is composed of sections called *lobes*. The right lung consists of three lobes, whereas the left has only two lobes (Fig. 25.2).

Because each lobe has its own bronchus and blood supply, the removal of one lobe (*lobectomy*) results in little or no damage to the rest of the lung. The left lung is longer and narrower. It has a distinct indentation in its center, known as the *cardiac notch*. This is where the left ventricle of the heart is located and where an apical pulse is heard.

Each lung is also enclosed by a double-folded, serous membrane called the *pleura*. The side of the membrane closest to the lungs is the *visceral pleura*. The side that lines the inner surface of the rib cage is the *parietal pleura*. Small amounts of pleural fluid fill the space between the two membranes and provide lubrication for the movement of the lungs during inhalation and exhalation.

The muscles responsible for normal, quiet respiration are the **diaphragm** and the **intercostal muscles**. On **inspiration**, the diaphragm is pulled down and flattened as it contracts, and the intercostal muscles expand, pulling air into the lungs. On **expiration**, the diaphragm relaxes and moves upward, pushing air out of the lungs.

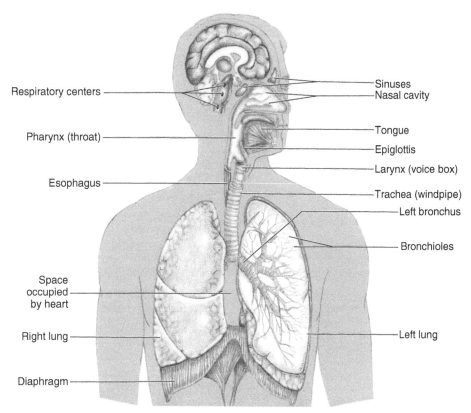

FIGURE 25.1 Anatomic structures of the respiratory system. (Modified from Solomon EP: *Introduction to human anatomy and physiology*, ed 3, St. Louis, 2009, Saunders.)

Life Span Changes

An infant has a narrow airway, with a shorter and softer trachea. If the neck is overextended, the airway can collapse. Infants tend to breathe through their noses, which means nasal congestions can make breathing difficult. Infants are abdominal breathers and have immature respiratory muscles, meaning fatigue with breathing difficulties can set in quickly. With a disproportionately larger tongue and epiglottis, infants and young children are at risk for airway obstruction.

At around age 20 to 25, the lungs reach maturity. By age 35, lung function starts to decline. People who smoke can increase the aging in their lungs. As a person ages, the following respiratory system changes occur:

- Chest wall and thoracic spine deformities cause increased work of breathing.
- The diaphragm grows weaker, leading to a decreased ability to inhale and exhale.
- Weakness in respiratory muscles causes the coughing reflex to be less effective.
- A decrease in tissue elasticity leads to an inability to keep the airway completely open.
- Alveoli lose their shape, which causes air to be trapped in the lungs. This leads to a decrease in gas exchange and lung capacity.

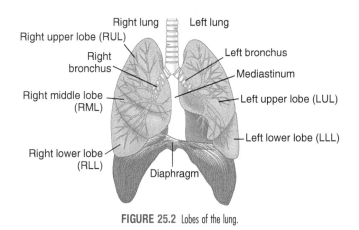

FIGURE 25.2 Lobes of the lung.

PHYSIOLOGY OF THE RESPIRATORY SYSTEM

The two primary functions of the respiratory system are to exchange O_2 from the atmosphere for CO_2 waste and to maintain the acid-base balance in the body. Both functions involve *ventilation* (breathing), which is the movement of gases between the lungs and the environment. Ventilation includes the process of inspiration (air moving into the lungs) and expiration (air moving out of the lungs).

Bronchioles and Alveoli

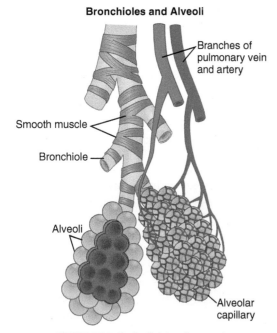

FIGURE 25.3 Alveoli with their capillary network.

Two types of respiration occur during the ventilation process.
- *External respiration* occurs when oxygenated air moves into the alveoli. Surrounding each alveolus is a pulmonary capillary network (Fig. 25.3). The alveoli and the pulmonary capillaries are made of single-celled walls. This allows the O_2 to move easily across the alveoli and capillaries into the blood. CO_2 and other wastes are forced out of the capillaries and move into the alveoli.
- *Internal respiration* occurs when O_2 is exchanged for CO_2 between the cells in the body and the blood.

Inspiration

A healthy person breathes when the blood CO_2 level increases. A person with chronic obstructive pulmonary disease (COPD) has a constantly elevated blood CO_2 level. At some point, the body no longer uses the elevated blood CO_2 level as a trigger to breathe. A secondary system kicks in. Breathing is triggered by a decreased blood O_2 level.

CRITICAL THINKING APPLICATION   25.1
Renee sees many patients with COPD who are using oxygen constantly. She realizes that the amount of oxygen is much lower than the amount providers order for patients without COPD. Confused, she asks John why patients with COPD use smaller amounts of supplemental oxygen. How would you answer this question?

When the breathing trigger is activated, it signals the medulla oblongata (the respiratory center) in the brainstem. The respiratory center causes a stimulus (i.e., signal) to be carried by the phrenic nerve to the diaphragm. When the diaphragm receives the signal, it flattens out and pulls downward. At the same moment, the intercostal muscles between the ribs contract, causing the ribs to move outward. The movement enlarges the chest cavity and causes the lungs to expand, increasing their volume. The greater the contraction, the deeper the inhalation and the greater the air volume.

When individuals are experiencing respiratory distress, they are unable to move enough air into the lungs. To help move additional air into their lungs, they use **accessory muscles.** To identify whether a person is using the accessory muscles, expose the chest and look for chest retractions with breathing. With intercostal retractions, the chest tissue in between the ribs is indrawn or pulled in during breathing. Upper airway obstructions can cause the following conditions:
- *Suprasternal retractions* (sucking in of the skin just above the sternum)
- *Supraclavicular retractions* (sucking in of the skin just above the clavicle)

Lower airway obstructions can cause the following:
- *Substernal retractions* (sucking in of the abdomen just below the sternum)
- *Subcostal retractions* (sucking in of the abdomen just below the ribs)

Using accessory muscles to breathe can tire a person. This can lead to **respiratory arrest**, a medical emergency. Typically, this occurs quicker in infants and young children.

CRITICAL THINKING APPLICATION   25.2
The pulmonologist asks Renee to review the signs of respiratory distress with the mother of an asthmatic patient. Discuss what Renee should review with the mother.

Expiration

The second half of ventilation is expiration. Once inspiration is complete, the diaphragm and intercostal muscles relax, which causes the diaphragm to move upward into the thoracic cavity and the ribs to move inward. This movement reduces the lung capacity and forces air out of the lungs. Typically, expiration requires very little energy. However, with some conditions (e.g., asthma and emphysema), the person has difficulty getting air out of the lungs. The accessory muscles are needed to help with complete exhalation.

Acid-Base Balance

The body attempts to keep the pH between 7.35 and 7.45. The respiratory system has an important role in acid-base balance. It regulates the amount of CO_2 in the blood. CO_2 in the blood can combine with water to form the buffer bicarbonate. If a person *hyperventilates* (breathes rapidly), the CO_2 and bicarbonate levels in the blood decrease. This causes the pH of the body to rise, resulting in *respiratory alkalosis*. This condition can be seen in patients with anxiety or an acute asthma attack. If hypoventilation occurs, the CO_2 in the blood increases (*hypercapnia*), and *respiratory acidosis* can occur. Respiratory alkalosis and respiratory acidosis are both life-threatening disorders if the underlying causes are not corrected.

DISORDERS OF THE RESPIRATORY SYSTEM

Many diseases affect the respiratory system. Table 25.1 defines terms related to signs and symptoms of respiratory conditions. The following

TABLE 25.1 Signs and Symptoms of Respiratory Conditions

MEDICAL TERM	DEFINITION
Apnea	Absence of breathing
Bradypnea	Abnormally slow breathing
Cheyne-Stokes respiration	Abnormal pattern of varying shallow and deep breathing; often seen in terminally ill patients
Clubbing	Abnormal enlargement of the distal phalanges (fingers and toes) associated with cyanotic heart disease or advanced chronic pulmonary disease
Cyanosis	Bluish discoloration of the skin and mucous membrane
Dyspnea	Difficulty breathing
Epistaxis	Nosebleed
Hemoptysis	Expectoration of blood
Hypercapnia	Greater than normal level of carbon dioxide in the blood
Hyperpnea	Deep, rapid, labored respiration that may occur because of exercise or pain and fever
Hypoxemia	Low level of oxygen in the blood
Orthopnea	The need to sit or stand to breathe comfortably
Pleurisy	Inflammation of the parietal pleura, causing dyspnea and stabbing pain; a friction rub may be auscultated
Rales	Bubbling or popping sound heard on auscultation; it is produced by the passage of air through bronchi that are constricted or contain secretions
Rhinorrhea	Excessive drainage from the nose
Rhonchi	Continuous rumbling sound heard on auscultation; it is caused by thick secretions or spasms
Shortness of breath (SOB)	Difficult or labored breathing; breathlessness
Stridor	High-pitched, noisy breathing
Tachypnea	Abnormally rapid rate of breathing
Wheezing	High-pitched whistling sound related to labored breathing

sections describe in detail some of the more common diseases seen in the ambulatory care setting.

Chronic Respiratory Diseases
Allergic Rhinitis
When a person is allergic to dust, animal dander, pollen, or foods, allergic rhinitis can occur. When due to a pollen allergy, the person is said to have hay fever, seasonal allergies, or allergic rhinitis.

The etiology of allergic rhinitis can be traced to an allergen that triggers an allergy in the person. When the allergen is breathed in, histamines in the body cause allergy symptoms to occur. The signs and symptoms include the following:
- Itchy nose, mouth, eyes, and throat; problems smelling; runny nose; sneezing; and watery eyes
- Later symptoms may include nasal congestion, coughing, decreased sense of smell, sore throat, dark circles and puffiness under the eyes, fatigue, and headache

The provider will perform a physical exam and ask about the patient's allergy history. Allergy testing, a complete blood count (CBC), and other allergy-related tests (e.g., the IgE radioallergosorbent test [RAST] test) may be done. Treatment consists of avoiding the allergen or reducing exposure. A nasal wash may be recommended to remove mucus from the nose. Medications such as antihistamines, **decongestants**, and **corticosteroids** may also be ordered. Depending on the severity, the provider may also refer the patient to an allergy department for evaluation. Allergy shots (immunotherapy) are sometimes recommended.

Asthma
Asthma is a chronic disease that affects the airway. Bronchospasms and airway swelling narrow the passageway. Mucus in the lungs clogs the airway (Fig. 25.4). Getting air into and out of the lungs becomes harder. The frequency of asthma episodes can vary. Severe asthma attacks are life-threatening and require immediate emergency care.

Common asthmatic triggers include allergens, environmental causes (chemical gases or fumes, dust, high humidity, and cold, dry air), strong emotional states, and strenuous physical exercise. Asthma symptoms can vary in type and frequency. Typical symptoms include shortness of breath (SOB), chest tightness or pain, coughing, and wheezing.

The provider may order peak flow monitoring, pulse oximetry, and spirometry tests for diagnostic testing. Peak flow monitoring can be used with at-home management of asthma. Treatment for asthma is based on the severity of the disease. Asthma medications can be taken orally or inhaled. Long-term control medications are usually taken daily and may include the following:
- Inhaled **corticosteroids**: fluticasone, budesonide, beclomethasone, and mometasone
- Leukotriene modifiers: montelukast, zafirlukast, and zileuton
- Long-acting beta agonists: salmeterol and formoterol
- Combination inhalers: fluticasone-salmeterol, budesonide-formoterol, and formoterol-mometasone

Quick-relief medications are usually taken during the asthma episode because they provide rapid, short-term relief. Quick-relief medications include short-acting beta agonists supplied by metered-dose inhalers (MDIs), such as albuterol and levalbuterol. If the quick-relief medications do not reduce the episode, immediate emergency care is required.

During asthma symptoms

Normal airway

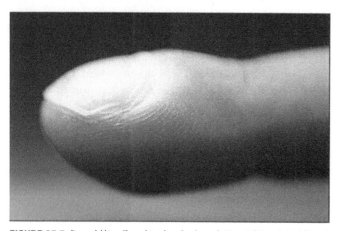

Airways

Lungs

Muscle

Airway wall

Muscle

Airway wall

A

B

Narrowed airway (limited air flow)

Tightened muscles constrict airway

Inflamed/thickened airway wall

Muscle

Mucus

C

FIGURE 25.4 Inflammation and bronchospasm.

FIGURE 25.5 Finger clubbing. The nail is enlarged and curved. (From Ball J, et al: *Seidel's guide to physical examination*, ed 9, St. Louis, 2019, Mosby.)

Chronic Obstructive Pulmonary Disease

More than 11 million Americans have chronic obstructive pulmonary disease (COPD). It is the third leading cause of death in the United States. But this condition is both treatable and preventable. COPD develops slowly, making it hard for the affected person to breathe. It includes two conditions:

- *Emphysema*: Thinning and eventual destruction of the alveoli. This usually accompanies chronic bronchitis.
- *Chronic bronchitis*: Inflammation of the bronchial tubes, excessive production of mucus, and diminished activity of the cilia.

The main cause of COPD is smoking tobacco. Other causes include secondhand smoke, air pollution, dust, and chemical fumes. COPD can also be caused by an alpha-1 antitrypsin (AAT) deficiency. The symptoms of COPD often appear after damage has already been done to the lungs. With chronic bronchitis, a long-term, daily productive cough is seen. Additional symptoms of COPD include shortness of breath, chest tightness, breathlessness, wheezing, cyanosis of the lips and nail beds, and clubbing (Fig. 25.5). The patient may experience a lack of energy and fatigue. Frequent respiratory infections are common.

> ### Alpha-1 Antitrypsin Deficiency
>
> Alpha-1 antitrypsin (AAT) deficiency is a rare inherited disorder that can increase a person's risk for developing lung disease and liver disease. The onset of lung disease occurs at a younger age than normal (around 30 to 40 years of age).
>
> AAT is a protein in the blood and lungs. It protects the lungs from chronic obstructive pulmonary disease (COPD). Sometimes a person may not make enough of this protein, or the AAT that is made is abnormal. Genetic testing is available to determine a person's risk. There is no cure for AAT deficiency, although the lung disease can be managed.

Typical diagnostic tests include lung function tests (i.e., spirometry and pulse oximetry), chest x-ray, and chest computed tomography (CT) scan. An arterial blood gas test may be done to identify the severity of the COPD. Because there is no cure for COPD, the goal of treatment is to slow the disease progression. Patients typically use **bronchodilators** and a bronchodilator-corticosteroid combination to reduce the inflammation. Patients may use low-level oxygen therapy. Adequate nutrition, vaccinations, and smoking cessation are also important in the treatment plan. With severe COPD, surgical options may be considered, such as lung volume reduction surgery (removal of damaged lung tissue) and lung transplantation.

Hazards of Tobacco Product Use. Tobacco smoke contains more than 7000 chemicals. Of these, 250 are harmful, and at least 69 can cause cancer. It is estimated that one in five deaths are related to smoking. According to the Centers for Disease Control and Prevention (CDC), smokers are more likely to develop heart disease, lung cancer, and strokes. Smoking can cause the following effects:

- *Respiratory system:* Pneumonia, COPD, tuberculosis, asthma, and cancer of the trachea, bronchus, and lung
- *Nervous system:* Stroke
- *Cardiovascular system:* Aortic aneurysm, early abdominal aortic atherosclerosis in young adults, coronary heart disease, atherosclerotic peripheral vascular disease, and acute myeloid leukemia

- *Sensory system:* Blindness, cataracts, and age-related macular degeneration
- *Digestive system:* Orofacial clefts (congenital defect from maternal smoking) and periodontitis; oropharynx, larynx, esophagus, stomach, liver, and colorectal cancers
- *Endocrine system:* Type 2 diabetes mellitus and pancreatic cancer
- *Musculoskeletal system:* Hip fractures and rheumatoid arthritis
- *Urinary system:* Cancer of the bladder, kidney, and ureters
- *Immune system:* Immune function issues
- *Reproductive system:* In women, reproductive effects (e.g., reduced fertility), ectopic pregnancy, and cervical cancer; in men, erectile dysfunction

Passive or *secondhand smoke*, which stays in the air and can be breathed in by others, causes lung cancer, strokes, low-birth-weight babies, and heart disease. Exposure to secondhand smoke increases a person's risk for lung cancer by 20%. Children exposed to secondhand smoke have an increased risk of sudden infant death syndrome (SIDS), ear infections, bronchitis, pneumonia, colds, and asthma. Secondhand smoke causes more than 53,000 deaths a year in the United States.

Thirdhand smoke is the residue or chemicals from the smoke that gets on skin, clothing, furniture, carpet, and so on. This can be harmful to little children and animals that spend time on the floor. Besides breathing in the residue, these chemicals can be ingested. They can transfer from the carpet, clothing, and so on to hands and then into the person's mouth.

The CDC reports that at least 28 cancer-causing chemicals have been found in smokeless tobacco (e.g., chew and dip). Smokeless tobacco can cause cancer of the mouth, pancreas, and esophagus.

E-cigarettes, which are used for vaping, are also considered tobacco products because they usually contain nicotine. E-cigarettes (also called e-cigs, vape pens, mods, or e-hookahs) are battery operated devices that heat liquids to form an aerosol that is then inhaled. The liquids typically contain nicotine, flavorings, and other additives. E-cigs can also be used for marijuana and other drugs. An e-cig may look like a cigarette, pipe, cigar, pen, or USB (flash) drive. When compared with cigarettes, e-cigs are safer, but they still can be harmful. The aerosol can contain nicotine, heavy metals (e.g., lead), volatile organic compounds, and cancer-causing substances. One example of a health risk comes from diacetyl, which is found in many e-cigarette flavors. It has been known to cause bronchiolitis obliterans, commonly called "popcorn lung." Diacetyl was an ingredient in microwave popcorn and food flavorings until it was linked to hundreds of cases of bronchiolitis obliterans. Like COPD, this disease can cause wheezing, persistent cough, shortness of breath, and death. The alveoli become scarred, and the airway becomes narrowed.

According to the CDC, advantages of giving up the use of tobacco products include the following:
- Blood pressure and heart rate begin to return to normal.
- Within a few hours, carbon monoxide levels in the blood decline.
- Within a few weeks, circulation improves and abnormal respiratory systems (e.g., cough, wheezing) decrease.
- One year after quitting, the cardiovascular risks decrease sharply.
- Two to five years after quitting, the risk for stroke returns to a nonsmoker's level.

- Five years after quitting, the risk of cancer of the esophagus, bladder, throat, and mouth is cut in half.
- Ten years after quitting, the lung cancer risk decreases by 50%.

Local resources and prescriptive medications are available if a person wants to quit using these products. Websites (e.g., https://smokefree.gov) and quit lines are also available (e.g., National Cancer Institute Smoking Quitline: 1-877-44U-QUIT).

Cystic Fibrosis

Cystic fibrosis (CF) is a life-threatening, congenital disease. Mucus builds up in the lungs, pancreas, and other organs. The mucus blocks the airways and increases the risk of infections. In the pancreas, the mucus interrupts the release of digestive enzymes used to break down food. More than 30,000 people in the United States have cystic fibrosis. Half of them are age 18 or younger. All states require newborn screening tests for cystic fibrosis. With improvements in treatments, people with CF can live, work, and play with a much greater quality of life than in the past.

CF is a genetic disease. The signs and symptoms of CF include the following:
- Higher than normal levels of salt in the sweat, electrolyte imbalances
- A persistent cough that produces a thick, sticky **sputum**; breathlessness, shortness of breath, wheezing, and frequent lung infections
- Poor growth and weight gain
- Intestinal blockage, severe constipation, foul-smelling and greasy stools

CF is diagnosed with either two positive sweat tests performed on different days or with a genetic test and one positive sweat test. There is no cure for CF. Treatment centers on reducing the complications and symptoms. Treatment can include O_2 therapy, antibiotics for lung infections, and anti-inflammatory medications to reduce the swelling in the lungs. Chest physical therapy, vest therapy (vibrating vest), bronchodilators, and mucus-thinning medication can help clear the lungs of mucus. Oral pancreatic enzymes are used to help with digestion. Surgical options for CF complications include lung transplantation and bowel surgery for obstructions.

Laryngeal Cancer

Laryngeal cancer is throat cancer, and it impacts the vocal cords and larynx (voice box). In most cases, laryngeal cancer develops in adults older than 50 years, and men are more likely to get it than women.

The causes of laryngeal cancer include tobacco and alcohol use. The signs and symptoms include constant sore throat, painful swallowing, ear pain, lump in the neck or throat, and hoarseness.

After a physical exam, the provider may order a biopsy with a laryngoscopy or endoscopy, CT scan, magnetic resonance imaging (MRI), positron emission tomography (PET) scan, bone scan, and barium swallow (or upper gastrointestinal series). Treatment consists of surgery, chemotherapy, and radiation therapy.

Lung Cancer

There are two main types of lung cancer, non–small cell and small cell. Non–small cell lung cancer is more prevalent. Lung cancer is the leading cause of cancer-related deaths in the United States.

The leading cause of lung cancer is cigarette smoking. The longer a person has smoked and the more a person has smoked, the more likely it is that he or she will contract lung cancer. High exposure levels of asbestos, radiation, and pollution can also increase a person's risk for lung cancer. Common signs and symptoms of lung cancer include a chronic, worsening cough with hemoptysis and constant chest pain. Lung cancer can cause wheezing, breathlessness, shortness of breath, clubbing, and more frequent respiratory infections. Fatigue, loss of appetite, weight loss, and swelling of the face and hands can also be seen with lung cancer.

Chest x-rays and CT scans, sputum cytology, bronchoscopy, and lung tissue biopsy are used to diagnose lung cancer. Treatment for lung cancer is based on the person's health, the stage of the disease, and the person's preferences. Treatments can include chemotherapy, radiation therapy, targeted drug therapy, and surgery.

Pneumoconiosis

Pneumoconioses are a group of interstitial lung diseases that lead to the inflammation and scarring of the lungs (*pulmonary fibrosis*). It becomes difficult for oxygen to pass into the bloodstream. Specific types of interstitial lung disease include the following:

- *Asbestosis* from inhaling asbestos fibers
- *Black lung disease* (or coal workers' pneumoconiosis [CWP]) from inhaling coal dust
- *Farmer's lung* from inhaling farm dust
- *Siderosis* from inhaling iron from mines or welding fumes
- *Silicosis* from inhaling silica dust

Its etiology can be traced to inhaling certain types of dust (e.g., aluminum, graphite, iron, talc, grain), droppings from birds and animals, molds, gases, or fumes. Signs and symptoms include shortness of breath at rest and with activity and a dry cough.

After an examination, a provider will order a chest x-ray and pulmonary function tests (e.g., spirometry) (Fig. 25.6). Treatment depends on the type of exposure and the stage of the disease. The patient may be put on medications and oxygen therapy. If the disease is severe, a lung transplant may be done.

Sleep Apnea

Sleep apnea occurs when a person stops breathing or the breathing becomes very shallow. Breathing pauses may last a few seconds to minutes and may occur 30 or more times an hour. The main types of sleep apnea are the following:

- *Obstructive sleep apnea (OSA):* The most common type of sleep apnea, it causes breathing to pause during sleep. OSA results from a blockage or narrowing of the airway when the throat muscles relax. It can be caused by excessive weight, a thicker neck circumference, a narrowed airway, smoking, and nasal congestions. Men are twice as likely to have it, and age increases the risk.
- *Central sleep apnea:* The breathing stops repeatedly during sleep. The brain temporarily stops sending signals to the muscles that control breathing. This condition can be caused by brainstem injuries (including infections and stroke), congestive heart disease, and narcotic **analgesics**.
- *Complex sleep apnea syndrome:* Occurs when a person has both obstructive sleep apnea and central sleep apnea.

The etiology varies depending on the type of sleep apnea the person has. The most common signs and symptoms of these conditions include loud snoring, breathing cessation during sleep, dry mouth, sore throat, morning headache, difficulty staying asleep, excessive daytime sleepiness, irritability, and attention problems.

After an examination, the provider may refer the patient to a sleep specialist or order a sleep study. Treatments may include weight loss or stopping the use of alcohol or medications that may be causing the condition. Continuous positive airway pressure (CPAP) therapy is the most common treatment for OSA (Fig. 25.7). It uses mild air pressure to keep the airway opened.

Acute Respiratory Diseases

There are many acute respiratory diseases. Tables 25.2 and 25.3 list several acute upper and lower respiratory diseases. In addition, the following sections describe commonly seen acute respiratory diseases.

Acute Bronchitis

Acute bronchitis is an inflammation of the lining of the bronchial tubes. The bronchial tubes become irritated and swollen, narrowing the airway. Excessive mucus is produced, leading to increased coughing.

Acute bronchitis is usually caused by a lower respiratory viral infection. Viral conditions, such as the common cold, influenza, and *pertussis* (whooping cough), can also cause acute bronchitis. In rare cases a bacterial infection causes the disease. In addition, breathing

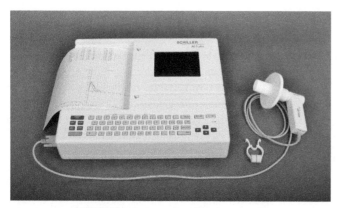

FIGURE 25.6 A spirometer is used for spirometry testing.

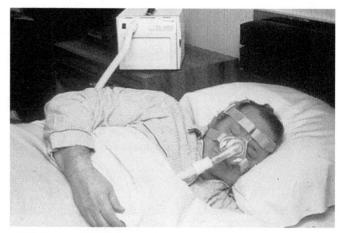

FIGURE 25.7 Patient with a CPAP machine. (Courtesy Respironics, Murrysville, Pennsylvania.)

TABLE 25.2 Acute Upper Respiratory Tract Diseases

Disease	Epiglottitis	Laryngitis	Sinusitis	Strep throat
Description	Life-threatening inflammation of the epiglottis	Inflammation of the larynx	Inflammation of the sinuses	Highly contagious bacterial infection of the throat
Etiology	*Hib, Streptococcus pneumoniae,* or viruses	Overuse, irritation, or infection	Structural abnormalities or a cold that may cause mucus to pool and pathogens to grow	Group A streptococcal bacteria are highly contagious
Signs and Symptoms	High fever, **pharyngitis**, stridor, cyanosis, drooling, difficulty breathing and swallowing, hoarseness	Hoarseness, weakened (or loss of) voice, tickling sensation, sore or dry throat, dry cough	Fever, weakness, fatigue, nasal and sinus congestion, cough, bad breath, or loss of smell	Rash, nausea and vomiting, fever, headache, painful swallowing, sore throat, tiny red spots at the back of the throat, or white pus patches
Diagnostic Procedures	History and physical exam, blood/throat cultures, CBC, neck x-ray	History and physical exam; for chronic problems, laryngoscopy, biopsy.	History and physical exam, x-rays	History and physical, rapid antigen test (CLIA waived), throat culture
Treatment	Hospitalization, humidified oxygen, antibiotics, corticosteroids	Antibiotics, corticosteroids, increase fluid intake, rest voice, breathe moist air	Antibiotics, decongestants, analgesics, heating pads, saline nasal sprays, vaporizers	Antibiotics, stay home until on antibiotics for 24 hours, analgesics

CBC, Complete blood count; *CLIA,* Clinical Laboratory Improvement Amendments; *Hib, Haemophilus influenzae* type b.

TABLE 25.3 Acute Lower Respiratory Tract Diseases

Disease	Croup	Influenza	Pertussis	Pleurisy	Pneumothorax
Description	Inflammation of the trachea and larynx	Acute viral infection; also called flu	Bacterial infection; also called whooping cough	Infection of the pleura	Air or gas in the pleural space, causing the lung to collapse (*atelectasis*)
Etiology	Variety of viruses, including influenza	Influenza viruses	*Bordetella pertussis* (bacteria)	Bacteria, fungus, parasites, or viruses; also caused by inhaled toxins	Rupturing of a small blister on the lung's surface; trauma
Signs and Symptoms	Harsh, barklike cough; hoarseness, fever, and inspiratory stridor	Fever, cough, sore throat, muscle aches, headaches, fatigue	Early stage: runny nose, low-grade fever, mild cough, and apnea in babies; later stage: fits of many, rapid coughs, followed by a whooping sound, vomiting, and exhaustion	Stabbing pain (especially with inspiration), cough, fever, chills, and dyspnea	Sudden, sharp pleuritic pain that increases with movement, breathing, or coughing; shortness of breath, cyanosis, rapid pulse, and respiratory distress
Diagnostic Procedures	Cultures to identify causative organism; neck and chest x-ray	History and physical exam, nasopharyngeal swab, and rapid influenza diagnostic tests (CLIA waived)	History of cold, physical exam, nasopharyngeal specimen culture, and PCR (rapid test)	Pleural friction rub is heard over the lung field, chest x-ray, ultrasound, and CT scan	Decreased breath sounds heard over the collapsed lung field, chest x-ray, CT scan, pulse oximetry, and arterial blood gases
Treatment	Antipyretics, humidifier, bed rest, increase fluid intake, and sitting may help child breathe easier; in severe cases, hospitalization with antibiotic and oxygen therapy	Bed rest, increased fluids, antiviral medications, and analgesics	Antibiotics, stay home, good hand washing, and humidifier	Analgesics, anti-inflammatory agents, bed rest, and **thoracentesis**	Treatment depends on cause of collapse; bed rest and monitoring of vital signs, chest tube, and surgical procedures to remove a portion of the pleura (*pleurectomy*)

CLIA, Clinical Laboratory Improvement Amendments; *CT,* computed tomography; *PCR,* polymerase chain reaction.

in irritants or inhaling food or vomit can cause acute bronchitis. Symptoms of acute bronchitis include a dry, hacking cough that can turn into a **productive cough**, a low-grade fever, fatigue, and weakness.

After obtaining a medical history and performing an examination, the provider may order a chest x-ray. Pulse oximetry may also be performed (Fig. 25.8). In most cases, acute bronchitis is viral, so no antibiotics are prescribed. At-home treatments include using cough drops and a humidifier to soothe a dry throat. Patients are encouraged to drink plenty of fluids and get adequate rest. Over-the-counter (OTC) medications are used for fevers and body aches. Patients are encouraged to stop smoking and using e-cigarettes.

Pneumonia

Pneumonia is an infection of the lungs. It may affect one or both lungs. The alveoli fill with fluid or pus. Young children, adults over 65 years of age, people who smoke, and those with chronic illnesses are at more risk for pneumonia. The severity of pneumonia can range from mild to life-threatening. In the United States, about 1 million people have pneumonia a year, and about 50,000 people die from the disease. Adults are at most risk. Globally, it is the leading infectious disease killer of children under age 5.

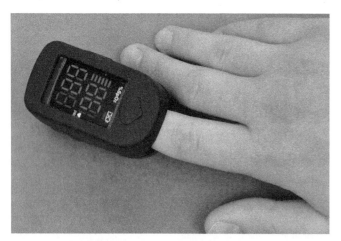

FIGURE 25.8 A pulse oximeter is used for pulse oximetry.

Pneumonia can be caused by bacteria, viruses, and fungi (Table 25.4). If a person has viral pneumonia, there is also a risk of getting bacterial pneumonia. Various chemicals can also cause pneumonia. Signs and symptoms of pneumonia vary based on the severity and type of pneumonia. Typical signs and symptoms include high fever and chills, productive cough, shortness of breath, chest pain with coughing or breathing, decreased appetite, and fatigue. Confusion can be seen in older adults.

Providers will listen to a patient's lungs for abnormal sounds. Chest x-rays, a CBC, a sputum culture, and pulse oximetry are typical diagnostic procedures used to check for pneumonia. Treatment for pneumonia is based on the type of pneumonia a person has. Antibiotics are used for bacterial pneumonia, and antiviral medications are used for viral pneumonia. Patients are encouraged to drink plenty of fluids and get rest. Over-the-counter **antipyretics** and **analgesics** (e.g., ibuprofen and acetaminophen) may be recommended.

CRITICAL THINKING APPLICATION   25.3

Renee is rooming Carl Bowden. He is here today for a recheck appointment. He was diagnosed 10 days ago with pneumonia. As Renee is gathering Carl's history, he tells her that he has smoked two packs a day for the past 30 years. He also states that he has had pneumonia six times over the past 2 years. He asks Renee if smoking might have something to do with that. Thinking back to the respiratory structures and functions you have learned about in this chapter, how would you answer his question?

Pulmonary Embolism

Pulmonary embolism (PE) is a condition in which one of the pulmonary arteries is blocked. PE is a medical emergency and can be life-threatening. Due to the blockage, blood flow may be interrupted to that section of the lung. This can lead to **pulmonary hypertension**. Oxygen can be limited to other body organs.

Often PE is a complication of deep vein thrombosis (DVT). Blood clots form in the veins, usually in the legs. Some of the clots break off and travel through the bloodstream. Eventually, the clot

TABLE 25.4	Examples of Pathogens That Cause Pneumonia	
TYPE OF PATHOGEN	PATHOGEN	DESCRIPTION
Bacteria	*Streptococcus pneumoniae*	Children under 2 years of age and adults 65 years and older are at most risk; pneumococcal vaccines are used for prevention
	Haemophilus influenzae	Haemophilus influenza type b (Hib) vaccine is used as a prevention
	Legionella pneumophila	Causes Legionnaires disease and Pontiac fever
	Mycoplasma pneumoniae	Called "walking pneumonia"
	Chlamydia pneumoniae	Most common in school-aged children
	Chlamydia psittaci	Causes psittacosis; comes from infected pet birds and poultry
Virus	Influenza virus	Prevention includes the yearly influenza vaccine
	Respiratory syncytial virus (RSV)	Most common cause of pneumonia in children under 1 year of age
Fungi	*Pneumocystis jirovecii*	More common in people with weakened immune systems

blocks a pulmonary artery. Signs and symptoms of pulmonary embolism include problems breathing or unexplained shortness of breath, chest pain, coughing or coughing up blood, arrhythmias, and rapid breathing. A patient may also feel lightheadedness and faint.

Besides a medical history and physical exam, the provider may order the following diagnostic procedures: ultrasound, CT scan with contrast, lung ventilation/perfusion scan (VQ scan), pulmonary angiography, chest x-ray, and chest MRI. Echocardiography and an electrocardiogram (ECG) may also be done. The goals of treatment include preventing more clots or larger clots from forming. Treatment includes the following:

- *Anticoagulants*: "Blood thinners" (e.g., warfarin [Coumadin] and heparin) to prevent clots from forming.
- *Thrombolytics*: Medications that break up the clot. These are used in emergencies. Thrombolytics can be delivered by a catheter to the site of the clot.
- *Compression stockings:* To help prevent blood from pooling and clotting in the legs.

Pulmonary Tuberculosis

Pulmonary tuberculosis (TB) is caused by bacteria that can affect the lungs. There are two TB-related conditions: latent TB infection and TB disease.

Tuberculosis is caused by *Mycobacterium tuberculosis,* which is spread through the air. Individuals at risk for TB include the following:

- Anyone who has lived in a country where TB is prevalent
- Anyone in frequent close contact with someone with TB disease
- Those working in healthcare, a homeless shelter, or a prison
- Those living in a nursing home, prison, or homeless shelter
- People who have latent TB infection and a weakened immune system, because TB can become active under these conditions

There are differences regarding the spread and the signs/symptoms of the two TB-related conditions. With latent TB infection, a person cannot spread TB bacteria to others and there are no signs or symptoms. With TB disease, a person can spread the disease by coughing, sneezing, singing, or talking. TB disease can cause a bad cough that lasts 3 or more weeks, pain in the chest, blood in the sputum, weakness, no appetite, weight loss, chills, fever, and night sweats.

Initially, the person is tested with either a Mantoux tuberculin skin test (TST) (also known as a purified protein derivative [PPD] test) or a TB blood test (e.g., QuantiFERON-TB Gold [QFT], T-SPOT.TB) (Fig. 25.9). If the test is positive, then the person will have additional testing (e.g., chest x-ray and sputum smear/culture) to determine if it is latent TB infection or TB disease. With latent TB infection, the chest x-ray is normal and the sputum smear/culture is negative. With TB disease, the chest x-ray is abnormal and the sputum smear/culture is positive. For treatment:

- For latent TB infections, isoniazid or rifapentine may be prescribed. The goal is to prevent TB disease; a weakened immune system can increase the risk of TB disease.
- For TB disease, isoniazid, rifampin, ethambutol, or pyrazinamide may be prescribed. With treatment, TB disease symptoms tend to diminish within 2 to 3 weeks, but medication treatment may last for 6 to 9 months.

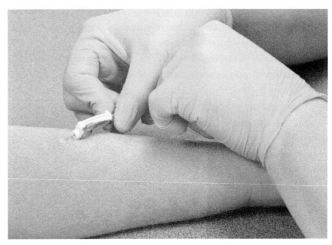

FIGURE 25.9 Administering a Mantoux tuberculin skin test.

CRITICAL THINKING APPLICATION   **25.4**

Renee is confused about the two different types of tuberculosis (TB). She asks John to summarize the difference between latent TB infection and TB disease. How would you summarize the differences?

Respiratory Syncytial Virus

Respiratory syncytial virus (RSV) produces upper respiratory "cold" symptoms in healthy older children and adults. For young children and adults with medical problems, it can cause pneumonia and severe breathing problems.

RSV spreads by coughing or sneezing. The virus can survive for several hours on infected surfaces. Typical outbreaks of RSV occur in winter and early spring. RSV can cause nasal congestion, low-grade fevers, a runny nose, and a mild cough. Complications can include a barking cough from swelling near the vocal cords, high fevers, wheezing, apnea, cyanosis, and difficulty breathing.

During the physical exam, the provider listens to the lungs, checking for wheezing and other abnormal lung sounds. Additional diagnostic procedures include pulse oximetry, chest x-rays, and laboratory tests (e.g., a CLIA–waived RSV test), viral cultures of the respiratory secretions from the nose). Treatment consists of over-the-counter medication (e.g., acetaminophen [Tylenol]) for the fever and plenty of fluids to prevent dehydration. People with severe cases of RSV are hospitalized. Supplemental oxygen, albuterol breathing treatments, and inhaled epinephrine may be given.

Additional Respiratory System Diseases

There are many respiratory diseases. The following list provides a brief description of several of them:

- *Acute respiratory distress syndrome*: A life-threatening condition that prevents enough oxygen from getting into the blood. Fluid buildup in the lungs decreases the ability for lung expansion and causes hypoxemia.
- *Bronchiectasis*: An infection or other conditions cause damage to the airway, leading to bronchial dilation and scarring.

- *Bronchiolitis*: A common viral infection in young children and infants. The bronchioles become inflamed, and mucus builds up in the airway, affecting breathing.
- *Bronchopulmonary dysplasia (BPD)*: Chronic respiratory condition that affects premature infants or infants who are on a *ventilator* (breathing machine). Infants require high concentrations of oxygen and assisted ventilation. They may have lung damage and are at greater risk for repeated respiratory infections.
- *Diphtheria*: A bacterial respiratory infection characterized by sore throat, fever, and headache.
- *Neonatal respiratory distress syndrome (RDS):* Often seen in premature babies born before 37 to 39 weeks. They lack enough surfactant in their lungs, which leads to respiratory distress. Infants are given warm, moist oxygen and may be put on a ventilator.
- *Pulmonary fibrosis*: Scarring of lung tissue, causing the tissues to get stiff and thick. Breathing can be difficult, and the person can have hypoxemia.
- *Pulmonary hypertension (PH):* The blood pressure is high in the pulmonary arteries, which affects the blood flow in the lungs. The blood vessels become hard and narrow, causing hypoxemia. PH may be related to genetics or other conditions, such as heart or lung disease.

THE MEDICAL ASSISTANT'S ROLE IN PULMONARY PROCEDURES

Assisting With the Examination

Preparing a patient for a respiratory examination includes having the patient disrobe to the waist. The patient should put on a gown with the opening in the front or back, depending on the provider's preference. To assess the status of the respiratory system, the provider uses inspection, palpation, percussion, and auscultation on the anterior thorax, then repeats the process on the posterior and lateral thorax.

The medical assistant is responsible for assisting the provider throughout the examination and for providing privacy and support for the patient.

Assisting With Diagnostic Procedures

Table 25.5 lists common diagnostic procedures for respiratory diseases. Some diagnostic procedures are done in the clinic, whereas others are done in other departments (e.g., medical laboratory and radiology). The medical assistant may be responsible for coaching patients on diagnostic procedures done in other departments. As with other diagnostic procedures, the medical assistant should coach the patient regarding the following:

- Patient preparation (e.g., dietary restrictions and medications to hold)
- Location and time of the test
- What to expect during the procedure
- Any follow-up required after the procedure

The following diagnostic procedures are performed by the medical assistant.

CRITICAL THINKING APPLICATION   **25.5**

Renee is working with a patient who needs to have a pulse oximetry measurement. The patient asks Renee what this test shows. Thinking back to what you have learned already in this chapter, how would you answer the patient?

Sputum Specimen Collection

Sputum cultures may be ordered when patients have symptoms that may be related to infectious respiratory diseases. Examples of other sputum tests include the following:

- *Legionella* testing for legionnaires' disease
- Acid-fast bacillus (AFB) testing for tuberculosis
- Gram stain for bacterial or fungal infections

The medical assistant may be responsible for coaching patients on how to collect sputum specimens. Many times, sputum specimens

---

TABLE 25.5	Common Diagnostic Procedures for Respiratory Diseases			
TYPE OF PROCEDURE	**PROCEDURE**	**DESCRIPTION**		**PATIENT PREPARATION AND COACHING**
Medical laboratory blood tests	*Arterial blood gas* (ABG)	A test in which a blood specimen is collected from the artery in the wrist, and the pH of the blood, carbon dioxide (CO_2), and oxygen (O_2) content are measured.		Usually no restrictions for tests. Typically done in the hospital setting.
Medical laboratory tests	*CLIA-waived tests*	• *Legionella* urinary antigen test: for legionnaires' disease • Influenza A & B test: for influenza • Rapid strep A test: for strep throat • RSV test: for respiratory syncytial virus pneumonia		Usually no restrictions for tests.
	Sputum cytology	Sputum is examined under a microscope for abnormal cells.		Provide patient with instructions on collecting sputum specimens.
	Sputum culture	Sputum is analyzed in the lab for bacterial growth over a period of days.		

TABLE 25.5   Common Diagnostic Procedures for Respiratory Diseases—*continued*

TYPE OF PROCEDURE	PROCEDURE	DESCRIPTION	PATIENT PREPARATION AND COACHING
Imaging procedures	Chest x-rays (CXRs)	Images taken from several directions, which provides a good outline of the heart and lungs. Abnormal air "pockets," fluid, and tumors can be seen on chest x-rays.	Metal must be removed (e.g., jewelry, glasses, cell phone). Patient should be screened for pregnancy and surgically implanted devices (e.g., heart valve and pacemaker).
	Computed tomography (CT)	An imaging technique can provide more information than chest x-rays.	Screen patient for pregnancy. All metal objects must be removed (e.g., glasses, dentures, jewelry). May have eating and drinking restrictions.
	Magnetic resonance imaging (MRI)	An imaging technique that can provide more information than chest x-rays.	Screen patient for pregnancy and implanted metal or electronic devices (e.g., pacemaker, valves, heart defibrillator, shrapnel, and cochlear implants). Darker inks used in tattoos may contain metal.
	Lung positron emission tomography (PET) scan	A tracer is given intravenously and after about an hour, a PET scan is taken.	Screen patient for pregnancy, claustrophobia, and an allergy to contrast dye or iodine. Patient may need to sign a consent form. May have eating and drinking restrictions.
	Pulmonary angiography	A procedure in which a catheter is inserted into the pulmonary blood vessels. Dye is injected, and x-ray pictures show the blood flow through the pulmonary vessels.	Screen patient for pregnancy and an allergy to contrast dye or iodine. Patient may need to sign a consent form. May have eating and drinking restrictions.
	Lung ventilation/ perfusion scan (VQ scan)	A procedure in which a radioisotope substance is inhaled and injected; then a special x-ray scanner creates a picture of the blood flow and airflow in the lungs.	Screen patient for pregnancy. Usually needs a recent chest x-ray.
Pulmonary Function Tests	Peak flow monitor	A handheld device that measures the exhaled air. Used in the clinic and at home to manage chronic respiratory conditions (e.g., asthma).	Need to loosen any restrictive clothing. Gum and loose dentures should be removed. Instruct patient on how to perform the test.
	Pulse oximetry	A noninvasive test used to measure the oxygen saturation of the blood. A probe is placed on the finger or on skin in other locations.	Remove nail polish or artificial nails to get an accurate reading.
	Spirometry test	Measures the volume of inhaled and exhaled air, and the time required for each one. Patient breathes multiple times through a tube that is connected to a computer.	Patient will need instructions regarding taking or holding respiratory medications. Need to loosen any restrictive clothing. Gum and loose dentures should be removed. Instruct patient on how to perform the test.
	Lung volume test	Determines lung volume after inhalation and exhalation. Also called plethysmography.	Patient may sit in a clear box and breathes in and out of a mouthpiece of the plethysmograph.
	Lung diffusion capacity	Determines how effectively gas travels from the lungs to the bloodstream.	Patient breathes in a *tracer gas* (harmless gas), and the concentration of the gas is measured in the exhaled air.
Endoscopy	Bronchoscopy	An instrument (bronchoscope) is inserted through the mouth to visualize the trachea and bronchi.	Patient may need to stop anticoagulants and NSAIDs prior to procedure. Patient should not eat or drink (NPO) after midnight. Someone must drive the patient home after the test. Patient may need to sign a consent form.

CLIA, Clinical Laboratory Improvement Amendments.

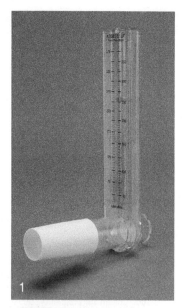

FIGURE 25.10 Manual peak flow meter.

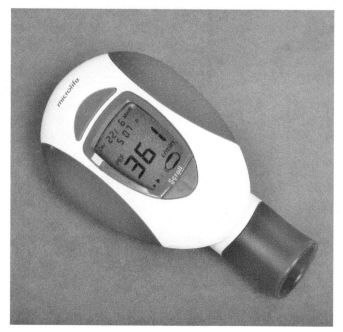

FIGURE 25.11 Digital peak flow meter.

are collected in the morning. For some tests, three sputum samples may be collected over 3 days. Patients should follow these directions when collecting a sputum specimen:

1. Avoid food for 1 to 2 hours before collecting the sputum specimen.
2. Rinse your mouth well to remove food particles.
3. Open the container, and avoid touching the inside of the container and cover.
4. Inhale two to three times, breathing out hard each time, then cough deeply.
5. Collect the sputum from the cough. Do not spit oral secretions in the cup.
6. Cover the container when enough sputum is collected.

The medical assistant should discuss how the specimen should be stored and brought to the healthcare facility for testing.

TABLE 25.6 Asthma Action Plan

ZONE	SYMPTOMS	ACTION TO TAKE
Green Zone: Doing well	No asthma symptoms; peak flow is more than 80% of normal peak flow.	Take prescribed long-term control medications.
Yellow Zone: Asthma is getting worse	Asthma symptoms are present, or waking at night, or person cannot do usual activities, or peak flow is 50%–79% of normal peak flow.	Add quick-relief medication to the Green Zone medication. Continue to monitor. Contact provider if not improving.
Red Zone: Medical alert	Very short of breath, or quick-relief medications have not helped, or peak flow is less than 50% of best peak flow.	Take short-acting beta agonist medication and/or oral steroid. Contact the provider immediately.

Adapted from the National Institutes of Health. Asthma Action Plan. www.nhlbi.nih.gov/health/public/lung/asthma/asthma_actplan.pdf. Accessed 06/26/2018.

CRITICAL THINKING APPLICATION 25.6

Renee needs to collect sputum from a patient who needs a sputum culture. Renee tells the patient that she needs the sputum to come from the lungs. The patient asks why she cannot just use "spit" from his mouth. How might you respond?

Peak Flow Rate

The peak flow meter measures the amount of air exhaled. A peak flow rate is measured using a manual or digital peak flow meter in an ambulatory care or home setting (Figs. 25.10 and 25.11). It is used to diagnose acute conditions and to manage chronic diseases, such as asthma. Procedure 25.1 on p. 646 describes the steps to take when measuring a peak flow rate. When a patient is performing a peak flow rate test, it is important that the medical assistant have three adequate readings.

For chronic disease management, providers encourage patients to use peak flow meters at home. The providers create Asthma Action Plans for the patients to follow (Table 25.6). Based on the patient's peak flow rate at home, the patient follows the directions on the plan.

CRITICAL THINKING APPLICATION 25.7

Renee is working with an adult patient newly diagnosed with asthma. She has just explained how to use a peak flow meter at home, and the patient's "normal" peak flow volume was identified. As Renee explains the Asthma Action Plan the pulmonologist has ordered, the patient begins to look confused. He asks, "Why can't I just call or come in if I don't feel good? Why do I need to bother with the Asthma Action Plan?" What might be the benefits to the patient of using the Asthma Action Plan? How might you respond to his question?

Spirometry

Spirometry evaluates lung function as it is affected by respiratory, cardiac, and neuromuscular diseases. It can be ordered if the provider identifies abnormalities in the respiratory system. A spirometer can evaluate the amount of air you exhale and inhale. It looks at how quickly the air is exhaled and the rate at which air is breathed in. Several different tests can be done with spirometry (Table 25.7).

With spirometry testing, it is important that the medical assistant enter accurate patient data into the spirometer computer. Besides the patient's name, medical record number, and date of birth, the medical assistant may need to enter the person's gender, age, race, height, and weight. The patient's current height and weight need to be obtained prior to the spirometry. The computer then pulls stored data and creates a "normal" person for those characteristics. After the patient has completed the test, the computer will print out the patient's results compared with the "normal" person's results. This helps the provider identify areas of concern.

Procedure 25.2 on 972 describes the spirometry procedure. When performing the spirometry procedure, the following steps should be taken:

- Adults should exhale 6 seconds and children should exhale 3 seconds for the forced vital capacity (FVC). For patients with obstructive breathing patterns, the FVC may take up to 15 seconds.
- Give the patient at least 30 seconds between blows. Have the patient indicate when he or she is ready for the next blow.
- Do a minimum of three blows and a maximum of eight blows (unless otherwise indicated by the facility's protocols).
- Make sure to follow the operator's manual for the machine you are using.
- Be encouraging yet respectful of the patient when coaching him or her through the procedure.

CRITICAL THINKING APPLICATION 25.8

Renee's last patient of the day is Janine Butler, who is seeing the provider because of her asthma. After the provider sees Janine, he orders a spirometry test. Renee prepares the equipment and brings Janine into the testing room. However, Janine refuses to have her height and weight measured. Renee explains to Janine the importance of getting an accurate height and weight. Discuss how you would explain the importance of obtaining accurate height and weight measurements when doing a spirometry test.

Assisting With Treatments

Patients with pulmonary conditions are prescribed a variety of medications. The following are some of the more common classifications:

- *Antihistamines*: Counteract the effects of histamine.
- *Antivirals*: Inhibit the growth or reduce the spread of viral cells
- *Antitussives*: Inhibit the cough center
- *Bronchodilators*: Relax the smooth muscles of the bronchi
- *Corticosteroids* (oral, nasal, and inhaled): Reduce airway inflammation and bronchial resistance

TABLE 25.7	**Spirometry Tests**	
TEST	**DESCRIPTION**	**PATIENT COACHING**
Tidal volume (TV)	Volume of air inhaled and exhaled during a normal respiration	Breathe in and out normally with lips pursed around the mouthpiece.
Forced vital capacity (FVC)	Amount of air that can be forcefully exhaled from a maximum inhalation	Inhale as deeply as possible, then quickly forcibly exhale as much as possible.
Forced expiratory volume in 1 second (FEV$_1$)	Volume of air exhaled in the first second of the FVC	
Expiratory reserve volume (ERV)	Maximal volume of air exhaled after normal exhalation	Breathe in and out normally, then exhale forcibly at the end of the TV.
Inspiratory reserve volume (IRV)	Maximal volume of air inhaled after normal inhalation	Breathe in normally, then forcibly inhale.
Vital capacity (VC)	Maximum amount of air that can be exhaled during a normal or slow exhalation after maximum inhalation	Inhale deeply and exhale completely.
Inspiratory capacity (IC)	Maximum amount of air that can be inhaled after a normal exhalation	Breathe in and out normally, then forcibly inhale at the end of the TV.
Functional residual capacity (FRC)	Amount of air remaining in the lungs at the end of a normal exhalation.	
Residual volume (RV)	Volume of air remaining in the lungs after a forced exhalation.	
Total lung capacity (TLC)	Maximum amount of air in the lungs with maximum inhalation	
Maximum voluntary ventilation (MVV)	Maximum volume that is breathed in and out in 1 minute	Breathe in and out as deeply and as frequently as possible for 15 seconds

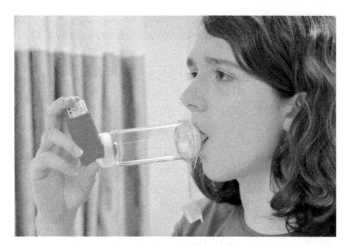

FIGURE 25.12 Using a metered dose inhaler with spacer.

- *Decongestants*: Relieve local congestion in the nasal and sinus tissues
- *Expectorants*: Thin the secretions in the bronchial tubes to make it easier to cough up the mucus
- *Leukotriene receptor antagonists*: Block the action of substances that cause asthma and allergic rhinitis

Refer to Table 25.8, Medication Classification, for information on the classification, including indication for use, desired effect, side effects, adverse reactions, and generic and trade names. Medical assistants should be familiar with medications that are prescribed to patients.

In the ambulatory care facility, common respiratory treatments include medication administration and oxygen therapy. Depending on the state's statutes and the facility's policies, the medical assistant may be able to administer nebulizer treatments and oxygen therapy when ordered by the provider. The medical assistant may also instruct patients on how to use metered-dose inhalers. The following sections cover metered-dose inhaler education, nebulizer treatments, and oxygen therapy.

Metered-Dose Inhalers

A metered-dose inhaler (MDI) provides aerosol medication that is breathed into the lungs. MDIs are typically ordered for conditions such as asthma and COPD.

In many cases the provider will order an MDI with a spacer. A *spacer* is a long tube that is attached to the mouthpiece of an MDI (Fig. 25.12). Spacers slow the delivery of medication from MDIs. Without a spacer, the MDI blasts the medication to the back of the throat and mouth. With inhaled corticosteroids, this can cause irritation and infections over time. When a spacer is used, the medication is blasted into the tube and over several breaths is pulled into the lungs. In an ambulatory care facility, the medical assistant may need to instruct the patient on the proper use of an MDI.

Nebulizer Treatment

Inhaled medication for asthma, COPD, and other lung diseases can be given using a nebulizer. A nebulizer treatment can be done in the ambulatory care setting and in the home. A nebulizer is a small machine that turns liquid medication into a fine spray that can be inhaled. Typically, the medication used for nebulizers is much

---

Using a Metered-Dose Inhaler (MDI)

1. Shake the MDI three or four times. Remove the cover from the MDI's mouthpiece.
   a. If using a spacer:
      - Attach the spacer. Breathe out. Place the mouthpiece between your lips, and close your lips around it.
      - Press the top of the canister on the MDI.
      - Breathe in very slowly, taking a full breath in. Some spacers will produce a whistle-like sound if you are breathing in too fast.
   b. If not using a spacer:
      - Breathe out. Place the inhaler 1 to 2 inches (about 2 finger widths) in front of your opened mouth.
      - Press the top of the canister on the MDI.
      - Breathe in very slowly, taking a full breath in.

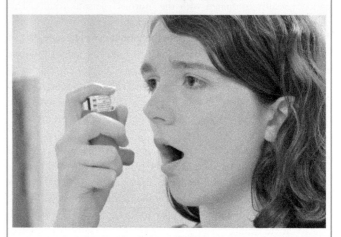

2. Hold your breath for 10 seconds (or count to 10), and then breathe out. If you are using inhaled, quick-relief medication (beta-agonists), wait 1 minute between puffs.
3. Repeat steps 1a or 1b and 2 until your dose is completed.

---

stronger than the same medication found in an MDI. Procedure 25.3 on p. 649 describes the steps for administering a nebulizer treatment.

Oxygen Therapy

When a patient comes to the ambulatory care facility with a cardiac or respiratory condition, the provider may order oxygen to be administered. Oxygen should be treated as a medication. The medical assistant must get the order from the provider for how much oxygen to administer and how to administer it. In the ambulatory care facility, oxygen may be available in the room by means of a wall-mounted flow meter or oxygen cylinders (portable tanks).

Room air is about 21% oxygen. Oxygen devices increase the concentration of oxygen for the patient to breathe in. Typically, a nasal cannula or a simple mask is used in the ambulatory care setting. Other masks that deliver higher oxygen concentrations may also be available (Fig. 25.13). Table 25.9 provides information on the more common oxygen delivery devices used in the ambulatory care setting. Procedure 25.4 on p. 650 presents the steps for administering oxygen.

TABLE 25.8 Medication Classifications

CLASSIFICATION	INFORMATION	GENERIC NAME (TRADE NAME)
Antihistamines	**Indications for use:** Relieve allergies. **Desired effects:** Blocks the action of histamine, which causes allergic symptoms. **Side effects and adverse reactions:** CNS depression, muscle weakness, GI distress, dry mouth.	• **loratadine** (Claritin, Alavert) • **diphenhydramine** (Benadryl, Unisom) • **cetirizine** (Zyrtec, Alleroff)
Antivirals	**Indications for use:** Treat viral infections, including oral and genital herpes, influenza, and HIV. **Desired effects:** Inhibit the growth or reduce the spread of viral cells. **Side effects and adverse reactions:** Confusion, diarrhea, headache, kidney disease, urticaria, vomiting.	• **oseltamivir** (Tamiflu) • **acyclovir** (Zovirax)
Bronchodilators	**Indications for use:** Treat asthma, bronchospasm; promote bronchodilation. **Desired effect:** Relax the smooth muscle of the bronchi. **Side effects and adverse reactions:** CNS stimulation, tremors, tachycardia, increased blood glucose level, hypertension.	• **albuterol** (Ventolin HFA, Proventil, ProAir HFA) • **tiotropium** (Spiriva Handihaler)
Corticosteroids (oral)	**Indications for use:** Used to treat chronic inflammatory diseases (e.g., arthritis) and acute conditions (e.g., poison ivy, asthma). **Desired effects:** Reduce inflammation. **Side effects and adverse reactions:** Headache, mood changes, difficulty falling asleep or staying asleep, increased sweating, vision problems, depression, and weight gain.	• **prednisone** (Prednisone Intensol, Sterapred) • **prednisolone** (Flo-Pred, Orapred, Pediapred) • **methylprednisolone** (Medrol)
Corticosteroids (nasal and inhaled)	**Indications for use:** Long-term relief of asthma symptoms; decrease frequency of asthma attacks; manage chronic obstructive pulmonary disease (COPD) and seasonal allergies. **Desired effects:** Reduce airway inflammation and bronchial resistance. **Side effects and adverse reactions:** Headache, pharyngitis, myalgia, hypersensitivity, oral candidiasis. Diskus products are contraindicated in patients with a milk allergy.	• **fluticasone and salmeterol** (Advair Diskus) • **fluticasone** (Flovent Diskus, Flovent HFA, Flonase nasal spray) • **budesonide** (Pulmicort Flexhaler, Pulmicort Respules, Rhinocort) • **budesonide and formoterol** (Symbicort) • **mometasone** (Nasonex)
Decongestants	**Indications for use:** Relieve nasal and sinus congestion caused by common cold, hay fever, or upper respiratory tract disorders. **Desired effect:** Relieve local congestion in the nasal and sinus tissues. **Side effects and adverse reactions:** Arrhythmias, hypertension, headache, nausea, dry mouth.	• **pseudoephedrine** (Sudafed) • **Phenylephrine** (Sudafed PE Congestion, PediaCare Children's Decongestant, Suphedrin PE)
Expectorants	**Indications for use:** Relieve upper respiratory tract congestion. **Desired effect:** Thin the secretions in the bronchial tubes to make it easier to cough up the mucus. **Side effects and adverse reactions:** GI distress.	• **guaifenesin**
Leukotriene receptor antagonists	**Indications for use**: Asthma, exercise induced bronchospasms **Desired effect**: Block the action of substances that cause asthma and allergic rhinitis **Side effects and adverse reactions:** headache, dizziness, heartburn, stomach pain, tiredness, hypersensitivity, numbness in arms and legs, swelling of the sinuses	• **montelukast** (Singulair)

TABLE 25.9   Common Oxygen Delivery Devices

TYPE	FLOW RANGE (LITERS/MINUTE [LPM])	OXYGEN DELIVERED	DESCRIPTIONS
Nasal cannula	1–2 2–4 4–6	24%–28% 28%–34% 34%–44%	• Soft tube with prongs that are placed in the nose; make sure prongs curve downward. • A humidification device is used if flow is over 4 LPM. • Allows patient to talk, drink, and eat. • Cannot be used with upper respiratory obstructions (e.g., nasal polyps); not helpful for mouth breathers.
Mask	5–10	30%–60%	• Used for mouth breathers. • Best used for short-term situations (e.g., ambulatory care). • Restrictive for communication, coughing, and eating. • Requires 5–6 LPM to avoid CO_2 accumulation in the mask.
Partial rebreathing mask	6–10	40%–70%	• Oxygen feeds into a reservoir bag attached to a mask. • About one-third of expired air enters reservoir bag, and the rest exits the mask through exhalation ports.
Non-rebreathing face mask	10–15	Up to about 90%	• Mask with a reservoir bag and one-way valve. • One-way valve allows patient to inhale oxygen from the reservoir bag but prevents expired air from entering bag. • Before applying to patient, occlude valve and allow reservoir bag to fill with oxygen.

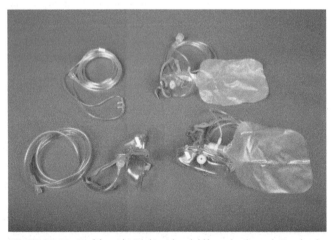

FIGURE 25.13 *(Top left to right)* Nasal cannula and child non-rebreather mask. Non-rebreather masks have one-way valves (e.g., yellow circle on the mask). *(Bottom left to right)* Simple face mask and adult non-rebreather mask.

CLOSING COMMENTS

Patient Coaching

Many patients who have chronic pulmonary conditions use MDIs as part of their treatments. It is important that patients learn how to clean their MDIs and spacers to prevent additional issues. A blocked or partially blocked MDI can prevent the patient from getting the proper dose of medication. To clean the MDI and spacer, do the following:

- Spacers can be taken apart, cleaned with mild soap and water, and then allowed to air dry.
- To clean the MDI inhaler, remove the medication canister and mouthpiece cover. Let warm water flow over the top and bottom of the MDI inhaler for about 30 seconds. Shake off the water, and let the MDI air dry overnight. When assembling, spray twice in the air before taking a dose. Clean the MDI weekly to prevent medication from building up and blocking the dose sprayed.
- Cleaning techniques can vary with medication products. Patients should be encouraged to check the product's website for directions.

Legal and Ethical Issues

Many times, with pulmonary disorders and treatments, patients may become dizzy. This can affect their balance or even cause them to faint. If a patient has a recent history of fainting, or "passing out," it is important for the medical assistant to keep the patient safe in the ambulatory care environment. Some ways to assist patients and prevent falls are the following:

- Warn the patient not to take continuous deep breaths during a nebulizer treatment.
- Assist the patient as needed when stepping on and off the scale.
- Assist the patient on and off the exam table.

- Do not leave the patient on the exam table unattended.
- Ask the patient if he or she would like a wheelchair.

Many lawsuits have been brought forward involving situations in which patients were injured from falls in the ambulatory care environment. Several cases involved medical assistants not helping patients on and off items like scales or having patients wait unattended on exam tables. Remember, safety is one of the most important issues when caring for patients.

Patient-Centered Care

To provide patient-centered care, medical assistants need to do the following:

- Provide patients with clear instructions on the pulmonary procedure being done.
- Perform the procedure correctly, so the patient's results are accurate.
- Be sensitive to patients' concerns and feelings regarding pulmonary diseases.
- Be respectful and empathetic when encouraging patients to breathe for spirometry tests. Remember, if the patient is short of breath or coughing due to an illness, blowing for a spirometry test can be difficult. Allow the patient to tell you when he or she is ready to do the next test.

Professional Behaviors

Part of being professional is one's appearance and grooming. When working with patients, it is essential that the medical assistant has no odors on his or her body. Wearing perfume or cologne or using scented lotions can trigger an allergic reaction in a patient. Patients with asthma can have flare-ups when they are around different scents, such as perfume, cologne, or scented lotions.

Medical assistants who smoke cigarettes need to be especially concerned with the odor. Research has shown that tobacco smoke contains more than 7000 chemicals, of which 250 are harmful. When the olfactory (sense of smell) system is exposed to these chemicals, reversible or permanent injuries can occur. The injury relates to the length of time the person has smoked and the tobacco toxicity. Ultimately, smoking tobacco can lead to a decrease in odor sensibility and recognition. This means people who smoke may not be able to smell the cigarette smoke on their clothing or body, yet it may be noticeable to others.

Many patients who have a chronic illness, like cancer or COPD, have quit smoking tobacco products. It is important that the healthcare professionals who care for these patients (and all other patients) do not smell of cigarette smoke.

SUMMARY OF SCENARIO

As Renee works with John, she realizes she has a lot more to learn. Pulmonary disease is common. Renee decides to research the diseases she encounters every week. She feels that to be professional, it is important to be up to date on the latest information. She likes to be confident in her skills and knowledge. This helps when patients have questions about diseases, procedures, or treatments.

Renee looks forward to her weekly pulmonary experiences. She is confident in rooming patients, performing pulse oximetry, and gathering sputum specimens. She is excited about learning how to do peak flow and spirometry tests in the coming weeks.

SUMMARY OF LEARNING OBJECTIVES

1. **Describe the organs of the respiratory system, including their function and anatomical location, and compare the structure and function of the respiratory system across the life span.**

   The upper respiratory tract is composed the nose, pharynx, and the larynx. These organs are located outside of the chest cavity. The main functions of the upper respiratory tract include warming and cleaning the inspired air, serving as a passageway for air, and providing the sense of smell.

   The lower respiratory tract consists of the trachea, bronchial tubes, and lungs. The trachea (windpipe) lies in the space between the lungs, called the mediastinum. Air travels from the larynx through the trachea, and then the trachea branches into the right and left bronchi. The bronchi divide into smaller branches, called bronchioles. These bronchioles end in microscopic ducts capped by air sacs, called alveoli, which are involved with gas exchange.

   An infant has a narrow airway, with a shorter and softer trachea and tends to breathe through the nose. Infants are abdominal breathers and have immature respiratory muscles, meaning fatigue with breathing

   difficulties can set in quickly. As a person ages, the diaphragm grows weaker. The respiratory muscles become weaker, and there is a decrease in tissue elasticity. The alveoli lose their shape.

2. **Discuss the physiology of the respiratory system, and explain the process of ventilation.**

   The two primary functions of the respiratory system are to exchange O_2 from the atmosphere for CO_2 waste and to maintain the acid-base balance in the body. Both functions involve ventilation (breathing), which is the movement of gases between the lungs and the environment. Ventilation includes the process of inspiration (air moving into the lungs) and expiration (air moving out of the lungs). Two types of respiration occur during the ventilation process, external respiration and internal respiration.

3. **Discuss common chronic and acute respiratory system disorders, including signs, symptoms, etiology, diagnostic procedures, and treatments. In addition, discuss the hazards of using tobacco products, including cigarettes, smokeless tobacco, and e-cigarettes (vaping).**

Continued

The chronic respiratory diseases discussed in this chapter include allergic rhinitis, asthma, chronic obstructive pulmonary disease (i.e., chronic bronchitis and emphysema), cystic fibrosis, laryngeal cancer, lung cancer, types of pneumoconiosis, and sleep apnea.

Acute respiratory conditions explained include acute bronchitis, croup, epiglottitis, influenza, laryngitis, pertussis, pleurisy, pneumonia, pneumothorax, pulmonary embolism, pulmonary tuberculosis, respiratory syncytial virus, sinusitis, and strep throat. Refer to each disease to learn about the signs, symptoms, etiology, diagnostic procedures, and treatments.

This chapter discussed the hazards of using tobacco products. Cigarette smokers are more likely to develop heart disease, lung cancer, and strokes. Smoking impacts all the body systems. Passive or secondhand smoke also causes health problems to others. Thirdhand smoke is the residue or chemicals from the smoke. This can be inhaled or ingested and can cause problems.

Smokeless tobacco (e.g., chew and dip) can cause cancer of the mouth, pancreas, and esophagus. When compared with cigarettes, e-cigarettes (vaping) are safer, but they still can be harmful. The aerosol can contain nicotine, heavy metals (e.g., lead), volatile organic compounds, and cancer-causing substances.

4. **Discuss the medical assistant's role in pulmonary procedures, including assisting with examination and diagnostic procedures such as measuring the peak flow rate and performing spirometry.**

Preparing a patient for respiratory examination includes having the patient disrobe to the waist. The medical assistant is responsible for assisting the provider throughout the examination and for providing privacy and support for the patient.

The peak flow meter measures the amount of air exhaled. A peak flow rate is measured using a peak flow meter in an ambulatory care or home setting. It is used to diagnose acute conditions and to manage chronic diseases, such as asthma. Procedure 25.1 describes the steps to measure a peak flow rate.

Spirometry is done to evaluate lung function as affected by respiratory, cardiac, and neuromuscular diseases. It can be ordered if the provider identifies abnormalities in the respiratory system. A spirometer can evaluate the amount of air inhaled and exhaled. Procedure 25.2 on p. 647 describes the spirometry procedure.

5. **Describe pulmonary treatments, including metered-dose inhalers, nebulizer treatments, and oxygen therapy.**

A metered-dose inhaler (MDI) provides aerosol medication that is breathed into the lungs. MDIs are typically ordered for conditions such as asthma and chronic obstructive pulmonary disease (COPD).

A nebulizer treatment can be done in the ambulatory care setting and in the home. A nebulizer is a small machine that turns liquid medication into a fine spray that can be inhaled. Typically, the medication used for nebulizers is much stronger than the same medication found in an MDI. Procedure 25.3 on p. 649 describes the steps for administering a nebulizer treatment.

When a patient comes to the ambulatory care facility with a cardiac or respiratory condition, the provider may order oxygen to be administered. Oxygen should be treated as a medication. The medical assistant must get the order from the provider for how much to administer and how to administer it. Procedure 25.4 on p. 650 presents the steps for administering oxygen.

PROCEDURE 25.1 Measure the Peak Flow Rate

Tasks: Perform a peak flow. Document the procedure in the patient's health record.

EQUIPMENT and SUPPLIES

- Peak flow meter
- Disposable mouthpiece
- Disinfection wipes
- Gloves
- Waste container
- Paper towel or denture cup (optional)
- Patient's health record

PROCEDURAL STEPS

1. Wash hands or use hand sanitizer.
   PURPOSE: Hand sanitization is an important step for infection control.
2. Assemble equipment and supplies needed for the peak flow procedure. Place the mouthpiece on the peak flow meter. Move the indicator to the bottom of the calibration scale (if not using a digital meter).

PURPOSE: Having the equipment ready reduces the patient's wait time. The indicator needs to be at the bottom of the scale before the test to get an accurate reading.

3. Greet the patient. Identify yourself. Verify the patient's identity with full name and date of birth. Explain the procedure to be performed in a manner that the patient understands. Answer any questions the patient may have about the procedure.
   PURPOSE: It is important to identify the patient in two different ways to ensure that you have the correct patient. Explaining the procedure can make the patient feel more comfortable and reduces anxiety.
4. Ask the patient to loosen any restrictive clothing. Have the patient remove any gum and loose dentures from his or her mouth. Make sure to provide a paper towel or denture cup if needed.
   PURPOSE: To get the most accurate results, the patient needs to be able to take a large breath in before the test. Normally, dentures can be left

PROCEDURE 25.1   Measure the Peak Flow Rate—*continued*

in the mouth, but loose-fitting dentures may affect the results of the test and must be removed.

5. With the patient in the seated position, ensure that his or her feet are flat on the floor and the legs uncrossed. The patient should sit straight up and against the back of the chair.
   PURPOSE: It is important for the patient to be in a position in which the lungs can fully expand.

6. Describe how the patient should do the test: "Take the deepest breath possible. Seal your lips around the mouthpiece. Blow as hard and as fast as you can." Encourage the patient to state when he or she is ready to start the test. Seal your lips around the mouthpiece (Fig. 1).

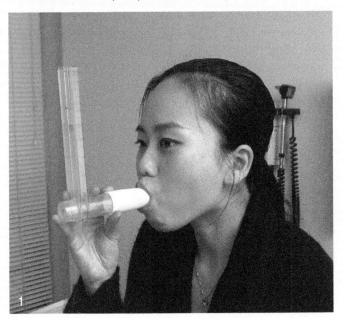

PURPOSE: Clear directions will help the patient understand what to do.

7. Coach the patient during the test. After the patient has blown through the meter, read the number next to the indicator. Write the number down. Reset the indicator to the bottom of the scale (if it is not a digital meter).
   PURPOSE: If the patient has breathing problems, it is important to allow the patient to indicate when he or she is ready.

8. Make any adjustments as needed. Repeat the test two additional times. Write down the last two numbers.
   PURPOSE: Three acceptable readings are needed for the peak flow procedure.

9. Put on gloves, and remove the mouthpiece. Discard the mouthpiece in the waste container. Disinfect the peak flow meter. Remove gloves, and dispose of them in the waste container. Wash hands or use hand sanitizer.
   PURPOSE: Wearing gloves and disinfecting the peak flow meter are important for infection control.

10. Notify the provider of the readings, and document the readings in the patient's health record. Indicate the name of the provider who ordered the test, the name of the test, the results of the test, and how the patient tolerated the test.
    PURPOSE: Indicating who ordered the test and what was done is important for insurance reimbursement and for legal reasons.

Documentation Example

08/07/20XX 1423 Per Dr. Angela Perez's order, a peak flow was performed. Pt stated she was "a little short of breath" on the third test. Peak flow readings: 200, 230, and 260 L/min. Dr. Perez was notified of results and patient's SOB complaint. _____ Renee Thomas, CMA (AAMA)

PROCEDURE 25.2   Perform Spirometry Testing

Tasks: Perform a spirometry test. Document the procedure in the patient's health record.

EQUIPMENT and SUPPLIES

- Spirometry machine with paper (and operator's manual if applicable)
- Disposable mouthpiece and tubing (if applicable)
- Nose clip
- Calibration equipment
- Disinfection wipes
- Gloves
- Waste container
- Paper towel or denture cup (optional)
- Patient's health record
- Scale (if no height and weight measurements were taken earlier that day)

PROCEDURAL STEPS

1. Wash hands or use hand sanitizer.
   PURPOSE: Hand sanitization is an important step for infection control.

2. Assemble equipment and supplies needed for the spirometry procedure. Calibrate the machine according to the operator's manual and the facility's procedures.
   PURPOSE: It is important to calibrate according to the facility's procedures. Calibration ensures that the results are accurate and reliable.

3. Greet the patient. Identify yourself. Verify the patient's identity with full name and date of birth. Explain the procedure to be performed in a manner that the patient understands. Answer any questions the patient may have about the procedure.

Continued

PROCEDURE 25.2 | Perform Spirometry Testing—*continued*

PURPOSE: It is important to identify the patient in two different ways to ensure that you have the correct patient. Explaining the procedure can make the patient feel more comfortable and reduces anxiety.

4. Enter the patient's name, medical record number, age (or date of birth), race, gender, weight, and height into the machine. Enter any additional required information.
PURPOSE: The information used for the spirometry calculations is current weight, height, age, race, and gender.

5. Ask the patient to loosen any restrictive clothing. Have the patient remove any gum and loose dentures from his or her mouth. Make sure to provide a paper towel or denture cup if needed.
PURPOSE: To get the most accurate results, the patient needs to be able to take a large breath in before the test. Loose-fitting dentures can affect the results of the test.

6. With the patient in the seated position, ensure that his or her feet are flat on the floor and the legs uncrossed. The patient should sit straight up and against the back of the chair.
PURPOSE: The patient may get dizzy during the test, so standing can be problematic. The seated position provides the maximum lung expansion for the test.

7. Describe how the patient should do the test: "Take the deepest breath possible. Seal your lips around the mouthpiece. Blow as hard and as fast as you can. Blow until you empty the air from your lungs."
PURPOSE: Clear directions will help the patient understand what to do.

8. Attach the mouthpiece to the machine. Explain the purpose of the nose clip to the patient. Apply the nose clip to the patient (Fig. 1). Have the patient state when he or she is ready to start. Start the test as directed by the operator's manual.
PURPOSE: The nose clip prevents air from leaking out through the nose. It provides a more accurate reading.

9. During the test, encourage the patient to empty the lungs. Repeat until three acceptable tests have been done. Allow the patient to rest between tests, if needed, and to indicate when he or she is ready for next test.
PURPOSE: Usually three test results are needed for comparison. If the patient is struggling and having difficulty breathing, ask the provider if three tests need to be done.

10. Put on gloves, and remove the mouthpiece. Discard the mouthpiece in the waste container. Disinfect the spirometer as indicated in the operator's manual. Remove gloves, and dispose of them in the waste container. Wash hands or use hand sanitizer.
PURPOSE: Wearing gloves and disinfecting the equipment is important for infection control.

11. Document that the test was performed. Indicate the name of the provider who ordered the test, the name of the test, how the patient tolerated the test, and what you did with the test results. Any patient instructions regarding follow-up can also be documented.
PURPOSE: Indicating who ordered the test and what was done is important for insurance reimbursement and for legal reasons.

Documentation Example

08/08/20XX 1423: Per Dr. James Martin's order, a spirometry test was performed. Pt stated she felt dizzy during the third attempt. The dizziness cleared within 5 minutes, and she stated she felt better. Pt was instructed to call the clinic tomorrow for the spirometry results. The spirometry results were given to Dr. Martin. _____ Renee Thomas, CMA (AAMA)

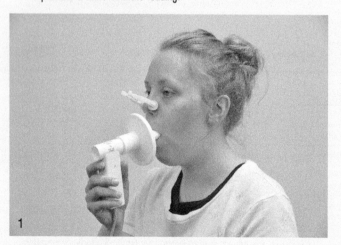
1

PROCEDURE 25.3 Administer a Nebulizer Treatment

Tasks: Administer a nebulizer treatment. Document the medication administration in the patient's health record.

Order: Levalbuterol 0.63 mg by nebulization

EQUIPMENT and SUPPLIES

- Nebulizer machine
- Disposable nebulizer patient kit (tubing, medication cup, mouthpiece or mask, flexible tube, and tee)
- Medication as ordered
- Provider's order
- Normal saline (as ordered or according to the facility's protocol)
- Disinfection wipes
- Gloves
- Waste container
- Patient's health record

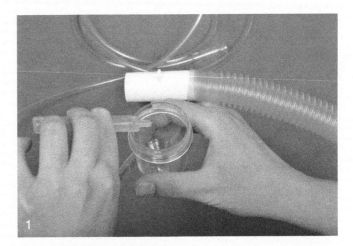

PROCEDURAL STEPS

1. Wash hands or use hand sanitizer. Using the drug reference information and the order, review the information on the medication if needed. Clarify any questions you have with the provider.
   PURPOSE: Hand sanitization is an important step for infection control. It is important to be knowledgeable about the medication you are giving.
2. Select the right medication from the storage area. Check to see if the medication is concentrated and requires normal saline to dilute it. Check the medication label (and normal saline label, if used) against the order. Check for the right name, form, and route. Check the expiration date to make sure the drug has not expired. Verify that it is the right dose and time.
   PURPOSE: A provider's order is required for the nebulizer treatment. The medication needs to be verified three times before it is given. The Nine Rights of Medication Administration also need to be followed.
3. Assemble equipment and supplies needed for the nebulizer treatment.
   PURPOSE: Having the equipment ready reduces the patient's wait time.
4. Perform the second medication check. Check the medication and normal saline label(s) against the order. Check for the right name, form, and route.
   PURPOSE: It is important to do the second check of the label(s) before pouring the medication into the medication cup.
5. Add the medication and, if required, the normal saline to the medication cup (Fig. 1). Secure the cover on the cup.
   PURPOSE: The medication cup holds the medication during the treatment.

6. Perform the third medication check. Check the medication label and normal saline label (if used) against the order. Check for the right name, form, and route. Verify that the amount of medication in the cup is correct according to the order. Clean up the area.
   PURPOSE: It is important to do the third check of the label before giving the medication.
7. Prior to entering the exam room, knock on the door and wait a moment. Greet the patient. Identify yourself. Verify the patient's identity with full name and date of birth. Make sure the patient's information matches the order and the record. Explain what you are going to do.
   PURPOSE: It is important to identify the patient in two different ways to ensure that you have the correct patient. Explaining the procedure can make the patient feel more comfortable and reduces anxiety.
8. Provide the right education to the patient. Explain the medication ordered, the desired effect, and common side effects; also identify the provider who ordered it. Answer any questions the patient may have. Use language the patient can understand. Ask the patient if he or she has any allergies. If the patient refuses the medication, notify the provider.
   PURPOSE: The patient needs to be aware of what you are giving, the action and side effects, and who ordered it. It is also important to double-check the patient's allergies before administering the medication.
9. Attach the mouthpiece (or mask). Attach the tubing to the medication cup and the machine.
   PURPOSE: Use a mask if ordered by the provider.
10. Perform the right technique. The patient should be sitting upright on a chair to allow for total lung expansion. Instruct the patient to hold the mouthpiece between the teeth and seal the lips around the mouthpiece. Encourage the patient to take slow, deep breaths through the mouth. The patient should hold each breath 2 to 3 seconds before exhaling.
    PURPOSE: Sitting upright allows for total lung expansion. If patients breathe too deeply and too fast, they will become dizzy and may hyperventilate. Holding the breath in allows the medication to disperse through the lungs.

Continued

PROCEDURE 25.3   Administer a Nebulizer Treatment—*continued*

11. Turn on the nebulizer, and give the medicine cup and mouthpiece to the patient to start the treatment. Instruct the patient to put it into his or her mouth. If using a mask, position it securely and comfortably over the patient's nose and mouth.
    PURPOSE: It is important to make sure the mask is comfortable over the patient's face. If it is not comfortable, the patient may not tolerate the treatment.

12. Continue the treatment until the mist has stopped (approximately 10 minutes) (Fig. 2). Turn off the nebulizer. Encourage the patient to take several deep breaths and cough.
    PURPOSE: After the treatment, it is common that patients will need to cough. Ensure that tissue is available if the patient needs it.

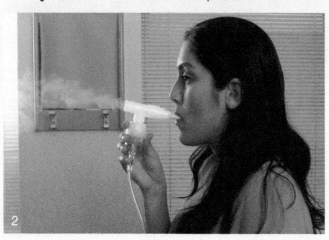

13. Put on gloves, and dispose of the used supplies. Disinfect the nebulizer machine. Remove gloves, and dispose of them in the waste container. Wash hands or use hand sanitizer.
    PURPOSE: To ensure infection control.

14. Document the procedure in the patient's health record. Include the name of the provider ordering the treatment, what was administered, how the patient tolerated the medication, and any follow-up assessments (e.g., vital signs).
    PURPOSE: Documentation is the last of the Nine Rights of Medication Administration.

Documentation Example

08/06/20XX 1120: P: 76 regular, strong; R: 26 regular, shallow. Per Dr. Angela Perez's order, Levalbuterol 0.63 mg administered by nebulizer. Pt stated she felt a little shaky after the treatment and her lungs felt less tight. Pt is resting on the exam table. P: 86 regular, strong; R: 20 regular, normal. Dr. Perez notified._____ Renee Thomas, CMA (AAMA)

PROCEDURE 25.4   Administer Oxygen Per Nasal Cannula or Mask

Tasks: Administer oxygen per nasal cannula or mask. Document the oxygen administration in the patient's health record.

Order 1: Administer 2 LPM of oxygen per nasal cannula.

Order 2: Administer 6 LPM of oxygen per simple mask.

EQUIPMENT and SUPPLIES

- Oxygen cylinder with oxygen regulator or oxygen flow meter (wall unit)
- Adult nasal cannula or simple mask
- Provider's order
- Patient's health record
- Mannequin (optional)

PROCEDURAL STEPS

1. Wash hands or use hand sanitizer.
   PURPOSE: Hand sanitization is an important step for infection control.

2. Assemble equipment and supplies needed for the provider's order. If an oxygen cylinder is used, identify the amount of oxygen left in the cylinder.

PURPOSE: The order will include the amount to give and the device (e.g., cannula) to use for the administration. It is important to make sure the cylinder has enough oxygen for the patient.

3. Verify the order if you have any questions.
   PURPOSE: A provider's order is required for oxygen administration.

4. Greet the patient. Identify yourself. Verify the patient's identity with full name and date of birth. Make sure the patient's information matches the order and the record. Explain the procedure in a manner that the patient understands. Answer any questions the patient may have about the procedure.
   PURPOSE: It is important to identify the patient in two different ways to ensure that you have the correct patient. Explaining the procedure can make the patient feel more comfortable and reduces anxiety.

PROCEDURE 25.4 Administer Oxygen Per Nasal Cannula or Mask—*continued*

5. Connect the nasal cannula or mask to the regulator or flow meter. Turn on the oxygen, and adjust the flow rate to the correct amount per the provider's order. The ball should be centered on the number of liters ordered.
   PURPOSE: Oxygen needs to be flowing through the tubing before the cannula is applied to the patient.

6. Apply the mask or nasal cannula:
   a. Place the mask over the patient's nose, mouth, and chin. Place the elastic over the head. Adjust the elastic strap to tighten the mask on the face. Adjust the metal nasal bridge clamp, making sure it fits without obstructing the nose. Ensure that the mask fits tightly on the face.
      PURPOSE: A poorly fitted mask can cause oxygen to be directed into the eyes, causing additional problems.
   b. Insert the tips of the cannula into the nostrils. If the tips are curved, the curves face downward toward the bottom of the nose (Fig. 1). Adjust the tubing around the back of the ears and then under the chin. Encourage the patient to breathe through the nose with the mouth closed.
      PURPOSE: The cannula needs to be inserted correctly into the nostrils. The cannula tips may be blocked by the top of the nostrils if they are inserted incorrectly. Breathing through the mouth when using a cannula is not as beneficial as breathing through the nose.

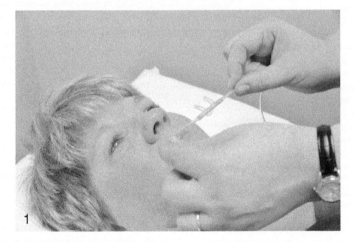

1

7. Make sure the patient is comfortable. Answer any questions he or she may have. Sanitize your hands.
   PURPOSE: Unanswered questions can cause anxiety. With breathing problems, it is important for the patient to be comfortable and calm.

8. Document the procedure. Include the name of the ordering provider, the number of liters of oxygen administered, the device used for administering the oxygen, and the patient's condition.
   PURPOSE: Indicating who ordered the oxygen and what was administered is important for insurance reimbursement and for legal reasons.

Documentation Example

08/07/20XX 1540: R: 28 regular, shallow. Per Dr. Angela Perez's order, 2 LPM of oxygen administered via nasal cannula. Pt resting on exam table.
———————————————————————— Renee Thomas, CMA (AAMA)

08/07/20XX 1555: R: 20 regular, normal. Pt stated she is "feeling better" with the oxygen and has less SOB. Dr. Angela Perez was notified.
———————————————————————— Renee Thomas, CMA (AAMA)

26

UROLOGY AND MALE REPRODUCTION

SCENARIO

Hannah Yang, a certified medical assistant (CMA) through the American Association of Medical Assistants (AAMA), was hired 4 months ago. She assists the specialists who hold outreach clinics at Walden-Martin Family Medical (WMFM) Clinic. She has been training with the urology staff that comes for the outreach clinics four times a month.

Hannah's role with the urology staff is to help room patients and assist the staff. To prepare for working with the specialists, Hannah spent some time reviewing her medical assistant textbook. She had forgotten the process of urine formation. She had to brush up on the way the urinary system impacts the

homeostasis of the body. Hannah knows that the urinary system is important and that if a person's kidneys are not functioning, he or she will need to go on dialysis. As part of her orientation to this specialty, she was able to spend 4 hours at the local dialysis clinic. There, the "regular" patients enjoyed telling her their experiences. Their experiences and the information from the dialysis technicians helped Hannah understand what patients go through with kidney disease.

When she assists the urologist, Dr. Ubert Riney, and his team, Hannah learns a great deal. She knows she has more to learn about this specialty.

While studying this chapter, think about the following questions:
- What terms relate to the urinary and male reproductive systems?
- What is the location of the urinary system structures?
- What is the location of the male reproductive system structures?
- What process is required to make urine?

- What are common urinary system diseases, including their etiology, signs and symptoms, diagnostic procedures, and treatments?
- What are common male reproductive system diseases, including their etiology, signs and symptoms, diagnostic procedures, and treatments?

LEARNING OBJECTIVES

1. Describe the anatomical location of the major organs of the urinary system.
2. Describe the anatomical location of the major organs of the male reproductive system, and explain the process of spermatogenesis.
3. Explain the physiology of the urinary system, and describe life span changes related to the urinary system.
4. Explain the physiology of the male reproductive system.
5. List common signs and symptoms of urinary and male reproductive systems diseases, and identify common disorders of the urinary and male reproductive systems.

6. Discuss the medical assistant's role in urology procedures, and demonstrate how to coach patients regarding health maintenance (e.g., testicular self-exam).
7. Describe diagnostic procedures used for urinary and male reproductive diseases.
8. Identify CLIA-waived tests associated with urinary disease, and describe treatments used for urinary and male reproductive diseases.

VOCABULARY

afferent (AF fur ent) Pertains to carrying toward a structure.

anticoagulant (an tee koe AG yoo lant) A substance (i.e., medication or chemical) that prevents the clotting of blood.

antihyperlipidemic (an tie hie per lip i DEE mik) A drug that lowers the lipid levels in the blood.

antihypertensive A drug that reduces high blood pressure.

arterioles (ar TEER ee ohlz) Small arteries.

arteriovenous Pertains to the arteries and veins.

arteriovenous fistula An abnormal joining of an artery and vein.

calculi (KAL kyuh lie) Stones formed in the kidneys, gallbladder, and other parts of the body.

catheter A hollow, flexible tube that can be inserted into a vessel, organ, or cavity of the body to withdraw or instill fluid, monitor information, and visualize a vessel or cavity.

corticosteroids A group of steroid hormones produced in the body or given as a drug; some have metabolic functions, and others decrease tissue inflammation. Glucocorticoids and mineralocorticoids are two types.

diuretic A drug that increases the amount of urine produced.

efferent (EF fur ent) Pertains to carrying away from a structure.

erythropoietin (eh rith roh POY eh tin) A hormone that is produced by the kidney cells and travels to the bone marrow to stimulate red blood cell formation.

filtrate Fluid and substances that are filtered out of the blood in the Bowman capsule.

graft Tissue taken from one area in the body and inserted into another area or person.

hydronephrosis (hie droh nuh FROH sis) A backup of urine that causes dilation of the ureters and calyces; can increase pressure on the nephron units.

hyperlipidemia (hie per lip i DEE mee ah) An elevated level of lipids in the blood.

hypoalbuminemia (hie poh al byoo mi NEE mee ah) A decreased level of albumin (protein) in the blood.

intermittent Occurring in intervals.

interstitial (in ter STISH uhl) Between the cells.

interstitial cells Testosterone-secreting cells of testes that are found in the spaces between the seminiferous tubules.

intravenous (IV) Through a vein; fluids and medications can be given through a vein.

metabolites (meh TAB uh lites) Byproducts of drug metabolism.

nephrectomy Surgical removal of a kidney.

neuropathy (nu ROP a thee) A nervous system disorder of the peripheral nerves that causes discomfort, numbness, and weakness, especially in the extremities.

peritoneum (per i tuh NEE um) A serous membrane lining of the abdominal cavity, which folds inward to enclose the viscera (internal organs).

peritubular (per i TOO bu lar) **capillaries** Blood capillaries surrounding the proximal and distal convoluted tubules in the kidneys.

permeability A quality or characteristic of a material that allows another substance to pass through it.

pruritus Itching.

puberty (PYOO bur tee) The stage of life in which males and females become functionally capable of sexual reproduction.

residual urine Urine that remains in the bladder after micturition or urination.

rugae (ROO gay) Folds in the wall of the organ; when the organ (e.g., stomach, bladder, uterus) fills or needs to expand, the rugae unfold.

septicemia (sep ti SEE mee ah) A systemic infection involving pathologic microbes in the blood as a result of an infection that has spread from elsewhere in the body.

spermatozoa (spur muh tah ZOH ah) (singular, spermatozoon) Mature male reproductive cells.

stoma (STOH mah) A temporary or permanent surgically created opening used for drainage (i.e., urine, stool).

stretch receptor A sensory nerve ending that responds to a stretch stimulus.

testis (TES tis) (plural, testes) The male gonad, also called a testicle (TES ti kul).

testosterone (tess TOS tuh rohn) Male sex hormone produced by the interstitial cells in the testes.

transitional epithelium A type of cell found in the lining of hollow organs. It has the ability to stretch with the contraction and distention of the organ.

urostomy (yoo ROS te mee) A surgically created opening on the abdominal wall used to drain urine.

vascular access A surgical procedure that creates a vein to remove and return blood during the hemodialysis procedure.

venule (VEN yuhl) A very small vein.

---

*U*rology is the healthcare specialty that deals with most urinary and male reproductive disorders. A *urologist* is a specialist involved in the diagnosis, treatment, and prevention of disorders of the urinary system and the male reproductive system.

It is common for patients with either urinary symptoms or men with reproduction-related concerns to see their primary care provider or an urgent care provider. All medical assistants should be familiar with the anatomy, physiology, and *pathology* (diseases) of both the urinary and male reproductive systems. Sexually transmitted infections (STIs), which can impact both the urinary and male reproductive systems, are discussed in Chapter 18.

ANATOMY OF THE URINARY AND THE MALE REPRODUCTIVE SYSTEMS

Urinary System

The urinary system is composed of two kidneys, two ureters, a urinary bladder, and a urethra (Figs. 26.1 and 26.2). The kidneys filter the blood and eliminate waste through the passage of urine. The ureters move urine from the kidneys to the bladder. The urinary bladder stores the urine until it is excreted. The urethra is the tube that conducts the urine out of the bladder.

Kidneys

The kidneys are bean-shaped organs, the size of a fist. The *hilum* (an indentation) is the location on the kidney where the ureter and renal vein leave the kidney and the renal artery enters. The kidneys are located posterior to the **peritoneum**, the muscles of the back, and between the T12 and L3 vertebrae. The left kidney is situated about 1 inch (2 cm) higher than the right because of the location of the liver.

The kidneys remove unwanted substances from the blood and form urine for excretion. Blood is delivered to the two kidneys by the renal arteries, which branch off the abdominal aorta (Fig. 26.3). Blood flows from the renal arteries into **afferent arterioles** (smaller arteries) and then through a network of capillaries called the *glomeruli*. Filtration of the blood occurs in the glomerulus. Blood from the glomerulus moves into the **efferent** arterioles and then into the **peritubular capillaries**. As the blood leaves the kidneys, it moves from the peritubular capillaries to **venules** and then empties into the

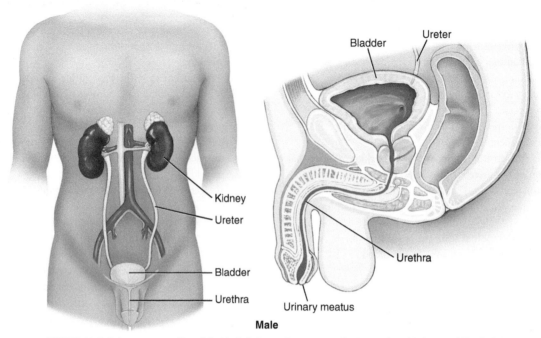

Male

FIGURE 26.1 Male urinary system. (From Shiland B: *Medical terminology & anatomy for ICD-10 coding*, ed 2, St. Louis, 2016, Mosby.)

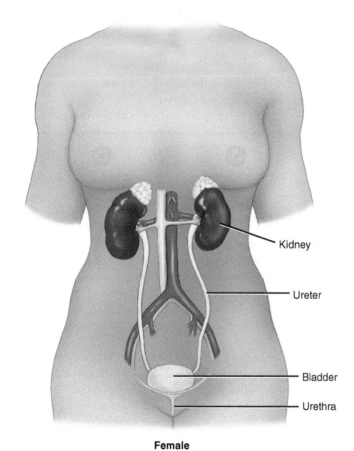

Female

FIGURE 26.2 Female urinary system. (From Shiland B: *Medical terminology & anatomy for ICD-10 coding*, ed 2, St. Louis, 2016, Mosby.)

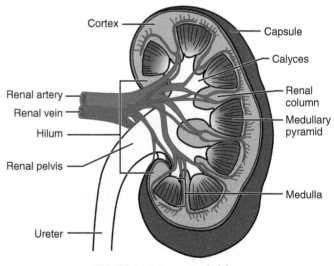

FIGURE 26.3 Cross section of a kidney.

renal veins. The renal veins take the blood out of the kidneys. Blood from the renal veins flows into the inferior vena cava as it heads to the heart to become oxygenated again (Fig. 26.4).

If a kidney were sliced open, you would see the following:

- *Capsule*: The fibrous outer covering of the kidney
- *Cortex*: The outer portion of the kidney
- *Renal column*: An extension of the cortex that dips down between the medullary pyramids
- *Medulla*: The inner portion that extends from the end of the cortex to the calyces

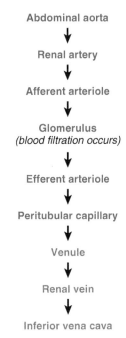

Abdominal aorta

↓

Renal artery

↓

Afferent arteriole

↓

Glomerulus
(blood filtration occurs)

↓

Efferent arteriole

↓

Peritubular capillary

↓

Venule

↓

Renal vein

↓

Inferior vena cava

FIGURE 26.4 Blood flow to and from the kidney.

- *Medullary pyramid*: A cone-shaped structure located in the medulla and containing straight tubular structures and blood vessels
- *Minor and major calyces and the renal pelvis*: Extensions of the ureter inside the kidney

Each kidney contains tissue with millions of microscopic units called *nephrons*. Nephrons are the functional units of the kidneys. They are located in the cortex and extend into the medulla. Each nephron is a very long tube, or *tubule*. One end of the nephron is the *renal corpuscle*, and the remaining section of the nephron is the *renal tubule*. The renal corpuscle consists of the following:

- *Bowman capsule*: A cup-shaped structure of the nephron that surrounds the glomerulus
- *Glomerulus*: A cluster of capillaries inside of the Bowman capsule

The afferent arteriole brings blood into the glomerulus, and the efferent arteriole takes blood away from the glomerulus. The diameter of the afferent arteriole is much larger than the diameter of the efferent arteriole. The importance of the narrowed diameter will be discussed in the Physiology of the Urinary and the Male Reproductive Systems section of this chapter.

The renal tubule is a long, thin, twisted tube that brings the **filtrate** (which will become urine) from the Bowman capsule to the renal pelvis. During the passage of filtrate from the Bowman capsule to the renal pelvis, water and electrolytes move between the urine and the blood to maintain homeostasis. The formation of urine will be discussed later in the chapter. The renal tubule is made up of the following:

- *Proximal (convoluted) tubule* (PCT): The first section of the renal tubule that is attached to the Bowman capsule.
- *Henle loop*: Follows the PCT and includes a straight descending section, a loop, and then a straight ascending section.
- *Distal (convoluted) tubule* (DCT): Follows after the ascending section of the Henle loop.

- *Collecting duct* (CD): Multiple distal tubules join and form this straight collecting duct, which empties into the calyx.

To summarize, the nephron begins on one end with the Bowman capsule, which is filled with the capillaries. The proximal tubule is the next section of the nephron. It is followed by the Henle loop, then the distal tubule, and finally the collecting duct. Many collecting ducts empty into one calyx. Many calyces merge into the renal pelvis, which is an extension of the ureter inside the kidney. The Bowman capsule, proximal tubules, and distal tubes are in the cortex. The Henle loop and the collecting ducts are in the medulla of the kidney.

CRITICAL THINKING APPLICATION   26.1

Hannah is working with Mrs. Green, a urology patient. Mrs. Green has kidney disease and asks Hannah what the kidneys do. How should Hannah explain the role of the kidneys to Mrs. Green?

Ureters

The bilateral ureters are thin, muscular tubes approximately 10 inches long. The tube's muscular layer creates peristaltic waves that help move the urine to the bladder. The ureters' walls are made of **transitional epithelium**, which allows the ureters to stretch to accommodate urine flow. Many nerve endings are also in the walls. A stone in the ureter can cause severe pain.

The point where the ureter enters the bladder is called the *ureterovesical junction*. The ureters enter the bladder at an angle. This creates a flap over the end of the ureter, which serves as a valve. Urine can empty into the bladder, but it cannot back up from the bladder and reenter the ureter. This mechanism also prevents bacteria from moving from the bladder up to the kidneys.

Bladder

The urinary bladder is a hollow organ in the pelvic cavity. It serves as a holding tank for urine. Urine enters the bladder through the ureters and leaves the bladder through the urethra. The triangular area in the bladder between the ureters' entrance and the urethral outlet is called the *trigone*.

Transitional epithelium creates the inner lining of the bladder. When the bladder is empty, it flattens, and the walls overlap in folds, also known as **rugae**. This creates a wrinkled appearance. As the bladder starts to fill with urine, the rugae and transitional epithelium allow for greater bladder volume. Think of a balloon that was blown up and then emptied of air. The balloon is smaller and wrinkly in appearance. When inflated, the wrinkles are gone, and it can accommodate a large volume of air. The same thing happens with the bladder and urine.

The bladder is also composed of smooth muscle fibers that make up the *detrusor muscle*. The detrusor muscle relaxes when the bladder fills. It contracts to push urine out of the bladder and into the urethra. Normally, the bladder holds about 1.5 to 2 cups (360 to 480 mL) of urine during the day and doubles that amount at night. As the bladder fills to about 150 mL, **stretch receptors** in the detrusor send a message to the central nervous system. As more urine enters the bladder, the urge to urinate increases. After urination or *micturition*, **residual urine** remains (usually less than 50 mL) in the bladder.

TABLE 26.1	Difference in the Urethra Between the Genders	
	FEMALE	**MALE**
Length	1–1.5 inches	8 inches
Function	Urination	Urination and ejaculation
Location of Internal Sphincter	None	At the proximal end (bladder end) of the urethra; may prevent semen from moving into the bladder
Location of External Sphincter	Extends up to the bladder, encircles the vagina and urethra	Under the prostate gland

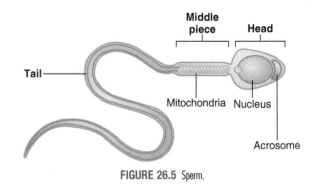

FIGURE 26.5 Sperm.

Urethra

The urethra is a mucous membrane–lined tube that drains urine out of the bladder. In males, the internal urethral sphincter is located at the bladder end (or proximal end) of the urethra. The sphincter is made of smooth involuntary muscles. The external sphincter is located in different places in males and in females (Table 26.1). The external sphincter is made of skeletal muscles and is a voluntary muscle. A voluntary muscle provides you with the ability to control when you urinate. The distal end of the urethra is called the *urinary meatus*. The urinary meatus is the final structure before the urine leaves the body.

CRITICAL THINKING APPLICATION   26.2
Hannah is working with Katrina, the urology medical assistant. Hannah asks Katrina what the major differences are between the male and female urinary systems. How would Katrina respond to Hannah's question?

Male Reproductive System

The primary reproductive organs in the male are testes. Each **testis** is oval in shape and about 4 cm (1.6 inches) long and 2.5 cm (1 inch) wide. The testes are surrounded by a white, fibrous capsule and are suspended together in a sac outside the body called the scrotum. Testes produce the gametes called **spermatozoa**. Spermatozoa are made up of three parts (Fig. 26.5):

- *Head*: Contains the chromosomes in the nucleus; the *acrosome* covers the head of the sperm and contains enzymes to help penetrate the ovum
- *Midpiece:* Contains mitochondria, which produce energy for movement
- *Tail* (or *flagellum*): Used for movement

The formation of sperm is called *spermatogenesis*. The spermatozoa are formed in a series of tightly coiled tiny tubes in each testis called the *seminiferous tubules*. From the seminiferous tubules, the formed spermatozoa travel to the *epididymis*, where they mature and are stored. The epididymis is a coiled tube that is almost 6 meters (20 feet) long and rests on top of and behind each testis.

From the epididymis, the spermatozoa move into the *vas deferens* (or *ductus deferens*) (Fig. 26.6). Each vas deferens is a muscular tunnel about 45 cm (18 inches) long that connects to the base of the epididymis and passes along the side of the testis. The vas deferens travels into the pelvic cavity to just behind the bladder. Spermatozoa can stay in the vas deferens for several months in an inactive state.

The *prostate gland* is the size of a walnut and found below the bladder in males. It surrounds part of the urethra. The prostate is considered a reproductive organ, but it also impacts the urinary system. When the prostate increases in size (as with benign prostatic hyperplasia [BPH]), it can obstruct the urethra, blocking the urine flow. The prostate gland, *seminal vesicles*, and *Cowper glands* provide fluid either to nourish or to aid in motility and lubrication. The sperm and the fluid together make up a substance called *semen*. The *ejaculatory duct* begins where the seminal vesicles join the vas deferens, and this "tube" joins the urethra. The urethra is found within the *penis* and transports the semen to the outside of the body. The urethra also transports urine to the outside of the body. The semen exits the body through the tip of the penis, the *glans penis*. At birth, the glans penis is surrounded by a fold of skin called the *prepuce* or *foreskin*, which can be removed by a *circumcision*.

CRITICAL THINKING APPLICATION   26.3
To review the anatomy of the male reproductive system, Hannah is writing down the process of spermatogenesis, including all of the structures needed from the formation of the sperm until it leaves the body in semen. Can you do the same?

CRITICAL THINKING APPLICATION   26.4
Hannah is working with Mr. Endl, who has BPH. He asks Hannah why the BPH impacts his urine flow. How should Hannah respond to Mr. Endl?

PHYSIOLOGY OF THE URINARY AND THE MALE REPRODUCTIVE SYSTEMS

Urinary System

The urinary system has several important roles that help regulate homeostasis in the body:

- *Maintains fluid volume.* The urinary system increases fluid loss in urine when fluid volume is high. It decreases the fluid loss when the fluid volume is low (e.g., with dehydration).

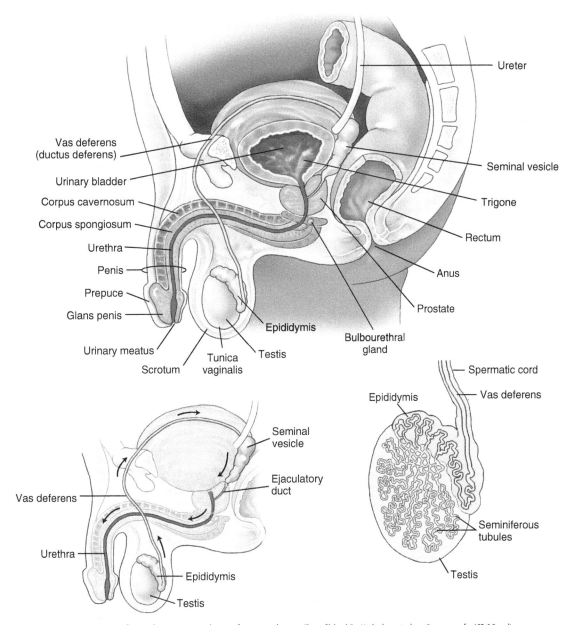

FIGURE 26.6 Male reproductive system with inset of sperm production. (From Shiland B: *Medical terminology & anatomy for ICD-10 coding,* ed 2, St. Louis, 2016, Mosby.)

- *Maintains the normal composition of body fluids.* The urinary system can increase or decrease the loss of certain electrolytes in the urine as it regulates the normal makeup of the body fluids. This helps to keep the pH of the blood within normal limits.
- *Maintains an adequate blood pressure.* Renin, an enzyme, is secreted in the urinary system and is involved with increasing the blood pressure.
- *Controls red blood cell production.* **Erythropoietin** is secreted by the urinary system, which triggers red blood cell production.
- *Activates vitamin D.* The kidneys are involved with the final step of vitamin D activation. Vitamin D is important in the absorption of calcium and phosphorus.

Many of these roles are performed during the formation of urine. The body rids itself of unneeded substances produced during the metabolic process. The process of urine formation includes three steps: filtration, reabsorption, and secretion. Each step will be described in more detail in the coming sections.

Filtration

Filtration is the first step in urine formation. It is a continual process that involves the renal corpuscle. If you recall, the renal corpuscle consists of a cup-shaped structure (Bowman capsule) that surrounds the network of capillaries (glomerulus).

The blood is brought to the kidneys by the renal arteries. The arteries branch into smaller vessels that transport the blood throughout the kidney. As the blood gets to the nephron, an afferent arteriole brings the blood into the glomerulus, and an efferent arteriole takes the blood away. Eventually the blood moves into the renal vein and out of the kidney.

Let us focus on what occurs in the glomerulus. The diameter of the afferent arteriole is larger than the efferent arteriole's diameter. This means the blood moves into the glomerulus faster than it leaves. The pressure inside the glomerulus is high, with the quantity of blood moving into the glomerulus. This forces water and dissolved substances through the one-celled wall of the capillary and into the Bowman capsule. The substance in the Bowman capsule is known as filtrate. (Think of a garden hose that is wide at one part and narrow at the other. The pressure builds up behind the narrowed section. Water can leak from any weakened areas in the wall. This is similar to what occurs in the glomerulus.)

Several dissolved substances can move through the capillary wall:
- Electrolytes (i.e., sodium, chloride, and potassium)
- Waste products (i.e., urea, **metabolites**)
- Other substances (i.e., amino acids and glucose)

White blood cells, red blood cells, and plasma proteins are too large to pass through the capillary wall. With normal kidney function, they remain in the capillary.

If the blood pressure falls (i.e., with hemorrhaging), the pressure in the glomerulus is not high enough to cause movement of the fluids, so little to no filtrate is created and the person will have little to no urine output.

Reabsorption

Reabsorption means substances move from the filtrate back into the blood in the peritubular capillaries. As the filtrate moves out of the Bowman capsule and into the proximal tubule, the reabsorption process starts. Water (H_2O) and solutes (e.g., sodium [Na^+] ions and glucose) move back into the blood (Fig. 26.7). See Table 26.2 for the list of solutes that move back into the blood.

In the Henle loop, the reabsorption process is a bit different. The Henle loop dips down into the medulla and then moves back up. The countercurrent flow occurs as the filtrate flows down and then moves back up. During this time, the chloride (Cl^-) and sodium ions move out of the filtrate and into the **interstitial** fluid and blood.

This creates a salty interstitial fluid, which then helps pull water from the distal tubule filtrate. Water, chloride, and sodium are reabsorbed back into the blood as the filtrate passes through the distal tubule.

In the distal tubules, some sodium and chloride ions are reabsorbed from the filtrate. The walls of the distal tubules do not allow water to move out of the filtrate without special help. With the help of

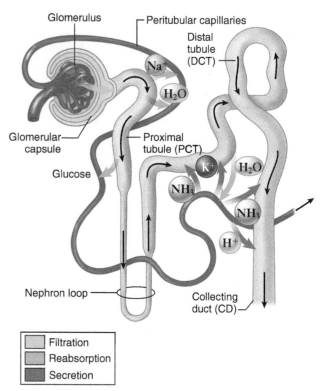

FIGURE 26.7 Formation of urine. Diagram shows examples of steps in urine formation in successive parts of a nephron: filtration, reabsorption, and secretion. (From Patton KT, Thibodeau G: *The human body in health and disease*, ed 7, St. Louis, 2019, Mosby.)

TABLE 26.2	Movement of Substances Between the Blood and Filtrate in the Nephron				
NEPHRON SECTIONS PROCESSES	RENAL CORPUSCLE *(BOWMAN CAPSULE AND GLOMERULUS)*	PROXIMAL TUBULE (PCT)	HENLE LOOP	DISTAL TUBULE (DCT)	COLLECTING DUCT (CD)
Filtration (moves from blood to create filtrate)	Water, electrolyte ions (sodium, chloride, potassium), urea, glucose, and amino acids				
Reabsorption (moves from filtrate to blood)		Water, glucose, amino acids, urea, and electrolyte ions (sodium, chloride, phosphate)	Water and electrolyte ions (chloride, sodium)	Electrolyte ions (chloride, sodium) and water (only in the presence of ADH)	Electrolyte ions (sodium), urea, water (only in the presence of ADH)
Secretion (moves from blood to filtrate)			Urea	Ammonium, potassium, hydrogen, some drugs	Ammonium, potassium, hydrogen, some drugs

ADH, Antidiuretic hormone.

antidiuretic hormone (ADH) (also called *vasopressin*), water moves out of the filtrate and into the bloodstream. ADH is a hormone stored in the posterior pituitary gland. ADH helps increase the water **permeability** of the walls of the distal tubule and collecting duct. Without ADH, a person would pass vast quantities of urine. An inadequate supply of ADH causes diabetes insipidus.

CRITICAL THINKING APPLICATION   **26.5**

Hannah is confused about diabetes insipidus. She always thought diabetes related to insulin and blood glucose. She does not recall learning about diabetes insipidus in school. She asks Katrina, the urology medical assistant, to explain how diabetes insipidus impacts the urinary system. How might Katrina respond to Hannah's question?

Besides ADH, another hormone, called *aldosterone*, works on the urinary system. Aldosterone is secreted by the adrenal cortex. This hormone increases the movement of sodium out of the filtrate in the distal tubule and collecting duct. See Table 26.2 for the complete list of substances reabsorbed in the distal tubule and collecting duct.

To maintain homeostasis, the kidneys retain (or reabsorb) what the body needs. Substances in excessive concentrations and metabolism waste products remain in the filtrate. The filtrate becomes more concentrated as water is reabsorbed into the bloodstream. The kidneys create about 48 gallons (about 182 L) of filtrate a day. By the time reabsorption occurs, they produce only 1 to 2 quarts (about 0.9 to 1.9 L) of urine a day.

Life Span Changes

At about 10 to 12 weeks after conception, the kidneys start producing urine. While the baby is in utero, the mother's placenta performs most of the kidneys' function until the last few weeks before birth. When babies are born, they have the same number of nephrons as an adult. The nephrons are immature and reach maturity by age 2. A baby's kidneys do not retain water like adult kidneys do. Thus, babies can lose water quickly, especially when they are hot or if they have diarrhea. During childhood, the bladder continues to grow. Bladder control is learned usually between age 2 and 3.

During pregnancy, the filtration rate increases in women. The number of nephrons remains the same, but the filtration surface increases. This increase allows the kidneys to filter more blood, which is useful with the increased blood flow during pregnancy. In late pregnancy, the bladder may be twice as big. The anatomical and physiological changes that occur during pregnancy put women at more risk for pyelonephritis at that time.

In older adults, the kidney tissue and number of nephrons are reduced by up to 20%. The renal arteries can harden. This causes the kidneys to filter blood slower. The kidneys become less able to regulate water balance. Older adults are at more risk of dehydration when the weather is hot or if they have diarrhea. The bladder wall becomes less stretchy with age. The bladder cannot hold as much urine as before. Bladder muscles weaken. The urethra may be obstructed by an enlarged prostate gland or a prolapse of the bladder or vagina. Older adults are at more risk for chronic kidney disease, UTIs, and incontinence.

Secretion

Secretion means that substances move from the blood to the filtrate. This allows the body to maintain homeostasis and move unneeded substances back into the filtrate. Urea moves back to the filtrate in the Henle loop. As the filtrate moves through the distal tubule and collecting duct, more adjustments are made. Ammonia (NH_3), certain drugs, hydrogen (H^+), and potassium (K^+) move from the blood into the filtrate. The movement of potassium into the filtrate can be caused by aldosterone. After the filtrate or urine leaves the collecting ducts, no more adjustments are made. The urine then flows to the calyces and to the ureter before going through the rest of the urinary system structures.

Renin and Blood Pressure

As mentioned before, the kidneys have an important role in maintaining blood pressure. The *juxtaglomerular cells* are smooth muscle cells in the afferent arterioles. These cells make and secrete the enzyme *renin*. When the arterial blood pressure decreases or when there is a decrease in sodium, renin is released. Secreting renin is one of the first steps in the complex renin-angiotensin aldosterone system (RAAS). Ultimately when renin is secreted, a series of events occur. The outcome increases the blood pressure two different ways: by creating more blood plasma volume and by constricting of blood vessels. Many hypertensive (high blood pressure) medications impact the RAAS at various points in the hope of lowering the blood pressure. Sometimes it takes more than one medication to lower a person's blood pressure to a safe level.

Erythropoietin

As the blood is moving through the kidneys, specialized kidney cells can detect low oxygen levels in the blood. When this occurs, a hormone called erythropoietin is released from the kidney cells. Erythropoietin travels to the bone marrow and stimulates the marrow to make more red blood cells.

Vitamin D

Vitamin D assists with calcium absorption and helps maintain calcium and phosphorus levels. These minerals are important for strong bones. We get vitamin D from exposure to sunlight, as well as from the consumption of supplements and food. The kidneys must convert vitamin D to an active form so that the body can use it.

Male Reproductive System

At **puberty**, the **interstitial cells** in the testicles begin to produce **testosterone**. Testosterone is responsible for maintaining reproductive structures and for the development of sperm cells. Testosterone also helps with the development of secondary sex characteristics (e.g., deep voice, broad shoulders, narrow hips, and additional body hair).

In addition to testosterone, the *follicle-stimulating hormone* (FSH), which is secreted by the pituitary gland, promotes the formation of spermatozoa. The pituitary gland also produces *luteinizing hormone* (LH), which stimulates the interstitial cells to produce testosterone.

Under the influence of these hormones, the sperm cells develop and move into the epididymis to mature. As described in the anatomy section, eventually the sperm reach the urethra and travel through the shaft, or body, of the *penis*. The penis is composed of three columns of highly vascular erectile tissue. There are two columns of *corpora cavernosa* and one of *corpus spongiosum* that fill with blood through the dorsal veins during sexual arousal. During ejaculation, the sperm exit through the enlarged tip of the penis, the *glans penis*.

DISORDERS OF THE URINARY AND THE MALE REPRODUCTIVE SYSTEMS

Urinary System

Urologic diseases are conditions that impact one or more of the urinary system structures. Common urinary signs and symptoms include the following:

- *Anuria* (no urination), *diuresis* (excretion of large amounts of urine), *dysuria* (painful urination), *enuresis* ("bed wetting"), *oliguria* (scanty urination), *nocturia* (urination during the night), and *polyuria* (excessive urination)
- *Urgency* (need to urinate immediately), *frequency* (urinating more often than normal), *urinary incontinence* (inability to hold urine), and *urinary retention* (inability to release urine)
- *Abnormal substances in the urine: Albuminuria* or *proteinuria* (albumin), *azoturia* (excessive urea), *bacteriuria* (bacteria), *glycosuria* (glycose [sugar]), *hematuria* (blood), and *pyuria* (pus)

Urinary diseases can include infections, stones, kidney problems, cancer, and bladder control problems. A urinary tract infection (UTI) is an infection in one or more of the urinary tract structures. Specific infections will be discussed in the following section, along with other diseases.

Bladder Cancer

Bladder cancer is the sixth most common cancer in the United States. Bladder cancer tends to recur, so follow-up testing is critical. Transitional cell carcinoma (also called urothelial carcinoma) is the most common type of bladder cancer in the United States.

Smoking, chemical exposure, family history of the disease, some chemotherapy medications, and chronic bladder infections can increase the risk of bladder cancer. People over 40 years of age, men, and Caucasians are also more at risk. Common signs and symptoms include hematuria, frequency, urgency, dysuria, pelvic pain, and low back pain.

The provider will do a physical exam. Urine testing, cystoscopy, and a biopsy may be done to diagnose bladder cancer. Additional imaging testing is done to check if the cancer has spread to other parts of the body. Treatments used for bladder cancer include surgery, radiation therapy, and chemotherapy. *Biologic therapy* or *immunotherapy* can be useful, as it increases the body's ability to help fight the cancer.

Cystitis, Acute

Acute cystitis is an inflammation of the bladder. Due to the shorter urethra, women are more at risk than men to get infections.

Typically, acute cystitis is caused by a bacterial infection, most commonly *Escherichia coli* (*E. coli*). Other causes of inflammation can include medications, radiation therapy, spermicidal jellies, and long-term catheterization. Being pregnant, going through menopause, a **catheter**, urinary tract procedure, urinary retention, an obstruction, bowel incontinence, or diabetes can increase the risk of cystitis. Signs and symptoms include the following:

- Nocturia, dysuria, urgency, and frequency
- Urinary retention; cloudy, bloody, or strong/foul-smelling urine
- Low abdominal pressure or cramping, low-grade fever
- With older adults: confusion, mental changes

Usually the provider will order a urinalysis and a urine culture and sensitivity (C&S) test (which is discussed in Chapter 31). The urinalysis provides information to help diagnose the cystitis, and the C&S may take up to 3 days to identify the organism. If the urinalysis and culture come back negative for an infection, the provider may do additional tests (e.g., cystoscopy) to try to identify the cause of the symptoms. Treatment for bacterial cystitis consists of antibiotics.

Home care treatments may include drinking plenty of liquids; avoiding coffee, alcohol, and soft drinks; and taking an analgesic, having a sitz bath, or using a heating pad to decrease the discomfort.

End-Stage Renal Disease

End-stage renal disease (ESRD), also called end-stage kidney disease and kidney failure, occurs when the kidneys are no longer filtering waste from the blood. Dangerous levels of electrolytes, waste products, and fluids build up in the bloodstream. More than 660,000 Americans have kidney failure. Over 44% of those patients are between the ages of 45 and 64.

The top two causes of ESRD are diabetes mellitus and *hypertension* (high blood pressure). Additional causes include glomerulonephritis, polycystic kidney disease, prolonged obstructions or recurrent kidney infections, and vesicoureteral reflux. Using tobacco increases the risk of ESRD. Men, African Americans, and being 45 years or older can also increase the risk. The kidneys can slowly stop functioning over the course of 10 to 20 years before ESRD occurs. A number of symptoms can signal renal failure:

- Loss of appetite, nausea, and weight loss
- Fatigue, headache, and feeling ill
- **Pruritus**, dry skin, changes in skin color and nails
- Numbness in extremities, twitching, and muscle cramps
- Difficulty concentrating and sleep problems

Besides a physical exam, providers will order a bone density test and blood work (e.g., complete blood count [CBC], electrolytes, albumin, and parathyroid hormone). The patient's blood pressure will be monitored closely. ESRD is often treated with a low-protein diet, fluid restrictions, **antihypertensive** medications, vitamin and mineral supplements, dialysis, and a kidney transplant. Dialysis works like a kidney by filtering out the waste products, extra fluids, and electrolytes. There are two different types of dialysis:

- *Peritoneal dialysis*: A catheter is surgically placed in the abdomen. The patient can then infuse a special sterile solution through the catheter into the abdomen. The peritoneal membrane is used as a natural filter, and waste from the blood moves into the infused solution. After a few hours, the patient drains the fluid out of the abdomen via the catheter (Fig. 26.8). New fluid is then infused into the abdomen. There may be four to six exchanges of fluid a day. This type of dialysis allows the person to work, travel, or sleep during the process.
- *Hemodialysis*: A **vascular access** (i.e., catheter, **arteriovenous graft**, **arteriovenous fistula**) is placed. Using the vascular access, the patient is hooked up to a dialysis machine. The person's blood flows through the special filter inside the machine (Fig. 26.9). The filter cleans the blood of waste products and extra

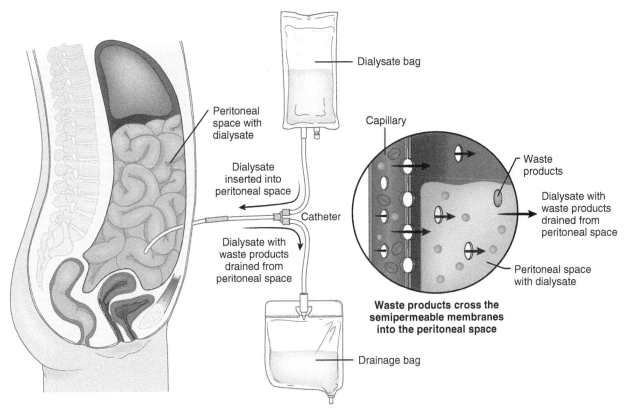

FIGURE 26.8 Peritoneal dialysis.

fluids. Typically, patients need to have hemodialysis three times a week for several hours at the dialysis center. This timely procedure impacts the person's life. Travelling can be an issue, because the person needs to be near a dialysis facility for treatments.

CRITICAL THINKING APPLICATION   **26.6**

With Hannah's experience in the dialysis unit, she learned that many people need to do hemodialysis three times a week for several hours each day. How might this impact a patient's lifestyle?

Glomerulonephritis

Glomerulonephritis is inflammation of the glomeruli and usually has an abrupt onset. Damage to the glomeruli can cause protein and red blood cells to leak into the urine.

The cause is often unknown, and it can follow a streptococcal infection. Signs and symptoms include puffy eyes, fatigue, low-grade fever, headache, and pain over the kidney region. Hematuria, cola-colored urine, proteinuria, and oliguria can also be seen.

After the physical exam, the provider may order a urinalysis, blood urea nitrogen (BUN), creatinine, erythrocyte sedimentation rate (ESR), imaging tests (e.g., computed tomography [CT] scan, x-ray, and ultrasound), and a renal biopsy. Treatment is based on the cause of the illness. Bed rest, hypertensive medications, antibiotics, **diuretics**, and dietary restrictions (e.g., protein, salt, and potassium) may be ordered.

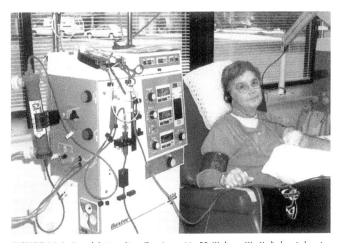

FIGURE 26.9 Hemodialysis machine. (From Ignatavicius DD, Workman ML: *Medical-surgical nursing: critical thinking for collaborative care,* ed 6, Philadelphia, 2011, Saunders.)

Kidney Cancer

Kidney cancer or primary kidney cancer occurs when a cancer starts in the kidney. There are three main types of primary kidney cancer:

- *Renal cell carcinoma* (RCC) (or *renal adenocarcinoma*): Most common type in adults; forms in the lining of the kidney tubules
- *Wilms tumor* (or *nephroblastoma*): Most common type in children younger than 5 years; occurs in the kidney tissue; improved treatments have increased the survival rate

TABLE 26.3   Common Types of Kidney Cancer

	RENAL CELL CARCINOMA	WILMS TUMOR	TRANSITIONAL CELL CANCER
Signs and Symptoms	Hematuria, lump in abdomen, side and back pain (below the ribs), loss of appetite, weight loss, anemia, **intermittent** fever	Hematuria, fever, and abdominal pain, mass and swelling	Hematuria, back pain, extreme fatigue, weight loss, dysuria
Diagnostic Procedures	Physical exam, CBC, blood chemistry tests, UA, liver function tests, CT, MRI, US, biopsy	Physical exam, CBC, blood chemistry tests, UA, US, CT, MRI	Physical exam, CBC, blood chemistry tests, UA, ureteroscopy, IVP, CT, US, MRI, biopsy
Treatment	Surgery (**nephrectomy**), radiation, chemotherapy, biologic therapy, targeted therapy	Surgery (nephrectomy), radiation, chemotherapy	Segmental resection of the ureter, nephroureterectomy, chemotherapy, radiation

CBC, Complete blood count; *CT*, computed tomography; *IVP*, intravenous pyelogram; *MRI*, magnetic resonance imaging; *UA*, urinalysis; *US*, ultrasonography.

- *Transitional cell cancer*: Occurs in adults; forms in the ureter and renal pelvis

It is unclear what causes the mutation of the kidney cell that leads to the tumor development. With kidney cancer, pain and hematuria can be key symptoms. See Table 26.3 for the symptoms for the three types of kidney cancer.

Diagnostic procedures for the three types of kidney cancer are similar (see Table 26.3). During the exam, the provider may identify a kidney mass. Urinalysis and blood work may be done to check for hematuria and the person's overall health. Once kidney cancer is diagnosed, imaging tests are done to check for cancer in other parts of the body. Treatment for kidney cancer can involve surgery. If no kidney function exists, then dialysis and a kidney transplant are done. If surgery is not an option, an arterial embolization can be done. A catheter is inserted through an incision and passed into the main blood vessel of the kidney. A special gelatin sponge is inserted through the catheter into the blood vessel, creating a blockage and preventing blood flow, thus killing the tumor.

Nephrotic Syndrome

Nephrotic syndrome consists of a collection of symptoms that indicate kidney damage. The syndrome is caused by other disorders that eventually lead to kidney tissue destruction.

Minimal change disease is the most common cause of nephrotic syndrome in children. Membranous glomerulonephritis is the most common cause in adults. Nephrotic syndrome can also occur as the result of cancer, chronic disease (e.g., diabetes, systemic lupus erythematosus), infections, immune and genetic disorders, and with the use of certain drugs. The most common sign is swelling of the face, extremities, and abdomen. Additional signs and symptoms can include poor appetite, weight gain, seizures, skin sores, and foamy appearing urine. Blood and urine tests show proteinuria, **hyperlipidemia**, and **hypoalbuminemia**.

Providers will do a physical exam, laboratory testing, and a kidney biopsy. Laboratory work includes blood testing (e.g., albumin, blood chemistry tests, BUN, and creatinine) and urine testing (e.g., creatinine clearance and urinalysis). The treatment goals are to reduce symptoms, delay kidney damage, and prevent additional complications. Antihypertensives, **corticosteroids**, **anticoagulants**, **antihyperlipidemics**, diuretics, and vitamin D supplements may be prescribed. Dietary changes (low fat, low cholesterol, low salt, and low protein) are also recommended.

Neurogenic Bladder

The central nervous system, nerves that supply the bladder, and muscles work together for bladder control. Damage or disorders that impact the bladder nerves or the central nervous system can cause neurogenic bladder. A person with neurogenic bladder lacks bladder control, causing it to be *overactive* (the bladder muscles contract controllably) or *underactive* (the person does not have the urge to go even though the bladder is filled).

The central nervous system disorders that can cause neurogenic bladder include birth defects, cerebral palsy, Alzheimer disease, brain or spinal cord tumors, multiple sclerosis (MS), Parkinson disease, stroke, and spinal cord injury. Damage and disorders of the bladder nerves can be caused by diabetes, syphilis, heavy alcohol use, **neuropathy**, nerve damage from pelvic surgery, herniated disk, or spinal canal stenosis. With overactive bladder, urgency and frequency to urinate are common. With an underactive bladder, the bladder fills but the person does not have the urge to go and incontinence (urine leakage) can occur. Problems with starting to urinate or completely emptying the bladder can also be experienced.

After a physical exam, additional procedures may be ordered, including a postvoid residual volume, blood tests to check kidney functioning (e.g., serum creatinine), renal ultrasonography, and cystoscopy. Treatment is aimed at managing the symptoms of neurogenic bladder. Possible treatments include the following:

- Medications: Antimuscarinic, anticholinergic, botulinum toxin, GABA supplements, and antiepileptics
- Surgical procedures: Artificial urinary sphincter, an implanted electronic device to stimulate bladder nerves, and urinary **stoma** (or **urostomy**)
- Additional procedures: Kegel exercises and a urinary catheter

---

CRITICAL THINKING APPLICATION   26.7

Dr. Riney asked Hannah to coach Mrs. Smith on doing Kegel exercises. How might Hannah explain the process of doing Kegels to Mrs. Smith?

Kegel Exercises

Kegel exercises are used to strengthen the pelvic floor muscles. Both males and females can do them. To use the right muscles, pretend you have to urinate but hold it. The muscles you tighten to stop urination help tighten the pelvic floor muscles. Muscles in the vagina (for females), rectum, and bladder should tighten. The muscles in the thighs, buttock, and abdomen should not be tightened. Kegel exercises should be done three times a day.

To perform Kegel exercises:
1. Empty your bladder.
2. You can be sitting or lying down during the exercises.
3. Tighten the pelvic floor muscles ("hold the urine"). Tighten as you count to 8.
4. Relax the muscles as you count to 10.
5. Repeat this sequence 10 times.

Polycystic Kidney Disease

Polycystic kidney disease (PKD) is an inherited condition. Cysts form in the kidneys, causing the kidneys to become enlarged (Fig. 26.10). A cyst-filled kidney may weigh up to 30 pounds. There are two types of PKD:

- *Autosomal dominant*: The gene is inherited from one parent, and the child will get the disease. This is the most common form of PKD and also the most common inherited kidney disorder. It is typically identified between the ages of 30 and 50, though it can occur in childhood.
- *Autosomal recessive*: To get the disease, a person must get a copy of the defected gene from both parents.

PKD is genetic. People with PKD may also have cysts in their liver and pancreas; aneurysms and diverticula of the colon may also be associated with it. The signs and symptoms of PKD may include nocturia, hematuria, drowsiness, nail abnormalities, and pain in the flank, abdomen, or joints.

During the physical examination, the provider may find pain or tenderness over the liver, an enlarged liver, a heart murmur, and high blood pressure. The provider may order a CBC, liver blood tests, and urinalysis (UA). To check for aneurysms, cerebral angiography may be done. An **intravenous** pyelogram (IVP), abdominal CT, magnetic resonance imaging (MRI), and ultrasound (US) may be ordered to check for cysts on the liver and other organs. The treatment goals are to control symptoms and prevent complications. Treatment often includes antihypertensive medications, diuretics, and a low-salt diet. PKD can increase the risk of urinary tract infections due to blockages. Surgery to remove one or both kidneys may be required, along with dialysis or a kidney transplant.

Pyelonephritis

Pyelonephritis is a urinary tract infection of one or both of the kidneys. Prompt treatment is required to prevent kidney damage and **septicemia**. The bacteria can spread to the bloodstream, causing an overwhelming infection that can be life-threatening.

Pyelonephritis is caused by a bacterium or virus. The pathogen can move from the bladder to the kidneys, or it can be carried by the bloodstream to the kidneys. Increased risk factors for pyelonephritis include structural defect, urinary reflux, obstruction, and bladder infection. The signs and symptoms consist of fever, chills, nausea, vomiting, dysuria, frequency, hematuria, bad-smelling urine, and low back, side (flank), or groin pain. Young children may only experience a fever, and some adults may have confusion and speech difficulties.

After the physical exam, the provider will usually order a urinalysis, urine culture, blood culture, and blood work. Imaging tests (ultrasound, CT scan), a voiding cystourethrogram, a digital rectal examination, and dimercaptosuccinic acid scintigraphy may be done. Initially the provider will treat the infection with a broad-spectrum antibiotic. When the blood and urine culture results are known, the provider may have the patient take an antibiotic that is known to kill the pathogen. For severely ill patients, hospitalization, intravenous fluids and antibiotics, and close observation may be required. Repeat cultures may be taken after the antibiotics have been completed to ensure that the infection is gone.

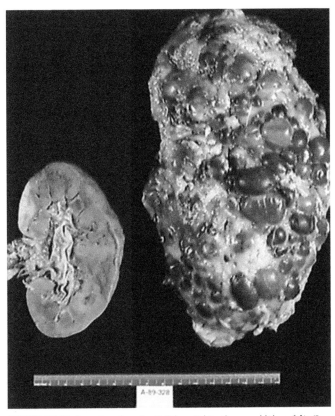

FIGURE 26.10 Comparison of a polycystic kidney *(right)* with a normal kidney *(left)*. (From Lewis SM: *Medical-surgical nursing: assessment and management of clinical problems*, ed 8, St. Louis, 2011, Mosby.)

CRITICAL THINKING APPLICATION   26.8

Hannah is working with Dr. Riney. He ordered an antibiotic for Mrs. Williams, who has a UTI. When the urine culture and sensitivity (C&S) report came back to the department, he asked Hannah to call Mrs. Williams regarding a change in the antibiotic. Why might the provider change the antibiotic once the urine C&S report became available?

Renal Calculi

Renal **calculi** or kidney stones are mineral pebbles that form in the kidney. Symptoms can occur if the calculi grow larger or move into the ureters or renal pelvis (Fig. 26.11). If a stone blocks the flow of urine, infection can develop from the backflow of urine. This blockage also can result in **hydronephrosis** (see Fig. 26.12).

Renal calculi can occur when high levels of certain minerals collect in the kidney. Common minerals include calcium, oxalate, and uric acid. Calculi can also form if fluid intake is low and the filtrate becomes highly concentrated. The tendency to develop kidney stones runs in families. With small stones, the person may not experience symptoms. With larger stones or stones that cause blockages, symptoms will be experienced. Signs and symptoms of kidney stones include dysuria, nausea, vomiting, fever, chills, and severe constant pain on either side of the lower back.

After the physical exam is concluded, a urinalysis, blood tests, and imaging tests are used to diagnose renal calculi. Treatment depends on the size, type, and location of the stones. Small stones may pass on their own. Analgesics may be encouraged for the pain and discomfort. Extra fluids are encouraged to flush the stone out. Typically, patients are asked to strain their urine. Kidney stone strainers should be supplied. If the patient finds a stone, it should be placed in a specimen container and be brought to the lab to be analyzed (Fig. 26.13). Additional procedures include the following:

- *Extracorporeal shock wave lithotripsy* (ESWL): Shock waves are used to break up the stones, so they pass without a problem (Fig. 26.14).
- *Ureteroscopy:* The ureteroscope is threaded up through the bladder and ureter. If the provider sees a stone, it can be removed during the procedure. Sometimes ESWL and ureteroscopy are both done. The stone is broken up before it is removed.
- *Nephrolithotomy:* A surgical incision is made, and the stones are removed by the tube. With *percutaneous nephrolithotripsy* (PNL), the stones are crushed up and removed using suction.

CRITICAL THINKING APPLICATION   26.9

Hannah received a call from Zach Backstrom. He stated that he has a kidney stone and wondered if he really needed to strain his urine and have it analyzed in the lab. What might be the benefits to Zach if he continued to strain his urine for the stone?

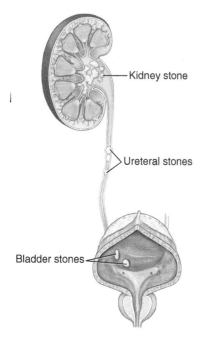

FIGURE 26.11 Locations of ureteral calculi. (From Shiland B: *Mastering healthcare terminology,* ed 5. St. Louis, 2016, Elsevier.)

Urinary Incontinence

Urinary incontinence (UI) is the loss of bladder control causing an accidental loss of urine. There are several types of urinary incontinence (Table 26.4).

UI can occur for many reasons, including damage to the nerves that control the bladder, weak or overactive bladder muscles, diseases that limit mobility, urethral blockages (e.g., enlarged prostate), increase in urine volume, UTI, and constipation. Persistent incontinence can come from pregnancy, childbirth, menopause, pelvic surgery, aging,

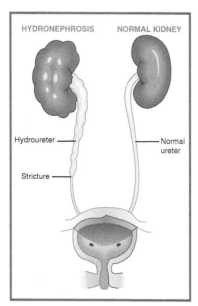

FIGURE 26.12 Hydronephrosis.

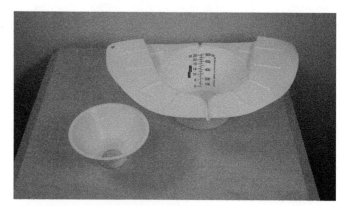

FIGURE 26.13 Urine strainer with a urine/stool collection container (also called hat or pan).

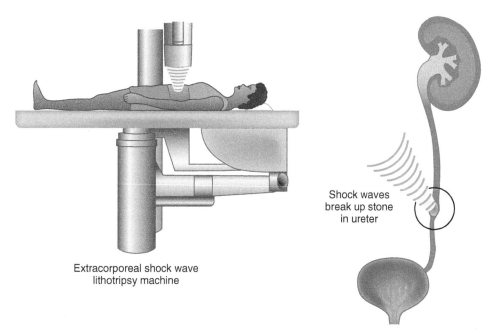

Extracorporeal shock wave
lithotripsy machine

Shock waves
break up stone
in ureter

FIGURE 26.14 Extracorporeal shock wave lithotripsy. (From Linton AD: *Introduction to medical-surgical nursing,* ed 6, Philadelphia, 2016, Saunders.)

TABLE 26.4	Types of Incontinence
TYPE	**DESCRIPTION**
Stress incontinence	Leakage of urine from stress on the bladder; caused by obesity, pregnancy, laughing, running, sneezing, coughing, or lifting heavy objects
Urge incontinence	Also called overactive bladder; strong sudden urge (urgency) before the accidental loss of urine
Overflow incontinence	Most often affects men; the person has difficulty emptying the bladder
Functional incontinence	Caused by a mental or physical disease; leakage occurs before the person can reach the toilet
Mixed incontinence	Typically impacts females; leakage of urine due to overactive bladder and stress incontinence
Total incontinence	Severest type; constant urine leakage
Bed wetting	Usually seen in children; bladder fills during the night and child does not get up to urinate

prostate diseases, obstructions, and neurologic disorders. Accidental leakage of urine, urgency, constant dribbling, and inability to empty the bladder are possible signs and symptoms.

Procedures used to diagnose incontinence include urinalysis, postvoid residual measurement, cystoscopy, cystogram, and pelvic ultrasound. The patient may keep a bladder diary, recording the amount of fluid consumed and urinated, number of incontinence episodes, and frequency and urgency feelings. *Urodynamic testing* may also be done, which involves the bladder being filled via a catheter while the bladder pressure is measured. Treatments can vary based on the type of incontinence. Behavior techniques, including bladder training, double voiding, scheduled toilet trips, and management of fluid and diet, may be done. Kegel exercises and electrical stimulation are used to strengthen pelvic floor muscles. Medications can also be used as part of the treatment for incontinence. Anticholinergics, mirabegron, alpha-blockers, Botox, and topical estrogen can also be used. Surgical procedures can also be performed to treat certain types of incontinence. Medical devices may be used as treatment, including the following:
- *Urethral insert:* A disposable device inserted into the urethra before activities that trigger incontinence
- *Pessary:* A stiff ring inserted into the vagina that holds up the bladder; used for incontinence due to prolapsed bladder
- *Nerve stimulator:* An implanted device that delivers electrical pulses to the nerves that control the bladder

Additional Urinary System Disorders
There are many urinary system disorders. The following list provides a brief description of additional urinary conditions:
- *Acute tubular necrosis:* Rapid destruction of the tubular sections of the nephrons due to blood flow impairment or toxins.
- *Anterior prolapse:* Also called cystocele, prolapse, or dropped bladder. Anterior prolapse is a bulging or dropping of the bladder into the vagina caused by weakening and stretching of supportive tissues and muscles (Fig. 26.15).
- *Bladder outlet obstruction* (BOO): Blockage at the opening of the bladder or in the urethra.
- *Diabetes insipidus:* Endocrine disorder that causes dehydration and vast quantities of urine to be excreted. (Discussed in Chapter 23.)

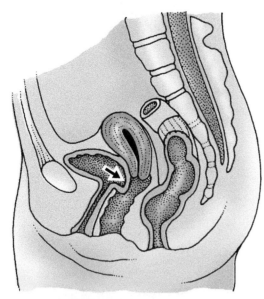

FIGURE 26.15 Anterior prolapse. The urinary bladder is displaced downward *(arrow)*, which causes bulging of the anterior vaginal wall. (From Ignatavicius DD, Workman ML: *Medical-surgical nursing: critical thinking for collaborative care*, ed 6, Philadelphia, 2011, Saunders.)

- *Hydronephrosis:* Distention of renal pelvis and calyces due to urinary tract obstruction; caused by a congenital defect or renal calculi.
- *Interstitial cystitis* (IC): Also called *painful bladder syndrome* (PBS); causes recurring bladder and pelvic region pain and discomfort, frequency, and urgency.
- *Membranous glomerulonephritis:* Inflammation occurs in the kidney due to glomerular changes, and large amounts of protein are excreted in the urine. The exact etiology is unknown.
- *Minimal change disease:* Damage occurs to the glomeruli, though the cause is unknown.
- *Nocturnal enuresis:* Also called bed wetting. The bladder fills up during the night, and the child is in too deep of a sleep to get up to urinate.
- *Prune belly syndrome* (PBS): Group of genetic birth defects usually occurring in boys; involves enlarged ureters and bladder, hydronephrosis (kidney swelling), poor development of the abdominal muscles, undescended testicles, and wrinkled skin over the abdomen.
- *Reflux nephropathy:* Urine backflows from the bladder, causing kidney damage. Can be due to a ureter defect, obstruction, or swelling.
- *Ureterocele:* End of ureter is malformed and bulges, creating a ureterocele, and may obstruct the ureter or bladder.
- *Ureteropelvic junction* (UPJ) *obstruction:* Blockage where the ureter joins the kidney, causing kidney swelling.
- *Urethritis:* Inflammation of the urethra due to bacteria, viruses, injury, or chemical sensitivity.
- *Vesicoureteral reflux* (VUR): Urine backs up into the ureter from the bladder due to a malformed or missing valve over the end of the ureter.

Male Reproductive Disorders

Male reproductive disorders can impact the urinary system. Common male reproductive disorder signs and symptoms include the following:
- Redness and swelling
- Changes in the urinary stream
- Lumps

The following sections discuss more common male reproductive disorders.

Benign Prostatic Hyperplasia

Benign prostatic hyperplasia (BPH) is a nonmalignant condition seen in about half of men over the age of 50 and in more than 90% of men in their 70s and 80s.

As men age, the cells of the prostate gland that surround the urethra can start to reproduce more rapidly, causing the organ to enlarge (*hyperplasia*). The enlarged prostate compresses the urethra, causing urgency, frequency, difficulty starting urination, urine retention, dribbling, hematuria, and repeated UTIs.

During the physical exam, the provider will do a digital rectal exam (DRE) by inserting a gloved finger in the rectum to palpate the prostate (Fig. 26.16). Blood tests (e.g., prostate-specific antigen [PSA], tests of kidney function), urinalysis, transrectal biopsy, urodynamic tests, and cystoscopy may also be done. Treatments include the following:
- *Lifestyle changes:* Bladder training, avoiding caffeine and alcohol, and preventing constipation.
- *Medications:* Used independently or combined with other medications:
  - *Alpha-blockers:* Relax the smooth muscles of the prostate and the bladder neck to improve urine flow and reduce the blockage. Examples include terazosin (Hytrin), doxazosin (Cardura), tamsulosin (Flomax), alfuzosin (Uroxatral), and silodosin (Rapaflo).
  - *5-Alpha reductase inhibitors:* Prevent growth of or shrinks the prostate. Examples include finasteride (Proscar) and dutasteride (Avodart).
- *Transurethral resection of the prostate (TURP) surgery:* A lighted scope is inserted into the urethra, and all but the outer part of the prostate is removed.
- *Laser therapy:* A high-energy laser is used to destroy the overgrown prostate tissue.

Erectile Dysfunction

Erectile dysfunction (ED), also called *impotence*, occurs when a male has trouble keeping or getting an erection. ED is an ongoing issue that impacts relationships, affects the male's self-confidence, and can cause stress.

Common conditions that lead to ED include heart disease, hypertension, tobacco use, alcoholism, diabetes, metabolic syndrome, Parkinson disease, prior pelvic surgeries and treatments, obesity, depression, and stress. Male arousal involves hormones, emotions, muscles, blood vessels, nerves, and the brain, thus any change in these may lead to ED. The sign of ED is trouble keeping or getting an erection firm enough for sex.

After the physical exam, the provider may order tests to identify the cause of ED. Treatment consists of a healthy lifestyle and oral erectile dysfunction medications, including avanafil (Stendra), sildenafil

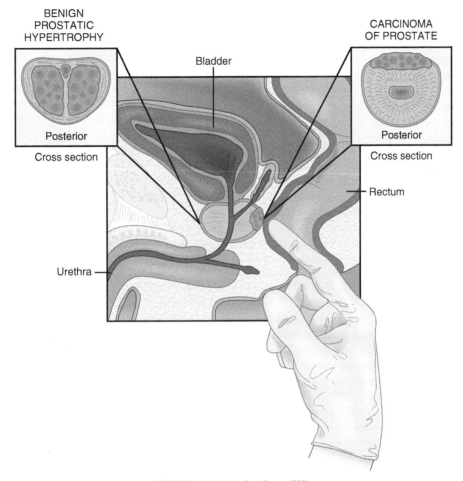

FIGURE 26.16 Digital rectal exam (DRE).

(Viagra, Revatio), tadalafil (Adcirca, Cialis), and vardenafil (Levitra, Staxyn).

Prostate Cancer

Prostate cancer is the second most common cancer among males, and the survival rate is very high. With prostate cancer, the gland can increase in size, obstructing the urethra and causing additional urinary complications About one in seven men will be diagnosed with prostate cancer.

Cells in the prostate mutate, causing the cancer. The risk for prostate cancer is increased in men over 60 years of age, African Americans, or those with a family history of the disease. Having a brother or father with the disease doubles the risk. This risk for the aggressive form of prostate cancer is increased in men who are tall, obese, lack exercise, have a family history of the disease, are African American, consume a high intake of calcium, and have been exposed to Agent Orange. Prostate cancer tends to be a silent disease in the early stages. It is not until the cancer grows large enough to obstruct the urethra that symptoms are noticeable. With advanced prostate cancer, the symptoms can include the following:

- Problems with urination: slow, weak stream; frequency, nocturia
- Hematuria, blood in the semen
- Difficulty getting an erection
- Hip pain, back pain
- Loss of bladder or bowel control

The provider completes a DRE during the examination and a prostate-specific antigen (PSA) blood test is done. If the DRE is abnormal or the PSA blood test level has increased from the baseline, a needle biopsy of the prostate may be done. If cancer is detected, additional imaging tests will be ordered to determine the extent of cancer. Treatment will be based on the type of prostate cancer. If the cancer is a nonaggressive type, the provider may suggest frequent checks to monitor any signs that the cancer is growing or changing. For aggressive prostate cancers, a *prostatectomy* (surgical removal of the prostate) and radiation may be done.

Agent Orange

Agent Orange was an herbicide used by the US military to remove dense foliage during the Vietnam War. It is presumed that any veteran who served in Vietnam was exposed to Agent Orange. The Veterans Administration has attributed several diseases to Agent Orange. These diseases include diabetes mellitus, Hodgkin disease, multiple myeloma, Parkinson disease, respiratory cancers, and prostate cancers. A 2013 study found that veterans exposed to Agent Orange had a higher risk for developing prostate cancer. They also have a greater risk for aggressive prostate cancer. Screening for prostate cancer is important in veterans exposed to Agent Orange. Male children of veterans with aggressive prostate cancer are also at greater risk of developing prostate cancer.

Prostate-Specific Antigen Blood Test

The prostate-specific antigen (PSA) blood test is used as a screening tool for prostate cancer. Both normal and cancerous prostate cells make the protein PSA. Often PSA levels increase in the blood with prostate cancer, prostatitis, and BPH. It is recommended for men to have a baseline PSA test at the age of 40. If the patient has an increased risk, the provider may decide to get a baseline PSA test earlier than age 40. The provider then checks the PSA level over time by comparing it to the baseline level. The higher the PSA level, the more likely it is that the patient has prostate cancer. However, because the PSA level can be elevated with other disorders, one abnormal screening value is not enough to diagnose cancer. The reliability of the PSA blood test is debated, but it is the only screening tool available at this time.

CRITICAL THINKING APPLICATION   26.10

Hannah is rooming Sam Fox, a 40-year-old father of three children. He is 6 feet tall. When Hannah obtains a family history on Sam, she learns that his father, a Vietnam veteran, was just diagnosed with aggressive prostate cancer. What risk factors does Sam have for prostate cancer?

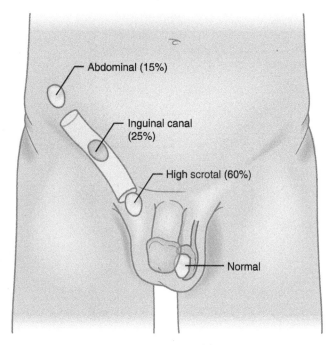

FIGURE 26.17 Cryptorchidism.

Testicular Cancer

Testicular cancer is rare and highly treatable. It is the most common cancer in males between 15 and 35 years of age. It is more common in men who had abnormal testicle development, an undescended testicle, and a family history of the cancer.

Many causes of testicular cancer are unknown. The patient usually discovers a lump or swelling in the testicle. There may also be complaints of a heavy sensation in the scrotum accompanied by a sudden collection of fluid; the patient may also experience pain in a testicle or the scrotum, abdomen, or groin.

To determine if a lump is testicular cancer, a provider may order the following:

- Ultrasound and CT scan
- Biopsy of testicular tissue
- Blood tests to check the testicular cancer markers (alpha fetoprotein [AFP], beta human chorionic gonadotropin [beta-hCG], and lactate dehydrogenase [LDH])

Treatment consists of surgery to remove the testicle (*radical inguinal orchiectomy*), radiation therapy, and chemotherapy.

Additional Male Reproductive Disorders

There are many male reproductive disorders. The following list provides a brief description of additional conditions:

- Penile disorders: Affecting the penis
  - *Balanitis:* Inflammation of the head and foreskin of the penis
  - *Peyronie disease:* Thick scar tissue develops in the penis, causing it to bend
  - *Priapism:* Painful erection that does not go away
  - *Penile cancer:* Rare form of cancer; highly curable in the early stages
- Disorders of the testicular, epididymis, breast, and other structures:

- *Epididymitis:* Inflammation of the epididymis; often caused by a bacterial infection that starts in the bladder, prostate, or urethra
- *Gynecomastia:* Enlargement of breast tissue in males caused by an estrogen and testosterone imbalance.
- *Orchitis:* Inflammation of one or both of the testicles, usually caused by bacteria or viruses (e.g., mumps)
- *Prostatitis:* Inflammation of the prostate that can obstruct urinary flow
- *Spermatocele:* A cystlike mass filled with fluid and dead sperm cells; located in the epididymis
- *Testicular torsion:* Twisting of the spermatic cord, causing the blood supply to be blocked off from the testicles; may occur after an injury to the area
- *Varicocele:* Enlargement of the veins in the scrotum; may cause low sperm production and quality, leading to infertility
- Congenital disorders:
  - *Anorchism:* The absence of one or both testes at birth
  - *Chordee:* Downward curve of the penis due to a congenital condition such as hypospadias
  - *Cryptorchidism:* Also called undescended testicle, or the testicle fails to descend into the scrotum (Fig. 26.17); the testicle develops in the abdomen and starts its descent into the scrotum in utero around the seventh month; treatment for this condition consists of gonadotropic hormones and surgery (*orchiopexy*).
  - *Epispadias:* Congenital malformation causing the urethra to open on top of the penis
  - *Hypospadias:* Congenital malformation causing the urethra to open on the underside of the penis
  - *Hydrocele:* Fluid-filled sac in the scrotum, common in newborn infants and may go away in a few months (Fig. 26.18); often caused by an inguinal hernia

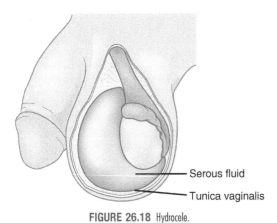

Serous fluid

Tunica vaginalis

FIGURE 26.18 Hydrocele.

- *Phimosis*: Tightening of the penile foreskin that may result in the closure of the urethra opening and the foreskin may not retract

THE MEDICAL ASSISTANT'S ROLE IN UROLOGY PROCEDURES

Assisting With the Examination

As with other physical examinations, a careful history provides the physician with valuable information. The medical assistant should ask specific questions to gather important information on the patient's chief complaint for the visit. For instance, if a patient states, "I think I have a bladder infection," the medical assistant should focus on what signs and symptoms the patient is experiencing and not just document what the patient stated. For this type of situation, the medical assistant may ask the following questions:

- What is occurring now? When did it start?
- Have you had a history of bladder infections?
- Are you experiencing pain or discomfort? Where? When?
- Any urgency or the need to go "now"? Are you going more frequently?
- Is there blood in the urine?
- Any fevers? Chills?

Remember to start with questions that are more "open ended"; in other words, use questions that encourage the patient to answer in more than just one or two words. To get specific details, the medical assistant can ask questions that are "closed ended," or those that require one- or two-word answers, such as yes or no.

Testicular Self-Exam

According to the American Cancer Society, males at any age can develop testicular cancer. About 50% of those diagnosed are between 20 and 34 years of age. It is estimated that 1 in 263 males will get testicular cancer. If the cancer is found early (before it has spread), there is a good chance of a cure.

The American Cancer Society recommends that providers perform a testicular exam as part of a routine physical exam. Some providers recommend that after puberty (around age 15), males should do a monthly testicular self-exam (TSE) after a shower (see Procedure 26.1, p. 675). The medical assistant may be involved in coaching a patient on how to do a TSE. Procedure 26.1 discusses how to coach a patient on the TSE. It is helpful for the patient to have a brochure

and to practice the technique on a TSE model during the coaching session.

Assisting With Diagnostic Procedures

The medical assistant assists with diagnostic procedures by scheduling and preparing patients for procedures. If tests require restrictions of food or fluids, the medical assistant should address the following points with the patient after talking with the provider:

- Can the patient have water prior to the test?
- Which medications should the patient take prior to the test, or when can the patient resume the current medications?

Table 26.5 describes common diagnostic procedures used for urinary conditions. The medical assistant may need to screen the patient for specific allergies, medications, and pregnancy prior to the scheduling of the procedure. For some procedures, a signed consent form is required. The patient should be notified of what he or she will experience during the procedure and any follow-up care required after the test. Table 26.6 lists common laboratory tests used for urinary conditions.

Assisting With Treatments

Patients with urinary conditions are prescribed a variety of medications. The following are some of the more common classifications of medications for urinary conditions:

- *Antibiotic*: Destroys or inhibits the growth of bacteria. Used to treat bacterial infections.
- *Anticholinergics*: Stimulates the bladder to contract, which helps with urination. Used to treat overactive bladder and urge incontinence.
- *Antimuscarinics*: Relaxes the bladder muscle and decreases bladder contraction. Used to treat overactive bladder.
- *Diuretics*: Used to treat a variety of diseases such as hypertension; increases urinary output
- *Electrolytes*: Mineral supplements used to treat certain diseases; they may also be used in combination with other medications, such as diuretics
- *Erectile dysfunction agents*: Used to facilitate an erection in patients with erectile dysfunction (impotence) and symptoms of benign prostatic hypertrophy (enlarged prostate)

Refer to Table 26.7, Medication Classifications, for information on the classification, including indication for use, desired effect, side effects, adverse reactions, and generic and trade names. Medical assistants should be familiar with medications that are prescribed to patients.

Vasectomy

A vasectomy is a surgical procedure that is considered a permanent form of male birth control. The procedure involves cutting and sealing the vas deferens, which carries the sperm from the testicles. A vasectomy offers no protection from sexually transmitted infections.

The patient must stop taking any over-the-counter and prescription medication that may prevent blood clotting, such as aspirin, ibuprofen (Motrin, Advil), and anticoagulants (heparin, warfarin [Coumadin, Jantoven], enoxaparin [Lovenox]). The patient should shower the morning of the procedure, washing the genital area thoroughly. The provider may have the patient bring an athletic supporter or a pair of tight-fitting underwear to wear after the procedure to support the scrotum and minimize swelling at the site. The patient will not be able

TABLE 26.5   Diagnostic Procedures for Urinary Conditions

PROCEDURE	DESCRIPTION	PATIENT PREPARATION
Cystoscopy and ureteroscopy	Cystoscopy is used to examine the urethra and bladder, and procedures like removing small tumors may be done. A cystoscope is inserted into the urethra and advanced into the bladder. Ureteroscopy can be done at the same time. A smaller endoscope is used to examine the ureters.	The patient may need to take antibiotics prior to the procedure. For procedures requiring sedation or general anesthesia, there will be food and liquid restrictions prior to the procedure. The patient will not be able to drive. A consent form will be completed prior to the start of the procedure. To help with discomfort, local anesthetic medications may be used to numb the urethra.
Digital rectal examination (DRE)	Done during the physical examination. The provider inserts a gloved, lubricated finger into the rectum to feel for abnormalities in the prostate, bladder, ovaries, or uterus. For urinary tract issues, the DRE may be done to check if the prostate gland is swollen and obstructing the urinary tract structures.	Done during the physical examination. No advance preparation usually required. The patient may feel some discomfort during the test. Usually, taking some deep breaths will help.
DMSA scan	A renal scan that uses the radioisotope, technetium-99m dimercaptosuccinic acid (DMSA), to evaluate the kidneys. The function, shape, position, size, and scarring can be observed. The radioisotope is injected, and a gamma camera is used to take pictures of the kidney.	If sedation is required, there will be food and fluid restrictions prior to the test. The medical assistant should screen the patient for allergies. An IV will be inserted, and the tracer will be injected. The patient may need to wait 2 to 4 hours before the test can occur. During the test, the person must remain still in a prone position.
Intravenous pyelogram (IVP)	An IV iodine contrast is given, and then x-ray images will be taken to see how the kidneys filter the contrast from the blood. The test can provide information on the functioning of the kidneys, bladder, and ureters.	The medical assistant will screen the patient for allergies (especially to iodine and shellfish), pregnancy, and a history of any reaction to x-ray dyes. Food and fluid restrictions prior to the test may be required. An IV will be placed, and the patient will need to be in a supine position on the exam table. The patient may be asked to urinate during the exam.
Postvoid residual (PVR) urine test	Measures the amount of urine in the bladder after urination. A straight catheter is inserted and drains the remaining urine. A portable ultrasound unit can also be used to scan and calculate the volume of residual urine.	The patient will be asked to urinate prior to the test. The patient will experience some discomfort if a catheter is used for the test. With a catheter, the risk of a urinary tract infection increases. There is no discomfort if the test is done with a portable ultrasound unit.
Urodynamic testing	Using x-rays or ultrasound (US) scans, pictures or videos are taken as the bladder fills and empties. A catheter will be inserted in the bladder and contrast medium (for x-rays) or warm water (for the US scan) will be used to fill the bladder.	The patient will be asked to urinate prior to the test. During the test, the patient may have some discomfort as the catheter is inserted and the bladder is filled. After the test, the patient may experience some discomfort with urination and may need to take an antibiotic.
Voiding cystourethrogram (VCUG)	A minimally invasive test that involves fluoroscopy to visualize the urinary tract and bladder. Images are taken while the bladder is full and during urination. Contrast medium is used to help visualize the urinary structures on the x-ray image.	The patient may be asked to urinate prior to the test. Sedation may be used with children, and food and fluid restrictions prior to the test may be required. During the test, the patient may have some discomfort as the catheter is inserted and the bladder is filled. After the test, the patient may experience some discomfort with urination and may need to take an antibiotic.

to drive after the procedure. A consent form needs to be signed after the provider discusses the procedure and alternatives with the patient.

Vasectomies are done in the ambulatory care facility, usually in urology or family medicine departments. They can also be done in ambulatory surgical centers under local anesthesia. The procedure may take about 30 minutes.

During the procedure, the provider will inject local anesthetic into the skin of the scrotum. A small incision or a small puncture is made in the scrotum. The provider will locate the vas deferens and withdraw part of the tube through the incision or puncture. The vas deferens is then cut and sealed either by tying it, cauterizing it with heat, or applying surgical clips (Fig. 26.19). The provider returns the ends of the vas deferens into the scrotum and may close the hole with glue or stitches.

After the procedure, the patient will experience swelling, pain, and bruising in the area. Applying ice packs, limiting activity, and

TABLE 26.6 Medical Laboratory Tests for Urologic Conditions

TEST(S)	DESCRIPTION
Blood urea nitrogen (BUN)	Urea is a waste product in the blood that is filtered out by the kidneys. If the kidney function is abnormal, the blood level of urea will be increased.
Creatinine and creatinine clearance	Creatinine is a waste product from normal muscle breakdown. Creatinine is filtered out of the blood by the kidneys. The blood creatinine level indicates kidney function. The creatinine clearance rate shows how the kidneys filter creatinine from the blood.
Urinalysis (UA)	A urine sample is collected in a special container. The urine is analyzed in the lab for abnormal levels of substances. Some of the substances that may be found in urine include blood, ketones, bilirubin, glucose, protein, and nitrites. The urinalysis is a CLIA-waived test. Specific CLIA-waived tests are also available, including glucose and ketones.
Urine culture	A urine sample is collected in a special container. The urine is analyzed in the lab for bacterial growth over a period of days (usually 1–3 days). Specific bacteria grown in the sample will be listed on the urine culture report.
Urine culture and sensitivity (C&S)	A urine culture is done as discussed above. The sensitivity results indicate if the pathogen is susceptible or resistant to specific antibiotics.

CLIA, Clinical Laboratory Improvement Amendments.

TABLE 26.7 Medication Classifications

CLASSIFICATION	INFORMATION	GENERIC NAME (TRADE NAME)
Antibiotics	**Indications for use:** Treat bacterial infections. **Desired effects:** Kill or inhibit bacteria growth. **Side effects and adverse reactions:** Hypersensitivity reaction, GI distress	*Penicillins*: • **amoxicillin** (Amoxil, Moxtag) • **amoxicillin and clavulanic acid** (Augmentin) *Cephalosporins*: • **cephalexin** (Keflex) • **cefuroxime** (Ceftin) *Macrolides*: • **erythromycin** (Ery-Tab) • **clarithromycin** (Biaxin) • **azithromycin** (Zithromax, Zithromax Z-Paks, Zmak) *Fluoroquinolones*: • **ciprofloxacin** (Cipro) • **levofloxacin** (Levaquin) *Sulfonamide*: • **co-trimoxazole** (Bactrim, Septra) • **trimethoprim** (Primsol) *Tetracyclines*: • **tetracycline** Sumycin) • **doxycycline** (Doryx, Oracea, Vibramycin) *Aminoglycosides*: • **gentamicin** (Garamycin) • **tobramycin** (Tobrex)
Anticholinergics	**Indications for use:** Dry secretions before surgery; prevent bronchospasm. **Desired effects:** Parasympathetic blocking agents; reduce spasms in smooth muscles. **Side effects and adverse reactions:** Blurred vision, confusion, reduced GI and genitourinary motility, dilation of pupils, fever, flushing, headache, increased heart rate.	• **dicyclomine** (Bentyl) • **propantheline** (Pro-Banthine) • **glycopyrrolate** (Cuvposa, Robinul)

Continued

TABLE 26.7   Medication Classifications—*continued*

CLASSIFICATION	INFORMATION	GENERIC NAME (TRADE NAME)
Antimuscarinics	**Indications for use:** Overactive bladder **Desired effects:** Relaxes the bladder muscles. **Side effects and adverse reactions:** Blurred vision, dry mouth and eyes, GI disturbances, headache, confusion, arrhythmias.	• **oxybutynin** (Ditropan) • **solifenacin** (VESIcare) • **fesoterodine** (Toviaz) • **tolterodine** (Detrol)
Diuretics	**Indications for use:** Increase urinary output; lower blood pressure. **Desired effects:** Inhibit reabsorption of sodium and chloride in the kidneys; promote excretion of excess fluid in the body. **Side effects and adverse reactions:** Dehydration, muscle weakness, fatigue, electrolyte imbalance.	• **triamterene** (Dyrenium) • **furosemide** (Lasix) • **hydrochlorothiazide** (HCTZ) (Microzide, Oretic)
Electrolytes	**Indications for use:** mineral supplement needed for certain diseases and medications. **Desired effect:** maintain normal electrolyte level; proper functioning of the body systems. **Side effects and adverse reactions:** (depends on medication) confusion, listlessness, gray skin, black stools.	• **potassium** (K-Tab, Klor-Con, K-Dur) • **ferrous sulfate** (Feosol, Fer-in-Sol, Slow-Fe)
Erectile Dysfunction agents	**Indications for use:** Facilitates an erection in patients with erectile dysfunction (impotence) and symptoms of benign prostatic hypertrophy (enlarged prostate). **Desired effect:** Facilitate an erection. **Side effects and adverse reactions:** Headache, flushing, nasal congestion, myalgia, prolonged erections, cerebrovascular accident (CVA), myocardial infarction (MI).	• **avanafil** (Stendra) • **sildenafil** (Viagra, Revatio) • **tadalafil** (Cialis, Adcirca) • **vardenafil** (Levitra, Staxyn)

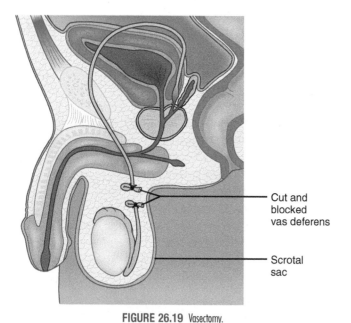

Cut and blocked vas deferens

Scrotal sac

FIGURE 26.19 Vasectomy.

wearing tight-fitting underwear for 48 hours can minimize the pain and swelling. Sexual activity is limited for at least 1 week.

It is important for the patient to follow up with the provider. The provider will do follow-up semen analysis 6 to 12 weeks after the surgery to ensure that no sperm exist in the semen. During this period of time, it is recommended that men use an alternative form of birth control.

A vasectomy reversal can undo a vasectomy by reconnecting the vas deferens. Success rates range from 40% to 90%. The surgery is usually done in an ambulatory care surgery center using general anesthesia.

CLOSING COMMENTS

Patient Coaching

Most men younger than 50 years of age have not seen a provider in years. Medical studies reveal that attitude, not biology, has a lot to do with the difference between men's and women's life spans. Men just do not go to the doctor as often as women do and tend to ignore symptoms of disease. The solution to maintaining good health is preventive care, and the first step is establishing a good rapport with a provider of choice. As a general rule, a man in good health should have three checkups in his 20s, three to four checkups in his 30s, and a checkup every other year in his 40s. After the age of 50, a yearly checkup is recommended. In addition to testing for conditions such as cancer, heart disease, and diabetes, patient education can help male patients make responsible healthcare decisions.

The urinary system is a very private, personal part of the patient's body. Patients often feel embarrassed to ask questions about how to obtain the requested urine or semen sample. The medical assistant can provide this information in a sincere, confidential manner to relieve the patient's anxiety and worry. Diagrams, models, and handouts help the patient understand disease processes and treatments and also encourage patient compliance.

Legal and Ethical Issues

When working in a urology office, the medical assistant must be very careful to ensure that patients have provided informed consent for ordered procedures. If the patient refuses a procedure, the assistant must have the patient sign the appropriate informed refusal forms, which are then included in the health record. All patient education should be done after the provider has completed the explanation and has given the assistant instructions to do so. Never diagnose, prescribe, or offer comments about a patient's condition. Medical assistants who overstep their professional boundaries may place the provider and themselves in legal jeopardy. Remember that the patient who is legally informed and satisfied with the care received is less likely to take legal action.

Patient-Centered Care

Respecting a patient's preference is a key element to patient-centered care. When a medical assistant gathers a medical history on a patient regarding a male reproductive or a urology concern, the patient may hesitate to give information. These topics are sensitive, and the patient may only want to discuss concerns with the provider. Telling the patient, "If you would rather share the information with the provider, I will let him know" can show sensitivity. It is important for the medical assistant to respect the patient's wishes and help put the patient at ease.

Professional Behaviors

A urology practice manages many sensitive patient issues that require strict adherence to confidentiality guidelines. This is especially true for a patient who has a functional disorder with the reproductive system. The Health Insurance Portability and Accountability Act of 1996 (HIPAA) protects the patient's confidential information, not just the paper or electronic records of that information. This means that verbal disclosure of a patient's information is limited to only the personnel who have the right to that information according to individual state laws.

SUMMARY OF SCENARIO

When Hannah started working with the urology team, she realized she knew very little about the urinary system. She had studied it during her medical assistant program, but she never appreciated what it might be like if her kidneys did not work. She was familiar with kidney cancer and UTIs, but she was amazed at all of the other urinary diseases. As she learned more, she realized that hypertension could lead to kidney disease and kidney disease could lead to hypertension.

Looking back over the last weeks, Hannah realized that one of her favorite experiences was working with Mr. Rodgers. He had been on dialysis for the past 5 years and never had a vacation. He wanted to see his new grandson who lived on the East Coast. Hannah found a dialysis unit in the city where he was going to stay. She was able to get him scheduled for 2 weeks' worth of dialysis during his stay. She still can recall Mr. Rodgers' excitement when he realized he could do dialysis while on vacation. He started talking about other trips he was dreaming of taking.

Hannah is excited to continue her work with the urology team. She has learned so much in the short time she has worked with the patients.

SUMMARY OF LEARNING OBJECTIVES

1. **Describe the anatomical location of the major organs of the urinary system.**

   The urinary system is composed of two kidneys, two ureters, a urinary bladder, and a urethra. The kidneys are located posterior to the peritoneum, the muscles of the back, and between the T12 and L3 vertebrae. They filter the blood and eliminate waste through the passage of urine. The ureters move urine from the kidneys to the bladder. The urinary bladder, in the pelvic cavity, stores the urine until it is excreted. The urethra is the tube that conducts the urine out of the bladder.

2. **Describe the anatomical location of the major organs of the male reproductive system, and explain the process of spermatogenesis.**

   With the male reproductive system, the testes are surrounded by a white, fibrous capsule and are suspended together in a sac outside of the body called the scrotum. The epididymis is a coiled tube that is almost 6 meters (20 feet) long and rests on top of and behind each testis. Each vas deferens is a muscular tunnel about 45 cm (18 inches) long that connects to the base of the epididymis and passes along the side of the testis. The vas deferens travels into the pelvic cavity to just behind the bladder. The *prostate gland* is the size of a walnut and is found below the bladder in males. It surrounds part of the urethra.

   The primary reproductive organs in the male are a pair of testes. Testes produce the gametes called spermatozoa. The formation of sperm is called spermatogenesis. The spermatozoa are formed in a series of tightly coiled tiny tubes in each testis called the seminiferous tubules. From the seminiferous tubules, the formed spermatozoa travel to the epididymis, where they mature and are stored. From the epididymis, the spermatozoa move into the vas deferens (or ductus deferens). Spermatozoa can stay in the vas deferens for several months in an inactive state.

Continued

The prostate gland, seminal vesicles, and Cowper glands provide fluid either to nourish or to aid in motility and lubrication. The sperm and the fluid together make up a substance called semen. The ejaculatory duct begins where the seminal vesicles join the vas deferens, and this "tube" joins the urethra. The urethra is found within the penis and transports the semen to the outside of the body. The semen exits the body through the tip of the penis, the glans penis.

3. **Explain the physiology of the urinary system, and describe life span changes related to the urinary system.**

The urinary system has several important roles that help regulate homeostasis in the body:
- Maintains fluid volume
- Maintains the normal composition of body fluids
- Maintains an adequate blood pressure
- Controls red blood cell production
- Activates vitamin D

Many of these roles are performed during the formation of urine. The body rids itself of unneeded substances produced during the metabolic process. The process of urine formation includes three steps:

a. *Filtration*: During this phase in the glomerulus, substances from the blood such as electrolytes, waste products, and other substances move through the capillary wall into the filtrate.

b. *Reabsorption*: This process starts as the filtrate moves out of the Bowman capsule and into the proximal tubule. Substances move from the filtrate back into the blood in the peritubular capillaries.

c. *Secretion*: This process allows substances from the blood to move into the filtrate. This allows the body to maintain homeostasis and move unneeded substances back into the filtrate.

When babies are born, they have the same number of nephrons as an adult, though the nephrons are not mature until age 2. During childhood, the bladder continues to grow. Bladder control is learned usually between ages 2 and 3.

During pregnancy, the filtration rate increases in women. The number of nephrons remains the same, but the filtration surface increases. This increase allows the kidneys to filter more blood, which is useful with the increased blood flow during pregnancy. In late pregnancy, the bladder may be twice as big.

In older adults, the kidney tissue and number of nephrons are reduced up to 20%. The renal arteries can harden, causing the kidneys to filter blood slower. The kidneys become less able to regulate water balance. Older adults are at more risk of dehydration when the weather is hot or if they have diarrhea. The bladder wall becomes less stretchy with age. The bladder cannot hold as much urine as before. Bladder muscles weaken. The urethra may be obstructed by an enlarged prostate gland or a prolapse of the bladder or vagina.

4. **Explain the physiology of the male reproductive system.**

At puberty, the interstitial cells in the testicles begin to produce testosterone. Testosterone is responsible for maintaining reproductive structures and for the development of sperm cells and secondary sex characteristics (e.g., deep voice, broad shoulders, narrow hips, and additional body hair).

In addition to testosterone, the follicle-stimulating hormone (FSH), which is secreted by the pituitary gland, promotes the formation of spermatozoa. The pituitary gland also produces luteinizing hormone (LH), which stimulates the interstitial cells to produce testosterone.

5. **List common signs and symptoms of urinary and male reproductive systems diseases, and identify common disorders of the urinary and male reproductive systems.**
- Common urinary signs and symptoms include the following:
  - Anuria, diuresis, dysuria, enuresis, oliguria, nocturia, and polyuria
  - Urgency, frequency, urinary incontinence, and urinary retention
  - Abnormal substances in the urine: Albuminuria or proteinuria, azoturia, bacteriuria, glycosuria, hematuria, and pyuria
- Common male reproductive disorder signs and symptoms include redness, swelling, changes in the urinary stream, and lumps.
- Common urinary system disorders include the following:
  - Bladder cancer, kidney cancer
  - Acute cystitis, glomerulonephritis, and pyelonephritis
  - End-stage renal disease, nephrotic syndrome, neurogenic bladder, polycystic kidney disease, renal calculi, and urinary incontinence
- Common male reproductive disorders include the following:
  - Benign prostatic hyperplasia and erectile dysfunction
  - Prostate cancer and testicular cancer

6. **Discuss the medical assistant's role in urology procedures, and demonstrate how to coach patients regarding health maintenance (e.g., testicular self-exam).**

As with physical examinations, a careful history provides the physician with valuable information, and the medical assistant should ask specific questions to gather important information on the patient's chief complaint for the visit.

The medical assistant can coach patients on doing the testicular self-exam. Procedure 26.1 on p. 675 outlines the steps followed to coach patients on the testicular self-exam. A TSE model and a brochure can be used to help with coaching. The patient should be given a TSE brochure to take home as a reference for the procedure.

7. **Describe diagnostic procedures used for urinary and male reproductive diseases.**

a. *Cystoscopy*: Used to examine the urethra and bladder and for procedures like removing small tumors.

b. *Ureteroscopy*: Can be done at the same time as cystoscopy. A smaller endoscope is used to examine the ureters.

c. *Digital rectal examination (DRE):* The provider inserts a gloved, lubricated finger into the rectum to feel for abnormalities in the prostate, bladder, ovaries, or uterus.

d. *DMSA scan:* A renal scan that uses the radioisotope, technetium-99m dimercaptosuccinic acid (DMSA), to evaluate the kidneys.

e. *Intravenous pyelogram (IVP):* An intravenous (IV) iodine contrast is given, and then x-ray images are taken to see how the kidneys filter the contrast from the blood.

f. *Postvoid residual (PVR) urine test:* Measures the amount of urine in the bladder after urination.

g. *Urodynamic testing:* Using x-rays or US scans, pictures or videos are taken as the bladder fills and empties.

h. *Voiding cystourethrogram (VCUG):* A minimally invasive test that involves fluoroscopy to visualize the urinary tract and bladder.

8. **Identify CLIA-waived tests associated with urinary disease, and describe treatments used for urinary and male reproductive diseases.**

The urinalysis is a CLIA-waived test. Specific CLIA-waived tests are also available, including tests for glucose and ketones.

Treatments vary for the different diseases. Medications commonly prescribed in urology include antibiotics, antimuscarinics, diuretics, electrolytes, and erectile dysfunction agents. Vasectomies, a permanent form of male birth control, are also done in urology and family practice departments.

PROCEDURE 26.1   Coach a Patient on Testicular Self-Exam

Tasks: Coach a patient to do a testicular self-exam (TSE) while considering the patient's developmental life stage. Document your teaching in the patient's health record.

Scenario: You are working with Dr. David Kahn. He has ordered you to provide Truong Tran (date of birth [DOB]: 05/30/1991) with TSE coaching.

EQUIPMENT and SUPPLIES

- Testicular self-examination brochure (optional)
- Testicular model
- Provider's order
- Patient's health record

PROCEDURAL STEPS

1. Wash hands or use hand sanitizer.
   UNDERLINE: PURPOSE: Hand sanitization is an important step for infection control.
2. Read the provider's order. Assemble the equipment.
   PURPOSE: It is important to know the provider's order before starting the procedure.
3. Greet the patient. Identify yourself. Verify the patient's identity with full name and date of birth. Explain the procedure to be performed in a manner that the patient understands. Answer any questions the patient may have about the procedure.
   PURPOSE: It is important to identify the patient in two different ways to ensure that you have the correct patient. Explaining the procedure can make the patient feel more comfortable and reduces anxiety.

4. Ask the patient what he knows about the self-exam. Clarify any inaccuracies. Build on the patient's prior knowledge of the topic during the session. Identify the patient's motivating factor for learning about the self-exam. Listen to the patient's concerns.
   PURPOSE: It is important to adapt the coaching to the patient's developmental stage. Because of the patient's age, identifying motivating factors is important.
5. Explain to the patient that the best time to do the self-exam is after a warm shower or bath.
   PURPOSE: The scrotal skin is more relaxed.
6. Demonstrate on the model while discussing the technique. Instruct the patient to examine each testicle gently with both hands. Roll the testicle between the thumb and fingers (Fig. 1). Show the patient the epididymis, the soft curved structure behind and on top of the testicle (Fig. 2). Then show the patient how to examine the vas deferens, which is the tube that runs up the epididymis (Fig. 3).
   PURPOSE: This allows the person to do a better self-exam.

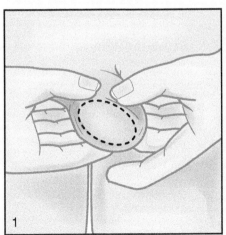
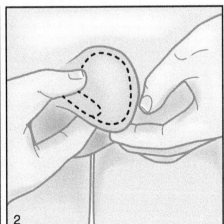
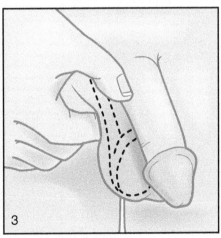

Continued

PROCEDURE 26.1   **Coach a Patient on Testicular Self-Exam**—*continued*

7. Instruct the patient to feel for any abnormalities and lumps. These could be painless or painful. Instruct the person to look for changes in the size, texture, or shape.
PURPOSE: Any changes should be reported to the provider for possible follow-up.

8. Have the patient demonstrate the technique on the model. Coach the patient on ways to improve the exam if needed.
PURPOSE: It is important to have the patient demonstrate the teaching to check for accuracy of technique and correct understanding.

9. Answer any questions the patient may have. Provide the patient with a brochure to take home (optional).
PURPOSE: It is important to answer any questions the patient has and, if possible, provide him with a brochure to take home.

10. Document the patient education in the patient's health record. Include the provider's name, the order, what was taught, how the patient responded, how the patient did the demonstration, and any handouts provided.
PURPOSE: It is important to document the patient education in the health record to show it was done.

Documentation Example
07/19/20XX 1505 Per Dr. Kahn's order, instructed pt on TSE. Instructed the patient on how to check for changes in the testes. Explained the technique, and encouraged the patient to do monthly checks after a warm shower/bath. Pt provided an accurate return demonstration. His questions were answered. Gave pt the "TSE" brochure. _____ Hannah Yang, CMA (AAMA)

OBSTETRICS AND GYNECOLOGY

27

SCENARIO

Peggy St. John has been working in the obstetrics and gynecology (OB/GYN) department for about 5 years. She loves what she does and feels grateful that she can be there for her patients as they go through the pregnancy process. She also gets a lot of satisfaction from working with patients who come in with gynecologic issues. She especially likes the patient education that she can do with all of her patients. Her supervisor recognizes that Peggy enjoys teaching and has asked her to mentor a medical assistant student, Jill Snow, who is just starting her practicum. Peggy is excited to share how she works with patients in the OB/GYN department.

While studying this chapter, think about the following questions:

- What is the basic anatomy and physiology of the female reproductive system?
- What does Jill need to learn about contraceptives to be able to answer patients' questions?
- Jill needs to become familiar with which gynecologic disorders?
- What are the primary malignancies of the female reproductive system?
- How should Peggy assist the provider with a Pap test?

- How can Peggy teach patients to perform breast self-examination?
- What are the stages of pregnancy and birth?
- How can Peggy help patients understand issues that can arise with menopause?
- What are the typical diagnostic procedures used in obstetrics and gynecology?

LEARNING OBJECTIVES

1. Describe the anatomic location of the major organs of the female reproductive system.
2. Explain the phases of the menstrual cycle, and discuss pregnancy and delivery.
3. Discuss sexually transmitted infections, and describe the common cancers of the female reproductive system.
4. Discuss endometriosis, and list the common infections of the female reproductive system.
5. Specify the signs, symptoms, and treatments for conditions related to menopause.
6. Outline the medical assistant's role in a gynecologic examination (including breast, abdominal, and pelvic examinations), and demonstrate how to assist with a gynecologic examination.
7. Prepare for and assist with the collection of specimens, including those for a Pap test, a maturation index, and tests for various types of vaginal infections.

8. Compare and contrast current contraceptive methods.
9. Discuss postexamination duties. Also, describe three of the most common gynecologic procedures performed in the medical office:
   - Cryotherapy
   - Colposcopy with or without a biopsy
   - Loop electrosurgical excision procedure (LEEP)
10. Summarize the process of pregnancy and postpartum care, including the prenatal record, the first prenatal examination, return prenatal visits, and the postpartum visit.
11. Describe the common specialized tests and procedures for obstetric patients.
12. Describe the possible signs of domestic abuse, and know how to report it.

VOCABULARY

adhesions (ad HEE zhuns) Bands of scar tissue that can bind anatomic structures together.
amenorrhea (ey men uh REE uh) Lack of menstrual flow.
anencephaly (an en SEF uh lee) Congenital absence of part or all of the brain.

anovulation Failure of the ovaries to release an ovum at the time of ovulation.
Bartholin (BAR thoh lin) **cyst** A fluid-filled cyst in one of the vestibular glands located on either side of the vaginal orifice.
clitoris (KLIT uh ris) Sensitive, erectile tissue.

colposcopy (kol PAW skoh pee) Using a microscope with a light source, the vagina and cervix are visually examined to locate and evaluate abnormal cells. A biopsy of abnormal cells may be taken during this procedure.

cone biopsy An extensive cervical biopsy during which a cone-shaped wedge of tissue is removed from the cervix and examined under a microscope. Abnormal tissue, along with a small amount of normal tissue, is removed.

curettage (kyoo r I TAZH) A small, spoon-shaped instrument (curette) or a thin brush is used to scrape a tissue sample from the cervix.

cystic fibrosis (CF) A disorder that affects all the exocrine cells, but affects the respiratory system the most. Mucus is abnormally thick and blocks the alveoli, causing dyspnea.

Down syndrome A genetic disorder in which abnormal cell division results in an extra chromosome 21.

dysmenorrhea (dis men uh REE uh) Painful menstrual flow, cramps.

dyspareunia (dis ph ROO nee ah) Painful or difficult intercourse.

ectopic (eck TAH pick) **pregnancy** Implantation of the embryo in any location other than the uterus.

gamete (GAM eet) A mature sexual reproductive cell; spermatozoa or ovum.

gonads (GOH nadz) Organs that produce sex cells in both males and females.

hemophilia (hee moh FEE lee ah) A group of inherited blood disorders characterized by a deficiency of one of the factors necessary for the coagulation of blood.

hysterectomy Surgical removal of the uterus and cervix. The ovaries and fallopian tubes may also be removed.

labia majora (LAY bee ah muh JOR ah) The larger external folds of skin surrounding the opening of the vagina.

labia minora (LAY bee ah min NOR uh) The smaller inner folds of skin surrounding the opening of the vagina.

laparoscopy (lap ar AW scoh pee) A procedure used to visually examine the abdomen.

loop electrosurgical excision procedure (LEEP) After an anesthetic has been injected into the cervix, a high-frequency electrical current running through a wire is used to remove

abnormal tissue from both the cervix and the endocervical canal.

lumpectomy (luhm PEK tuh mee) Removal of the breast tumor and a small amount of the surrounding tissue.

mastectomy (ma STEK tuh mee) Removal of the entire breast.

meningocele (meh NING goh seel) The protrusion of the meninges through an opening in the spinal column or skull.

menometrorrhagia (men oh meh troh RAH zsa) Excessive menstrual flow and uterine bleeding other than that caused by menstruation.

menorrhagia (men or RAH zsa) Abnormally heavy menstrual flow or prolonged menstrual periods.

necrosis (nuh KROH sis) Tissue death.

orifice (ORE ih fis) The vaginal opening.

osteoporosis (os tee oh phuh ROH sis) Abnormal thinning of the bone structure, causing bones to become brittle and weak.

ovulation (OV yuh ley shun) The release of the ovum from the ovarian follicle.

perineum (pair ih NEE um) The area between the opening of the vagina and the anus.

phenylketonuria (PKU) A deficiency in the enzyme phenylalanine hydroxylase, which is responsible for converting phenylalanine into tyrosine.

preeclampsia (pree eh KLAMP see ah) An abnormal condition of pregnancy of unknown cause, marked by hypertension, edema, and proteinuria.

purulent (PYOOR yoo lent) Pus like.

salpingo-oophorectomy (sal ping goh oh of or EK toh mee) Surgical removal of the fallopian tube and ovary.

sentinel node biopsy Removal of a limited number of lymph nodes to determine if the cancer has spread to the lymph nodes.

sickle cell anemia An inherited anemia characterized by crescent-shaped red blood cells (RBCs). It causes RBCs to block capillaries, reducing the oxygen supply to the cells.

spina bifida (SPY nah BIF id dah) A condition in which the spinal column has an abnormal opening that allows protrusion of the meninges or the spinal column.

symmetry (SIM i tree) Similarity in size, form, and arrangement of parts on opposite sides of the body.

viability Ability to live.

The branch of medicine that deals with pregnancy, labor, and the postpartum period is known as *obstetrics*, and the branch of medicine that deals with diseases of the reproductive system in women is called *gynecology*. Frequently, a provider practices both specialties and is known as an *OB/GYN provider*. Assessment of the female reproductive system is an important part of healthcare. Patients are often hesitant and uncomfortable talking about sexual matters, so they wait until the symptoms are uncomfortable or until the disease is advanced before they seek medical care. The medical assistant needs to be familiar with signs and symptoms of the diseases and conditions related to this specialty. In addition, the medical assistant must be aware of the patient's emotional state and must give support when needed.

In this chapter, we will review the anatomy and physiology of the female reproductive system and diseases and disorders of the reproductive system. We will also discuss the medical assistant's role in gynecologic and obstetric procedures. A medical assistant has two roles in these situations:

• Assist the provider in any way needed
• Be there for the patient by helping her to be as comfortable as possible during her time in the healthcare facility

When we make patients feel comfortable, we help to establish a trusting relationship where patients will be able to share the information the provider needs to give them the best possible care.

ANATOMY OF THE FEMALE REPRODUCTIVE SYSTEM

The anatomy of the female reproductive system can be divided into two parts. *Parenchymal* or *primary tissue* produces sex cells for reproduction. *Stromal*, or *secondary tissue* includes all of the glands, nerves, ducts, and other tissues that serve a supportive function in producing, maintaining, and transmitting these sex cells.

In females, the **gonads** are the *ovaries*. They produce *ova*, the female **gametes**. From *menarche*, the first menstrual period, to *menopause*, the cessation of menstruation, mature ova are produced. The ovaries are small, almond-shaped, paired organs located on either side of the uterus in the female pelvic cavity. They are attached to the uterus by the ovarian ligaments. The ovaries lie close to the opening of the *fallopian tubes*, the ducts that convey the ova from the ovaries to the *uterus*. Fallopian tubes are also called *oviducts* or *uterine tubes*.

Once the mature ovum has been released, it is drawn into the *fimbriae*, the feathery ends of the fallopian tube. These tubes are about 1 cm in diameter and about 10 to 12 cm long. The ovum travels down the fallopian tube to the uterus. The fallopian tubes and the ovaries make up what is called the *uterine adnexa*, or accessory organs, of the uterus.

Once the ovum has moved down the fallopian tube, it is secreted into the uterus, or womb. The uterus is a pear-shaped organ that is designed to nurture a developing embryo/fetus. The uterus is composed of three layers:

- Outer layer, called the *perimetrium*
- Middle or muscle layer, called the *myometrium*
- Lining, called the *endometrium*

As a whole, it can be divided into several areas:

- *Corpus* or body: the large central area
- *Fundus*: the raised area at the top of the uterus between the outlets for the fallopian tubes
- *Cervix*: the narrowed lower area, often referred to as the neck of the uterus; the opening of the cervix is called the *cervical os*

CRITICAL THINKING APPLICATION 27.1

Many anatomic structures are involved in the ovulation process. Can you list them in order, starting with the structure that holds the ovum?

The *vagina* is a 10-cm (4-inch) muscular tubelike structure that extends from the uterine cervix to the vulva (the external genitalia). It connects the internal reproductive structures with the external reproductive structures (Fig. 27.1B). The vagina serves as the passageway for endometrium during menstruation, receives the penis during intercourse, and is the birth canal during the delivery of a baby.

The external female genitalia collectively are called the *vulva*; it consists of the **orifice**, *hymen*, **labia majora**, **labia minora**, **clitoris**, and **perineum**. The paired glands in the vulva that secrete a mucous lubricant for the vagina are the *Bartholin glands*. The *mons pubis* is a fatty cushion of tissue over the pubic bone (Fig. 27.1A).

The *breasts*, or *mammary glands*, function to secrete milk. The breast tissue is composed of glandular, milk-producing, fatty, and fibrous tissue. The *nipple* of the breast is the *mammary papilla*, and the darker colored skin surrounding the nipple is the *areola*.

PHYSIOLOGY OF THE FEMALE REPRODUCTIVE SYSTEM

When a girl enters puberty, one of the many changes that occur is menarche. *Menstruation* is a normal body process that occurs in every female. It is the physiologic means by which the body rids itself of the thickened endometrial wall that develops during the average 28-day cycle. The menstrual cycle involves a series of events controlled by hormones from the pituitary gland and the ovaries. The cycle is divided into the follicular phase, the luteal phase, and the menstrual phase.

The follicular phase is also called the proliferative phase. In this phase, hormones are secreted to mature a graafian follicle in an ovary that contains an ovum. The mature ovarian follicle secretes estrogen, which stimulates the growth of the endometrium. It takes approximately 9 days for the graafian follicle to ripen and bulge out from the ovarian wall. The ovarian wall becomes thinner as the follicle enlarges until it bursts, releasing the ovum into the abdominal cavity. Expulsion of the ovum ends the follicular phase. The fallopian fimbriae begin their wavelike motion to fan the ovum into the fallopian tube. The rupture spot on the ovary, now called the *corpus luteum*, begins to secrete progesterone. **Ovulation** causes a rise in body temperature, and some women experience cramping and tenderness in the lower abdominal area at this time as a result of the rupture of the graafian follicle.

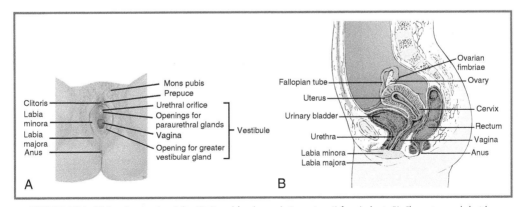

FIGURE 27.1 (A) Female external genitalia. **(B)** Normal female reproductive system. (A from Applegate EJ: *The anatomy and physiology learning system,* ed 4, Philadelphia, 2011, Saunders; B from Frazier MS, Drzymkowski JA: *Essentials of human diseases and conditions,* ed 5, St. Louis, 2013, Saunders.)

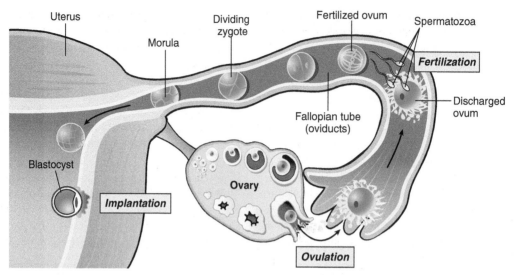

FIGURE 27.2 Ovulation, fertilization, and implantation. (From Salvo SG: *Massage therapy*, ed 3, St. Louis, 2007, Saunders.)

The luteal phase is also called the secretory phase. Once ovulation is complete, the luteal phase begins. During this phase, progesterone secreted by the corpus luteum causes extensive growth of the endometrium as it prepares for a possible pregnancy. If conception occurs, the corpus luteum continues to secrete progesterone until the placenta is well established. The corpus luteum can secrete progesterone and human chorionic gonadotropin (hCG) to maintain the pregnancy. If conception does not occur, hCG is not secreted, and the corpus luteum atrophies. Without increased levels of progesterone and hCG, the endometrium breaks down, and menstruation begins.

In the menstrual phase, the uterus contracts to shed the lining of the uterus, made up of necrotic endometrial tissue, mucus, and the blood from endometrial engorgement. A woman may experience cramping pain, and irritability. This phase usually lasts approximately 5 days.

Pregnancy and Delivery

Pregnancy begins with the fertilization of an ovum by a sperm, often in the fallopian tube, as the ovum travels toward the uterus (Fig. 27.2). Conception is usually the result of sexual intercourse. However, other methods of conception are possible if the couple has difficulty conceiving. These methods are discussed in the Disorders of the Female Reproductive System section.

CRITICAL THINKING APPLICATION   **27.2**

After Peggy and Jill reviewed the female reproductive anatomy, Jill asked Peggy to help her recall the phases of the menstrual cycle. Write down the different phases of the menstrual cycle and what occurs during each phase.

The fertilized egg, or *zygote*, divides as it moves through the fallopian tube to the uterus. In the first few days after fertilization, when the zygote has become a solid ball of cells from repeated divisions, it is called a *morula*. As it continues to develop, it moves from the fallopian tube into the uterus and implants into the uterine wall. At this point, it is called a *blastocyst*.

During implantation, the zygote functions as an endocrine gland by secreting hCG. The function of the hormone is to stop the corpus luteum from deteriorating. The corpus luteum allows the continued production of estrogen and progesterone to support the pregnancy and prevent menstruation. From the third to the eighth week of development, the organism is called an *embryo*. From the ninth through the thirty-eighth week of development (a normal length for *gestation*, or pregnancy), it is called a *fetus*.

At the same time that the embryo is developing, extraembryonic membranes are forming to sustain the pregnancy:

- The *amnion* and the *chorion* form the inner and outer sacs that contain the embryo.
- The fluid that forms inside the amnion is the *amniotic fluid*. It cushions the embryo, protects it against temperature changes, and allows it to move.
- The *placenta* is a highly vascular structure that acts as a physical communication between the mother and the embryo.
- The *umbilical cord* is the tissue that connects the embryo to the placenta (and hence to the mother). When the baby is delivered, the umbilical cord is cut, and the baby is then dependent on his or her own body for all physiologic processes. The remaining "scar" is the *umbilicus*, or navel. The delivery of an infant is termed *parturition*.

DISORDERS OF THE FEMALE REPRODUCTIVE SYSTEM

Sexually Transmitted Infections

Many pathogens cause sexually transmitted infections (STIs), but what they have in common is that all of them are most efficiently transmitted by *sexual contact*. Sexual contact refers to intercourse or to any contact between the genitals of one person and the body of another person. No one is immune to these diseases. An individual can be infected with more than one STI at a time. No cure is available for viral STIs, such as human immunodeficiency virus (HIV) infection, herpes, and venereal warts. Bacterial infections are increasingly becoming resistant to antibiotic therapy.

STIs frequently are asymptomatic in men, although they can cause serious health problems and are infectious regardless of whether symptoms are present. More information about STIs can be found in Chapter 18.

Cancers of the Female Reproductive System

Breast Cancer

Breast cancer is the second leading cause of cancer deaths in women. According to the American Cancer Society, 1 in 8 women have a lifetime risk of developing breast cancer, and 1 in 28 risk of dying from the disease.

It is not known what causes breast cancer. Risk factors include being female, a family history of breast cancer, inherited genes, radiation exposure, obesity, menarche at a younger age, menopause at an older age, having your first child at an older age, having never been pregnant, postmenopausal hormone therapy, and drinking alcohol. Signs and symptoms include a breast lump or thickening; change in the size, shape or appearance of a breast; changes to the skin over the breast, such as dimpling, a newly inverted nipple, peeling, scaling, or flaking of the pigmented area of the skin surrounding the nipple (areola) or breast skin; and redness or pitting of the skin over the breast.

Diagnostic procedures start with a breast examination by the provider and may also include a mammogram, breast ultrasound, biopsy, or breast magnetic resonance imaging (MRI). Surgical treatment could consist of a **lumpectomy**, **mastectomy**, or **sentinel node biopsy**. Some women with cancer in one breast choose to have the other breast removed (contralateral prophylactic mastectomy). Treatment could also include radiation, chemotherapy, and/or hormone therapy.

Cervical Cancer

Almost all cervical carcinomas are caused by the human papillomavirus (HPV). The first stage of cervical cancer is asymptomatic, but early diagnosis of cervical cellular changes is possible with a Papanicolaou (Pap) test, and HPV can be detected with HPV testing.

It is not known what causes cervical cancer, but it is known that HPV plays a role. Risk factors include many sexual partners, early sexual activity, having other STIs, a weak immune system, and smoking. In the early stages of cervical cancer the patient is asymptomatic. In the advanced stages signs and symptoms include vaginal bleeding after intercourse, between periods, or after menopause; watery, bloody vaginal discharge that may be heavy and have a foul odor; and pelvic pain or pain during intercourse.

A Pap test is the most common screening test. From the same sample an HPV test can be done. Diagnostic tests include a punch biopsy, endocervical **curettage**, **colposcopy**, and **loop electrosurgical excision procedure** (LEEP). The LEEP procedure can also be a treatment that removes all of the cancer cells. Other treatment options include **cone biopsy**, **hysterectomy**, radiation, and chemotherapy.

Ovarian Cancer

Ovarian cancer causes more deaths than any other cancer of the female reproductive system, but it accounts for only about 3% of all cancers in women. Most of the time the cancer has already metastasized before the tumor is diagnosed.

It is not known what causes ovarian cancer. Risk factors include age, inherited gene mutation, estrogen hormone replacement therapy, menarche at a young age, menopause at an older age, having never been pregnant, fertility treatment, smoking, use of an intrauterine device, and polycystic ovary syndrome. In the early stages of ovarian cancer, the patient is asymptomatic. In the advanced stages, signs and symptoms can include abdominal bloating, quickly feeling full when eating, weight loss, discomfort in the pelvis area, changes in bowel habits, and a frequent need to urinate.

Diagnostic procedures include pelvic examination, ultrasound, or computed tomography (CT) scan, cancer antigen 125 (CA-125) blood test (looks for certain proteins in the blood), and a biopsy. Surgical treatments include hysterectomy, unilateral **salpingo-oophorectomy**, or bilateral salpingo-oophorectomy. Chemotherapy may also be used in the treatment of ovarian cancer.

CRITICAL THINKING APPLICATION   **27.3**

A patient was seen in the OB/GYN department after there was an abnormal Pap test and Dr. Walden had recommended a LEEP procedure. Jill was wondering why a LEEP was recommended instead of a cone biopsy. Can you explain the difference between the two procedures?

Endometriosis

With endometriosis, functional endometrial tissue is located outside of the uterus. It is commonly found attached to the ovaries, urinary bladder, fallopian tubes, uterosacral ligaments, intestines, and peritoneum. The endometrial tissue continues to act as it normally would during a menstrual cycle. It will thicken, break down, and bleed just like the endometrium found in the uterus. This can cause inflammation at the implantation site that will recur with each cycle. Scar tissue and **adhesions** may form. Endometriosis can cause infertility and put women at higher risk for ovarian cancer.

The exact cause of endometriosis is not known, although there are some possible explanations: retrograde menstruation (the menstrual blood containing endometrial cells flows back through the fallopian tubes instead of leaving the uterus through the cervix), endometrial cells are transported through the blood vessels or lymphatic system to other parts of the body, and an immune system disorder in which the immune system does not recognize and destroy the endometrial tissue that is growing outside the uterus. Risk factors for endometriosis include never giving birth, menarche at a younger age, short menstrual cycles, low body mass index, alcohol consumption, family history of endometriosis, and uterine abnormalities. Common signs and symptoms of endometriosis include **dysmenorrhea**, **dyspareunia**, pain with bowel movements or urination, **menorrhagia**, **menometrorrhagia**, infertility, fatigue, diarrhea, constipation, bloating, and nausea.

To diagnose endometriosis, oftentimes an ultrasound will be done. The ultrasound could be done through the abdomen or transvaginally. Another method of diagnosing endometriosis is **laparoscopy**. The surgeon will look inside the abdomen for signs of endometriosis. There are two methods for treating endometriosis: medications or surgery. Medications might include over-the-counter medications such as ibuprofen or naproxen sodium for pain; hormone therapy including contraceptives, gonadotropin-releasing hormone (GN-RH) agonists and antagonists, which block the production of ovarian-stimulating hormones, lowering estrogen levels and preventing menstruation; or progestin therapy, during which a progestin-only contraceptive such as an intrauterine device is used to stop menstrual periods and the growth of endometrial implants. Surgical options might include removal of the endometrial implants, which can be done laparoscopically or through an abdominal incision and will preserve the uterus and ovaries, or hysterectomy, which is removal of the uterus, cervix, and both ovaries.

Infections

The female genitalia provide an excellent environment for infections to occur. There is moisture, warmth, and plenty of nutrients that permit the infectious agents to flourish. The most common infections of the female reproductive system are discussed next.

Candidiasis

Commonly called a yeast infection. *Candida* organisms are part of the normal flora of the mouth, skin, intestinal tract, and vagina. Overgrowth of the organism can be caused by antibiotic use, high estrogen levels, oral contraceptive use, diabetes mellitus, pregnancy, and immunosuppressive disorders, including acquired immunodeficiency syndrome (AIDS).

This infection is caused by *Candida albicans* (fungus). Signs and symptoms include vulvovaginal itching; dry, bright red vaginal tissue; and an odorless, white, "cottage cheese" like vaginal discharge.

Diagnosis is made by means of a pelvic examination and a test of the vaginal secretions. Treatment includes antifungal medications, cream, ointments, tablets, and suppositories; some of these treatments may be available over the counter.

Cervicitis

Cervicitis is an inflammation of the cervix caused by an invading organism. This is caused by sexually transmitted infections, an allergic reaction, or a bacterial overgrowth. Signs and symptoms include thick, **purulent** discharge with odor, dysuria, dyspareunia, and vaginal bleeding after intercourse.

Diagnosis is made by means of a pelvic examination and test of the vaginal secretions. Treatment may not be needed unless the cervicitis is caused by an STI; then both the patient and her partner must be treated for the STI.

Pelvic Inflammatory Disease

Pelvic inflammatory disease (PID) is any acute or chronic infection of the reproductive system that ascends from the vagina, cervix, uterus, fallopian tubes, and ovaries. These infections may cause the fallopian tubes to fill with pus, and chronic episodes can result in scarring of the fallopian tubes and the formation of adhesions.

PID is most often caused by gonorrhea or chlamydia (see Chapter 18), but many types of bacteria can cause PID. Initially the patient may be asymptomatic. When signs and symptoms do occur, they could include fever, abdominal or pelvic pain, vaginal discharge, dysuria, and dyspareunia.

Diagnosis is made by means of a pelvic examination and test of the vaginal secretions. Treatment includes antibiotics for the patient and her partner and analgesics.

Additional Female Reproductive System Diseases/Disorders

There are additional female reproductive system diseases, and Table 27.1 provides information on many of them. Table 27.2 provides information on pregnancy-related conditions.

TABLE 27.1	Female Reproductive System Diseases
DISEASE	**DESCRIPTION**
Dysfunctional uterine bleeding (DUB)	Abnormal uterine bleeding not caused by a tumor, inflammation, or pregnancy.
Menopause	The cessation of menses.
Ovarian cyst	Benign, fluid-filled sac. Can be either a follicular cyst, which occurs when a follicle does not rupture at ovulation, or a cyst of the corpus luteum, which is caused when it does not continue its transformation.
Polycystic ovary syndrome	Bilateral presence of numerous cysts, caused by a hormonal abnormality leading to the secretion of androgens. Can cause acne, facial hair, and infertility.
Premenstrual dysphoric disorder (PMDD)	Mood disorder that includes depression, irritability, fatigue, changes in appetite or sleep, and difficulty in concentrating; occurs 1 to 2 weeks before the onset of the menstrual flow.
Premenstrual syndrome (PMS)	Poorly understood group of symptoms that occur in some women on a cyclical basis: breast pain, irritability, fluid retention, headache, and a lack of coordination are some of the symptoms.
Tumors fibroid/myoma	Fibroids are smooth muscle tumors of the uterus. They are usually nonpainful growths that may be removed surgically. Theses tumors may also be referred to as myomas.

TABLE 27.2 Pregnancy-Related Conditions

DISEASE	DESCRIPTION
Abruptio placentae	Premature separation of the placenta from the uterine wall; may result in a severe hemorrhage that can threaten both infant and maternal lives.
Eclampsia	Extremely serious form of hypertension secondary to pregnancy. Patients are at risk for coma, convulsions, and death.
Hemolytic disease of the newborn (HDN)	A mother with Rh− blood will develop antibodies to an Rh+ fetus during the first pregnancy. If another pregnancy occurs with an Rh+ fetus, the antibodies can destroy the fetal blood cells.
Hyperemesis gravidarum	Excessive vomiting that causes weakness, dehydration, and fluid and electrolyte imbalance.
Placenta previa	Placenta that is positioned in the uterus so that it covers the opening of the cervix.
Preeclampsia	Abnormal condition of pregnancy with unknown cause, marked by hypertension, edema, and proteinuria.
Zika virus	A mosquito-borne virus that typically causes a mild fever, rash, and joint pain. The virus can be passed to a fetus and is associated with certain birth defects such as microcephaly.

CRITICAL THINKING APPLICATION   27.4

As Jill was working with more pregnant patients, she was becoming more familiar with the complications that can occur. She was still a bit confused between preeclampsia and eclampsia. How would you describe the differences?

Menopause

Conditions and disorders related to the menstrual cycle are a big part of a gynecologic specialty. *Menopause* is the permanent ending of menstruation as a result of the end of ovarian function. It usually occurs between 45 and 55 years of age but can occur as early as the 30s and as late as the 60s. Menses may stop suddenly, flow may decrease over time, or the time between menses may lengthen until menstruation completely stops. Menopause can be diagnosed only retrospectively. Only after 12 months of **amenorrhea** is a woman said to be in menopause, and the years after this are called *postmenopause.*

Perimenopause begins when hormone-related changes start to appear, and it lasts until the final menses; this can be as long as 10 years before menopause. During this time, women are still ovulating, but the uneven rise and fall of estrogen and progesterone may cause symptoms. Some women experience few or no symptoms, whereas others may have symptoms such as the following:

- Hot flashes
- Concentration problems
- Mood swings
- Irritability
- Migraines
- Vaginal dryness
- Urinary incontinence
- Dry skin
- Sleep disorders

Treatment focuses on relieving these signs and symptoms. The provider may prescribe very-low-dose oral contraceptives to balance estrogen and progesterone levels or short-term hormone replacement therapy (HRT) to treat symptoms. The provider also may recommend that the patient consume soy products or take soy supplements for a plant source of estrogen. Vitamin E may help ease hot flashes, and vitamin B_6 helps create natural serotonin, a neurotransmitter that affects mood. Other methods that help with symptoms include the following:

- Avoiding caffeine and spicy foods (to reduce hot flashes)
- Using relaxation techniques (to aid with sleep disorders)
- Consuming a low-fat diet high in calcium and vitamin D
- Performing regular weight-bearing exercise (to help prevent **osteoporosis** and heart disease)

Medical treatment of menopause focuses on managing uncomfortable symptoms and preventing conditions associated with a drop in blood levels of estrogen, such as osteoporosis and coronary artery disease. Providers traditionally treated perimenopause and menopause with long-term HRT for most women; however, studies indicate that although HRT does protect the menopausal woman from osteoporosis, hip fracture, and colon cancer, at the same time it increases the risk of heart attack, stroke, breast cancer, and blood clotting. It is now recommended that providers prescribe HRT to meet individual patient needs over a short term (i.e., no longer than 5 years) rather than as routine treatment for all menopausal women. Studies show that the risk for heart disease and other complications increases after 5 years of HRT. The medical assistant must be aware of the provider's recommendations regarding HRT.

Other medications that may be prescribed include antidepressants to prevent hot flashes. Gabapentin and clonidine also may be prescribed to reduce the frequency of hot flashes. Because the development of osteoporosis is a concern in perimenopausal and postmenopausal women, the provider may prescribe alendronate, risedronate, or ibandronate to reduce bone loss and the risk of fracture. Another drug that may be used to improve postmenopausal bone density is raloxifene; however, hot flashes are a common side effect of this medication. Vaginal dryness can be treated with estrogen administered locally by vaginal tablet, ring, or cream, or the patient can use K-Y Jelly or some other vaginal moisturizer as a lubricant.

LIFE SPAN CHANGES

Pediatrics

A review of the most recent national statistics for all diagnoses for hospital inpatients who were newborns or children under the age of 17 revealed some surprises. For neonates (28 days old and younger), diagnoses that included complications of delivery were common. Meconium staining and cord entanglement were high on the list. However, for fertile females between the ages of 1 and 17, the delivery of a single live born is second only to hypovolemia for all diagnoses. (Pneumonia and asthma follow closely behind.) Still within the top 50 diagnoses are a large number of complications of delivery.

Geriatrics

Later in life, senior women are seen most often for neoplasms of the breast, uterus, cervix, and ovaries. Breast cancer alone will be diagnosed in one in eight women in their lifetime in the United States.

THE MEDICAL ASSISTANT'S ROLE IN OBSTETRICS AND GYNECOLOGY PROCEDURES

In this section, we will discuss the medical assistant's role in gynecologic and obstetric procedures. A medical assistant has two roles in these situations:

- Assist the provider in any way needed
- Be there for the patient by helping her to be as comfortable as possible during her time in the healthcare facility

When we make the patient feel comfortable, we help to establish a trusting relationship with her. This enables her to share the information the provider needs so as to give her the best possible care.

The Gynecologic Examination

The need for an annual pelvic examination is being debated in the medical community. Currently the American College of Obstetricians and Gynecologists (ACOG) recommends that pelvic and breast examination be performed when indicated by medical history or symptoms. This examination is done to evaluate the reproductive organs and to diagnose and treat any abnormalities of those organs.

A breast examination is considered part of the gynecologic examination. A clinical breast examination should be done every 1 to 3 years. The provider examines the breast, underarm area, and just below the clavicle.

Setting Up for a Gynecologic Examination

A medical assistant is responsible for setting up the examination room and making sure that all of the supplies are available for a gynecologic examination. The following is a list of supplies needed for a routine gynecologic examination:

- Patient's health record
- Laboratory requisition slips
- Patient gown and drape
- Lubricant
- Examination light
- Cervical spatula or cytobrush
- Microscope slides (direct smear method)
- Fixative (direct smear method)
- Plastic-fronded broom (liquid-based method)
- Liquid preparation container (liquid-based method)
- Vaginal speculum
- Sterile swabs
- Fecal occult blood test cards with developer
- Biohazard waste container

All items should be placed within easy reach for the provider and organized in a logical manner.

Preparation for the Gynecologic Examination

At the time the appointment was made, the patient should have been advised not to douche or have sexual intercourse for 24 hours before the examination. This allows the vaginal discharge to be properly evaluated and ensures accurate results of cytologic studies. Before the provider begins the pelvic examination, the medical assistant should obtain a complete gynecologic history. After documenting the patient's history and chief complaint, the medical assistant should prepare the room and the patient for the examination (see Procedure 27.1, p. 701).

The following should be included in the gynecologic history:

- Age at menarche
- Details about the regularity of the menstrual cycle, the amount and duration of menstrual flow, and a history of menstrual disturbances and their treatment
- Any current indicators of infection, including vaginal discharge, pelvic pain, and urinary difficulties
- Description of any breast abnormalities and the date of the patient's last mammogram
- Date of the last Pap test
- Sexual history; sexually transmitted infection (STI) history
- Number of times pregnant and the number of pregnancies carried to more than 20 weeks
- Date of last menstrual period (LMP)
- Lifestyle factors, including diet, exercise, smoking, and alcohol use

Assisting With an Examination

The pelvic and breast examination can be an embarrassing and emotionally difficult medical experience. In our society, reproduction is not openly talked about. Aside from the embarrassment, many women fear the provider's findings. By behaving in a professional manner, explaining what is going to happen, and showing a genuine interest in the patient's concerns, the medical assistant can help lay to rest most of the patient's anxieties and fears.

The medical assistant is responsible for supporting the patient and assisting the provider during the procedure. To prevent unnecessary embarrassment and discomfort, the procedure should be fully explained to the patient. During the explanation, the medical assistant has the opportunity to provide patient education. This should be done using terms that are easy for the patient to understand. The medical assistant should remain in the examination room to provide reassurance to the patient and legal protection for the provider.

The patient should be instructed to empty her bladder, completely disrobe, and put on an examination gown. Some providers prefer that the patient put the gown on with the opening in the front, whereas others prefer the opening in the back. As the medical assistant, you should be aware of your provider's preference and instruct the patient accordingly.

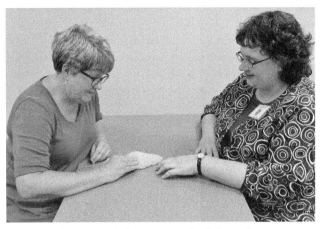

FIGURE 27.3 Coaching a patient regarding the breast self-exam.

Pap Test and Other Guidelines for Women

- Women ages 21 to 29 should have a Pap test alone every 3 years. HPV testing is not recommended
- Women ages 30 to 65 should have a Pap test and an HPV test (co-testing) every 5 years (preferred). It also is acceptable to have a Pap test alone every 3 years.
- If you have had a hysterectomy, you still may need screening. The decision is based on whether your cervix was removed, why the hysterectomy was needed, and whether you have a history of moderate or severe cervical cell changes or cervical cancer. Even if your cervix is removed at the time of hysterectomy, cervical cells can still be present at the top of the vagina. If you have a history of cervical cancer or cervical cell changes, you should continue to have screening for 20 years after the time of your surgery.
- You should stop having cervical cancer screening after age 65 years if the following conditions apply:
  - You do not have a history of moderate or severe abnormal cervical cells or cervical cancer, and
  - You have had either three negative Pap test results in a row or two negative co-test results in a row within the past 10 years, with the most recent test performed within the past 5 years.

Cervical cancer screening. Patient Education FAQ085. Washington, DC: ACOG: 2017. Available at https://www.acog.org/Patients/FAQs/Cervical-Cancer-Screening. Accessed October 16, 2018.

Breast Examination. The first part of the gynecologic examination is the breast examination. The exam begins with the patient in the sitting position for a visual check of the breasts. The gown should be adjusted so that the breast tissue can be easily exposed. After the visual inspection, the patient will be placed in the supine position. The medical assistant should be prepared to help the patient to lie down on the examination table. The footrest should be extended, and a small pillow may be placed under the patient's head for comfort. If needed, the gown and drape should be adjusted to protect the patient's modesty. Palpation will be used to determine if there is thickening or lumps in the breast and collar bone area. The provider will instruct the patient to place her arms above her head to allow assessment of the underarm area using palpation. When the examination is complete, the gown is readjusted to cover the breasts. The

provider may choose to discuss breast self-examination with the patient at this time or may inform the patient that the medical assistant will be explaining the technique at the end of the examination.

According to the American Cancer Society, research has not shown a benefit for a patient or provider breast exam when women are also getting mammograms. It is recommended for women with an average risk of breast cancer to start having yearly mammograms by age 45. It is optional to start earlier.

It is important for all women to know what is normal with their breasts. Any abnormality should be reported to their provider. Some providers still recommend monthly breast self-exams (BSEs) to be done after the menses. Procedure 27.2 on p. 701 describes how to perform a BSE. It is helpful for the medical assistant to provide the patient with a brochure showing the technique. It is also recommended to show the technique on a model (Fig. 27.3). If possible, the patient should demonstrate the technique back to the medical assistant. This practice helps the medical assistant to determine if the patient understood the coaching.

Warning Signs of Breast Cancer

- Change in the skin (redness, warmth, darkening of the color, dimpling, puckering)
- Lump or hard area inside the breast or in the axilla area
- Change in the size or shape of the breast
- Change in the nipple (inverted or pulling in appearance, rash, sore, or drainage)
- Pain that does not go away

Abdominal Examination. While the patient is in the supine position, the provider will palpate the abdomen. This is done to confirm normal **symmetry** of the pelvic organs and to detect any masses. The provider also watches for any signs of discomfort or pain that could indicate a problem.

Pelvic Examination. For the pelvic examination, the patient is placed in the lithotomy position. This can be an awkward position for the patient to assume without assistance, and it may be embarrassing to the patient. If needed, the medical assistant should be available to help the patient into this position. Never place the patient in the lithotomy position until the provider is ready to begin the examination.

When you assist the patient into the lithotomy position, always keep her totally covered.

You should stand at the patient's side so that you can observe her, yet still be able to move quickly (if needed by the provider). First, the provider inspects the external genitalia and palpates the perineal area. The patient may be asked to bear down to show any muscular weaknesses that may be the result of lacerations of the perineal body during childbirth. A third-degree laceration may have involved the rectal sphincter and may cause rectal incontinence.

Next, the vaginal speculum is inserted for examination of the cervix and the vaginal canal to obtain the Pap specimen. The speculum should be prewarmed with warm water. Have the patient take some deep breaths to help relax the abdominal muscles. The normal cervix points posteriorly and has smooth, pink, squamous epithelium. Abnormalities most frequently seen are ulcerations (erosions), **Bartholin cysts**, and cervical polyps. Because erosions cannot be palpated, inspection is the only method of detecting them. Healed lacerations from childbirth are common in a patient who has had multiple deliveries. Pregnancy increases the size of the cervix, and hormone deficiency causes it to atrophy. The vaginal wall is reddish pink and has a corrugated appearance from the overlapping tissue (rugae) lining. Vaginal infections change the appearance of the vaginal mucosa.

After inspecting the vaginal wall, the provider may collect a specimen for a Pap test. When the specimen has been obtained, the medical assistant may be responsible for labeling the specimen and preparing it for transport to the cytology laboratory. Be sure to follow laboratory instructions during the preparation to avoid having to repeat the examination.

After removal of the vaginal speculum, the provider does a bimanual examination. For a bimanual examination, two gloved fingers are lubricated with a water-soluble jelly (lubricant) and inserted into the vaginal canal, and the other hand palpates the abdomen over the pelvic organs and the mons pubis (Fig. 27.4). The uterus is examined for shape, size, and consistency, and its position is noted. A normal uterus is freely movable with limited discomfort. A laterally displaced uterus is usually the result of pelvic adhesions or displacement caused by a pelvic tumor. The fallopian tubes and ovaries are evaluated. Normal tubes and ovaries are difficult to palpate, which is why the provider may have to press firmly in the pelvic area, causing minor discomfort for the patient. A digital rectal exam may be done at this time. This involves the insertion of a gloved finger into the rectum. A small amount of stool is left on the glove and can be used for a fecal occult blood test.

Specimen Collection

During a pelvic examination, several types of specimens may be collected. If the pelvic exam is part of a wellness examination, a specimen for a Pap test may be collected. If the provider wants to evaluate endocrine function, a maturation index may be ordered. If the pelvic examination is for a possible vaginal infection, a specimen may be collected for culture or observation under a microscope.

Pap Test. The two methods of specimen collection for a Pap test are the direct smear method and the liquid-based method.

Direct Smear Method
1. The specimen is collected with a cervical spatula.
2. The cells are placed (smeared) directly on a microscope slide.
3. A fixative must be applied immediately to the slide before it is sent to the laboratory.

Liquid-Based Method
1. The specimen is collected with a plastic-fronded broom.
2. Cells are suspended in a bottle of preservative by rinsing the broom in the specimen vial.
3. The results of the Pap test are often reported using the Bethesda System.

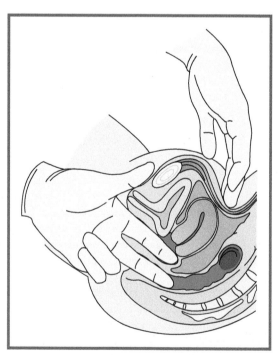

FIGURE 27.4 Bimanual examination.

Pap Test Results

The Bethesda System is often used to report the results of a Pap test. This system looks at the squamous cells and the glandular cells separately.

Squamous Cells
- Negative for intraepithelial lesion of malignancy: normal epithelial cells, no precancerous findings.
- Atypical squamous cells (ASC).
  - Atypical squamous cells of undetermined significance (ASC-US): Squamous cells do not appear completely normal but do not clearly suggest precancerous cells. Most often means there is an infection.
  - Atypical squamous cells, cannot exclude a high-grade squamous intraepithelial lesion (ASC-H): Minor changes with unknown causes that are at risk of progressing to high-grade lesion (HSIL).
- Low-grade squamous intraepithelial lesions (LSILs): Mild cell changes that may be classified as mild dysplasia. These abnormalities are often caused by human papillomavirus (HPV) infection.
- High-grade squamous intraepithelial lesions (HSILs): Severe abnormalities that have a higher likelihood of progressing to cancer if left untreated. May be classified as moderate or severe dysplasia.
- Squamous cell carcinoma: Cervical cancer.

Glandular Cells

- Atypical glandular cells (ACG): Glandular cells do not appear normal, but it is not clear what is causing the changes.
- Endocervical adenocarcinoma in situ (AIS): Severely abnormal cells are found, but they have not spread beyond the glandular tissue of the cervix.
- Adenocarcinoma: Cancer of the endocervical canal and possibly endometrial, extrauterine, and other cancers.

Maturation Index. A *maturation index* is an endocrine evaluation that can assist in the diagnosis and treatment of infertility issues, amenorrhea, menopause, or postmenopausal bleeding. Cells are collected from the vaginal wall and treated much like a Pap test specimen. If the provider orders a maturation index, it must be indicated on the cytology request form.

Vaginal Infections. Earlier in this chapter, common vaginal infections were discussed. To collect a specimen to determine what type of vaginal infection is occurring, a pelvic exam needs to be done. For many vaginal infections, a sterile swab is used to collect a sample of the discharge. The secretion is then swabbed on the microscope slide, and the provider looks at it under a microscope. Common infections, the infectious agents, and the type of specimen and test used to identify each include the following:

- *Candidiasis (yeast infection):* The provider tests for the presence of *Candida albicans*. A small amount of discharge is placed on a slide, and a drop of a 10% solution of potassium hydroxide (KOH) is added. The KOH dissolves other cellular debris so that the provider can see the yeast buds.
- *Trichomoniasis:* A small amount of discharge is placed on a slide, and a drop of saline is added. The provider is looking for *Trichomonas vaginalis,* which appears as a pear-shaped organism with a flagellum (tail) that moves it around.
- *Chlamydia:* A sterile swab is used to collect a specimen from the endocervical canal. The swab is then placed in a tube containing a transport medium and sent to the lab for testing. The causative organism frequently is *Chlamydia trachomatis.*

Contraception

At the time of a gynecologic examination, a provider may discuss contraception with the patient. A woman's choice of a contraceptive method is based on many factors. To make an informed choice, a patient should know the risks, benefits, side effects, costs, failure rates, and convenience of each available method. In addition, although condoms are only moderately successful at preventing pregnancy, they should be used consistently to prevent the transmission of STIs. The medical assistant may help provide patient education on contraceptive methods. Table 27.3 summarizes the characteristics of various contraceptive methods.

Barrier Methods. Barrier methods of contraception either kill sperm (through the use of a chemical spermicide) or prevent them from entering the cervical os. These methods, which are relatively inexpensive, include the condom, diaphragm, and cervical cap or sponge. Each method must be used every time the person has intercourse,

which means the patient must be motivated to follow through on using it. Patient education on the use of a diaphragm includes the following instructions:

- Examine the diaphragm before each use by holding it up to a bright light to check for holes or cracks.
- Place 1 to 2 tablespoons of spermicidal jelly or cream into the diaphragm dome before insertion.
- Leave the diaphragm in place for 6 hours after intercourse; do not douche until after you have removed it.
- Before repeated intercourse, add spermicide to the outside of the diaphragm with an applicator. Do not remove the diaphragm until 6 hours after the last intercourse.
- After removal, wash the diaphragm with soap and water, allow it to air dry, and inspect it for breaks or holes before storing.
- Have the diaphragm refitted if the following occurs:
  - You gain or lose more than 10 to 15 pounds
  - You have a miscarriage, give birth, or undergo any type of pelvic surgery
  - You have difficulty voiding or moving your bowels with the diaphragm in place

The cervical cap is a thimble-sized, domed barrier device that fits over the end of the cervix. It also is used with spermicidal jelly (Fig. 27.5).

If used properly, the cervical cap is 92% to 96% effective. An advantage of this barrier method is that the cap can be inserted up to 12 hours before intercourse and can stay in place up to 72 hours without a decrease in effectiveness or safety. The cervical sponge contains spermicide and can also be inserted hours before intercourse and is effective for 24 hours. If always used as directed, the sponge is 80% to 91% effective.

Hormonal Contraceptives. Hormonal contraceptives are a highly effective and reversible form of contraception. They work by preventing ovulation, changing the cervical mucosa, affecting sperm mobility, and preventing thickening of the endometrial wall. Hormonal contraceptives include the following:

- Birth control pills or patch
- Vaginal ring
- Depo-Provera injections
- Hormonal implants

Besides being a highly effective method of birth control, oral contraceptives can be used to treat a wide range of gynecologic conditions, including menstrual irregularities, premenstrual syndrome (PMS) symptoms, and **anovulation**. They also can be used to prevent ovarian cysts and may be prescribed to increase bone density. However, to be effective, the pills must be taken daily, at the same time each day. Failure rates are associated with noncompliance and can range from less than 1% (in highly compliant women) to greater than 15% (in those who do not take the pills as prescribed). Oral contraceptive pills (OCPs) can have serious side effects. Patients should be informed of conditions that require immediate medical attention. These can be remembered with the mnemonic ACHES: *a*bdominal pain (new and severe), *c*hest pain (new and severe), *h*eadaches (new or more frequent), *e*ye problems (blurred vision or vision loss), and *s*evere leg pain. These symptoms may indicate the formation of a blood clot in the abdomen, chest, or leg. They may also be signs of a stroke. Blood clot formation and stroke are the most serious complications of OCPs.

TABLE 27.3   Commonly Used Contraceptive Methods

	FAILURE RATE	CHARACTERISTICS	CONTRAINDICATIONS	SIDE EFFECTS
Male or female condom (barrier method)	2%–10%	No prescription or examination needed; easily available; inexpensive	Latex allergy in either partner	Possible allergic response to latex or spermicide
Diaphragm, cervical cap, cervical sponge (barrier method)	2%–19%	Must be fitted by clinician; requires instruction on how to insert and remove; spermicide must be used each time; diaphragm and sponge must be left in place for 6 hours after intercourse	Latex, rubber, or spermicide allergy; uterine prolapse; severe cystocele or rectocele	Increased risk for UTI (diaphragm); increased risk of abnormal Pap test result (cap)
Intrauterine device (IUD)	2%–6%	Copper type releases copper, which slows sperm in the cervix; hormonal type releases progestin, which reduces sperm mobility and prevents thickening of the endometrial wall	Cervicitis, vaginitis, endometriosis, pelvic infection, history of STI or ectopic pregnancy	Copper type may temporarily increase vaginal bleeding and menstrual pain; hormonal IUDs decrease menstrual flow and cramping
Birth control implants	1%	Flexible plastic implant inserted under skin of upper arm; releases progestin to prevent ovulation, thickens cervical secretions to block semen, thins endometrial wall; effective for up to 3 years	Certain antibiotics, HIV drugs, seizure medications may make it less effective; history of blood clots, liver disease, or breast cancer	Irregular bleeding in first 6–12 months; nausea, headache, sore breasts, scarring at implantation site
Depo-Provera (DMPA)	0.5%	Requires 150-mg intramuscular injection every 3 months	Intention of becoming pregnant within 1 year, breast cancer, liver disease	Return of fertility may be delayed 10–18 months; should not be used more than 2 years in a row because it can cause a temporary loss of bone density; headache, weight gain, possibly depression
Oral contraceptives (OCPs) Hormonal patch Vaginal ring	1%	Suppress ovulation; atrophy of the endometrium	Thrombolytic, liver, or coronary artery disease; breast, liver, reproductive tract cancer; smoker over age 35; diabetes; sickle cell disease	Nausea, breakthrough bleeding, breast tenderness, fluid retention; hypertension, elevated lipid levels, blood clots, strokes

A type of oral contraception, the extended cycle pill, limits the number of menstrual periods to four a year. Patients are more likely to have spotting and breakthrough bleeding with this hormone therapy than with the traditional 28-day birth control pill. The extended cycle pill is designed to be taken once a day for 84 days, and then an inactive dose is taken for a week, during which the woman would menstruate. A combination birth control pill that contains both estrogen and progestin may be prescribed for women suffering from premenstrual dysphoric disorder (PMDD); it also is useful for treating acne in female patients at least 14 years of age who have started menstruating.

As mentioned, hormonal contraception also can be delivered via a transdermal patch. The patch is a 1¾-inch square that slowly releases estrogen and progestin through the skin into the bloodstream. It is considered as effective as oral contraceptives in women who weigh less than 198 pounds; however, the patch is still a very effective method for women who weigh more than this. Current research shows that the risk of blood clots with the contraceptive patch is similar to the risks observed with oral contraceptives. However, cigarette smoking increases the risk of serious cardiovascular side effects, especially if the patient is over age 35. Patients should be told not to apply any creams or oils at the application site, to change the patch weekly for 3 consecutive weeks, and to go patch free the fourth week, allowing menstruation to occur. The patch can be applied to the buttocks, lower abdomen, and upper body, but not to the breasts. The woman can bathe, shower, and swim while wearing the patch, but if it comes off, it should be replaced immediately.

The vaginal ring contraceptive device is made of flexible plastic and is inserted into the vagina. The ring slowly releases estrogen and progestin in order to prevent pregnancy and provide effective contraceptive action for 1 month after insertion. The device is 2 inches in diameter and can be inserted anywhere in the vagina; however,

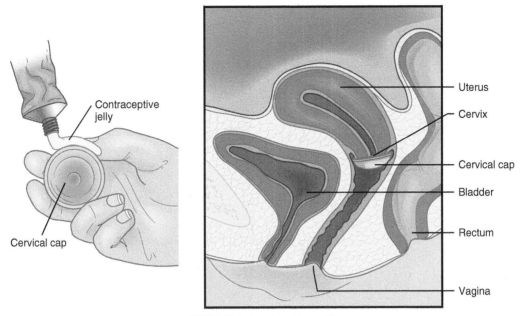

FIGURE 27.5 Cervical cap with spermicide.

the deeper it is placed, the less likely it is to be felt after insertion. Side effects of the vaginal ring are similar to those of other hormonal contraceptives, and it may increase the risk of heart attack, stroke, and blood clots. When the patient first starts using the ring, an additional method of birth control must be used for the first week. If the ring falls out, it should be rinsed with warm water and reinserted within 3 hours. If it is out for longer than 3 hours, contraception is not certain, and the patient should use another birth control method for 1 week.

Depo-Provera is an injectable contraceptive that contains high doses of progestin. Each dose prevents pregnancy for up to 3 months, but women must be compliant in returning to the healthcare facility for follow-up and repeat doses every 9 to 13 weeks. The first injection should be administered within the first 5 days of the menstrual period for birth control coverage. This is a highly effective method of contraception and is ideal for women who either do not comply with a birth control regimen or do not want to take a pill every day. However, using Depo-Provera for 2 years or longer may increase the risk of bone loss and the eventual development of osteoporosis. Almost all patients using the injections experience some menstrual irregularities, but these usually subside after two doses. Women using this form of hormonal contraception are not at risk for the side effects of estrogen exposure, such as increased risk of blood clots and cardiovascular disease.

A birth control implant is a single, flexible rod, about the size of a match, that is inserted under the skin of the upper arm. The birth control implant releases a low, steady dose of progestin. This suppresses ovulation, thickens cervical mucus to block the passage of sperm, and thins the endometrial wall to prevent implantation. It prevents pregnancy for up to 3 years after insertion. Hormonal implants have risks and contraindications similar to those of other hormonal types of contraception.

Intrauterine Devices. The intrauterine device (IUD) (Fig. 27.6) is a T-shaped plastic frame with threads attached that the provider inserts into the uterus to prevent pregnancy. Two general types of IUDs are available: the copper type and the hormonal type. Both

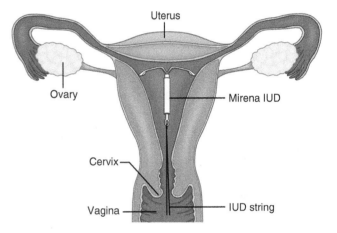

FIGURE 27.6 Intrauterine device.

products inhibit fertilization by blocking the sperm's journey to the fallopian tubes, and, if fertilization does occur, they prevent the embryo from implanting into the uterine wall. In addition, the copper type of IUD releases copper, which acts to slow sperm in the cervix. The hormonal types of IUDs release progestin, which reduces sperm mobility and prevents the thickening of the endometrial wall during the menstrual cycle. Both types of IUDs are extremely effective at preventing pregnancy (over 99%); the copper type can remain in place as long as 12 years, whereas the hormonal type must be replaced every 3 to 5 years. The copper IUD may temporarily increase vaginal bleeding and menstrual pain. The hormonal IUD results in both decreased menstrual flow and cramping. To remove an IUD, the provider gently withdraws it by pulling on the IUD string. In rare instances, it must be removed surgically.

Permanent Methods. Both male and female patients can undergo surgical procedures that are considered permanent contraceptive methods. Vasectomies in the male were addressed in Chapter 26. For the female, a bilateral tubal ligation can be performed in which a portion of both fallopian tubes is excised or ligated. The cost and rate of complications are higher for tubal ligations than for vasectomies. In addition, tubal ligations must be done on an outpatient basis with general anesthesia, so the woman has that additional risk. Both procedures can be reversed, but not always successfully.

CRITICAL THINKING APPLICATION   **27.6**

When directed by the provider, Peggy provides patient education regarding contraceptives. She has asked Jill to create a reference sheet that covers all birth control options, their characteristics and side effects, and any patient education details that might be appropriate. What should Jill include?

Postexamination Duties

When the examination is finished, help the patient into a sitting position and into the dressing room if needed. Following the Standard Precautions established by the Occupational Safety and Health Administration (OSHA), remove the examination equipment and supplies while the patient is dressing so that when the provider returns to talk to the patient, the room is neat and clean. Once the patient has left, the room should be sanitized, disinfected, and restocked as necessary so it is ready for the next patient.

Special Procedures

There are a number of gynecology-related special procedures that a patient may undergo related to an abnormal Pap test result. Let's look at the three most commonly performed procedures:

- Cryotherapy
- Colposcopy with or without a biopsy
- Loop electrosurgical excision procedure (LEEP)

Cryotherapy. Depending on the condition of the cervix, *cryotherapy*, or the application of freezing temperatures, may be used to treat chronic cervicitis and cervical erosion. Freezing causes cellular **necrosis**, and in approximately 1 month, the dead cells are replaced with healthy cells. The procedure involves placing a probe against the problem area on the cervix and applying liquid nitrogen to the area for approximately 3 to 4 minutes or until the site is frozen. The patient may experience some pain for 30 minutes or so after the procedure, and a slight watery discharge for up to a week. If any signs of infection, foul discharge, or pain develop, the patient should call the provider's office. Advise the patient not to engage in sexual intercourse for 1 month and to expect a heavier than usual menstrual flow for the first cycle after the procedure.

Colposcopy With or Without a Biopsy. *Colposcopy* is the visual examination of the vagina and cervical surfaces with a colposcope (Fig. 27.7). The *colposcope* is a microscope with a light source and a magnifying lens that can be used during a vaginal examination to do the following:

- Locate and evaluate abnormal cells
- Detect cancer of the cervix in the early stages
- Examine tissue from which an abnormal Pap test result has been obtained
- Monitor areas of the cervix where malignant lesions have been removed

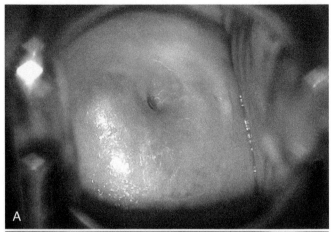
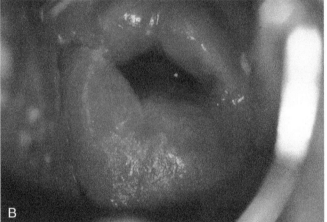

FIGURE 27.7 Colposcopic appearance of normal cervix **(A)** and abnormal cervix **(B)**.

In combination with a colposcopy, a cervical biopsy may be performed. A major advantage of obtaining a biopsy during colposcopy is that the instrument permits visualization of the suspicious area so that the biopsy can be taken from the most atypical site. Multiple biopsies may be taken. The provider is looking for abnormalities on the cervix and will take a biopsy specimen when one is seen. You may be receiving the sample from the provider. It is very important to accurately label each specimen container with the location of the biopsy. The provider uses the face of a clock for determining the location of the biopsy. The specimen container label should indicate that location (e.g., 2:00).

Colposcopy is a relatively safe, painless procedure performed in the provider's office. Discomfort may occur when the speculum is inserted into the vagina to improve visualization of the tissue. Discomfort and bleeding can occur when tissue is taken in a biopsy.

Loop Electrosurgical Excision Procedure. Depending on the results of the cervical biopsy, the patient may need a more extensive procedure, *conization*, in which a cone-shaped wedge of cervical tissue is removed for treatment or further analysis. More often a less-invasive LEEP is performed. With this technique, a local anesthetic is injected into the cervix, and a wire loop is inserted into the vagina. A high-frequency electrical current running through the wire is used to remove abnormal tissue from both the cervix and the endocervical canal. Like conization, LEEP can be used as a diagnostic tool to collect biopsy samples and as a treatment to remove abnormal tissue (Fig. 27.8).

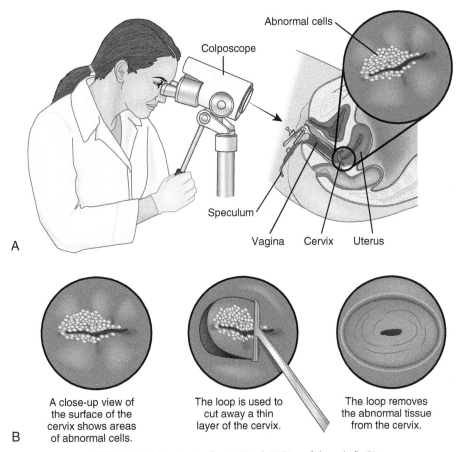

FIGURE 27.8 Colposcopic view of cervix **(A)** and LEEP biopsy of abnormal cells **(B)**.

Obstetrics

Pregnancy can be the most exciting and most terrifying experience for a patient, especially the first time around. As a medical assistant working in obstetrics, it is important to be able to reassure the patient while remaining professional. The next section discusses the examinations and procedures related to prenatal and postpartum care.

Prenatal Record

At the first prenatal examination, an extensive health history will be taken. This history can help to identify any risk factors for the patient. Frequently, the first prenatal visit is the first comprehensive physical examination that the patient has had in a long time. The health history can point out pregnancy-related risk factors and overall health-related risk factors that can also be addressed. The following information should be collected when creating the prenatal record for a patient:

- Demographic information
- Menstrual history
- Obstetric history
- Medical and surgical history
- Family and social history

Demographic Information. The healthcare facility must have accurate and up-to-date demographic information, including the following:

- Address and phone numbers (land line and cellular)
- Employment

- Insurance
- Emergency contact
- Language
- Self-identified ethnicity
- Religious preference

This information is necessary for billing purposes and for preauthorization of services. It also can help to ensure that we are providing all of the services needed for the patient by making sure that we have an interpreter available (if needed, based on language) and having any special dietary needs met for the patient at the hospital.

Menstrual History. The prenatal record should include the first day of the last menstrual period. This is used to determine the estimated date of delivery (EDD). It is also important to know the normal cycle length for the patient and if this last menstrual period was "normal." The medical assistant should also ask if the patient was using contraception when she became pregnant. If she was, the method being used should be documented.

Obstetric History. The provider will need to have a complete history of previous pregnancies. This will help to determine any risk factors for the current pregnancy. The following information should be included in the obstetric history (Fig. 27.9):

- Dates of deliveries
- Types of deliveries (vaginal or cesarean); if cesarean, the type of incision should be noted
- Birth weight and gestational age of previous infants
- Complications of previous pregnancies

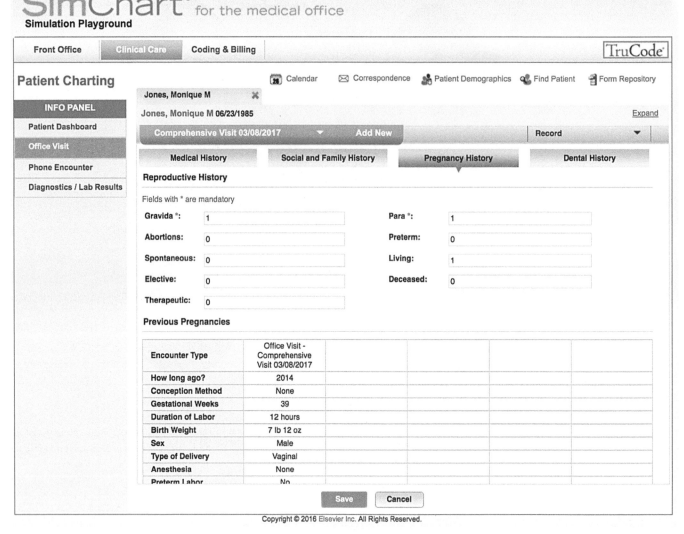

FIGURE 27.9 Pregnancy history form from SimChart for the Medical Office.

There are some specific terms related to an obstetric history that you should be familiar with. Table 27.4 lists those terms and their definitions.

A prenatal record includes documenting the gravida, para, and abortion information. As a medical assistant, you should be able to determine those numbers after obtaining the obstetric history from a patient. It is important to remember that gravida and para refer to the number of pregnancies and not the number of babies. A twin pregnancy is considered just one pregnancy. If this was the first pregnancy for the patient and the pregnancy went to term (38 to 40 weeks), she would be gravida: 1 and para: 1.

CRITICAL THINKING APPLICATION   27.7

Jill is interviewing a new OB patient. The patient tells Jill that this is her fourth pregnancy, and she has two children. She had two early miscarriages. What would her gravida number be? What would her para number be? What would her abortion number be?

Medical and Surgical History. There are medical and surgical conditions that could affect a patient's current pregnancy. Common chronic conditions, such as diabetes, hypertension, asthma, and mitral valve prolapse, should be included in the prenatal record. The management of these conditions could change with pregnancy. Less common conditions, such as thyroid disorders, systemic lupus erythematosus, and bleeding disorders, can also affect the patient and the fetus. To help both, the provider needs to be aware of these conditions and the treatment that is being followed.

Certain infections can affect a pregnancy. A history of certain STIs can put the patient at risk for complications. Pelvic inflammatory disease (PID) can cause scarring of the fallopian tubes, which increases the risk of an **ectopic pregnancy**. Genital herpes and other infections can be transmitted to the newborn during delivery. If the provider is aware of those conditions, plans can be made to protect both the mother and the baby.

If the patient has had any type of abdominal surgical procedure, it could affect the pregnancy or delivery. If there is a history of a prior ectopic pregnancy, this would be a risk factor for another one.

TABLE 27.4 Obstetric History Terms

TERM	DEFINITION
Gravida	Number of pregnancies
Primigravida	A woman who is pregnant for the first time
Multigravida	A woman who has been pregnant two or more times
Nulligravida	A woman who has never been pregnant
Para	Number of pregnancies that have gone to the age of fetal **viability** (20 weeks' gestation)
Primipara	A woman who has carried one pregnancy to the age of fetal viability
Multipara	A woman who has carried two or more pregnancies to the age of fetal viability
Nullipara	A woman who has not carried a pregnancy to the age of fetal viability
Abortion	Termination of a pregnancy before the fetal age of viability Miscarriage, spontaneous, elective
Spontaneous abortion	Natural death of an embryo or fetus before the fetal age of viability; also called a miscarriage
Therapeutic or elective abortion	A procedure for the planned termination of a pregnancy
Stillbirth	Fetal death after 20 weeks' gestation; also called intrauterine fetal death (IUFD)

If there is a history of a uterine puncture or any uterine incision, the patient and provider will need to talk about a possible cesarean section.

Family and Social History. Many conditions have a genetic component. Obtaining an accurate family history can help to determine if the patient or the infant is at risk. With this knowledge, the patient and the provider can be prepared. Additional testing may be included during the prenatal period for a patient with certain factors in the family history. Conditions that could be of concern include the following:

- Diabetes
- Hypertension
- Heart disease
- Autoimmune disorders (e.g., lupus, rheumatoid arthritis)
- Kidney disease
- Seizures
- Depression
- Thyroid disease
- **Preeclampsia**

A family history of genetic disorders should also be documented in the patient's family history. These disorders can include the following:

- **Down syndrome**
- Neural tube defects (**spina bifida, meningocele, anencephaly**)
- **Hemophilia**
- **Sickle cell anemia**
- **Cystic fibrosis (CF)**
- **Phenylketonuria (PKU)**

Other family history information that should be noted would include a history of twins in the family, food allergies, and a family history of recurrent miscarriages or stillbirths.

The social history includes tobacco, alcohol, and recreational drug use. This information can be used for patient education as it relates to pregnancy. Nutrition and exercise are an important part of pregnancy. Finding out if the pregnant patient follows a particular diet, such as vegan or vegetarian, will provide the opportunity for patient education regarding nutritional needs during pregnancy. Employment is also part of a social history. This can point out any occupational duties that could be affected by pregnancy, such as working with certain chemicals, or physical activities that should not be done when pregnant.

Collecting all of the components discussed previously is a great start to completing the patient's prenatal record, in addition to supplying the provider with the information needed to provide excellent care during the patient's pregnancy.

The prenatal record will continue to be updated throughout the pregnancy. Clinical data will be added at each prenatal visit. The medical assistant will also be checking with the patient to see if there have been any changes or additions to the initial demographic and history information.

First Prenatal Examination

The physical examination during a first prenatal visit includes an overall assessment of the woman's health status. This would include vital signs, weight, and urinalysis. The medical assistant must prepare the patient. The patient should be asked if she needs to empty her bladder. If she does, she should collect a urine specimen for a routine urinalysis and a possible pregnancy test. The medical assistant should also prepare the exam room, ensuring that the supplies and equipment necessary to obtain pelvic measurements, perform serologic tests, and prepare for laboratory tests are available. The provider will assess the heart, lung, and thyroid. A physical examination will be done to rule out any other abnormalities. Next, the provider performs an obstetric examination that includes measurement of the height of the uterus and an internal or pelvic examination. A Pap test may be performed if one has not been done in the past year.

Pregnancy Test

There are two types of pregnancy tests. One is done with a urine sample and the other one is done with a blood sample. Both tests are looking for hCG levels. Blood tests are usually performed at the provider's office or laboratory. Urine tests can be performed at the provider's office, or the patient may do a home pregnancy test.

Whether the test is performed at home or in the office, the process is very much the same. A sample of the urine is placed on the test stick and then the user waits for the results. Some test sticks will show a plus sign for a positive test and negative sign for a minus test. Other tests will actually display the term *pregnant* for a positive test or *not pregnant* for a negative test.

The estimated date of delivery, or due date, will be determined at this visit. There are a number of ways to determine the due date. One method is using a gestational wheel (Fig. 27.10). With this method, the arrow is lined up with the first date of the LMP, and the EDD is shown at the 40-week mark. The EDD may also be calculated by the electronic health record (EHR) or determined by ultrasound.

A series of blood tests also is performed during the initial prenatal visit. Prenatal blood and laboratory tests include the following:
- Hematocrit and hemoglobin levels, to check for anemia.
- Blood type and Rh with antibody screening for possible Rh incompatibility (Fig. 27.11).
- Rubella titer to determine whether the mother is immune to German measles; rubella infection during pregnancy can cause

multiple birth defects, including deafness, vision disorders, and intellectual disability.
- Syphilis screening; if the result is positive, antibiotic treatment is initiated to protect the fetus from congenital syphilis.
- Hepatitis B screening, because this virus can be passed to the fetus in utero.
- Human immunodeficiency virus (HIV) screening is suggested; if the result is positive, treatment of the mother greatly reduces the risk of transmission to the fetus.
- Gonorrhea and chlamydia cultures to prevent infection of the baby at birth.
- Urinalysis to detect protein, white blood cells, or glucose.

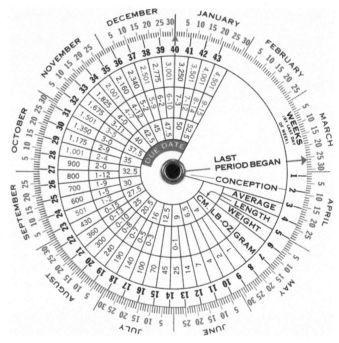

FIGURE 27.10 Gestational wheel. (From Jarvis C: *Physical examination and health assessment,* ed 6, St. Louis, 2012, Saunders.)

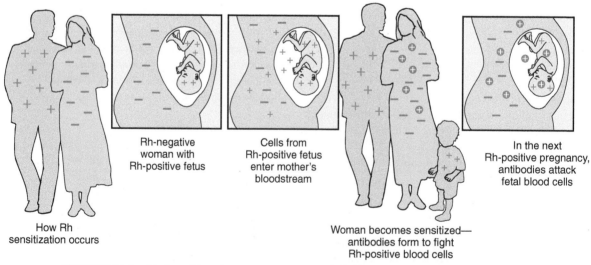

FIGURE 27.11 Hemolytic disease of the newborn. (From Hagen-Ansert SL: *Textbook of diagnostic sonography,* ed 7, St. Louis, 2012, Mosby)

Hemolytic Disease of the Newborn (HDN)

To determine if someone's blood type is Rh positive or Rh negative, the blood is tested for the presence of D antigens. Rh-positive blood has D antigens; Rh-negative blood does not. If the blood type with Rh factor shows that the mother has Rh-negative blood, there is a concern that hemolytic disease of the newborn (HDN) could develop if the fetus is Rh positive. HDN is also known as *erythroblastosis fetalis*. If the mother is Rh negative and her fetus is Rh positive, the mother will form antibodies to the Rh-positive factor. Future Rh-positive pregnancies will be in jeopardy because the mother's anti-Rh antibodies will cross the placenta and destroy fetal blood cells (Fig. 27.11).

HDN can be prevented by giving the mother Rh immune globulin products. RhoGAM, or anti-D immune globulin, is given at 28 to 30 weeks of gestation to Rh-negative mothers, regardless of the father's Rh type. After delivery, the cord blood is tested, and a dose of RhoGAM is given within 72 hours of delivery only if the baby is Rh positive. RhoGAM is also given for miscarriages or abortions. The immune globulin prevents the infant's Rh-positive cells from stimulating the mother's immune system, thus preventing HDN.

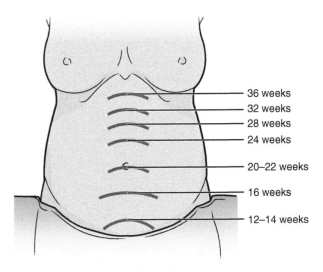

FIGURE 27.12 Fundal height measurement.

Any concerns that the patient has should be noted and reported to the provider. The medical assistant should be prepared to suggest community resources that can provide assistance to new parents, such as the following:
- Childbirth and parenting classes
- Infant cardiopulmonary resuscitation (CPR) courses
- Nutritional counseling, if needed
- Contact information for the Special Supplemental Nutrition Program for Women, Infants, and Children (WIC), which helps lower-income expectant mothers get nutritious food

Return Prenatal Visits

The return prenatal visits follow a regular schedule:
- Every 4 weeks through 28 weeks' gestation
- Every 2 weeks through 35 weeks' gestation
- Every 1 week until delivery

In follow-up prenatal visits, the medical assistant should collect a urine specimen for urinalysis, weigh the patient, measure her blood pressure, and answer questions about diet and health habits. The mother should gain approximately 10 to 12 pounds in the first half of pregnancy and another 15 to 17 pounds during the second half. Experts believe that a healthy weight gain is somewhere between 25 and 35 pounds.

Fetal Heart Tones. A Doppler monitor may be used to hear the baby's heart tones somewhere between 9 and 12 weeks' gestation. Once recorded, the fetal heart rate is assessed at each subsequent visit. It is important to remember that a fetal heart rate should be between 120 and 160 beats per minute. If you get a reading of between 60 and 100 beats per minute, you may be assessing the patient's heart rate and not the fetal heart rate.

Fundal Height Measurement. Fundal height measurement is routinely done during the return prenatal visit. As the uterus grows during pregnancy, it will rise into the abdominal cavity. Between week 8 and week 13, the fundus (the top of the uterus) can be palpated above the symphysis pubis. The fundal height measurement is taken with a flexible tape measure, measuring from the symphysis pubis to the fundus of the uterus. The height is measured in centimeters (cm) and most often matches the number of weeks the patient has been pregnant. For example, if the patient is 25 weeks pregnant, the provider would expect to see a fundal height measurement of 25 cm (Fig. 27.12). This is only considered accurate for the first and second trimesters. If the fundal height measurement does not match the number of weeks pregnant, this could signal an issue with the pregnancy. Fundal height measurements that either are larger or smaller than expected could indicate the following:
- Slow fetal growth (intrauterine growth restriction)
- A significantly larger than average baby (*fetal macrosomia*)
- Too little amniotic fluid (*oligohydramnios*)
- Too much amniotic fluid (*polyhydramnios*)

If the provider suspects an issue, an ultrasound would likely be ordered to determine what was causing the unusual measurements.

Postpartum Visit

The patient should return about 6 weeks after delivery for a postpartum visit. At this visit, the provider will do a pelvic examination to make sure that everything is healing. If a cesarean section was done, the incision site also will be checked for healing. If the patient is interested in using contraceptives, the provider will talk about contraceptive choices. If the patient previously used a diaphragm, the fit will need to be checked. There may also be a discussion about how breast-feeding is going. Any of the patient's questions about care for the baby should be answered at this visit.

The postpartum visit is also an opportunity to see how the patient is doing emotionally. The provider will ask questions related to the patient's moods and check for signs of postpartum depression.

Postpartum Depression

- The incidence of postpartum depression (PPD) is not clear, but an estimated 10% to 20% of women struggle with major depression before, during, and after delivery of a baby. Fewer than half of these are diagnosed in routine office visits.
- Postpartum depression can be diagnosed a month to a year after childbirth. Women with a history of depression during pregnancy should be monitored for signs of postpartum depression for a minimum of 4 months.
- Risk factors include a history of depression, abuse, or mental illness; smoking or alcohol use; anxiety during pregnancy and fears over child care; lack of financial resources and secure relationships; a fussy or colicky infant; and lack of social support.
- Symptoms of postpartum depression include anorexia and insomnia; irritability and anger; overwhelming fatigue; loss of interest in sex and lack of a feeling of joy in life; feelings of shame, guilt, or inadequacy; severe mood swings; difficulty bonding with the baby; withdrawal from family and friends; and thoughts of harming one's self or the baby.
- Postpartum depression must be detected as soon as possible so that treatment can begin; untreated postpartum depression may last for a year or longer. Treatment includes both counseling and antidepressant medication.

The 10-question Edinburgh Postnatal Depression Scale (EPDS) is a valuable and efficient way of identifying patients at risk for *perinatal* depression (between the 28th week of pregnancy and the 28th day after birth). Healthcare professionals working with the perinatal population should use the EPDS as a routine part of postnatal care, because the EPDS is a valid and reliable means of detecting PPD. This screening tool is user-friendly, easy to administer, and easy to score. A score of 9 to 13 is considered the cutoff for PPD; the mother should be referred for further evaluation or treatment. Users may reproduce the scale without further permission, providing they respect the copyright by quoting the names of the authors and the title and the source of the paper in all reproduced copies. The EPDS can be accessed at the American Academy of Pediatrics website:

https://www.aap.org/en-us/advocacy-and-policy/aap-health-initiatives/practicing-safety/Documents/Postnatal%20Depression%20Scale.pdf.

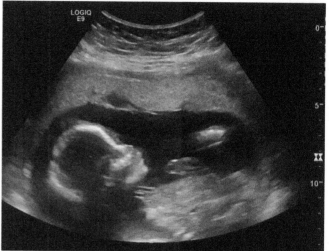
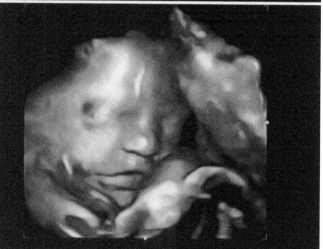

FIGURE 27.13 Ultrasound of a fetus. (Courtesy of Megan Pepper.)

Medical assistants should set up for this visit just as they would set up for a pelvic examination. You should also be aware of the patient's mood and body language. These can alert you to potential issues with postpartum depression. You should also have a list of provider-approved resources for the patient regarding postpartum depression or breast-feeding issues.

Special Tests and Procedures

Throughout the pregnancy, there are special tests and procedures that may done to assess the status of the pregnancy. In the next section we will explore some of the more common tests and procedures.

Ultrasound. Ultrasound exams are typically done once during the first trimester and then again between weeks 18 and 20 in order to assess fetal development and thereby confirm the age of the fetus and proper growth (Fig. 27.13). The sex of the baby can also be determined at that time. It is best if the patient has a full bladder for the ultrasound. The full bladder provides a great "window" for the sound waves to travel through, allowing for the best possible images. The patient should be instructed to drink two or three 8-ounce glasses of water 1 hour before the scheduled ultrasound.

Laboratory Testing. Between weeks 15 and 18 of pregnancy, the provider may suggest that the patient have a maternal blood screen in order to detect any risk of fetal and chromosomal disorders. This could be a triple screen test (also known as AFP Plus and multiple marker screening) or a quad screen test. Both tests screen for the following:

- Alpha-fetoprotein (AFP)
- Human chorionic gonadotropin (hCG)
- Estriol

The quad screen also tests for inhibin-A. These tests are used to evaluate if there is an increased chance of certain chromosomal conditions, such as Down syndrome. The alpha-fetoprotein evaluates the chances of neural tube defects, such as spina bifida.

If the patient is at risk for gestational diabetes, the provider will likely order a glucose challenge test. Risk factors for gestational diabetes include the following:

- A body mass index (BMI) before pregnancy of 30 or higher
- Mother, father, sibling, or child with diabetes

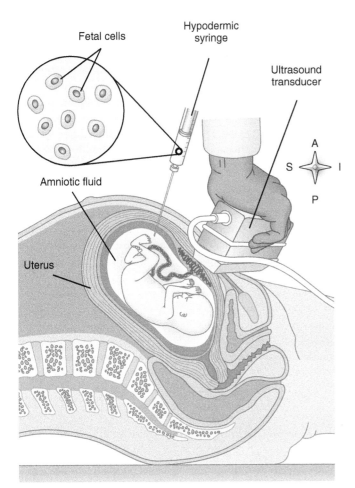

FIGURE 27.14 Amniocentesis. (From Shiland B: *Mastering healthcare terminology*, St. Louis, 2016, Elsevier.)

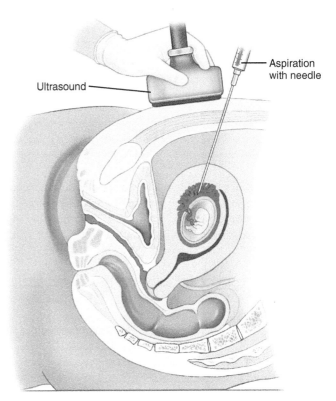

FIGURE 27.15 Chorionic villus sampling (CVS). (From Shiland B: *Medical terminology and anatomy for ICD-10 coding*, St. Louis, 2012, Mosby.)

For a glucose challenge test, the patient must drink a glucose solution. One hour later, a blood test will be done to measure the glucose level. A blood glucose level of 130 to 140 milligrams per deciliter (mg/dL) is considered normal. If the result is higher than that, a glucose tolerance test may be ordered. The glucose tolerance test involves having the patient fast overnight before coming in for a blood glucose reading. The patient will then drink another glucose solution and have her blood glucose level checked every hour for the next 3 hours. If two out of the three readings are higher than normal, the patient would be diagnosed with gestational diabetes.

Group B streptococcus is a common bacterium found in the intestines. It is usually harmless in adults, but in newborns it can cause group B strep disease. This is a serious illness for newborns. A group B streptococcus culture of the lower vagina can be performed between weeks 32 and 36. If the result is positive, the mother is treated with intravenous (IV) antibiotics to prevent fetal exposure during vaginal birth.

Amniocentesis. Amniocentesis involves needle aspiration of approximately 2 tablespoons of amniotic fluid after week 14 of pregnancy. The aim is to detect genetic and chromosomal abnormalities or inherited metabolic disorders (Fig. 27.14). Potential complications include the following:

- Miscarriage
- Fetal injury

- Infection
- Premature labor
- Maternal hemorrhage

Results take up to 2 weeks.

Chorionic Villus Sampling. *Chorionic villi* are tiny placental projections, the cells of which have the same genetic material found in fetal cells. Chorionic villus sampling (CVS) involves the removal of a small piece of the chorionic villi, either transvaginally or through a small incision in the abdomen (Fig. 27.15). Cellular screening at 8 to 12 weeks' gestation provides early detection of genetic or chromosomal disorders. Potential complications include the following:

- Accidental abortion
- Infection, bleeding
- Fetal limb deformities

Results are available within several days.

Recognizing Domestic Abuse

There are federal laws in place that require many insurance plans to provide coverage for certain preventive health services without any cost-sharing for the patient. Included in the preventive health services is screening and counseling for interpersonal and domestic violence. Working in healthcare gives us an opportunity to provide support and resources for someone who is dealing with domestic violence. As a medical assistant, you should be looking for possible signs of abuse, such as the following:

- Unusual or frequent bruises or fractures
- Attempts to hide the bruises with makeup or clothing
- Low self-esteem

- Being extremely apologetic and meek
- References to the partner's temper

If you notice any of these signs, you should make the provider aware of them. Even a patient who shows no signs of abuse should be asked if he or she feels safe in the home.

The healthcare facility should put together a list of resources for patients who may be victims of domestic abuse. Having a list of shelters, advocacy groups, emergency contact phone numbers, and transportation services to give to patients may provide them with the resources they need to make the decision to leave the abusive situation.

Abuse does not just happen in marriages or committed relationships; it can also occur in a dating relationship. We should be observing all patients for possible signs of abuse. Here are three national help lines with websites that patients could be referred to:

- National Domestic Violence Hotline: 800-799-SAFE (7233) or TTY 800-787-3224; https://www.thehotline.org
- National Dating Abuse Helpline: 866-331-9474 or TTY 866-331-8453; https://www.loveisrespect.org (live chat is available); text "loveis" to 77054
- Office on Women's Health: https://www.womenshealth.gov/relationships-and-safety/relationships-and-safety-resources

CLOSING COMMENTS

Patient Coaching

A woman who is planning a pregnancy or who has just found out that she is pregnant may benefit from some simple guidelines for healthy living:

- *Nutrition:* Before pregnancy, emphasize the need for folic acid to prevent neural tube defects. The woman can take a supplement or can eat dark green, leafy vegetables. Many women have iron-deficiency anemia, and eating foods high in iron (red meat, spinach, or enriched cereal) is helpful. A pregnant woman must meet the calcium needs of both herself and her fetus; therefore, she needs about 1000 mg of calcium a day. Most pregnant women should consume about 1800 calories per day during the first trimester, 2200 per day during the second trimester, and 2400 calories per day during the third trimester. Women of average weight should gain 25 to 35 pounds, but underweight women should gain 35 to 45 pounds for a healthy infant.
- *Alcohol:* Alcohol passes through the placenta to the fetus and can cause serious problems. No one knows how much is safe, so it is a good idea for pregnant women to avoid alcohol completely.
- *Smoking:* Smoking can cause premature birth and low-birth-weight full-term infants. Smoking is linked to an increased risk of otitis media, heart problems, and upper respiratory infection in infants, and also to sudden infant death syndrome (SIDS). Pregnant women should not smoke and should not be exposed to secondhand smoke.

- *Medicine:* All chemicals pass through the placenta; therefore, a pregnant woman should never take any medicine (even over-the-counter drugs) without the knowledge and approval of her provider. If the medical assistant is managing telephone screening, having a list of provider-approved medications next to the phone helps in answering patients' questions.
- *STI screening:* STI screening should be done before a woman becomes pregnant. Many STIs are asymptomatic in women but treatable. Infants are at risk for serious health problems if exposed to certain STIs in utero or during the birth process.

Legal and Ethical Issues

Many ethical and legal issues arise as a result of missed communication. Listen to what every patient reports, and write down any information that will assist the provider in treating the patient. The issue may appear to be an insignificant problem, but to the patient, it may be a major concern. Let the provider be the judge of whether the problem is relevant. As the patient's advocate and the provider's assistant, the medical assistant plays an important role in establishing good communication as a vital link in patient care.

Confidentiality is crucial in dealing with obstetric and gynecologic disorders. Only healthcare professionals directly involved in the patient's care should know the purpose of the patient's visit, diagnosis, or treatment. Maintaining patient confidentiality is not just an ethical responsibility, it is a legal requirement.

Patient-Centered Care

When providing patient-centered care while working in obstetrics and gynecology, a medical assistant should do the following:

- Behave in a professional manner at all times, because an OB/GYN visit can be an uncomfortable and embarrassing situation for the patient.
- During patient education sessions, make sure that the patient truly understands the content.
- Stay current with the new topics and technology related to obstetrics and gynecology.
- Treat all patients as you would want to be treated.

Professional Behaviors

When working in obstetrics and gynecology, it is important to remain nonjudgmental when dealing with different patient circumstances. Patients can present with situations that you have strong personal feelings about. It could be a young patient who is asking about birth control. It could be a patient who is being seen repeatedly for STIs. It could be a patient who is not following the prenatal care plan. In any of those situations, we must always do what is best for the patient and follow office policies and procedures. We cannot give our opinion on how we think the patient should behave. We do have a responsibility to inform the provider of any patient issues that are presented.

SUMMARY OF SCENARIO

Jill Snow has enjoyed her time in the OB/GYN department and has learned a lot from Peggy. She was able to observe several procedures and saw how Peggy prepped the patient and the exam room for those procedures. Peggy has been an amazing mentor for Jill. She has taken the time to explain the reasons for how each procedure is done. Peggy's knowledge and expertise in OB/GYN

along with her willingness to teach others has made Jill decide to pursue a position in this field after she graduates. Peggy's supervisor recognizes her talents in this area and has asked her to take over the practicum program for their department.

SUMMARY OF LEARNING OBJECTIVES

1. **Describe the anatomic location of the major organs of the female reproductive system.**

   There are two parts to the anatomy of the female reproductive system: parenchymal and stromal. Parenchymal or primary tissue produces sex cells for reproduction. The stromal or secondary tissues serve a supportive function for those sex cells.

   The ovaries, fallopian tubes, uterus, vagina, vulva, and breasts are the major organs of the female reproductive system.

2. **Explain the phases of the menstrual cycle, and discuss pregnancy and delivery.**

   The menstrual cycle is divided into follicular, luteal, and the menstrual phases. In the follicular phase, hormones are secreted to mature a graafian follicle in the ovary. The mature follicle secretes estrogen that stimulates the growth of the endometrium. This phase ends when the ovum is released. In the luteal phase, progesterone is secreted to prepare the endometrium for a possible pregnancy. If pregnancy does not occur, the menstrual phase begins and uterus sheds the lining.

   Pregnancy begins with the fertilization of an ovum by a sperm. During implantation, the zygote functions as an endocrine gland by secreting hCG. At the same time that the embryo is developing, extraembryonic membranes are forming to sustain the pregnancy.

3. **Discuss sexually transmitted infections, and describe the common cancers of the female reproductive system.**

   Sexually transmitted infections (STIs) are typically asymptomatic in men, although they can cause serious problems. Many pathogens cause STIs, but what they have in common is that all of them are most efficiently transmitted by *sexual contact*.

   Breast cancer is the second leading cause of cancer deaths in women. The cause of breast cancer is not known, but risk factors include being female, a family history of breast cancer, inherited genes, radiation exposure, obesity, menarche at a younger age, menopause at an older age, having your first child at an older age, having never been pregnant, postmenopausal hormone therapy, and drinking alcohol. Patients should be aware of any changes in the breast and report to the provider. Diagnostic procedures include a breast examination by the provider and possibly a mammogram, breast ultrasound, a biopsy, or a breast MRI.

   HPV is the most common cause of cervical cancer; other risk factors include many sexual partners, early sexual activity, having other

   STIs, a weak immune system, and smoking. A Pap test is the most common screening test for cervical cancer. Diagnostic tests include a punch biopsy, endocervical curettage, colposcopy, and loop electrosurgical excision procedure (LEEP).

   Ovarian cancer has often metastasized before the tumor is diagnosed. The causes of ovarian cancer are not known, but risk factors include age, inherited gene mutation, estrogen hormone replacement therapy, menarche at a young age, menopause at an older age, having never been pregnant, fertility treatment, smoking, use of an intrauterine device, and polycystic ovary syndrome. Diagnostic procedures include a pelvic examination ultrasound or CT scan, a CA-125 blood test (looks for certain proteins in the blood), and a biopsy.

4. **Discuss endometriosis, and list the common infections of the female reproductive system.**

   With endometriosis, functional endometrial tissue is located outside the uterus. It is commonly found attached to the ovaries, urinary bladder, fallopian tubes, uterosacral ligaments, intestines, or peritoneum. Common signs and symptoms of endometriosis include dysmenorrhea, dyspareunia, pain with bowel movements or urination, menorrhagia, menometrorrhagia, infertility, fatigue, diarrhea, constipation, bloating, and nausea.

   Common infections of the female reproductive system include candidiasis, cervicitis, and pelvic inflammatory disease (PID).

5. **Specify the signs, symptoms, and treatments for conditions related to menopause.**

   Menopause is the permanent ending of menstruation caused by the cessation of ovarian function. Perimenopause begins when hormone-related changes start to appear and lasts until the final menses. Some women experience few or no symptoms, whereas others have hot flashes, concentration problems, mood swings, irritability, migraines, vaginal dryness, urinary incontinence, dry skin, and sleep disorders. The provider may prescribe low-dose oral contraceptives or HRT, weight-bearing exercise, soy products or vitamin supplements, dietary changes, and medication to manage hot flashes, mood swings, vaginal dryness, and to prevent osteoporosis.

6. **Outline the medical assistant's role in a gynecologic examination (including breast, abdominal, and pelvic examinations), and demonstrate how to assist with a gynecologic examination.**

   The medical assistant prepares the patient for the examination, equips the room, makes sure supplies are available and properly prepared,

Continued

positions and drapes the patient as needed, assists with the Pap smear or any other procedures, and provides support and understanding for the patient. (See Procedure 27.1.)

7. Prepare for and assist with the collection of specimens, including those for a Pap test, a maturation index, and tests for various types of vaginal infections.

A specimen for a Pap test can be collected in two ways. In the direct smear method, the cells are collected from the cervix with a cervical spatula and placed directly on a microscope slide and a fixative is applied. For the liquid-based method, a plastic-fronded broom is used to collect the cells from the cervix and the broom is then rinsed in the specimen vial. The cells are prepared for viewing at the laboratory.

For a maturation index, cells are collected from the vaginal wall and are treated like a Pap test specimen.

For vaginal infections, a swab is used to collect a sample of the discharge. The sample is then placed on a microscope slide. If the provider suspects candidiasis, a drop of a 10% solution of potassium hydroxide (KOH) is added. If the provider is looking for trichomoniasis, a drop of saline is added. For chlamydia, the swab is sent to the lab for testing.

8. Compare and contrast current contraceptive methods.

Barrier contraceptive methods include the use of condoms, a diaphragm, a cervical cap, or a cervical sponge; all of these are relatively inexpensive and reversible, but they must be used with each instance of intercourse. Two general types of IUDs are available to inhibit fertilization and prevent the embryo from implanting in the uterine wall. Hormonal contraceptives include Depo-Provera injections, Implanon or Nexplanon implants, oral and patch contraceptives, and the vaginal ring, all of which are very effective but have side effects and contraindications. (See Table 27.3.)

9. Discuss postexamination duties. Also, describe three of the most common gynecologic procedures performed in the medical office:

The patient should be helped into the sitting position and assistance offered for dressing. The examination room should be cleaned following OSHA Standard Precautions.

Three of the most common gynecologic procedures performed in the medical office are as follows:

- Cryotherapy

Cryotherapy involves the application of freezing temperature to the cervix. This causes necrosis, and dead cells are replaced with healthy cells.

- Colposcopy with or without a biopsy

Colposcopy is the visual examination of the vagina and the cervical surfaces. A colposcope is used to locate and evaluate abnormal cells, detect cancer in the early stages, and monitor areas of the cervix where malignant lesions have been removed. If the provider identifies an area of concern, a biopsy will be obtained. Correct labeling of the biopsy specimen container is very important.

- Loop electrosurgical excision procedure (LEEP)

In a LEEP procedure, a wire loop with electrical current running through it is used to remove abnormal tissue from the cervix and the endocervical canal. This procedure can also be used to collect a biopsy sample.

10. Summarize the process of pregnancy and postpartum care, including the prenatal record, the first prenatal examination, return prenatal visits, and the postpartum visit.

At the first prenatal visit, a prenatal record will be created. It includes the following: demographic information, menstrual history, obstetric history, medical and surgical history, and family and social history.

The first prenatal examination includes an overall assessment of the woman's health status. A series of lab tests will be done, including a urinalysis and multiple blood tests. Return prenatal visits will follow a regular schedule and will include a check of vital signs, a test of hemoglobin, and a urinalysis.

The patient will return at about 6 weeks after delivery for a postpartum visit. A pelvic examination will be done to assess healing; if the patient is interested in contraception, the options will be discussed.

11. Describe the common specialized tests and procedures for obstetric patients.

An ultrasound is usually performed in the first trimester to assess fetal development, which is used to confirm the age of the fetus. The sex can also be determined at between 18 and 20 weeks' gestation.

A number of laboratory tests can be ordered for an obstetric patient, including a triple screen test or a quad screen test. These tests are used to determine if there is an increased chance of certain chromosomal conditions, such as Down syndrome. The alpha-fetoprotein evaluates the chances of neural tube defects, such as spina bifida. If the patient is at risk for gestational diabetes, a glucose challenge test may be ordered. For this test, the patient must drink a glucose solution. One hour later, a blood test will be done to measure the glucose level. A blood glucose level of 130 to 140 milligrams per deciliter (mg/dL) is considered normal. If the result is higher than that, a glucose tolerance test may be ordered.

An amniocentesis may be done after week 14 of pregnancy to detect genetic and chromosomal abnormalities or inherited metabolic disorders. Chorionic villus sampling is another test that can be done to detect genetic or chromosomal disorders.

12. Describe the possible signs of domestic abuse, and know how to report it.

Signs of abuse include the following: unusual or frequent bruises or fractures, attempts to hide the bruises with makeup or clothing, low self-esteem, being extremely apologetic and meek, and references to the partner's temper. Medical assistants should be aware of the laws in their state regarding the reporting of domestic abuse.

PROCEDURE 27.1 Set Up for and Assist the Provider With a Gynecologic Examination

Task: Prepare equipment for a gynecologic examination, and assist the provider by placing the patient in the appropriate positions.

EQUIPMENT and SUPPLIES

- Disposable examination gloves
- Fecal occult blood test kit
- Water soluble lubricant
- Vaginal speculum
- Slide and fixative or liquid preparation container
- Cervical spatula or plastic-fronded broom
- Laboratory requisition form
- Cotton-tipped applicator
- Patient gown
- Patient drape sheet
- Tray or Mayo stand

PROCEDURAL STEPS

1. Sanitize hands.
   PURPOSE: Hand sanitization is an important step for infection control.
2. Assemble equipment needed for the gynecologic examination. Place on a tray or Mayo stand in a logical order.
   PURPOSE: Having the equipment in a logical order allows you to assist the clinician in an efficient manner.
3. Change the table paper if needed.
   PURPOSE: Clean table paper prevents the transmission of microorganisms from one patient to another.
4. Greet the patient. Identify yourself. Verify the patient's identity with full name and date of birth. Explain the procedure to be performed in a manner that the patient understands. Answer any questions the patient may have.
   PURPOSE: It is important to identify the patient in two different ways to ensure that you have the correct patient. Explaining the procedure can make the patient feel more comfortable and reduces anxiety.

5. Ask if the patient needs to empty her bladder, and collect a urine specimen if needed.
   PURPOSE: An empty bladder will make the pelvic examination more comfortable for the patient.
6. Instruct the patient to undress and put on the gown.
   PURPOSE: The patient will need to be completely undressed for the examination.
7. Assist the patient onto the examination table; she should remain in the sitting position. Place the drape across her lap.
   PURPOSE: The first position used for the gynecologic examination is the sitting position. While the patient is in this position, the provider will visually inspect the breasts.
8. Assist the patient into the supine position, and provide a pillow to be placed under her head for comfort. Pull out the leg extension on the examination table.
   PURPOSE: For the rest of the breast examination and the abdominal examination, the patient will need to be in the supine position.
9. With the stirrups in place on the examination table, assist the patient into the lithotomy position. The leg extension should be pushed in.
   PURPOSE: The lithotomy position is used for the pelvic examination.
10. When the examination is complete, assist the patient into the sitting position. Instruct the patient that she can get dressed.
    PURPOSE: At the end of the examination, the patient can get dressed.
11. After the patient has dressed and left the exam room, clean the room and prepare specimens for transport to the laboratory.
    PURPOSE: By cleaning the examination room, you are preparing it for the next patient. It is the medical assistant's responsibility to properly prepare specimens for transport to the laboratory.

PROCEDURE 27.2 Coach a Patient on Breast Self-Examination

Tasks: Coach a patient to do a breast self-exam (BSE) while considering the patient's cultural beliefs and developmental life stage. Document teaching in the patient's health record.

EQUIPMENT and SUPPLIES

- Breast self-examination brochure (optional)
- Breast model
- Provider's order
- Patient's health record

Scenario: You are working with Dr. David Kahn. He has ordered you to show Bihn, an 18-year-old Vietnamese patient, how to do a breast self-exam. She has a strong family history of breast cancer. The patient is fluent in speaking and understanding English.

PROCEDURAL STEPS

1. Wash hands or use hand sanitizer.
   PURPOSE: Hand sanitization is an important step for infection control.
2. Read the provider's order. Assemble the equipment.
   PURPOSE: It is important to know the provider's order before starting the procedure.
3. Greet the patient. Identify yourself. Verify the patient's identify with full name and date of birth. Explain obsteture procedure to be performed in a manner that the patient understands. Answer any questions the patient may have.
   Continued

PROCEDURE 27.2 | **Coach a Patient on Breast Self-Examination**—*continued*

PURPOSE: It is important to identify the patient in two different ways to ensure that you have the correct patient. Explaining the procedure can make the patient feel more comfortable and reduces anxiety.

4. Provide privacy and independence during the session. Encourage the patient to ask questions and discuss her concerns.
   PURPOSE: It is important to adapt the coaching to the patient's developmental stage. Because she is 18, privacy and independence are important to her. Encouraging questions and discussions is also effective.

5. Ask the patient if she is familiar with breast self-examinations. Discuss with her thoughts on illness and what she does for alternative therapies. Explain the importance of doing a self-exam.
   PURPOSE: In the Vietnamese culture, illness is often explained by mystical beliefs. Asking the patient her thoughts might be helpful to the medical assistant during the coaching session.

6. Explain to the patient that she will need to undress and look at her breast in the mirror to identify any changes. She will need to check to see if they are the usual size, shape, and color and should look for any swelling, redness, rash, dimpling, puckering, or bulging of the skin. She will also need to see if the nipple position or appearance has changed. Also explain that she should check to see if any fluid is coming from the nipple by placing her thumb and index finger on the tissue by the nipple and pulling outward toward the end of the nipple (Fig. 1).
   PURPOSE: Changes in the appearance may indicate an issue.

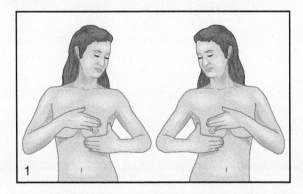

7. Instruct the patient that she needs to change positions and continue to check the appearance of the breast. She needs to place her hands on her hips and press down. This tightens the chest muscle under the breast. While in this position, she should turn from side to side to see the outer part of the breasts. Instruct her to clasp her hands behind her head or raise her arms and look at the outer part of the breast again (Fig. 2).
   PURPOSE: Sometimes changing the arm position may cause an abnormality to appear.

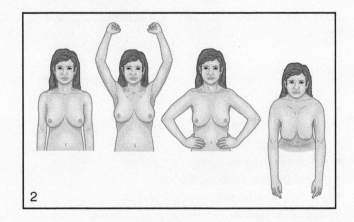

8. Instruct the patient to then bend forward and to roll her shoulders and elbows forward while tightening her chest muscles. While in this position, she can check for changes in the shape.
   PURPOSE: Sometimes changing the arm position may cause an abnormality to appear.

9. Instruct the patient to palpate the breast using one of the two techniques. Use the model as you explain each technique.
   a. *Lying down technique*: Instruct the patient to check the breast while lying down. She should tuck a small pillow under the side being checked; then she can tuck one arm under the head and with the other hand check the opposite breast (e.g., the right hand checks the left breast). Instruct the patient to use the first two or three finger pads. With fingers together, she can use a circular motion and a firm, smooth touch to check the entire breast. Explain that she should start at the top of the breast and move around it in a circular pattern. When the top of the breast is reached again, she can move in 1 inch toward the nipple and complete another circle around the breast. Instruct her to work in a systematic method to cover the entire breast from armpit to the cleavage. She can then place her fingers flat on the nipple and feel for any changes beneath the nipple. Explain that she will repeat this procedure on the other breast.
   b. *Shower technique*: Instruct the patient to place her right hand on her right hip. With a soapy left hand, she can feel for changes in the right axilla area. Describe how she can use two or three finger pads to press on the breast. She will be moving in an up-and-down pattern over the breast tissue. Remind her to make sure to cover the area from the bra line to the collar bone. Explain that she will repeat this procedure on the opposite side.
   PURPOSE: This position allows the patient to check the entire breast for changes, including under the arm and up to the collarbone.

10. Have the patient select a technique that she will use. Encourage the patient to demonstrate the technique on the breast model. Coach the patient on ways to improve the exam if needed.
    PURPOSE: It is important to have the patient demonstrate the teaching to check for accuracy of technique and correct understanding.

PROCEDURE 27.2 | **Coach a Patient on Breast Self-Examination**—*continued*

11. Answer any questions the patient may have. Provide the patient with a brochure to take home (optional).
    PURPOSE: It is important to answer any questions and, if possible, provide the patient with a brochure to take home.

12. Document the patient education in the patient health record. Include the provider's name, the order, what was taught to the patient, how the patient responded, how the patient did the demonstration, and any handouts provided.
    PURPOSE: It is important to document the patient education in the health record to show it was done.

07/19/20XX 1505 Per Dr. Kahn's order, instructed pt on the BSE. Instructed the patient on how to check for changes in the breast. Explained the lying and showering techniques. Pt opted for the showering technique. She demonstrated how to palpate the breast tissue correctly using a breast model. All her questions were answered. Provided her with the "BSE" brochure and encouraged her to perform it monthly. _____ Peggy St. John, CMA (AAMA)

28

PEDIATRICS

Allison Kwong, who has 2 years of experience as a certified medical assistant (CMA) through the American Association of Medical Assistants (AAMA), has accepted a new position with the pediatric department of the Walden-Martin Family Medical (WMFM) Clinic. Allison's primary responsibility will be to assist in the clinical area, but she also will have to rotate through the message screening center in the office. Office policy states that telephone screening employees should manage problems as much as possible. However, if patient callbacks are needed, they are to be referred to the provider on call that day by noon for morning calls and no later than 5 p.m. for afternoon calls. Although Allison has worked in the healthcare field for 2 years, she does not have much experience with pediatrics. She is glad that she has been assigned a mentor for the first few weeks.

While studying this chapter, think about the following questions:

- What are the expected growth and developmental patterns for children?
- When screening telephone calls from patients, which medical conditions should the screener call to the provider's attention right away and why?
- How does the Centers for Disease Control and Prevention (CDC) schedule of immunizations affect patient care?
- What is the importance of Vaccine Information Statements (VISs)?
- What information is needed when documenting immunizations?

LEARNING OBJECTIVES

1. Describe childhood growth patterns.
2. Discuss developmental patterns and therapeutic approaches for infants, toddlers, preschoolers, school-aged children, and adolescents.
3. Describe Erickson's developmental theory.
4. List and describe common pediatric diseases and disorders.
5. Do the following related to the pediatric patient examination:
   - Describe the medical assistant's role in pediatric procedures.
   - Cite reference ranges for pediatric vital signs.
   - Describe how the Apgar scoring system works.
   - List the recommendations of the American Academy of Pediatrics when it comes to the frequency of well-child visits.
- Discuss sick-child visits, as well as important questions for telephone screening of an older child who can communicate symptoms.
- Describe how to measure the circumference of an infant's head and how to obtain an infant's length and weight.
6. Assist with diagnostic procedures, including obtaining a urine sample.
7. Discuss the current immunization schedule for children from newborn to 18 years old. Also, detail guidelines for childhood immunization, and document immunizations.
8. Discuss the unique challenges and needs of the adolescent patient.
9. Specify child safety guidelines for injury prevention and management of suspected child abuse.

VOCABULARY

attenuated (uh TEN yoo ayt ed) Weakened or changed.

autonomy (aw TON uh mee) The ability to function independently.

epiphyseal plate (eh pi FIZ ee uhl) A thin layer of cartilage located at the ends of a long bone where new bone forms.

excoriation (ik skawr ee AY shun) Inflammation and irritation of the skin.

fontanelle (fon tah NEL) A space covered by thick membranes between the sutures of an infant's skull; called the baby's "soft spots"; there are both anterior and posterior fontanelles.

hydrocephaly (hye droh SEF ul lee) Enlargement of the cranium caused by abnormal accumulation of cerebrospinal fluid in the cerebral system.

lethargy (LETH er jee) The state of being drowsy and dull, listless and unenergetic.

microcephaly (mie kroh SEF ul lee) Abnormally small head associated with incomplete brain development.

nonorganic (nahn or GAN ik) Not having an organic or physiologic cause; a disorder that does not have a cause that can be found in the body.

serous (SEER uhs) A thin, watery, serum-like drainage.

suppurative (SUHP yuh ray tiv) Characterized by the formation or discharge of pus.

urticaria (ur ti KAYR ee ah) Hives.

Pediatrics is the medical specialty that deals with the development and care of children and with the treatment of childhood diseases. Pediatric patients range in age from newborn to puberty. Some practices continue to see the child until he or she graduates from high school. Subspecialties within pediatrics include surgery, cardiology, and psychiatry.

Approximately 50% of the patients in a pediatric office are there for well-baby or well-child visits. The roles of the provider and the medical office staff are to supervise and help maintain the health of these patients. The medical assistant can help by encouraging therapeutic communication among the patient, parents, caregivers, and medical staff. The trust that a child develops in these relationships and the consideration the family receives in the provider's office form the basis of good medical care.

Pediatric care actually starts before the child is born, with good prenatal care. The confidence and enthusiasm of the parents can have a significant impact on an infant's physical and emotional well-being.

NORMAL GROWTH AND DEVELOPMENT

The terms *growth* and *development* are often used together. They refer to the combination of changes a child goes through as he or she matures. *Growth* refers to measurable changes, such as height and weight. The first determinant of these physical characteristics is the genetics inherited from the parents; however, a child's growth can be influenced by many factors, including nutritional status, environmental factors, and the presence of disease. *Development* refers to the stages of physical, cognitive, and social growth. A provider looks at how the child is progressing in motor, mental, social, and language skills. A child's development is determined by a combination of prenatal, environmental, and caregiver factors. Each child has his or her own pattern of growth and development. Pediatric assessments are individualized for each child according to age, developmental level, health condition, family characteristics, and past experiences with healthcare professionals. National standards are used to help pinpoint irregularities in growth and development. The child's physical, intellectual, and social levels are compared with published national standards. This comparison indicates whether the child is at the appropriate stage of growth and development for his or her chronologic age.

Growth Patterns

Physical growth is one of the most visible changes in childhood. The average birth weight is 7 to 7½ pounds, and in 6 months, the baby's birth weight doubles. Growth then slows slightly over the next 6 months and even more over the next couple of years (Table 28.1). Between ages 2 and 3, most children slim down, so that by the time the third birthday arrives, the potbellied toddler has become the characteristic preschooler.

By age 4, the child usually has doubled the birth length. During this time, the legs are the fastest growing part; fatty connective tissue continues to increase slowly until approximately age 7. This same growth rate continues through the school-aged period (6 to 12 years), and as this period of development ends, the child usually is into a growth spurt that indicates impending puberty.

The growth spurt continues for approximately 2 years, and the child then reaches adolescence (ages 12 to 18 years). During this period, the adolescent gains almost half of his or her adult weight,

TABLE 28.1	Growth Patterns
6 months	Birth weight doubles
1 year	Birth weight triples, length increased by 50%
2 years	Gains 6 pounds in 1 year
3 years	Gains 3–5 pounds in 1 year and grows 2–2½ inches
3–6 years	Gains 3–5 pounds per year, grows 1½–2½ inches per year

and the skeleton and organs double in size. Weight increases in girls by 20 to 25 pounds and in boys by 15 to 20 pounds. Girls grow 5 to 6 inches, and boys grow 4 to 5 inches. As the growth spurt is completed, the teenager reaches sexual maturity. In girls, sexual maturity is signaled by the onset of the menstrual cycle; in boys, it is determined by the presence of sperm in the semen. The timing of sexual maturity in both genders varies greatly.

Skeletal growth is complete in girls between 15 and 16 years of age and in boys between ages 17 and 18. Skeletal growth is considered complete when the **epiphyseal plates** (growth plates) of the long bones of the extremities have completely fused.

Growth charts are used to compare the child's individual growth pattern with national standards. The CDC has developed growth charts that can track growth continuously through the age of 20. The growth charts are gender-specific. Length, weight, and head circumference are tracked on the birth to 36 months growth chart. Stature and weight are tracked on the 2 to 20 years growth chart. There are also CDC growth charts used to track body mass index (BMI) in infants and young adults 2 to 20 years of age, giving providers another weapon in the fight against childhood obesity. BMI is a means of assessing the relationship between height and weight. BMI conversion charts typically are available, or they are calculated automatically in electronic health record (EHR) programs. The actual formula to calculate BMI is as follows:

$$\text{BMI} = \frac{\text{Weight (kg)}}{\text{Height (m)}^2}$$

For adults, the BMI itself is used as the screening tool. In pediatrics, the BMI needs to be plotted on the gender-specific growth chart, and the growth chart percentile is the screening tool. The CDC has developed four weight status categories.

Centers for Disease Control and Prevention (CDC) Weight Status Categories

WEIGHT STATUS CATEGORY	PERCENTILE RANGE
Underweight	Less than the 5th percentile
Normal or healthy weight	5th percentile to less than the 85th percentile
Overweight	85th percentile to less than the 95th percentile
Obese	Equal to or greater than the 95th percentile

Source: https://www.cdc.gov/healthyweight/assessing/bmi/childrens_bmi/about_childrens _bmi.html. Accessed October 18, 2018.

Developmental Patterns

General patterns of child development occur rapidly during the first year of life as the infant progresses from reflex activities (e.g., grasping fingers and sucking) to learning to manipulate simple objects (e.g., pulling open drawers or throwing toys out of the crib). In addition to these motor skills, the child learns verbal patterns, progressing from cooing and crying for attention to speaking his or her first words.

By age 3, the child is showing increased **autonomy**. Now the child can walk, is toilet trained, sits at the table and eats with the family, can make simple sentences, understands the word *no*, and even imitates the parent by using verbal gestures that he or she has seen used. The child's vocabulary consists of up to 900 words.

Therapeutic Approaches for Infants (Newborn to 12 Months)

- Crying is normal; use distraction, but do not overstimulate.
- It is important to keep the infant close to the caregiver; either have the parent hold the infant or keep the parent in the child's line of vision.
- Involve the parent as much as possible, depending on the task and the parent's level of comfort.
- Place a familiar object near the infant, and keep frightening ones out of view.
- An infant's negative response to strangers usually develops at approximately 8 months; do not take the rejection personally.
- Do not restrain the infant any more than necessary, but be ready to use restraint at times (e.g., when giving an injection) to keep the infant safe.
- Encourage the caregiver to cuddle and hug the child after the procedure is complete.
- Unpleasant procedures are associated with other objects, so do not use play areas for treatment, and do not use a favorite toy or object during the procedure; offer it afterward for comfort.

During the preschool stage, the child becomes increasingly independent and initiates activities. Preschoolers have mastered many gross motor skills and are perfecting their fine motor development. Verbal communication has increased to full simple and even complex sentences but remains quite literal. For example, if you tell a preschool child that you are going to fly to visit Aunt Sue, the child thinks you are going to flap your arms and fly. Nonverbal communication skills are also being mastered. The vocabulary now includes more than 2000 words. During this period, children need to develop social skills, such as sharing and taking part in peer group activities.

Therapeutic Approaches for Toddlers and Preschoolers (2 to 6 Years)

- Toddlers and preschoolers often fear visits to the doctor; ignore temper tantrums and negative behavior.
- Praise the child as much as possible.
- Perform unpleasant procedures as quickly as possible; the fear of the procedure is worse than the actual discomfort.
- Allow the child to keep on as much clothing as possible for security and comfort.
- Use words familiar to the child, and do not use words the child could misinterpret. For example, "The test uses dye" (the child may think you mean "die"); "The doctor will put you to sleep so that it doesn't hurt" (the family dog may have been put to sleep).
- Explain a procedure as the child would sense it — that is, what it will look like, how it will smell, how it will feel, and so on.
- Allow the child to handle equipment when possible.
- Do not use the child's favorite doll or stuffed animal to demonstrate; the child may believe the toy feels pain.
- Explain procedures to the parents away from the child when possible; the child may misinterpret the information.

CRITICAL THINKING APPLICATION 28.1

Allison receives a call from the mother of a 6-month-old child. The woman is concerned that her child may not be reaching his developmental milestones. What type of information about the child's growth and development should Allison gather? If Allison is unable to answer the mother's questions, what should she do?

School-aged children have perfected fine motor skills and can paint, draw, and play an instrument. They enjoy team activities and are expanding their reading and writing skills. Their intellectual skills are developing, and social skills are going through refinement as a sense of self-achievement and self-worth is developed. During this time, the child learns and tests the rules for socializing outside the immediate family as an independent individual.

Therapeutic Approaches for School-Aged Children (7 to 11 Years)

- Allow choices when possible, such as which arm to use for an injection.
- A parent or caregiver should always be present during examinations.
- Remove only as much clothing as needed for the examination or procedure.
- Explain procedures in concrete terms; use pictures and diagrams when possible.
- Give the child time to ask questions.
- School-aged children often are curious, and they can be cooperative if they know what is expected of them.
- Address the conversation to the child; involve the child in decision making as much as possible.
- Provide privacy.

Adolescence, or the transition stage, is the time when the individual attempts to establish an adult identity. The teenager proceeds by trial and error, experimenting with adult roles and behavior patterns. Traditional values learned in childhood may be questioned, and peer relationships take on new importance. During this time, teenagers must develop the emotional maturity and motivation to make reasonable decisions. They look to family members for encouragement and guidance in making decisions that will help them develop self-confidence and to become patient, in addition to becoming less impulsive and self-centered.

Therapeutic Approaches for Adolescents (12 to 18 Years)

- Adolescents are self-conscious and strongly influenced by peers.
- Privacy is very important to them.
- Address how a procedure might affect the adolescent's appearance.
- Do not be judgmental; listen without condemning.
- Encourage the adolescent to verbalize his or her concerns and fears.
- The adolescent may regress to more childish behaviors when sick.
- Teenagers want to be treated as adults; they want to know what is being done and why.
- To promote an honest discussion about lifestyle issues, encourage the teenager to see the provider without the parent present.

CRITICAL THINKING APPLICATION   28.2

Based on what you have learned about therapeutic approaches for the pediatric patient, what would be the best way to deal with the following patient situations?

1. A crying 3-month-old being seen for a well-child visit
2. A 10-month-old with otitis media
3. A 2-year-old who needs the dressing changed on an infected wound
4. A 5-year-old scheduled for vision and hearing screening
5. An 8-year-old who needs a throat culture to rule out a strep infection
6. A 12-year-old who needs a penicillin injection in the vastus lateralis site
7. A 15-year-old girl who complains of abdominal pain and is accompanied by her mother

Developmental Theory

Psychologists have been researching and developing theories about human behavior since the beginning of the 20th century. Erik Erikson, a developmental psychologist, expanded on Sigmund Freud's work. Erikson's theory recognizes the cultural and social influences on individual development. His theory is based on stages of development that the individual must pass through and master. Each stage focuses on a developmental crisis, starting in infancy and ending in old age. According to Erikson, children must master the following stages:

- *Trust versus mistrust:* Infants learn to rely on caregivers; mistrust occurs if needs are not met.

- *Autonomy versus shame and doubt:* Toddlers learn language skills and gain independence; they may feel shame and doubt if they cannot meet parental expectations or are overprotected.
- *Initiative versus guilt:* Preschoolers actively seek out new experiences; children become hesitant if restrictions or reprimands make them feel guilty or afraid to try more challenging skills.
- *Industry versus inferiority:* School-aged children enjoy finishing projects and receiving recognition; they develop feelings of inferiority if they are not accepted by peers or if they cannot please their parents.
- *Identity versus role confusion:* Adolescents face many physical and hormonal changes in this stage. Teenagers work at figuring out who they are and where they fit; they are seeking a direction for their lives. If they are unable to establish an identity and sense of direction, they become role-confused.

When working in pediatrics, it can be helpful to understand Erikson's stages and how you can help someone master those stages.

PEDIATRIC DISEASES AND DISORDERS

The disease process in pediatric patients poses special problems, because children are constantly changing both physically and functionally. As a child grows and develops, the immune system matures, and with the aid of routine prophylactic immunizations, the child acquires long-term protection against certain infectious diseases.

Colic

Colic usually is seen in the newborn period or in early infancy. The problem is intermittent. The classic situation is an infant between 2 weeks and 4 months of age who has crying episodes that occur at least three times a week for longer than 3 hours a day and lasting 3 weeks. During an attack, the infant draws up the legs, clenches the fists, and cries inconsolably. The abdominal distress of colic usually occurs in the late afternoon and evening. Many theories have been suggested for why infants have colic, but none has been proven correct. If the baby is fed infant formula, providers recommend switching formulas to a non–cow's milk type, because this may help relieve the infant's discomfort. Treatment consists of determining the cause; however, the child frequently outgrows the condition before the causative agent can be identified. Drugs have not been found to be helpful. Parents need reassurance that they are not responsible for the child's discomfort, and they may find counseling and assistance in developing coping techniques helpful.

Diarrhea

Diarrhea can be caused by a variety of microorganisms, including bacteria, viruses, and parasites. However, children sometimes can have diarrhea without having an infection. It could be caused by food allergies or by certain medications, such as antibiotics. Diarrhea is diagnosed when the child has two or more watery or apparently abnormal stools within 24 hours. The child may not show other signs of illness or may have nausea, vomiting, stomach aches, headache, or fever. If the diarrhea continues for longer than 2 days, medical intervention is needed. Prolonged diarrhea can cause dehydration and an electrolyte imbalance because of excessive fluid loss. In addition, diarrhea can cause diaper rash and **excoriation**, which can be very painful.

Pediatric diarrhea needs to be followed closely. In the case of bloody stools, laboratory analysis should be ordered to determine the cause. If the patient is an infant or small child, a follow-up telephone call should be made after 12 hours and then daily until the diarrhea has stopped. Parents should know the indications of dehydration:

- Lack of tears when crying
- **Lethargy**
- Fewer wet diapers or decreased urination
- Dry mouth and lips
- Weight loss

The provider may recommend the use of oral rehydration therapy, such as Pedialyte or Enfalyte; small amounts (approximately 2 tablespoons) are offered at a time (i.e., every 15 minutes) to prevent vomiting. Soft drinks, juices, sports drinks, and tea should be avoided because they lack electrolytes and may lead to even more diarrhea. Parents should be informed that the child's diarrhea may not stop when the child is given oral rehydration therapy, but the fluids prevent the child from becoming dehydrated. It is important to continue to feed the child because lack of food can damage the villi in the small intestine. If breast-fed, the baby should continue to nurse because breast milk has been shown to protect the gastrointestinal lining.

The banana, rice, applesauce, and toast (BRAT) diet has been the traditional approach to treat children with diarrhea, but it is no longer recommended because there is no evidence that it is useful. In fact, the poor protein content of the BRAT diet may contribute to continued diarrhea and poor nutrition. Providers now recommend that children resume their prediarrhea diet as soon as possible so that they continue to eat something they prefer while the intestine heals. Probiotics found in certain yogurt products can also help to stabilize the child while the intestinal tract gets back to normal. The child should not be given over-the-counter (OTC) antidiarrheal medications, such as Pepto-Bismol, Kaopectate, Imodium, or Lomotil, because these can cause serious side effects, including decreased motility of the bowel, respiratory depression, and drowsiness. The provider may prescribe antibiotics if stool cultures test positive for pathogens. Children with severe dehydration require hospitalization and intravenous (IV) hydration to replace electrolytes and fluids.

Failure to Thrive

Failure to thrive refers to children whose current weight or rate of weight gain is much lower than that of other children of similar age and gender. It is a symptom more than a disease. An infant or a young child whose weight is consistently below the 3rd percentile on standardized growth charts, or who is 20% below the ideal body weight for length, may be diagnosed with failure to thrive. Physical, mental, and social skills also are delayed in these children. This could include failure to roll over, smile, coo, stand, or walk at age-appropriate developmental levels. Failure to thrive can be caused by a physiologic factor (e.g., malabsorption disease or cleft palate), or it may be related to a problem with the parent-child relationship. The provider needs an accurately recorded history of the child's birth weight and subsequent length, weight, and head circumference measurements. A comprehensive family history is important to rule out genetic growth abnormalities or a history of malabsorption problems, such as cystic fibrosis or celiac disease.

Children with failure to thrive need more calories than usual—approximately 150% of their normal calorie load—to catch up to their target weight. Both medical and social factors are evaluated in the treatment of children with this problem. Experts believe that infants may suffer from this problem if they are being neglected; however, low weight gains also are possible with extremely attentive and cautious parents. The family must be considered as a whole to treat **nonorganic** causes effectively. Treatment may include the use of support groups and parental counseling.

Obesity

Just as with adult weight patterns, children are assessed according to their BMI. A child's level of body fat varies as the child grows; for example, children normally slim down as they reach school age, and very often their weight increases as they mature from adolescence to adulthood. In addition, body fat levels vary between boys and girls as they reach puberty. Providers use growth charts that plot the child's BMI-for-age to determine whether the child's weight, in comparison with height, is within healthy limits. Obesity now affects nearly 20% of all children and adolescents in the United States. Children who are overweight or obese as preschoolers are five times as likely as normal-weight children to be overweight or obese as adults. Studies have shown that a child who is obese between the ages of 10 and 13 has an 80% chance of becoming an obese adult.

The reasons for childhood obesity vary; they include a family history of obesity, inactivity, high-calorie diets, and stress. In rare cases, childhood obesity may be caused by metabolic or endocrine disorders. Overweight and obese children are at greater risk of developing serious health conditions, including asthma, diabetes mellitus type 2, sleep apnea, and hypercholesterolemia, which increases the risk of cardiovascular disease and hypertension. The psychosocial impact of obesity can be overwhelming for many children because isolation, loneliness, and lack of self-esteem are common. The provider can recommend a comprehensive diet and exercise program that emphasizes healthy living. The medical assistant can help by providing educational materials, encouragement for the child and parents, and referral to community education and support programs.

Otitis Media

Infection or inflammation of the middle ear usually is a side effect of a cold or other upper respiratory tract disorder, but it also can be

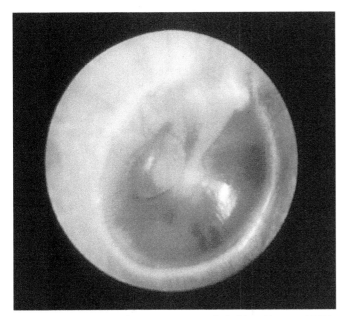

FIGURE 28.1 Serous otitis media. (From Swartz MH: *Textbook of physical diagnosis*, ed 5, Philadelphia, 2006, Saunders.)

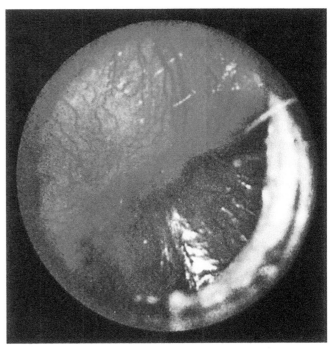

FIGURE 28.2 Suppurative otitis media. (Courtesy Dr. Richard A. Buckinham and Dr. George E. Shambaugh, Jr.)

caused by allergies. Otitis media usually occurs in children younger than 3 years of age. Signs include inflammation of the middle ear, with fluid building up behind the tympanic membrane. The child may cry persistently, tug at the ear, have a fever, be irritable, and have diminished hearing in the affected ear. These symptoms sometimes may be accompanied by diarrhea, nausea, and vomiting.

Otitis media is classified as either **serous** (Fig. 28.1) or **suppurative** (Fig. 28.2), depending on the fluid in the middle ear. In Fig. 28.2, pus is in the middle ear and shows up as white in the image. Because otitis media may be caused by bacteria or a virus, determining the most appropriate treatment can be difficult.

In 2013 the American Academy of Pediatrics (AAP) and the American Academy of Family Physicians (AAFP) released an updated clinical practice guideline for the diagnosis and management of otitis media in children age 6 months to 12 years. Antibiotics (typically amoxicillin or azithromycin [Zithromax]) should be prescribed for children 6 months or older who have severe signs and symptoms. Antibiotics can also be prescribed for patients younger than 24 months of age who are experiencing nonsevere bilateral infections. However, in children older than 6 months with nonsevere symptoms, observation and a follow-up within 48 to 72 hours before initiating antibiotics may be offered to assess patient improvement. If no improvement is noticed or symptoms have worsened, antibiotic therapy should be initiated. In all cases, if the child has not improved in 48 to 72 hours, the current antibiotic should be switched. Because antibiotics do not provide immediate relief from symptoms, children can be given oral acetaminophen or ibuprofen for pain relief.

If fluid in the middle ear persists for longer than 3 months or if the child experiences hearing loss, the provider may recommend a *myringotomy*; in this operation, a small incision is made in the tympanic membrane and a tube is inserted to drain the fluid and balance the pressure between the outer and middle ear. The tube typically stays in the eardrum for 6 to 12 months and falls out as the child grows.

Common Childhood Diseases

- Conjunctivitis—also called *pinkeye*, is a common infection in children and is highly contagious, especially in day care centers and schools. It can be caused by a bacterial or viral infection that produces white or yellowish pus, which may cause the eyelids to stick shut in the morning.

- Fifths disease—also called *erythema infectiosum, parvovirus infection,* or *slapped cheek disease,* is an infection caused by parvovirus B19. Outbreaks are most common in the winter and spring. Symptoms begin with a mild fever and general malaise. After a few days, the cheeks take on a flushed appearance, making the face look as if it has been slapped. A lacy rash also may be seen on the trunk, arms, and legs, but not all those infected develop the rash.

- Hand-foot-and-mouth disease—caused by the coxsackievirus, which is transmitted by direct contact with nose and throat drainage, saliva, or the stool of an infected individual. The disease is seen most often in day care settings, where children can easily come in contact with infected bodily secretions. Symptoms include a combination of fever; sore throat; painful red blisters on the tongue, mouth, palms, and soles; headache; anorexia; and irritability (Fig. 28.3).

- Reye syndrome—the cause of Reye syndrome is unknown, but the disorder has been linked to the use of aspirin during a viral illness. Reye syndrome is an acute and sometimes fatal illness characterized by fatty invasion of the inner organs, especially the liver, and swelling of the brain. It most often is seen in children from infancy through puberty (age 16). Prevention is the best treatment, which means children up to age 14 should never be given aspirin unless prescribed by a provider for a chronic condition such as juvenile rheumatoid arthritis.

Autism Spectrum Disorder

- Children diagnosed with autism spectrum disorder (ASD) show a wide range of neurologic and developmental behaviors. The most severe form is autism, or classical ASD; a milder form may present as Asperger syndrome; and sometimes a child cannot be categorized into a specific diagnosis and so is labeled as a pervasive developmental disorder (PDD).
- ASD occurs in all ethnic and socioeconomic groups and affects every age group.
- The Centers for Disease Control and Prevention (CDC) estimate the prevalence of ASD to be 1 in 68; it is almost five times more common among boys (1 in 42) than among girls (1 in 189).
- Children with autism have impaired social interaction, do not respond to their name, avoid eye contact, and show limited interest in their surroundings. They rarely communicate with others and display repetitive movements or mannerisms, such as rocking or twirling. They may also have self-abusive behaviors, such as biting and head banging. Many children with autism have a very high pain tolerance but are extremely sensitive to noise, touch, or other sensory stimulation.
- The cause of this developmental disorder is unknown, but researchers believe it is due to a combination of genetic errors and environmental factors, perhaps a problem with fetal brain development. Although many parents are concerned about a connection with vaccines, extensive studies have failed to show a link between the two.
- The American Academy of Pediatrics (AAP) recommends a general developmental screening at every well-child visit and a developmental screening using a standardized tool at 9, 18, and 30 months, or whenever a caregiver expresses concern. In addition, autism-specific screening is recommended for all children at the 18- and 24-month visits.
- Treatment involves coordinated educational and behavioral interventions to help the child develop social and language skills. Medications may be prescribed to treat depression, anxiety, and obsessive-compulsive behaviors.

From https://www.aap.org/en-us/about-the-aap/Committees-Councils-Sections/Council-on-Children-with-Disabilities/Pages/Autism.aspx. Accessed October 21, 2018.

ROLE OF THE MEDICAL ASSISTANT IN PEDIATRIC PROCEDURES

The medical assistant is responsible for the following:
- Assisting the provider with examinations
- Updating patient histories
- Performing ordered screening tests (e.g., vision, hearing, urinalysis, and hemoglobin checks)
- Measuring and weighing children as needed
- Administering immunizations
- Providing patient and caregiver support

A medical assistant must develop a relationship with the pediatric patient that encourages cooperation and compliance with tests and treatment plans.

Interacting with children requires special techniques, depending on the child's age. A calm, unhurried manner is essential to gaining cooperation. The tone of voice should be gentle but confident. Using

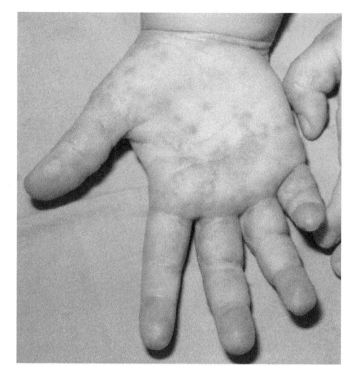

FIGURE 28.3 Vesicular palm lesions in hand-foot-and-mouth disease. (From Schachner LA, Hansen RC: *Pediatric dermatology*, ed 4, St. Louis, 2011, Mosby.)

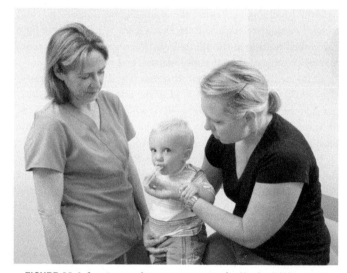

FIGURE 28.4 Sometimes a pediatric patient is more comfortable when held by a parent.

a firm, direct approach about expected behavior is important to gain the cooperation of older children. Offer reasonable choices when possible, such as "Would you like your shot in your left leg or your right leg?" not "Are you ready for your shot now?" Offering sincere praise for the child during the examination or procedures helps ease anxiety and builds self-esteem. If the child is having an unusually difficult time, try to discover the reason. If he or she had a bad medical experience in the past, the child may be afraid of what might happen. Each step should be explained in a language the child (and parent) can understand. Children younger than age 2 feel better when the parent holds them or remains very close (Fig. 28.4). Preschool children enjoy playing, so making a game out of the situation is helpful (Fig. 28.5). Whatever the child's age, the medical

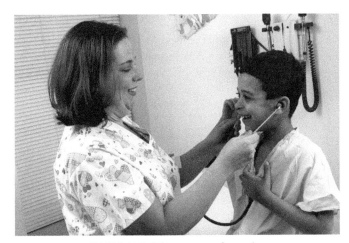

FIGURE 28.5 *Making a game out of a procedure.*

TABLE 28.2	Reference Ranges for Pediatric Vital Signs	
VITAL SIGN	**REFERENCE RANGE**	
Temperature		
• Oral	98.6°F (37°C)	
• Tympanic	99.6°F (37.6°C)	
• Axillary	97.6°F (36.4°C)	
Pulse		
• Newborn	100–180 beats per minute	
• 3 mo–2 yr	80–150 beats per minute	
• 2–10 yr	65–130 beats per minute	
Respirations		
• Newborn	• 30–50 breaths per minute	
• 1–3 yr	• 25–30 breaths per minute	
• 4–6 yr	• 23–25 breaths per minute	
• 7+ yr	• 16–20 breaths per minute	
Blood pressure		
• Newborn	• Systolic 90 mm Hg; diastolic 70 mm Hg	
• 1–5 yr	• Systolic 100 mm Hg; diastolic 70 mm Hg	
• 6–12 yr	• Systolic 120 mm Hg; diastolic 84 mm Hg	
• 13+ yr	• Systolic, 100 mm Hg + age; diastolic, 30–40 mm Hg less	

assistant should be sensitive to his or her individual needs and should adapt the examination and procedures as much as possible to meet those needs.

The sequence of the provider's examination varies and frequently is based on the child's cooperation. The provider will probably leave procedures and tests that are likely to cause the most objections until the end of the appointment. The provider is constantly evaluating the child's growth and development. A child's alertness and responses tell the provider a considerable amount. With infants and young children of preschool age, the parent is closely questioned about the child's eating, sleeping, and elimination habits. A school-aged child is usually a little more cooperative during an examination and can answer most questions without parental assistance. Adolescent patients should be given the option of not having parents present during an examination. This may permit teenagers to respond more honestly about lifestyle factors, and it also protects their privacy.

Assisting With the Examination

The provider will have a designated set of procedures that the medical assistant completes before the provider sees the child. Vital signs are measured first (Table 28.2). Depending on the child's age and level of cooperation, the temperature may be obtained by the axillary, oral, rectal, tympanic, or temporal artery method. The rectal and temporal artery methods are considered most accurate in infants; however, the temporal artery method is easiest, quickest, and less invasive. It is important to remember that the younger the child, the more immature the ability to regulate body heat. Therefore, the temperature of an infant may fluctuate easily and rapidly. The child's pulse rate is affected similarly to that of an adult; it can increase as a result of activity, anxiety, illness, and environmental temperature. If the child is younger than age 2, the pulse is measured apically by placing the stethoscope on the left side of the chest medial to the nipple. Always count the beats for 1 full minute for accuracy.

An alternative method of obtaining the pulse of a very young child is to use the brachial artery in the upper arm. After age 2, the child's pulse may be taken at the radial pulse site. Anticipate a pulse rate higher than that of an adult; the younger the child, the faster the pulse. The respiratory rate is easily obtained in a child because the chest can be readily observed. Expect the rate to be increased

according to the child's age (the younger the child, the faster the normal respiratory rate) and health. The ratio of 4 pulse beats to 1 respiration should remain constant in a healthy child.

It is recommended that blood pressure be checked for children aged 3 years or older. The cuff must be the appropriate width to obtain an accurate reading, and the bell of the stethoscope must be small enough to seal over the site. It is best to use a pediatric stethoscope with a pediatric bell when obtaining an infant's pressure. Blood pressure readings in a young child are lower than those in an adult (see Table 28.2).

To prevent a small child or infant from rolling the head from side to side during the provider's examination, stand at the head of the table and support the child's head between your hands, taking care not to press on the ears or on the anterior or posterior **fontanelles**. An infant need not be draped, but privacy is important to an older child. Sincere respect and friendly conversation at the child's level accomplish a great deal. Always be patient with children. Make sure they understand what is expected. Always involve the parents or caregivers as much as possible.

Accurately judging the level of pain a young patient is experiencing can be difficult. If the child is able to communicate, the Wong-Baker FACES Pain Scale could be used, which shows simple drawings of faces that express varying levels of pain on a 0-to-10 scale (Fig. 28.6).

An infant's first physical assessment comes at the time of delivery, when the provider assesses the newborn's ability to thrive outside the uterus. The Apgar score is a system for evaluating the infant's physical condition at 1 and 5 minutes after birth (Table 28.3). Developed by pediatrician Virginia Apgar, the scoring system evaluates the following: *a*ppearance (color), *p*ulse (heart rate), *g*rimace (reflex; response to stimuli), *a*ctivity (muscle tone), and *r*espiration (breathing). These parameters are each rated 0, 1, or 2. The maximum total score is 10. Infants with low scores require immediate medical attention.

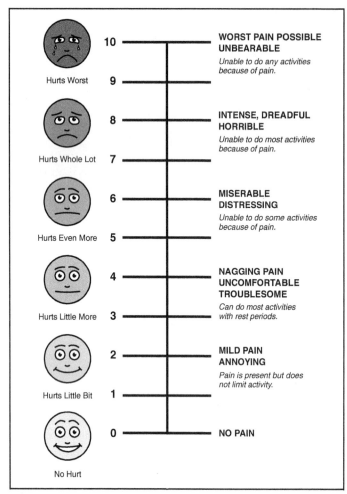

FIGURE 28.6 Wong-Baker FACES pain scale.

Well-Child Visits

The frequency of well-child visits varies with the provider and the community. The American Academy of Pediatrics recommends the following pattern:

- 2 to 5 days
- 1 month
- 2 months
- 4 months
- 6 months
- 9 months
- 12 months
- 15 months
- 18 months
- 2 years
- Annually

These visits focus on maintaining the child's health through basic system examinations, immunizations, and updating of the child's medical history record.

The decision on whether the child is to be seen alone or with the parent depends on the provider and the child's age. Often the child looks to the parent for approval before answering or performing a skill; for this reason, the provider may want to assess the child alone. If this is the case, explain to the parent that the provider wants to evaluate the child's independent abilities and that as soon as testing is complete, the provider will explain the results of the tests.

The medical history is an essential guide to the pediatric examination. With an infant, the provider depends on the caregiver for the history, but as the child gets older, some history may be obtained from the child and clarified or amplified by the parent. When asking about things like lead paint, the child may not understand the question and the parent may have to answer. Close observation also gives the provider considerable information.

Lead Paint Exposure

Children are especially vulnerable to lead levels in their environment. High blood lead levels can result in serious brain injury, including seizures, coma, and death. Lower levels can cause learning problems, stunted growth, and behavior disorders. The most common causes of lead exposure are lead-based paint in homes and on imported toys, and chronic exposure to lead-contaminated dust and water. The Centers for Disease Control and Prevention (CDC) recommend a screening blood test for lead levels in all children between 1 and 2 years of age. For children who show elevated levels, follow-up should include home and school environmental testing to determine the cause of lead exposure.

TABLE 28.3	Apgar Scoring System[a]		
	ASSIGNED SCORE		
CLINICAL SIGN	**0**	**1**	**2**
Heart rate	Absent	<100 beats per minute	>100 beats per minute
Respiratory effort	Absent	Slow and irregular	Good and crying
Muscle tone	Limp	Some flexion of the arms and legs	Active movement
Reflex irritability	No response	Grimace	Coughing, sneezing, or vigorous cry
Color	Blue and pale	Body pink and extremities blue	Pink all over

[a]Readings are taken by the provider at 1 minute and 5 minutes after birth. At *1 minute:* If the score is 7 or lower, some nervous system problems are suspected. If the score is below 4, resuscitation usually is necessary. At *5 minutes:* If the score is at least 8, the child probably is reacting normally.

Sick-Child Visits

Sick-child visits occur whenever needed, usually on short notice. For this reason, most pediatric offices keep open appointments in the schedule to accommodate calls for sick-child visits. The length and frequency of this type of visit depends entirely on the child and the illness. The medical assistant is frequently the first point of contact for a sick child and the child's caregiver.

Determining whether the child should be seen immediately or if the problem can wait for an opening in the schedule is crucial to pediatric care. The medical assistant should follow established office policies, but when in doubt about the seriousness of the problem, he or she should ask the office manager or provider for advice. Usually the provider prefers to see the child rather than delay seeing a patient with a potentially serious condition. The child should be seen right away if the child is young (under 2 years old) and the parent reports any of the following:

- Frequent cycles of crying, lethargy, or vomiting that has persisted longer than 24 hours
- Diarrhea (more than six stools in the past 12 hours)
- Fever of 101°F (38.3°C) or higher
- The child cannot verbalize associated pain or problems

Table 28.4 summarizes some important questions for telephone screening of an older child who can communicate symptoms. It is important to focus on the *onset* (when symptoms first started), *frequency* (whether symptoms are constant or cycle through recurrences), and *duration* (how long the episodes last) of the problem, in addition to attempted treatments and their effectiveness. As with any other patient,

all telephone communication should be documented to record the reason for the call; the information gathered; the action taken, including whether the provider was consulted; any orders given; and whether and when an appointment was scheduled.

Measurements

Examination of the child during routine well-child care includes measurement of the circumference of the infant's head to determine normal growth and development (see Procedure 28.1, p. 723). The size of the child's head reflects the growth of the brain. Brain growth is 50% complete by 1 year of age, 75% by age 3, and 90% by age 6. Routine head measurement is recommended in children until 36 months of age and in older children whose head size is not within norms. If the circumference of the head deviates greatly from normal measurements, **hydrocephaly** or **microcephaly** may be suspected. It is important to discover any congenital problem as early as possible so that appropriate treatment can be started.

Along with the head circumference, the medical assistant should record the child's length (or height) and weight (Procedure 28.2 on p. 724) on growth charts so that the provider can compare the child's measurement statistics with national standards. Growth charts consist of a series of percentile curves that illustrate the distribution of selected body measurements.

The CDC has gender-specific growth charts for the following:
- Birth to 36 months (Figs. 28.7 and 28.8)
  - Length for age
  - Weight for age

TABLE 28.4	Important Questions for Telephone Screening of Pediatric Problems
COMPLAINT	**SCREENING QUESTIONS**
Pain	• What are the onset, frequency, and duration of the pain? • On a scale of 1 to 10, how severe is the pain? • Where is the exact location? • Was any accident involved (include details)? • Has the pain gotten worse over time? • Has the pain interfered with sleep? • Is there associated fever, vomiting, diarrhea, or rash?
Gastrointestinal	• What are the onset, duration, and frequency of the symptoms? Has the child been vomiting longer than 24 hours without improvement? • Is the child drinking and/or eating? • Is the child dehydrated (e.g., dry mouth, no urination in 8–10 hours, listless)? • If the child has diarrhea, have there been more than five or six watery stools in 12 hours? • Does the child have other symptoms (e.g., vomiting, fever of 101°F [38.3°C], rapid breathing)?
Respiratory	• What are the onset, duration, and frequency of the symptoms? • How would you describe the child's breathing? • Has the child been diagnosed with a breathing disorder? • Is a prescribed treatment being used? • Are any other signs or symptoms present (e.g., severe headache, stiff neck, fever, cough)? • If the child is coughing, what does it sound like? • Are there signs of a sore throat or earache?

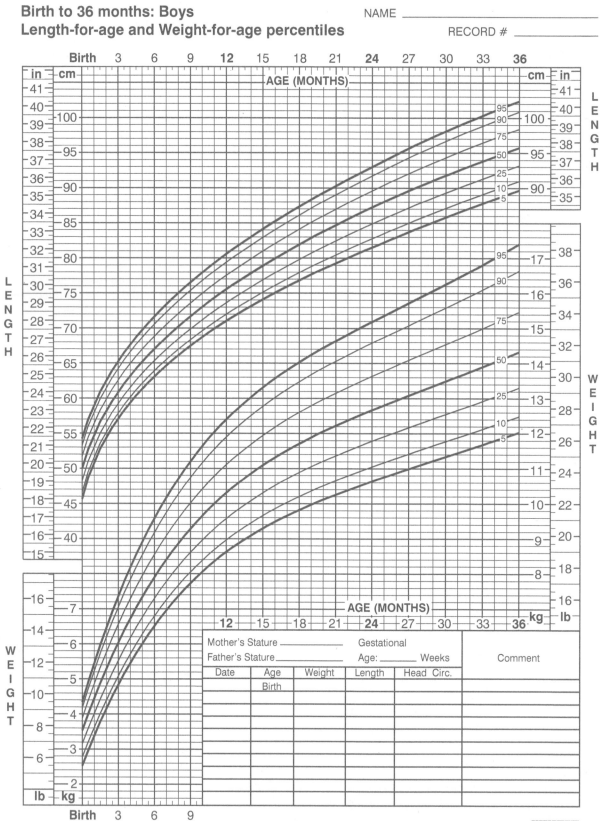

Birth to 36 months: Boys
Length-for-age and Weight-for-age percentiles

NAME _____

RECORD # _____

Published May 30, 2000 (modified 4/20/01).
SOURCE: Developed by the National Center for Health Statistics in collaboration with
the National Center for Chronic Disease Prevention and Health Promotion (2000).
http://www.cdc.gov/growthcharts

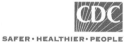

FIGURE 28.7 Growth chart: boys (birth to 36 months).

2 to 20 years: Girls
Stature-for-age and Weight-for-age percentiles

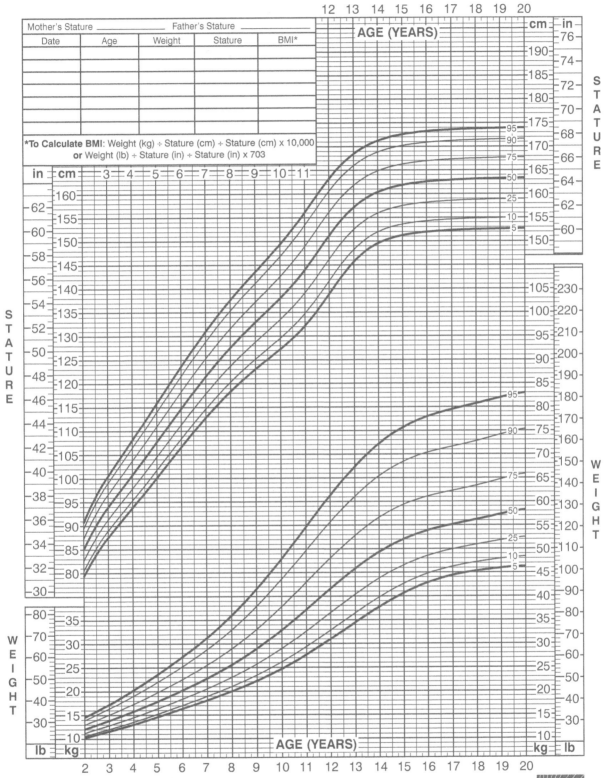

FIGURE 28.8 Growth chart: girls (2 to 20 years).

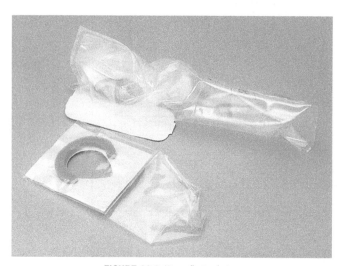

FIGURE 28.9 Urine collection devices.

- Head circumference for age
- Weight for length
- 2 to 20 years
  - Stature for age
  - Weight for age
  - BMI for age

There are 20 CDC charts (10 for boys and 10 for girls). As mentioned previously, the BMI is the recommended method of determining whether children or adults are overweight or obese. The BMI growth charts can be used beginning at 2 years of age, when height can be measured accurately.

EHRs may automatically plot the measurements on the appropriate growth chart and calculate the percentile.

Assisting With Diagnostic Procedures
Obtaining a Urine Sample

The easiest way to obtain a urine sample from a child who is toilet trained is to give the parent the container and instructions ahead of time. Then, when the child arrives at the office for the examination, the sample is available to be tested. If the sample is needed while the child is at the office, consult with the parent for the best method to use. If the child is not toilet trained, a pediatric urine collection device can be put on him or her to collect the sample (Fig. 28.9). This device is placed as soon as the child is checked in to increase the chance of obtaining the needed sample before the child leaves. Once the device is in place, the child can be diapered to help hold it properly. Make sure the adhesive sticks tightly so that the specimen collects in the device when the child urinates.

In some cases, the child may need to be catheterized to obtain the specimen. Pediatric catheterization kits contain all the supplies needed for this procedure. When preparing the kit, always remember that this is a sterile procedure. The provider usually asks the parent to help with the infant while the medical assistant labels and prepares the specimen for the laboratory. In some practices, a registered nurse or a specially trained medical assistant may perform a catheterization procedure to collect a pediatric urine sample.

Assisting With Treatments
Immunizations

Over the years, immunization has helped dramatically reduce potentially lethal childhood infections. Fig. 28.10 shows the 2018 immunization schedule from the CDC for children 0 through 18 years of age. All of the immunization schedules can be found at the CDC's website at http://www.cdc.gov/vaccines/schedules/downloads/child/0-18yrs-child-combined-schedule.pdf.

The schedules are updated periodically as new vaccines become available or research indicates a better method for giving the vaccine. The CDC recommends immunization against infectious diseases for all children, except those for whom a particular vaccination would pose a risk. However, each state develops its own immunization program and methods of enforcement. Parents/guardians do have the right to refuse immunizations.

The vaccines consist of a suspension of **attenuated** organisms or their toxins, which is administered to stimulate an active immune response in the body. This results in the production of antibodies against the specific pathogens. Booster doses are usually equivalent to a single dose of the initial immunization. For some immunizations (e.g., tetanus) boosters are prescribed at designated intervals to ensure maintenance of immune levels.

Vaccine manufacturers have trade names for each product and have established protocols to ensure potency and stability. All vaccines are tested for safety and effectiveness. Every vaccine package has an insert that fully describes the following:
- The vaccine and its use
- The route of administration
- Adverse reactions
- Signs and symptoms the parent might observe after immunization that would indicate a potential problem

Unfavorable responses include high fever, swelling at the site of the injection, **urticaria**, breathing difficulties, severe headache, and convulsions. Any of these should be immediately reported to the provider. Vaccine storage should follow the manufacturer's guidelines (e.g., some vaccines must be refrigerated; others must not be exposed to sunlight).

Some vaccines are grown in birds' eggs or in a medium made of animal organs, or they are weakened with chemicals. Therefore, a child who is allergic to eggs cannot receive some of the vaccines, such as influenza. The medical assistant must know the potential allergic problems, common symptoms, and adverse reactions to immunizations and must make sure the parent is informed. Table 28.5 details guidelines for childhood immunizations.

Before a child or adult receives a vaccine, the healthcare provider is required by the National Childhood Vaccine Injury Act (NCVIA) to provide a copy of a Vaccine Information Statement (VIS) to either the adult patient or the child's parent or legal guardian. A VIS provides information about the risks and benefits of each vaccine. If providing the parent or guardian with the VIS is the medical assistant's responsibility, he or she should do the following (see Procedure 28.3, p. 725):
- Before administering the vaccine, give the parent the most current VIS available for that particular vaccine. Give the parent enough time to review the information, and then answer any questions or refer the parent's concerns to the provider before

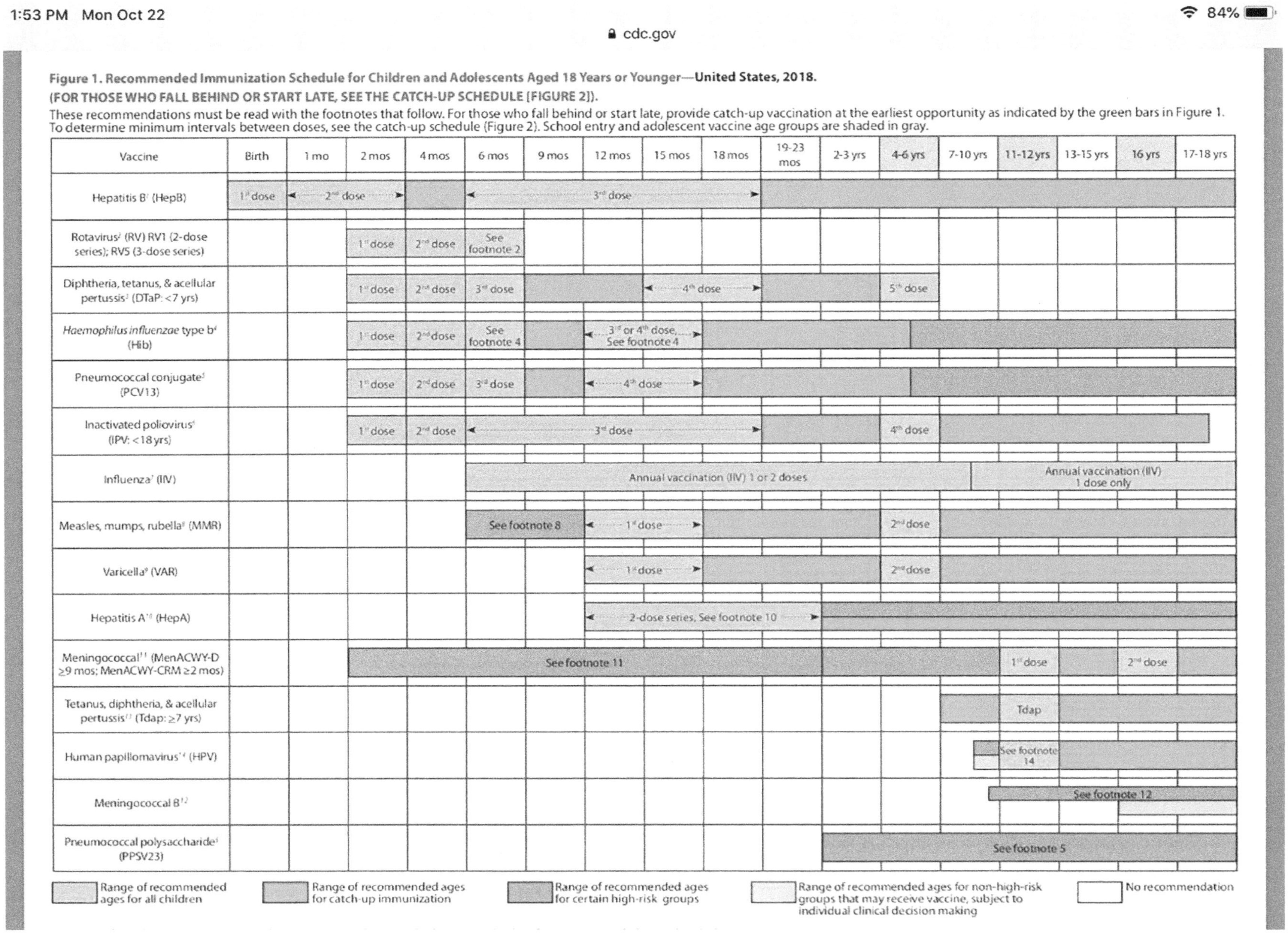

Figure 1. Recommended Immunization Schedule for Children and Adolescents Aged 18 Years or Younger—United States, 2018.
(FOR THOSE WHO FALL BEHIND OR START LATE, SEE THE CATCH-UP SCHEDULE [FIGURE 2]).

These recommendations must be read with the footnotes that follow. For those who fall behind or start late, provide catch-up vaccination at the earliest opportunity as indicated by the green bars in Figure 1. To determine minimum intervals between doses, see the catch-up schedule (Figure 2). School entry and adolescent vaccine age groups are shaded in gray.

Vaccine	Birth	1 mo	2 mos	4 mos	6 mos	9 mos	12 mos	15 mos	18 mos	19-23 mos	2-3 yrs	4-6 yrs	7-10 yrs	11-12 yrs	13-15 yrs	16 yrs	17-18 yrs
Hepatitis B¹ (HepB)	1ˢᵗ dose	←—— 2ⁿᵈ dose ——→			←————————————— 3ʳᵈ dose —————————————→												
Rotavirus² (RV) RV1 (2-dose series); RV5 (3-dose series)			1ˢᵗ dose	2ⁿᵈ dose	See footnote 2												
Diphtheria, tetanus, & acellular pertussis³ (DTaP: <7 yrs)			1ˢᵗ dose	2ⁿᵈ dose	3ʳᵈ dose			←——— 4ᵗʰ dose ———→				5ᵗʰ dose					
Haemophilus influenzae type bᵈ (Hib)			1ˢᵗ dose	2ⁿᵈ dose	See footnote 4		←— 3ʳᵈ or 4ᵗʰ dose, See footnote 4 —→										
Pneumococcal conjugate⁵ (PCV13)			1ˢᵗ dose	2ⁿᵈ dose	3ʳᵈ dose		←— 4ᵗʰ dose —→										
Inactivated poliovirus⁶ (IPV: <18 yrs)			1ˢᵗ dose	2ⁿᵈ dose	←————————————— 3ʳᵈ dose —————————————→							4ᵗʰ dose					
Influenza⁷ (IIV)					See footnote 8		Annual vaccination (IIV) 1 or 2 doses						Annual vaccination (IIV) 1 dose only				
Measles, mumps, rubella⁸ (MMR)							←— 1ˢᵗ dose —→					2ⁿᵈ dose					
Varicella⁹ (VAR)							←— 1ˢᵗ dose —→					2ⁿᵈ dose					
Hepatitis A¹⁰ (HepA)							←— 2-dose series, See footnote 10 —→										
Meningococcal¹¹ (MenACWY-D ≥9 mos; MenACWY-CRM ≥2 mos)							See footnote 11							1ˢᵗ dose		2ⁿᵈ dose	
Tetanus, diphtheria, & acellular pertussis¹² (Tdap: ≥7 yrs)														Tdap			
Human papillomavirus¹³ (HPV)														See footnote 14			
Meningococcal B¹²														See footnote 12			
Pneumococcal polysaccharide⁵ (PPSV23)												See footnote 5					

Range of recommended ages for all children

Range of recommended ages for catch-up immunization

Range of recommended ages for certain high-risk groups

Range of recommended ages that may receive vaccine, subject to individual clinical decision making

No recommendation

FIGURE 28.10 Recommended immunization schedule for children ages birth to 18 years. (From http://www.cdc.gov/vaccines/schedules/downloads/child/0-18yrs-child-combined-schedule.pdf . Accessed October 22, 2018.)

TABLE 28.5   Guidelines for Childhood Immunizations

VACCINE	TRADE NAME	ROUTE OF ADMINISTRATION	CONTRAINDICATIONS[a]	SIDE EFFECTS
DTaP Diphtheria, tetanus, pertussis (whooping cough)	Daptacel, Infanrix	IM; Td (tetanus and diphtheria) boosters at 11–12 yr if at least 5 yr since last dose; subsequent booster every 10 yr	Moderate or severe acute illness; neurologic problem; complication after previous dose (e.g., fever, convulsions)	Mild fever, anorexia, irritability, drowsiness
HAV Hepatitis A (can use either Havrix or Vaqta)	Havrix, Vaqta	IM; all children 1 yr; 2 doses 6 mo apart	Hypersensitivity to product, acute infection or fever	Localized injection site reaction, fever, headache
HBV Hepatitis B	Engerix-B, Recombivax HB	IM; may give with all other vaccines but at a separate site; requires 3 injections	Moderate or severe acute illness; yeast allergy; severe cardiovascular disease	Fever, pain at injection site, headache, malaise, vomiting
Hib *Haemophilus influenzae* serotype B meningitis	COMVAX, PedvaxHIB, ActHIB, Hiberix	IM; may give with all other vaccines but at a separate site. Three doses of ActHIB, MenHibrix, or Pentacel at 2, 4, and 6 months or 2 doses of PedvaxHib or COMVAX at 2 and 4 months of age; booster dose at 12 through 15 months	Not routinely given to children older than 5; moderate or severe acute illness	Minimal
HPV Human papillomavirus	HPV2 (Cervarix) females only; HPV4 (Gardasil), HPV9 (Gardasil 9) males and females	IM; routine vaccination at age 11 or 12 years; second dose 1 to 2 months after first dose; third dose 16 weeks after second dose	Hypersensitivity to ingredients; pregnancy	Relatively few; mild headache and GI upset
Influenza Trivalent inactivated vaccine for 6 months; at 2 years, use live, attenuated vaccine	Afluria, Fluad, Flublok, Flucelvax, FluLaval, Fluarix, Fluvirin, Fluzone, FluMist (nasal spray)	IM; annually each fall	Allergy to eggs; recent fever	Uncommon; fever, local irritation at injection site, general malaise
IPV Inactive poliovirus for polio	Ipol	SC or IM; 4 doses; may give with all other vaccines but at a separate site	Moderate or severe acute illness; egg allergy	Uncommon
Meningococcal vaccine for meningitis (MCV4)	Menactra, Menomune, MenHibrix, Bexsero, or Trumenba	IM; single dose of Menactra or Menveo vaccine at age 11 through 12 years, with a booster dose at age 16 years; aged 16 through 23 years vaccinated with a 2-dose series of Bexsero or a 3-dose series of Trumenba vaccine to provide short-term protection	Moderate or severe acute illness; history of allergic reaction to MCV4	Uncommon
MMR Measles, mumps, rubella	M-M-R II	SC; may give with all other vaccines but at a separate site	Moderate or severe acute illness; immunocompromised patients (may be given if HIV positive); pregnancy or possible pregnancy in 3 mo; egg allergy	Fever

TABLE 28.5   Guidelines for Childhood Immunizations—*continued*

VACCINE	TRADE NAME	ROUTE OF ADMINISTRATION	CONTRAINDICATIONS[a]	SIDE EFFECTS
Pneumococcal (PCV) Pneumococcal pneumonia	Pneumovax 23, Prevnar 13	IM or SC; all children 2–23 mo; administer every 6 yr for high-risk patients	Moderate or severe acute illness; hypersensitivity	Drowsiness, local irritation at site, mild fever
Rotavirus (Rota) RotaTeq for prevention of rotavirus gastroenteritis	Rotarix	PO; 3 doses at 6–12 wk; subsequent doses at 4–10 wk intervals	Hypersensitivity	GI upset and blood disorders
Varicella (chickenpox)	Varivax	SC; may give with all other vaccines but at a separate site; 2-dose series at ages 12 through 15 mo and 4 through 6 yr	Confirmed history of chickenpox; pregnancy or possible pregnancy in 1 mo; moderate or severe acute illness; immunocompromised patients; egg allergy	No salicylates for 6 wk afterward to prevent risk of Reye syndrome
May give combination vaccine: measles, mumps, rubella, varicella (MMRV)	ProQuad	SC; may give with all other vaccines but at a separate site; all susceptible children 12 mo or older	Confirmed history of chickenpox; pregnancy or possible pregnancy in 1 mo; moderate or severe acute illness; immunocompromised patients; egg allergy	No salicylates for 6 wk afterward to prevent risk of Reye's syndrome

[a]Mild illness is not a contraindication.
GI, Gastrointestinal; *HIV*, human immunodeficiency virus; *IM*, intramuscular; *PO*, oral; *SC*, subcutaneous.

administering the vaccine. VIS forms are available online in a number of languages to meet the needs of a diverse patient population.

- Document in the child's health record the date the VIS was given and the publication date of the VIS (which appears on the bottom of the form).
- To make sure the office has the most current VIS forms, either call the state health department or refer to the CDC's website at www.cdc.gov/vaccines/hcp/vis/current-vis.html. Forms can be printed directly from the site.
- If an informed consent form is required in your state, it must be signed and attached to the child's health record or electronically signed in the child's EHR before immunizations are given. Documentation of immunization administration must include the date the vaccine was administered, the manufacturer of the vaccine, the manufacturer's lot number, the type of vaccine, the exact site of administration if an injection was given, any reported or observed side effects, the name and title of the person who administered the vaccine, and the address of the medical office where the vaccine was administered.
- An immunization record should be given to the parent. If it is in paper form (e.g., a booklet), it should be updated as needed to reflect the child's current immunization status. Most EHRs allow for the immunization record to be printed after each immunization. The medical assistant should not only document the required details in the patient's health record, but he or she should also complete the parent's immunization record each time the child receives another vaccination or booster. These parent records help schools and day care centers

determine the child's immunization status. Some states are developing computerized immunization record systems.

- It is very important that vaccine vials are handled and stored properly to maintain the compound's ability to fight disease. The CDC's recommendations for vaccine management practices can be found at its website at http://www.cdc.gov/vaccines/recs/storage/.

Safe Handling and Storage of Vaccines

The Centers for Disease Control and Prevention (CDC) has devised a list of important rules and steps to ensure safekeeping of a practice's vaccine supply. This list can be used as a checklist in the office.

_____ 1. One person should be in charge of the handling and storage of vaccines at the facility, with a backup person to ensure proper management.

_____ 2. A vaccine inventory log should be maintained that includes the following:

_____ (1) Vaccine name
_____ (2) Number of doses
_____ (3) Date vaccine was received
_____ (4) Condition of vaccine on arrival
_____ (5) Manufacturer
_____ (6) Lot number
_____ (7) Expiration date

____ 3. Vaccines should be stored in separate, self-contained units that refrigerate or freeze only. A household-style combination unit can be used to store only refrigerated vaccines; frozen vaccines must be kept in a separate, stand-alone freezer.

____ 4. The vaccine refrigerator and freezer should not be used for food or drinks.

____ 5. Vaccines should be stored in the middle of the refrigerator or freezer, not in the door.

____ 6. New supplies should be placed behind the vials with the closest expiration date; the vials with the nearest expiration date should be used first.

____ 7. A sign should be posted on the refrigerator door identifying which vaccines should be stored in either the refrigerator or the freezer.

____ 8. One thermometer should be kept in the refrigerator and one in the freezer; the refrigerator temperature should be maintained at 35° to 46°F (2° to 8°C) and the freezer temperature at −58° to 5°F (−50° to 15°C) or colder.

____ 9. Containers of water should be kept in the refrigerator and ice packs in the freezer to help maintain cold temperatures.

____ 10. A temperature log should be kept on the refrigerator door; the refrigerator and freezer temperatures should be recorded twice a day: first thing in the morning and at the end of the day.

____ 11. A "Do Not Unplug" sign should be posted next to the refrigerator's electrical outlet.

____ 12. If the refrigerator or freezer stops working, the following steps should be taken:
- Immediately place the vaccines in another refrigerator or freezer, and mark them so that they can be separated from vaccines that were not affected.
- Record the temperature of the refrigerator or freezer, and contact the vaccine manufacturer or state health department. Follow their instructions on the use, alteration of expiration dates, or disposal of the vaccines.

____ 13. The facility should have a copy of the health department's general and emergency vaccine management policies.

CRITICAL THINKING APPLICATION   28.5

Allison will be administering pediatric immunizations during the well-baby visits scheduled for today. To prepare for this responsibility, she looked up the primary vaccinations, their routes of administration, contraindications, and possible side effects. The first child arrives for her 4-month checkup. She has received all of her previous immunizations on schedule. What immunizations should the child receive, and how should they be administered? The baby's father asks whether she will get sick from the vaccines. What should Allison tell him? What does Allison need to do to meet the requirements of the National Childhood Vaccine Injury Act?

THE ADOLESCENT PATIENT

The adolescent patient may present the greatest challenge to health education and disease management. Adolescence begins with the onset of puberty, a time when the child's reproductive system matures. This is a period marked by rapid changes in the endocrine and musculoskeletal systems. The adolescent undergoes rapid growth spurts and the development of secondary sexual characteristics.

Health examinations for patients in this age group should include the following:
- Screening for height and weight
- Gathering details about diet and exercise routines
- Screening for sexually transmitted infections (STIs)
- Pap test (for sexually active female adolescents), especially to screen for infection with the human papillomavirus [HPV])
- Reviewing the vaccination history and administering boosters as indicated
- Assessing for high-risk behaviors, such as substance abuse, smoking, and sexual behavior

Health problems most frequently seen in adolescent patients include eating disorders (anorexia nervosa and bulimia nervosa), obesity, and injury-related problems. Accidents are the leading cause of death and injury in adolescence, and suicide is the third leading cause of death. All healthcare personnel should be on the alert for indicators of suicide, including the following:
- Signs of depression, such as headaches, abdominal discomfort, anorexia, fatigue, aggressiveness, drug or alcohol abuse, and sexual promiscuity
- Verbal statements that hint at the adolescent's intention to commit suicide; talking about dying
- Actions such as giving away prized objects, withdrawing from social groups, suddenly changing normal behavior patterns, or writing a suicide note

CLOSING COMMENTS

Patient Coaching

Unintentional injuries are the leading cause of death and disability in children in the United States. Injuries cause more childhood deaths than all diseases combined. The primary causes of childhood injuries are the following:
- Motor vehicle accidents
- Drowning
- Burns
- Falls
- Poisoning
- Aspiration with airway obstruction
- Firearm accidents

Childhood injuries are linked to the child's growth and development level and usually are preventable. Young children are totally dependent on caregivers to keep them safe, so constant supervision and a childproof environment are essential for this age group. Older children need to be aware of health hazards and should be encouraged to protect themselves from injury (e.g., they should use bike helmets, protective padding when skateboarding, seat belts, and so on). The highest incidence of accidental injuries is seen in children under age 9, but as children grow older, the percentage of deaths from injuries increases. In the United States, more than 9000 children die each year—about 25 deaths a day—from injuries. Healthcare workers play a major role in injury prevention. The medical assistant is responsible for making sure the ambulatory care office is safe and parents are educated about potential hazards.

Legal and Ethical Issues

The Child Abuse Prevention and Treatment Act states that all threats to a child's physical and/or mental welfare must be reported. This means that every teacher, healthcare worker, and social worker—in fact, every citizen—who suspects that a child is being neglected, abused, or exploited must report this to the proper authority. The agency must record the report, and after three similar reports, the agency must investigate.

When suspected abuse, neglect, or exploitation is reported, the individual must provide his or her name. This is considered confidential information and is not given to the child's parent or guardian, nor is it given to the investigating officer. The individual making the report is also protected under the law from any liability for reporting suspicions of child abuse.

If the medical assistant suspects that a child is a victim of abuse, neglect, or exploitation, he or she should consult with the provider immediately. In most states, the medical assistant and the provider can make separate reports to the authorities. However, state laws vary, so state and local reporting protocols should be outlined in the office procedures manual.

Signs of Child Abuse

Obvious Signs
- Previously filed reports of physical or sexual abuse of the child
- Documented abuse of other family members
- Different stories from the parents and the child on how an accident happened
- Stories of incidents and injuries that are suspicious
- Injuries blamed on other family members
- Repeated visits to the emergency department for injuries

Examination Findings
- Trauma to the nervous system
- Internal abdominal pain
- Discolorations/bruising on the buttocks, back, and abdomen
- Elbow, wrist, and shoulder dislocations

Changes in Child's Behavior
- Too eager to please the parent
- Overly passive and too compliant
- Aggressive and demanding
- Parenting the parent (role reversal)
- Delays in the normal growth and development patterns
- Erratic school attendance

Physical Indicators
- Poor hygiene
- Malnutrition
- Obvious dental neglect
- Neglected well-baby procedures (e.g., immunizations)

Patient-Centered Care

In a pediatric practice, the child usually is joined by one or both parents during visits to the provider. Parents need reinforcement, praise, and understanding in dealing with the health and welfare of their child. Provide parents with information to help them understand their children's behavior and improve their parenting skills. Understanding the normal behavioral characteristics of a particular developmental stage may increase the parents' confidence and reinforce expectations for the child.

The waiting room is an ideal place for parent education. Use the space and resources available to provide up-to-date information on child health issues and on local resources for support and assistance. If the provider has pamphlets available, discuss them with the parents. Answer questions when possible, or alert the provider so that questions can be answered during the office visit. Every opportunity should be taken to teach parents about sound healthcare. Because so many ambulatory care visits involve infectious disorders, educating children and parents on the following infection control measures may reduce the spread of disease:

- Children should cover their mouth with a disposable tissue when they cough, or they should cough into their bent arm rather than their hands.
- A tissue should be used only once and then immediately thrown away.
- Children should not be allowed to share toys they have put in their mouth.
- After a child has discarded a toy that was in the mouth, it should be placed in a bin for dirty toys that is out of the reach of others. Wash and disinfect these toys before allowing children to play with them again.
- Make sure all children and adults follow good handwashing practices. Have pump hand sanitizers available throughout the office.

Professional Behaviors

Working as a medical assistant in a busy pediatric practice can be very challenging. In essence, you are faced with two clients: a child who may be frightened and not feeling well, and a caregiver who typically is stressed. When you are dealing with emotionally charged situations, it is easy to lose patience and act out yourself. Continuing to act professionally can help you manage these difficult situations. Consider the following suggestions:

- Routinely use active listening to get as much information as possible from the parents. Paying attention not only to the parents' words, but also to their feelings helps the parents feel valued.
- Focus on age-appropriate methods for communicating with the child. Interacting with children on a level that they can understand helps them feel more comfortable and hopefully promotes cooperative behavior.
- Use time management techniques to handle the work challenges you face each day. Staying organized keeps you from feeling overwhelmed.

SUMMARY OF SCENARIO

After working with the telephone screening staff, Allison has come to realize the importance of becoming familiar with childhood diseases and disorders and the management policy of her provider-employers. Many times Allison has had to refer to the office procedure manual to make sure she is asking the right questions and gathering all the information needed for the provider who will make the daily response calls. From working in the clinical area, Allison has also realized that a pediatric practice actually has two groups of patients: the child and the caregivers. She must be sensitive to the needs of both groups and develop communication

skills that build trust with the child and his or her parents. Allison is working on developing a comprehensive education site in the office for interested parents and is creating a community resource guide for interested caregivers. She recognizes the need to stay up to date on the CDC's recommendations for childhood immunizations, and she routinely refers to the CDC's website to make sure the office has the most recently published VIS forms. Allison regularly attends her local American Association of Medical Assistants (AAMA) chapter meetings to maintain her certification and to continue to learn about the pediatric practice specialty.

SUMMARY OF LEARNING OBJECTIVES

1. **Describe childhood growth patterns.**

   By 6 months of age, the child's birth weight has doubled; at 1 year it has tripled, and the child's length has increased by 50%. By age 2, the child has reached approximately 50% of adult height. This same growth rate continues throughout the school-age period, ages 6 to 12 years, which leads into a growth spurt that indicates impending puberty. In adolescence, ages 12 to 18 years, the adolescent gains almost half of his or her adult weight and the skeleton and organs double in size.

2. **Discuss developmental patterns and therapeutic approaches for infants, toddlers, preschoolers, school-aged children, and adolescents.**

   Using therapeutic approaches for infants, toddlers, school-age, and adolescent patients improves communication with a variety of patient age groups and promotes quality patient care. Unnumbered boxes in the text discuss therapeutic approaches for pediatric patients.

3. **Describe Erickson's developmental theory.**

   Erik Erickson's developmental theory focuses on five stages that an individual must pass through and master: trust versus mistrust, autonomy versus shame and doubt, initiative versus guilt, industry versus inferiority, and identity versus role confusion.

4. **List and describe common pediatric diseases and disorders.**

   Pediatric gastrointestinal disorders include infant colic; diarrhea, which can be caused by a variety of microorganisms and is treated medically when it continues for longer than 2 days; failure to thrive caused by a physiologic factor (e.g., malabsorption disease or cleft palate) or a nonorganic cause that is associated with the parent-child relationship; and obesity if the child's BMI is equal to or greater than the 95th percentile.

   The common cold may lead to secondary bacterial infections, including strep throat or otitis media; croup is a viral disorder that affects the larynx; pertussis, commonly known as whooping cough, is caused by bacteria that attach to the cilia of the upper respiratory system and can cause violent, rapid coughing and apnea in infants; bronchiolitis is a viral infection of the bronchioles that causes acute onset of wheezing and dyspnea; RSV is a virus that infects the lungs and bronchioles; asthma causes bronchospasms and inflammation of the bronchioles; and influenza is an acute, highly contagious viral infection of the respiratory tract.

   Pediatric infectious diseases include conjunctivitis, caused by a bacterial or viral infection; tonsillitis, typically caused by beta-hemolytic

streptococci; fifth disease, also called *erythema infectiosum*, a mild infection caused by parvovirus B19; hand-foot-and-mouth disease, caused by the coxsackievirus, which leads to multiple symptoms, including painful blisters on the tongue, mouth, palms of the hands, and soles of the feet; and Reye syndrome, which is linked with the use of aspirin during a viral illness.

5. **Do the following related to the pediatric patient examination:**
   Describe the medical assistant's role in pediatric procedures.
   - The medical assistant assists the pediatrician with examinations; maintains patient histories; performs ordered screening tests, such as vision, hearing, urinalysis, and hemoglobin checks; administers immunizations; measures and weighs children as needed; documents accurately; and provides support to patients and caregivers.

   Cite reference ranges for pediatric vital signs.
   - Refer to Table 28.2.

   Describe how the Apgar scoring system works.
   - Apgar is used to evaluate a newborn's physical condition at 1 and 5 minutes after birth. The newborn is evaluated on appearance, pulse, grimace, activity, and respiration. Table 28.3 describes the scoring system.

   List the recommendations of the American Academy of Pediatrics when it comes to the frequency of well-child visits.
   - Well-child visits are typically scheduled from age 2 weeks through 15 years to focus on maintaining the child's health with physical examinations, immunizations, and upgrading of the child's medical health history record.

   Discuss sick-child visits, as well as important questions for telephone screening of an older child who can communicate symptoms.
   - Sick-child visits occur whenever the child needs to be seen because of illness or injury. Table 28.4 summarizes important questions for telephone screening of pediatric problems.

   Describe how to measure the circumference of an infant's head and how to obtain an infant's length and weight.
   - Procedure 28.1 on p. 723 outlines the steps for measuring an infant's head.
   - Procedure 28.2 on p. 724 outlines the steps for measuring an infant's length and weight and documenting on the child's growth chart.

SUMMARY OF LEARNING OBJECTIVES—*continued*

6. **Assist with diagnostic procedures, including obtaining a urine sample.**
   The easiest way to obtain a urine sample from a child who is toilet trained is to give the parent the container and instructions ahead of time. In some cases, the child may need to be catheterized to obtain the specimen. Pediatric catheterization kits contain all the supplies needed for this procedure. When preparing the kit, always remember that this is a sterile procedure.

7. **Discuss the current immunization schedule for children from newborn to 18 years old. Also, detail guidelines for childhood immunization, and document immunizations.**
   The CDC's recommendations for childhood immunization are summarized in Table 28.5 and Fig. 28.10.
   Procedure 28.3 on p. 725 summarizes how to document immunizations in both the official vaccination record and the parent's immunization booklet. Documentation of immunization administration on the VIS form must include the date the vaccine was administered, the vaccine's manufacturer, the manufacturer's lot number, the type of vaccine, the route of administration and exact site if an injection is given, any reported or observed side effects, the name and title of the person administering the vaccine, the address of the medical office where the vaccine was administered, and the date.

8. **Discuss the unique challenges and needs of the adolescent patient.**
   Adolescents are going through extreme physical and emotional changes, and an extra measure of patience and understanding is required to establish therapeutic interactions. Ensuring their privacy, giving them the option of being seen without parents, and providing pertinent education materials all are important factors in patient-centered adolescent care.

9. **Specify child safety guidelines for injury prevention and management of suspected child abuse.**
   The medical assistant should be involved in parent education on injury prevention for children. Childhood injuries are linked to the child's growth and development level and therefore are often predictable and many times are preventable. If the medical assistant suspects that a child is a victim of abuse, neglect, or exploitation, he or she should consult with the pediatrician immediately. In most states, the medical assistant and the physician can make separate reports to the authorities.

PROCEDURE 28.1   Measure the Head Circumference of an Infant

Task: Obtain an accurate measurement of the circumference of an infant's head, and plot the result on the patient's growth chart.

EQUIPMENT and SUPPLIES

- Patient's record
- Flexible disposable tape measure
- Age- and gender-specific growth chart
- Pen

PROCEDURAL STEPS

1. Wash hands or use hand sanitizer.
   PURPOSE: Hand sanitization is necessary to ensure infection control.
2. Greet the patient and the parents or caregivers. Identify yourself. Verify the patient's identity with full name and date of birth. Explain the procedure to be performed in a manner that the patient (if old enough) or the parent or caregiver understands. Answer any questions. If the child is old enough, gain his or her cooperation through conversation.
   PURPOSE: It is important to alleviate anxiety and gain the child's trust.
3. Place an infant in the supine position, or the infant may be held by the parent. An older infant may sit on the examination table.
4. Hold the tape measure with the zero mark against the infant's forehead, slightly above the eyebrows and the top of the ears. Ask the parent for assistance if necessary.
5. Bring the tape measure around the head, just above the ears, until it meets (Fig. 1).
6. Read to the nearest 0.5 centimeter or quarter inch.
7. Record the measurement on the growth chart and in the patient's health record.
   PURPOSE: A procedure is not done until it is recorded.

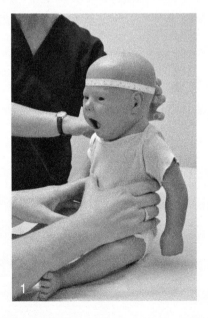

8. Dispose of the tape measure.
9. Wash hands or use hand sanitizer.
   PURPOSE: Hand sanitization is necessary to ensure infection control.

Documentation Example

10/21/20XX 10:20 am HC 39.5 cm _____
_____A. Kwong, CMA (AAMA)

PROCEDURE 28.2	**Measure an Infant's Length and Weight**

Task: Measure an infant's length and weight accurately so that growth patterns can be monitored and recorded.

EQUIPMENT and SUPPLIES

- Patient's record
- Infant scale with paper cover
- Flexible measuring tape
- Examination table paper
- Pen
- Pediatric length board, if available
- Gender-specific infant growth chart
- Waste container

PROCEDURAL STEPS

Measuring an Infant's Length

1. Wash hands or use hand sanitizer; assemble the necessary equipment.
   PURPOSE: Hand sanitization is necessary to ensure infection control.
2. Greet the patient and parents or caregivers. Identify yourself. Verify the patient's identity with full name and date of birth. Explain the procedure to be performed in a manner that the patient (if old enough) and the parent or caregiver understands. Answer any questions.
   PURPOSE: It is important to alleviate anxiety and gain the child's trust.
3. Undress the infant. The diaper may be left on.
4. Cover the examination table with smooth, flat paper. Ask the caregiver to place the infant on his or her back on the examination table. If using a pediatric table with a headboard, ask the caregiver to hold the infant's head gently against the headboard while you straighten the infant's leg and note the location of the heel on the measurement area. If there is no headboard, ask the caregiver to gently hold the infant's head still while you draw a line on the paper at the top of the baby's head and at the heel after extending the leg (Fig. 1).

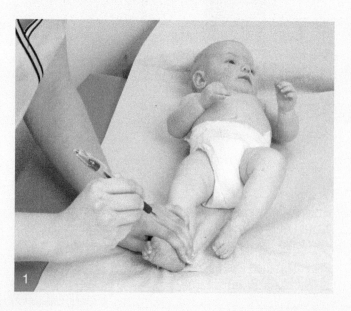

5. Measure the infant's length with the tape measure, and record it.
6. Document the results in either inches or centimeters, depending on office policy, on the infant's growth chart, in the progress notes, and in the caregiver's record if requested.

Weighing an Infant

1. Wash hands or use hand sanitizer, assemble the necessary equipment, and explain the procedure to the infant's caregiver.
   PURPOSE: Hand sanitization is necessary to ensure infection control.
2. Greet the patient and parents or caregivers. Identify yourself. Verify the patient's identity with full name and date of birth. Explain the procedure to be performed in a manner that the patient understands. Answer any questions the parents or caregivers may have.
   PURPOSE: It is important to alleviate anxiety and gain the trust of the child and the parents or caregivers.
3. If the scale is not a digital model, prepare it by sliding weights to the left; line the scale with disposable paper to reduce the risk of pathogen transmission.
4. Completely undress the infant. If the diaper is clean and dry, it can remain on.
   PURPOSE: It is important to get the most accurate weight possible, and a wet diaper will add to the total weight.
5. Place the infant gently on the center of the scale, keeping your hand directly above the infant's trunk for safety (Fig. 2).
   PURPOSE: This position will protect the infant from possible injury.

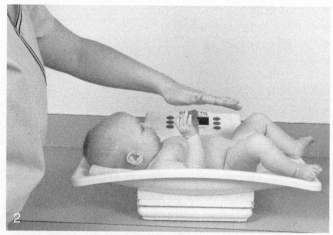

6. If the scale is not a digital model, slide the weights across it until balance is achieved. Read the infant's weight while he or she is still.
7. If the scale is not a digital model, return the weights to the far left of the scale and remove the baby. Discard the paper lining the scale. If the scale became contaminated during the procedure, follow Occupational Safety and Health Administration (OSHA) guidelines for use of gloves and disposal of contaminated waste. Disinfect the equipment according to the manufacturer's guidelines.
   PURPOSE: These steps will provide infection control.

PROCEDURE 28.2 | Measure an Infant's Length and Weight—*continued*

8. Wash hands or use hand sanitizer.
9. Document the results in either pounds or kilograms, depending on office policy, on the infant's growth chart, in the progress notes, and in the caregiver's record if requested.

Documentation Example
8/24/20XX 10:20 am Wt 17 lb 4 oz. Length 27 in. _____
_____ A. Kwong, CMA (AAMA)

PROCEDURE 28.3 | Document Immunizations

Task: Document accurately the administration of a pediatric immunization.

EQUIPMENT and SUPPLIES

- Patient's record
- Vaccine administration record (VAR)
- Parent's immunization record (if used in the medical practice)
- Vaccine Information Statement (VIS) for hepatitis B (the current VIS forms can be accessed at this website: http://www.cdc.gov/vaccines/hcp/vis/current-vis.html)

Scenario: Samantha Anderson, a 5-week-old infant, has just received her second dose of the hepatitis B (HBV) vaccine. Document the administration of the vaccine.

PROCEDURAL STEPS

1. Gather the necessary forms.
2. Make sure the provider obtained informed consent from the parent (if required by your state), that the hepatitis B VIS form was given, and that all the parent's questions were answered before the vaccine is dispensed and administered.
   PURPOSE: It is important to follow risk management practices.
3. Administer the vaccine intramuscularly (see Chapter 15, Administering Medications).
4. Complete the information required on the VAR, including the name of the vaccine, the date given, the route of administration and site, the vaccine lot number and manufacturer, the date on the VIS form, the date it was given to the parent, and your signature or initials.

PURPOSE: This level of documentation is necessary to meet the legal requirements of the National Childhood Vaccine Injury Act.
5. In the parent's copy of the immunization record, record the date of administration, the name and address of the provider's practice, and the type of vaccine administered.
   PURPOSE: It is important to maintain an accurate and comprehensive parental record of childhood immunizations for school or day care purposes.
6. After administering the HBV vaccine, record the following details in the child's health record:
   - Date the vaccine was administered
   - Vaccine's manufacturer, batch and lot numbers, and expiration date
   - Type of vaccine administered and dose
   - Route of administration and exact site if an injection was given
   - Any reported or observed side effects
   - Publication date of the VIS form given to the parent (on the bottom of the form)
   - Parent education about possible side effects of the vaccine
   - Name and title of the person who administered the vaccine

Documentation Example
4/2/20XX 3:25 pm Mother given VIS form for Hep B. Had no questions. Administered second dose of Hep B IM to Ⓛ vastus lateralis per Dr. Walden's order. No problems noted after injection. _____
_____ A. Kwong, CMA (AAMA)
Continued

PROCEDURE 28.3   **Document Immunizations**—*continued*

Vaccine Administration Record for Children and Teens

(Page 1 of 2)

Patient name: _____

Birthdate: _____ Patient ID number: _____

Clinic name and address

Before administering any vaccines, give copies of all pertinent Vaccine Information Statements (VISs) to the child's parent or legal representative and make sure he/she understands the risks and benefits of the vaccine(s). Always provide or update the patient's personal record card.

Vaccine	Type of Vaccine[1]	Date given (mo/day/yr)	Funding Source (F,S,P)[2]	Route & Site[3]	Vaccine		Vaccine Information Statement (VIS)		Vaccinator[5] (signature or initials & title)
					Lot #	Mfr.	Date on VIS[4]	Date given[4]	
Hepatitis B[6] (e.g., HepB, Hib-HepB, DTaP-HepB-IPV) Give IM.[3]									
Diphtheria, Tetanus, Pertussis[6] (e.g., DTaP, DTaP/Hib, DTaP-HepB-IPV, DT, DTaP-IPV/Hib, Tdap, DTaP-IPV, Td) Give IM.[3]									
Haemophilus influen-zae type b[6] (e.g., Hib, Hib-HepB, DTaP-IPV/Hib, DTaP/Hib, Hib-MenCY) Give IM.[3]									
Polio[6] (e.g., IPV, DTaP-HepB-DTaP-IPV/Hib, DTaP-IPV) Give IPV SC or IM.[3] Give all others IM.[3]									
Pneumococcal (e.g., PCV7, PCV13, con-jugate; PPSV23, polysac-charide) Give PCV IM.[3] Give PPSV SC or IM.[3]									
Rotavirus (RV1, RV5) Give orally (po).[3]									

See page 2 to record measles-mumps-rubella, varicella, hepatitis A, meningococcal, HPV, influenza, and other vaccines (e.g., travel vaccines).

How to Complete This Record

1. Record the generic abbreviation (e.g., Tdap) or the trade name for each vaccine (see table at right).

2. Record the funding source of the vaccine given as either F (federal), S (state), or P (private).

3. Record the route by which the vaccine was given as either intramuscular (IM), subcutaneous (SC), intradermal (ID), intranasal (IN), or oral (PO) and also the site where it was administered as either RA (right arm), LA (left arm), RT (right thigh), or LT (left thigh).

4. Record the publication date of each VIS as well as the date the VIS is given to the patient.

5. To meet the space constraints of this form and federal requirements for documentation, a healthcare setting may want to keep a reference list of vaccinators that includes their initials and titles.

6. For combination vaccines, fill in a row for each antigen in the combination.

Abbreviation	Trade Name and Manufacturer
DTaP	Daptacel (sanofi); Infanrix (GlaxoSmithKline [GSK]); Tripedia (sanofi pasteur)
DT (pediatric)	Generic DT (sanofi pasteur)
DTaP-HepB-IPV	Pediarix (GSK)
DTaP/Hib	TriHIBit (sanofi pasteur)
DTaP-IPV/Hib	Pentacel (sanofi pasteur)
DTaP-IPV	Kinrix (GSK)
HepB	Engerix-B (GSK); Recombivax HB (Merck)
HepA-HepB	Twinrix (GSK), can be given to teens age 18 and older
Hib	ActHIB (sanofi pasteur); Hiberix (GSK); PedvaxHIB (Merck)
Hib-HepB	Comvax (Merck)
Hib-MenCY	MenHibrix (GSK)
IPV	Ipol (sanofi pasteur)
PCV13	Prevnar 13 (Pfizer)
PPSV23	Pneumovax 23 (Merck)
RV1	Rotarix (GSK)
RV5	RotaTeq (Merck)
Tdap	Adacel (sanofi pasteur); Boostrix (GSK)
Td	Decavac (sanofi pasteur); Generic Td (MA Biological Labs)

Technical content reviewed by the Centers for Disease Control and Prevention

For additional copies, visit www.immunize.org/catg.d/p2022.pdf • Item #P2022 (4/14)

This form was created by the Immunization Action Coalition • www.immunize.org • www.vaccineinformation.org

GERIATRICS

29

SCENARIO

Bill Novelli, CMA (AAMA), works at Walden-Martin Family Medical (WMFM) Clinic. Although patients of all ages are seen in the practice, many patients are age 65 or older. Through his work with Dr. Angela Perez, Bill has learned to recognize the unique communication needs of aging individuals and the importance of using family and community resources to maintain optimum health in this special population.

While studying this chapter, think about the following questions:

- Do myths about aging and stereotypes about aging people negatively affect older individuals?
- What are the most common changes that occur in the aging body and what recommendations can be made for health promotion in this age group?
- What suggestions can be made to aging patients and their families to optimize older adults' health and protect them from injury and disease?
- How is Alzheimer disease diagnosed and what are the stages of its development?
- Why is depression so common in aging individuals and how is it diagnosed and treated?
- How can the medical assistant most effectively communicate with an older person?
- Why is the use of community resources such an important factor in the care of aging people?

LEARNING OBJECTIVES

1. Do the following related to the cardiovascular, endocrine, gastrointestinal, integumentary, and musculoskeletal body systems:
   - Explain the changes in the anatomy and physiology caused by aging.
   - Summarize the major related diseases and disorders faced by older patients.
2. Do the following related to the nervous system, pulmonary system, sensory organs, urinary system, and reproductive systems:
   - Explain the changes in the anatomy and physiology caused by aging.
- Summarize the major related diseases and disorders faced by older patients.
- Describe various screening tools for dementia, depression, and malnutrition in aging adults.
3. Summarize the role of the medical assistant in caring for aging patients.
4. Describe the principles of effective communication with older adults.
5. Differentiate among independent, assisted, and skilled nursing facilities.

VOCABULARY

collagen (KAHL ah jen) The most abundant structural protein found in skin and other connective tissues. It provides strength and cushioning to many parts of the body.

decubitus ulcers (deh KYOO bi tus) Sores or ulcers that develop over a bony prominence as the result of ischemia from prolonged pressure; also called *bed sores* or *pressure sores*.

dermatome (DUR mah tome) Skin surface areas supplied by a single afferent spinal nerve.

elastin (ih LAS tin) A highly elastic protein in connective tissue that allows tissues to resume their shape after stretching or contracting; found abundantly in the dermis of the skin.

explicit (ek SPLIS it) Fully and clearly expressed or demonstrated; leaving nothing merely implied.

insidious (in SID ee uhs) Proceeding in a gradual, subtle way, but with harmful effects.

lacrimation (lak ri MAY shun) The secretion or discharge of tears.

Ménière's disease (mayn YAIRZ) Chronic disease of the inner ear causing recurrent episodes of vertigo, progressive sensorineural hearing loss, and tinnitus.

mortality (mohr TAL i tee) The relative frequency of deaths in a specific population.

nocturia (nok TOOR ee uh) Frequent urination at night.

orthostatic hypotension (or thuh STAT ik) A temporary fall in blood pressure when a person rapidly changes from a recumbent position to a standing position.

oophorectomy (oo for ECK tuh mee) Surgical removal of the ovaries.

osteoporosis (os tee oh puh ROH sis) Abnormal thinning of the bone structure, causing bones to become brittle and weak.

ototoxic A medicine or substance capable of damaging cranial nerve VIII or the organs of hearing and balance.

peristalsis (per uh STAHL suhs) Rhythmic contraction of involuntary muscles lining the gastrointestinal tract.

postherpetic neuralgia (noo RAL juh) Nerve pain that occurs after a shingles outbreak and may become chronic.

According to the National Institutes of Health, the aging population in the United States (those age 65 or older) is expected to nearly double over the next 30 years. By 2050, it is projected that there will be 88 million people age 65 or over.

The average life expectancy of an individual who reaches age 65 is an additional 19.3 years (20.6 years for females and 18 years for males). A child born in 2014 can expect to live 78.9 years, about 30 years longer than a child born in 1900. Older women outnumber older men; 25.1 million women are over age 65, as are 19.6 million men. About 30% of older people who live outside of institutions live alone; half of women over age 75 live alone. More than half a million grandparents over the age of 65 are the primary caregivers for their grandchildren, who live with them. Most older people have at least one chronic medical condition, and many have multiple conditions. Hypertension, arthritis, heart disease, cancer, and diabetes are the health problems most commonly seen in the elderly, and a significant number also suffer from strokes, asthma, emphysema, and chronic bronchitis. Many of these conditions require medications. If a patient has multiple conditions, she or he could be on multiple medications. Pillbox organizers are a great tool for patients to keep those medications straight (Fig. 29.1). Some pharmacies will fill the pillbox organizers for patients. Medication bottles can be a challenge for the elderly to open, especially when they have childproof caps on them. Patients can ask the pharmacy to use non-childproof caps (Fig. 29.2).

What does all this mean to those who have chosen careers in healthcare? As the aging population expands, it will affect all aspects of society. One area in particular will be these individuals' increased use of health services. To provide quality care to aging patients, medical assistants must understand the aging process, including the physical and sensory changes that occur with aging (see Procedure 29.1, p. 742). This knowledge enables medical assistants to recognize the special needs of the aged and to develop therapeutic management and communication skills that can help them effectively care for the older patient. Ongoing research and education about the aging process have dispelled many of the old stereotypes.

Aging is a complex physiological, psychological, and social process. Old age is not an illness, but rather a normal life process that people experience in different ways. Lack of exercise, poor nutrition, substance abuse, continual stress, and air pollutants are all factors that cause a person to show the effects of aging decades earlier than someone who has practiced healthy living habits.

As people age, changes occur in their physical appearance and abilities, along with sensory changes in vision, hearing, taste, and smell. These changes do not occur at the same time in everyone; however, sensorimotor changes can have a profound effect on the individual's ability to interact with his or her environment.

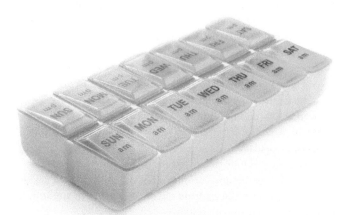

FIGURE 29.1 Pillbox organizer.

Stereotypes and Myths About Aging

- *Most aging people will develop dementia.* Dementia is not part of the normal aging process. However, the older the person, the greater the risk of dementia. About 6% of those over age 65 and almost 50% of those over age 85 are diagnosed with significant memory and disorientation issues.

- *Disease is a normal and an unavoidable part of the aging process.* Recent research verifies that individuals who have established healthy lifestyles as they age remain healthy well into their older years. Aging people are more likely to have health issues, but these are not inevitable for all persons over age 65.

- *Older workers are less productive than younger ones.* Individuals with a strong work ethic continue to perform in this way. It may take aging people longer to learn new material, but they continue to be capable of learning and applying new knowledge.

- *Most older people end up in long-term care facilities.* At any given time, approximately 5% of the aging population lives in long-term care facilities; 80% of aging individuals live independently, with or without a partner.

- *Most aging people have no interest in or capacity for sexual relations.* Sexual interest does not change significantly with age; a decrease in sexual activity is usually related to the loss of a partner.

- *Damage to health because of lifestyle factors is irreversible.* It is never too late to benefit from healthy lifestyle choices.

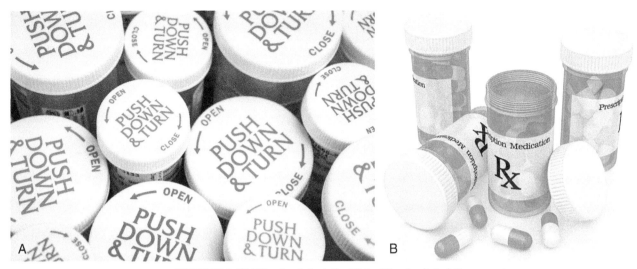

FIGURE 29.2 **(A)** Childproof medication bottles. **(B)** Non-childproof medication bottles.

CRITICAL THINKING APPLICATION 29.1

When Bill first started working with aging patients, he believed many of the stereotypes about people over age 65. Through his work with Dr. Perez, he has come to realize that many of these myths have no foundation in actual practice. Based on the myths mentioned in the text, what do you think about these beliefs on aging? Share your thoughts with your classmates.

CHANGES IN ANATOMY, PHYSIOLOGY, AND DISEASES

The aging process brings about changes in all of the body's systems. Table 29.1 summarizes these changes and what can be done to promote healthy aging.

Cardiovascular System

Cardiovascular disease is the most frequent cause of illness and disability in the aging population, and congestive heart failure (CHF) (see Chapter 24, Cardiology) is the most common reason for hospitalization. Age-related changes can occur in the cardiovascular system. Disease and lifestyle habits such as lack of exercise, poor diet, and stress can greatly contribute to these changes. Heart disease is ranked as the leading cause of death among men and women. Proper management of cardiovascular disease can help maintain the health of an aging population and reduce **mortality** rates.

The aging process causes structural changes in the heart. Myocardial cells enlarge, and deposits of fat and connective tissue increase. These combine to make the myocardial wall stiffer and to increase the time needed for the relaxation phase of the cardiac cycle. As a result, cardiac output declines, making aging people more susceptible to CHF. The reduction in cardiac output leads to pooling of blood in the legs, cold extremities, and edema. In addition, the heart cannot respond as quickly or as forcefully to an increased workload. Exercise, sudden movements, and changes in position can result in dizziness and loss of balance. Aging typically brings with it an increase in blood pressure, requiring the heart to work harder to pump blood into the systemic circulation. Hypertension increases the workload of the left ventricle, and this may result in hypertrophy of the chamber and weakening of the myocardial wall. The valves of the heart tend to thicken and become more rigid, making it more difficult for blood to circulate through the cardiopulmonary vessels. With these cardiovascular problems, arrhythmias become more common.

Aging causes the walls of the veins to weaken and stretch. This damages the valves, especially in the veins of the legs, where the walls are subject to greater pressure as blood struggles to return to the heart against the force of gravity. As a result, edema and varicose veins of the lower extremities are common in the elderly, increasing the risk of phlebitis and the formation of thrombi in the deep veins, or *deep vein thrombosis* (DVT).

Arteriosclerosis is considered part of the aging process. The vessel walls thicken and become less elastic as a result of the calcification and buildup of connective tissue. In addition, the artery's ability to dilate and contract diminishes. To maintain an adequate blood supply throughout the body, the heart must work harder to overcome the resistance caused by stiffened vessels. Older adults have a higher incidence of **orthostatic hypotension**. The clinical criterion for alterations in blood pressure from sitting to standing is:
- a drop of 20 mm Hg or more in the systolic pressure, or
- 10 mm Hg or more in the diastolic pressure, or
- experiencing lightheadedness or dizziness

When a person with orthostatic hypotension stands, gravity causes blood to pool in the legs, resulting in a drop in the amount of blood returning to the heart for circulation. This decrease in circulating blood volume causes a sudden drop in blood pressure. The provider may have the medical assistant take orthostatic blood pressures as part of the routine intake protocol for aging patients. To perform this procedure, have the patient lie down for 5 minutes, apply a blood pressure cuff, and take the individual's blood pressure and pulse while the patient is lying down. Leave the cuff in place, have the patient stand, take the blood pressure and pulse after 1 minute of standing, and then again after 3 minutes. Record

TABLE 29.1   System Changes With Aging and Measures to Promote Health

SYSTEM	AGE-RELATED CHANGES	HEALTH PROMOTION
Cardiovascular system	Arteriosclerosis and atherosclerotic plaque buildup reduces blood flow to major organs; 50% of the aging population have hypertension; CVD is the number one killer of women and men in their 60s.	Regular exercise; weight control; diet rich in fruits, vegetables, and whole grains; cholesterol, blood glucose monitoring
Central nervous system	Brain shrinks by 10% between ages 30 and 90; takes longer to learn new material; attention span and language remain the same; signs and symptoms may be caused by depression, vascular disease, and drug reactions.	Aerobic exercise to increase blood flow to CNS; maintaining mental activities (e.g., reading, interacting with others)
Endocrine system	After age 50, women have a sharp decline in estrogen; men have a more gradual decline in testosterone.	Possible hormone replacement therapy or natural soy supplements
Gastrointestinal system	Decline in gastric juices and enzymes by age 60; decreased peristalsis with increased constipation; some nutrients are not absorbed as well.	High-fiber diet and adequate fluid intake; regular exercise to prevent constipation
Musculoskeletal system	Muscle mass decreases; tendency to gain weight; gradual loss of bone density; deterioration of joint cartilage.	Strength training to increase muscle mass; stretching to remain limber; exercise; vitamin D and calcium supplements
Pulmonary system	At age 55 the lungs become less elastic and the chest wall gradually stiffens, making oxygenation more difficult.	Quit smoking; regular aerobic exercise
Sensory organs	Hearing is intact through the mid-50s but declines by 25% by age 80; oral problems are common; skin thins and loses elasticity; presbyopia after age 40; cataracts common after age 60.	Avoid exposure to loud noise, use hearing aids; good dental hygiene; prevention of sun damage to the skin; annual eye examinations; diet rich in dark green, leafy vegetables to prevent cataracts and macular degeneration
Urinary system	Kidneys become less efficient; bladder muscles weaken; one-third of seniors experience incontinence; prostate enlargement is common.	Pelvic exercises, drugs, or surgery for incontinence; annual PSA with digital rectal exam monitoring for men
Sexuality	*Men:* Impotence is not a symptom of normal aging; men over age 50 may have some altered function. *Women:* Menopause causes vaginal narrowing and dryness, resulting in painful intercourse.	*Men:* Maintenance of cardiovascular health with exercise, weight control, no smoking, diabetes management *Women:* Use of vaginal lubricants or estrogen cream

the blood pressure immediately, including the position for each of the readings.

Endocrine System

Hormonal changes that occur with aging are related to a general decrease in hormone production combined with changes in tissue receptor binding. The most common endocrine system disorder seen in aging patients is *diabetes mellitus (DM) type 2*. As a person ages, insulin production by the beta cells in the pancreas decreases and insulin resistance at the tissue level increases. According to the National Institutes of Health, more than half of the 16 million Americans diagnosed with diabetes type 2 are over age 65. Elderly patients with diabetes are at increased risk of developing vascular disease, including:

- renal disorders
- retinopathy
- neuropathy
- myocardial ischemia
- angina
- myocardial infarction
- cerebrovascular accidents
- peripheral vascular disease, such as lower extremity ulcers

Older patients do not always experience the classic symptoms of diabetes, which are polyuria, polydipsia, and polyphagia. They may show a variety of problems, including:

- unexplained weight loss
- slow wound healing
- recurrent bacterial or fungal infections
- changes in mental state
- cataracts
- macular disease
- muscle weakness and pain

- angina
- foot ulcers
- uremia

The range of symptoms is due to the **insidious** onset of diabetes in older people, who may have been gradually developing hyperglycemia for years before diagnosis.

The treatment protocol for aging patients with diabetes is the same as for other age groups; however, special consideration must be given to the patient's ability to understand and comply with the therapeutic plan. In addition, the person may have other health problems that are being treated with medications. Therefore, an aging patient newly diagnosed with diabetes may face a complicated treatment plan that requires **explicit** instruction and continual follow-up in the ambulatory care setting.

The medical assistant must be aware of any sensory abnormalities, such as diminished vision or problems with fine motor skills, that may interfere with the patient's ability to follow treatment guidelines. Coaching and treatment plans must be adapted to meet the individual needs of each patient. For example, if the patient has vision difficulties, an injector pen, with audible clicks, can be used to deliver a preset amount of insulin.

Factors That Can Affect Diabetes Management in Older People

- Modifying lifestyle risk factors may be more difficult because of poor nutrition, inability to exercise, and long-standing habits, such as smoking and a diet high in saturated fats and calories.
- Previously diagnosed health conditions, such as hypertension and heart disease, in addition to an age-related decline in kidney and liver function, increase the challenge of treating diabetes.
- Older people are more likely to be prescribed multiple medications, which increases the risk of adverse drug interactions.
- Elderly patients with diabetes are more prone to hypoglycemia and may not recognize and respond quickly to the signs of low blood glucose levels.
- Diabetic complications can develop quickly because of a long history of prediabetes before diagnosis.
- Older people may have decreased physical and/or mental abilities that make it difficult for them to understand and adhere to a complicated treatment regimen.
- Older patients may not be able to afford the medications and supplies needed to maintain health.

CRITICAL THINKING APPLICATION   29.2

Quite a few of the elderly patients at WMFM have diabetes type 2. Based on what you have learned about the difficulty of managing diabetes in aging people, what factors do you need to consider when conducting patient education for an elderly person with diabetes? Are there any community resources that might be useful for patients and their families?

Gastrointestinal System

Age-related changes in the gastrointestinal system begin in the mouth with dental problems:

- a decrease in the number of taste buds
- a decrease in the production of saliva
- a diminishing sense of smell

Older people generally find eating less pleasurable, have a reduced appetite, and are unable to chew and lubricate their food as well as younger people. This makes *dysphagia* (difficulty swallowing) a common age-related problem. Aging also brings a decrease in the production of hydrochloric acid, which affects the digestion of calcium and iron. Secretion of intrinsic factor, a protein that is needed for the absorption of vitamin B_{12}, also declines. This affects the function of the nervous system. It also affects the formation of red blood cells, resulting in excessive fatigue. It is not unusual for aging patients to be on regular vitamin B_{12} replacement therapy, either by oral dosage or by injection.

Food passes more quickly through the small intestine, resulting in poorer absorption of vitamins and minerals. **Peristalsis** in the colon decreases, making aging patients more susceptible to constipation and diverticular disease. Poor eating habits, a reduced fluid intake, and some medications (e.g., antidepressants, diuretics, antacids containing aluminum or calcium, and medications for Parkinson disease) also contribute to constipation. The liver decreases in size and weight after age 70. It is still able to perform vital functions, but more time is required to metabolize drugs and alcohol. All of these factors combine to increase the potential for adverse drug reactions in older adults.

Aging individuals have a higher incidence of several gastrointestinal system diseases, such as:

- gastroesophageal reflux disease (GERD)
- peptic ulcers
- diverticulosis (related to lack of dietary fiber and constipation)
- cholelithiasis
- colorectal cancer

Dietary counseling and annual screenings should be part of the routine care of aging patients.

Integumentary System

The skin is the body's first line of protection against infection, and it also is responsible for preventing the loss of body fluids and regulating body temperature. Changes in the appearance and function of the integumentary system are usually caused by a combination of ordinary age-related changes and environmental factors, especially the amount of sun exposure over time. Exposure to ultraviolet light from the sun frequently is the cause of:

- wrinkles
- age spots
- blotches
- leathery, dry, loose skin

All of which are associated with aging. Changes caused by the ultraviolet light from the sun or by the normal aging process can affect all three layers of the skin: the epidermis, dermis, and subcutaneous tissue.

The cells in the epidermis reproduce more slowly as people age, and this slower regeneration causes the skin to appear thinner. The skin becomes more prone to tearing and blistering. The risk of infections increases, the healing process takes longer, and older people are more susceptible to bruising. Because the skin can be easily torn, it is important to be very careful when performing phlebotomy or covering a wound on an older patient. The use of tape should be avoided. Vitamin D synthesis, a major function of the epidermis, significantly declines in aged skin, and a decrease in the number of melanocytes increases photosensitivity.

The dermis loses 20% of its mass during the aging process, resulting in the paper-thin or transparent skin seen in older adults. The number of **collagen** cells in the dermis also declines with age, causing the skin to sag and wrinkle. Because both sweat and sebaceous glands decrease in number, aging people have difficulty tolerating higher temperatures because they perspire less. At the same time, the blood supply to the dermis decreases; this makes it difficult to regulate the body temperature and leads to an increased susceptibility to both hypothermia and heat stroke in aging individuals. Any situation in which an older adult would be exposed to extremes of cold or heat should be avoided. Make sure a blanket is available in the examining room if the air conditioning is on. Ask the person if he or she is too cold or too hot and take the necessary steps to make the patient feel more comfortable.

Atrophy of the subcutaneous layer increases the skin's susceptibility to trauma, so patients bruise much more easily. The skin is denied natural lubrication, and dry skin is one of the most common complaints among older people. In addition, fat deposits increase in the abdomen in men and in the abdomen and thighs in women as they age.

Suggestions that might help older people prevent and treat dry skin include:

- Use a room humidifier to moisten the air
- Bathe less frequently and use warm rather than hot water
- Use a mild soap or cleansing cream (e.g., Aveeno, Basis, or Dove)
- Wear protective clothing in cold weather
- Moisturize dry skin

Pain receptors are distributed throughout the skin. Because of age-related changes in the receptors, older people have a higher pain threshold. They may not notice a cut or burn as quickly as a younger person would, so a more serious burn may occur before it is noticed. In addition, wound healing becomes a problem because of decreased blood flow to dermal tissues.

Other changes occur in the skin's appendages. Hair changes in color, growth, and distribution. Hair grays because of the decreased rate of melanin production and the replacement of pigmented hair with nonpigmented hair. Women lose hair on the trunk and have increased facial hair. Although *alopecia* (loss of hair) is caused by an inherited trait, aging also causes hair loss. Hair on the eyebrows and in the nose and ears becomes coarser and longer in men. The nails of older people take longer to grow and are more brittle. Nails, particularly toenails, thicken as a result of trauma or nutritional deficiencies. It is not unusual for nails to split, making them more susceptible to fungal infections.

Seborrheic keratoses, usually referred to as "age spots," are one of the most common benign skin disorders found in the aging population. They appear as waxy, scaly papules that vary from tan to dark brown (Fig. 29.3) and typically are found in areas of sun exposure, such as the trunk, back, face, neck, extremities, and scalp. They are not dangerous but may be removed for cosmetic purposes.

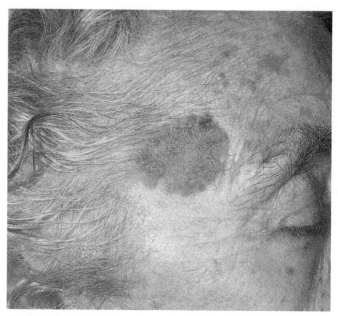

FIGURE 29.3 Seborrheic keratosis. (From Habif TP: *Clinical dermatology: a color guide to diagnosis and therapy*, ed 6, St Louis, 2016, Mosby.)

Shingles is another condition that shows up on the skin. It is caused by the same virus that causes chickenpox. A person who has had chickenpox in the past is at risk for developing shingles.

Shingles Risk Reduction

The varicella-zoster virus causes both shingles and chickenpox. After an active chickenpox infection, the virus lies dormant in a nerve **dermatome**. As people age, their risk increases that the virus will reactivate, causing the formation of blisters and varying degrees of pain along the affected nerve pathway. It is estimated that 1 in 3 adults will develop shingles in their lifetime. There are currently two shingles vaccines approved in the United States.

The older vaccine, Zostavax, was developed to reduce the risk of shingles in people age 60 and older. Zostavax is a live virus vaccine that boosts immunity against the varicella-zoster virus. The vaccine is administered as a single subcutaneous injection. Studies have shown that the vaccine reduces the risk of shingles by about half (51%) and the risk of **postherpetic neuralgia** by 67%; it is most effective in people ages 60 to 69 years.

The newer vaccine, Shingrix, also reduces the risk of shingles. Shingrix is a recombinant vaccine that also boosts immunity against the varicella-zoster virus. This vaccine is administered as an intramuscular injection. It is recommended that the two doses should be given 6 months apart. This vaccine is recommended for healthy adults 50 years and older. The two doses are 90% effective at preventing shingles and postherpetic neuralgia.

For individuals who develop shingles even though they were immunized, the duration of symptoms is shorter. The vaccine is recommended even if an individual has had shingles in the past, to help prevent future occurrences of the disease.

A shingles vaccination can be quite expensive ($200 to $300). Therefore, it is important that the patient or the medical assistant first check with the individual's insurance carrier to see whether the injection is covered.

Rose Deluca, a 71-year-old patient of Dr. Martin, is unhappy about the changes in her skin that have occurred in the past several years. Based on what Bill knows about the normal changes that occur in the skin as people age, how can he explain these changes to Mrs. Deluca, and what can he suggest to help with dryness and other typical aging changes?

Musculoskeletal System

As the body ages, changes occur in the muscles, bones, and joints that affect the individual's appearance, strength, and mobility. The extent of change depends on the person's diet, exercise pattern, and heredity. Cartilage loss and degeneration, which produce osteoarthritis, commonly occur in the weight-bearing joints of older people. Joint range of motion is affected, and the intervertebral disc spaces are decreased, causing loss of height as a person ages. A breakdown in joint structures may lead to inflammation, pain, stiffness, and deformity.

Suggestions for Helping the Older Adult With Mobility, Dexterity, and Balance Problems

- Encourage the person to use assistive devices, such as adaptive silverware, a tub seat or shower chair, electric razor, and reaching devices.
- Assist the person with gripping devices as needed (wait for the patient to place his or her hand around a cup or help him or her with it before letting go).
- Provide older adults with enough time to complete tasks independently.
- For a post-stroke patient who is ambulatory but has one weak side, use a gait belt when transferring the patient from a chair to an examination table.
- The provider may recommend physical therapy for range-of-motion exercises.
- Encourage activity approved by the provider; lack of activity results in a decline in the ability to function.

Aging brings a decrease in the strength and speed of muscle contractions in the extremities but only a slight decline in overall muscle endurance. Muscular changes in the aging patient are directly related to the individual's activity level. Research shows that musculoskeletal disease is not an inevitable result of the aging process; however, 40% to 50% of women over age 50 have a serious problem with bone demineralization. Men also experience bone loss, but at a later age, and at a much slower rate than women.

Osteoporosis

Osteoporosis is the primary cause of hip fractures, which can lead to a loss of independence and also to complications that ultimately can end in death. The spinal vertebrae also can collapse, producing the stooped posture associated with "dowager's hump." Sometimes bones break because of the sheer weight of the body on them. Often people say they fell and broke a bone, when in reality the bone fractured, causing them to fall. Multiple factors contribute to the development of osteoporosis, but it is most common in postmenopausal women. Risk factors for osteoporosis include:

- Female gender (women have a five times greater risk than men)
- Thin; small-boned frame
- Family history of osteoporosis
- Estrogen deficiency before age 45, either from early menopause or **oophorectomy**
- Estrogen deficiency resulting from an abnormal absence of menses (eating disorders, excessive aerobic exercise, fibrocystic ovaries)
- Racial background (Caucasian and Asian women have the highest risk)
- Aging
- Extended use of anticonvulsant drugs, prednisone, and excessive thyroid hormone medications
- Sedentary lifestyle, smoking, excessive alcohol intake, and lack of calcium and vitamin D when growing up

Weight-bearing exercises and calcium and vitamin D supplements are recommended to prevent demineralization of the bones. Medications used to prevent and/or treat osteoporosis include:

- alendronate (Fosamax) and risedronate (Actonel), which reduce the rate of demineralization
- raloxifene (Evista) and ibandronate (Boniva), which slow bone thinning and cause some increase in bone thickness
- denosumab (Prolia), an injectable medication, which helps increase bone mass
- calcitonin (Calcimar, Miacalcin), which is either injected or inhaled as a nasal spray and results in a decrease in the rate of bone thinning and relieves the pain associated with spinal compression

Another option is an intravenous (IV) medication, zoledronic acid (Reclast), for the once yearly treatment of postmenopausal women with osteoporosis. Reclast helps increase bone density in the spine and hip, thus reducing the risk of fractures.

Falls

The risk of injuries from falls increases with age; falls cause the greatest number of injuries in people over age 70. Aging individuals are at greater risk of falling because of sensorimotor changes in vision and mobility, osteoporosis, and cerebrovascular accidents (CVAs). Falls in older patients usually result in fractures because a large percentage of these individuals have osteoporosis. Serious fractures, such as those of the hip, require the patient to be immobile for extended periods, and this opens the door to a wide range of debilitating complications, such as:

- **decubitus ulcers**
- pneumonia
- placement in long-term care facilities
- even death

Falls are largely preventable. The medical assistant can play an active role in helping family members and patients become aware of risk factors and safety measures. Suggestions that can help patients prevent falls are:

- Have regular vision tests.
- Understand the side effects of medications, especially those that cause vertigo.

- If you experience orthostatic hypotension, rise slowly and stand still for a moment with support before moving.
- Limit the use of alcohol.
- If needed, consistently use assistive devices, such as a cane or walker, for support.
- Wear low-heeled, rubber-soled shoes with good support.
- Avoid going outside in icy weather.
- Engage in regular weight-bearing exercise for muscle and bone strength.
- Keep hallways, stairs, and bathrooms well lit.
- Assess the home for possible danger areas; remove throw rugs; use handrails on steps and grab bars in bathrooms; keep emergency numbers handy.

CRITICAL THINKING APPLICATION   29.4

The family of Rita Schaeffer, a 73-year-old patient, is concerned about the risk of falls. Mrs. Schaeffer recently was diagnosed with osteoporosis, and she lives alone. What information should Bill give the family to help them prevent accidents in their mother's home? Also, Mrs. Schaeffer's 45-year-old daughter is concerned about developing osteoporosis. What steps should the daughter take to prevent the disease?

Nervous System

Cognitive ability (i.e., the ability of a person to think) is influenced by many factors, including a person's general state of health, educational background, and genetic code. The normal process of aging may contribute to a change in the thinking process. The brain begins to get smaller at approximately age 50 and continues to get smaller as we age because of a loss of fluid within the neurons and shrinkage of dendrites. Thinning of the dendrites makes transmitting messages from one neuron to the next more difficult. As a result of all these factors, the aging brain is smaller, weighs less, and has started to pull away from the sheath or cortical mantle. Older neurons process information more slowly, so retrieving old information and learning new information takes longer. Reaction time also slows, and aging individuals are distracted more easily; however, recent research shows that the loss of brain cells is minimal and that the older brain is still capable of generating new neurons. Researchers believe that continued, moderate physical and mental activity can maintain the cognitive abilities of aging individuals.

Dementia, the severe loss of intellectual ability, is not an inevitable part of aging but rather the result of an organic disorder. Most men and women remain mentally competent until the end of their lives. Sudden loss of memory, disorientation, and trouble performing the daily tasks of life indicate a problem that should be investigated. Many conditions can cause signs and symptoms of dementia, including:

- depression
- reactions to prescription and over-the-counter (OTC) drugs
- alcoholism
- malnutrition
- thyroid, liver, heart, and vascular disorders
- Parkinson disease

Multiple factors can interfere with mental judgment and motor skills, giving the impression of decreased mental status.

The best way to ensure mental functioning in later life is to remain mentally and physically stimulated. Exercise improves memory and thinking because of its positive effect on vascular health, increasing the amount of oxygen delivered to the aging brain. Other ways to maintain mental function are to keep socially active; practice stress-reduction activities; quit smoking; drink alcohol in moderation; use hearing aids and glasses if needed to stay in touch with the world; and receive treatment for depression, diabetes, hypertension, and high cholesterol levels. Risk factors for cognitive decline include:

- Hypertension, diabetes, and heart disease (these reduce blood flow to the brain)
- Environmental exposure to lead
- High stress levels
- Sedentary lifestyle and lack of social interaction
- Low education level
- Smoking and substance abuse

Alzheimer Disease

Alzheimer disease (AD) is a progressive deterioration of the brain caused by the destruction of central nervous system (CNS) neurons, leading to problems with memory, language, thinking, and behavior. Three major changes occur in the brain:

- Amyloid plaques form.
- Neurofibrillary tangles clump together, affecting neuron function (neurons eventually die).
- The connections between neurons that are responsible for memory and learning are lost, resulting in neuron destruction; as neurons die throughout the brain, the affected regions begin to atrophy, or shrink. By the final stage of AD, damage is widespread and brain tissue has shrunk significantly.

Patients who show signs and symptoms of dementia are first evaluated for organic causes, such as systemic disease or depression. AD has no definitive diagnostic test because it can be confirmed only through examination of the brain at autopsy. If the patient shows a gradual onset of progressive difficulty with memory, functional abilities, and behavior, and has no evidence of other causes of these disturbances, the provider makes the diagnosis of AD. Imaging studies, including computed tomography (CT), magnetic resonance imaging (MRI), and positron emission tomography (PET), may help show the structural and functional changes in the brain associated with AD.

Researchers estimate that about 5 million Americans suffer from AD. The disease typically begins after age 60, and the risk of developing the disorder increases with age, although younger people as early as age 30 have been diagnosed with AD. Research shows that 1 in 10 Americans over age 65 have AD; almost 50% of people age 85 or older are diagnosed with the disease. Despite these statistics, AD is not considered a normal part of the aging process. AD is the sixth leading cause of death (across all ages) in the United States and the fifth leading cause of death for those age 65 to 85.

AD is a slowly progressive disease that begins with mild memory problems and ends with severe brain damage. The course the disease takes and how fast changes occur varies among individuals, but on average, patients live for 8 to 10 years after they have been diagnosed. Currently no treatment can stop the progression of the disease.

TABLE 29.2   Medications Approved for the Treatment of Alzheimer Disease

DRUG	STAGE OF TREATMENT	COMMON ADVERSE EFFECTS
Cholinesterase Inhibitors		
donepezil (Aricept) galantamine (Razadyne) rivastigmine (Exelon) – tablet, liquid, or topical patch	All stages Mild to moderate All stages	• Appetite loss • Dizziness • Fatigue • Increased frequency of bowel movements and diarrhea • Insomnia • Muscle cramps • Nausea, vomiting • Weight loss
Receptor Antagonist		
memantine (Namenda) – prescribed alone or in combination with donepezil	Moderate to severe	• Confusion • Constipation • Diarrhea • Dizziness • Headache

However, a great deal of research on the diagnosis and treatment of AD is under way.

The goal of treatment is to maintain normal activities as long as possible. Currently no medicines can slow the progression of AD, but the U.S. Food and Drug Administration (FDA) has approved four medications for the treatment of AD symptoms (Table 29.2). These drugs help individuals carry out the activities of daily living by maintaining thinking, memory, or speaking skills. They can also help with some of the behavioral and personality changes associated with AD. However, they will not stop or reverse AD, and they appear to help individuals for only a few months to a few years. Cholinesterase inhibitors improve the production of neurotransmitters in the brain, which helps prevent memory loss from becoming worse for a limited time. These drugs do not help everyone; as many as 50% of patients show no improvement in mental function. Memantine (Namenda) was the first drug to be approved for the treatment of moderate to severe AD, although it also has limited effects. Individuals with AD frequently experience changes in behavior, so medications may be prescribed to help control sleeplessness, agitation, wandering, anxiety, and depression. Treating these problems helps make the patient more comfortable while easing the burden on caregivers.

Supportive care for family members is absolutely essential because they are faced with caring for a loved one who is suffering progressive memory loss. The medical assistant can be especially helpful in recommending educational workshops, support groups, and stress management skills for caregivers. Multiple resources are available, including online information and support groups, which family members may find helpful.

Sleep Disorders

Complaints of sleeping difficulties increase with age. The amount of time spent sleeping may be slightly longer than in a younger person, but the quality of sleep declines. Older people are often light sleepers and have periods of wakefulness in bed. Rapid eye movement (REM) sleep is the stage of sleep in which people experience dreaming. Non-REM sleep is the period of deepest sleep. The amount of time spent in the deepest stages of sleep decreases with age. Sleep that is disturbed or that leaves the person feeling tired is not part of the aging process and may indicate some underlying emotional or physical problem. Lack of sleep can result in restlessness, disorientation, "thick" speech, and mispronounced words. Often, these symptoms are mistaken for signs of dementia. Other factors that might influence sleep patterns are medications, caffeine, alcohol, depression, and environmental or physical changes.

Common sleep problems in older adults include dyssomnias, such as periodic limb movement disorder (PLMD), in which periodic jerking of the legs occurs during sleep, and sleep apnea. This is common among overweight individuals and can occur frequently during the night, interrupting sleep. Numerous medical conditions can interfere with sleep, including:
- joint and bone pain
- Parkinson disease (because of difficulty changing positions)
- congestive heart failure
- chronic obstructive pulmonary disease (COPD)
- diabetes mellitus, which increases **nocturia**
- depression
- certain medications (e.g., beta blockers can cause nightmares, antidepressants increase PLMD, and barbiturates may result in nightmares or hallucinations)

It is important to be aware of the effect of sleep problems because often these can be confused with dementia. Patients who are experiencing difficulty with sleeping should be encouraged to document their sleeping patterns, napping patterns, medications, diet, exercise routines, and any events that have resulted in a change of lifestyle. They should discuss this problem with their provider. Simple modification of behavioral patterns may resolve the problem. Taking fewer naps, completing exercise several hours before bedtime, changing eating times, reducing the amount of alcohol and caffeine ingested, drinking a glass of milk before bedtime, or changing medications or the time they are taken all are suggestions that might alter the factors responsible for sleep disturbances.

If behavioral approaches are not effective, medications may be considered for short-term use only, because they have a high incidence of physical and psychological dependence. Elderly people are especially susceptible to side effects from these drugs, such as next-day drowsiness and temporary memory loss. Sedatives or hypnotics that may be prescribed include zolpidem (Ambien), eszopiclone (Lunesta), zaleplon (Sonata), and ramelteon (Rozerem).

Pulmonary System

Maximum lung function decreases with age. The rate of airflow through the bronchi slowly declines after age 30, and the maximum force one is able to achieve on inspiration and expiration declines. The lungs lose their elasticity because of changes in **elastin** and collagen. They become smaller and flabbier. The alveoli enlarge, their walls become thinner, and the number of capillaries is reduced. As a result, the area for gas exchange in the lungs is reduced. The chest wall may stiffen from osteoporosis of the ribs and vertebrae and calcification of the costal cartilage. The respiratory muscles become weaker, making it harder to move air into and out of the lungs. To compensate, older adults rely more on accessory muscles, such as the diaphragm. Weakening of the respiratory muscles and stiffening of the chest wall make it harder to cough deeply enough to clear mucus from the lungs. Pulmonary function tests reveal a decrease in vital capacity and an increase in residual volume. The incidence of sleep apnea and sleep disorders increases, causing a potential problem with nocturnal hypoxemia. All these factors combine to put the older adult at greater risk for pneumonia and aspiration and for reactivation of tuberculosis.

The larynx also changes with aging, causing a change in the pitch and quality of the voice. The voice sounds quieter and slightly hoarse. The individual's voice may sound weaker, but it should not interfere with the ability to effectively communicate.

Sensory Organs
Vision

By the time a person reaches age 50, structural and functional changes in the eye become noticeable (Table 29.3). The eyebrows and eyelashes start to gray. The skin around the eyelids wrinkles, and the loss of orbital fat allows the eye to sink deeper into the orbit. The cornea increases in thickness and has reduced refractive power. A yellow-gray ring (arcus senilis) may develop on the periphery of the cornea. The iris loses pigmentation, and as a result older people appear to have gray eyes.

The lens of the eye continues to grow. As new lens fibers grow, old lens fibers are compressed and pushed to the center, causing the lens to become denser. The lens becomes flatter, thicker, less elastic, and more opaque, progressively yellowing with age. By age 70, the

lens has tripled in mass. Clouding of the lens causes light rays to scatter, creating glare.

The pupil is designed to adjust to control the amount of light entering the eye. The ciliary muscle that causes the pupil to dilate weakens during the aging process. As a result, a reduction in the size of the pupil occurs, limiting the amount of light available to reach the retina. Tear production normally decreases. Tear glands do not make enough tears, or the tears are of poor quality and do not keep the eyes wet enough. Eye irritation and excessive tearing are a result of decreased **lacrimation**.

By the early to mid-40s, *presbyopia* develops, which makes it difficult to focus in detail on objects close at hand. This requires the use of corrective lenses to accommodate age-related farsightedness. The ability to refocus quickly from far to near or near to far decreases. Also, the ability to follow a moving object is decreased. The yellowing of the lens causes it to act like a filter, making it difficult to distinguish certain color intensities. Blues, greens, and violets are hard to differentiate, whereas yellows, reds, and oranges are easier to identify. The loss in the ability to discriminate closely related colors can affect the older person's ability to judge distances or his or her depth perception. This increases an aging person's susceptibility to falls and accidents. Stairs become a potential hazard because the edges of the steps cannot be seen clearly.

Older people need as much as six times more light to read; however, increasing the level of light does not completely compensate for visual decline because the elderly also experience an increased sensitivity to glare. Glare is probably one of the most painful experiences for the aging eye. Exposed light bulbs, such as those used in chandeliers, and light from highly reflective surfaces, such as glass tables and floors, can produce excessive glare. The eye has a decreased ability to respond to abrupt changes from light to dark or dark to light. Going from a well-lit waiting room into a dim hallway or negotiating the way down dimly lit aisles in a movie theater could be treacherous for an older person.

Cataracts, Glaucoma, and Macular Degeneration. Eye diseases and disorders that occur frequently in older individuals are:

- cataracts
- glaucoma
- macular degeneration

Cataracts are cloudy or opaque areas in the lens that cause blurring of vision; rings or halos around lights and objects; and a blue or yellow tint to the visual field (Fig. 29.4). Surgical lens extraction and implantation with an artificial lens improves vision in 95% of cases. The procedure, which is performed in an outpatient facility, involves a small incision to remove the lens, laser therapy, or *phacoemulsification* (ultrasonic vibrations), which breaks up the lens and removes it without the need for an incision. After the procedure, patients must avoid bending or lifting heavy objects for 3 to 4 weeks; wearing an eye shield at night and glasses during the day helps protect the eye until it heals. Recovery takes about 2 weeks.

Glaucoma is a result of blockage of the outflow of aqueous humor, which causes an increase in intraocular pressure and damage to the optic nerve. If not treated, glaucoma can cause progressive loss of peripheral vision and ultimately lead to blindness; however, it can be treated with medication.

The *macula* is the part of the eye responsible for sharp vision and color. Damage to or breakdown of the macula is called *macular*

TABLE 29.3   Age-Related Changes in the Anatomic Structures of the Eye

STRUCTURE	AGE-RELATED CHANGE	EFFECTS
Lens	Thickens, becomes more opaque	Decreased refraction, causing blurred vision; decreased color acuity; cataracts
Anterior chamber	Decrease in size and volume	May develop increased intraocular pressure and glaucoma
Ciliary muscles	Affects pupil constriction and dilation	Limits light accommodation; night blindness
Cornea	Thickens, curve decreases	Problems with refraction
Retina	Decrease in number of rods and cones	Decreased clarity; requires increase in minimum amount of light needed to see clearly

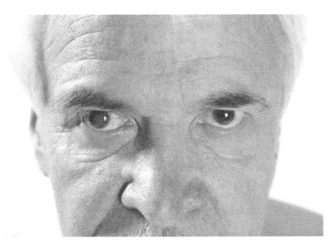

FIGURE 29.4 Cataracts. (https://www.mayoclinic.org/diseases-conditions/cataracts/symptoms-causes/syc-20353790)

degeneration, which causes progressive loss of the central field of vision. Macular degeneration is the leading cause of blindness in aging people. (All three of these eye disorders are discussed in more detail in Chapter 16, Ophthalmology and Otolaryngology.)

Suggestions for Helping the Visually Impaired Older Adult

- Ask the person if he or she wants assistance.
- When escorting an older person, regardless of whether he or she is visually impaired, allow the patient to place his or her hand above your elbow. It is easier for the person to follow your movements. This method also provides a source of support and security.
- Use high levels of evenly distributed, glare-free light.
- Ask the pharmacist to use large lettering when labeling medicine bottles.
- Use paper that has a non-glare finish and large print for forms and educational materials.
- Make distinct differences (e.g., size of containers or color coding with bright primary colors) for pills that are similar in size and color.
- Place all objects within the visual field and prevent clutter.

Hearing

Hearing loss can have a profound psychological effect on aging people, causing depression, social withdrawal, and feelings of isolation. Hearing loss occurs gradually over a long period and may go undetected by the older person and healthcare providers. Lack of attention when addressed, inappropriate responses, asking to have statements repeated, and speaking too loudly or too softly often are signs of hearing loss. Changes in hearing begin around age 30. By age 65, one out of three people has a hearing loss, and the number increases to 65% of those over age 80. Age-related hearing loss usually is caused by a dysfunction or loss of cochlear cilia, resulting in an inability to hear high-frequency sounds and difficulty understanding speech. Hearing impairment is compounded by impacted cerumen, otitis media, otosclerosis, **Ménière's disease**, long-term exposure to intense noise, and certain **ototoxic** drugs, such as aspirin.

Presbycusis is associated with normal aging and causes a decreased ability to hear high frequencies and to discriminate sounds. Parts of a conversation may be missed because the sound of the word goes above the 2000-cycle frequency. Often words that sound similar are difficult to differentiate. Consonants such as *g, f, s, sh, t,* and *z* produce high-pitched sounds that are more difficult to hear and differentiate. Low-frequency pitched sounds, such as the vowels *a, e, i, o,* and *u,* may be more easily heard by people with presbycusis. Inability to hear different frequencies combined with low background noise from groups of people talking, noise from appliances, or busy public places compromises an older person's ability to hear clearly. Hearing aids, which can be used to amplify speech, may increase background noises, resulting in sensory overload.

Another hearing disorder common among older people is *tinnitus*, a ringing or buzzing in the ear. It can be caused by:

- impacted cerumen
- ear infection
- use of antibiotics
- reaction to a medication
- nerve disorder

Tinnitus can cause difficulty understanding conversational speech and can make sleeping difficult because of the continuous sensation of ringing in the ears.

Hearing loss, with its resultant isolation, is directly related to the development of depression in older adults. Treatable depression often is overlooked in elderly people because of coexisting physical illnesses that mask the symptoms of depression. The medical assistant may be able to contribute to information about depression in elderly patients through conversations with the individual and family members. The provider may use or may train the medical assistant to use the Geriatric Depression Scale Short Form, which includes questions for the patient about daily activities, interests, and feelings to help diagnose depression in the ambulatory setting (Fig. 29.5).

Suggestions for Helping the Hearing-Impaired Older Adult

- Stand in the patient's direct line of vision and gently touch the person to get his or her attention.
- Use gestures, pictures, and large, bold print to communicate.
- Talk in short sentences into the ear with better hearing.
- Do not increase the volume of your speech; this also raises the frequency of the voice, which is the hearing most impaired in aging people. Use expanded speech; lower the tone of your voice and talk in distinct syllables.
- Avoid background noise. Give instructions in a quiet room with the door closed. If the patient has a hearing aid, make sure it is on.

Taste and Smell

During the aging process the abilities to taste and smell decline subtly. Deterioration and atrophy of the taste buds are part of the aging process. The ability to taste salt and sweet flavors is reduced, whereas the ability to detect bitter and sour flavors remains relatively the same. As a result, food frequently tastes bland and unappetizing. Patients on salt-restricted diets and patients with diabetes must be

GERIATRIC DEPRESSION SCALE (SHORT FORM)

Choose the best answer for how you have felt over the past week:

1. Are you basically satisfied with your life? YES / **NO**
2. Have you dropped many of your activities and interests? **YES** / NO
3. Do you feel that your life is empty? **YES** / NO
4. Do you often get bored? **YES** / NO
5. Are you in good spirits most of the time? YES / **NO**
6. Are you afraid that something bad is going to happen to you? **YES** / NO
7. Do you feel happy most of the time? YES / **NO**
8. Do you often feel helpless? **YES** / NO
9. Do you prefer to stay at home, rather than going out and doing new things? **YES** / NO
10. Do you feel you have more problems with memory than most? **YES** / NO
11. Do you think it is wonderful to be alive now? YES / **NO**
12. Do you feel pretty worthless the way you are now? **YES** / NO
13. Do you feel full of energy? YES / **NO**
14. Do you feel that your situation is hopeless? **YES** / NO
15. Do you think that most people are better off than you are? **YES** / NO

Answers in **bold** indicate depression. Although differing sensitivities and specificities have been obtained across studies, for clinical purposes a score >5 points is suggestive of depression and should warrant a follow-up interview. Scores >10 almost always indicate depression.

FIGURE 29.5 Geriatric Depression Scale.

cautioned about the use of excessive amounts of salt and sugar. A decrease in the sense of smell accompanies the decrease in taste. Not only does this affect the individual's enjoyment of food, it also puts him or her at risk of environmental dangers, such as gas leaks, smoke, and other dangerous odors that may go undetected. Checking for gas leaks around stoves and heaters and using smoke alarms reduce some of the danger. Also, dating food when it is put in the refrigerator is a good idea.

Nutritional Status. Because of the many environmental, social, economic, and physical changes of aging, older people are at greater risk for poor nutrition, which can adversely affect their health and energy level. It is estimated that 25% of the aging population suffers from malnutrition. Nutrition screening should be part of routine primary care, to identify nutritional deficiencies and correct them before a disease process develops or to assist in the treatment of chronic disease. Patients with chronic conditions, such as cardiovascular disease, hypertension, and diabetes, can benefit from nutrition assessments and interventions. Malnourished older patients get more infections; their injuries take longer to heal; surgery is riskier for them; and their hospital stays are longer and more expensive.

The most effective method of assessing a patient's nutritional status is through a comprehensive patient interview that considers all potential stumbling blocks to adequate nutrition. The medical assistant can help determine the nutritional status of older patients by considering the following factors when conducting patient interviews:

- *Oral health:* Does the patient wear dentures, and if so, do they fit properly? Does the patient have mouth pain? Can he or she swallow without difficulty?
- *Gastrointestinal complaints:* Does the patient have anorexia, nausea, vomiting, diarrhea, or constipation? Is the patient lactose-intolerant (the incidence increases with age)?
- *Sensorimotor changes:* Does the patient have loss of vision or hearing or changes in taste and smell? Can the patient feed herself or himself? Does the patient need adaptive utensils?
- *Diet influences:* Can the patient afford, shop for, and prepare food? Are ethnic or religious influences a factor? Does the patient have any disease-related diet restrictions? What is the patient's alcohol consumption?
- *Social and mental influences:* Is the patient depressed, lonely, or isolated? Are support systems available?

CRITICAL THINKING APPLICATION   **29.5**

Multiple sensory changes occur as people age. Dr. Perez asks Bill to develop a handout for patients and family members to help them understand these normal, age-related sensorimotor changes and also adaptations that can improve communication. What information should Bill include?

Urinary System

As the body ages, structural changes in the kidneys cause the urinary system to become less efficient. Between the ages of 40 and 80, the kidney loses about 20% of its mass. The number of functional nephron units decreases. Blood flow to the kidneys is reduced because of a decrease in cardiovascular efficiency. Because of the reduction of blood flow to the kidneys and the decreased number of nephrons, the kidneys become less efficient at filtering waste from the blood. This results in a more diluted, less concentrated urine. The kidneys require more water to excrete the same amount of waste. Medication takes longer to be removed from the body. Older adults are at increased risk for toxic levels of medication in the bloodstream because of this reduced filtration rate.

Fibrous connective tissue replaces the smooth muscle and elastic tissue in the bladder. This thickening of the bladder wall reduces the bladder's ability to expand. The bladder's capacity to store fluid comfortably is reduced from 400 to 250 mL. These structural changes lead to increased frequency of urination and urinary retention. Older adults are at increased risk of urinary tract infections because of residual urine. Sleep is interrupted by the need to void during the night. The sensation of bladder fullness is not recognized as quickly by the older brain. Reduced time between awareness of the need to void and involuntary urination can cause anxiety. Often, older adults reduce their fluid intake to prevent possible embarrassment. Unfortunately, this causes dehydration and an increased risk of urinary tract infections. Another change is loss of muscle tone in the urethra. In addition, the pelvic floor muscles in an aging woman relax as a result of decreased estrogen levels or previous pregnancy and childbirth.

Despite these changes, the kidneys have great reserve capacity and are able to continue functioning normally. *Urinary incontinence*, the involuntary loss of urine, is a significant problem for aging patients but is not a normal part of the aging process. Changes in the urinary system make older people more vulnerable to incontinence, but factors such as infection, confusion, difficulty with mobility, and side effects of medications contribute to the development of the problem. Incontinence is both an emotional and a physical problem. To avoid the risk of an embarrassing accident, people with this problem may avoid social occasions or activities they enjoy. Often people are too embarrassed to admit they have this condition, or they believe it is just part of aging. Once the condition has been diagnosed by a urologist, pelvic floor muscle exercises, medication, or surgery may be recommended.

Reproductive System

Aging brings a decrease in circulating levels of the female hormones estrogen and progesterone, whereas androgen levels increase. The results of this decrease are changes in the genital tract. The vagina diminishes in width and length and becomes less elastic. The cervix, uterus, and ovaries decrease in size. Vaginal secretions decline; therefore, lubrication diminishes, resulting in vaginal dryness. Bacterial or yeast infections may occur because vaginal secretions are less acidic. Estrogen cream applied to vaginal tissue may be prescribed by the provider for help with dryness and thinning of the vaginal tissue. The patient should discuss the benefits and risks of estrogen replacement therapy with the provider to determine whether it should be used.

Even though sperm production may decline in men over age 50, men remain virile well into old age. However, they experience a change in hormonal levels of testosterone, and these changes can affect the prostate gland. The prostate enlarges over time and presses down on the urethra, causing difficulty with urination. Surgery may be required to remove excess portions of the gland. Unfortunately, the operation may cause impotence, which can be treated medically with erectile dysfunction medications.

Men experience some changes in sexual functioning as they age. It takes longer for the penis to become erect, longer for an orgasm to occur, and longer to recover. Direct stimulation may be required before an erection occurs, and when it does, it may be less firm than in younger years.

Some drugs and illnesses can interfere with sexual function. Drugs used to control high blood pressure, antihistamines, antidepressants, and some stomach acid blockers, in addition to the diseases diabetes, arthritis, and arteriosclerosis, can have an adverse effect on sexual function. Often people who have had heart surgery or a heart attack are concerned about sexual activity. Patients need to feel comfortable and should not be embarrassed to discuss their concerns openly with their provider. It is important for healthcare practitioners to dismiss the myth that older patients have lost the desire for and interest in sexual intercourse.

THE MEDICAL ASSISTANT'S ROLE IN CARING FOR THE OLDER PATIENT

Elderly patients in the ambulatory care setting present a specific set of needs that require a certain amount of accommodation by the staff. For example, aging patients typically require more time to perform tasks and have questions answered. The office staff may want to hurry them so that the day's schedule can be maintained. In the best interests of the patient, however, he or she should be treated with respect and given whatever time is needed to prepare for examinations, ask questions and receive answers, and have procedures explained. A system that is sensitive to the needs of older patients:

- schedules longer periods for appointments
- has adequate lighting in the waiting room
- provides forms in large print
- has an examination room equipped with furniture, magazines, and treatment folders especially designed for older adults
- invites a professional in the management of older patients for in-service training

The primary issue in elder care is effective communication. How you communicate with people is often influenced by what you know or do not know about them. Older people are subject to many changes that affect how they are able to interact with their environment. It is important to recognize these changes and to investigate one's personal perception of older people to break down the barriers that prohibit effective communication.

As people age, they frequently experience a loss of control over their lives because of physical disabilities, economic constraints, and institutional living. Part of the medical assistant's job is to help aging people maintain their dignity and independence while in the ambulatory care setting. Remember, each patient, regardless of his or her education, socioeconomic status, or age, deserves to be treated with compassion and respect. Ask the patient directly what is wrong rather than discussing the patient with family members. It also is important to listen carefully and to be specific and sincere when responding. When a patient is talking, take time to allow him or her to complete the sentence; do not finish it for the person. Give the patient your full attention rather than continuing with other tasks while he or she is speaking. Older people may take a little longer to process information, but they are capable of understanding. Do not hurry through explanations or questions; rather, take time to review a form or give instructions as needed.

Suggestions for Effective Communication With Aging Patients

- Address the patient as Mr., Mrs., or Ms. unless the patient has given you permission to use his or her first name.
- Introduce yourself and explain the purpose of a procedure before performing the procedure.
- Face the aging person and softly touch the individual to get his or her attention before beginning to speak.
- Use expanded speech, gestures, demonstrations, or written instructions in block print.
- If the message must be repeated, paraphrase or find other words to say the same thing.
- Observe the patient's nonverbal behavior for cues indicating whether he or she understands.
- Provide adequate lighting without glare.
- Allow patients time to process information and take care of themselves unless they ask for assistance.

- Conduct communication in a quiet room without distractions.
- Involve family members as needed for continuity of care.
- When leaving a telephone message, remember to speak slowly and clearly and repeat the message in the same manner. It is difficult to interpret a message, and even more difficult to write it down, if the message was delivered in a hurried manner.
- Use referrals and community resources for support, such as:
  - Alzheimer's Association: *http://www.alz.org/* (1-800-272-3900).
  - American Council of the Blind: *http://acb.org/* (1-800-424-8666): Provides referrals to state and other organizations that provide services and equipment for the blind.
  - American Speech-Language-Hearing Association: *http://www.asha.org/* (1-800-638-8255): Offers information on hearing aids, hearing loss, and communication problems in older people and provides a list of certified audiologists and speech pathologists.
  - Arthritis Foundation Information Line: *http://www.arthritis.org* (404-872-7100): Makes referrals to local chapters and provides information on various types of arthritis.
  - American Diabetes Association: *http://www.diabetes.org/* (1-800-342-2383): Provides information and support for those with diabetes.
  - Eldercare Locator: *http://www.eldercare.gov/Eldercare.NET/Public/Index.aspx* (1-800-677-1116): Run by the National Association of Area Agencies on Aging; help line provides information on contacting local chapters that oversee services to older adults.
  - National Institute on Aging Information Center: *http://www.nia.nih.gov/* (1-800-222-2225): Provides information on aging health issues for patients, families, and healthcare professionals.
  - National Meals-on-Wheels Foundation: *http://www.mowaa.org/* (1-888-998-6325).

CLOSING COMMENTS

Patient Coaching

The medical assistant must keep in mind the sensorimotor changes that accompany aging, and also respectful patient communication, when conducting patient education with older patients. Remember, the aging process does not affect a person's ability to learn; it just may take longer to process the information, and the material may need to be repeated for understanding. Showing sensitivity to the needs of aging learners ensures successful patient education and improves compliance with prescribed treatment plans. The current aging population generally is respectful toward authority; therefore, if the medical assistant cannot gain the patient's cooperation, the provider may be able to provide authoritative reinforcement of material. General guidelines for effective patient education with older adults include:

- The patient may have short-term memory loss, so you may need to repeat the information using different words.
- The patient may be distracted more easily, so learning in a group may be difficult.

- The patient may take longer to process information, so teach at a pace that matches the patient's needs.
- Provide the patient with handouts that have large print and block letters for reviewing information at home.
- Involve family members as needed for continuity of care; supply provider-approved websites for reference.

Legal and Ethical Issues

One legal issue in the care of aging patients is the possibility of elder abuse, neglect, and exploitation. Mistreatment of aging people occurs at all social, racial, and economic levels. The abuse may be physical, mental, sexual, material, or financial; it may involve neglect or failure to provide adequate care, or it may involve self-neglect when aging people are unable or refuse to care for themselves. Abuse, neglect, and exploitation of elders by their caregivers may be difficult to identify. The aging victim could feel embarrassed, guilty, or afraid to report the abuse. Indications that a patient may be a victim of elder abuse, neglect, or exploitation are:

- Poor general appearance and poor hygiene
- Pattern of changing doctors and frequent emergency department visits
- Skin lesions, signs of dehydration, bruises (signs of new and old bruising together), abrasions, welts, burns, or pressure sores
- Recurrent injuries caused by accidents
- Signs of malnutrition and weight loss without related illness
- Any injury that does not fit the given history

If abuse, neglect, or exploitation is suspected, interviewing the caregiver and questioning the demands of care and self-reported perceptions of stress levels may help the provider detect the problem. Many states now have laws that require reporting of suspected elder abuse, neglect, or exploitation. Check your state laws to determine the requirements for healthcare workers.

Patient-Centered Care

When medical assistants work with the geriatric population, the subject of living arrangements will likely come up. At any given time, only 5% of the elderly population lives in long-term care facilities. According to information published by the National Institute on Aging, older people live close to their children and are in frequent contact with them. People prefer to age in place; that is, they want to live in their own home environment as long as possible. Individuals are admitted to nursing homes because they are no longer able to perform activities of daily living, such as bathing, dressing, eating, walking, and maintaining bladder and bowel continence. They also have difficulty with grocery shopping, housekeeping, and money management. Chronic health conditions and accidents interfere with the older person's ability to perform these tasks.

Many resources are available to help seniors maintain their independence. Outreach programs, such as Meals on Wheels, deliver nutritious meals to the homes of older adults. Senior centers serve as a focal point for many activities and as a source of information. Transportation services provide rides to doctors' appointments, day care centers, shopping centers, and community events. Home health agencies provide several types of services, including personal care, shopping, transportation, and meal preparation. Some home health agencies provide a range of activities, from patient education to IV therapy; medical-social services; physical, speech, and occupational therapies; and nutrition and dietary counseling. Advanced technology allows people to receive services at home that formerly were provided only in a hospital or a physician's office.

Adult day care centers provide socialization, recreation, meals and, in some centers, physical therapy, occupational therapy, and transportation. These centers offer supervision for older adults who may be taken care of by family members in the evening but need care during the day. They also serve as respite for a caregiver.

Assisted-living facilities can be retirement homes or board-and-care homes. These facilities are appropriate for older adults who need assistance with some activities of daily living, such as bathing, dressing, and walking. Skilled nursing facilities provide 24-hour medical care and supervision. In addition to medical care, residents receive care that may include physical, occupational, and speech therapies. The objective of treatment is to improve or maintain the person's abilities.

Professional Behaviors

Your future employers will expect you to use problem-solving techniques, including recognizing and defining a problem, analyzing the issue, and developing a plan of action. Elderly patients typically have multiple health problems that are frequently complicated by physical, psychological, and environmental factors. To provide quality care for these individuals, you must look at their health issues in a holistic way, taking into consideration all the factors that affect their eventual ability to follow treatment plans and improve their health status. Part of the process involves identifying resources that might help the aging person be better equipped to take care of himself or herself. Consistently using community and online resources may mean the difference between an aging person being able to stay in the home or having to go to long-term care. The professional medical assistant can play a crucial role in providing assistance to aging clients.

SUMMARY OF SCENARIO

Bill has learned to understand the special needs of aging patients. He used to think that most older people were chronically sick and would ultimately end up in long-term care facilities. Now he understands that most aging people lead healthy, active lives and that the disorders that occur in later life usually are the result of lifestyle factors, such as diet and lack of exercise. Bill also has learned how to communicate effectively with older patients and to conduct patient interviews so as to evaluate the patient's physical, mental, emotional, and nutritional health.

SUMMARY OF LEARNING OBJECTIVES

1. **Do the following related to the cardiovascular, endocrine, gastrointestinal, integumentary, and musculoskeletal body systems:**
   - *Explain the changes in the anatomy and physiology caused by aging.*
     Table 29.1 summarizes changes associated with aging that occur across all body systems. Normal age-related changes are expected, and the individual can compensate for them. However, these changes intensify with poor health habits and chronic disease. Age-related changes can be managed through regular exercise, a healthy diet, prevention of sun damage, and annual physical examinations with health screening.
   - *Summarize the major related diseases and disorders faced by older patients.*
     Major health issues of older people are related to an increase in atherosclerosis and potential cardiovascular disease; hypertension; diabetes mellitus type 2; integumentary system changes; arthritis; osteoporosis; and an increased risk of injury from falls.
2. **Do the following related to the nervous system, pulmonary system, sensory organs, urinary system, and reproductive systems:**
   - *Explain the changes in the anatomy and physiology caused by aging.*
     Cognitive ability is influenced by many factors, including the aging process. Maximum lung capacity also decreases with age. By the age of 50, structural and functional changes in the eye become noticeable. Hearing loss occurs gradually over a long period and

can go undetected. The ability to taste and smell declines subtly as a person ages. The structural changes in the kidney also cause the urinary system to become less efficient. Finally, aging brings a decrease in circulating levels of the female hormones estrogen and progesterone and an increase of androgen.
   - *Summarize the major related diseases and disorders faced by older patients.*
     Alzheimer disease is a progressive deterioration of the brain caused by the destruction of CNS neurons; it develops in three stages. Various structures of the eye are affected by aging. Presbycusis, which is associated with normal aging, diminishes the older person's ability to hear high frequencies and to discriminate sounds.
   - *Describe various screening tools for dementia, depression, and malnutrition in again adults.*
3. **Summarize the role of the medical assistant in caring for aging patients.**
   The medical assistant's role in caring for the older patient is to develop effective communication skills that accommodate age-related sensorimotor changes; to allow time for longer appointments; to provide adequate lighting and forms in large print; and to develop appropriate in-service training as requested by the provider. Examination rooms should have furniture and treatment folders especially designed for the elderly patient. Referrals and community resources should be used for patient and family support.

Continued

SUMMARY OF LEARNING OBJECTIVES—*continued*

4. Describe the principles of effective communication with older adults.

Effective communication with aging patients includes addressing the patient with an appropriate title; introducing yourself and explaining the purpose of a procedure before touching the patient; establishing eye contact and getting the patient's attention before beginning to speak; using expanded speech, gestures, demonstrations, or written instructions in block print; repeating the message as needed for understanding; observing the patient's nonverbal behaviors for cues that indicate whether he or she understands; allowing time to process information; preventing distractions; and involving family members as needed.

5. Differentiate among independent, assisted, and skilled nursing facilities.

Aging people prefer to remain in their home environment for as long as possible. Adult day care centers can provide supervision for older adults who may be taken care of by family members in the evening but need care during the day. Assisted-living facilities are appropriate for older adults who need assistance with some activities of daily living. Skilled nursing facilities provide 24-hour medical care and supervision.

PROCEDURE 29.1   Understand the Sensorimotor Changes of Aging

Task: To role-play an older adult so as to better understand the needs of aging people.

EQUIPMENT and SUPPLIES

- Yellow-tinted glasses, ski goggles, or laboratory goggles
- Pink, white, yellow "pills" (e.g., various colors of Tic Tac mints)
- Petroleum jelly (e.g., Vaseline)
- Cotton balls
- Eye patches
- Tape
- Utility gloves
- Tongue depressors
- Elastic bandages
- Medical forms in small print
- Pennies
- Button shirts
- Walker

PROCEDURAL STEPS

1. Role-play vision and hearing loss.
   - Put two cotton balls in each ear and an eye patch over one eye. Follow your partner's instructions.
   - *Partner:* Stand out of the line of vision (to prevent lip-reading). Without using gestures or changing your voice volume, tell your partner to cross the room and pick up a book.
2. Role-play yellowing of the lens of the eye.
   - Line up "pills" of different pastel colors.
   - *Partner:* Pick out the different colors while wearing the yellow-tinted glasses.

3. Role-play difficulty with focusing.
   - Put on goggles smeared with petroleum jelly and follow your partner's directions.
   - *Partner:* Stand at least 3 feet in front of your partner and motion for him or her to come to you (your partner is deaf, so talking will not help).
4. Role-play loss of peripheral vision.
   - Put on goggles with black paper taped to the sides.
   - *Partner:* Stand to the side, out of the field of vision, and motion for your partner to follow you.
5. Role-play aphasia and partial paralysis.
   - You are unable to use your right arm or leg. Place tape over your mouth. Let your partner know you need to go to the bathroom.
   - *Partner:* Stand at least 3 feet away with your back to your partner and wait for instructions.
6. Role-play problems with dexterity.
   - Put thick gloves on your hands and try to sign your name, button a shirt, tie your shoes, and pick up pennies.
7. Role-play problems with mobility.
   - Use the walker to cross the room.
   - *Partner:* After your partner starts to use the walker, hand him or her a book to carry.
8. Role-play changes in sensation.
   - Put on a rubber utility glove; turn on very warm water; test the difference in temperature between the gloved hand and the ungloved hand.
9. Summarize and share with the group your impressions of the effects of age-related sensorimotor changes.

INTRODUCTION TO THE CLINICAL LABORATORY

30

SCENARIO

Greg Stuart, a certified medical assistant (CMA) through the American Association of Medical Assistants (AAMA), graduated from a medical assisting program 4 years ago and has been working at Walden-Martin Family Medical (WMFM) Clinic ever since. He enjoys working with patients and providers, but recently WMFM Clinic decided to expand its physician office laboratory (POL). A few weeks ago, Greg transferred into the phlebotomy/laboratory area, and he has really enjoyed it so far. He loves the patient contact during the phlebotomy procedures, and every day is just a little different. He really liked the laboratory portion of his medical assistant coursework in school and wanted a new challenge at work. It has been fun to brush up on his phlebotomy skills, and he has found that he has a real talent for putting people at ease.

He is working with another laboratory CMA, Julie Salter, as he trains in the laboratory. Julie has worked in the POL for about 8 years and is happy to expand the services that are provided at WMFM Clinic. Today she is going to reintroduce Greg to the laboratory.

While studying this chapter, think about the following questions:
- What is the role of the clinical laboratory in patient care?
- What is the medical assistant's role in coordinating laboratory tests and results?
- What are the three regulatory categories established by the Clinical Laboratory Improvement Amendments (CLIA)?
- Why is it important to have quality assurance practices in the laboratory?
- What is a laboratory flow sheet and how is it used?
- What is a Safety Data Sheet (SDS), and why is it important?
- Why is it important to know safety techniques to minimize physical, chemical, and biologic hazards in the clinical laboratory?
- Why is specimen collection, including the importance of sensitivity to patients' rights and feelings when collecting specimens, important in the laboratory?
- What are the metric units used for measuring liquid volume, distance, and mass?
- What are the parts of a microscope?

LEARNING OBJECTIVES

1. Discuss the role of the clinical laboratory personnel in patient care and the medical assistant's role in coordinating laboratory tests and results.
2. Describe the divisions/departments of the clinical laboratory.
3. Explain the three regulatory categories established by the Clinical Laboratory Improvement Amendments (CLIA), and identify CLIA-waived tests associated with common diseases.
4. Identify quality assurance practices in healthcare, document the results on a laboratory flow sheet, and discuss quality control guidelines.
5. Discuss laboratory safety and the governing agencies involved in safety standards.
6. Discuss the purpose of a Safety Data Sheet (SDS), and summarize safety techniques to minimize physical, chemical, and biologic hazards in the clinical laboratory.
7. Describe the essential elements of a laboratory requisition.
8. Discuss specimen collection, including the importance of sensitivity to patients' rights and feelings when collecting specimen. Also, discuss the eight steps to follow when collecting specimens and informing patients of their results.
9. Explain the chain of custody and why it is important.
10. Discuss the measurement of time and temperature, and name the metric units used for measuring liquid volume, distance, and mass.
11. Name the parts of a microscope, and describe their functions. Also, summarize selected microscopy tests that may be performed in the ambulatory care setting.
12. Describe the safe use of a centrifuge.
13. Discuss the use of an incubator.

VOCABULARY

analyte (AN e lit) The substance or chemical being analyzed or detected in a specimen.

anticoagulants (an tee koh AG yuh lunts) Category of medication or a chemical that prevents clotting of blood.

aseptically (ay SEP tick ah lee) Free from living pathogenic organisms.

aspirate (AS puh rayt) To withdraw fluid using suction; the material removed using suction. Example: a specimen that has been removed from the body using a needle and syringe.

calibration (kal uh BRAY shun) Determining the accuracy of an instrument by comparing its output with that of a known standard or another instrument known to be accurate.

caustic (KAW stik) Capable of burning, corroding, or damaging tissue by chemical action.

control materials Manufacturer-prepared samples that have a known quantity of a specific analyte. Used for quality control purposes. Testing results should fall within a manufacturer-defined range of results. Also called controls or quality controls.

corrosive (kuh ROH siv) Causing or tending to cause the gradual destruction of a substance by chemical action.

culture media A solid, liquid, or semisolid medium designed to support the growth of microorganisms, especially bacteria and fungus.

cytology (sie TOL oh jee) The study of cells using microscopic methods.

exudates (EKS yoo dayts) Fluids with high concentrations of protein and cellular debris that have escaped from the blood vessels and have been deposited in tissues or on tissue surfaces.

forensic (fuh REN sik) Scientific tests or techniques used regarding the detection of crime.

hemolyzed (HEE muh liezd) A blood sample in which the red blood cells have ruptured.

histology (hi STOL oh jee) The study of tissues.

inhalant (in HAY lunt) Any substance that can be breathed into the lungs.

INR International Normalized Ratio; also called prothrombin time (PT). Used to test the effectiveness of blood-thinning medication.

in vitro Latin term meaning "in glass" and commonly known as "in the laboratory."

pathologist (pah THOL uh jist) A physician specially trained in the nature and cause of disease.

pure culture The growth of only one microorganism in a culture or on a nutrient surface.

quality control A process to ensure the reliability of test results, often using manufactured samples with known values.

reagent (re AY jent) A substance for use in a chemical reaction.

referral laboratory A laboratory that performs testing for another laboratory. Testing varies from high-volume routine testing to low-volume unique or unusual testing. Also called reference, diagnostic, or commercial testing laboratories. Often privately owned.

sharps Medical term for devices with sharp points or edges that can puncture or cut skin. Examples include needles, scalpels, or broken glass.

standard operating procedures Also known as SOP, a set of step-by-step instructions to help employees carry out routine operations with efficiency, high quality, and uniformity of performance.

sterile Free from all living organisms

toxicology (tok si KOL oh jee) The study and science that deal with the effects, antidotes, and detection of poisons or drugs.

Laboratory medicine is the medical discipline that applies clinical laboratory science to the care and diagnosis of patients. Patient *specimens* can be collected at the laboratory or in an ambulatory care facility. A specimen is a sample of body fluid, waste product, or tissue collected for analysis. Once in the laboratory, the specimen is processed and directed to the proper laboratory department. Each department of the lab will analyze and evaluate the specimen based on specific tests ordered by the provider. Tests can be performed *manually* (by hand) or through a variety of specialized automated instruments. Once test results are completed, they are reported to the provider.

PERSONNEL IN THE CLINICAL LABORATORY

Medical laboratories are in hospitals, ambulatory care facilities, public health departments, health maintenance organizations, and **referral laboratories**. The clinical laboratory is staffed with a variety of professionals, including the following:

- A director, who may be a **pathologist** or a clinical laboratory scientist with a doctorate degree

- Certified medical technologists (MTs) and certified medical laboratory technicians (MLTs)
- Medical laboratory assistants (MLAs), medical assistants (CMAs, RMAs), and phlebotomists

Phlebotomists and laboratory assistants have received specialized training in the collection of blood samples and the preparation of laboratory specimens. The agencies granting certifications and titles are listed in Table 30.1.

In ambulatory care facilities, the lab director may be the physician. This type of lab is referred to as a *physician office laboratory* (POL). Medical assistants are trained to properly collect patient specimens and perform specific testing procedures within the POL. They are also trained to properly collect specimens that are sent to outside reference laboratories for testing.

Laboratory tests are used for four main purposes:

- To document the good health of a patient
- To screen patients for diseases and conditions such as diabetes, high cholesterol, or urinary tract infections (UTIs)
- To help the provider diagnose a medical disease, disorder, or condition

TABLE 30.1 Certifying Agencies for Laboratory Personnel

AGENCY	TITLE	POSITION
American Society for Clinical Pathologists (ASCP)	MT (ASCP) MLT (ASCP) MLT-AD (ASCP)	Medical technologist Medical laboratory technician—certificate Medical laboratory technician—associate's degree
American Medical Technologists (AMT)	MT (AMT) MLT (AMT) MLA RMA	Medical technologist Medical laboratory technician Medical laboratory assistant Registered medical assistant
Department of Health and Human Services (DHHS)	CLT (HHS)	Clinical laboratory technologist
National Certification Agency for Medical Laboratory Personnel (NCA)	CLS (NCA) CLT (NCA)	Certified laboratory scientist Certified laboratory technician
International Society for Clinical Laboratory Technology (ISCLT)	RMT (ISCLT) RLT (ISCLT)	Registered medical technologist Registered laboratory technician
American Association of Medical Assistants (AAMA)	CMA (AAMA)	Certified medical assistant
National Healthcareer Association (NHA)	CCMA CPT CMLA	Certified clinical medical assistant Certified phlebotomy technician Certified medical laboratory assistant

From Proctor D, et al: *Kinn's the medical assistant*, ed 13, St. Louis, 2017, Elsevier.

- To help the provider decide the most appropriate treatment, to monitor the effects of medications and treatments, and to monitor a disease process

Only healthcare providers can request laboratory testing for a patient. The medical assistant is involved in the process of laboratory testing. To assume this responsibility, the medical assistant must know the following:

- Proper patient preparation
- Testing procedures common to the provider's practice
- Normal range of results for common testing

The medical assistant must carefully follow all laboratory instructions. This includes properly collecting and labeling patient specimens. Sending specimens to be tested to a laboratory will also require the medical assistant's attention to detail. Excellent communication between the team members and the patient is very important. The medical assistant should make the patient feel at ease with these procedures and hopefully gain the patient's cooperation and trust.

Clinical Laboratory Testing

Clinical laboratory testing is used in conjunction with a thorough health history and physical examination to obtain essential data for screening, diagnosis, or management of a patient's condition. The body is healthy when a state of equilibrium exists in the internal environment. This healthy state of equilibrium, called *homeostasis,* occurs when the physical and chemical characteristics of body substances are within a certain acceptable range, known as the *normal range,* or *reference range.* A normal or reference range is a numeric range of test values for which the general population consistently

shows similar results 95% of the time. A change in the internal environment of the body often results in abnormal test values that are outside the population's reference range. When a provider uses a laboratory test for diagnosis, the patient's results are compared with the reference range of values. Reference values are also useful for assessing the progress of a patient's course of treatment.

Abnormal values for a test may be seen with more than one pathologic condition. For example, a decrease in a patient's hemoglobin level is seen in iron-deficiency anemia, but also in hyperthyroidism and cirrhosis of the liver. Therefore, providers cannot rely solely on one laboratory test to make a diagnosis. They must use a combination of results obtained from the history and physical exam, and a number of diagnostic and laboratory tests.

Tests performed in a clinical laboratory range from simple screening tests of one **analyte** (e.g., measuring glucose to diagnose or monitor diabetes) to complex *profile testing*, where more than one analyte is tested from a single sample. The tests are all associated with an organ or disease (e.g., performing a lipid profile to determine the various fats in the blood). A *screening test* examines a specimen for the presence of an analyte that may indicate a disease state. Screening tests are not necessarily diagnostic for one disease; rather, they indicate that a disease state may exist. Screening tests are done routinely on patients based on their age, history, or gender. The results are often *qualitative,* which means that a numeric value is not attached to the result. Qualitative tests are reported as positive or negative. A *fecal occult blood* (FOB) test, which looks for blood in a stool specimen, is an example of a screening test; if the test is positive, further testing is needed to diagnose the cause of the condition.

TABLE 30.2 Comparison of Qualitative and Quantitative Testing

	QUALITATIVE TEST	QUANTITATIVE TEST
Definition	A numeric value is not attached to the test results; may be used as a screening test	Test results represent the amount or quantity of an analyte in a certain volume of specimen
Reported as	Positive or negative	Test result expressed as a number with units of measure attached
Example	Negative fecal occult blood (FOB)—normal result; no blood found in the stool Positive FOB—abnormal result; blood is found in the stool; could indicate a cancerous colon lesion; additional testing needed	RBCs, 5 million per cubic millimeter ($5 \times 10^6/mm^3$) Hemoglobin 15 g per deciliter (15 g/dL) Hematocrit 45%

In a *quantitative* test, the test result is expressed as a number, usually with units of measure attached to numeric values. It is essential that the quantitative test results be reported with the units of measure. See Table 30.2 for a comparison of qualitative and quantitative testing.

CRITICAL THINKING APPLICATION   **30.1**

Julie and Greg have been going over general information on laboratory testing this morning. It is important to know some terms used in the laboratory. Julie asks Greg to define a qualitative test and a quantitative test in his own words. Take a few moments to write down these definitions in your own words. Be ready to share them with your classmates.

Departments of the Clinical Laboratory

Large laboratories are divided into various departments, which may include urinalysis, hematology, chemistry, microbiology, specimen collection and processing, blood bank (immunohematology), coagulation, immunology/serology, **histology**, **cytology**, **toxicology**, and special chemistry. A POL generally performs test procedures in urinalysis, hematology, chemistry, and microbiology.

Urinalysis

Urinalysis includes the physical, chemical, and microscopic examination of urine. As part of the physical examination, the color, clarity, and specific gravity are noted. The specimen's temperature may also be measured to verify that the sample is at body temperature and, therefore, recently collected. Urine is tested with a multiple test strip, also called a *dipstick*, which tests the following analytes in urine: glucose, protein, ketones, blood, bilirubin, urobilinogen, nitrites, and pH. We will go into the details of urinalysis in Chapter 31. Microscopically, the provider may examine urine for the presence of RBCs, WBCs, and epithelial cells; mucus, casts, crystals, and microorganisms. Additional quantitative tests may be performed in the urinalysis department of a reference laboratory to confirm routine screening test results.

Hematology

Hematology is the study of blood cells and coagulation. Laboratory testing in the hematology department may be qualitative or quantitative. In a POL, screening tests for hemoglobin, hematocrit, and the

International Normalized Ratio (**INR**, a coagulation test) are typically performed in the ambulatory setting. Reference laboratories will perform blood cell counts that determine the number of RBCs, WBCs, and platelets in a blood sample. Microscopic tests determine the characteristics of cells, such as size, shape, and maturity. In addition, the hematology department performs tests to determine the coagulating ability of blood.

Chemistry

The clinical chemistry department analyzes the chemicals found in blood, cerebrospinal fluid, urine, and joint fluid (synovial fluid). Specimen testing may be done manually or with complex chemistry instruments. In a POL, procedures may include single analyte tests (of blood glucose) or multitest profiles. Chemistry profiles include tests for a number of related analytes. Lipid profiles, for example, include assessments of total cholesterol, triglycerides, and low-density lipoprotein (LDL) and high-density lipoprotein (HDL). POL chemistry analyzers are becoming more common in ambulatory care as technology becomes more compact and easier to use.

Microbiology

Microbiology involves the study of very small, infectious organisms such as bacteria, fungi, yeasts, parasites, and viruses. Specimens used in microbiology include blood, urine, sputum, cerebrospinal fluid (CSF), stool, wound material, and other biologic sources. Specimens used for microbiology testing must be collected **aseptically** in **sterile** containers.

The goal of the microbiology department is to identify the microorganism that is causing the infection. The staff will also determine the most effective antimicrobial medications, which include antibiotics. This process is called identification and sensitivity (or susceptibility) testing.

Microbiology specimens may be grown on **culture media**. Once the organism is growing and in **pure culture**, it can be identified. Organism identification tests have changed with technology and will continue to change in the future. A variety of methods and technologies are applied to identify the microorganism. Methods include biochemical, molecular, and antigen-antibody complex testing.

Sensitivity testing is performed on organisms to establish an appropriate antibiotic therapy for specific bacterium or fungi. Once again, a variety of techniques and technologies may be used to help determine which antibiotic would be most effective. In a POL this may include the following:

- Rapid strep testing may be performed to screen for strep throat
- Microbiologic specimens may be aseptically collected and then sent to a reference laboratory
- Some microscope slides may be prepared for the provider to examine

Identification and sensitivity testing are usually performed in larger centralized ambulatory care, hospital, or reference laboratories.

CRITICAL THINKING APPLICATION   **30.2**

Greg and Julie have reviewed the different areas that are common in a POL. WMFM is now doing testing in microbiology, a new area that has been added to the POL in the past 6 months. As they talk about microbiology, Julie asks the question, "Why do microbiology samples need to be collected aseptically in a sterile container?" How would you answer this question?

GOVERNMENT LEGISLATION AFFECTING CLINICAL LABORATORY TESTING

In 1988, Congress passed the *Clinical Laboratory Improvement Amendments* (CLIA). This law established quality standards for all clinical laboratory testing, and it is designed to ensure the accuracy, precision, reliability, and timeliness of patient test results, regardless of which laboratory performed the testing. A clinical laboratory is defined as any facility that performs laboratory testing on human specimens to provide information about the diagnosis, prevention, and treatment of disease or the impairment of health.

Clinical Laboratory Improvement Amendments

Under CLIA, all laboratories that perform even one type of test must meet certain federal requirements. They must register with the Centers for Medicare and Medicaid Services (CMS) as a laboratory. The registration application must be submitted to the CMS with information about the laboratory's operations. The type of certificate that is issued is based on the information provided in the application. (Note that most POLs are registered as CLIA-waived laboratories.)

The US Food and Drug Administration (FDA) is responsible for categorizing commercially marketed tests performed **in vitro**, based on the CLIA guidelines. The FDA has assumed primary responsibility for determining the CLIA complexity of all laboratory tests. Every laboratory test product is assigned to one of three CLIA categories based on the product's potential risk to public health. The CLIA categories are as follows: waived tests, moderate-complexity tests, and high-complexity tests.

CLIA-Waived Tests and Laboratories

CLIA-waived tests are defined as laboratory tests and procedures that have been approved by the FDA for home use or that are simple laboratory tests and procedures to perform. Waived tests are designed to have straightforward directions and procedures so that they have a minimal risk of incorrect results. Waived tests include tests that do the following:

- Use methodologies that are simple and accurate so that the likelihood of incorrect user results is negligible
- Pose no unreasonable risk of harm to the patient if it is performed incorrectly

Table 30.3 shows some common CLIA-waived tests performed in ambulatory care facilities registered as CLIA-waived laboratories.

The FDA's CLIA-waived database of tests is available to the public on the Internet. This database contains the commercially marketed laboratory test systems categorized by the FDA since January 31, 2000, and tests categorized by the Centers for Disease Control and Prevention (CDC) before that date. The database can be searched by test system name, specialty or subspecialty, analyte, document number, qualifier, effective date, and complexity.

Moderate- and High-Complexity Tests and Laboratories

The CLIA program oversees the quality of nearly 200,000 different laboratory procedures. Most laboratory tests are categorized by the FDA as moderate-complexity tests. Some moderate-complexity tests performed in POLs include the following:

- Hematology and chemistry: testing done on an automated analyzer
- Microbiology: Gram stain procedures
- Urinalysis: microscopic analysis of urine sediment

Moderate-complexity tests must be performed by qualified personnel as described by CLIA. High-complexity tests are generally not performed in a POL, but rather in a hospital or reference laboratory.

Laboratories that perform moderate- to high-complexity testing must meet rigorous CLIA regulations and are subject to surprise inspections every 2 years. Each laboratory that performs these tests must do the following:

- Establish a system to maintain the identification of patients' specimens throughout the testing process and ensure accurate reporting of results.
- Establish and follow written quality assurance, **quality control**, and **standard operating procedures** (SOPs).
- Participate in *proficiency testing*, which is a form of external quality control. Three times a year, the laboratory must test samples provided by an approved proficiency-testing agency. The proficiency samples are tested in the same way as patient samples. Results are then reported to the proficiency-testing agency, and the accuracy of testing is verified.
- Employ personnel that meet CLIA regulations and specific qualifications for a moderate- to high-complexity laboratory. Requirements are most rigorous for high-complexity testing.

Medical assistants can perform all CLIA-waived tests and some specific moderate-complexity tests. Additional training will be required to perform moderate-complexity tests, depending on the certification of the POL where they work. Although medical assistants cannot perform high-complexity tests, they can be involved in patient preparation, provider-directed patient education, specimen collection, and documenting results in the patient's health record.

CRITICAL THINKING APPLICATION   **30.3**

The laboratory at WMFM is a registered waived facility. List five commonly performed waived tests. What is the difference between waived testing and moderate- or high-complexity testing? List three differences, and be ready to share them with your classmates.

TABLE 30.3   CLIA-Waived Tests and Their Purposes

SPECIMEN AND TEST	PURPOSE
Dipstick or tablet reagent urinalysis (manual or automated)	Urine screening to assess or diagnose diseases such as diabetes mellitus, kidney disease, and urinary tract infection
Urine pregnancy tests: visual color comparison tests	Diagnose pregnancy
Fecal occult blood	Colorectal screening to detect hidden blood in the stool
Erythrocyte sedimentation rate, nonautomated	Diagnoses inflammatory process; increases in arthritis, infection, leukemia, and most cancers
Spun microhematocrit	Measures red blood cells; screening for certain types of anemia
STAT-CRIT hematocrit	Screening for certain types of anemia
Hemoglobin	Measures hemoglobin level in whole blood
Blood glucose by glucose-monitoring devices cleared by the FDA specifically for home use	Monitor blood glucose levels
Hemoglobin A_{1c} by single analyte instruments with self-contained or component features to perform specimen-reagent interaction	Measure A_{1c} levels to assess and manage long-term care of patients with diabetes
Cholestech LDX	Measures total blood cholesterol, triglycerides, HDL, and glucose levels
Whole-Blood i-STAT Chem8+ Cartridge	Measures ionized calcium, carbon dioxide, chloride, creatinine, glucose, potassium, sodium, urea nitrogen, and hematocrit in whole blood
Whole-blood thyroid-stimulating hormone (TSH) assay	Qualitative determination of thyroid-stimulating hormone (TSH) in whole blood
Blood mononucleosis antibodies	Rapid whole-blood test to detect heterophile antibodies to help diagnose infectious mononucleosis
Helicobacter pylori antibodies	Rapid whole-blood test to detect *H. pylori* antibodies to determine the cause of peptic ulcer
Borrelia burgdorferi antibodies	Rapid whole-blood test to detect *B. burgdorferi* antibodies to diagnose Lyme disease
Trinity Biotech Uni-Gold Recombigen HIV Test	Detects HIV-1 in a blood specimen
Nasal influenza A and B	Quick qualitative diagnosis of influenza antigens in nasal secretions or swab
Streptococcus A throat swab	Rapid strep test
Urine or blood drug tests	Multiple tests for the presence of a variety of substance abuse agents
Urine fertility and menopause tests	Detect follicle-stimulating hormone in urine
Ovulation tests; visual color comparison tests for luteinizing hormone	Detect ovulation

CLIA, Clinical Laboratory Improvement Amendments; *FDA,* US Food and Drug Administration; *HDL,* high-density lipoprotein; *HIV-1,* human immunodeficiency virus type 1.
Information summarized from the Centers for Medicare and Medicaid Services. Accessed on July 10, 2018, www.cms.gov/CLIA/downloads/waivetbl.pdf.

QUALITY ASSURANCE GUIDELINES

Quality assurance (QA) is a set of written policies and procedures that ensure the monitoring of all the processes involved before, during, and after a laboratory test is performed in order to produce reliable patient test results. It is the promise of healthcare professionals to achieve the highest degree of excellence in the care given to every patient. QA includes a comprehensive set of policies developed to

ensure excellent documentation and reliability of laboratory testing. These policies benefit the provider by reducing the liability for inaccurate reporting of test results. QA also focuses on establishing a series of operating procedures for the benefit of the patient and the medical assistant who does the laboratory testing. The QA system enables the laboratory to assess, verify, and document the quality of the laboratory process. This documentation is a way of comparing *what is happening* with *what should be happening.*

As mandated by law, QA programs monitor all aspects of laboratory activity, from specimen collection through processing, testing, and reporting steps. Programs check supplies, reagents, machinery, and actual test performance. QA includes quality control, personnel orientation, laboratory documentation, knowledge of laboratory instrumentation, and enrollment in a proficiency testing program (if the lab performs moderate- or high-complexity tests).

The Three Stages of Quality Assurance in the Laboratory

The overall process required to ensure QA in the laboratory is divided into three stages. These three stages must be applied to each test or procedure that is performed in the laboratory. If any of these steps are missed or performed incorrectly, QA has been broken.

Preanalytic Stage

1. The provider orders a test to screen, monitor, or diagnose a patient's condition.
2. A written or electronic requisition is filled out, showing the test requested, the specimen required, and where the specimen will be tested.
3. The specimen is collected, labeled, and processed.
4. The specimen is transported to the laboratory in the POL or properly prepared for offsite laboratory pickup.

Analytic Stage

1. Instruments are maintained and calibrated.
2. Controls are run and analyzed for each test method (part of ongoing quality control).
3. The specimen is tested, and the results are compared with reference ranges.
4. The test results are logged and documented in the patient's health record.

Postanalytic Stage

1. Specimens are properly discarded.
2. Analyses of control results are compared over time.
3. Patient reports from outside laboratories are logged or documented.
4. The provider interprets and signs all lab reports.
5. The patient is notified of the results in the office or is contacted by laboratory personnel.
6. The final report and all communication with the patient is documented in the patient's health record.

Accurate record keeping is one of the key responsibilities of a medical assistant. Various formats are available to record laboratory information. Most providers document patient information and testing results in electronic health records (EHRs). Some POLs still use paper records. In the case of paper records, the primary source of documentation is the *laboratory master logbook*. The logbook contains a written record for each procedure performed, the patient identification number, results obtained, the date performed, and personnel initials. The results are then sent to the provider for verification.

POLs are also required to have a procedure manual that describes how each test is performed and how the patient results are reported to the provider. Personnel are required to perform **calibration** or *optics checks* on laboratory instruments that use light detection or color change as part of the reaction process. An optics check is a specific type of calibration that assesses the optics of an electronic testing instrument or system. In addition, they must run quality control or **control materials** each day before patient testing. Each manufacturer will include instructions for running control materials for their kit, procedure, or instrument. Quality control results must be documented and readily accessible. If errors or problems occur while completing quality control, the POL must perform and document remedial actions to correct errors or problems as they are identified.

Finally, *preventive maintenance* schedules must be followed and documented. Preventive maintenance is regularly scheduled care of equipment that will decrease the likelihood of failure. It is performed and documented at regular intervals while the equipment is in good working order. Preventive maintenance includes daily cleaning and adjustment, as well as replacement of parts when necessary. Each instrument should have a paper or electronic log or worksheet for recording all changes, including daily maintenance details.

Ready? Set? Test! is an excellent online resource provided by the CDC for setting up and maintaining a CLIA-waived laboratory. Fig. 30.1 shows the checklist summary of the steps needed to assure proper CLIA-waived testing in a POL.

QUALITY CONTROL GUIDELINES

A crucial step in the QA process is running quality control (QC) specimens (see Procedure 30.1, p. 765). The purpose of QC in the laboratory is to ensure the reliability of test results while detecting and eliminating error. It is important to remember a few important terms:

- *Accuracy* is a measure of how close a test result is to the true value of the control material, as established by the manufacturer.
- *Precision* is the ability to consistently reproduce a test result.

When a series of control results show both accuracy and precision, the test is considered *reliable* and may be used for testing patients. QC monitoring is crucial because patient treatment is often based on or reinforced by the results of laboratory tests. Without QC monitoring, laboratory error is difficult to detect. Undetected laboratory errors may result in harm to the patient.

Prepared control samples are tested daily, along with patient samples. Control test results must fall within a preestablished range of results before patient results can be reported. QC samples are called *controls*. They are usually supplied with the manufacturer's prepackaged kits and are intended for use in a POL. Controls should be analyzed at specified intervals as recommended by the manufacturer.

Quality Control Examples

Examples of routine quality control testing in a POL include the following:

- Positive and negative controls supplied with pregnancy test kits are performed with each patient specimen or batch of patient specimens
- Urinalysis dipstick controls (used for chemical examination of urine) should be checked daily before patient testing and each time a new **reagent** container is opened
- Controls for automated chemistry analyses should be performed before patient testing and at specified intervals during the day, depending on the number of tests run per day and the manufacturer's recommendations

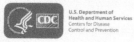

FIGURE 30.1 Summary checklist from Ready? Set? Test!

Every day that patient tests are performed, QC tests must also be performed and the results entered onto a paper or electronic graph or flow sheet. When new control materials are opened and used, the results and dates must be entered on a new flow sheet, along with the expiration dates of the controls. These records must be retained for several years; the exact number of years is determined by state law and CLIA mandates.

Another part of quality control is routine preventive maintenance. All laboratory equipment should be on a routine preventive maintenance schedule so that equipment is serviced before a breakdown occurs. Any time equipment cannot be used is an inconvenience to the patient.

Preventive Maintenance Program for Laboratory Equipment

- Follow the manufacturer's instructions for calibrating instruments.
- Read and understand the instructions for routine instrument care.
- Perform all preventive maintenance specified by the manufacturer's instructions.
- Keep spare parts available for immediate use.
- Record the name, address, and phone number of the contact person for maintenance or repair.
- Create a maintenance form, or use one provided by the manufacturer.

CRITICAL THINKING APPLICATION   30.4

As Greg and Julie are reviewing quality assurance and quality control, Greg asks Julie to clarify the differences between QA and QC. In your own words, define QA and QC. How are they different? Be ready to discuss your answer with your classmates.

LABORATORY SAFETY

The importance of safety in the laboratory cannot be overemphasized. Most laboratory accidents can be prevented using proper techniques and common sense. Following safe practices in the laboratory requires a personal commitment and concern for others. An unsafe act may also harm an innocent bystander without harming the person who performs the act.

Using a Graph for Quality Control Results

Many laboratories will use a graph to display daily quality control results. A paper graph or electronic graph file can be updated with daily QC values. Graphing advantages include the following:

- A graph is a physical representation of the QC results that can display data irregularities in an easy-to-see format.

- It displays possible *trends* (data that continue to go upward or downward in value) and *shifts* (data results that show an abrupt change in value) over time.

See the labeled graph that follows.

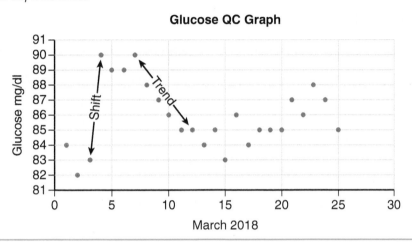

Glucose QC Graph

Safety Standards and Governing Agencies

The US government created a system of safeguards and regulations under the Occupational Safety and Health Act of 1970. This system affects nearly every worker in the United States because the regulations apply to all businesses with one or more employees (the regulations are discussed in detail in Chapter 4 in the main text). Two programs have been mandated by the Occupational Safety and Health Administration (OSHA) to ensure the safety of personnel working in clinical laboratories. One covers occupational exposure to chemical hazards; the other covers exposure to bloodborne pathogens.

The CDC also has established recommendations and resources in Standard Precautions and Transmission Precautions as they relate to specimen collection. (These recommendations were discussed in Chapter 4.)

Chemical Hazards

The clinical laboratory may have chemicals that are flammable, **caustic**, and potentially poisonous. Exposure to these dangerous chemicals can occur by breathing in fumes, direct absorption by contact with the skin, ingestion, direct contact with a mucous membrane, or entry through a cut, abrasion, or burn in the skin. OSHA is involved in regulating the standards directed at minimizing occupational exposure to hazardous chemicals in laboratories. OSHA's Hazard Communication Standard (HCS; known as the employee "right to know" rule) became law in 1991. It ensures that laboratory workers are made fully aware of the hazards associated with their workplace. The law requires the development of a comprehensive plan to put in place safe practices throughout the laboratory regarding chemicals. All workers must be provided with information and training. A Safety Data Sheet (SDS) must also be on file for all chemicals used in the laboratory. OSHA requires the manufacturer of the chemical to make

these sheets available, usually as a package insert or online. Employers must ensure that SDSs are readily accessible to employees. SDSs supply information about chemical safety and hazard information in case of an accident, spill, or fire to the user or emergency personnel.

Since June 2015, OSHA has required all SDSs to use a uniform format that includes the following section numbers, headings, and information:

Section 1. Identification
Section 2. Hazard(s) identification
Section 3. Composition/information on ingredients
Section 4. First-aid measures
Section 5. Fire-fighting measures
Section 6. Accidental release measures
Section 7. Handling and storage
Section 8. Exposure controls/personal protection
Section 9. Physical and chemical properties
Section 10. Stability and reactivity
Section 11. Toxicologic information
Section 12. Ecologic information
Section 13. Disposal considerations
Section 14. Transport information
Section 15. Regulatory information
Section 16. Other information

Please note that Sections 12 through 15 are regulated by agencies other than OSHA and are required of the manufacturers, not the employees.

In the POL, the most common hazardous chemicals are as follows:

- Sodium hypochlorite, commonly known as bleach, which is used for disinfecting laboratory work areas
- Caviwipes and glutaraldehyde, which are disinfectants
- Acetone and dyes, which are used for staining slides

It should be noted that all of these disinfectants and dyes are available in premixed sprays or wipes to reduce chemical exposure during dilution.

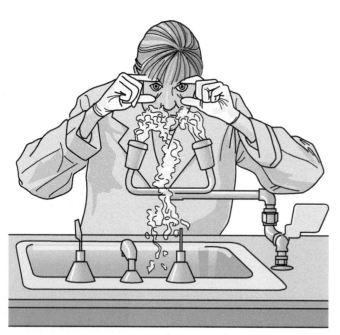

FIGURE 30.2 Eyewash station.

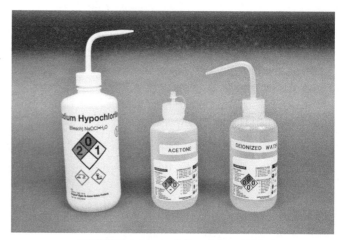

FIGURE 30.3 Laboratory bottles with chemical labels.

Following principles of proper chemical handling reduces the risk of harmful effects. The following are examples of proper chemical handling:

- If a chemical produces toxic or flammable vapors, work under a fume hood that exhausts air to the outside.
- In case of accidental exposure of the skin, rinse the affected area under running water for at least 5 minutes. Remove any contaminated clothing.
- If chemicals are splashed in the eyes, flush the eyes with water from an eyewash station (Fig. 30.2) for a minimum of 15 minutes. (See complete instructions on how to use an eyewash station in Procedure 30.2 on p. 766.)

Prompt medical attention must be given to victims of chemical exposure.

Chemical Labels

Chemicals should be tightly sealed and properly marked with the original manufacturer's labels. A hazard identification system, developed by the National Fire Protection Association (NFPA), provides information at a glance on the potential health, flammability, and chemical reactivity hazards of materials. This identification system consists of four small, diamond-shaped, colored symbols grouped into a larger diamond shape (see Fig. 30.3):

- The top diamond is red and indicates flammability (the potential to catch on fire).
- The diamond on the left is blue and indicates a health hazard such as a dangerous **inhalant** or **corrosive** acid.
- The bottom diamond is white and provides special hazard information, including recommended personal protective equipment (PPE) if biohazards are present, and other dangerous situations.
- The diamond on the right is yellow and indicates a reactivity or stability hazard. An example of reactivity is mixing an acid (e.g., bleach) with a base (e.g., ammonia), creating a dangerous gas.

The four-color system also indicates the severity of the hazard by using numbers imprinted in the diamonds from 0 to 4, with 0 representing no hazard and 4 representing an extremely hazardous substance (Fig. 30.3).

CRITICAL THINKING APPLICATION   **30.5**

Greg has a few hours to review WMFM's current laboratory safety policies and procedures on his own. There are a number of policies that apply to the laboratory only, but also many policies that apply to the entire facility. Why is it so important for employees to be aware of safety policies and procedures? Write down five reasons for being safety aware in the laboratory, and be ready to discuss your thoughts with the class.

Biohazards and Infection Control

Biohazards, or biologic hazards, are materials or situations that present the possible risk of infection (Fig. 30.4). Infection with biohazard material can occur during specimen collection, handling, transportation, or testing. Specimens with the potential to be infectious include blood, body fluids, biologic specimens, **exudates**, bacterial cultures, and smears. Infection can be introduced into the body in many ways; a few examples include the following:

- Breathing in a pathogen
- Accidental inoculation by a needlestick or **sharps** injury
- Aerosols created by uncapping specimen tubes
- Centrifuge accidents
- Entry of pathogens through a cut, abrasion, burn, or break in the skin

Standard Precautions

As described in Chapter 4, the CDC continuously monitors infection and disease in the United States. The CDC has also recommended preventive practices called Standard Precautions. These precautions apply to all patient care, regardless of the suspected or confirmed infection status of the patient. The precautions also apply to any setting where healthcare is delivered. The precautions are designed both to protect the healthcare provider and to prevent the healthcare provider from spreading infections among patients.

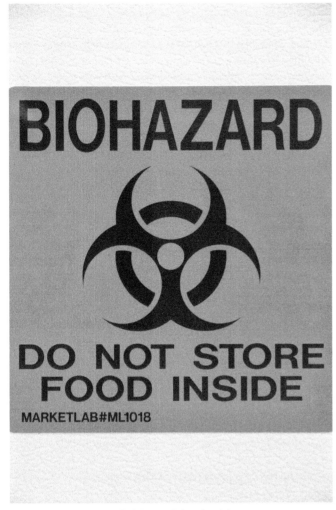

FIGURE 30.4 Biohazard symbol.

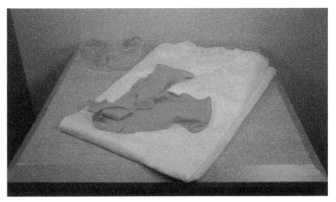

FIGURE 30.5 Personal protective equipment (PPE).

- Before and after eating
- Before and after using the restroom

After bloodborne pathogens were identified in the 1970s and 1980s, the CDC stepped up its infection control recommendations. The CDC acknowledged that all blood in all patients is potentially infectious. Therefore, they required additional monitoring and regulation for the safety of both healthcare providers and patients. These guidelines became known as *Universal Precautions.* Regulation of the new law, referred to as the Bloodborne Pathogens Standard (BBPS), was delegated to OSHA (see Chapter 4 in the main text, for additional information).

Bloodborne Pathogens Standard

OSHA's Bloodborne Pathogens Standard has been law since 1992. It regulates the handling of blood and blood products, but it also includes *other potentially infectious materials* (OPIM) that may contain bloodborne pathogens. Urine is the only fluid not specifically included in the standard. However, because blood and blood elements are frequently associated with urine, it must be included and considered a possible source of exposure.

The Bloodborne Pathogens Standard covers all employees who could "reasonably anticipate contact with blood and other potentially infectious materials as the result of performing their job duties." HBV, HCV, and HIV are a constant hazard to clinical laboratory personnel. Bloodborne pathogens are transmitted through exposure to blood and body fluids, which are the primary substances handled in the laboratory. The Bloodborne Pathogens Standard requires that the laboratory employer have a written exposure control plan that proves the following steps have been taken to protect employees:

- Written job categories of employees at risk of exposure to blood (laboratory workers are considered "high risk")
- HBV vaccination guidelines and records for each employee at risk
- Record of initial and annual Universal Precautions training for bloodborne pathogens and safety training for each employee (including proper use of safety needles)
- Definition and listing of safe work practices: personal protective equipment (PPE) for all lab personnel (fluid-impermeable lab coats that do not leave the laboratory area, gloves, face protection [Fig. 30.5]) and labeling of biohazard sharps and waste containers and their proper disposal

Standard Precautions

Standard Precautions include the following five elements:
- Hand hygiene
- Use of PPE (e.g., gloves, gowns, masks, eye protection)
- Safe needle practices
- Safe handling of potentially contaminated equipment or surfaces in the patient environment
- Respiratory hygiene/cough etiquette

According to the CDC, hand washing is the single most effective means of preventing infection. It is also the single most effective way of preventing the spread of infections. Proper hand sanitation protects you, your patient, and your co-workers, because it removes or kills potentially pathogenic organisms from the skin surface. In the laboratory, it is essential to wash your hands with soap and water or use hand sanitizer in the following situations:

- When entering the laboratory or before leaving the laboratory
- Before putting on gloves and after removing gloves
- After contact with body fluid

- Sharps injury log of all work-related needlesticks and exposures to blood, with medical intervention after exposure incidents
- Written plan to maintain privacy of the individual exposed to blood
- Documentation of employee input on new safety devices

Safety Guidelines for Other Potentially Infectious Materials

The following guidelines are required for handling other potentially infectious materials (OPIMs):

- Handle and process all specimens as if they contained infectious material.
- Wipe the outside of specimen containers with a germicide.
- Dispose of all infectious materials according to state and federal guidelines.
- Clean up spills using a disinfectant (see Chapter 4).
- Immediately dispose of any chipped or broken glassware into a sharps container using appropriate safety methods to prevent accidental punctures.

Physical Hazards

Physical hazards in the laboratory can be classified as electrical, fire, and mechanical hazards. Electric shock is a threat when any electrical equipment is in use. It is imperative to keep all electrical equipment in proper repair and always to follow manufacturers' instructions.

For electrical hazards, do the following:

- Use surge protectors.
- Inspect all cords and plugs frequently.
- Never use extension cords.
- Do not overload circuits.

Unplug the electrical device before servicing, and never operate electrical instruments with wet hands. If a sink is nearby, make sure electrical cords do not come in contact with the water supply. Signs and labels should be placed on specific electrical hazards (Fig. 30.6).

Open flames are rarely used in a laboratory anymore, but the potential for fire still exists. Fires may be ignited by smoking, heating elements, and sparks from electrical connections. Flammable materials should not be stored near any source of ignition. All laboratory personnel should be familiar with the locations of fire extinguishers and fire safety blankets. Fire extinguishers should be the carbon dioxide (CO_2), dry chemical, or halon type, known as the ABC type of extinguisher. ABC extinguishers can be used on all types of fires. Extinguishers should be inspected regularly by a licensed inspector and replaced or recharged if used. The medical assistant may be responsible for maintaining records on the care and maintenance of fire extinguishers (see Procedure 30.3, p. 767).

Fire safety blankets can be used to smother flames on burning clothing. However, a victim should not be wrapped in a fire blanket, because this may intensify burns. Instead, the flames should be patted out or the victim directed to stop, drop, and roll on the blanket.

Emergency phone numbers should be posted on the wall near the telephone, and all personnel should know the locations of fire alarms, the fire escape routes, and procedures to follow if exits are blocked. Periodic fire drills should be conducted, and hallways and exits should be kept free of clutter.

Mechanical hazards arise from the use of laboratory equipment. Care should be exercised when using equipment with moving parts, such as a centrifuge. A laboratory centrifuge is a device that separates liquids from solids by rotating samples in a test tube at a high rate of speed. This forces heavier constituents of the sample to the bottom of the test tube and allows lighter constituents to remain at the top of the sample. Centrifuges present a hazard not only from moving parts but also from glassware that might break during centrifugation and from aerosols that might be created if tubes are not capped tightly.

Care should also be exercised when using equipment that relies on pressure, such as autoclaves. Autoclaves are used to sterilize metal instruments, microbiologic media, and some microbiologic waste. Autoclaves present a danger if opened prematurely before the pressure has come down to a safe level.

Although centrifuges and autoclaves often have built-in safeguards, such as locks that prevent entry until the environment is safe, improper care of the equipment can cause safety measures to fail.

SPECIMEN COLLECTION, PROCESSING, AND STORAGE

Laboratory Requisitions and Reports

When the provider orders laboratory testing, an electronic or paper requisition must be generated. Patient information on the requisitions must be complete, accurate, and legible. The patient is then directed to the POL, or the specimen is collected, prepared, and sent to an outside laboratory.

Fig. 30.7 shows the electronic lab requisition form used in *SimChart for the Medical Office*. The following information typically is required on the requisition when specimens are sent to a reference laboratory:

- Provider's name, account number, address, and phone number
- Patient's full name, age, date of birth, gender, address, and insurance information
- Source of specimen
- Date and time of collection, and initials of the person collecting the specimen
- Specific test (or tests) requested
- Medications the patient is taking
- Whether the patient fasted or followed dietary restrictions if required; time of last intake
- Possible diagnosis
- Indication of whether the test is to be performed STAT

When the results of the tests are obtained, a laboratory report is sent to the office. The laboratory reports can be sent in two ways:

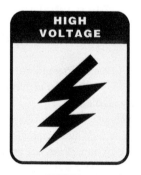
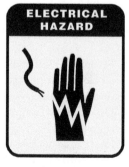

FIGURE 30.6 High voltage and electrical hazard labels.

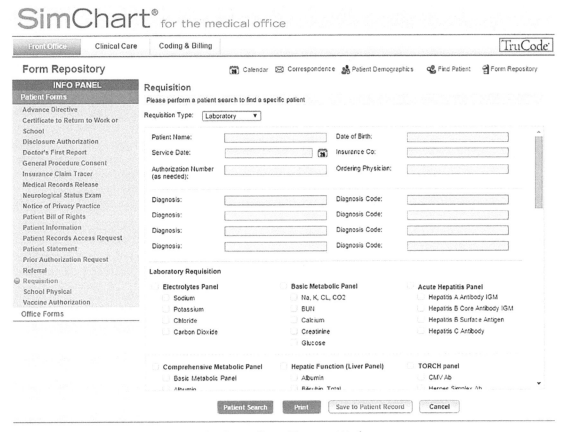

FIGURE 30.7 Electronic laboratory requisition form.

- Directly from the referral laboratory to the patient's EHR
- Electronically to the facility and then staff upload the electronic document to the EHR or print it out for the paper medical record

A medical assistant is frequently responsible for making sure that all outside laboratory reports have been received and given to the provider for review. Testing results cannot be given to a patient until the provider has reviewed them. Any testing that is completed outside the POL at a reference lab must be tracked. This can be done by maintaining a master laboratory specimen log sheet or electronic file. This tracks patient specimens, tests ordered, designated lab, results, and provider response.

Specimen Collection

The medical assistant is responsible for the collection of many different types of specimens. It is important to recognize that laboratory results are only as good as the specimen collected. The importance of proper specimen collection cannot be overemphasized. To ensure that test results are accurate indicators of the patient's state of health, it is critical that proper specimen collection procedures are understood and followed exactly. The most common specimens are blood, urine, and swab samples collected from wounds or mucous membranes. Specimens that may be collected less frequently include feces, gastric contents, CSF, tissue samples, semen, and **aspirates**.

Verifying the patient's identity before the specimen collection is a critical step in the collection process. Patient identification should follow the written procedure for your institution. Using a minimum of two patient identifiers before specimen collection is standard. If the patient is not identified properly, the laboratory results that are generated will be useless.

Tips for Labeling a Patient Specimen and Sample Label

When labeling a sample container, make sure you only use a black waterproof marker or pen, *never* pencil! All labels should include the following information, at a minimum:

- Patient name: surname, first name, then middle initial
- Identification number
- Date (MM/DD/YYYY) and time of collection
- Phlebotomist or collector's initials

If affixing a computer-generated label, make sure to write the time and initial the specimen after the venipuncture has been completed.

Another important step in specimen collection is the proper choice of a collection container. For example, blood may be collected using a vacuum tube system. Blood collection tubes are available in a variety of sizes, depending on the collection needs. Blood collection tubes

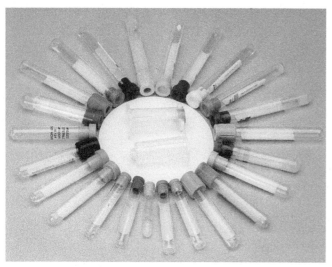

FIGURE 30.8 Vacutainer tubes with colored stoppers. (From Proctor D, et al: *Kinn's The Medical Assistant*, ed 13, St. Louis, 2017, Elsevier.)

are also available with and without preservatives and **anticoagulants**. The tube stoppers are color coded. The color of the stopper indicates which additive is present, if any (Fig. 30.8). Collection in an incorrect colored tube may result in an unacceptable specimen, and re-collection may be necessary.

If a specimen will be tested for the presence of microorganisms, a sterile container must be used. When a nonsterile container is used, it could cause contamination of the specimen. If patients are to collect the specimen at home, they should be provided with the appropriate container and complete instructions for collection. Patient education is an important role for the medical assistant. Each patient should receive clear instructions for proper home collection. Make sure your patients listen to the directions, and ask them to repeat the instructions back to you so that you know they understand the information. Remember to be sensitive to individual patient factors (e.g., hearing, sight, primary language, cognitive capacity). These can affect the patient's understanding of the instructions, as well as his or her ability to follow through. Giving patients written directions to take home can also be helpful and reassuring.

CRITICAL THINKING APPLICATION   30.6

As Greg has been working in phlebotomy, he has been reminded of the importance of patient identification. Write down three reasons why patient identification is critical to laboratory specimens. Be ready to share your reasons with the class.

The medical assistant should always check the laboratory's specimen requirements manual or reference laboratory website for any unfamiliar tests. A clear understanding of the specimen and collection requirements is very important. Any unanswered questions should be resolved by calling the reference laboratory before collecting the specimen. The container must be labeled properly at the time of collection. Unlabeled containers are not acceptable for laboratory testing and must be rejected. Labels should include the patient's full name, the

date and time of collection, the initials of the person collecting the specimen, and the specimen type.

Most offices have a laboratory courier service that picks up specimens periodically throughout the day. Specimens should be properly stored (some may require refrigeration) until the courier arrives. Instructions for properly obtaining, processing, and preparing a specimen for transport are usually supplied by the testing laboratory. If the instructions are not clear, or if you have a question about a particular test collection, the reference laboratory should be able to answer the question over the phone. Criteria for safe shipping of specimens include the following:

- Length of time acceptable for transport
- Recommended temperature range to maintain the specimen
- Appropriate material packaging if the specimen needs to be protected from light

If the specimen is to be mailed, it must be carefully packaged to prevent breakage, damage, or contamination during handling. Follow the instructions for transport supplied by the reference laboratory. Do not ship specimens without proper packaging and labeling as specified by the test laboratory.

Preventing Contamination

Medical assistants must take care to prevent contamination of specimens and themselves. Expiration dates on swabs, tubes, transport media, and other collection containers should be checked before the items are used. Any expired materials should not be used and should be properly discarded. An improperly handled specimen may become contaminated or may contaminate the surrounding environment. Standard Precautions should be followed. Blood and body fluids from all patients should be considered infectious.

The specimen collected must be a true representative sample. A swab for a wound culture collected from the surface of the wound generally does not yield the same results as one taken from the depths of the wound. A **hemolyzed** blood specimen shows marked differences in many tests (Fig. 30.9). If a large volume of specimen is collected (e.g., a 24-hour urine specimen), the total volume or weight must be carefully measured and recorded. The specimen must be well mixed before an *aliquot* is removed and submitted for testing.

Handling, Processing, and Storing Specimens

Specimens must be handled, processed, and stored according to test manufacturer's guidelines to prevent any changes that would affect test results. In Chapters 31 through 34, specimen handling, processing, and storage will be discussed for each specific area of the laboratory. Each department in the lab has unique testing and specimen requirements. Some general guidelines to keep in mind include the following:

- The storage temperature of the specimen should follow manufacturer's testing requirements.
- Serum must be separated from red blood cells as soon as possible after the specimen has clotted to prevent changes caused by the metabolism of the blood cells.
- Specimens for chemistry and liver panels may need to be protected from light.
- Specimens may need to be frozen to prevent chemical constituents from changing. Follow manufacturer's guidelines for freezing a specimen.

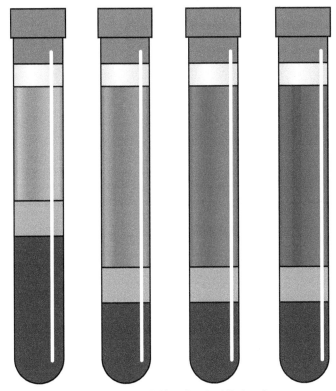

FIGURE 30.9 Normal (left) and hemolyzed blood samples.

TABLE 30.4 Greenwich Time and Military Time	
GREENWICH TIME	MILITARY TIME
1:00 a.m.	0100 hours
3:00 a.m.	0300 hours
5:00 a.m.	0500 hours
7:00 a.m.	0700 hours
9:00 a.m.	0900 hours
11:00 a.m.	1100 hours
1:00 p.m.	1300 hours
3:00 p.m.	1500 hours
5:00 p.m.	1700 hours
7:00 p.m.	1900 hours
9:00 p.m.	2100 hours
11:00 p.m.	2300 hours
12:00 a.m. (midnight)	2400 hours

• Manufacturer's package inserts or reference laboratory specimen requirements should be consulted to ensure that each specimen is handled and processed properly.

Chain of Custody

When a specimen may be needed as evidence in a court case, certain procedures must be followed when collecting and handling the specimen. **Forensic** or legal specimens should be collected, handled, and stored in a manner consistent with established standards designated by law. Specimen processing must be documented precisely, ensuring that no tampering with evidence has occurred. *Chain of custody* refers to the stepwise method used to collect, process, and test a specimen. The documentation must be signed by every person who has any contact with the specimen, from collection to the final reporting of results. Blood alcohol level testing and drug screening often require chain of custody handling. Everything needed for collection of the specimen is provided in a kit—the gloves, the vacuum tube, and the needle used to collect the blood specimen. Documentation is included and must be signed by all personnel. Medical assistants and phlebotomists can be subpoenaed to testify in court about specimens they have collected. It is always in your best interest to follow chain of custody procedures exactly.

CRITICAL THINKING APPLICATION   **30.7**

What is the difference between a patient specimen and a forensic specimen? In your own words, describe *chain of custody*.

LABORATORY MATHEMATICS AND MEASUREMENT

All laboratory testing relies on the accurate use of values, units, and measurements. For example, values are used for reporting the time the sample was collected, the volume of the specimen, the amount of analyte found in a specimen, and dilutions used in sample preparation and for recording QC results.

Measuring Time

Time of day is a critical factor in patient care. Medications must be administered, diets must be followed, and specimens must be collected on a timed schedule. Many laboratories use the 24-hour clock when recording time; this method avoids the confusion that comes with the *Greenwich clock*, which uses a.m. (morning) and p.m. (afternoon) designations.

The 24-hour clock system, also known as *military time*, is expressed with four digits in terms of "hundred hours." Noon is referred to as 1200 (twelve hundred) hours; midnight is 0000 (zero hundred), or 2400 hours. The military clock is based on 24 60-minute hours, as is the Greenwich clock; therefore, 5:35 p.m. is expressed as 1735 (seventeen thirty-five) hours (Table 30.4).

CRITICAL THINKING APPLICATION   **30.8**

If the time on the clock is 10 a.m., how would you write that in military time? If the time is 10 p.m., how would you write the time in military time? If the time on a document is written as 1900 hours, how would you write it in Greenwich time? How would you write it if it had been documented as 0800 hours?

Measuring Temperature

Two scales are currently used for measuring temperature; each is divided into units called *degrees* (Table 30.5). The Fahrenheit scale is considered part of the *English system* of measurement and is the scale most commonly used in the United States. The *Celsius scale*, formerly called the centigrade scale, is used in countries that apply the *metric system*. On the Celsius (C) scale, water freezes at 0°C and boils at 100°F. On the Fahrenheit (F) scale, water freezes at 32°F and boils at 212°F. Almost all laboratories in the United States use the Celsius scale for temperature.

Units of Measurement

The units of measurement that we commonly use in the United States differ from those used in the laboratory. In everyday life, we use the English system of measurement:

- Weight is measured in ounces and pounds.
- Length is measured in inches and feet.
- Volume is measured in cups and quarts.

In the laboratory, the metric system and the Système International (SI) are used. It is important that medical assistants memorize and practice these systems so that they can communicate professionally (Table 30.6).

The metric system is based on a decimal system, which consists of basic units and prefixes that indicate a system of division in multiples of 10. Prefixes are added to each symbol to reduce or enlarge them by units of 10. See Tables 30.7 and 30.8 for an overview of metric system measurements.

International organizations, such as the World Health Organization (WHO), officially recognize SI units. Many countries have adopted this system, but the United States has not completely converted to it. The SI is an adaptation of the metric system that uses several of the basic units, although some units are different for reporting results. For example, blood glucose is reported in millimoles per liter (mmol/L)

Converting Temperatures

To change from Fahrenheit to Celsius:
98.6°F = _____ °C
Step 1: Subtract 32 from F temp
Step 2: Divide number by 1.8

SOLUTION:
98.6 − 32 = 66.6
66.6 / 1.8 = 37°C

To change from Celsius to Fahrenheit:
100°C = _____ °F
Step 1: Multiply C temp by 1.8
Step 2: Add 32 to that number

SOLUTION:
100 × 1.8 = 180
180 + 32 = 212°F

TABLE 30.5 Common Laboratory Temperature Settings

	FAHRENHEIT	CELSIUS
Refrigerator	35°–46°	2°–8°
Freezer	32°	0°
Room	59°–86°	15°–30°
Incubator	98.6°	37°
Body temperature	98.6°	37°
Autoclave	254°	121°

TABLE 30.6 Comparing the English System of Measurement With the Metric System

	ENGLISH SYSTEM OF MEASUREMENT	METRIC SYSTEM
Weight	Ounces (oz) and pounds (lb)	Grams (g)
Length	Inches and feet	Meters (m)
Volume	Cups and quarts	Liters (L)

TABLE 30.7 Metric System: Prefixes of Measurements

PREFIXES	SIZE	OR ANOTHER WAY TO LOOK AT IT	
Kilo (k)	1000 base units	1 kilo = 1000 base units	Larger than the base unit
Hecto	100 base units	1 hecto = 100 base units	
Deka	10 base units	1 deka = 10 base units	
Base Units (Meter, Liter, or Gram)			
Deci	0.1 unit	10 deci = 1 base unit	Smaller than the base unit
Centi (c)	0.01 unit	100 centi = 1 base unit	
Milli (m)	0.001	1000 milli = 1 base unit	
Micro (mc)	0.000001	1,000,000 micro = 1 base unit	

TABLE 30.8 Common Units of Measure Seen in Healthcare		
VOLUME	**LENGTH**	**WEIGHT**
Liter (L)	Meter (m)	Gram (g)
Milliliter (mL or ml)	Centimeter (cm)	Kilogram (kg)
Cubic centimeter (cc)	Millimeter (mm)	Milligram (mg)
cc = mL		Microgram (mcg)

using the SI system, but it is reported as mg/dL using the metric system. Therefore, it is very important for the medical assistant to double-check the laboratory's standard and include the appropriate units of measurement when reporting test values.

CRITICAL THINKING APPLICATION   **30.9**

If you had 3.2 Grams of salt and you wanted to express it in milligrams, how would you write it? If the length of an item were 455 centimeters and you wanted to express it in meters, how would you write it?

Measuring Liquid Volume

Test tubes are used to test or hold liquid reagents, samples, or aliquots. Test tubes come in many sizes and are typically disposable. Test tubes may be sterile for use in microbiology. When liquids are measured into test tubes, the most common piece of glassware used is the *pipet*. A pipet is a hollow tube that can be made from glass or plastic. Pipets often have lines to indicate volume on the length of the tube. Some plastic pipets have a built-in bulb to help transfer fluids and are known as transfer pipets. This type of pipet usually does not have any measurement lines on the tube. Fig. 30.10 shows a variety of transfer pipets that are used in the laboratory. Micropipets are used to deliver very small volumes of liquid (Fig. 30.11). These pipetting devices must be fitted with an appropriate disposable tip. The device is equipped with a piston at the top, which must be depressed before the pipet is filled and when the pipet is drained. It is important to follow the manufacturer's instructions for use with all pipets and micropipets. Each type of pipet may be slightly different.

LABORATORY EQUIPMENT

Microscope

Nearly every medical laboratory is equipped with a *microscope*. This indispensable instrument is used to view objects too small to be seen with the naked eye (Fig. 30.12). The microscope is used to evaluate stained blood smears, urine sediment, vaginal secretions, and smears made from body fluids and microorganisms.

Microscopic procedures are not considered CLIA-waived because they require judgment and additional training. In addition, an error in reading microscopic tests may have a detrimental effect on the patient's care. Providers petitioned the CMS to create a new laboratory category that would allow them to perform a set of simple microscopic tests that could be performed in the ambulatory setting (Table 30.9).

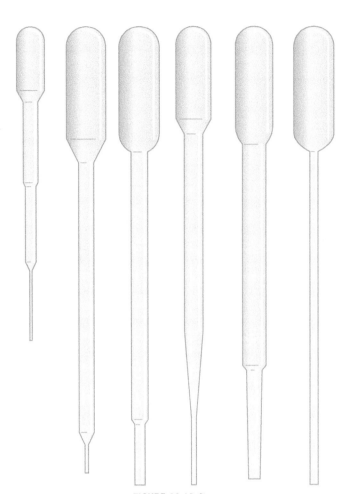

FIGURE 30.10 Pipets.

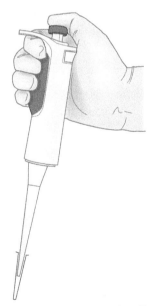

FIGURE 30.11 Micropipet with disposable tip.

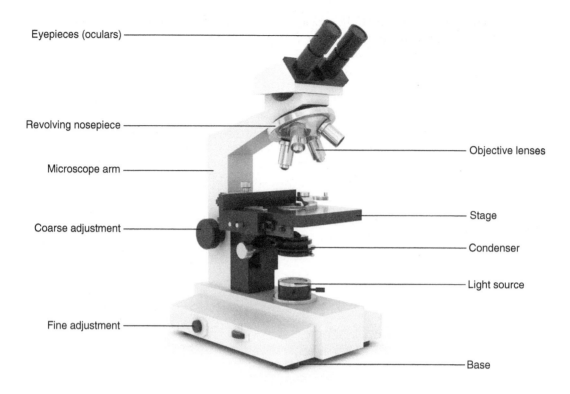

Eyepieces (oculars)

Revolving nosepiece

Microscope arm

Coarse adjustment

Fine adjustment

Objective lenses

Stage

Condenser

Light source

Base

FIGURE 30.12 The parts of a microscope. (Courtesy urfinguss/iStock/thinkstock.)

TABLE 30.9	CLIA-Approved Procedures for Provider-Performed Microscopy (PPM)	
TEST NAME	**DESCRIPTION**	**EXAMPLE**
Direct wet mount	Examination of specimens for the presence or absence of bacteria, fungi, parasites, and human cellular elements	Observing vaginal secretions for the presence of yeast to assist with diagnosis of vulvovaginal candidiasis
KOH preparation	Any preparation using potassium hydroxide	Observing skin scrapings for the presence of fungi
Fecal leukocyte examination	Simple stain of fecal specimen; assists in diagnosis of diarrheal disease	Leukocytes are found in stool in antibiotic-associated colitis, ulcerative colitis, shigellosis, and salmonellosis
Pinworm examination	Preparations are observed for the presence or absence of *Enterobius vermicularis* eggs	Performing a cellulose tape collection for pinworms
Postcoital direct, qualitative examinations	Vaginal or cervical mucus is examined 4–10 hours after intercourse for the presence of live, motile sperm	Assists in the diagnosis of infertility
Qualitative semen analysis	Semen is examined for the presence or absence of spermatozoa; motility of the sperm is noted	Assists in postvasectomy semen analysis and in the diagnosis of infertility
Urine sediment examination	Urine sediment is examined for the presence or absence of formed elements	Part of a routine urinalysis (see Chapter 31, Procedure 31.6 [see p. 797], Prepare a Urine Specimen for Microscopic Examination).

CLIA, Clinical Laboratory Improvement Amendments; *KOH,* potassium hydroxide.

The CMS approved the list and created an additional CLIA category called *provider-performed microscopy procedures* (PPMP). Certified CLIA-PPMP laboratories must meet the same quality standards as laboratories that perform moderate-complexity tests, including passing three proficiency tests from an outside agency per year. The medical assistant is taught how to prepare the microscope slide and bring it into focus. The final analysis of a microscope slide must be made by one of the following personnel:

- *Physician* (medical doctor, doctor of osteopathy, or doctor of podiatric medicine)
- *Midlevel practitioner* (nurse midwife, nurse practitioner, or physician's assistant)
- *Dentist* (doctor of dental surgery or doctor of dental medicine) trained as a laboratory professional with CLIA moderate- or high-complexity training

Microscopes have three components:

- The magnification system, which focuses the image
- The illumination system, which brings the image from the slide to the viewer
- The framework, which includes all components responsible for positioning the slide.

The magnification system includes the ocular and the objective lenses, plus the fine and coarse knobs to adjust the clarity. Microscopes may be monocular or binocular. A monocular microscope has one eyepiece for viewing, and a binocular microscope has two. The eyepiece, or ocular, is located at the top of the microscope and contains a lens to magnify what is being viewed.

The usual ocular magnification is 10 times (10×). In addition to the ocular, compound microscopes have objective lenses that increase the magnification of the specimen. The objectives are attached to the revolving nosepiece. Most microscopes have four objectives, each with a different magnifying power:

- The shortest objective has the lowest power (4×) and is called the *scanning lens*. This lens is used to scan the field of interest and then focus on a particular object.
- Greater detail is observed with the next longest objective, which is low power (10×).
- The high or high dry objective usually has a magnification of 40× or 45×
- The longest objective, oil immersion (100×), allows the finest focusing of the object and requires the use of a special oil that is placed directly on the slide. This special oil, called *immersion oil,* prevents refraction of the light and improves the resolution (clarity) of the magnified image. Oil immersion is used to view cells and extremely small materials (e.g., bacteria and platelets) and to examine stained specimens.

The total magnification of the specimen is determined by multiplying the magnification of the objective lens by 10 (the magnification of the ocular lens). Therefore, if you have the 10× objective in place when observing blood cells, you are magnifying the image 100 times. Just above the base are the focusing knobs. The coarse adjustment is used only with scanning and low-power lenses, and the fine adjustment is used with high-power and oil immersion lenses.

The arm of the microscope connects the objectives and the oculars to the base, which supports the microscope and contains its light source. The stage of the microscope holds the slide to be viewed. Under the stage is the light source, the condenser, and the iris diaphragm, which make up the illumination system. The condenser directs light up through the slide, and the iris diaphragm regulates the amount of light passing through the specimen.

Microscopes are very precise and expensive instruments that require careful handling. The amount of routine maintenance required depends on the amount of daily use. Dirt is the enemy of the microscope, which must be kept very clean at all times. Oil, makeup, dust, and eye secretions can all obstruct vision through the lens and may transmit infective organisms. The microscope should always be stored in a plastic dust cover when not in use. Lenses should be cleaned before and after each use with lens paper and lens cleaner. Any other type of tissue scratches the lenses or leaves lint residue behind. Routine use of solvent cleaners, such as xylene, is not recommended, because these cleaners may loosen a lens. The body of the microscope should be dusted with a soft cloth.

The microscope should be placed in a permanent location in the laboratory, on a sturdy table, in an area where it cannot be bumped. If a microscope must be moved, it should be carried securely, with one hand supporting the base and the other holding the arm. When the microscope is stored, it should be left covered and with the low-power objective in the highest position. The stage should be centered.

Using a microscope involves focusing and illumination (see Procedure 30.4, p. 767). The image is focused by moving the objectives closer to the specimen using the fine and coarse knobs. Proper focusing begins with the objective at lowest power. The coarse adjustment moves the objective quickly. This knob is used first to bring the specimen into approximate focus. The fine adjustment focus knob then brings the specimen into precise focus. The fine focus moves the objective more slowly to allow the viewer to zero in on the specimen with greater accuracy. Illumination is accomplished by raising or lowering the condenser and by opening and closing the diaphragm on the condenser.

If the microscope is a binocular model, the eyepieces may need to be adjusted to accommodate the distance between the pupils and the individual's point of greatest visual acuity. A gentle push inward or pull outward adjusts the distance between the eyepieces.

Centrifuge

A centrifuge is an instrument that is used to separate solids from liquids. A centrifuge works by rapidly spinning the specimen, which increases the gravitational force. The increased force pushes the heavier solids to the bottom of the specimen and lets lighter liquids remain at the top of the specimen. Centrifugation is used to separate blood cells from serum or plasma. It is also used to separate solid materials, such as cells and crystals, in urine specimens.

Centrifuges (Fig. 30.13) are designed for specific uses. They may be bench-top or floor models; some may be refrigerated. Some may have rotating parts or members known as *rotors* or heads that are interchangeable to accommodate different-sized sample tubes. Centrifuge configurations vary with the laboratory task that needs to be done. The three common configurations used in the clinical laboratory are:

- A centrifuge that has a fixed-angle *rotor,* where specimen cups are held in a rigid position at a fixed angle.
- A centrifuge that has a horizontal head with buckets that swing out horizontally during centrifugation.

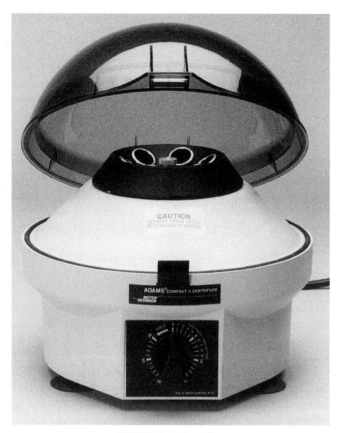

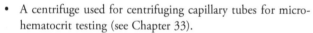

FIGURE 30.13 A centrifuge.

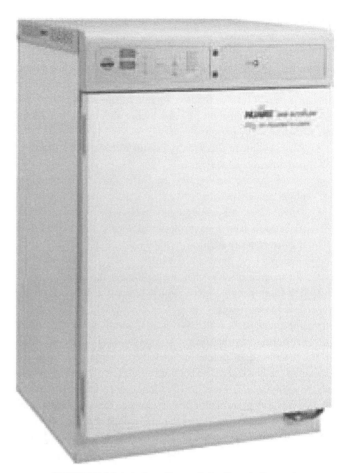

FIGURE 30.14 An incubator. (Courtesy NuAire, Plymouth, Minnesota.)

- A centrifuge used for centrifuging capillary tubes for microhematocrit testing (see Chapter 33).

Directions for using a centrifuge usually are given in terms of revolutions per minute (rpm). Spinning generates centrifugal force, causing the heaviest particles in a liquid to migrate to the bottom of the tube. Centrifuges can be dangerous if not used correctly. The most important rule is to ensure that the centrifuge is balanced so that tubes of equal size and containing equal volume are directly across from one another in the rotor holders or buckets. Therefore, there must always be an even number of tubes in the centrifuge. If a second specimen of the same volume in the same-sized tube is not available for balance, a tube of water may be used to balance the load. Tubes being centrifuged should be capped to prevent samples from creating aerosols during spinning. Rubber cups should be placed in the bottom of the carrier cups to prevent breakage of glass tubes.

Centrifuges should never be opened while they are in operation, nor should you attempt to slow a centrifuge with your hands. Most centrifuges are equipped with a brake, which should be used only in an emergency, the most common of which is a broken glass tube. In this case, wait until the centrifuge comes to a complete stop and follow the manufacturer's instructions for disinfecting the unit; also follow Standard Precautions to prevent injury and disease transmission.

Centrifuges should be checked, cleaned, and lubricated regularly to ensure proper operation. A certified technician must ensure the centrifuge's speed to comply with quality assurance guidelines set forth by the College of American Pathologists (CAP).

Incubator

Incubators are cabinets that maintain constant temperatures (Fig. 30.14). Generally used in the microbiology laboratory, an incubator can be set to a specific temperature. Microbiology departments usually maintain a constant temperature of 35° to 37°C (95° to 98.6°F), although other temperatures may also be appropriate. Incubators usually have warning alarms that sound if the temperature exceeds or falls below a specified range. The temperature should be checked daily, and the cabinets should be cleaned regularly with a disinfectant approved by the manufacturer.

See Table 30.10 for an example of a laboratory maintenance log. All laboratory equipment that is temperature-sensitive should have temperatures checked and recorded daily.

CLOSING COMMENTS

Patient Coaching

For many testing procedures, patients must be given a specific set of instructions to follow. The provider often communicates the instructions to the patient but may also ask the medical assistant to reinforce the information. For example, patients may be required to fast 8 to 12 hours before blood samples are collected.

Often, the medical assistant is responsible for communicating provider directions that need to be followed before laboratory testing.

TABLE 30.10   Laboratory Maintenance Log

	MEDICAL CLINIC							
	DAILY MAINTENANCE CONTROL CHART							
MONTH		**YEAR**						
	DAILY					**MONTHLY**		
	Refrig	Freezer	Room	Incubator	Bleach	Eyewash	Shower	BY
DAY	2°–8°C	–0°–20°C	15°–30°C	34°–36°C	Counters	Checked	Checked	
1								
2								
3								
4								
5								

Make sure you have reviewed the provider's orders correctly before explaining the procedure to the patient. The patient should be given verbal and written instructions prior to testing. Also include a phone number on the instruction sheet so that the patient can call if he or she has questions after returning home.

Legal and Ethical Issues

If disease did not exist, there would be little need for clinical laboratories. The fact that the human body is susceptible to disease necessitates the existence of laboratory testing. All health and safety risks cannot be anticipated or eliminated, but the risks are greatly reduced when everyone who works in the laboratory is conscious of safety guidelines.

Use common sense, and document everything. If you are in doubt about the safety of a procedure, ask your supervisor. If you are aware of a potential safety problem, report it to the person in charge. Your welfare, the welfare of the patient, and the welfare of your co-workers may depend on your commitment to safety.

Before the patient receives test results, the medical assistant must make sure the provider has reviewed and signed the results and has given permission for the patient to be told about them. Most providers personally inform patients of laboratory results, but some providers may delegate this duty to office staff. Regardless of who informs the patient of test results, the individual must make sure the specific guidelines for communication are followed as stipulated in the patient's Health Insurance Portability and Accountability Act (HIPAA) release form. Maintaining a patient's privacy and confidentiality are crucial factors that must be considered when dealing with test results.

Patient-Centered Care

All health and safety risks to laboratory workers cannot be anticipated or eliminated, but the risks are greatly reduced when everyone who works in the laboratory is conscious of safety guidelines. Use common sense, and document everything. If it is not documented, in the eyes of the law it did not happen. If you have questions about a safety procedure, ask the supervisor. If you are aware of a potential safety problem, report it to the person in charge. Your welfare, the welfare of the patient, and the welfare of co-workers may depend on your commitment to safety.

Professional Behaviors

The next four chapters discuss the most common CLIA-waived tests performed in the POL. They cover patient education, preparation, specimen collection, and testing procedures, which are all aspects of professionalism you must develop as you work with others and document your results appropriately. Look over the Professionalism evaluation form in your study guide to see what actions you should take to become a professional in the laboratory classroom. At the end of the laboratory chapters, your instructor may meet with you one-on-one to discuss your evaluation results, and/or you may do a self-evaluation of your performance.

SUMMARY OF SCENARIO

Greg has had a busy day in the laboratory. He has reviewed safety policies and procedures, reacquainted himself with waived laboratory testing, and had a refresher on units of measure. He is looking forward to another day training in the lab tomorrow, when he will be running some urinalysis tests.

There is a lot to remember and learn, but with some extra effort, review with Julie, and hands-on testing practice, Greg will become more comfortable in his new department. He thinks the change will be a good move for him.

SUMMARY OF LEARNING OBJECTIVES

1. **Discuss the role of the clinical laboratory personnel in patient care and the medical assistant's role in coordinating laboratory tests and results.**
   Clinical laboratory personnel are responsible for analyzing blood and body fluids and sending the provider the test results, which become part of the essential data for diagnosing and managing a patient's condition. Medical assistants are responsible for collecting specimens, instructing patients, and performing CLIA-waived and some moderately complex testing.

2. **Describe the divisions/departments of the clinical laboratory.**
   Most physician offices that perform laboratory testing do so in the areas of urinalysis, hematology, chemistry, and microbiology. Routine urinalysis, complete blood counts, glucose tests, and throat cultures are some of the tests that might be performed in a POL.

3. **Explain the three regulatory categories established by the Clinical Laboratory Improvement Amendments (CLIA), and identify CLIA-waived tests associated with common diseases.**
   A CLIA-waived test is one that has been approved by the FDA for over-the-counter sales and that may be performed in certified CLIA-waived laboratories (i.e., POLs). The test has been determined to pose no unreasonable risk of harm if performed incorrectly. More complex tests that require additional training or education may be performed only in CLIA-certified moderate- or high-complexity laboratories.
   Note: Providers may perform certain microscopic exams if they are certified to perform provider-performed microscopy (PPM) procedures.
   CLIA established the standards of quality for laboratory testing. Medical assistants are allowed to perform and monitor all CLIA-waived tests. Table 30.3 summarizes the CLIA-waived tests that may be performed in a registered CLIA-waived laboratory and the common diseases or conditions in which they are used.

4. **Identify quality assurance practices in healthcare, document the results on a laboratory flow sheet, and discuss quality control guidelines.**
   QA involves all the procedures undertaken to ensure that each patient is provided excellent care. QC, which determines whether a laboratory test is accurate, precise, and reliable, is one part of a QA program. Procedure 30.1 on p. 765 outlines the steps for analyzing the reliability of a test based on the results of running its control and documenting the results on a laboratory flow sheet.

5. **Discuss laboratory safety and the governing agencies involved in safety standards.**
   The importance of safety in the laboratory cannot be overemphasized. The US government created a system of safeguards and regulations under the Occupational Safety and Health Act of 1970. Two programs have been mandated by OSHA to ensure the safety of personnel working in clinical laboratories; one covers occupational exposure to chemical hazards, and the other covers exposure to bloodborne pathogens.

6. **Discuss the purpose of a Safety Data Sheet (SDS), and summarize safety techniques to minimize physical, chemical, and biologic hazards in the clinical laboratory.**

All workers must be provided with information and training, and a Safety Data Sheet (SDS, formerly MSDS) must be on file for all chemicals used in the laboratory. OSHA requires the manufacturer of the chemical to make these sheets available, usually as a package insert or online.
The medical facility must do the following: provide an annual formal safety training program to review and update physical, biologic, and chemical hazards that apply to the laboratory; maintain an up-to-date safety procedures manual; provide safety equipment (e.g., fire blankets, fire extinguishers, eyewash stations, and personal protective equipment) to all employees; make sure chemicals are clearly marked with the National Fire Protection Association (NFPA) diamond; make sure SDSs are bound in an accessible manual; and reinforce the principles of Standard Precautions when any biologic material is handled.
Note: Risks can be minimized in all areas of the laboratory by using common sense.

7. **Describe the essential elements of a laboratory requisition.**
   The laboratory requisition must include all information needed to identify the patient, the ordering provider, the test ordered, insurance information, and the specific details of collection of the specimen (e.g., time and source).

8. **Discuss specimen collection, including the importance of sensitivity to patients' rights and feelings when collecting specimens. Also, discuss the eight steps to follow when collecting specimens and informing patients of their results.**
   Identification of the patient is the first essential step. If the patient is to collect the specimen at home, he or she should be provided with the appropriate container and complete instructions for collection. Bear in mind the principles of patient education, and be sensitive to factors that can affect the patient's understanding of the instructions for specimen collection. Review the eight steps to follow when collecting specimens and informing patients of their results.

9. **Explain the chain of custody and why it is important.**
   Chain of custody is a method used to ensure that a specimen provided by a patient who may be involved in a legal matter is handled in a fashion that does not compromise the test results. All individuals who handle or test the specimen must be identified in writing and must provide a signature.

10. **Discuss the measurement of time and temperature, and name the metric units used for measuring liquid volume, distance, and mass.**
    Many laboratories use the 24-hour clock when recording time, which avoids the confusion that comes with the Greenwich clock. Two scales are used for measuring temperature: Fahrenheit and Celsius. Almost all laboratories in the United States use the Celsius scale for temperature.
    Liquid volume is measured in liters, distance is measured in meters, and mass is measured in Grams. Prefixes commonly used in the clinical laboratory include *deci-* (0.1), *centi-* (0.01), *milli-* (0.001), *micro-* (0.000001), and *kilo-* (1000).

11. **Name the parts of a microscope, and describe their functions. Also, summarize selected microscopy tests that may be performed in the ambulatory care setting.**

SUMMARY OF LEARNING OBJECTIVES—*continued*

The parts of the microscope can be divided into the illumination system (light source, condenser, and iris diaphragm lever), the frame (base, adjustment knobs, arm, stage, and stage control), and the magnification system (objective lenses on the revolving nosepiece and oculars). The illumination system controls the light that passes through the specimen to the eye, the frame provides the structure for the instrument and the components that allow for adjustment of the sample, and the magnification system provides the ground-glass lenses that magnify the specimen.

Refer to Table 30.9 to see a list of microscopy tests that may be performed in the ambulatory care setting.

12. **Describe the safe use of a centrifuge.**

To use a centrifuge safely, the proper tube must be used and it must be protected from breakage. Centrifuge loads must be carefully balanced, and specimens must be capped to prevent aerosols. Under no circumstances should a centrifuge be opened while it is in operation.

13. **Discuss the use of an incubator.**

Incubators are cabinets that maintain constant temperatures. They generally are used in a microbiology laboratory. The temperature should be checked daily.

PROCEDURE 30.1	Perform a Quality Control Measure on a Glucometer and Record the Results on a Flow Sheet

Task: Test and analyze the results of glucometer controls to see whether a glucometer is producing reliable test results, and record the results on the laboratory flow sheet.

EQUIPMENT and SUPPLIES

- Fluid-impermeable lab coat, gloves, and protective eyewear
- Glucometer
- Coded test strips designed for the glucometer used
- Control solution provided by the manufacturer
- Package insert showing directions on how to run the glucometer
- Biohazard waste container
- Glucose test control flow sheet

The three color-coded bottles of controls (1, 2, and 3) in the figure will produce high, low, and normal test results. The test strip is to the right of the glucometer, and the container for the test strips is on the far right (Fig. 1).

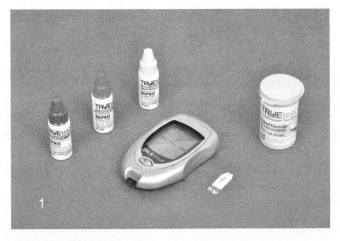

PROCEDURAL STEPS

The following can be a class exercise in which all the students participate.

1. Wash hands or use hand sanitizer. Put on lab coat, gloves, and eye protection.
   PURPOSE: Hand sanitization is an important step for infection control. PPE is necessary when working with any control or specimen material.

2. Take a coded strip out of the bottle, and note the control level and range listed on the control bottle or the strip container.

3. Review the directions on the glucometer package insert, and calibrate the meter by inserting the precoded test strip into the monitor or by manually inserting the code number into the monitor (Fig. 2).
   PURPOSE: Manufacturers must provide directions on how to calibrate light-sensitive meters every time a new container of test strips is used. Note: The newer test strips will code themselves when inserted into the meter.

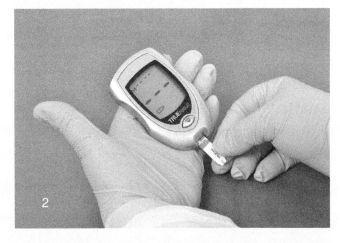

4. Check the expiration date on the liquid control bottle, and mix well by inverting and rolling the bottle between the palms of your hands.
   PURPOSE: If the date on the control bottle shows that it has expired, the control cannot be run. And it is crucial to have all the reagents in the bottle in suspension to produce reliable results.

5. Complete the top portion of the control log sheet with the test name, control lot number, expiration date, and the control's reference range based on whether it is a low-level, normal, or high-level control.

Continued

PROCEDURE 30.1	**Perform a Quality Control Measure on a Glucometer and Record the Results on a Flow Sheet**—*continued*

PURPOSE: All of this information is checked each time a control is run to compare the results of the same control.

6. Insert the strip into the glucometer, and apply a drop of the liquid control to the strip according to the directions.
   PURPOSE: The manufacturer must supply clear directions that ensure consistency every time a control or patient specimen is run.

7. Record the result on the glucose test control flow sheet, and note whether it falls within the manufacturer's reference range. If not, the test should be repeated with a new strip.
   PURPOSE: An occasional "out of range" result can occur. If the repeated test with a new strip is back in range, proceed with patient testing. If the second strip falls outside of the range, the patient may not be tested until the cause of the error is determined.

8. When you have finished running the controls, properly dispose of the strips as recommended by the manufacturer. Remove and dispose of gloves. Wash hands or use hand sanitizer. Remove protective eyewear.
   PURPOSE: This is necessary to ensure infection control.

9. Observe all the results obtained by the students, and compare them to the control ranges provided on the test strip bottle or liquid control bottle. Discuss the following:
   • *Accuracy:* Did all the results fall near the middle of the reference range?
   • *Precision:* Were the results consistently close to each other (without extreme highs and lows)?
   • *Reliability:* If both of the previous points are affirmed, the test result is reliable and may be used to test patients.

GLUCOSE TEST CONTROL FLOW SHEET					
Control Lot #: _____			Expiration Date: _____		
Control Range: _____			Level: Low/Normal/High		
DATE	STUDENT/MA INITIALS	RESULT	ACCEPT	REJECT	CORRECTIVE ACTION

PROCEDURE 30.2	Use of the Eyewash Equipment: Perform an Emergency Eyewash

Task: Minimize the risk of occupational exposure to pathogens if body fluids contact the eyes.

EQUIPMENT and SUPPLIES

• Plumbed or self-contained eyewash unit
• Gloves

PROCEDURAL STEPS

1. Wash hands or use hand sanitizer. Remove contact lenses or glasses. Put on gloves.
   PURPOSE: These actions will ensure flushing of all material in the eyes.

2. Following the manufacturer's directions, turn on the eyewash unit. If it is a plumbed unit, the control valve should remain on until the unit is manually shut off.
   PURPOSE: The unit must be plumbed so that it can remain on until manually turned off.

3. Hold the eyelids open with the thumbs and index fingers to ensure adequate rinsing of the entire eye and eyelid surface (see Fig. 30.2).

PURPOSE: The normal reflex is to close the eyes tightly, which prevents removal of all the contaminated material.

4. Avoid aiming the water stream directly onto the eyeball.
   PURPOSE: A direct water stream may cause discomfort or damage the eye.

5. Flush the eyes and eyelids for a minimum of 15 minutes, rolling the eyes periodically to ensure complete removal of the foreign material.
   PURPOSE: It is essential to completely remove the potentially dangerous substance from the eyes.

6. Properly remove and dispose of gloves. Wash hands or use hand sanitizer.
   PURPOSE: Proper infection control practices should be followed at all times.

7. After completion of the eyewash, follow postexposure follow-up procedures.
   PURPOSE: Depending on the type of exposure, the facility's policies may include provider completion of an exposure incident form and provider follow-up.

PROCEDURE 30.3   Evaluate the Laboratory Environment

Tasks: Evaluate the laboratory environment, and identify unsafe working conditions. Identify compliance with safety signs, symbols, and labels.

EQUIPMENT and SUPPLIES

- Laboratory environment evaluation form
- Pen

PROCEDURAL STEPS

1. Observe the use of safety signs, symbols, and labels in the laboratory setting. Document your findings on the work environment evaluation form.
   PURPOSE: Safety signs, symbols, and labels must be used in the laboratory setting.

2. Explain if the laboratory personnel are complying with the safety signs, symbols, and labels.

3. Observe the environment for safety risks. Document your findings.
   PURPOSE: Identifying and correcting safety risks is important in the workplace environment.

4. Based on your observations, summarize your findings. If risks are present, create a list of issues that need to be addressed. Describe what needs to be done for each risk.

PROCEDURE 30.4   Perform Routine Maintenance on Clinical Equipment (Microscope)

Task: Focus the microscope properly using a prepared slide under low power, high power, and oil immersion, then perform routine maintenance on the microscope before storing it.

EQUIPMENT and SUPPLIES

- Microscope
- Lens cleaner
- Lens tissue
- Slide containing specimen
- Immersion oil

PROCEDURAL STEPS

Note: Refer to Fig. 30.12 if needed.

1. Wash hands or use hand sanitizer.
   PURPOSE: Hand sanitization is necessary to ensure proper infection control practices.

2. Gather the needed materials.
   PURPOSE: Being prepared for the task will allow efficient use of your time.

3. Clean the lenses with lens tissue and lens cleaner.
   PURPOSE: Dust on lenses can obscure elements in the microscopic field.

4. Adjust the seating to a comfortable height.
   PURPOSE: Proper seat height will reduce back and neck strain.

5. Plug the microscope into an electrical outlet, and turn on the light switch. Place the slide specimen on the stage and secure it.

6. Turn the revolving nosepiece to engage the 4× or 10× lens.
   PURPOSE: It is important to always begin microscopic observations at low power.

7. Carefully raise the stage while observing with the naked eye from the side.
   PURPOSE: Observing from the side prevents breaking of the slide if the coarse adjustment knob is advanced too far.

8. Focus the specimen using the coarse adjustment knob.
   PURPOSE: The coarse adjustment knob quickly brings the specimen into focus.

9. Adjust the amount of light by closing the iris diaphragm, by bringing the condenser up or down, or by adjusting the light from the source.
   PURPOSE: Too much light when the low-power objective is used can irritate the eyes.

10. Switch to the 40× lens. Use the fine adjustment knob to focus the specimen in detail.

11. Turn the revolving nosepiece to the area between the high-power objective and oil immersion. Place a small drop of oil on the slide.
    PURPOSE: Immersion oil has nearly the same refractive index as glass and prevents refraction of the light, thus improving resolution.

12. Carefully rotate the oil immersion objective into place. The objective will be immersed in the oil. Adjust the focus with the fine adjustment knob.
    PURPOSE: The fine adjustment knob moves the objective slowly, preventing damage to the microscope and the slide.

13. Increase the light by opening the iris diaphragm and raising the condenser.
    PURPOSE: Lighting is crucial to microscopy; the higher the magnification, the more light that is needed.

14. Identify the specimen.

15. Return to low power, but do not drag the 40× lens through the oil. Remove the slide, and dispose of it in a biohazard sharps container.
    PURPOSE: Getting oil on the 40x lens will cause blurriness the next time it is used. It will have to be cleaned again.

Continued

PROCEDURE 30.4   **Perform Routine Maintenance on Clinical Equipment (Microscope)**—*continued*

16. Lower the stage. Center the stage.
    <u>PURPOSE:</u> Returning the microscope to this position protects it during storage.

17. Switch off the light, and unplug the microscope. Clean the lenses with lens tissue, and remove oil with lens cleaner.
    <u>PURPOSE:</u> Dust and oil must be removed from the lenses after a procedure.

18. Wipe the microscope with a cloth. Cover the microscope.
    <u>PURPOSE:</u> Exposing the microscope to a minimum of dust will help maintain the equipment.

19. Sanitize the work area. Wash hands or use hand sanitizer.
    <u>PURPOSE:</u> Sanitization is necessary in order to follow proper infection control practices.

31

URINALYSIS

SCENARIO

Becca Rundle is a medical assistant student who is observing at the Walden-Martin Family Medical (WMFM) Clinic physician office laboratory (POL) today. As part of an assignment, Becca needs to shadow an experienced medical assistant in an area that interests her. Becca is curious about the laboratory, so she will be spending a few hours with Julie Salter, a certified medical assistant (CMA) through the American Association of Medical Assistants (AAMA). Julie is going to explain the tests that she will be performing in the urinalysis department. She has even saved a few interesting samples that came in earlier in the week.

While studying this chapter, think about the following questions:

- How would you describe urine collection procedures and common choices of collection containers?
- What would you say to instruct a patient in the proper collection of a 24-hour urine specimen and a clean-catch midstream urine specimen?
- How would you examine and report the physical and chemical aspects of urine?
- How would you test and record quality control and chemical urinalysis using CLIA-waived methods?
- How would you prepare a urine specimen for microscopic evaluation?
- How would you explain the following CLIA-waived urine tests: Clinitest, urine pregnancy test, ovulation and menopause tests, and toxicology/drug tests?

LEARNING OBJECTIVES

1. Describe the anatomy and physiology of the urinary tract and discuss the formation and elimination of urine.
2. Show sensitivity to patients' rights and feelings when collecting specimens. Also, discuss collection containers, and instruct a patient on the collection of a 24-hour urine specimen.
3. Explain the various means and methods used to collect urine specimens. Also, instruct a patient on the collection of a clean-catch midstream urine specimen.
4. Discuss handling and transporting specimens.
5. Complete the following related to the physical examination of urine:
   - Examine and report the physical aspects of urine.
   - Assess urine for color and turbidity.
   - Perform quality control measures and differentiate between normal and abnormal results while determining the reliability of chemical reagent strips.
6. Examine and report on the chemical aspects of urine, and test urine with chemical reagent strips.
7. Discuss the limitations of reagent strip testing and explain quality control and quality assurance related to urinalysis.
8. Prepare a urine specimen for microscopic evaluation, and understand the significance of casts, cells, crystals, and miscellaneous findings in the microscopy report.
9. Explain or perform the following CLIA-waived urine tests:
   - Glucose testing using the Clinitest method
   - Urine pregnancy test
   - Ovulation and menopause tests
   - Urine toxicology and drug tests
10. List the means by which urine could be adulterated before drug testing and discuss chain of custody rules for drug testing.

VOCABULARY

artificial insemination The injection of semen into the vagina or uterus using a catheter or syringe. Nonsexual.

catheter A hollow, flexible tube that can be inserted into a vessel, organ, or cavity of the body to withdraw or instill fluid, monitor information, and visualize a vessel or cavity.

creatinine clearance rates Result from a procedure used to evaluate the glomerular filtration rate of the kidneys.

crystals Solid substances with a regular shape that is due to the structure of molecules.

decanting Pouring a liquid gently so that it does not disturb the remaining sediment.

esterase Any enzyme that breaks down esters (a type of organic molecule) into alcohols and acids.

follicle-stimulating hormone (FSH) A glycoprotein hormone secreted by the anterior pituitary gland. It stimulates the growth of ova (eggs) in the ovary and induces the formation of sperm in the testis.

glomerulonephritis A kidney disease affecting the glomeruli of the nephron. Characterized by albumin in the urine, edema, and high blood pressure.

graduated cylinder A narrow, tube-shaped container marked with horizontal lines to represent units of measurement. Used to precisely measure the volume of liquids.

homeostasis The internal environment of the body that is compatible with life. A steady state that is created by all the body systems working together to provide a consistent and unvarying internal environment.

ion An electrically charged atom or the smallest component of an element. (A cation has a positive charge, and an anion has a negative charge.)

jaundice Yellow discoloration of the skin, whites of the eyes, and mucous membranes due to an increase of bilirubin in the blood.

luteinizing hormone (LH) A hormone produced by the anterior pituitary gland. LH stimulates ovulation and the development of the corpus luteum in females and the production of testosterone in males.

meatus A body opening or passage, especially the external opening of a structure.

myoglobin Type of hemoglobin found in the muscle.

nephrotoxic Damaging or destructive to the kidneys.

normal flora Microorganisms (mostly bacteria and yeast) that live on or in the body. Normal microscopic residents of the body.

phenylalanine An essential amino acid found in milk, eggs, and other foods.

protozoa Single-celled organisms that are the most primitive form of animal life. Most are microscopic. Examples are amoebas, ciliates, flagellates, and sporozoans.

quantitative Describes a test result that is expressed as a number, usually with units of measure attached to numeric values.

renal ischemia A blood flow deficiency to the kidney(s).

renal threshold The blood level of a substance, above which the kidneys fail to reabsorb it, so the substance will appear in the urine.

sediment An insoluble material that settles to the bottom of a liquid specimen and to the bottom of a centrifuged sample.

supernatant The clear liquid above the sediment in a centrifuged urine specimen.

Urine is the second most common specimen analyzed in the laboratory. Only blood is tested more frequently. Urine is analyzed for several reasons:

- To detect diseases or disorders in which the kidneys are working normally but are excreting abnormal substances that are the result of an imbalance of **homeostasis** in the body. An example would be an individual with diabetes mellitus who is excreting glucose.
- To detect diseases or disorders of the kidneys or urinary tract. Examples would be the presence of kidney stones or a urinary tract infection (UTI).
- To detect medications or drugs that are excreted by the kidneys.

URINE FORMATION

Medical assistants must have a basic knowledge of kidney structure and urine formation to understand the results of a urinalysis (UA). For a helpful review of the urinary system, see Chapter 26.

The urinary tract consists of two kidneys, two ureters, one bladder, and one urethra. Blood passes through microscopic structures in the kidneys called *nephrons* (Fig. 31.1). In the nephrons blood is filtered to form a *filtrate*. The composition of the filtrate is adjusted as it passes through the renal tubules of the nephron. Selective reabsorption and secretion occur in the renal tubules until the filtrate reaches its final composition. The final filtrate is known as *urine*.

Elimination of Urine

Urine flows through a series of collection areas until it leaves the kidney through the ureter and is stored in the urinary bladder.

Urine remains in the bladder until it is voided through the urethra. The average person voids about 1 to 2 liters of urine per day.

The largest component of urine is water. Normal waste products found in urine include urea, uric acid, creatinine, and electrolytes (sodium, chloride, potassium). Abnormal waste products that can be found in urine include protein, glucose, ketones, red blood cells (RBCs), white blood cells (WBCs), bacteria, nitrites, bilirubin, and urobilinogen. Protein and blood cells are too large to be filtrated by the glomerulus, so when these substances appear in the urine, it may indicate kidney damage.

COLLECTING A URINE SPECIMEN

The request for a urine specimen may create an uneasy moment for the patient. The request should be made in a private area, such as the exam room if possible. The patient should be given clear instructions so that he or she understands what is expected. The medical assistant should clearly communicate and explain the details of the procedure.

Be observant and ask the patient to repeat the directions so you know he or she understands the procedure. Answer any questions with patience and clear directions to avoid confusion. If a language barrier exists, be creative but respectful of the patient's needs. Use an interpreter if one is available. Posting a picture with directions in a variety of languages in the patient restroom could also help.

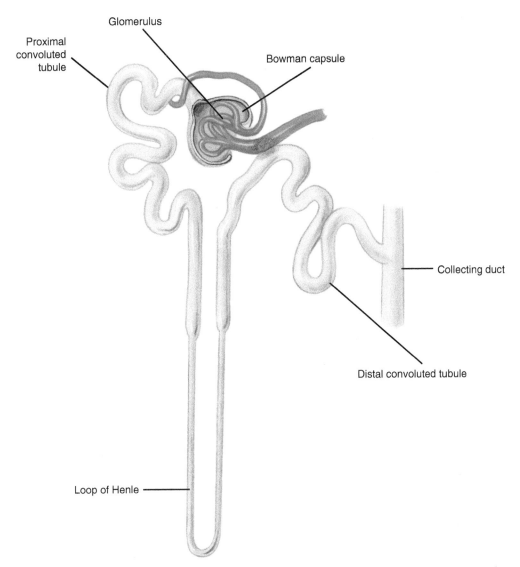

Proximal convoluted tubule

Glomerulus

Bowman capsule

Collecting duct

Distal convoluted tubule

Loop of Henle

FIGURE 31.1 Nephron. Notice the blood vessels entering and exiting the glomerulus, where the small particles in the blood are filtered out of the blood into the surrounding capsule of the nephron. Then, follow the filtrate through the proximal convoluted tubule, the descending limb, the loop of Henle, and the ascending limb of the nephron. This is where water and substances from the filtrate are reabsorbed back into the blood vessels. Finally, in the distal convoluted tubule of the nephron, additional waste products are selectively secreted into the filtrate by the blood vessels. The collection duct continues to concentrate the filtrate to form urine ready for excretion. (From Applegate EJ: *The anatomy and physiology learning system*, ed 4, Philadelphia, 2011, Saunders.)

CRITICAL THINKING APPLICATION   31.1

Becca and Julie meet in the reception area and walk back to the POL. They talk about the need for proper personal protective equipment (PPE), and Julie gives Becca a lab coat and protective eyewear. She also shows Becca where the gloves are near the UA counter. Becca will not be performing tests today, but anyone in the lab should wear proper PPE even if they are observing.

There are a few specimens on the counter, and Julie asks Becca if she has practiced giving instructions for UA collection procedures in any of her classes. Becca replies that she has, but thought it was a bit silly. Julie talks about how patients can be embarrassed about collecting specimens and may not want to ask too many questions. Julie asks Becca to write down three items that are important to include when explaining a UA collection procedure. Write down your own answer and be ready to share with your class.

Containers

The POL should provide the appropriate urine container for the patient. Patients should not use containers from home. Disposable, nonsterile, plastic, or coated paper containers are the most frequently used and are available in many sizes with tight-fitting lids. Most routine UA tests, pregnancy tests, and tests for abnormal analytes are performed on urine collected in nonsterile containers. Special flexible polyethylene bags with adhesive are used to collect urine from infants and children who are not toilet trained (see Chapter 28). For specimens that must be collected over a stated time (24-hour urines), large, wide-mouth plastic containers with screw-cap tops are used (see Procedure 31.1, p. 791).

If the sample is being sent to the microbiology department of the laboratory for culture, it must be collected in a sterile container. Explain the collection procedure to the patient and make sure the

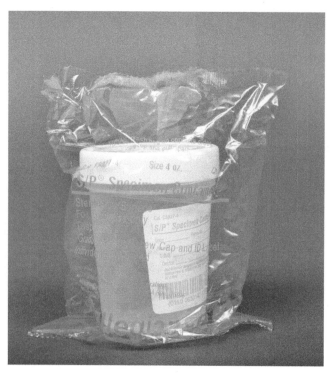

FIGURE 31.2 Sterile urine container.

patient understands how to collect the specimen and how to handle the sterile specimen cup. Sterile containers have a paper seal over the cap. If the seal is broken, the specimen cup may not be sterile and should be discarded. (Fig. 31.2).

The label on all specimens must be printed in permanent marker or ink and must include the patient's name, the date and time of collection, and the type of specimen. If available, computer-generated labels should be placed on the container so that the information is easy to read. Always put on gloves before handling filled specimen containers.

Additional Labeling Information

A note about specimen labels: When a clinic sends specimens to multiple laboratories, it is important to have a system in place that meets the labeling and collection needs of all facilities. Each laboratory may require specific information and specific specimen containers. To avoid mistakes and possible specimen recollection issues, double-check the laboratory name and specimen requirements before patient collection. Patient insurance may direct laboratory usage or affiliation.

Methods of Specimen Collection

Most tests are performed on freshly collected urine in clean containers; this is called a *random specimen*. If the specimen ordered should be collected when the patient first wakes up in the morning, it is called a *first morning specimen*. This type of specimen is more concentrated than a random sample and is best used when testing for nitrite, protein, or pregnancy and for microscopic examination. First morning samples are also the preferred sample for possible UTI testing, but

this is not a requirement. *Two-hour postprandial urine specimens*, collected 2 hours after a meal, are used in diabetes screening and for home diabetes testing programs. A *24-hour urine specimen* is collected over 24 hours to provide a **quantitative** chemical analysis, such as hormone levels and **creatinine clearance rates**. The patient must understand the proper way to collect a 24-hour urine specimen (see Procedure 31.1, p. 791).

Additional Patient Instructions for At-Home 24-Hour Urine Collection

- Do not put anything but urine into the container.
- Do not pour out any liquid or powdered preservative from the container.
- If you accidentally spill some of the preservative on yourself, immediately wash with water and call the POL, provider's office, or testing laboratory.
- Always keep the collection container cool. Refrigerate the container or keep it in an ice-filled cooler or pail.
- Keep the cap on the container.

A *second-voided specimen* usually is collected to determine glucose levels in urine. The first void of the morning is discarded, and the second void of the day is collected for testing. For a catheterized specimen, the provider, nurse, or specially trained medical assistant inserts a sterile **catheter** into the bladder to collect the specimen.

A *clean-catch midstream specimen* (CCMS) is ordered when the provider suspects a urinary tract infection. When a UTI is possible, the provider will order a urine *culture and sensitivity* (C&S). For a C&S procedure the specimen is cultured on microbiologic media to detect bacterial or fungal growth. This is followed by screening the bacteria that grows for antibiotic sensitivity. C&S is performed in the microbiology department of a referral laboratory.

The clean-catch technique is used to eliminate microorganisms from the urinary **meatus**. In the medical facility, collection of CCMS samples starts by instructing the patient to thoroughly cleanse around the meatus and then urinate a small amount into the toilet. This is done to flush out the distal portion of the urethra, where **normal flora** can accumulate. The patient then collects a CCMS specimen. Prior to collection, the medical assistant needs to give complete, understandable instructions to the patient on the method of collection (see Procedure 31.2, p. 792). Failure to do so may mean that the patient will have to return to the office to provide another specimen. For a urine C&S, the urine is collected either by catheterization or by the clean-catch method into a sterile container.

CRITICAL THINKING APPLICATION   **31.2**

As Julie and Becca review the different types of UA specimens, Julie asks, "Why is it so important that a CCMS be collected midstream? Why not start collecting the sample as soon as the void starts?" What would your answer be to that question? Write down your answer and be ready to share in class.

TABLE 31.1 Changes in Urine After 1 Hour at Room Temperature

CONSTITUENT	CHANGE
Clarity	Urine becomes cloudy as crystals precipitate and bacteria multiply
Color	May change if pH becomes alkaline
pH	Becomes alkaline as bacteria form ammonia from urea
Glucose	Decreases as it is metabolized by bacteria
Ketones	Decrease because of evaporation
Bilirubin and urobilinogen	Undergo degradation in light
Blood	May hemolyze; false-positive results are possible because of bacterial enzymes
Nitrite	Test result may change from negative to positive as bacteria multiply and reduce nitrates to nitrites
Casts	Lyse or dissolve in alkaline urine
Cells	Lyse or dissolve in alkaline urine
Bacteria	Multiply twofold approximately every 20 minutes
Yeasts	Multiply
Crystals	Precipitate as urine cools; may dissolve if pH changes

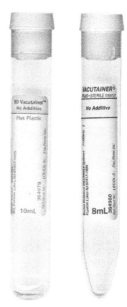

FIGURE 31.3 Urine transport tubes. (Courtesy Becton, Dickinson & Co., Franklin Lakes, NJ.)

- Patient's name and the date
- Type of urinalysis ordered
- Name of the provider requesting the examination
- Appropriate *Current Procedural Terminology* (CPT) code for the diagnosis
- A line on which the provider signs after he or she has reviewed the results

Specimens are sent to the laboratory in a plastic biohazard bag that zips closed and has an outside pocket, where a paper laboratory request is placed. After the test has been performed, the lab physically sends a paper report or electronically sends the results to the provider.

ROUTINE URINALYSIS

The minimum volume needed for a routine UA usually is about 10 to 12 mL, but more is preferred. A complete UA is an assessment of the following:

- Physical properties of the urine
- Selected chemical measurements that are important in the diagnosis of disease (Table 31.2).
- Microscopic contents of the urine and its **sediment**

Physical Examination of Urine: Appearance

The physical examination of urine involves observations regarding the appearance of the specimen (see Procedure 31.3, p. 794). This does not involve chemical analysis but rather observation of the characteristics of color, *turbidity* (cloudiness), volume, presence of foam and/or odor, and specific gravity.

Color

Normal urine is a shade of yellow that ranges from pale straw to yellow to amber (Fig. 31.4). The color depends on the concentration of the pigment *urochrome*, a yellow pigment normally found in urine, and the amount of water in the specimen. A dilute specimen should

Handling and Transporting a Specimen

Proper handling of specimens is essential. The chemical and cellular components of urine change if the urine warms to room temperature (Table 31.1). Urine specimens should therefore be kept refrigerated and should be processed within 1 hour of collection. If the specimen must be transported to a referral laboratory, evacuated transport tubes are available (Fig. 31.3). These tubes contain preservatives and look like blood collection tubes. The preservatives in the tube prevent the overgrowth of bacteria and will prevent chemical changes in the urine that may affect test results. Chemical reagent strip testing can be performed on preserved specimens within 72 hours. Tubes may be held at room temperature during this time.

A different preservative must be used for urine culture specimens. The preservative used for culture specimens helps maintain the number of bacteria present at the time of collection. This type of transport system should be used only for urine specimens that will be cultured. Results on the chemical reagent strip may be altered by the alternative preservatives. Culture and sensitivity testing should be performed within 72 hours. The C&S tubes can be held at room temperature.

A laboratory request form, paper or electronic, must be completed for all specimens that will be transported to another site for analysis. Typical forms include the following information:

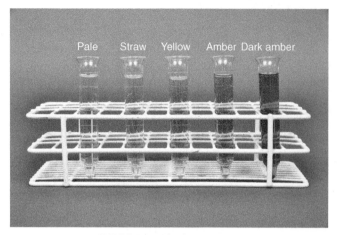

FIGURE 31.4 Color of urine specimens.

be a pale straw color, and a more concentrated specimen should be a darker yellow or amber color. First morning specimens will likely be amber in color due to the concentration of the urochrome during the night. Variations in color may also be caused by diet, medication, and disease. Abnormal colors may be related to pathologic or non-pathologic factors (Table 31.3).

Turbidity

Both normal and abnormal urine specimens may range in appearance from clear to very cloudy (Fig. 31.5). Turbidity may be caused by cells, bacteria, yeast, vaginal contaminants, or **crystals**. It is possible for a urine specimen to be clear when voided, but then as crystals form and precipitate out of the liquid, this causes the urine to become cloudy as it cools.

Volume

The amount of urine is rarely measured in a random specimen. With a timed specimen, volume is measured by pouring the complete collection into a large, **graduated cylinder**. It is not accurate enough to use the markings on the side of the collection container. Once the volume has been measured and recorded, a portion of well-mixed specimen, called an *aliquot,* is removed for testing. The remainder is discarded or stored, depending on the preference of the laboratory.

The normal volume of urine produced every 24 hours varies according to the age of the individual. Infants and children produce smaller volumes than adults. The normal adult volume of urine produced is approximately 800 to 2000 mL in 24 hours. Excessive production of urine is called *polyuria.* This is common in those who have diabetes mellitus, diabetes insipidus, and certain kidney disorders. *Oliguria* is an insufficient production of urine, which can be caused by dehydration, decreased fluid intake, shock, renal disease, or urinary tract infections. The absence of urine production, *anuria,* occurs when there is renal obstruction and renal failure.

TABLE 31.2 Components of Physical and Chemical Urinalysis	
PHYSICAL PROPERTY	**CHEMICAL COMPONENT**
Color	Protein
Clarity	Glucose
Specific gravity	Ketones
Volume[a]	Bilirubin
Odor[a]	Blood
Foam[a]	Nitrite
	pH
	Urobilinogen
	Leukocyte enzyme

[a]Not always assessed.

TABLE 31.3	Possible Causes of Urine Colors	
COLOR	**PATHOLOGIC CAUSE**	**NONPATHOLOGIC CAUSE**
Straw	Diabetes	Diuretics; high fluid intake (coffee, beer)
Amber	Dehydration	Concentrated first morning specimen; excessive sweating; low fluid intake
Bright yellow	—	Carotene, vitamins
Red	Blood, porphyrins	Menstruation, beets, drugs, dyes
Orange-yellow	Bile, hepatitis	Phenazopyridine (fen az oh PEER i deen) (Pyridium, Uristat), dyes, drugs
Greenish yellow	Bile, hepatitis	Senna (laxative), cascara (laxative), rhubarb
Reddish brown	Old blood, methemoglobin	—
Brownish black	Methemoglobin, melanin	Carbidopa-levodopa (kar bi DOH puh—lee vuh DOH puh) (Sinemet, Parcopa)
Salmon pink	—	Amorphous urates
White (milky)	Fats, pus	Amorphous phosphates
Blue-green	Biliverdin, infection with *Pseudomonas* organisms	Vitamin B, drugs, dyes

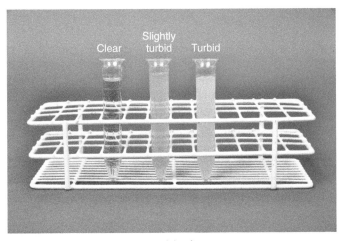

FIGURE 31.5 Turbidity of urine specimens.

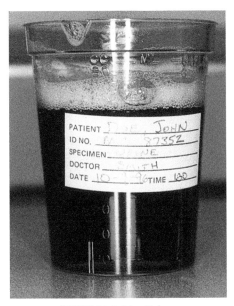

FIGURE 31.6 Urine with foam.

CRITICAL THINKING APPLICATION   31.3

Write down in your own words definitions for these terms: anuria, oliguria, and polyuria. Be ready to share with your class.

Foam

Normally the presence of foam is not recorded, but careful observation of this property can detect a significant clue to an abnormality. Foam consists of small bubbles that persist for a long time after the specimen has been swirled to mix. Foam must not be confused with any bubbles that rapidly disappear. White foam can indicate the presence of increased protein (Fig. 31.6). Greenish-yellow foam may indicate bilirubin in the urine. Care should be taken in handling such urine specimens because the greenish-yellow color may indicate that the patient has viral hepatitis, which is highly contagious. Always observe Standard Precautions and wear appropriate personal protective equipment (PPE) when handling specimens. If foam is observed and seems significant, add a note in the Comments field of a paper or electronic test report.

Odor

As with foam, odor is not normally recorded but can be an important clue to metabolic disorders. Normal urine is said to be *aromatic* or having a distinct or fragrant smell. Changes in the odor of urine may be caused by disease, the presence of bacteria, or diet. A patient with diabetes may pass urine that has a fruity odor if he or she is excreting ketones in the urine. An ammonia or a *putrid* (foul or decaying) smell in the urine can be caused by an infection. An ammonia smell may also be noticed in urine that has been at room temperature for too long before it is tested. Foods such as asparagus and garlic also can produce an abnormal odor in the urine. Urine from a child with *phenylketonuria* (PKU) may smell "mousy." If the odor seems significant, add a note in the Comments field of a paper or electronic test report.

Phenylketonuria

Phenylketonuria (PKU) is a rare hereditary condition in which the amino acid **phenylalanine** is not properly metabolized or broken down in the body. PKU that is undiagnosed or untreated can lead to severe cognitive disabilities. Accumulation of phenylalanine in the blood and urine gives body fluids the odor of wet fur. (Blood sampling for PKU is discussed in Chapter 32.)

Specific Gravity

Specific gravity is defined as the weight of a substance compared with the weight of an equal volume of distilled water. In UA, specific gravity is the approximate measurement of the concentration of substances dissolved in the urine. The specific gravity of distilled water is 1.000. The normal specific gravity of urine ranges from 1.005 to 1.030, depending on the patient's fluid intake. Most samples fall between 1.010 and 1.025. The urine's specific gravity indicates whether the kidneys can concentrate the urine. A change in specific gravity is one of the first indications of kidney disease. Conditions such as **glomerulonephritis**, chronic renal insufficiency, or diabetes may lower the specific gravity. To measure specific gravity, laboratories may use a refractometer, but most use Clinical Laboratory Improvement Amendments (CLIA)-waived chemical reagent strips.

A *refractometer* measures the *refraction* (bending) of light through solids in a liquid. The result is called the *refractive index*, which, for our purposes, is the same as *specific gravity*. The refractometer requires only a drop of urine. One drop of well-mixed urine is placed under the hinged cover of the instrument. Then the value is read directly from a scale viewed through the eyepiece. Fig. 31.7 shows the refractometer on the left and the visual results of the urine in the circle on the right. The scale on the left side of the circle shows a urine specific gravity of 1.020. The refractometer must be calibrated daily with distilled water, which should read 1.000. Note that specific gravity carries no unit of measure after the number.

The analysis that uses a reagent strip, also called a urine *dipstick*, is a CLIA-waived test. A reagent strip test is the most common method used for measuring specific gravity in the POL. The pad on the strip contains a chemical that is sensitive to positively charged **ions**, such as sodium (Na^+) and potassium (K^+). The pad detects the

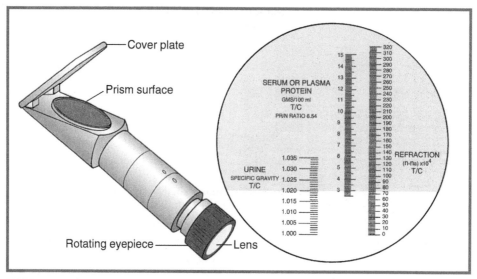

FIGURE 31.7 Refractometer. A drop of urine is placed on the prism surface of the refractometer *(left)*, and the cover plate is closed. When the examiner looks through the lens, two graphs are seen in the circular field of vision *(right)*. The urine specific gravity (SG) is read from the left scale, where the blue shadow meets the lighted bottom. The SG is 1.020.

urine's specific gravity. Various color changes indicate values between 1.000 and 1.030 (see the *specific gravity* row of colors in Procedure 31.5, Fig. 2).

Chemical Examination of Urine

Tests can be performed on urine to detect the presence of certain chemicals, which can provide valuable information to the provider. In certain situations, these chemical test results can be critical to a diagnosis. Also, some urine dipstick results will turn positive before a patient has specific symptoms of a disease or disorder. That is one reason a routine urinalysis can be a screening test for many conditions.

Reagent strip testing is the most widely used technique for detecting chemicals in the urine (see Procedure 31.5, p. 796). These strip tests are available in a variety of types (Fig. 31.8). Dipsticks are plastic strips with paper pads attached. The paper pads contain chemical reagents. The reagents react chemically with analytes in the urine. The chemical reaction is read by looking for a color change on each individual pad. The presence or absence of these chemicals in the urine provides information on the status of carbohydrate metabolism, liver and kidney function, and the patient's acid-base balance.

Reagent strips are designed to be used once and then discarded in a biohazard waste container. The directions for each type of reagent strip test are included inside the package. Instructions must be followed exactly if accurate results are to be obtained. A color comparison chart is provided on the label of the container. In addition to reagent strips, a few tablet tests are available for chemically testing urine.

All strips and tablets must be kept in tightly closed containers in a cool, dry area and should be removed just before testing. To prevent contamination of the bottle, never touch a strip that has been exposed to urine against the color comparison chart on the bottle. If both a UA and a C&S have been ordered for a specimen, separate the sample. The original sample in the sterile container will go to microbiology and be used for the C&S. Pour off an aliquot into a

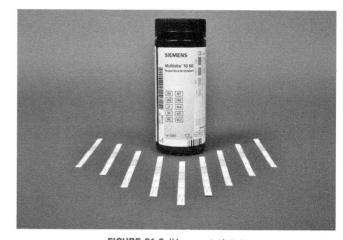

FIGURE 31.8 Urine reagent strip test.

nonsterile urine tube for the UA. If you were to introduce a reagent strip into the sterile urine sample, it would contaminate the specimen and make it unfit for C&S testing.

pH

The pH is a measurement of the acidity or alkalinity of the urine. A urine specimen with a pH of 7 is neutral. A value below 7 indicates acidity, and a value above 7 indicates alkalinity. Normal, freshly voided urine may have a pH range of 5.5 to 8 (Fig. 31.9). The urinary pH varies with an individual's metabolic status, diet, drug therapy, and disease. In the case of bacteria in the urine, the urine pH is usually alkaline. Knowing the pH of the sample also helps when identifying crystals that may be found in the urine sediment.

Glucose

Glucose is filtered out of the blood in the glomerulus, and, under normal conditions, most glucose is reabsorbed in the tubules of the

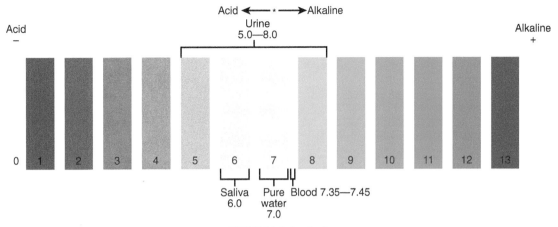

FIGURE 31.9 The pH scale.

nephron. Detectable *glycosuria* (glucose in the urine) occurs when the filtered glucose in the renal tubules is so high it cannot be reabsorbed into the blood. A positive urine glucose may be the first indication that a patient is diabetic. The glucose pad on a reagent strip test is based on a specific enzyme reaction in which glucose, and no other sugar, causes a positive reaction.

Glucose Reabsorption

The reabsorption of glucose depends on its **renal threshold**. The renal threshold for blood glucose is below 160 mg/dL. This means that all the glucose will be reabsorbed into the blood if the blood glucose level is below 160 mg/dL. If the blood glucose level is higher than 160 mg/dL, the blood will not reabsorb the glucose. The filtered glucose then remains in the urine, which will show up as a positive test result for glucose during urinalysis.

Ketones

Ketones are the end product of fat metabolism in the body. *Ketonuria* (ketones in the urine) is commonly seen in patients with diabetes mellitus that is not well controlled; in persons on a very-low-carbohydrate diet; or after excessive vomiting. Because ketones evaporate at room temperature, urine should be tested immediately, or the specimen should be tightly covered and refrigerated. Examples of ketones include acetoacetate and acetone.

CRITICAL THINKING APPLICATION   31.4

- Julie performs routine urinalysis as Becca observes. One sample has a high glucose level and a low ketone level. Becca knows that both analytes are associated with diabetes. How would you explain a high urine glucose and low urine ketone result? Write down your answer. Could there be more than one explanation? Discuss this question with your class.

Protein

Protein in the urine in detectable amounts is called *proteinuria* and is one of the first signs of renal disease. We normally excrete a very small amount of protein every day that is undetectable.

Some causes of proteinuria may include the following:
- *Orthostatic proteinuria*: protein is excreted only when the patient is in an upright position.
- Pregnancy: a common finding in pregnancy and must be monitored along with excessive weight gain and increased blood pressure (three possible symptoms of preeclampsia; see Chapter 27).
- After heavy exercise

The reagent strip is highly sensitive to urinary albumin and is less sensitive to the other proteins.

Blood

The presence of blood in urine may indicate infection or trauma to the urinary tract. The blood test pad on the reagent strip reacts with three different blood constituents: *intact* (whole) red blood cells, hemoglobin from *lysed* (broken) red blood cells, and **myoglobin**.

Hematuria is the presence of intact red blood cells in urine. The color reaction on the reagent strip ranges from yellow to green to dark green when hematuria is present, revealing a speckled appearance. Hematuria can be caused by irritation of the kidneys, ureters, bladder, or urethra. It also is a common finding in *cystitis* (inflammation of the urinary bladder) and in individuals passing kidney stones. A random specimen may contain blood from vaginal contamination if the woman is menstruating.

Hemoglobinuria is the presence of *hemolyzed* (ruptured, broken) red blood cells in urine (Fig. 31.10). True hemoglobinuria is not common. But urine specimens that contain blood may test positive for hemolyzed blood for a few reasons:
- The urine specimen has sat for too long at room temperature, causing the RBCs to lyse. Freshly collected specimens give the most accurate testing results.
- The pH of the urine is highly alkaline, which can cause RBCs to lyse.
- The specific gravity of the sample is below 1.010; this can also cause RBCs to lyse.
- Bacteria in the urine can also cause a false-positive hemolyzed blood test result.

Finding blood or hemolyzed blood on the urine dipstick should be confirmed by microscopic examination of the urine. If intact RBCs are seen microscopically, this should be noted on the UA report to the

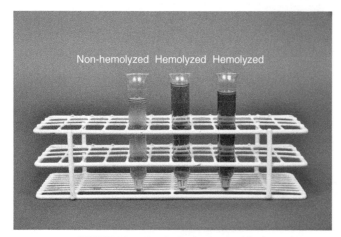

FIGURE 31.10 Hemolyzed and nonhemolyzed blood.

TABLE 31.4   Normal Urine Reference Ranges for Reagent Strips

PROPERTY	REFERENCE RANGE
Color	Pale yellow to amber
Clarity	Clear to slightly turbid
Specific gravity	1.001–1.035
pH	4.6–8
Protein (mg/dL)	NEG
Glucose (mg/dL)	NEG
Ketone (mg/dL)	NEG
Bilirubin (mg/dL)	NEG
Blood (mg/dL)	NEG
Nitrite (mg/dL)	NEG
Urobilinogen (Ehrlich units)	0.1–1
White blood cells	NEG

NEG, Negative.

provider. True hemoglobinuria is the result of intravascular red blood cell destruction and can be caused by blood transfusion reactions, malaria, drug reactions, snakebites, and severe burns.

Myoglobinuria (myoglobin in the urine) occurs when muscle tissue is damaged or injured. This can occur with crushing injuries, myocardial infarctions, contact sports, or strenuous exercise. Patients with muscular dystrophy often have myoglobinuria. Hemoglobinuria cannot be distinguished from myoglobinuria by reagent strip testing. Both cause a uniform change in color from light green to dark green on the strip.

Bilirubin and Urobilinogen

Bilirubin is a product of the breakdown of hemoglobin. Hemoglobin is released from old red blood cells and is gradually converted to bilirubin in the liver. The liver continues to convert bilirubin to *urobilinogen,* which is sent to the intestines for excretion. Bilirubin is a bile pigment not normally found in urine. Its presence in urine is one of the first signs of liver disease or other diseases in which the liver may be involved.

Bilirubin in the urine (*bilirubinuria*) can occur even before **jaundice** or other symptoms of liver disease are evident. It is the result of liver cell damage or obstruction of the common bile duct by stones or tumors. Excessive bilirubin colors the urine yellow-brown to greenish orange. Because direct light causes bilirubin to break down, urine samples must be protected from light until testing is complete.

Urobilinogen normally is present in urine in small amounts. Elevated urobilinogen is seen with increased red blood cell destruction, liver disease, or total obstruction of the bile duct.

Nitrite

Nitrate is a common component of normal urine. *Nitrites* occur in urine when bacteria break down nitrate. A positive nitrite test result may indicate the presence of a UTI. However, not all bacteria are able to break down nitrate to nitrite. A negative nitrite test can occur when bacteria are in small numbers or when the urine has not been in the bladder long enough for the chemical breakdown to occur. *Escherichia coli* (*E. coli*), the bacteria that is the most common cause of UTIs, does break down nitrate to nitrite. A positive reaction is any pink color on the nitrite dipstick pad.

Leukocyte Esterase

Leukocytes (white blood cells) are present in urine when a person has a UTI. The leukocyte **esterase** test pad on the reagent strip takes 2 minutes to release esterase from white blood cells. Wait a full 2 minutes before reading the leukocyte esterase result. The test does not react with small numbers of white blood cells found in normal urine. A false-positive result could be caused by WBC contaminants from the vagina, especially if the sample is allowed to sit at room temperature. Urine specimens should be tested as soon as possible after collection. If this is not possible the specimen should be refrigerated.

CRITICAL THINKING APPLICATION   **31.5**

One of yesterday's samples that Julie saved in the laboratory refrigerator is ready to test. The sample gives a bright pink positive result for nitrites and a moderate positive result for leukocytes on the reagent strip test. What condition would give this result on a dipstick UA? Could there be more than one answer?

Limitations of Reagent Strip Testing

The reagent strip is a reliable method of testing urine if used properly. The normal urine reference ranges for a reagent strip are presented in Table 31.4. Errors can arise from several sources:

- The test strip is soaked in the specimen, and chemicals in the pads may be overly diluted.
- The test strip is not held horizontally while read, and colors from one pad may bleed onto another.
- The test pads on the strip are not read at the proper time, or the chemical reaction may be read incorrectly.

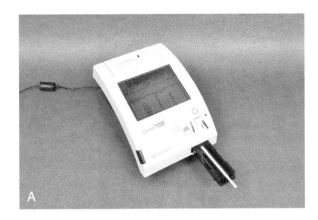

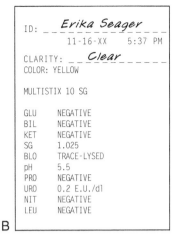

ID: _Erika Seager_ _ _ _ _ _
            11-16-XX   5:37 PM
CLARITY: _ _Clear_ _ _ _ _ _ _
COLOR: YELLOW

MULTISTIX 10 SG

GLU   NEGATIVE
BIL   NEGATIVE
KET   NEGATIVE
SG   1.025
BLO   TRACE-LYSED
pH   5.5
PRO   NEGATIVE
URO   0.2 E.U./dl
NIT   NEGATIVE
LEU   NEGATIVE

FIGURE 31.11 (A) Clinitek 50 Urine Chemistry Analyzer. The reagent strip is placed on the tray before the test is begun. **(B)** Sample of the Clinitek results.

- Certain chemicals, such as vitamin C, also called *ascorbic acid*, may affect the results of nitrite, glucose, bilirubin, and blood tests. Normal levels of vitamin C do not interfere with routine urinalysis, but large amounts can alter test results.

Visual interpretation of the color on the reagent strip pads is likely to vary among individuals. Some laboratories use automated instruments to read the strips. Several companies manufacture instruments that detect the color change in the analysis of the reagent strip. Once the strip has been placed in the instrument, a microprocessor controls the movement of the strip into the instrument. Light of a specific wavelength is beamed onto each of the test areas on the strip. The color change on each pad is analyzed by the microprocessor and converted into a digital reading, and the results are printed out (Fig. 31.11). The advantage of this method is that timing and color interpretation are consistent. The disadvantage is that the instrument is not able to identify and adjust for highly colored urine, leading to false results. The medical assistant should be aware of this and should manually test urine specimens that are darkly colored.

Assurance and Quality Control in Urinalysis

The US Food and Drug Administration (FDA) categorizes the chemical analysis of urine performed by an instrument or a reagent strip as a CLIA-waived test. The chemical analysis includes the reagent strip (dipstick) tests for bilirubin, glucose, hemoglobin or blood, ketones, leukocyte esterase, nitrite, pH, protein, specific gravity, and urobilinogen. A commercially available control strip should be used to determine the reliability of the reagent strips used in chemical analysis. One such control strip is the Chek-Stix. The plastic control strip has seven pads, each of which contains synthetic ingredients that mimic human urine when reconstituted in water. After reconstitution, a reagent test strip is immersed in the control solution, and the results are compared with a chart that accompanies the Chek-Stix. Both positive and negative Chek-Stix controls are available (see Procedure 31.4, p. 795). The positive reconstituted control shows positive (abnormal) results when a test strip is inserted and read, whereas the negative reconstituted control shows normal urinalysis results along its test strip. It is important to observe and record the abnormal and normal results produced by the positive and negative controls.

Also, make sure the test results are consistent with the Chek-Stix charts provided by the manufacturer before testing patient urine specimens.

The Chek-Stix is one type of commercial control, but other strips and prepared liquid controls are also available. Each POL should investigate the best commercial control for its needs and quality control program.

MICROSCOPIC PREPARATION AND EXAMINATION OF URINE SEDIMENT

Microscopic examination of urine consists of categorizing and counting cells, casts, crystals, and miscellaneous constituents in the sediment of a urine sample. The sediment is obtained after a measured portion of urine is centrifuged. The sediment will be pushed to the bottom of the tube containing urine. The sediment will be prepared for a microscopic exam, and the remaining liquid urine will be poured off and disposed of properly.

Many formed elements are found in the urine. Some are significant, and others are not. Most important, the microscopic examination should correlate with the physical and chemical analyses. For example, if the physical examination of the urine showed a reddish color and the chemical reagent strip tested positive for blood, then seeing red blood cells during the microscopic examination would be consistent with the physical and chemical results. Medical assistants should be familiar with the preparation of urine specimens for this test and with the possible test results (see Procedure 31.6, p. 797).

Microscopic Preparation of Urine

To perform the microscopic UA procedure, a laboratory must be certified to perform CLIA Provider-Performed Microscopy Procedures (PPMPs), a subcategory of CLIA moderate-complexity laboratories. Quality assurance is just as important in the microscopic examination as in the chemical analysis of urine. To ensure consistency and standardization, commercially available systems can be used, such as the KOVA System or the UriSystem. These systems may include specially designed, graduated centrifuge tubes with devices or pipets that allow easy **decanting** of **supernatant** and retention of an exact amount of sediment. They also use specially designed plastic slides with wells or coverslips that accept only a given volume of sediment. Control solutions containing preserved cells are also available from KOVA. This type of solution also provides quality control for cell identification. Whatever system is used, the Clinical and Laboratory Standards Institute (CLSI) recommends the following:

- The urine volume should be 12 mL.
- The specimen should be centrifuged for 5 minutes at a relative centrifugal force of 400 *g* (i.e., 400 times normal gravity).
- A standardized slide should be used to view the sediment.
- A consistent reporting format should be used.

When a urine sample is centrifuged, the clear upper portion of the specimen is called the *supernatant.* It is poured off, and a drop of the well-mixed sediment at the bottom of the centrifuged tube is examined under a microscope. The sediment may be stained to give greater contrast to the formed elements. The stain assists in the identification of formed elements by improving the detail of cellular structures.

Microscopic Examination of Urine

The examination of urine is not categorized as CLIA-waived; therefore it cannot be performed by a medical assistant without additional training, additional supervision, and rigid compliance with CLIA quality assurance protocols for the laboratory. Periodic proficiency testing must be successfully completed to maintain a PPMP laboratory certification. (See Chapter 30 for CLIA moderate-complexity approved personnel.)

The three main categories of microscopic findings are casts, cells, and crystals.

Casts

Casts are created when protein accumulates and precipitates in the kidney tubules and is then washed into the urine. The protein takes on the size and shape of the tubules, forming the casts. Casts are cylindric, with flat or rounded ends, and are classified according to the substances observed inside them. Certain types of casts are connected to specific renal diseases and disorders. Other casts are physiologic and are generally caused by strenuous exercise. Casts can dissolve in alkaline urine if the sample is not examined promptly. The microscopic exam should take place as soon as possible after specimen collection. The following paragraphs describe some of the casts that may be seen, but these are not all the possible casts.

Hyaline casts are pale, transparent, cylindric structures that have rounded ends and parallel sides (Fig. 31.12). They are formed when urine flow through individual nephrons is diminished. They can be found in the urine of individuals with kidney disease, but also in the urine of people without such disease who have exercised heavily. Hyaline casts will be missed entirely if the light is not adjusted properly. Occasionally, hyaline casts have granular or cellular inclusions.

White blood cell casts are hyaline casts that contain leukocytes. White blood cells seen in casts usually have a multilobed nucleus. White blood cell casts are seen in pyelonephritis (Fig. 31.13).

Red blood cell casts always indicate a pathologic condition and are highly diagnostic. These casts occur in glomerulonephritis. They are hyaline casts with embedded red blood cells. Their presence indicates damage to the glomerulus. They may appear brown due to the color of the red blood cells present (Fig. 31.14).

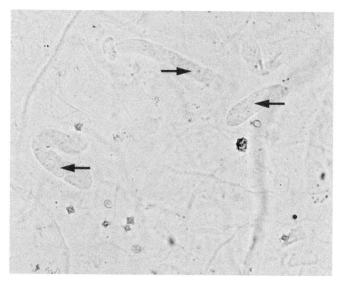

FIGURE 31.12 Hyaline cast. (From Brunzel NA: *Fundamentals of urine and body fluid analysis,* ed 3, Philadelphia, 2013, Saunders.)

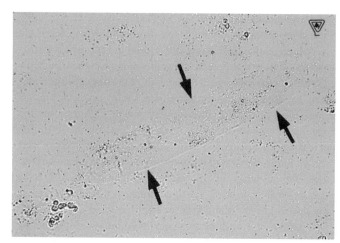

FIGURE 31.13 White blood cell cast. (From Stepp CA, Woods MA: *Laboratory procedures for medical office personnel,* Philadelphia, 1998, Saunders.)

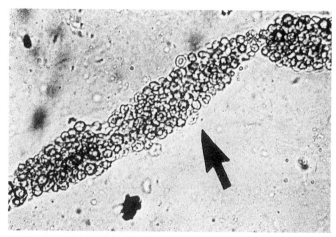

FIGURE 31.14 Red blood cell cast. (From Stepp CA, Woods MA: *Laboratory procedures for medical office personnel,* Philadelphia, 1998, Saunders.)

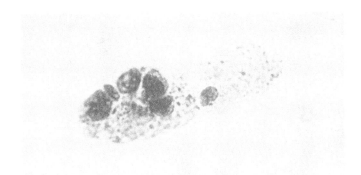

FIGURE 31.15 Renal tubular epithelial cell cast. (From Brunzel NA: *Fundamentals of urine and body fluid analysis*, ed 3, Philadelphia, 2013, Saunders.)

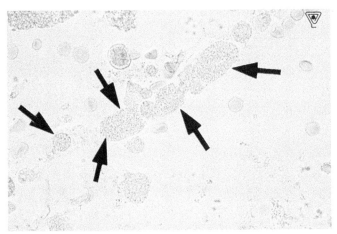

FIGURE 31.16 Granular cast. (From Stepp CA, Woods MA: *Laboratory procedures for medical office personnel*, Philadelphia, 1998, Saunders.)

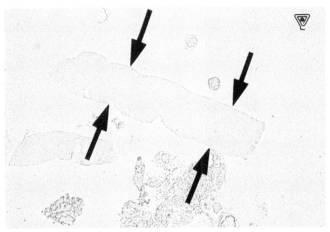

FIGURE 31.17 Waxy cast. (From Stepp CA, Woods MA: *Laboratory procedures for medical office personnel*, Philadelphia, 1998, Saunders.)

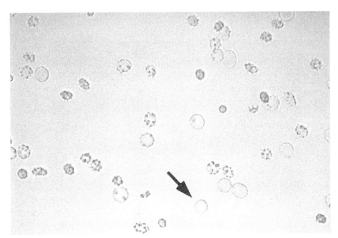

FIGURE 31.18 Red blood cells in urine. (From Stepp CA, Woods MA: *Laboratory procedures for medical office personnel*, Philadelphia, 1998, Saunders.)

Renal tubular epithelial cell casts contain embedded renal tubular epithelial cells. These casts are easily confused with white blood cell casts, particularly if the cells have started to degenerate. Renal tubular epithelial cell casts are found when excessive damage has occurred in the kidney. Causes include shock, **renal ischemia**, heavy-metal poisoning, certain allergic reactions, and **nephrotoxic** drugs (Fig. 31.15).

Finely and coarsely granular casts may indicate renal disease. On close examination, granular casts show a hyaline cast with coarse or fine granular inclusions. The granules are thought to be caused by protein clusters or the breakdown of cellular inclusions (Fig. 31.16).

Waxy casts are rarely seen. They appear as glassy, brittle, smooth, homogeneous structures. They usually are yellowish, have cracks or fissures, and have squared or broken ends. They are considered to be cellular casts that have broken down and are found in individuals with severe renal disease (Fig. 31.17).

Occasionally more than one type of cell is found in a single cast. Mixed cellular casts have been reported, and absolute identification of the cell types present may be difficult. Cast identification is not a CLIA-waived procedure.

Cells

Cells found in the urine include epithelial cells, which come from the lining of the genitourinary tract. Red blood cells and white blood cells, which come from the bloodstream, also may be seen. Cells are classified and counted under high-power magnification.

Red blood cells may enter the urinary tract at any point of inflammation or injury. They may be found in normal urine in small numbers. Persistent hematuria should be investigated. Red blood cells are smaller than white blood cells and have no nucleus (Fig. 31.18). If they are in *hypotonic* (dilute) urine, they swell and burst. In *hypertonic* (concentrated) urine, they may be bumpy or wrinkle.

CRITICAL THINKING APPLICATION   31.6
Becca is excited to look in the microscope and see a urine sediment that has been prepared for the nurse practitioner at WMFM, Jean Burke. As Becca looks in the microscope's eyepiece, she sees quite a few red blood cells. What could cause red blood cells to be present in the urine? Discuss your thoughts with the class.

Yeast cells in the urine may indicate vaginal contamination or a urinary yeast infection (Fig. 31.19). Yeast is common in the urine of patients with diabetes. Yeast cells are oval shaped and may show budding.

White blood cells may occasionally be found in normal urine, but increased numbers are associated with a UTI or with vaginal

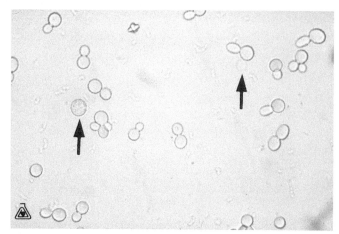

FIGURE 31.19 Yeast cells in urine. (From Stepp CA, Woods MA: *Laboratory procedures for medical office personnel,* Philadelphia, 1998, Saunders.)

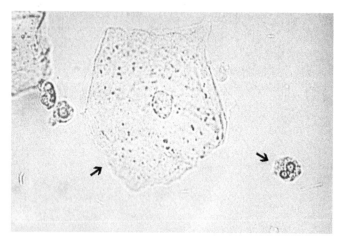

FIGURE 31.20 A large squamous epithelial cell *(left arrow)* and a white blood cell *(right arrow)* in urine. (From Ringsrud KM, Linne JJ: *Urinalysis and body fluids: a color text and atlas,* St Louis, 1995, Mosby.)

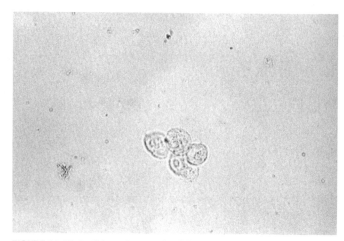

FIGURE 31.21 Small cluster of transitional epithelial cells in urine. (From Ringsrud KM, Linne JJ: *Urinalysis and body fluids: a color text and atlas,* St Louis, 1995, Mosby.)

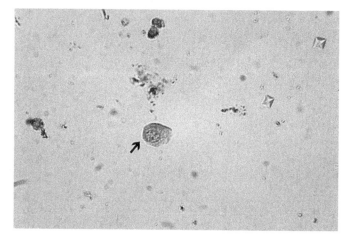

FIGURE 31.22 Renal tubular cell *(arrow)* in urine. (From Ringsrud KM, Linne JJ: *Urinalysis and body fluids: a color text and atlas,* St Louis, 1995, Mosby.)

contamination during specimen collection. White blood cells are larger than red blood cells and have a granular appearance. They may have a multilobed nucleus. Most white blood cells in the urine are neutrophils (Fig. 31.20).

Squamous epithelial cells line the lower portion of the genitourinary tract. When present in large numbers in female patients, they usually indicate vaginal contamination. Squamous epithelial cells are large, flat, and irregular. They have a single, small, round, centrally located nucleus and often occur in sheets or clumps (see Fig. 31.20).

Transitional epithelial cells line most of the urinary tract. They are round or oval and may have a tail. Occasionally, two nuclei are seen. They may be seen in diseases of the urinary system (Fig. 31.21).

Renal tubular epithelial cells are somewhat larger than white blood cells, are round or oval, and have a nucleus that is single, large, oval, and sometimes eccentric. A few may be found in normal urine specimens, but their presence in increased numbers indicates tubular damage of the nephrons (Fig. 31.22).

Crystals

Crystals are common in urine specimens, particularly if the specimen has been allowed to cool. Cooling causes solid crystals to precipitate

out of the urine, which changes the urine's appearance from clear to cloudy. The presence of most crystals is not clinically significant unless the crystals are found in large numbers. With only rare exceptions, abnormal crystals are seen in acidic urine. Abnormal crystals may be present because of certain disease states or an inherited metabolic condition. They may also be *iatrogenic,* which means they are present because of medication or treatment. Identification of crystals begins with noting the pH of the urine specimen. A history of medications and recent diagnostic testing may be helpful too.

Crystals are reported as occasional, few, moderate, or many per high-power field (Table 31.5). At times, crystals can be *amorphous,* or lacking a defined shape. Frequently crystals are difficult to identify without additional chemical testing.

Miscellaneous Findings

Oval fat bodies are formed when renal tubular epithelial cells or macrophages absorb fats. The fat droplets in the cells vary in size. They are characteristic of kidney distress (Fig. 31.23).

A few *bacteria* may be found in normal urine specimens. High bacterial counts in a urine specimen without white blood cells may indicate that the specimen sat at room temperature and the bacteria

TABLE 31.5 Normal and Abnormal Crystals Found in Urine

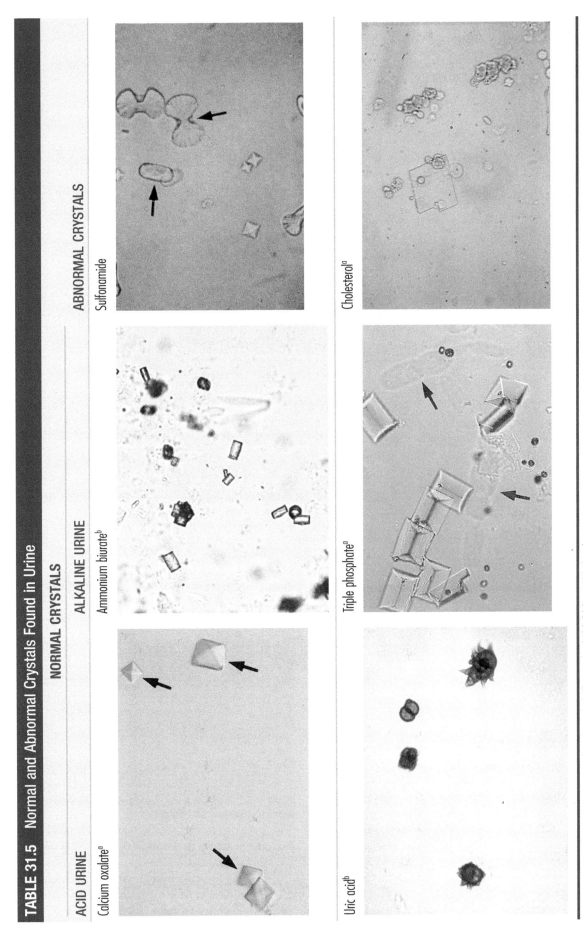

NORMAL CRYSTALS

ACID URINE

Calcium oxalate[a]

Uric acid[b]

ALKALINE URINE

Ammonium biurate[b]

Triple phosphate[a]

ABNORMAL CRYSTALS

Sulfonamide

Cholesterol[a]

[a]From Stepp CA, Woods MA: *Laboratory procedures for medical office personnel,* Philadelphia, 1998, Saunders.
[b]From Brunzel NA: *Fundamentals of urine and body fluid analysis,* ed 3, Philadelphia, 2013, Saunders.

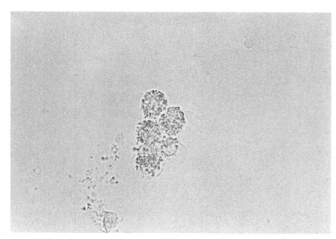

FIGURE 31.23 Small cluster of oval fat bodies in urine. (From Ringsrud KM, Linne JJ: *Urinalysis and body fluids: a color text and atlas*, St Louis, 1995, Mosby.)

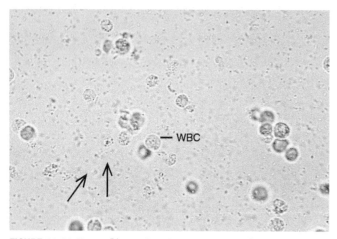

FIGURE 31.24 Many small bacteria *(arrows)* in urine. (From Ringsrud KM, Linne JJ: *Urinalysis and body fluids: a color text and atlas*, St Louis, 1995, Mosby.)

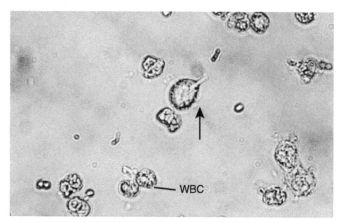

FIGURE 31.25 *Trichomonas* sp. *(arrow)* in urine. (From Stepp CA, Woods MA: *Laboratory procedures for medical office personnel*, Philadelphia, 1998, Saunders.)

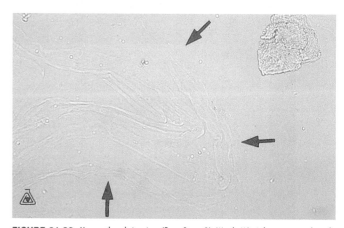

FIGURE 31.26 Mucous threads in urine. (From Stepp CA, Woods MA: *Laboratory procedures for medical office personnel*, Philadelphia, 1998, Saunders.)

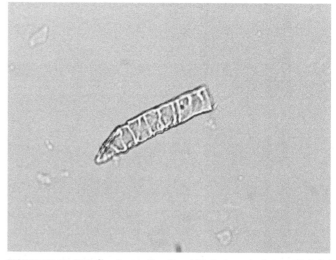

FIGURE 31.27 Diaper fibers in urine. (From Brunzel NA: *Fundamentals of urine and body fluid analysis*, ed 3, Philadelphia, 2013, Saunders.)

multiplied. Urine specimens with a putrid odor, numerous white blood cells, and bacteria (Fig. 31.24) are common in UTIs. Bacteria are seen under high-power magnification. They are often *motile* (moving).

Spermatozoa can be found in the urine specimens of both male and female patients. In a specimen from a female, their presence represents vaginal contamination. Sperm usually have pointed, oval heads and long, whip-like tails. They may be motile in fresh urine.

Trichomonas vaginalis is the most commonly encountered **protozoan** in urine (Fig. 31.25). It is frequently a vaginal contaminant but may also be found in urine specimens from male patients. When urine is fresh and warm, trichomonas may be motile and move rapidly when viewed under the microscope. Trichomonas organisms are pear-shaped protozoa with four *flagella*, or whip-like tails. They are larger than round epithelial cells but smaller than squamous cells. Trichomonas organisms die when the specimen cools.

Mucous threads can be found in most urine specimens. They appear as pale, irregular, threadlike structures with tapered ends. Beginners often confuse hyaline casts with mucous threads. They are frequently seen in patients with inflammation and in specimens contaminated with vaginal secretions (Fig. 31.26).

Artifacts and contaminants are often found in urine sediment. Training is required to tell them apart from significant structures.

Fibers are common in the sediment and come from clothing, diapers, or digested plant material:

- Clothing fibers often are long and twisted and sometimes are colored. Diaper fibers can be confused with casts (Fig. 31.27).
- Plant fibers appear in the urine because of fecal contamination (Fig. 31.28).

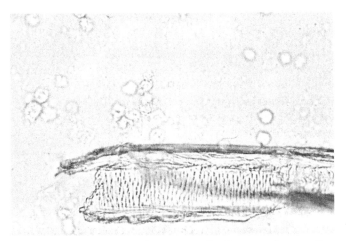

FIGURE 31.28 Plant fibers from fecal contamination; cells and bacteria are also present. (From Ringsrud KM, Linne JJ: *Urinalysis and body fluids: a color text and atlas,* St Louis, 1995, Mosby.)

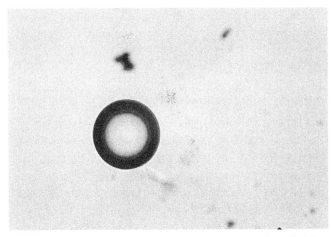

FIGURE 31.30 Large air bubble in urine. (From Ringsrud KM, Linne JJ: *Urinalysis and body fluids: a color text and atlas,* St Louis, 1995, Mosby.)

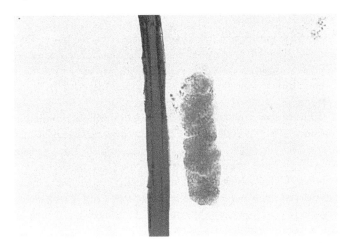

FIGURE 31.29 Fiber, probably hair *(left)* and waxy cast *(right)* in urine. (From Ringsrud KM, Linne JJ: *Urinalysis and body fluids: a color text and atlas,* St Louis, 1995, Mosby.)

- Hair is distinct not only because of the visible rough look to the strand but also because of the large size (Fig. 31.29).
- Air bubbles are common if the coverslip was improperly placed over the sediment. Air bubbles are structureless and *refractile* (refracting light, causing a glow) and have a dark outline (Fig. 31.30).

Understanding the Results of Microscopic Examination

The medical assistant should understand how the microscopic findings of the sediment are reported. First, the sediment is examined under the low-power objective and low light to locate casts, which generally are found around the edges of the coverslip. From 10 to 15 low-power fields are scanned, and the number of casts is counted and reported.

Red and white blood cells, epithelial cells, yeasts, bacteria, and crystals are identified using the high-power objective and increased light. From 10 to 15 high-power fields should be scanned and the number counted, averaged, and reported. The method of counting varies considerably among laboratories. It is important that all workers in the same laboratory use the same counting and reporting systems.

The numbers of casts, RBCs, and WBCs are counted, totaled, and averaged. They are reported using numeric ranges based on the average seen (e.g., range of 0–1, 1–2, 2–5, 5–10, 10–20, and so

forth; also, too numerous to count [TNTC]). Microscopic examination of epithelial cells is similar. Epithelial cells are counted, totaled, and averaged. Then they are reported as occasional, few, moderate, or many per high-power field (e.g., 1–3 occasional, 4–6 few, 7–12 moderate, >12 many). Miscellaneous elements seen in urine are counted, averaged, and estimated. Reports will be estimated as occasional – not seen in every field; few – covers less than one-fourth of the field; moderate – covers approximately one-half of the field; and many – covers the entire field.

ADDITIONAL CLIA-WAIVED URINE TESTS

Clinitest

The glucose test on the reagent strip detects only glucose, the most common sugar found in the urine. However, sugars other than glucose also can appear in the urine. Certain metabolic disorders can result in the excretion of sugars such as galactose, fructose, lactose, maltose, or pentose. Galactosemia, a rare pathologic condition, is a congenital deficiency in the body's ability to metabolize galactose to glucose; galactosemia results in excretion of galactose in the urine. Seen in infants, it results in failure to thrive, vomiting, and diarrhea. If detected early, galactose can be eliminated from the diet, and the child develops normally. Lactose may be found in the urine of pregnant women or premature infants. Maltose may be excreted in patients with diabetes. Of the many sugars in the body, only the presence of glucose or galactose indicates possible pathologic conditions.

The Clinitest is based on the chemical reduction of copper. It is used to detect reducing substances (sugars) in the urine (see Procedure 31.7, p. 799). Copper reduction tests are based on the principle that reducing substances can chemically convert one form of copper into another form of copper. The chemical reaction produces a color change. The Clinitest uses a reagent tablet that is dropped directly into a test tube containing diluted urine. A heat-releasing reaction occurs and causes the Clinitest contents to boil. The reaction only takes a few seconds and then the boiling stops. After the reaction is complete, the color of the reaction is compared with the color chart supplied by the manufacturer. *Clinitest Reaction Note:* If the color change reaches the orange maximum color during the reaction and then ends in a lower color range, the test result is reported as "greater than" the highest positive result.

The Clinitest has traditionally been done in the POL, but new methods of testing are becoming more common. It is likely that the Clinitest will not be done in the near future as technology and testing methods change and improve.

CRITICAL THINKING APPLICATION   31.7

Julie has three specimens on which she needs to run a Clinitest, but first she needs to complete the quality control samples: one positive control and one negative control. She has Becca read the procedure and then put on gloves and protective eyewear. Julie performs the quality control tests, and Becca watches as the tests bubble and boil. Why is it important for Becca to have on PPE during this test and during her whole time in the lab? Share your thoughts with your class.

Urine Pregnancy Testing

All pregnancy tests detect the presence of human chorionic gonadotropin (hCG), a hormone produced by the placenta and present in urine during pregnancy (see Procedure 31.8, p. 800). After the fertilized egg has implanted in the uterus, the hCG levels in serum double every few days. This rapid rise occurs for approximately 7 weeks, and then the level begins to decline. Within 72 hours of delivery, the hormone disappears.

The most common type of test for pregnancy is the lateral flow immunoassay test. Many brands are available for laboratory use and are also available over the counter (OTC) for home use. These tests are sensitive enough to detect the presence of hCG in urine as early as 1 week after implantation, or 4 to 5 days before a missed menstrual period. The tests can be performed in as little as 5 minutes and are easy to interpret. CLIA-waived pregnancy tests or home pregnancy tests are read following the manufacturer's instructions. Tests are easy to read and often are as simple as reading a color change. For optimum results, the test should be performed on a first morning urine specimen because it is the most concentrated urine of the day.

The test is based on reactions that occur between *antibodies* and *antigens*. Antibodies are proteins formed in response to a specific antigen (e.g., paired like a lock and key). Antigens are foreign substances that initiate the production of antibodies. When antibodies and antigens come in contact, the antibody binds to the antigen. This makes the antigen unable to cause disease. (See Chapter 18 for more information on antibodies and antigens.)

The pregnancy test cartridge contains a membrane with an absorbent pad. The urine sample is pipetted into the sample well of the test cartridge. The urine then moves along the absorbent pad, reaching the test area on the membrane. The following reactions can occur:

- All samples (positive or negative) cause the control zone (C) line to turn blue. The presence of this line indicates that the test has been carried out correctly. If the C control zone does not show a color reaction, the test is considered invalid (incorrect) and must be repeated using another test device.
- In a positive sample, the hCG antigen attaches to the antibodies in the test zone (T), forming a pink line.
- In a negative sample, there is no hCG antigen to attach to the antibodies in the test zone (T), and no line forms.

The Quick Vue test (see Procedure 31.8, p. 800) is a lateral flow pregnancy test that can be performed on urine. It is used routinely in many POLs.

Ovulation Testing

CLIA-waived lateral flow urine tests are available to predict ovulation for women attempting to conceive either naturally or using **artificial insemination**. During the menstrual cycle, **luteinizing hormone (LH)** remains at a relatively stable level. Approximately 14 days before menstruation, the body experiences the "LH surge," a brief, rapid increase in LH. This surge triggers the release of an ovum (egg) from the ovary. Two to 3 days after the surge, the LH level returns to the base level. Conception is most likely to occur within 36 hours after the LH surge. The principle behind this test is similar to that of the pregnancy test. The absorbent membrane contains anti-LH antibodies. A positive test result indicates a urine LH level of 20 mIU/mL or higher. Testing usually is performed for 5 consecutive days in the middle of a woman's cycle. Once the surge is detected, ovulation can be expected within 2 to 3 days.

Menopause Testing

A woman is said to have reached *menopause* when she has not had a menstrual period for at least 12 months. The time before menopause, called *perimenopause,* can last for years, bringing with it uncomfortable symptoms such as irregular periods, hot flashes, vaginal dryness, and sleep problems.

Some of this may be due to an increase in **follicle-stimulating hormone (FSH)**. Levels of FSH increase temporarily each month to stimulate the ovaries to produce an ovum (egg). When a woman enters menopause, the ovaries stop producing eggs, and the levels of FSH rise. CLIA-waived lateral flow tests detect FSH in the urine. A positive test result indicates that a woman may be in menopause; a negative test result, along with symptoms of menopause, may indicate that a woman is in perimenopause.

The qualitative lateral flow test should never be used to direct a woman to stop using birth control methods if she does not want to conceive. Pregnancy is still possible during perimenopause.

CRITICAL THINKING APPLICATION   31.8

Becca thinks the immunoassays are so fun, watching the quality control samples flow through the kit and the results develop right in front of her. Take a few moments and in your own words describe how a lateral flow immunoassay works. What substances interact to create the reaction in the test kit?

Urine Toxicology

Toxicology is the study of poisonous substances and drugs, and their effects on the body. The clinical laboratory performs testing on body fluids and tissues to monitor the use of therapeutic drugs such as; antibiotics, anticonvulsants, antidepressants, and barbiturates. They may also test for poisoning by herbicides, metals, animal toxins, and poisonous gases (e.g., carbon monoxide)

Laboratory testing for illegal drugs or alcohol is also done, most commonly due to an employment, insurance, or legal requirement (Table 31.6). A urine specimen is the most reliable choice for most routine screening procedures. Urine drug tests detect drug *metabolites* and not the drug themselves. A metabolite is a byproduct of drug metabolism. Urine samples will remain positive even after the effects of the drugs are gone (see Procedure 31.9, p. 801). For routine screening, a random specimen is usually collected.

TABLE 31.6   Commonly Abused Drugs and Body Retention Times

DRUG	RETENTION TIME
Alcohol	2–10 hours
Amphetamine	24–48 hours
Methamphetamine	3–5+ days
Barbiturates	
Phenobarbital	2–6 days
Secobarbital	24 hours
Cocaine, cocaine metabolites	12 hours–3 days
Opiates, heroin, morphine	3–4 days
Phencyclidine (PCP)	3–7+ days
Marijuana (tetrahydrocannabinol metabolites)	2 days up to 11 weeks (for daily users)
Oxycodone	3 days

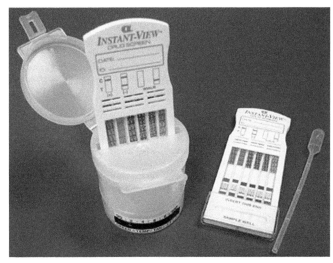

FIGURE 31.31 Instant View drug screening test. (Courtesy Alfa Scientific, Poway, CA.)

Often, the following safeguards are used to ensure that a specimen is fresh and is truly from the patient:
- Water may be temporarily unavailable in the restroom.
- Bluing agents may be added to the toilets.
- A sealed container with a temperature-sensitive strip may be provided for collection.
- Someone of the same gender may accompany the patient into the restroom during the collection.

The *chain of custody* protocol is required for any legal specimen. This means that everyone handling the specimen must document their interaction with the sample. The drugs and their metabolites often remain in urine much longer than the physical impairment lasts. This is one reason urine screening is favored over blood screening.

As a medical assistant, you may be responsible for collecting specimens for toxicology tests and for performing certain laboratory tests. Rapid drug screening devices are about the size and shape of a credit card (Fig. 31.31). The device is dipped into a urine sample, or urine is directly applied to the device. The results are read according to the manufacturer's instructions in just minutes. Negative results indicate that none of the targeted drugs were found in the urine sample at a detectable level. Inconclusive results indicate that the device reacted with something in the urine and confirmatory testing is needed.

Urine multidrug screening tests are a type of lateral flow immunoassay that tests for urine metabolites of a variety of drugs. Common drugs tested include amphetamines, barbiturates, benzodiazepines, cocaine, morphine, methadone, phencyclidine (PCP), tricyclic antidepressants, marijuana, Ecstasy, methamphetamines, methadone, oxycodone, and opiates. This type of testing is also an immunoassay in which antibodies and antigens react to form a readable test result. By using antibodies specific to different drug classes, some test cartridges can simultaneously detect up to 10 different drugs from a single sample in 5 minutes.

Note: Unlike with the lateral flow tests for pregnancy, ovulation, and menopause, the appearance of a line in the T band during a drug screening test indicates a negative test result.

Adulteration Testing and Chain of Custody

Drug testing has legal consequences; therefore additional testing may be necessary to ensure that samples have not been *adulterated*. Adulteration is the intentional manipulation of a urine sample that allows someone to falsely pass a drug screening test. It may involve using urine from another person or an animal, diluting the sample with water, or adding other substances that would compromise the test procedure.

Sensitivity limits for drug screening are set by the US Substance Abuse and Mental Health Services Administration (SAMHSA), the National Institute on Drug Abuse (NIDA), and the US Department of Health and Human Services (DHHS). Positive results on urine drug samples should be confirmed with more specific confirmatory testing methods.

Chain of Custody Rules.
1. The individual being tested must provide a photo identification.
2. Indirect observation of specimen collection is important to make sure the patient being tested has provided the sample. Indirect methods of observation include:
   - Measuring the specimen's temperature
   - Securing water faucets in the restroom so that urine cannot be diluted
   - Having the patient remove outer clothing and leave personal belongings in the examination room
   - Not allowing water to be run or the toilet to be flushed in the restroom during the collection

Note: If you suspect the sample has been adulterated, the patient may be asked to provide another specimen.
3. Within 4 minutes of receiving the specimen, check its temperature (range should be 32° to 38°C [90° to 100°F]). Sample volume should be a minimum of 30 to 45 mL. Inspect the sample for any indications of adulteration (e.g., an unusual color, the presence of foreign materials).
4. Pour the specimen into a specimen bottle and seal the lid with the tamper-evident label/seal provided at the bottom of the chain of custody form. The donor should be present when this is done and should see you write the date and your initials on the label (Fig. 31.32).
5. Ship the specimen to the testing laboratory as soon as possible. It must be sent the same day it was collected.

FEDERAL DRUG TESTING CUSTODY AND CONTROL FORM

|||||||||||||||||||||||||||

SPECIMEN ID NO.   **1234567**   LAB ACCESSION NO.

OMB No. 0930-0158

STEP 1: COMPLETED BY COLLECTOR OR EMPLOYER REPRESENTATIVE

A. Employer Name, Address, I.D. No.   B. MRO Name, Address, Phone and Fax No.

C. Donor SSN or Employee I.D. No. _____

D. Reason for Test: ☐ Pre-employment   ☐ Random   ☐ Reasonable Suspicion/Cause   ☐ Post Accident
                                 ☐ Return to Duty   ☐ Follow-up   ☐ Other (specify)_____

E. Drug Tests to be Performed: ☐ THC, COC, PCP, OPI, AMP   ☐ THC & COC Only   ☐ Other (specify)_____

F. Collection Site Address:

Collector Phone No. _____

Collector Fax No. _____

STEP 2: COMPLETED BY COLLECTOR

| Read specimen temperature within 4 minutes. Is temperature between 90° and 100° F? ☐ Yes   ☐ No, Enter Remark | Specimen Collection: ☐ Split   ☐ Single   ☐ None Provided (Enter Remark) | ☐ Observed (Enter Remark) |

REMARKS

STEP 3: Collector affixes bottle seal(s) to bottle(s). Collector dates seal(s). Donor initials seal(s). Donor completes STEP 5 on Copy 2 (MRO Copy)

STEP 4: CHAIN OF CUSTODY - INITIATED BY COLLECTOR AND COMPLETED BY LABORATORY

I certify that the specimen given to me by the donor identified in the certification section on Copy 2 of this form was collected, labeled, sealed and released to the Delivery Service noted in accordance with applicable Federal requirements.

X _____   AM
Signature of Collector   Time of Collection   PM ▶

_____   __/__/__
(PRINT) Collector's Name (First, MI, Last)   Date (Mo./Day/Yr.) ▶

SPECIMEN BOTTLE(S) RELEASED TO:

Name of Delivery Service Transferring Specimen to Lab

RECEIVED AT LAB:

X _____
Signature of Accessioner

_____   __/__/__
(PRINT) Accessioner's Name (First, MI, Last)   Date (Mo./Day/Yr.) ▶

Primary Specimen Bottle Seal Intact
☐ Yes
☐ No, Enter Remark Below

SPECIMEN BOTTLE(S) RELEASED TO:

STEP 5a: PRIMARY SPECIMEN TEST RESULTS - COMPLETED BY PRIMARY LABORATORY

☐ NEGATIVE   ☐ POSITIVE for: ☐ MARIJUANA METABOLITE   ☐ CODEINE   ☐ AMPHETAMINE   ☐ ADULTERATED
    ☐ DILUTE   ☐ COCAINE METABOLITE   ☐ MORPHINE   ☐ METHAMPHETAMINE   ☐ SUBSTITUTED
    ☐ REJECTED FOR TESTING   ☐ PCP   ☐ 6-ACETYLMORPHINE   ☐ INVALID RESULT

REMARKS _____

TEST LAB (if different from above) _____

I certify that the specimen identified on this form was examined upon receipt, handled using chain of custody procedures, analyzed, and reported in accordance with applicable Federal requirements.

X _____   _____   __/__/__
Signature of Certifying Scientist   (PRINT) Certifying Scientist's Name (First, MI, Last)   Date (Mo./Day/Yr.)

STEP 5b: SPLIT SPECIMEN TEST RESULTS - (IF TESTED) COMPLETED BY SECONDARY LABORATORY

| Laboratory Name | ☐ RECONFIRMED   ☐ FAILED TO RECONFIRM - REASON |
| Laboratory Address | I certify that the split specimen identified on this form was examined upon receipt, handled using chain of custody procedures, analyzed, and reported in accordance with applicable Federal requirements. |

X _____   _____   __/__/__
Signature of Certifying Scientist   (PRINT) Certifying Scientist's Name (First, MI, Last)   Date (Mo./Day/Yr.)

PEEL ||||||||||||||||||||
1234567   A
SPECIMEN ID NO.

PLACE OVER CAP

1234567
SPECIMEN BOTTLE SEAL

__/__/__
Date (Mo. Day Yr.)

_____
Donor's Initials

PEEL ||||||||||||||||||||
1234567   B (SPLIT)
SPECIMEN ID NO.

PLACE OVER CAP

1234567
SPECIMEN BOTTLE SEAL

__/__/__
Date (Mo. Day Yr.)

_____
Donor's Initials

COPY 1 - LABORATORY

PRESS HARD - YOU ARE MAKING MULTIPLE COPIES

0000-0000-0225

Drug Form Part 1
Face Inks: 000 BLK / 000 RED
Date: 05/09/00
Not To Use For Colormatch
Follow PMS Guide For Colors

FIGURE 31.32 First page of the Federal Drug Testing Custody and Control Form.

6. Individual testing method results may vary. Some tests have lower limits of detection, which can make some results positive at lower substance levels. Also, a person's diet, the volume of urine flow, and recent fluid intake can affect some results.

7. Because of the legal implications of drug testing, chain of custody must be strictly followed. Each step from collection of the specimen to reporting the test results must be strictly monitored and documented. Requirements include sealed specimen containers, supervised laboratory analysis throughout the process, and authorized signatures at each step.

CLOSING COMMENTS

Patient Coaching

Frequently a medical assistant is called on to explain specimen collection techniques to the patient. Patients want to do the procedure correctly but often lack the knowledge of urinary terminology. They may be embarrassed or may not know how to ask questions about cleaning the genital area. When explaining a urinary collection procedure, you should use pictures and words that the patient will understand. As you explain the procedure in terms the patient knows, he or she will feel comfortable telling you or asking you about pertinent details that may have a definite effect on treatment of the problem. Providing the patient with a clearly written instruction sheet also is helpful. The instruction sheet should be personalized with the patient's name, the time to begin collection or testing (if applicable), what supplies should be used, and a phone number to call if questions arise.

Legal and Ethical Issues

Similar to all other procedures, the test is only as valid as the specimen and the procedure performed on that specimen. You, as the provider's agent, are responsible for that validity when you instruct the patient and when you perform the test.

A medical assistant responsible for office laboratory testing must clearly understand the basic concepts of laboratory medicine. Therefore, you must stay current with the rapid technologic advances in laboratory medicine and help establish a protocol of the tests best suited to your provider-employer.

You are responsible for properly collecting specimens and testing them accurately. In addition, you are responsible for strict adherence to protocol when collecting and testing specimens, especially when legal ramifications are associated with the test results. Patient confidentiality is paramount when drug testing is performed, as is rigid conformation to all established rules and regulations.

Patient-Centered Care

Urine testing is frequently done in an ambulatory care setting. Knowing laboratory procedures helps the medical assistant ask informed and useful questions of their patients. Vitamin C can affect urine reagent strip testing, so asking a patient if he or she takes a vitamin C supplement is useful for obtaining correct testing results. If a person consumes large amounts of vitamin C, a special strip can be used to detect interfering levels of vitamin C. If an elevated level is found, the patient should be instructed to discontinue vitamin C intake for 24 hours, and then another urine specimen should be collected for testing.

Professional Behaviors

Attributes of a laboratory professional performing urinalysis include:
- A discreet, respectful attitude when communicating with patients, co-workers, and supervisors
- Good eyesight and manual dexterity
- Accountability, honesty, and integrity when unsure of any procedure
- Ability to multitask, manage his or her time, pay attention to details, and problem-solve if test results are unexpected

---

SUMMARY OF SCENARIO

Becca has had a fun and busy time in the laboratory at WMFM. She has enjoyed learning about the laboratory. She has had a chance to see some of the testing, PPE, quality assurance, and quality control processes that are part of a day in the lab. It was also nice to see the general workflow of the lab and the need for organization, attention to detail, and manual dexterity in laboratory testing.

With these observations fresh in her mind, Becca will finish her assignment later today. She is looking forward to graduating soon and working as a medical assistant. There are so many areas within ambulatory care to work as a medical assistant. Becca is excited for the future.

SUMMARY OF LEARNING OBJECTIVES

1. **Describe the anatomy and physiology of the urinary tract and discuss the formation and elimination of urine.**

   The urinary tract consists of two kidneys, two ureters, one bladder, and one urethra. The functional unit of the kidney is the nephron, and each nephron interacts with the blood by filtration, reabsorption, and secretion. Urine passes from the pelvis of the kidney down the ureter and into the bladder, where it remains until it is voided through the urethra.

2. **Show sensitivity to patients' rights and feelings when collecting specimens. Also, discuss collection containers, and instruct a patient on the collection of a 24-hour urine specimen.**

   - *Show sensitivity to patients' rights and feelings when collecting specimens.*

     Requesting a urine specimen from a patient may be an embarrassing moment for the patient. The request should be made in private,

Continued

and the patient should be given explicit instructions so that he or she understands what is expected.

- *Discuss collection containers.*

  The most important requirement for a collection container is that it be scrupulously clean. The physician's office laboratory should provide the container.

- *Instruct a patient in the collection of a 24-hour urine specimen.*

  Timed urine specimens are collected to determine the amount of a particular analyte in the urine during a given time frame. Proper patient instruction is necessary to obtain an acceptable specimen (see Procedure 31.1, p. 791).

3. **Explain the various means and methods used to collect urine specimens. Also, instruct a patient on the collection of a clean-catch midstream urine specimen.**

   - *Explain the various means and methods used to collect urine specimens.*

     Some urine collections, such as the 2-hour postprandial specimen, must be timed around meals or fasts. Routine UA requires no special preparation, whereas a CCMS requires cleansing of the external genitalia. Only urine that will be cultured must be collected in a sterile container. Urine to be sent to a referral laboratory may require the addition of preservatives.

     Proper patient instruction is necessary for an acceptable CCMS. Both men and women are given instructions in cleaning the external genitalia to prevent contamination of the urine. Urine must be collected in a sterile container and refrigerated if it cannot be tested within 1 hour (see Procedure 31.2, p. 792).

4. **Discuss handling and transporting specimens.**

   Urine specimens should be kept refrigerated and should be processed within 1 hour of collection. If the specimen must be transported to a referral laboratory, evacuated transport tubes are often used. These tubes contain preservatives that prevent the overgrowth of bacteria and will prevent chemical changes in the urine that may affect test results. Chemical reagent strip testing can be performed on preserved specimens within 72 hours. Tubes may be held at room temperature during this time. A different preservative must be used for urine culture specimens. The preservative used for culture specimens helps maintain the number of bacteria present at the time of collection.

5. **Complete the following related to the physical examination of urine:**

   - *Examine and report the physical aspects of urine.*

     Physical examination of the urine involves determination of the color, turbidity, and specific gravity. Odor and foam color also may be noted (see Procedure 31.3, p. 794).

     - *Assess urine for color and turbidity.*

       Color. Normal urine is a shade of yellow that ranges from pale straw to yellow to amber. The color depends on the concentration of the pigment urochrome and the amount of water in the specimen. Variations in color may also be caused by diet, medication, and disease.

Turbidity. Both normal and abnormal urine specimens may range in appearance from clear to very cloudy. Turbidity may be caused by cells, bacteria, yeast, vaginal contaminants, or crystals.

- *Perform quality control measures and differentiate between normal and abnormal results while determining the reliability of chemical reagent strips.*

  The medical assistant should analyze and differentiate the normal and abnormal control results for the reagent strips before running the patient's chemical urinalysis (see Procedure 31.4, p. 795).

6. **Examine and report on the chemical aspects of urine, and test urine with chemical reagent strips.**

   The chemical examination of urine involves determination of the pH level and the levels of glucose, protein, ketones, blood, bilirubin, urobilinogen, and nitrite, in addition to specific gravity and leukocyte esterase, using a reagent strip. Most chemical urine testing requires reagent strips. It is essential that these supplies be stored in a dark, cool, moisture-free area (see Procedure 31.5, p. 796).

7. **Discuss the limitations of reagent strip testing and explain quality control and quality assurance related to urinalysis.**

   - *Reagent strip testing limitations can arise from several sources:*
     - The test strip is soaked in the specimen, and chemicals in the pads may be overly diluted.
     - The test strip is not held horizontally while read, and colors from one pad may bleed onto another.
     - The test pads on the strip are not read at the proper time, or the chemical reaction may be read incorrectly.
     - Certain chemicals may affect the results of nitrite, glucose, bilirubin, and blood tests.
     - Visual interpretation of color on the reagent strip pads is likely to vary among individuals.

   - *Quality assurance and quality control.*

     A commercially available control strip should be used to determine the reliability of chemical analysis. One such control strip is the Chek-Stix. After reconstitution, a reagent test strip is immersed in the control solution, and the results are compared with a chart that accompanies the Chek-Stix. Both positive and negative Chek-Stix controls are available (see Procedure 31.4, p. 795). It is important to observe and record the abnormal and normal results produced by the positive and negative controls. Also, make sure the test results are consistent with the Chek-Stix charts provided by the manufacturer before testing patient urine specimens. There are many manufactured QC liquids and strips that can be used for QC testing. The Chek-Stix is just one example.

8. **Prepare a urine specimen for microscopic evaluation, and understand the significance of casts, cells, crystals, and miscellaneous findings in the microscopy report.**

   A complete UA involves physical, chemical, and microscopic assessment. The results of these three assessments must correlate with one another. Refer to Procedure 31.6, p. 797.

SUMMARY OF LEARNING OBJECTIVES—*continued*

9. **Explain or perform the following CLIA-waived urine tests:**
   - *Glucose testing using the Clinitest method*
     The Clinitest detects reducing sugars in the urine, including glucose and galactose. It is superior to the reagent strip test because it detects sugars other than glucose (see Procedure 31.7, p. 799).
   - *Urine pregnancy test*
     Pregnancy tests detect hCG, a hormone produced by the placenta. Urine moves through the test (T) and control (C) areas of the test device by lateral absorption. Anti-hCG antibodies embedded in the test cartridge bind to hCG in the urine, causing a color change in the test area (see Procedure 31.8, p. 800).
   - *Ovulation and menopause tests*
     Fertility can be assessed using lateral flow tests that detect LH, which increases in concentration in the urine shortly before ovulation.

   Menopause can be assessed using lateral flow tests that detect FSH, which increases as menopause approaches.
   - *Urine toxicology and drug testing*
     Drug testing with lateral flow technology is similar to pregnancy testing except that it uses a competitive binding principle. Unlike with the pregnancy test, a line in the T region indicates a negative test result (see Procedure 31.9, p. 801).

10. **List the means by which urine could be adulterated before drug testing and discuss chain of custody rules for drug testing.**
    Drinking excessive water before urinating, adding water to a urine specimen, and adding chemicals or products sold specifically to adulterate urine all can render a drug test invalid. Adulteration test strips can detect most methods of adulteration.

PROCEDURE 31.1   Instruct a Patient in the Collection of a 24-Hour Urine Specimen

Task: Collect a 24-hour urine sample to test for creatinine clearance.

EQUIPMENT and SUPPLIES

- Patient's health record
- 2-L urine collection container
- Plastic cup or specimen collection pan for collecting urine (which is then poured into the collection container)
- Printed patient instructions
- Laboratory requisition
- Fluid-impermeable lab coat, protective eyewear, and gloves

PROCEDURAL STEPS

1. Greet the patient. Identify yourself. Verify the patient's identity with full name, ask the patient to spell the first and last name, and give his or her date of birth. Explain the procedure to be performed in a manner that the patient understands. Answer any questions about the procedure.
   PURPOSE: It is important to identify the patient in two different ways to ensure that you have the correct patient. Explaining the procedure can make the patient feel more comfortable and reduces anxiety.

2. Label the container with the patient's name and the current date, identify the specimen as a 24-hour urine specimen, and include your initials. Check for preservative if needed.
   PURPOSE: Labeling the container prevents a possible mix-up of specimens.

3. Explain the following instructions to adult patients or to the guardians of pediatric patients.

Patient Instructions: Obtaining a 24-Hour Urine Specimen

(1) Empty your bladder into the toilet in the morning without saving any of the specimen. Record the time you first emptied your bladder on the label.

(2) For the next 24 hours, each time you empty your bladder, all the urine should be collected into the plastic cup or collection pan that is placed on the toilet (also called a nun's cap or toilet hat). Then pour all the collected urine directly into the large specimen container (see the following figure).
   PURPOSE: Do not urinate directly into the large specimen container. It may contain a preservative that could be caustic. You do not want to splash any of the preservative while urinating.

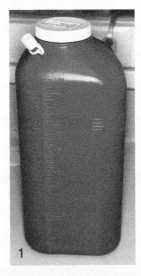

(3) Put the lid back on the container after each urination and rinse out the plastic cup or collection pan; store the container in the refrigerator or at room temperature, as directed, throughout the 24 hours of the study.
   PURPOSE: Refrigeration or the preservative inhibits microbial growth in the specimen.

Continued

PROCEDURE 31.1   Instruct a Patient in the Collection of a 24-Hour Urine Specimen—*continued*

(4) If at any time you forget to collect your specimen or if some urine is accidentally spilled, you must begin the test over again with a new container and a newly recorded start time.
PURPOSE: The test will be inaccurate if you fail to collect all urine produced during the designated 24-hour period.

(5) Collect the final urine specimen at the same time you started the collection process on the previous day. This last collected specimen is placed in the large container. Collection ends with the voided morning specimen on the second day, which completes the 24-hour period.

(6) As soon as possible after completing collection, return the specimen container to the provider's office or the designated laboratory.

4. Give the patient the specimen container and supplies with written instructions to confirm understanding.
PURPOSE: Ensuring correct supplies and instructions is essential to proper specimen collection.

5. Document details of the patient education session in the patient's record.
PURPOSE: Documentation confirms patient education was completed.

Processing a 24-Hour Urine Specimen

1. Ask the patient whether he or she collected all voided urine throughout the 24-hour period or whether any problems occurred during the collection process.
PURPOSE: To confirm the accuracy of the specimen.

2. Complete the laboratory request form. Make sure that all the information is filled out on the container label.
PURPOSE: Proper labeling ensures specimen identification.

3. Wash hands or use hand sanitizer. Put on a fluid-impermeable lab coat, protective eyewear, and gloves before preparing the specimen for transport.
PURPOSE: To ensure infection control.

4. Store the specimen in the refrigerator until it is picked up by the laboratory.
PURPOSE: Proper storage ensures the quality of the specimen.

5. Remove gloves and discard them appropriately. Remove protective eyewear and lab coat. Wash hands or use hand sanitizer.
PURPOSE: To ensure infection control.

6. Document that the specimen was sent to the laboratory, including the type of test ordered, the date and time, the type of specimen, and your initials.
PURPOSE: Properly documenting specimen collection and transport are an essential part of the process.

PROCEDURE 31.2   Collect a Clean-Catch Midstream Urine Specimen

Task: Collect a contaminant-free urine sample for culture or analysis using the clean-catch midstream specimen (CCMS) technique.

EQUIPMENT and SUPPLIES

- Patient's record
- Sterile container with a lid and label
- Antiseptic towelettes
- Fluid-impermeable lab coat, protective eyewear, and gloves

PROCEDURAL STEPS

1. Greet the patient. Identify yourself. Verify the patient's identity with full name, ask the patient to spell the first and last name, and give his or her date of birth. Explain the procedure to be performed in a manner that the patient understands. Answer any questions about the procedure.
PURPOSE: It is important to identify the patient in two different ways to ensure that you have the correct patient. Explaining the procedure can make the patient feel more comfortable and reduce anxiety.

2. Label the sterile sealed container (not the lid) and give the patient the towelette supplies (see the following figure) and patient instruction form, if needed.
PURPOSE: Labeling the container prevents a possible mix-up of specimens.

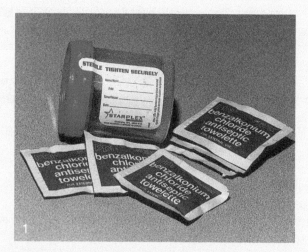

3. Explain the following instructions to adult patients or to the guardians of pediatric patients, making sure you show sensitivity to privacy issues.
PURPOSE: Instructions must be understood if they are to be followed correctly. By talking to the patient, you can determine whether the patient understands or has any questions.

PROCEDURE 31.2 | Collect a Clean-Catch Midstream Urine Specimen—*continued*

Patient Instructions: Obtaining a Clean-Catch Midstream Specimen (Female Patient)

(1) Wash your hands and open the towelette packages for easy access.
   PURPOSE: To wash away any contaminating bacteria from the hands

(2) Remove the lid from the specimen container, being careful not to touch the inside of the lid or the inside of the container. Place the lid, facing up, on a paper towel.
   PURPOSE: The lid and the container must be handled carefully to maintain the internal sterility of the container and prevent contamination of the urine sample.

(3) Lower your underclothing and sit on the toilet.

(4) Expose the urinary meatus by spreading apart the labia with one hand (see the following figure, part A).
   PURPOSE: To allow for adequate cleansing.

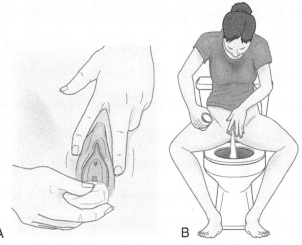

2 A   B

(5) Cleanse each side of the urinary meatus with a front-to-back motion, from the pubis toward the anus. Use a separate antiseptic wipe to cleanse each side of the meatus.
   PURPOSE: Cleansing the area around the urinary meatus prevents contamination of the urine sample. Wiping in one stroke from front to back prevents the passage of microorganisms from the anal region to the area around the urinary meatus.

(6) Cleanse directly across the meatus, front to back, using a third antiseptic wipe (see the preceding figure, part A).

(7) Hold the labia apart throughout this procedure.
   PURPOSE: To avoid specimen contamination.

(8) Void a small amount of urine into the toilet (see the preceding figure, part B).
   PURPOSE: Allowing the initial flow of urine to pass into the toilet flushes the opening of the urethra.

(9) Move the specimen container into position and void the next portion of urine into it. Fill the container halfway. Remember, this is a sterile container. Do not put your fingers on the inside of the container.
   PURPOSE: To avoid specimen contamination

(10) Remove the cup and void the last amount of urine into the toilet. (This means that the first part and the last part of the urinary flow have been excluded from the specimen. Only the middle portion of the flow is included.)
   PURPOSE: To avoid specimen contamination

(11) Place the lid on the container, taking care not to touch the interior surface of the lid. Wipe in your usual manner, redress. Wash your hands and return the sterile specimen to the place designated by the medical facility.
   PURPOSE: To avoid specimen contamination. To ensure infection control.

Patient Instructions: Obtaining a Clean-Catch Midstream Specimen (Male Patient)

(1) Wash your hands and expose the penis.

(2) Retract the foreskin of the penis (if not circumcised).
   PURPOSE: To allow for adequate cleansing.

(3) Cleanse the area around the glans penis (tip of the penis) and the urethral opening (meatus) by washing each side of the glans with a separate antiseptic wipe (see the following figure, part A).

Continued

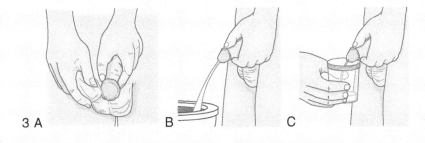

3 A   B   C

PROCEDURE 31.2   Collect a Clean-Catch Midstream Urine Specimen—*continued*

(4) Cleanse directly across the urethral opening using a third antiseptic wipe.
   PURPOSE: To cleanse the area of normal flora that may contaminate the specimen.

(5) Void a small amount of urine into the toilet or urinal (see the preceding figure in step (3), part B).

(6) Collect the next portion of the urine in the sterile container, filling the container halfway without touching the inside of the container with the hands or the penis (see the preceding figure in step (3), part C).
   PURPOSE: To avoid specimen contamination

(7) Void the last amount of urine into the toilet or urinal.

(8) Place the lid on the container, taking care not to touch the interior surface of the lid. Wipe in your usual manner, redress. Wash your hands and return the sterile specimen to the place designated by the medical facility.
   PURPOSE: To avoid specimen contamination. To ensure infection control.

(9) Return the specimen to the designated area.

Processing a Clean-Catch Urine Specimen

1. Document the date, time, and collection type.
   PURPOSE: Essential information for specimen documentation.

2. Wash hands or use hand sanitizer. Put on the fluid-impermeable lab coat, protective eyewear, and gloves.
   PURPOSE: Hand sanitization is an important step for infection control. PPE is part of Standard Precautions.

3. Process the specimen according to the provider's orders. Perform urinalysis in the office or prepare the specimen for transport to the laboratory. If it is to be sent to an outside laboratory, complete the following steps:
   (1) Make sure the label is properly completed with the patient's information and the date, time, test ordered, and your initials.
   (2) Place the specimen in a biohazard specimen bag.
   (3) Complete a laboratory requisition and place it in the outside pocket of the specimen bag.
   (4) Keep the specimen refrigerated until pickup.
      PURPOSE: Proper labeling, storage, and transport ensure the correct patient specimen and specimen quality.

4. Remove gloves, protective eyewear, and lab coat. Dispose of gloves appropriately. Wash hands or use hand sanitizer. Document that the specimen was sent.
   PURPOSE: To ensure infection control. A procedure is not completed until it is documented.

PROCEDURE 31.3   Assess Urine for Color and Turbidity: Physical Test

Task: Assess and record the color and clarity of a urine specimen.

EQUIPMENT and SUPPLIES

- Patient's record
- Urine specimen
- Centrifuge tube
- Fluid-impermeable lab coat, protective eyewear, and gloves
- Biohazard waste container

PROCEDURAL STEPS

1. Wash hands or use hand sanitizer. Put on the fluid-impermeable lab coat, protective eyewear, and gloves.
   PURPOSE: Hand sanitization is an important step for infection control. Wearing PPE is part of Standard Precautions.

2. Mix the urine by gently swirling the specimen.
   PURPOSE: Suspended substances settle when urine stands. If urine is not mixed before its appearance is assessed, the finding will be incorrect.

3. Label a centrifuge tube if a complete urinalysis is to be done.
   PURPOSE: If a complete urinalysis is to be done, a portion of the specimen will be centrifuged for microscopic examination. The centrifuged specimen must be labeled to prevent specimen confusion.

4. Pour the specimen into a standard-sized centrifuge tube.
   PURPOSE: Standard-sized containers are better for assessing color and clarity results.

5. Assess and record the color (see Fig. 31.4):
   - Pale straw or straw
   - Yellow
   - Amber or dark amber

6. Assess the turbidity (see Fig. 31.5) by placing a piece of white paper with fine, dark black print behind the specimen and see if you can see the print:
   - *Clear* — Able to read through the specimen; no cloudiness
   - *Slightly turbid* — Can barely see fine print on white paper through the tube

PROCEDURE 31.3	Assess Urine for Color and Turbidity: Physical Test—*continued*

- *Turbid* – Cannot see fine print, dark print possibly seen through the tube, or see no print at all through the tube

7. Clean the work area and dispose of procedure supplies in the biohazard waste container.
   PURPOSE: To ensure infection control.

8. Dispose of gloves. Remove lab coat and protective eyewear. Wash hands or use hand sanitizer.
   PURPOSE: To ensure infection control.

9. Record the results in the patient's record.
   PURPOSE: A procedure is not considered completed until it is documented.

PROCEDURE 31.4	Perform Quality Control Measures: Differentiate Between Normal and Abnormal Test Results While Determining the Reliability of Chemical Reagent Strips

Task: Reconstitute a control sample and test the reliability of the urinalysis chemical testing strip.

EQUIPMENT and SUPPLIES

- Chek-Stix Control Strips with reference ranges for urinalysis
- Distilled water
- Capped tube with milliliter markings
- Test tube rack
- Forceps
- Timer
- Urine chemical strips for urine testing
- Color chart for interpreting the chemical strip results
- Fluid-impermeable lab coat, protective eyewear, and gloves
- Biohazard waste container
- Control reference sheet and control flow sheet

PROCEDURAL STEPS

1. Assemble the equipment and supplies. Record the lot number and the expiration date of the Chek-Stix on the control log sheet.
   PURPOSE: Chek-Stix cannot be used if the expiration date has passed. Recording the lot number and expiration date is an important part of quality assurance.

2. Wash hands or use hand sanitizer. Put on the fluid-impermeable lab coat, protective eyewear, and gloves.
   PURPOSE: To ensure infection control. PPE is part of Standard Precautions.

3. Place a conical tube in a test tube rack, and remove the cap.

4. Pour 15 mL of distilled water into the tube.

5. Using forceps, remove one strip from the Chek-Stix bottle. Inspect the strips for mottling or discoloration.
   PURPOSE: The control strips have chemicals that you should not handle or contaminate with your hands. Any mottling or discoloration may mean that the strips have been exposed to moisture, light, or solvents. Improperly stored control strips should not be used.

6. Place the strip into the water, and tightly cap the tube.

7. Invert the tube for 2 minutes.
   PURPOSE: Chemicals embedded in the pads must be thoroughly dissolved in the water.

8. Allow the tube to sit in the test tube rack for 30 minutes.

9. Invert the tube one time and remove the strip with forceps.

10. Discard the strip in the biohazard waste container. Once reconstituted, the control solution is stable for 8 hours at room temperature.
    PURPOSE: To ensure infection control.

11. Perform quality control of the chemical reagent strip by dipping it into the control solution (see Procedure 31.5, p. 796).
    PURPOSE: Quality control is an essential step in assuring quality patient results.

12. Read and record the results.
    PURPOSE: Proper documentation is a necessity in all quality control procedures.

13. Compare the results with the control reference ranges provided on the Chek-Stix package insert.
    PURPOSE: Results should fall within a given range provided by the manufacturer. If they do not, the chemical reagent strips cannot be used to test patients' urine.

14. Discard the chemical reagent strip and the control solution in the biohazard waste container.

15. Clean up the work area, and appropriately dispose of supplies and gloves in a biohazard waste container.
    PURPOSE: To ensure infection control. To maintain a proper work area.

16. Remove protective eyewear and lab coat. Wash hands or use hand sanitizer.
    PURPOSE: To ensure infection control.

PROCEDURE 31.5   Test Urine With Chemical Reagent Strips

Task: Perform chemical testing on a urine sample, and reassure the patient of its accuracy.

EQUIPMENT and SUPPLIES

- Patient's record
- Urine specimen
- Reagent strips
- Timer
- Fluid-impermeable lab coat, protective eyewear, and gloves
- Biohazard waste container

PROCEDURAL STEPS

1. Wash hands or use hand sanitizer. Put on the fluid-impermeable lab coat, protective eyewear, and gloves.
   PURPOSE: To ensure infection control. PPE is part of Standard Precautions.
2. Check the time of collection, the container, and the mode of preservation.
   PURPOSE: Proper specimen identification and screening of specimens for appropriate collection containers and collection procedures prevent the testing of inappropriate specimens.
3. If the specimen has been refrigerated, allow it to warm to room temperature.
   PURPOSE: Certain tests are temperature-dependent. Testing cold specimens may cause false-negative results.
4. Check the reagent strip container for the expiration date.
   PURPOSE: Do not use expired reagents.
5. Remove the reagent strip from the container. Hold it in your hand or place it on a clean, dry paper towel. Recap the container tightly.
   PURPOSE: Test strips are sensitive to moisture and light and must be stored in tightly sealed containers. Contamination from chemical residues on countertops can affect results.
6. Compare nonreactive test pads with the negative color blocks on the color chart on the container.
   PURPOSE: Discolored pads indicate that the product has not been properly stored and must not be used for testing.
7. Thoroughly mix the specimen by gently swirling the container.
   PURPOSE: If settling occurs, certain elements may not be detected.
8. Following the manufacturer's directions, note the time, dip the strip into the urine, and then remove it.
   PURPOSE: Tests are time dependent. Some pads darken over time.

9. Quickly remove the excess urine from the strip by pulling the back of the strip across the lip of the specimen container and then blotting the edge of the strip on a clean, dry paper towel or the side of the specimen container.
   PURPOSE: Excess urine on the strip or prolonged dipping time affects test results.
10. Hold the strip horizontally (see the following figure). At the required time, compare the strip with the appropriate color chart on the reagent container. *Do not touch the strip to the bottle.*

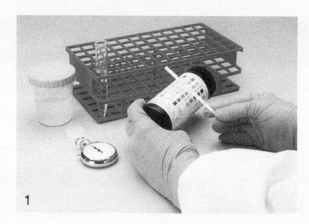

1

11. Alternately, the strip can be placed on a clean, dry paper towel.
    PURPOSE: Holding the strip horizontally prevents runover from one test pad to another and prevents interference from mixing chemicals in the test pads.
12. Read and record the first two results 30 seconds after dipping the strip (the indicated time to read the "Glucose" and "Bilirubin"). Compare the two reagent pads closest to your hand with the bottom two rows of the color chart (see the following figure). Continue reading and recording each row of possible results with its appropriate reagent pad at its designated time.

| PROCEDURE 31.5 | Test Urine With Chemical Reagent Strips—*continued* |

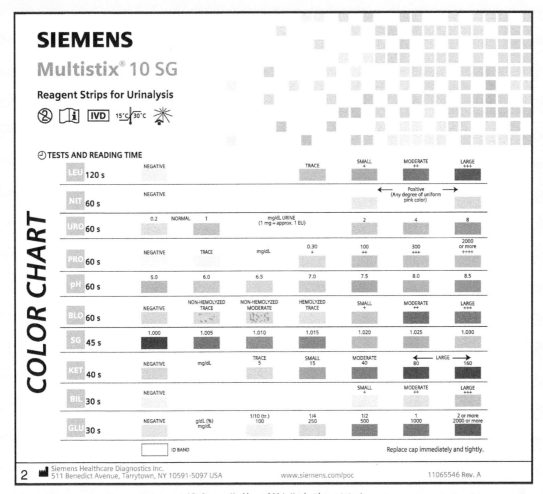

(© Siemens Healthcare 2016. Used with permission.)

PURPOSE: Timing is critical. Allowing the strip to touch the bottle contaminates the bottle.

13. Clean the work area. If a paper towel was used, dispose of it and the reagent strip in an appropriate biohazard waste container.
PURPOSE: To ensure infection control.

14. Remove gloves and dispose of them appropriately. Remove protective eyewear and lab coat. Wash hands or use hand sanitizer.
PURPOSE: To ensure infection control.

15. Document the results in the patient's paper record or EHR.
PURPOSE: A procedure is not complete until it has been documented.

| PROCEDURE 31.6 | Prepare a Urine Specimen for Microscopic Examination |

Task: Prepare a urine specimen for the provider's microscopic examination to determine the presence of normal and abnormal elements.

EQUIPMENT and SUPPLIES

- Patient's record
- Urine specimen
- Centrifuge tube
- Centrifuge
- Disposable pipet
- Sedi-Stain
- Microscope slide and coverslip
- Microscope
- Permanent marker
- Fluid-impermeable lab coat, protective eyewear, and gloves
- Biohazard waste container

Continued

| PROCEDURE 31.6 | **Prepare a Urine Specimen for Microscopic Examination**—*continued* |

PROCEDURAL STEPS

1. Wash hands or use hand sanitizer. Put on the fluid-impermeable lab coat, protective eyewear, and gloves.
   PURPOSE: To ensure infection control. PPE is part of Standard Precautions.

2. Gently mix the urine specimen by swirling the covered specimen container.
   PURPOSE: If the urine is not well mixed, elements that have settled to the bottom of the specimen container will be missed.

3. Pour 12 mL of urine into a labeled centrifuge tube and cap the tube.
   PURPOSE: Label to ensure proper specimen identification.

4. Place the tube in the centrifuge (see the following figure).

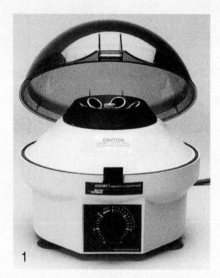

(From Stepp CA, Woods MA: *Laboratory procedures for medical office personnel,* Philadelphia, 1998, Saunders.)

5. Place another tube containing 12 mL of urine or water in the opposite cup.
   PURPOSE: For proper operation, centrifuges must be carefully balanced. If not properly balanced, damage to the instrument can occur.

6. Secure the lid and centrifuge for 5 minutes or for the time specified for your instrument.
   PURPOSE: Timing varies according to the speed and the size of the centrifuge head.

7. Remove the tube from the centrifuge after the instrument has come to a full stop.
   PURPOSE: Wait for a full stop to safely operate the centrifuge.

8. Pour off the clear supernatant from the top of the specimen by inverting the centrifuge tube over the sink drain while allowing the running water from the faucet to flush the urine down the drain.
   PURPOSE: Decanting the supernatant creates a good sediment specimen.

9. Turn the tube upright when the supernatant has been decanted, allowing a small amount to return to the sediment on the bottom of the tube without losing sediment down the drain (see the following figure).
   PURPOSE: The sediment will be examined under the microscope.

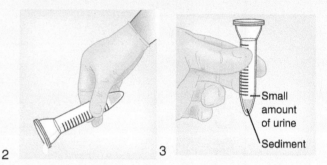

10. Thoroughly mix the sediment with a drop of Sedi-Stain by grasping the tube near the top and rapidly flicking it with the fingers of the other hand until all sediment is thoroughly resuspended.
    PURPOSE: Elements centrifuge at different rates. Failure to mix the entire sediment completely may result in evaluation errors. Sedi-Stain colors the sediment for easier viewing.

11. Transfer 1 drop of sediment to a clean, labeled slide using a clean, disposable transfer pipet.
    PURPOSE: A clean slide will not contaminate the specimen. Labeling ensures the correct patient specimen.

12. Place a clean coverslip over the drop and place the slide on the microscope stage. Remove eye protection.
    PURPOSE: The coverslip allows the specimen to be properly focused on the microscope.

13. Focus under low power and reduce the light.
    Note: Once the slide is focused under low power, the remaining steps of this procedure are performed by the trained healthcare provider or moderate/highly complex trained laboratory personnel.

PROCEDURE 31.7   Test Urine for Glucose Using the Clinitest Method

Task: Perform confirmatory testing for glucose and other simple sugars in the urine using the Clinitest procedure for reducing substances.

EQUIPMENT and SUPPLIES

- Patient's record
- Urine specimen
- Clinitest tablet, glass test tube, and transfer pipet (Note: When performing a Clinitest, always use glass test tubes.)
- Distilled water
- Test tube rack
- Appropriate-sized plastic or metal forceps
- Color chart
- Timer
- Fluid-impermeable lab coat, protective eyewear, and gloves
- Biohazard waste container

PROCEDURAL STEPS

1. Wash hands or use hand sanitizer. Put on fluid-impermeable lab coat, protective eyewear, and gloves.
   PURPOSE: To ensure infection control. PPE is part of Standard Precautions.
2. Holding a transfer pipet vertically, add 10 drops of distilled water and then 5 drops of urine to a test tube.
   PURPOSE: Holding the transfer pipet vertically prevents alteration of the size of the drops.
3. Place the prepared tube in the test tube rack (see the following figure).
   PURPOSE: The tube will become too hot to hold after the tablet is placed in the tube.

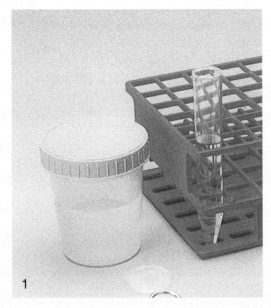

4. Remove a Clinitest tablet from the bottle by shaking a tablet into the bottle cap.
   PURPOSE: Clinitest tablets react with moisture and become caustic.

Note: Do not handle Clinitest tablets with your hands or gloved hands. Always use forceps to transfer the tablet to the test tube.

5. Using a metal or plastic forceps, pick up the Clinitest tablet from the bottle cap, and drop the tablet into the prepared test tube. Recap the container.
   Note: Use caution when performing a Clinitest because the reaction boils. Always use glass test tubes — plastic tubes may melt!
   PURPOSE: Clinitest tablets should always be handled with a forceps.
6. With the test tube in the rack, observe the entire reaction to detect the rapid pass-through phenomenon, which indicates that the glucose level in the urine is very high.
   Note: If an orange color briefly develops during the reaction and then converts to a lower, darker color, rapid pass-through has occurred, meaning that the glucose was greater than the highest reading; this is recorded as "greater than 2%."
   PURPOSE: If pass-through occurs but is not detected, the reading will be falsely low.
7. When boiling stops, time exactly 15 seconds and then gently shake the tube to mix all of the contents.
8. Immediately compare the color of the specimen with the 5-drop color chart and record your findings (see the following figure). See the *Note* in step 6.
   PURPOSE: For accurate results, wait 15 seconds and then quickly read results. Color results will continue to darken over time.

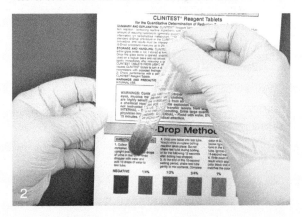

9. Record the results.
   PURPOSE: A procedure has not taken place until it is documented.
10. Clean up the work area, dispose of supplies in appropriate waste containers, then remove your gloves.
    PURPOSE: To ensure infection control.
11. Remove the fluid-impermeable lab coat and protective eyewear.
12. Wash hands or use hand sanitizer.
    PURPOSE: To ensure infection control.
13. Record the results in the patient's record.
    PURPOSE: A procedure is not considered finished until it is recorded.

| PROCEDURE 31.8 | Perform a CLIA-Waived Urinalysis: Perform a Pregnancy Test |

Task: Perform a pregnancy test on urine using the QuickVue pregnancy test method.

EQUIPMENT and SUPPLIES

- Patient's record
- Urine specimen
- QuickVue test kit
- Fluid-impermeable lab coat, protective eyewear, and gloves
- Biohazard sharps container
- Biohazard waste container

PROCEDURAL STEPS

1. Wash hands or use hand sanitizer. Put on fluid-impermeable lab coat, protective eyewear, and gloves.
   PURPOSE: Hand sanitization is an important step for infection control. PPE is part of Standard Precautions.
2. Prepare the testing equipment (see the following figure). Check the expiration date of the kit before proceeding.
   PURPOSE: Expired kits should not be used for quality control or patient samples.

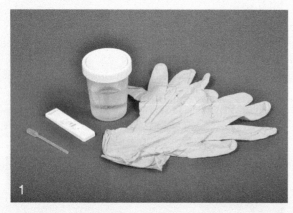

3. Obtain the proper patient specimen (preferably a first morning specimen).
4. Remove the test cassette from the foil pouch.
5. Add 3 drops of urine using the transfer pipet (dropper) that accompanies the kit (see the following figure).
   PURPOSE: To ensure accurate test results, the specimen amount must be added as indicated by the manufacturer's written procedure.

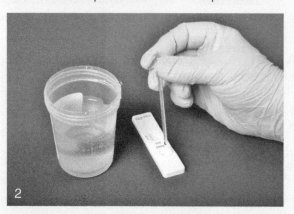

6. Dispose of the pipet in a biohazard sharps container.
   PURPOSE: To ensure infection control.
7. Wait 3 minutes. Read the test results at 3 minutes.
   PURPOSE: To ensure accurate test results, timing must be accurate.
8. Interpret the results as follows (see the following figure):
   Negative: A blue control line is next to the letter C; no line is seen next to the letter T (see the cassette in the middle).
   Positive: A blue control line is next to the letter C; a pink line is next to the letter T (see the cassette on the right).
   Invalid: If a blue line does not appear in the C area, the test is invalid and the specimen must be retested using another kit. Check the expiration date of the kit before proceeding (see the cassette on the left).

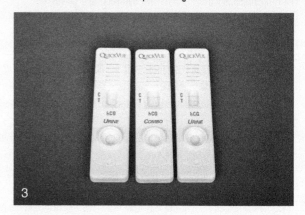

9. Discard the test cassette in the biohazard waste container, clean up the testing area, then remove and discard gloves in a biohazard waste container. Remove lab coat and protective eyewear.
   PURPOSE: To ensure infection control.
10. Wash hands or use hand sanitizer.
    PURPOSE: To ensure infection control.
11. Record the results in the patient's record as either positive or negative for pregnancy.
    PURPOSE: A procedure is not considered completed until it is documented.

10/2/20XX 3:45 p.m.: Last menstrual period (LMP) 9/16/20XX.
QuickVue pregnancy test: Positive._____Julie Salter, CMA (AAMA)

PROCEDURE 31.9	Obtain a Specimen and Perform a CLIA-Waived Urinalysis: Perform a Multidrug Screening Test on Urine

Task: To screen a urine specimen for drugs or drug metabolites at their specified cutoff levels.

EQUIPMENT and SUPPLIES

- Patient's record
- Multi-Drug Screen Urine Test in a sealed container
- Freshly voided urine sample
- Timer
- Fluid-impermeable lab coat, eye protection, and gloves
- Biohazard waste container

PROCEDURAL STEPS

1. Wash hand or use hand sanitizer. Put on the fluid-impermeable lab coat, eye protection, and gloves.
   PURPOSE: To ensure infection control and use of Standard Precautions.
2. Assemble the equipment and specimen. Check the expiration date on the test kit.
   PURPOSE: An expired test strip may yield inaccurate results.
3. Determine the temperature of the urine (within 4 minutes of voiding). The temperature should be between 32° and 38°C (90° and 100°F).
   PURPOSE: If the urine temperature is below or above this range, the sample may have been adulterated. Once it has been determined that the sample is at the correct temperature, it may be stored at room temperature for 8 hours or in the refrigerator for up to 3 days before testing.
4. Bring the specimen and the testing device to room temperature.
   PURPOSE: Both the specimen and the device must be at room temperature to ensure accurate results.
5. Remove the device from the foil pouch and label it with the specimen identification.
   PURPOSE: To ensure correct specimen identification

Dip Method

6. Remove the cap of the specimen and dip the device into the specimen for 10 seconds, making sure the surface of the urine is above the sample well and below the arrowheads in the window (see the following figure).
   PURPOSE: The pads must be saturated with urine.

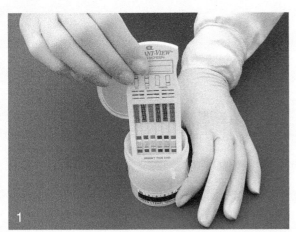

(Courtesy Alfa Scientific, Poway, CA.)

Alternate Method

7. Remove the pipet from the pouch and fill it to the line on the barrel with urine. Dispense the entire volume onto the sample well on the testing device (see the following figure).
   PURPOSE: If insufficient urine is available in the cup to use the dip method, this method applies urine directly to the device.

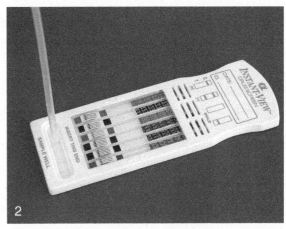

(Courtesy Alfa Scientific, Poway, CA.)

8. Recap the urine specimen.
   PURPOSE: To ensure no specimen spills.
9. Set the timer for the designated time. Do not read the results until after maximum time as stated in the manufacturer's instructions.
   PURPOSE: Correct timing is essential for reliable, accurate test results.
10. Interpret the results (see the following figure):
    Positive: If the C line appears but the T line does not, the result is positive for that drug.
    Negative: If both the C line and the T line appear, the level of the drug or its metabolites is below the cutoff level (i.e., negative for that drug).
    Invalid: If no C line develops within 5 minutes on any test strip, the assay is invalid. Repeat the assay with a new test device if invalid.

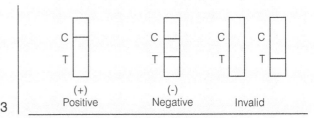

11. Discard the urine and the device in the biohazard container.
    PURPOSE: To ensure infection control.
12. Disinfect the area. Remove your gloves and dispose in biohazard container. Remove lab coat, and wash hands or use hand sanitizer.
    PURPOSE: To ensure infection control.
13. Record the results in the patient's record.
    PURPOSE: A procedure is not considered complete until it is documented.

32

BLOOD COLLECTION

SCENARIO

Maggie Brandt, a certified medical assistant (CMA) through the American Association of Medical Assistants (AAMA), has been a medical assistant with the Walden-Martin Family Medical (WMFM) Clinic for about 15 years. She has worked in many areas of the clinic, but for the past 8 years she has been the primary phlebotomist each morning from 8 a.m. until noon. Maggie has the right combination of skills to be a wonderful phlebotomist:

- She is warm, friendly, and can easily talk to patients.
- She is detail-oriented, a stickler for safety practices, and very organized.

- She has good small motor skills and a certain quality that seems to make her venipunctures so smooth that patients hardly feel the needle go through the skin.
- She can explain procedures well in understandable terms and is willing to listen to her patients and put them at ease.

It is Monday morning, and the phlebotomy area is usually busy with patients who have scheduled venipunctures in advance. Let's see what is happening in the phlebotomy area today.

While studying this chapter, think about the following questions:

- What equipment is needed to perform a venipuncture and a capillary puncture?
- What is different about each colored stopper venipuncture tube, and what is the correct order of the draw?
- What types of safety needles and collection devices are used in phlebotomy?
- What steps should be followed for postexposure management of accidental needlesticks?

- How do you properly perform a venipuncture using evacuated tubes? How do you properly perform a venipuncture using a syringe or butterfly equipment? How do you properly perform a capillary puncture?
- What are problem-solving strategies related to blood collection?
- How is pediatric phlebotomy unique? Include patient behavior, parental involvement during phlebotomy, and general guidelines for pediatric blood collection.

LEARNING OBJECTIVES

1. Discuss venipuncture equipment and personal protective equipment. Also, explain the purpose of a tourniquet, how to apply it, and the consequences of improper tourniquet application.
2. Discuss antiseptics, explain why the stopper colors on vacuum tubes differ, and state the correct order of the draw.
3. Discuss the needles and supplies used in phlebotomy.
4. Discuss needle safety and postexposure needlestick follow-up.
5. Complete the following related to routine venipuncture:
   - Discuss patient preparation for routine venipuncture.
   - List in order the steps of a routine venipuncture.
   - Detail patient preparation for venipuncture that shows sensitivity to the patient's rights and feelings.

- Perform a venipuncture using the vacuum tube method, syringe, and winged-infusion (butterfly) assembly.
6. Discuss possible solutions to venipuncture complications.
7. List situations in which capillary puncture would be preferred over venipuncture, and discuss the equipment used.
8. Perform a capillary puncture.
9. Discuss pediatric phlebotomy, including typical childhood behavior and parental involvement during phlebotomy, and general guidelines for pediatric venipuncture.
10. Describe handling and transport methods for blood after collection.

VOCABULARY

anticoagulant (an tee koh AG yuh lant) A substance (i.e., medication or chemical) that prevents clotting of blood.

antiseptic (an tuh SEP tik) Substances that inhibit the growth of microorganisms on living tissue (e.g., alcohol and

povidone-iodine solution [Betadine]); they are used to cleanse the skin, wounds, and so on.

aspirating (AS puh rayt ing) To draw off or remove by suction.

blood culture A microbiologic procedure ordered when a provider suspects a bacterial infection is causing a fever of unknown origin (FUO). A blood sample is collected into a nutrient media and held at body temperature. If bacteria are in the blood sample, the culture media should encourage the growth of the infecting bacteria in the laboratory.

clot activators Substances added to a venipuncture tube to enhance and speed up blood clotting.

evacuated Absence of air to create a vacuum in a tube, flask, or reaction vessel.

g-force A force acting on an object because of gravity. Example: A centrifuge spins and exerts g-force.

glycolysis (glie KOL uh sis) The chemical breakdown of carbohydrates (glucose) by enzymes, with the release of energy.

hematoma (hee mah TOH mah) An abnormal buildup of blood in an organ or tissue of the body, caused by a leak or cut in a blood vessel.

hemoconcentration (hee muh kon sun TRAY shun) A condition in which the concentration of blood cells is increased in proportion to the plasma.

hemolysis (hee MOL i sis) The breakdown of red blood cells with the release of hemoglobin.

interstitial (in ter STISH ul) Between the cells.

lymphostasis (lim foh STAY sis) Obstruction or interruption of normal lymph flow.

nosocomial (nos uh KOH mee ul) Also known as healthcare-acquired infections (HAI).

petechiae (peh TEE kee ah) A very small, round hemorrhage in the skin or mucous membrane.

plasma (PLAZ muh) The liquid portion of a whole blood sample that has not clotted due to an anticoagulant. Liquid portion of blood that contains clotting factors. Liquid portion of the blood found in the body.

serum (SEER um) The liquid portion of a clotted blood specimen. It no longer contains active clotting agents.

suction (SUHK shun) The production of a partial vacuum by the removal of air in order to force fluid into a vacant space.

syringe (suh RINJ) A device with a slender barrel and needle used to withdraw blood from a vein or artery.

Phlebotomy is performed primarily to do the following:
- Assist the provider in diagnosing disease
- Monitor a patient's condition, treatment, or medication levels
- Document the existing good health of a patient

According to the American Society of Clinical Pathologists (ASCP), nearly 80% of providers base at least part of their diagnostic decisions on the results of laboratory tests. The most common specimen used in the laboratory is blood. *Phlebotomy* is the process of acquiring blood from a patient. Phlebotomy involves highly developed skills, procedures, and equipment to ensure the patient's comfort and safety.

When it comes to phlebotomy, safety is an important concern. There are several bloodborne viral diseases that can be spread by exposure to infected blood and body fluids. The viruses identified as possible bloodborne pathogen risks are hepatitis B virus (HBV), hepatitis C virus (HCV), and human immunodeficiency virus (HIV).

These viruses are not the only diseases that can be spread by contaminated blood or body fluids, but they are considered a risk for healthcare workers and public safety personnel (such as firefighters, police, and first responders). The high standards necessary for the safe practice of phlebotomy led to the creation of the Bloodborne Pathogens Standard (overseen by the Occupational Safety and Health Administration [OSHA]) and by different organizations that develop additional standards for training (see Chapter 4).

Medical assistants are trained to perform phlebotomy as part of their education. They can choose to become certified phlebotomists by completing additional training, coursework, and passing a national certification examination. Phlebotomy certifying agencies include the American Society of Clinical Pathologists (ASCP), the International Academy of Phlebotomy Sciences (IAPS), the National Certification Agency (NCA), the National Phlebotomy Association (NPA), the National Healthcare Association (NHA), and the American Medical Technologists (AMT). Continuing education often is required to maintain a phlebotomy certification. It is important that medical assistants become familiar with the guidelines of the states in which they work, because not all states require a certificate to perform phlebotomy.

The most common method of obtaining a blood specimen is by *venipuncture*, which is when blood is taken directly from a surface vein. The vein is punctured with a needle, and the blood is collected directly into a stoppered vacuum tube, or into a **syringe**, and then transferred into the vacuum tube. The procedure is safe when performed by a trained professional, but it must be performed with care. Practice is required to become skilled and confident in the technique of venipuncture.

VENIPUNCTURE EQUIPMENT

Proper collection of blood requires specialized equipment. Phlebotomists in hospitals generally carry the equipment in a portable tray (Fig. 32.1). A physician office laboratory (POL) often has a permanent location where the same supplies are stored and venipuncture is performed. In such cases, you may use a phlebotomy chair, which has an adjustable locking armrest to protect the patient if he or she should faint (Fig. 32.2). However, if the patient has a history of *syncope* (fainting), it is best to perform phlebotomy while the patient is lying on an examination table or in a reclining phlebotomy chair.

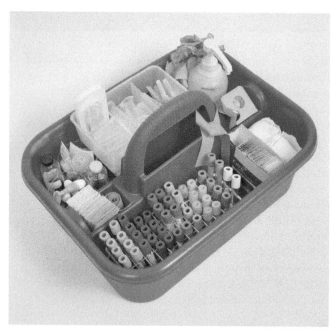

FIGURE 32.1 A stocked venipuncture tray.

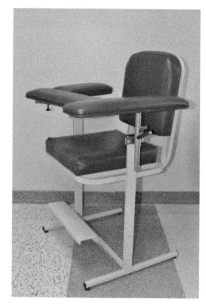

FIGURE 32.2 A phlebotomy chair.

Equipment Used in Routine Venipuncture

Personal protective equipment (PPE): gloves, fluid-impermeable lab coat, and protective eyewear, or face shield (if necessary)
- Permanent marker
- Alcohol wipes
- Gauze
- Hypoallergenic self-stick wrap, tape, or bandages
- Nonlatex tourniquets
- Double-pointed safety needles
- Winged infusion sets (butterfly needles)
- Disposable needle holders
- Evacuated, stoppered tubes
- Syringes and removable needles with safety devices
- Biohazard sharps container
- Biohazard waste container

Personal Protective Equipment

Employers must provide employees with personal protective equipment (PPE), such as gloves, disposable fluid-impenetrable lab coats, protective eyewear, and face shields. All facilities must stock only latex-free supplies because of the potential for allergic responses in workers and patients. Some people with latex allergies can have life-threatening reactions with latex exposure.

CRITICAL THINKING APPLICATION   32.1

Maggie is in a little early on a Monday morning. She knows that Monday is usually busy, and she wants to make sure all her supplies are adequately stocked. Maggie cleans her protective eyewear and has it ready at the phlebotomy station. Why is it important to wear protective eyewear whenever drawing blood? Can you think of a few reasons and share them with your class?

OSHA requires healthcare workers to wear gloves during venipuncture. Because veins can be difficult to locate with gloved fingertips, the site may be palpated before gloves are put on, as long as the hands have been washed or sanitized. According to the standard procedure for venipuncture established by the Clinical and Laboratory Standards Institute (CLSI), gloves may be put on after vein palpation but before preparation of the site. Those who need the final assurance of one last palpation before the needle is inserted must remember that touching the prepared site, even with gloves, contaminates the area. To help yourself find the vein after the area has been cleansed, make note of any skin markers, such as creases, freckles, or scars. If the area is touched, *it must be cleansed again.* Keep in mind that the tourniquet should be tied for no longer than 1 minute at a time.

Tourniquets

Before blood can be drawn, a vein must be located. Most venipunctures are done in the *antecubital region*, or inner bend in front of the elbow. Application of a *tourniquet* is very helpful in locating veins in the antecubital region and any other area that may be drawn for venipuncture. Tourniquets prevent the venous blood flow out of the site, causing the veins to bulge or plump up. If the antecubital area is drawn, a tourniquet is tied around the upper arm so that it is tight but still comfortable and can be easily released with one hand. Single-use, nonlatex tourniquets are available (Fig. 32.3) and currently are recommended to do the following:
- Reduce cross-contamination between patients and healthcare workers
- Help prevent **nosocomial** infections
- Prevent latex exposure

Other types of tourniquets with quick-release closures are available, but they must be disinfected after each use.

Tourniquets are applied 3 to 4 inches above the elbow immediately before the venipuncture procedure begins. Because a tourniquet slows blood flow, leaving it on for longer than 1 minute greatly increases the possibility of **hemoconcentration** and altered test results. The tourniquet should not be tied so tightly that it restricts arterial blood

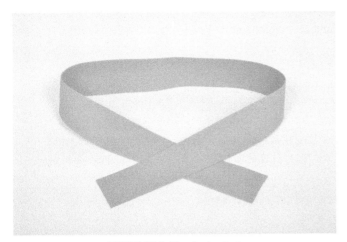

FIGURE 32.3 A latex-free tourniquet.

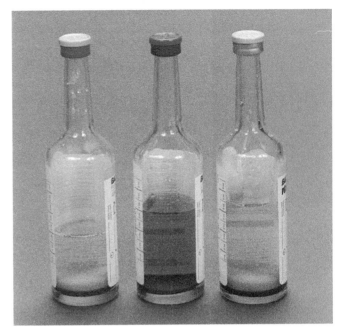

FIGURE 32.4 Blood culture bottles.

flow. If arterial blood flow is restricted, then venous blood return is also restricted. As a result, veins will not plump up. Checking the pulse at the wrist ensures that arterial flow is not restricted. Tourniquets also are used when blood is drawn from hand and foot veins and are tied on the wrist or ankle, respectively.

Tourniquets can be uncomfortable for patients, especially those with heavy-set or hairy upper arms, if they are not applied correctly. Make sure the tourniquet is flat against the skin, and, if necessary, tie it over the clothing if it is causing the patient discomfort. This may be especially important when blood is drawn on an older adult because of the thinness or fragility of the skin.

Antiseptics

To prevent infection, a venipuncture site must be cleansed with an **antiseptic**. The most commonly used antiseptic is 70% isopropyl alcohol, also known as *rubbing alcohol*. Prepackaged alcohol wipes are the product used most often. An alcohol wipe is used to clean the puncture site, which is then allowed to air dry. Alcohol does not sterilize the skin, but it kills many of the existing bacteria that might contaminate the sample. To be most effective, the alcohol should remain on the skin for 30 to 60 seconds and allowed to air dry. As the alcohol dries, it breaks open the bacterial cells and kills the bacteria. Alcohol wipes should not be used when collecting a blood alcohol sample. Sterile soap pads, benzalkonium chloride, or povidone-iodine (Betadine) can be used instead.

If a provider suspects a fever of unknown origin (FUO), a **blood culture** is frequently ordered. Additional preparation is needed at the venipuncture site to eliminate contaminating bacteria. First, 70% isopropyl alcohol wipes are used to clean the area, which is allowed to air dry. Then an iodine solution is used, such as povidone-iodine. Chlorhexidine gluconate or benzalkonium chloride can be used for patients who are allergic to iodine. The iodine prep is also allowed to air dry. Once the venipuncture site is properly prepared, the blood cultures must be drawn into a sterile tube or bottle specifically designed for the test (Fig. 32.4).

Evacuated Collection Tubes

The most common collection system is the **evacuated** tube system (these tubes are also called *vacuum tubes;* a particular brand of vacuum tubes is the Vacutainer). It consists of evacuated tubes of various sizes

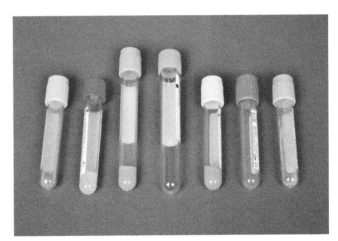

FIGURE 32.5 Hemogard tube stoppers.

that have color-coded stoppers. The colored stoppers indicate the tube's contents (Table 32.1). Venipuncture tubes must be either shatter-resistant glass or plastic. More traditional rubber tube stoppers have been replaced by safer plastic *Hemogard* colored tops. Hemogard tops have the advantage of not splattering blood when removed from the tube (Fig. 32.5). Table 32.1 lists the colored stoppers and the chemical additives, **anticoagulants**, **clot activators**, or thixotropic gel that are contained in each type of tube. The different stopper colors indicate the unique contents of that color-coded tube. The vacuum in each tube draws a measured amount of blood into the tube. Tube volumes range from 2 to 15 mL.

CRITICAL THINKING APPLICATION   32.2

It is important to use a tourniquet to properly locate veins for phlebotomy. List three advantages of using a tourniquet to help locate veins. Be ready to share them with your class.

TABLE 32.1	Common Color-Coded Stoppers and Their Additives and Laboratory Uses			
VACUUM TUBE COLOR[a]	COLOR	HEMOGARD COLOR[b]	ADDITIVE AND ITS FUNCTION[c]	LABORATORY USE
Blood culture bottles	No color for blood culture bottles (see Fig. 32.4)	Yellow	Sodium polyanethole sulfonate (SPS); prevents blood from clotting and stabilizes bacterial growth. Yellow-topped tubes have specific uses. They cannot be used to collect all blood culture specimens.	Blood culture bottles—blood or body fluid cultures Yellow-topped tubes—mycobacteria, fungus, or acid-fast bacilli (AFB) blood cultures
Light blue		Light blue	Sodium citrate; removes calcium to prevent blood from clotting.	Coagulation testing
Red		Red	None.	Serum tests; chemistry studies, blood bank, immunology
Red-gray (marbled)		Gold	No anticoagulant, but contains silica particles to enhance clot formation; usually contain gel for serum separation.	Serum tests; chemistry studies, immunology
Green		Green	Heparin; inhibits thrombin formation to prevent clotting.	Chemistry tests
Green-gray (marbled)		Light green	Lithium heparin and gel; for plasma separation.	Plasma determinations in chemistry studies
Lavender		Lavender	Ethylenediaminetetraacetic acid (EDTA); removes calcium to prevent blood from clotting.	Hematology tests
Gray		Gray	Potassium oxalate and sodium fluoride; removes calcium to prevent blood from clotting; fluoride inhibits **glycolysis**.	Chemistry testing, especially glucose and alcohol levels

[a]Stopper colors are based on BD Vacutainer tubes.
[b]Hemogard closures provide a protective plastic cover over the rubber stopper as an additional safety feature.
[c]Additives, additive functions, and laboratory uses are the same for both pediatric and adult tubes.

The size of the tube to be drawn depends on several factors. Each test performed in the laboratory requires a specific amount of blood. Blood volumes can often be combined, which reduces the number of tubes that must be drawn. For example, both a complete blood count and an erythrocyte sedimentation rate test (discussed in Chapter 33) are performed on a sample from a lavender-topped tube. The combined volume for both tests can be drawn with one lavender-topped tube, so you do not need to draw two tubes. When in doubt, call the laboratory. Keep in mind that blood is approximately half cells and half liquid. If a test requires 2 mL of serum, at least 4 mL of blood must be collected.

Tube Additives

Most vacuum tubes contain an additive. The plain red-topped tube contains nothing! It is a plain tube with no additives and no anticoagulants or clot enhancers. A gold-topped tube contains silica to activate clotting and an inert thixotropic gel to separate serum and cells after the sample is centrifuged. Most other color-topped plastic tubes contain some form of anticoagulant, which prevents blood from clotting. The additive may be a powder, a liquid visible in the tube, or a liquid sprayed inside the tube by the manufacturer and allowed to dry. The choice of anticoagulant depends on the test to be completed.

Anticoagulant additives prevent blood from clotting, which allows the contents of the tube to be used in two ways. First, the sample can be used as whole blood; second, the sample can be centrifuged, and the liquid portion, called **plasma**, can be used for testing. An example of a test that uses whole blood would be a complete blood count (CBC). An example of a test that uses plasma would be a coagulation study.

Ethylenediaminetetraacetic acid (EDTA) is the anticoagulant found in the lavender-topped tube. It prevents platelet clumping and preserves the appearance of blood cells for microscopic examination.

Clot activators promote blood clotting in the tubes with either a marbled red-gray or a gold top. For example, silica particles in the gold tubes enhance clotting by providing a surface for platelet activation. Thrombin from the platelets quickly promotes clotting and is used in tubes drawn for chemistry testing or in the event a sample is needed from a patient taking a prescribed anticoagulant, such as heparin.

If blood clots and then is centrifuged, the liquid portion is referred to as **serum**. Without a clot activator, blood clots in 15 to 60 minutes, after which it must be centrifuged. The serum must be quickly separated from the cells because cells may continue to metabolize glucose or may release substances that interfere with testing.

Thixotropic gel can be found in some tubes, including *serum separator tubes* (SSTs). SST tubes are identified by the marbled red-gray rubber stopper or the gold Hemogard top. The *plasma separator tube* (PST) also contains thixotropic gel. The tubes have a marbled green-gray top, and the Hemogard tubes have a light green top. Thixotropic gel, a synthetic, chemically neutral gel, has a density between that of red cells and plasma or serum. The gel settles between the plasma/serum and cells during centrifugation. The gel forms a barrier that makes it easy to pour off the liquid portion of the sample without cells contaminating the specimen.

It is important to avoid a "short draw" (i.e., a tube that is not completely filled). Table 32.2 lists the consequences of underfilling tubes. Some tubes are designed to fill only partially, according to their preset vacuum. Having the proper ratio of blood to additive is crucial. Always check the tube for the expiration date. Outdated tubes may have a diminished vacuum, or the additive may have degraded and not be as effective.

CRITICAL THINKING APPLICATION   32.3

In your own words, define *plasma* and *serum*.

ORDER OF THE DRAW

If more than one tube must be drawn during a venipuncture, a specified order must be followed. Carryover of additives from one tube to the next could cause sample alteration and incorrect results. CLSI has established a set of standards outlining the order to follow for a multitube draw. The same order applies to the filling of tubes when blood is collected in a syringe.

1. *Blood culture bottles:* These bottles are filled first because they are sterile and should not be contaminated by the other tubes. In addition to blood culture bottles, a yellow-topped tube can be drawn for blood cultures for mycobacteria, fungi, and

TABLE 32.2 Effects of Underfilling Collection Tubes

STOPPER COLOR	EFFECTS OF UNDERFILLING
Yellow	Reduces possibility of bacterial recovery
Light blue	Coagulation test results falsely prolonged
Red	Insufficient sample
Marbled red-gray, and gold (SST tubes)	Poor barrier formation; insufficient sample
Green	False results because of excess heparin
Marbled green-gray, and light green (PST tubes)	False results because of excess heparin
Lavender	Falsely low blood cell counts and hematocrits; morphologic changes to red blood cells; staining changes
Gray	False results

acid-fast bacilli. These tubes are not drawn frequently in an ambulatory setting. If they are ordered, they would be drawn in the same place as blood culture bottles in the order of the draw.

2. *Light blue* top: These tubes, which contain sodium citrate, are next because other anticoagulants might contaminate the sample collected for coagulation studies. If no blood culture has been ordered, CLSI recommends that blood for the light blue–topped tube be drawn first if routine coagulation testing has been ordered. Examples of coagulation tests include prothrombin time (PT) and activated partial thromboplastin time (APTT). See Chapter 33 for more details about coagulation testing. Some laboratories recommend that a red-topped "waste" tube with no additives be partially filled before the light blue–topped tube. This is done to remove any tissue thromboplastin that may be released during the venipuncture. Thromboplastin interferes with coagulation testing. CLSI also recommends that, when a winged infusion (butterfly assembly) is used, blood should be drawn into the red-topped tube even if the order does not call for it. This is done to fill the tubing's dead air space with blood before drawing the light blue–topped sodium citrate tube. A light blue tube must have an exact blood-to-citrate dilution. It is not necessary to completely fill the waste tube, because it will be discarded.

3. *Red* top or *gold* top: Red serum tubes without clot activator, or gold serum tubes with clot activator, are filled next. These tubes are drawn to test serum after the specimens have clotted and been centrifuged. SSTs with thixotropic gel are also drawn at this time. SST tubes have a marbled red-gray stopper or a gold Hemogard stopper.

4. *Green* top: These tubes are drawn next because the plasma in their anticoagulated specimen is used for testing when STAT results are needed (usually in chemistry). The dark green tops

contain no thixotropic gel. The tubes with marbled green-gray tops and light green Hemogard tops both contain gel to help separate the plasma from the cells when centrifuged.

5. *Lavender* top: These tubes are drawn next. They contain an EDTA anticoagulant that preserves blood cell morphology. EDTA tubes are drawn near the end of the draw because the additive interferes with chemistry and coagulation specimens.

6. *Gray* top: This tube is drawn last, and the blood is used to test glucose or blood alcohol levels. Its additives may elevate electrolyte levels and damage cells if passed into the other tubes.

It is important to gently mix the contents of the tubes after collection by inverting them (do not shake the tubes). Most tubes should be inverted eight times, but clot activator tubes should be inverted five times, and sodium citrate three to four times.

CRITICAL THINKING APPLICATION   **32.4**

Sometimes making up a saying or sentence can help you remember the order of a process. Here are a few sayings that might help the medical assistant to remember the order of the draw.

The order of the draw is as follows: **st**erile (blood culture bottles/tubes)—light **b**lue—**r**ed/gold—**g**reen—**l**avender—**g**ray. Use the first letter for each tube color and make up a sentence that helps you remember the order of the draw.

Examples:
1. Stop light red. Green light go.
2. Stan's light red glasses look gray.
3. Stella's lecture reading gives little giggles.
4. Street lights reveal green little gardens.

Can you make up your own saying to remember the order of the draw? Share your saying with your classmates!

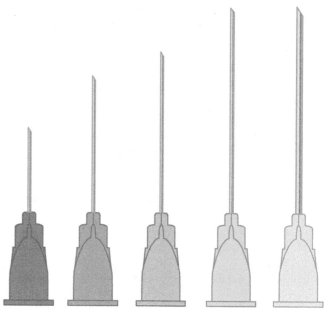

FIGURE 32.6 Venipuncture needles.

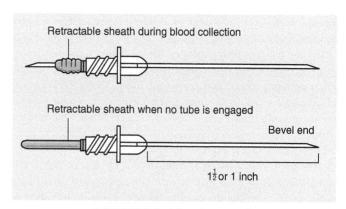

Retractable sheath during blood collection

Retractable sheath when no tube is engaged

Bevel end

$1\frac{1}{2}$ or 1 inch

FIGURE 32.7 Bevel of a venipuncture needle.

NEEDLES AND SUPPLIES USED IN PHLEBOTOMY

A critical part of phlebotomy is knowing which needle and which tube, or syringe, should be used in each situation. All needles used in phlebotomy are sterile and have a safety device that is activated immediately after withdrawal from the vein. The needle is then discarded in a biohazard sharps container. Each needle is housed in a protected cover, which should be inspected before use to ensure that sterility has not been compromised (i.e., the seal should be intact) and that the needle has no manufacturing defects, such as burs, nicks, or bends.

Needles have two parts, the hub and the shaft. The hub of the needle is designed to attach the needle to the vacuum tube needle holder or a syringe. Shafts differ in length, ranging from ¾ inch to 1½ inches (Fig. 32.6). The length of the shaft has no bearing on the venipuncture procedure. Some phlebotomists prefer a longer needle, and others prefer a shorter needle because it makes patients less uneasy. One end of the shaft is cut at an angle and forms the *bevel*, which creates a very sharp point. The bevel of the needle makes the entry into the skin much smoother (Fig. 32.7)

The bore, or hollow space, inside the needle is called the *lumen*. Lumen size is important and is referred to as the *gauge*. A numeric value designates the gauge of the needle. The higher the gauge number, the smaller the lumen. Be sure to match the needle gauge to the size of the tube. A large vacuum tube is more likely to hemolyze the blood if a high-gauge needle (i.e., small lumen) is used. For example, blood banks use a large, 16-gauge needle to collect pints of blood for transfusions. The lumen is wide, which reduces the chance of **hemolysis**. A small, 23-gauge needle is used to collect blood from small or fragile veins, such as those in older adults and very young patients. Routine adult venipuncture requires a 20- to 21-gauge needle.

Multisample Needles

Multisample needles are commonly used in routine adult venipuncture. They are used when several tubes need to be drawn during a single venipuncture. These needles are double pointed (see Fig. 32.7). One point enters the patient's vein, and the other punctures the stopper of the collection tube. The point that enters the tube is sheathed with a retractable rubber sleeve that allows tubes to be changed without blood leaking into the needle holder or tube holder.

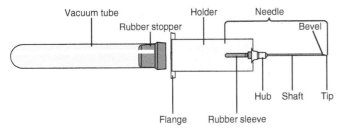

FIGURE 32.8 Venipuncture assembly. (From Hunt SA: *Saunders fundamentals of medical assisting*, revised reprint, St. Louis, 2007, Saunders.)

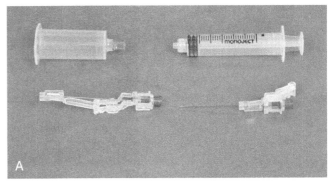

CRITICAL THINKING APPLICATION   32.5

Maggie has a few different gauge needles to use in phlebotomy. Why would she need different sized needles? If the process is the same for each patient, why would the needle size be important? Share your ideas with the class.

Needle Holders

Double-pointed needles must be firmly placed into a needle holder (Fig. 32.8). Usually needle holders are translucent cylinders, and they come in different sizes to accommodate different-sized tubes. The holders often have a ring that indicates how far the tube can be pushed onto the needle without losing the vacuum. To prevent accidental needlesticks, OSHA requires that the needle holder, with its safety-activated needle still attached, must be discarded into a biohazard sharps container immediately after completing the venipuncture.

Syringes

Syringes are used when there is concern that the strong vacuum in a stoppered vacuum tube might collapse the vein. The syringe needle fits on the end of the syringe barrel. Syringe needles also come in different gauges. The amount of blood drawn into the syringe barrel depends on how much blood needs to be collected for testing. When blood is drawn into a syringe, it must be transferred immediately to the evacuated tube(s). Blood that sits in the syringe barrel could clot if not transferred quickly. The syringe needle safety device must be activated and discarded in the sharps container. A special transfer tube device is then used to transfer the blood to the vacuum tubes. This device connects to the top of the syringe; it contains an enclosed needle that punctures the vacuum tube's stopper and delivers the blood into the tube (Fig. 32.9).

Winged Infusion Sets (Butterfly Assembly)

Butterfly assemblies (Fig. 32.10) are designed for use on small veins. Butterfly needles are often used to draw veins in the back of the hand or when drawing a pediatric patient. The most common butterfly needle size is a 22 or 23 gauge with a needle length of $\frac{1}{2}$ to $\frac{3}{4}$ inch. A butterfly needle has a plastic, flexible, butterfly-shaped grip attached to a short length of tubing. The hub end is fitted into a syringe or a needle holder tube adapter. Syringes are frequently paired with butterfly needles because the syringe can create a gentle vacuum that can easily be controlled by the phlebotomist. The syringe blood sample must be transferred to the evacuated tubes using the transfer device described previously.

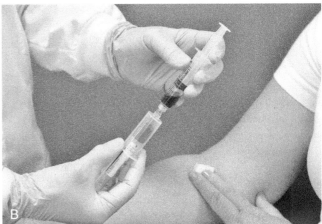

FIGURE 32.9 Syringe assembly. **(A)** Syringe, syringe safety needle, and safety transfer tube device. **(B)** Using a syringe safety transfer tube device.

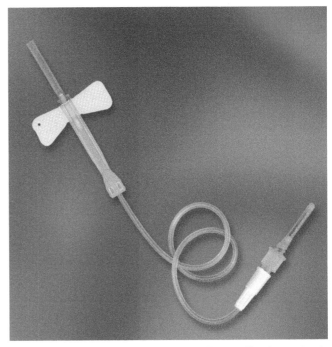

FIGURE 32.10 Butterfly assembly. (Courtesy Becton, Dickinson, Franklin Lakes, New Jersey.)

CRITICAL THINKING APPLICATION   32.6

Describe the difference between a syringe and a winged infusion assembly. List two situations when each type of equipment may be used.

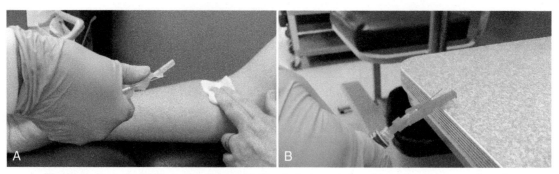

FIGURE 32.11 One-handed safety needles. (A) Activated by sliding the thumb up at the base of the guard, causing it to cover the needle. (B) Activated by pressing the orange guard against a solid surface, causing it to cover the needle.

NEEDLE SAFETY

Healthcare workers who use or may be exposed to needles are at increased risk of needlestick injury. Such injuries can lead to serious or fatal infections with blood-borne pathogens, such as HBV, HCV, and HIV. Needlestick injuries account for most accidental exposures to blood. As is discussed in Chapter 4, used needles should never be recapped. After use, needles should be covered with the appropriate engineered safety device that is part of the needle assembly.

According to OSHA, the best practice for preventing needlestick injuries after phlebotomy is to use safety needles that are activated with one hand immediately after use. The US Food and Drug Administration (FDA), which is responsible for approving medical devices marketed and sold in the United States, recommends devices that provide a barrier between the hands and the needle, after use, in which the phlebotomist's hands remain behind the needle at all times. Safety shields that can be activated before or immediately after removal of the needle from the vein and that remain in effect after disposal should also be an integral part of the device. Finally, these devices should be as simple as possible, requiring little or no training to use. Some examples of needle safety devices are as follows:

One-handed vacuum tube needle: After the needle has been used and removed from the vein, the thumb holding the vacuum tube holder slides under the base of the pink safety device, causing it to snap over the contaminated needle (Fig. 32.11A). Or an orange needle shield on the holder is activated by pressing the device against a hard, flat surface (Fig. 32.11B).

Protect Against Needlestick Injuries

OSHA's Bloodborne Pathogens Standard emphasizes that phlebotomists should have direct input on the type of safety needles they will be using. The following steps should be taken to protect against needlestick injuries:

- Help your employer evaluate and select devices with safety features.
- Use devices with safety features provided by your employer.
- Never recap a contaminated needle except with a safety device.
- Plan for safe handling and disposal before beginning any procedure using needles.
- Dispose of used needles and needle holders promptly in appropriate biohazard sharps containers.

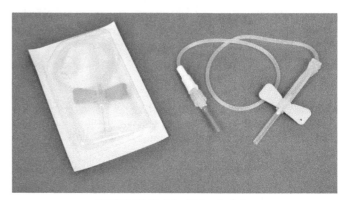

FIGURE 32.12 Safety-Lok butterfly needle.

- Report all needlestick and other sharps-related injuries promptly to ensure that you receive appropriate follow-up care.
- Tell your employer about hazards from needles that you observe in your work environment.
- Participate in bloodborne pathogen training, and follow recommended infection prevention practices, including vaccination against hepatitis B virus (HBV).

Syringe needle safety devices (see Fig. 32.9): These devices have a spring-activated shield attached to a disposable syringe needle. After the venipuncture, the phlebotomist activates the device with the thumb holding the syringe, and a spring locks a protective plastic tip into place, protecting the needle. The needle can then be removed and discarded. The syringe is attached to the safety transfer device to deliver the collected blood into the appropriate vacuum tubes (see Fig. 32.9).

Butterfly needle safety lock (Fig. 32.12): After the venipuncture, the dominant hand holds the butterfly tail while the nondominant hand pulls back on the tubing, causing the needle to slide into the tubing and lock into place.

Push-button butterfly safety device (Fig. 32.13): With the needle still in the arm, the medical assistant grasps the tail of the butterfly with the dominant hand while the nondominant hand presses the button just below the wings, causing the needle to retract into the butterfly body as it leaves the vein.

Needle-blunting butterfly set (Fig. 32.14): A third "wing" is rotated after collection and before removal of the needle from the vein. As the third wing is rotated, it moves the blunt needle down the shaft before it is removed from the patient.

OSHA requires employers to establish and maintain a sharps injury log for recording injuries from contaminated sharps. This log should contain information about the device involved in the incident and the department or work area where the incident occurred, in addition to an explanation of the incident. Employee confidentiality must be maintained.

Postexposure Needlestick Follow-Up

An accidental needlestick is a medical emergency. OSHA-recommended management procedures are discussed in Chapter 4. Effective management of an accidental sharps exposure includes the following measures:

- Immediately after injury, the wound is inspected and washed for 10 minutes with soap, 10% iodine solution, or chlorine-based antiseptic.
- The injury is reported to the supervisor, and an incident report is completed.
- The employee is referred to a physician for confidential assessment and follow-up. Baseline testing for HBV, HCV, and HIV is recommended for both the employee and the source individual. If the employee has been immunized for HBV and has a positive postimmunization titer, there is no risk of acquiring HBV and no source testing is needed. If the worker has not been immunized or the postimmunization titer is negative, source testing for infection with HBV is recommended if the source is known and can be located. If the source patient tests positive for HBV, the employee should receive HBV immune globulin (HBIG), and the series of HBV immunizations should

be initiated. If the source tests negative, no treatment is indicated. If the source patient cannot be tested, the employee should be treated as if the source patient were positive for HBV. The source should also be tested for HCV. If the source is positive, the employee should be monitored for signs and symptoms of hepatitis for 6 months. No postexposure prophylaxis is recommended for HCV infection. For HIV exposure, most employers recommend a 4-week regimen of antiretroviral drugs. To best protect the victim, antiretroviral therapy should be administered within hours of exposure. Early HIV drug therapy is now recommended for anyone who may be at risk of infection. Because these medications have side effects, the employee is the one who decides whether the medications are started. If the source is found to be negative, antiretroviral therapy can be discontinued.

- Interim testing may be performed if the healthcare worker experiences symptoms of acute HIV exposure or hepatitis. For HIV, antibody testing should be repeated at 6 weeks, 12 weeks, and 6 months if the source was HIV positive or the source's status remains unknown. Confidential follow-up care must include provisions for emotional support and counseling for the healthcare worker.

ROUTINE VENIPUNCTURE

Venipuncture involves a series of steps that are vital to collecting a good sample. In addition to learning good technique, we also want to be able to make our patients as comfortable as possible. As you read through the information, you will start to become familiar with the venipuncture procedure and the details of the process.

The first step of the procedure is to select the proper method for venipuncture (evacuated tube, syringe, or butterfly assembly). Next, prepare your patient for the procedure. Then you are ready to collect the sample and process the specimen appropriately.

Patient Preparation

All blood collections begin with a requisition, a form from the patient's provider requesting a test. Requisitions may be computer-generated or handwritten, and at a minimum they must include the following information:

- Patient's name
- Patient's date of birth
- Patient's identification number
- Name of the provider submitting the order
- Type of test requested
- Test status (timed, fasting, STAT, and so forth)

Begin the venipuncture procedure by greeting the patient and verifying his or her identity. According to CLSI, proper identification includes asking outpatients to (1) state and spell their first and last name, and (2) state their birth date. All the information must be

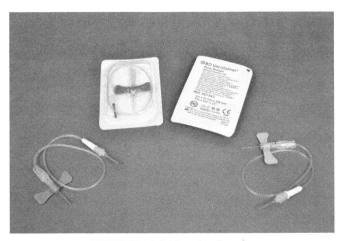

FIGURE 32.13 Push-button butterfly needle.

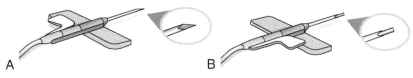

FIGURE 32.14 Needle-blunting butterfly needle.

compared and verified with the patient requisition. If communication with the patient is not effective due to any circumstances, a family member, guardian, or medical translator must provide the needed information. The name of the person assisting should be documented in the patient's medical record. Always follow your institution's procedures for assisted communication before completing the venipuncture procedure.

Briefly explain the venipuncture procedure to your patient, and make sure to ask him or her the following questions:

- Do you have any questions or concerns?
- Do you have an arm, vein, or site preference?
- Were you given any special instructions prior to the venipuncture (e.g., does the person need to be fasting)?
- Have you ever experienced any problems or complications with a routine venipuncture in the past?

Answer questions and concerns, and take steps to prevent any past problems from recurring. If you cannot answer all the patient's questions, ask if he or she would like to talk to the provider for clarification. Obtain verbal consent to perform the venipuncture simply by asking whether you have permission to draw blood from the patient.

Your self-confidence in the procedure will help put your patient at ease. Act and speak professionally. Treat your patient with kindness and respect. Being pleasant and friendly is important. It makes your patients feel comfortable and shows that you take your role in their care seriously.

CRITICAL THINKING APPLICATION   **32.7**

Why is patient identification so important in phlebotomy? List four reasons, and be ready to share them with the class.

Preparing for the Venipuncture

Seat the patient in a phlebotomy area. Ask the patient to extend an arm and position his or her other hand under the elbow to help straighten the elbow, if necessary. Inspect both arms, and ask whether the patient has an arm or site preference. Veins in the antecubital area are most commonly used for venipuncture (Fig. 32.15). According to CLSI standards, the veins in the center of the antecubital area should be located as a first choice before alternative veins within the antecubital area are considered. The puncture site should be carefully selected after both arms have been inspected. Alternative sites may be chosen if the area is scarred, bruised, burned, or swollen. You may use the veins on the back of the hand if the patient gives permission. For any other alternative site, consult the provider, and do not proceed without supervision.

When choosing the best available vein, palpate the area. Feel for a vein that has "bounce" when lightly palpated. Consider the 3 Ds of vein selection; **d**epth below the surface, **d**iameter of the vein, and **d**irection through the antecubital region. Choosing a vein correctly is one of the most important aspects of a venipuncture.

The medial veins generally run at a slight angle to the fold in the antecubital area. The cephalic veins are on the thumb side of the antecubital area. These veins are the veins of choice. The basilic vein, which lies on the inside of the antecubital area (the little finger side), is very close to the brachial artery and median nerves and should *not*

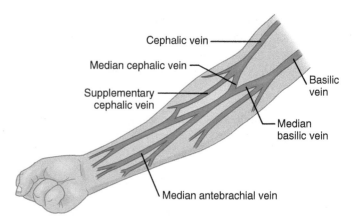

FIGURE 32.15 The veins of the forearm. (From Stepp CA, Woods MA: *Laboratory procedures for medical office personnel*, Philadelphia, 1998, Saunders.)

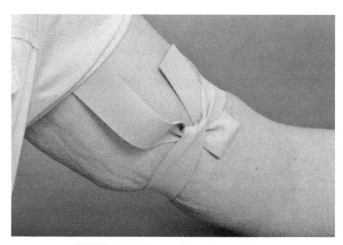

FIGURE 32.16 Placement of the tourniquet on the arm.

be used! If the medial or cephalic veins are not accessible, consult the provider. Only the most experienced phlebotomists should ever attempt a basilic venipuncture. The chance of injury to the patient is too great.

The tourniquet should be placed about 3 to 4 inches above the patient's elbow. Make sure it is not twisted because that will cause discomfort to your patient (Fig. 32.16). Grasp the tourniquet ends, one in each hand, close to the patient's skin. Pull the ends apart to gently stretch the tourniquet, then cross one end over the other while maintaining the tension. Tuck the top portion of the tourniquet underneath the bottom portion, creating a loop with the upper flap free. The free end will be tugged on to release the tourniquet later in the draw. The tourniquet should be tight without being uncomfortable or pinching the patient's skin. Both ends of the tourniquet should be pointing upward on the arm. This way, the end of the tourniquet does not contaminate the venipuncture site.

When the tourniquet is in place, ask the patient to place his or her other hand or fist under the elbow of the arm that will be drawn if this aids in palpating the vein. Ask the person to just relax the arm. Palpate for an acceptable vein using your gloved index finger. It is more efficient to put on gloves at the beginning of the procedure and continue. Also, if you learn to palpate veins with your gloves on, you will train your finger to recognize the veins through the gloves from the beginning.

According to the Clinical and Laboratory Standards Institute (CLSI), you can palpate veins without gloves on as long as the venipuncture site has not yet been cleaned. After locating the vein, clean the area with a 70% isopropyl alcohol wipe. While the site is drying, resanitize your hands, put on gloves, and continue with the rest of the procedure.

Performing the Venipuncture

When you have located a vein, remove the tourniquet. A tourniquet can remain in place for 1 minute. After its removal, wait 2 minutes before reapplying it. During this time, sanitize your hands and put on gloves (if they are not already on). Then cleanse the antecubital area with a 70% alcohol wipe. Clean the area by using a back-and-forth motion. CLSI guidelines recommend cleansing the site with friction and not a circular motion. Do not touch this area after cleaning with alcohol. Assemble the equipment, and place it within easy reach of the patient's arm.

Reapply the tourniquet. Do not have the patient clench or pump the fist. If the fist is relaxed, the venipuncture will feel less painful. Visually relocate the vein, do not retouch the cleaned area. Anchor the vein by gently stretching the skin downward, about 2 to 3 inches below the collection site with the thumb of the nondominant hand. Smoothly and quickly insert the needle into the vein at about a 15-degree angle, depending on the depth and position of the vein. The bevel should be facing up. Push the evacuated tube onto the double-pointed needle, or pull back on the syringe plunger with your nondominant hand.

Angle of Needle Entry

Why is the angle of the needle so important? If the needle is inserted at an angle greater than 15 degrees, it penetrates the vein quickly and may pass through the back side of the vein and enter other structures. Formation of a hematoma is more likely then.

If the angle is less than 15 degrees, the needle may skim on the top of the vein and not create a clean puncture. If the vein is just skimmed or scratched, there is a greater chance of creating a hematoma on the front of the vein.

The depth and position of the vein may require angle adjustment, but a 15-degree angle is a good place to start. The angle of entry is very important to a successful venipuncture.

CRITICAL THINKING APPLICATION 32.8

Maggie is drawing Ken Thomas this morning. The provider has ordered three different tests, so Maggie will need to draw three different-colored tubes. As Maggie puts on the tourniquet to locate a vein, Ken pumps his fist a few times to try to make the veins stand out. But Maggie asks him to just relax his hand. Why would relaxing his hand be better. List one or two reasons, and be ready to share them with the class.

Completing the Venipuncture

Continue to draw the specimens, checking periodically on the patient's condition. As you remove each tube from the needle holder, gently invert it several times before placing it in a collection rack. Tubes

with sodium citrate should be inverted three to four times. Tubes with clot activator should be inverted five times. Tubes with anticoagulant should be inverted eight times. If the tubes are not inverted immediately after collection, small clots can form in the specimen. When the last tube has started to fill, carefully release the tourniquet. Gently tug on the short portion of the tourniquet, and it should just fall open. Remove the final vacuum tube. Cover the venipuncture area with gauze, then smoothly and quickly remove the needle. Once the needle is out of the arm, apply pressure to the site. At the same time, activate the safety device to cover the needle. Dispose of the entire venipuncture assembly into a sharps container. Ask the patient to apply direct pressure to the gauze. *Do not* bend the arm.

While the patient applies pressure to the site, label the tubes with computer-generated labels or by writing the information in permanent marker. Make sure the label contains the following minimum information:

- Patient's last name, then first name
- Patient's date of birth
- Patient's ID number or medical insurance number
- Date and time of the draw, and the phlebotomist's initials
- Provider's name; also indicate if the patient was fasting (optional)

Before putting on a bandage, perform a two-point check to make sure the site is not leaking. Observe the site for 5 to 10 seconds after releasing pressure and removing the gauze. If visible bleeding occurs or if the tissue around the puncture site rises, continue applying pressure until the bleeding has stopped. Special precautions must be taken for patients taking anticoagulants because the phlebotomy site will bleed longer than normal. Put on a pressure bandage by placing a folded gauze (not a cotton ball) over the site and then applying hypoallergenic self-stick wrap, stretchy gauze, or a bandage. Never leave the room or release an outpatient until all the tubes have been labeled. Make sure the patient is doing well, then escort him or her to the exit or to the reception area.

CRITICAL THINKING APPLICATION 32.9

At the end of Ken's venipuncture, Maggie asks Ken to hold pressure on the draw site. She puts the computer-generated labels on the three tubes she drew and writes her initials and time of collection on the labels. Then Maggie checks Ken's arm and wraps a gauze around the site.

Why is it important to label the tubes immediately after finishing the venipuncture? List two reasons this is a good practice for a phlebotomist.

Procedures 32.1 and 32.2 on pp. 822–825 outline the proper procedures for venipuncture using the evacuated tube method and the syringe method. Some patients may have small veins, and using a syringe or butterfly for venipuncture may work better than the standard evacuated assembly. Young children, chemotherapy patients, older adult patients, and people with veins that are difficult to draw may require syringe or butterfly equipment. Alternative equipment is always used to draw blood from hand veins (see Procedure 32.3, p. 828).

PROBLEMS ASSOCIATED WITH VENIPUNCTURE

Failure to obtain blood can occur because of several factors. Determining the cause of the problem may help you decide whether a second attempt would be successful. The first rule is to remain calm and professional. Remaining calm helps you think clearly about the situation and about the potential causes for not getting blood.

Hematoma

A **hematoma** is a large, painful, bruised area at the puncture site caused by blood leaking into the tissue, which causes the tissue around the puncture site to swell. The most common causes of hematoma formation during the draw are excessive probing with the needle to locate a vein, failure to insert the needle far enough into the vein, and passing the needle through the vein. A hematoma can also form after a draw if the tourniquet is not removed before removing the needle, if the vacuum tube is not removed from the hub of the needle before the needle is withdrawn, if adequate pressure is not applied at the puncture site, or if the elbow is bent while pressure is applied. If a hematoma forms, discontinue the procedure STAT, apply pressure to the area for a minimum of 3 minutes, and then apply an ice pack to the area. Notify the provider, and observe the site to determine whether the bleeding has stopped. Depending on the facility's policy, an incident report may have to be completed and documented in the patient's record. A hematoma may also occur if the puncture reopens and bleeds into the tissue due to heavy lifting with the venipuncture arm. Instruct the patient to be careful with the arm for several hours after the procedure.

Nerve Damage and Other Complications

Nerve damage can be a consequence of venipuncture, but the risk is very small. Preventive measures include the following:

- Avoiding the basilic vein for phlebotomy
- Refraining from *blind probing* (moving the needle in the arm with the hope of finding a vein) if the vein is missed with the initial draw

Table 32.3 lists some workable solutions to complications. As a rule, it is wise to limit yourself to two venipuncture attempts for a patient. If a second attempt is unsuccessful, ask whether the patient would allow another phlebotomist to look at his or her arms. If another phlebotomist feels confident to attempt a venipuncture, that person will need to get permission from the patient first. If the patient does not give permission, it may be better to reschedule the venipuncture for another time. This strategy lets patients know that they have input into their care and some measure of control of the situation. At one time or another, everyone is unsuccessful in obtaining a blood sample, so do not have bad feelings about it. Make the best of the situation, learn from the experience, and treat the patient with kindness. We are all human, and our patients are usually quite understanding.

Fainting

Fainting, or syncope, can have serious consequences, so the phlebotomist must always be prepared to take action quickly. Positioning the patient in a blood collection chair (by turning the armrest pad in front of the patient) prevents bodily injury if the person faints. Making eye contact and observing the patient before phlebotomy can help you estimate his or her level of comfort with the procedure. Constant light conversation with the patient during the venipuncture can help identify if the patient is distressed or anxious. As you finish the venipuncture, observe the patient's face, and assess the breathing

TABLE 32.3	Managing Possible Blood Draw Complications
COMPLICATION	**MANAGEMENT STRATEGIES**
Burned area	Choose another site because these areas are prone to infection.
Convulsions	Stay calm. Remove the needle and quickly dispose of it in a sharps container. Then help guide the patient to the floor, protecting him or her from injury. Call for help.
Damaged or scarred veins or infected areas	Look for an alternative site; do not draw blood from scarred or infected areas.
Edema	Avoid the area; look for an alternative site.
Hematoma	Adjust the depth of the needle, or remove the needle and apply pressure.
Intravenous (IV) therapy or blood transfusion sites	Blood samples should not be drawn from an arm that is also the site for IV infusion or blood transfusion because of the dilution factor.
Mastectomy	Do not draw blood from the side of the mastectomy, because mastectomy surgery causes **lymphostasis**, which may produce false results.
Nausea	Place a cold cloth on the patient's forehead, give the patient a basin in case of vomiting, and instruct him or her to take deep breaths. Alert the provider.
No blood	Manipulate the needle slightly or remove the vacuum tube, and perform the blood draw again using a syringe or butterfly setup.
Petechiae	Loosen the tourniquet because this complication usually results from the tourniquet being in place longer than 2 minutes.
Syncope	Position the patient's head between the knees (if in a sitting position). Check and record the patient's pulse, blood pressure, and respiration rate, and continue to observe the patient. Never leave the patient unattended.

rate if he or she seems anxious. Safety comes first. Make sure the patient is not in a position in which he or she can be hurt.

According to CLSI, the procedure for a fainting patient or one who is nonresponsive is as follows:

- If the patient begins to faint, quickly remove the tourniquet and needle from the arm, immediately activate the needle safety device, apply pressure to the site, and dispose of the unit in a sharps container to prevent an accidental exposure.
- Notify staff members for assistance.
- Lay the patient flat or lower the head if the patient is sitting.
- Loosen tight clothing.
- Do not use ammonia inhalants/capsules because these are associated with adverse effects and are no longer recommended.
- Apply a cold compress or washcloth to the patient's forehead and back of the neck.
- Stay with the patient until recovery is complete.
- Document the incident according to facility policies.

- When the patient regains consciousness, he or she must remain in the facility for at least 15 minutes and should not operate a vehicle for at least 30 minutes.

See Chapter 12 for information on what to do if a patient faints.

Specimen Re-collection

Sometimes problems with a sample cannot be determined until the specimen is analyzed in the laboratory. Rejected specimens must be re-collected. The laboratory may reject a specimen for reasons that include the following:

- Unlabeled or mislabeled specimen
- Insufficient specimen quantity
- Defective tube
- Incorrect tube used for the test ordered (incorrect stopper color)
- Hemolysis (Table 32.4)
- Clotted blood in an anticoagulated specimen
- Improper handling

TABLE 32.4 Major Causes of Hemolysis During Collection

CAUSE	EXPLANATION	PREVENTION
Alcohol preparation	Transfer of alcohol into the specimen causes hemolysis.	Allow the venipuncture site to dry completely.
Incorrect needle size	A high-gauge needle causes the blood to go through a small lumen with great force, causing hemolysis. A very-low-gauge needle causes a large amount of blood to suddenly enter the tube with great force, causing frothing.	Choose the correct needle for the job, aiming for a 19- to 23-gauge needle.
Loose connections on the vacuum tube assembly	If the connection between the needle holder and the double-pointed needle or the syringe and the needle is loose, air can enter the sample and cause frothing.	Make sure all connections are tight before beginning the venipuncture.
Removing the needle from the vein with the tube intact	The remaining vacuum in the tube can cause air to be drawn forcefully into the tube, causing frothing.	Remove the final tube from the needle holder before withdrawing the needle from the patient's vein.
Underfilled tubes	Underfilling tubes leads to an improper blood/additive ratio.	Permit blood to flow into the tubes until no more movement can be seen.
Syringe collections	Pulling back too rapidly on the plunger draws blood too quickly through the needle. This causes hemolysis.	Loosen the plunger before use. Use the smallest syringe possible. Gently draw the plunger so no more than 1 mL of air space is present. When transferring blood into the vacuum tube, use a transfer device. *Never* push on the plunger when transferring blood.
Mixing tubes too vigorously	All tubes should be gently inverted. (See Table 32.3.)	Gently invert tubes immediately after the draw. Vigorous mixing can hemolyze cells.
Temperature and transport problems	Trauma and temperature extremes can damage cells. Freezing will cause hemolysis.	Tubes should be transported in the upright position with as little trauma as possible. Control the temperature.
Separation of plasma or serum from red blood cells	Removing the serum/plasma from cells lowers the risk of contaminating the specimen with red blood cells (RBCs).	Blood samples that are centrifuged should have cells and plasma/serum separated as soon as possible.
Prolonged tourniquet time	**Interstitial** fluid can leak into the veins and hemolyze RBCs.	Only leave the tourniquet on for no longer than 1 minute.
Poor collection; blood flowing too slowly into the tube	The needle lumen may be blocked because it is too close to the inner wall of the vein.	Withdraw the needle slightly to center it within the vein.

Hemolysis is the major cause of specimen rejection. It cannot be detected until the blood cells are separated from the plasma or serum. It is crucial to take steps to prevent red blood cell damage during collection. Hemolyzed serum or plasma appears rosy to bright red because of the release of hemoglobin from the cells. Some routine tests that are adversely affected by hemolysis are chemistry tests for electrolytes (e.g., potassium, sodium), bilirubin, total protein, and liver enzymes.

CAPILLARY PUNCTURE

Capillaries are small blood vessels that connect small arterioles to small venules. A capillary puncture is an efficient means of collecting a blood specimen when only a small amount of blood is needed. Capillary punctures are also used when a patient's condition makes venipuncture difficult, such as in a patient undergoing chemotherapy. Also, capillary punctures are performed on infants (as a heelstick) and some young children. The test requisition may not specify a capillary collection, so be familiar with the advantages, limitations, and appropriate uses of this technique. Capillary puncture is warranted for the following patients:

- Older adult patients
- Pediatric patients (especially younger than age 2)
- Patients who require frequent glucose monitoring
- Patients with burns or scars in venipuncture sites
- Obese patients
- Patients receiving intravenous (IV) therapy or chemotherapy
- Patients who have had a mastectomy
- Patients at risk for venous thrombosis
- Patients who are severely dehydrated
- Patients who are undergoing tests that require a small volume of blood (i.e., some CLIA-wiaved tests)

Capillaries are connections between arteries and veins, so capillary blood is a mixture of the two. Small volumes of tissue fluid also are present in capillary blood, especially in the first drop. Analyte levels are usually the same in capillary and venous blood, with a few exceptions. Hemoglobin and glucose values are higher in capillary blood; potassium, calcium, and total protein are higher in venous blood.

Equipment

Capillary punctures are performed with specialized equipment. A look at the equipment is useful and can help you decide when a capillary puncture should be performed instead of a venipuncture.

Skin Puncture Devices

The device used to perform a dermal puncture is the *lancet*, which delivers a quick puncture to a preset depth (Fig. 32.17). OSHA has directed that lancets must have retractable blades. Safety lancets only puncture once and cannot be reused. Lancets are available as needle lancets and blade lancets. The choice of lancet should follow CLSI standards for puncture depth. Lancets should always be discarded in a sharps container immediately after use.

CRITICAL THINKING APPLICATION   **32.10**

A capillary puncture is also called a fingerstick. What other term is used for this procedure?

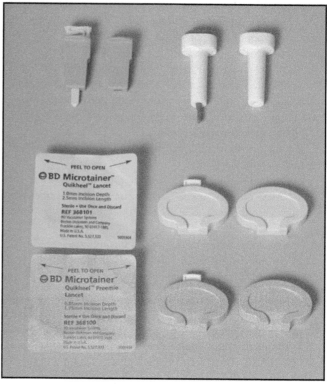

FIGURE 32.17 Dermal puncture devices. (Courtesy Becton, Dickinson, Franklin Lakes, New Jersey.)

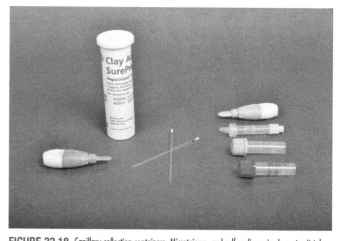

FIGURE 32.18 Capillary collection containers, Microtainers, and self-sealing microhematocrit tubes.

Collection Containers

Different types of containers and collection devices are available, and the ones used depend on the test to be performed. Microcollection tubes and Microtainers (Fig. 32.18) are available with a variety of anticoagulants and additives. Their color-coded tops indicate the same additives as evacuated tubes. Blood drops are collected into the Microtainers through a funnel-like device.

Capillary tubes are another type of blood collection tube used to get a capillary sample. A capillary tube is a glass tube surrounded by a protective plastic coating for safety. The blood is pulled into the tube by *capillary action*; this means that the blood fills these

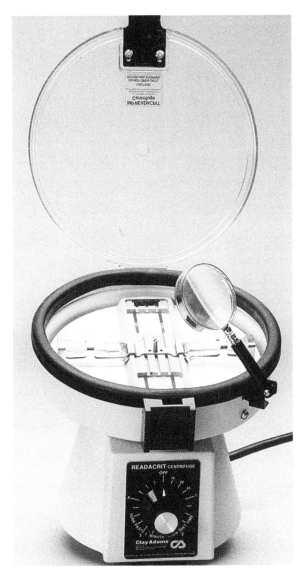

FIGURE 32.19 Microhematocrit centrifuge with indicators for capillary tube placement.

small, narrow tubes without the help of **suction**. If the capillary tube is coated with the anticoagulant heparin, a red band will be seen at the top of the tube. A common, heparin-coated capillary tube is the microhematocrit tube. Microhematocrit tubes are used to determine the percentage of packed red blood cells in the blood (discussed in Chapter 33). Fig. 32.19 shows a microhematocrit tube and centrifuge. Self-sealing capillary tubes are used in the microhematocrit test.

Manufacturers often provide collection devices for obtaining small amounts of blood for point-of-care testing (POCT), such as glucose, hemoglobin A1c, and cholesterol (see Chapter 33). Blood is pulled into the collecting device by capillary action after the puncture, or it is applied to a reagent strip that has been inserted into the instrument to be analyzed.

Blood from a capillary puncture may also be deposited on paper cards. The Guthrie card (Fig. 32.20) is used to test babies for certain metabolic disorders, such as phenylketonuria (PKU). Blood is deposited into circles on biologically inactive filter paper and is

sent to a referral laboratory for analysis within 24 hours of sampling. Federal postal regulations for mailing biohazard material must be followed.

ROUTINE CAPILLARY PUNCTURE

Site Selection

In adults and children (older than 1 year), capillary puncture sites include the ring or middle finger. Why do we collect capillary samples only from the middle and ring fingers? The thumb usually is too callused or thick-skinned, and the index finger has nerve endings that make the puncture more painful. The fifth finger (pinky finger) has too little tissue for a successful puncture.

Dermal puncture of an infant should be done on the heel of the foot (see Fig. 32.21). A capillary puncture is made on the palmar surface of the finger, near the tip and slightly to the side of the finger. Punctures should be made across to the whorls of the finger. This helps to create a nice drop of blood to collect. Avoid areas that are callused, scarred, burned, infected, cyanotic, or edematous.

For children younger than 2 years of age, dermal puncture is performed on the medial or lateral areas of the *plantar surface* (bottom) of the heel or on the *palmar surface* of the ring or middle finger. Areas other than these are unsafe, and bone or nerve damage to an infant may occur. Blood flow from an infant's heel can be increased by applying a warm, moist towel (or other warming device) at a temperature no higher than 108°F (42°C) for 3 to 5 minutes. Never place bandages on the heel or anywhere on infants younger than age 2, because they may peel off and become a choking hazard.

Patient Preparation

Preparation for a capillary puncture is similar to that for a venipuncture. Put on a fluid-impermeable lab coat, wash your hands or use hand sanitizer, and put on gloves and protective eyewear. If the patient's hands are excessively soiled, ask the person to wash them before the procedure. If the patient's hands are cold, warm them in warm water and dry them thoroughly, or ask the person to rub or shake them vigorously. Cleanse the finger well with a 70% alcohol wipe.

You must work efficiently when performing a capillary puncture because blood flow stops quickly. Be sure to have the supplies organized and within easy reach. Press the lancet firmly against the skin and quickly depress the plunger.

Collecting the Specimen

After the skin has been punctured, it is important to wipe away the first drop of blood with gauze. This drop contains tissue fluid that could interfere with test results. Fill the sampling containers according to the manufacturer's directions. Touch the container to the drop of blood as it is released from the puncture site, but do not touch the skin. If blood flow stops, wiping the site with gauze may restart the flow. Because you are working with blood that is free-flowing, make sure there are spare gloves, extra gauze, and disinfectant nearby. Be prepared if your gloves become contaminated with blood. After the containers have been filled, ask the patient to apply pressure to the gauze placed over the puncture site. Seal and mix the containers by gently inverting the tubes as recommended by the manufacturer.

FIGURE 32.20 (A) Guthrie card used in neonatal screening. **(B)** Correctly and incorrectly filled cards. (From Warekois RS, Robinson R: *Phlebotomy: work text and procedures manual*, ed 4, St Louis, 2016, Saunders.)

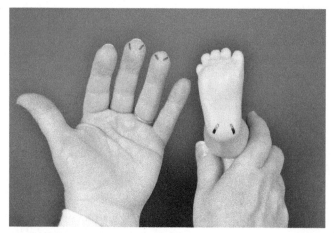

FIGURE 32.21 Dermal puncture site selection and lancet placement.

CRITICAL THINKING APPLICATION   32.11

Maggie is performing a capillary puncture on Johnny Parker, who is 7 years old. She is looking at his fingers to choose a site, and his hands are chilly. Which fingers would be the best choice for a child? If Johnny's hands are chilly, what can Maggie do to make sure they warm up?

Specimen Handling

Capillary collection containers are often too small for a label to be applied to the tube. The most efficient way to transport capillary tubes is to remove the stopper from a red-topped venipuncture tube, insert the capillary tubes, sealed-end down, replace the stopper, and label the red-topped tube. Microtainer tubes have plastic plugs that fit over the top. They may be placed in a labeled tube or in a labeled

TABLE 32.5 Childhood Behavior and Parental Involvement During Phlebotomy

AGE	TYPICAL MENTAL STATE	SUGGESTED PARENTAL INVOLVEMENT
Newborns (0–12 months)	Trust that adults will respond to their needs	Parent should assist by cradling and comforting child.
Infants and toddlers (1–3 years)	Minimal fear of danger but fear of separation; limited language and understanding of procedure	Parent should assist by holding the child and providing emotional support.
Preschoolers (3–6 years)	Fearful of injury to body; still dependent on parent	Parent may be present to provide emotional support and to assist in obtaining child's cooperation.
School-aged children (7–12 years)	Less dependent on parent and more willing to cooperate; fear of loss of self-control (crying)	Child may not want parent present.
Teenagers (13–18 years)	Fully engaged in the process; embarrassed to show fear and may show hostility to cover emotions	Teen may not want parent present.

zipper-lock bag for transport. Always decontaminate collection containers before delivering them to the laboratory if blood was deposited on the surface during collection. The procedure for routine capillary collection is outlined in Procedure 32.4 on p. 830.

PEDIATRIC PHLEBOTOMY

Obtaining blood from children and infants may be difficult and potentially hazardous. The procedure should be performed by personnel trained in pediatric phlebotomy. Successfully obtaining blood from children requires skill and an understanding of children and their development. Good communication skills are essential when dealing with children. The phlebotomist must gain the child's trust and often that of the parent or guardian. Parents frequently ask the phlebotomist to explain the tests being done and the reasons for testing. Be respectful when talking to parents. Defer to the provider if questions come up about specific information regarding possible diseases or conditions the child may have.

A parent or guardian may be helpful during phlebotomy. Ask the parent or guardian about the child's previous phlebotomy experiences and how cooperative the child has been in the past. Respectfully determine whether the parent or guardian seems comfortable assisting in restraint of an uncooperative child. Parental behavior greatly influences the child's behavior during the procedure. Children should never be restrained in a way that might cause physical injury or pain. If the parent or guardian is unable or unwilling to assist with the procedure, always refer to the office or laboratory policy on procedural holds for phlebotomy. Table 32.5 provides information on the typical fears and concerns of children during the procedure and suggested parental involvement.

Removing large amounts of blood, especially from premature infants, may result in anemia (Table 32.6). The amount of blood withdrawn must be recorded in the child's chart. Puncturing deep veins in children may result in serious complications, such as cardiac arrest, hemorrhage, venous thrombosis, damage to surrounding tissues, and infection.

In addition, the child could be harmed during restraint. To prevent these problems, blood should be collected only by dermal puncture from children younger than age 2 unless the procedure warrants

TABLE 32.6 General Guidelines for Pediatric Venipuncture

WEIGHT (LB)	SINGLE DRAW LIMIT
8–10	3.5 mL
11–15	5 mL
16–40	10 mL
41–60	20 mL
61–65	25 mL
66–80	30 mL

venous collection (lead levels or blood culture). Venipuncture on children younger than age 2 should be performed only on surface veins, including the dorsal hand vein, using a 23-gauge winged infusion set coupled to a syringe or a pediatric vacuum tube collection set.

When required to perform pediatric phlebotomy, the medical assistant should remember to do the following:

- Wear a colorful, fluid-impermeable jacket lab coat, if possible.
- Be truthful about the discomfort the child will feel.
- Provide tokens and praise for bravery.
- Try to lessen the child's fears.

Topical anesthetics (e.g., ethyl chloride [EC] spray or EMLA cream) may be used to reduce pain at the puncture site. In most cases a calm, professional phlebotomist who understands children and relates to them on their level can gain the trust needed. Work to perform a successful venipuncture or capillary puncture with a minimum of restraint and frustration.

HANDLING THE SPECIMEN AFTER COLLECTION

The results of laboratory testing are only as good as the specimen sent for testing. Specimens handled improperly after collection may provide incorrect results. They may even compromise the patient's health. From the moment a specimen is collected, analytes in the blood begin to break down. By testing specimens as soon as possible, the laboratory tries to provide results that accurately represent the patient's condition at the time of blood collection. After collection, blood may need to be processed before the sample is tested. This may include separation of plasma or serum from the red blood cells. If the venipuncture tube contains no anticoagulant (i.e., tubes with a red, a marbled red-gray, or a gold stopper), blood starts the clotting process when it touches the tube. The "clot" tubes should sit upright in a rack for 30 to 60 minutes at room temperature while a solid clot forms. Tubes with clot accelerator should form a dense clot within 30 minutes. The presence of anticoagulants in the patient's blood, such as warfarin (Coumadin) or heparin, may delay clotting. Once the clot has formed, every effort should be made to remove the clot from the serum within 2 hours.

Removing the serum from a clot tube requires centrifugation. For thixotropic gel to form a barrier between the clot and the serum, certain requirements must be met. The tube must be centrifuged at a specified **g-force**, time, and temperature. A clinical centrifuge instruction manual should provide the appropriate settings for spinning blood specimens. The serum does not have to be removed from the tube after centrifugation because the gel has formed a barrier over the red blood cells. Once a tube with thixotropic gel has been centrifuged, it cannot be centrifuged again. The serum, however, can be decanted and centrifuged in another tube.

For tests that require plasma, the plasma should be removed from the cells as soon as possible. This can be done by centrifuging the tube and then **aspirating** the plasma off the cells. The plasma is then transferred to another tube using a disposable transfer pipet. You can also use a PST tube with a marbled green-gray top or a PST tube with a light green top. Both contain lithium heparin anticoagulant and a thixotropic gel, which form the necessary barrier when centrifuged.

Certain blood tests, such as a CBC, require whole blood. It is wise to check the specimen requirements of the laboratory that will perform the test and follow the lab's instructions for transport and storage. The College of American Pathologists (CAP) recommends that whole blood for automated blood counts be refrigerated and tested within 72 hours.

Often specimens must be transported by courier to other facilities. The Hazardous Materials Shipping Regulations, established by the Department of Transportation, apply to the packaging and shipping of hazardous materials by ground transportation. POLs that ship human specimens must be trained to properly handle, pack, and ship biohazard materials. Reference labs will frequently have couriers who pick up specimens. The specimens and their requisitions are typically placed in individual biohazard bags and sorted according to which reference lab is affiliated with the patient's insurance.

Chain of Custody

Blood samples may be collected as evidence in legal proceedings. Blood may be drawn for drug and alcohol testing, DNA analysis, or paternity testing. These samples must be handled according to special procedures to prevent tampering, misidentification, or interference with the test results.

Chain of custody is a legal term that refers to the ability to guarantee the identity and integrity of the specimen from collection to reporting of test results. It is a process used to maintain and document the history of a specimen. Documents should include the name or initials of the individual collecting the specimen, each person who tests or transports the specimen, the date the specimen was collected or transferred, the employer or agency, the specimen number, the patient's or employee's name, and a brief description of the specimen.

Collection kits are available that contain everything needed for the venipuncture, including the tube, the needle, the chain of custody forms and seals, the antiseptic, and even the tourniquet. Familiarize yourself with these kits before using them. Phlebotomists may be required to testify at legal proceedings if they are involved in the collection or testing of a legal sample.

CLOSING COMMENTS

Patient Coaching

Phlebotomy can be a stressful event for some patients. Helping patients to remain calm and at ease is a high priority for the phlebotomist. Patients often express great concern when several tubes of blood must be drawn. It seems like they are losing a lot of blood. You can put their fears to rest by explaining that the average adult has a little less than 5 L of blood (10 pints). Most adults can relate to donating a unit of blood, which is about 500 mL (1 pint). Because a large red-topped tube contains 10 mL of blood, you would have to draw about 50 tubes to remove 500 mL of blood.

Provide as much explanation as needed to ease the patient's anxiety. Often the patient can help by identifying the site of the last successful blood venipuncture. When it is appropriate, follow the patient's suggestion in choosing the site for a venipuncture. When patients become active participants in the procedure, they remain more relaxed, talkative, and confident in your expertise as a phlebotomist.

Legal and Ethical Issues

Phlebotomy is an invasive procedure in which a sterile needle or lancet is inserted through the skin. Because the skin is penetrated, drawing blood becomes a surgical procedure and is subject to the laws and regulations of surgery. When a venipuncture is performed, the rules and regulations must be obeyed with no exceptions. Be sure to follow the written procedures in the laboratory. Become familiar with the regulations and standards established by CLSI and OSHA, and by state and local agencies. Deviations from the standards leave the medical assistant open to malpractice. Document any situations in which the standard of care comes into question.

Patient-Centered Care

You may want to ask your patients how they would prefer to be addressed: By their first name? A nickname? Dr. Smith, Mr. Jones, Mrs. Blake, or Ms. Washington? Don't assume that patients want to be called by their first name. Also, do not call patients "sweetie," "honey," or "dear." Be respectful, professional, and patient-focused.

Professional Behaviors

Your appearance and actions reflect your laboratory or facility. A patient's first impression of the facility often comes from the medical assistant. Clean fluid-impermeable laboratory coats and scrubs tell the patient the facility is clean; sanitizing your hands in front of the patient and wearing gloves tells the patient you will treat him or her with care; and speaking knowledgeably provides the impression that the facility is staffed with professionals.

Medical assistants who perform venous and capillary blood collection must maintain a professional attitude yet remain sympathetic to the patient's fears and anxiety about the procedure. Establishing an environment that encourages

the person to relax can minimize the patient's pain and discomfort during the procedure. Always remember to verify your patient's identity and explain what you are going to do. Answer any questions the patient may have, and then make every effort to perform the procedure skillfully, quickly, and efficiently.

If your patient has a history of syncope when blood is drawn or if you suspect the patient may be very anxious during the procedure, have the person lie down. Assemble your equipment, and alert the provider before beginning the procedure. This type of professional care may help the patient get through the procedure without feeling anxious.

SUMMARY OF SCENARIO

Maggie has had a busy morning in the phlebotomy area. She likes it when it is busy. The morning seems to fly by. After the morning rush, Maggie restocks a few supplies and then is ready to sit down and take her lunch break. As she relaxes in the lunchroom for a few minutes, she thinks back on the morning with satisfaction. She helped a number of patients today. Norma Washington was in, she is in her fourth week of chemotherapy. She was nervous about

today's venipuncture. Maggie calmed her fears and was able to do a capillary puncture instead of a venipuncture. That made Norma's day!

Every patient who came into the phlebotomy area this morning left with a smile. That does not happen every day, but Maggie was so happy that this Monday morning went well.

SUMMARY OF LEARNING OBJECTIVES

1. **Discuss venipuncture equipment and personal protective equipment. Also, explain the purpose of a tourniquet, how to apply it, and the consequences of improper tourniquet application.**

   Venipuncture requires a double-pointed safety needle, evacuated collection tubes, a needle holder or a syringe fitted with a safety needle, a tourniquet, an alcohol prep pad, gauze or cotton, a sterile bandage, nonlatex gloves, a fluid-impermeable lab coat, protective eyewear, and a biohazard sharps container.

   A tourniquet is used to hold back venous flow out of the site, which causes the veins to bulge. The tourniquet makes veins easier to locate and puncture. Tourniquets are applied snugly around the upper arm (or wrist for a hand draw) in a fashion that permits easy release. Leaving the tourniquet on a prolonged time results in hemoconcentration; applying the tourniquet too tightly results in unnecessary discomfort to the patient and the release of tissue fluid into the blood.

2. **Discuss antiseptics, explain why the stopper colors on vacuum tubes differ, and state the correct order of the draw.**

   To prevent infection, a venipuncture site must be cleansed with an antiseptic. The most commonly used antiseptic is 70% isopropyl alcohol or *rubbing alcohol*. Alcohol kills many of the existing bacteria that might contaminate the sample. To be most effective, the alcohol should remain on the skin for 30 to 60 seconds and allowed to air dry.

   The various colors of vacuum tube stoppers indicate the contents of the tube. Certain additives are compatible with certain laboratory tests. The phlebotomist must be knowledgeable about blood tests and

   the types of tubes needed. Consulting literature provided by the manufacturer ensures the proper choice of a collection tube. The correct order of draw is (1) pale yellow (sterile or sodium polyanethole sulfonate [SPS]), (2) light blue, (3) red, red-gray marbled, or gold plastic top, (4) green, (5) lavender, and (6) gray. Vacuum tubes are collected in a specific order to prevent carryover of tube additives.

3. **Discuss the needles and supplies used in phlebotomy.**

   The venipuncture needle has a shaft with one end cut at an angle (bevel). The other end (the hub) attaches to the syringe or to a needle holder. The inner bore or space in the needle is called the *lumen*. It is measured in gauge numbers (the higher the gauge number, the smaller the lumen). Double-pointed needles are used for the evacuated tube method in which the blood flows directly from the vein into the evacuated tube. Removable safety needles are used with disposable syringes. The collected blood in the syringe is then transferred to the appropriate evacuated tubes using a safety transfer device. Safety lancets are used for dermal puncture.

4. **Discuss needle safety and postexposure needlestick follow-up.**

   OSHA requires employers to have a postexposure plan in place for accidental sharps exposures. These plans generally include a means to cleanse the wound with an appropriate antiseptic cleanser; evaluation of the exposure to determine whether the employee is at risk for contracting HBV, HCV, or HIV, depending on the circumstance of the injury; gathering of information about the source of the blood involved;

Continued

prophylactic care if necessary; confidential counseling for the injured; and follow-up on the exposure.

5. **Complete the following related to routine venipuncture:**
   - **Discuss patient preparation for routine venipuncture.**
     Start the venipuncture by greeting the patient and verifying his or her identity. According to CLSI, proper identification includes asking outpatients to (1) state and spell their first and last name, and (2) state their birth date. All the information must be compared and verified with the patient requisition. Briefly explain the venipuncture procedure to your patient, and make sure to ask him or her the necessary questions. Answer questions and concerns and take steps to prevent any past problems from recurring. If you cannot answer all the patient's questions, ask if he or she would like to talk to the provider for clarification. Obtain verbal consent to perform the venipuncture simply by asking whether you have permission to draw blood from the patient.

   - **List in order the steps of a routine venipuncture.**
     A routine venipuncture begins with greeting the patient and verifying his or her identity. The medical assistant then sanitizes his or her hands, assembles the equipment and PPE, locates the vein, disinfects the area over the vein, allows the alcohol to dry, draws the blood into the correct vacuum tubes in the proper order of draw, removes and properly disposes of the needle, tends to the puncture site, labels the tubes, and delivers them to the laboratory. Standard Precautions are followed during the procedure.

   - **Detail patient preparation for venipuncture that shows sensitivity to the patient's rights and feelings.**
     The medical assistant must be sensitive to the needs and concerns of patients both before and during the phlebotomy procedure. The procedure should be explained to the patient, and all questions

should be answered. The patient should be observed for any problems during the procedure, and the medical assistant should use therapeutic communication techniques throughout the intervention.
   - Perform a venipuncture using the vacuum tube method, syringe, and winged-infusion (butterfly) assembly.
     Refer to Procedures 32.1, 32.2, and 32.3 on pp. 822–828

6. **Discuss possible solutions to venipuncture complications.**
   Refer to Table 32.3 for a list of solutions to possible complications.

7. **List situations in which capillary puncture would be preferred over venipuncture, and discuss the equipment used.**
   Capillary puncture is preferred over venipuncture for certain point-of-care tests, such as hematocrit or hemoglobin analysis. It is performed routinely on children younger than age 2.

8. **Perform a capillary puncture.**
   Refer to Procedure 32.4 on p. 830.

9. **Discuss pediatric phlebotomy, including typical childhood behavior and parental involvement during phlebotomy and general guidelines for pediatric venipuncture.**
   Obtaining blood from children and infants may be difficult and potentially hazardous. Refer to Table 32.5 for information on typical fears and concerns of children during the procedure and suggested parental involvement. Refer to Table 32.6 for general guidelines for pediatric venipuncture.

10. **Describe handling and transport methods for blood after collection.**
    From the moment the specimen is collected, analytes in the blood begin to decay, and it is a race against time to provide results that accurately represent a patient's condition at the time of the blood collection. There are various procedures based on the type of test performed.

PROCEDURE 32.1   Perform a Venipuncture: Collect a Venous Blood Sample Using the Vacuum Tube Method

Task: Collect a venous blood specimen by the vacuum tube technique.

EQUIPMENT and SUPPLIES

- Patient's health record
- Provider's order or lab requisition
- Vacuum tube needle, needle holder, and proper tubes for requested tests
- 70% isopropyl alcohol wipes
- Gauze
- Tourniquet
- Hypoallergenic self-stick wrap, tape, or bandage

- Permanent marking pen or printed labels
- Fluid-impermeable lab coat, protective eyewear, and gloves
- Biohazard sharps container
- Biohazard waste container

PROCEDURAL STEPS

1. Check the provider's order or requisition form to determine the tests ordered. Gather the appropriate tubes and supplies. Put on a fluid-impermeable lab coat.

PROCEDURE 32.1 | **Perform a Venipuncture: Collect a Venous Blood Sample Using the Vacuum Tube Method**—*continued*

PURPOSE: Each test requires a specific tube color that is indicated on the requisition. Donning a lab coat is part of ongoing infection control.

2. Greet the patient. Identify yourself. Verify the patient's identity with full name; ask the patient to spell the first and last names and to give his or her date of birth. Explain the procedure to be performed in a manner that the patient understands. Answer any questions the patient may have. Obtain permission for the venipuncture.
   PURPOSE: Verifying the patient's identity ensures that you have the right patient. Explanations help gain the patient's cooperation and show awareness of a patient's concerns related to the procedure being performed.

3. Wash hands or use hand sanitizer, then put on gloves and protective eyewear.
   PURPOSE: It is important to ensure infection control.

4. Have the patient sit with the arm well supported in a slightly downward position. Ask if he or she has a preference regarding which arm is used for the venipuncture.
   PURPOSE: The veins of the antecubital area are more easily located when the elbow is straight. Asking about a patient preference gives the patient a chance to participate in the procedure.

5. Apply the tourniquet 3 to 4 inches above the elbow on the patient's preferred arm. The tourniquet should never be tied so tightly that it restricts blood flow in the artery (Fig. 1). Tourniquets should remain in place no longer than 60 seconds.
   PURPOSE: The tourniquet is used to make the veins more prominent.

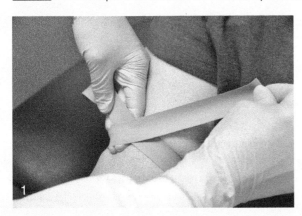

6. Select the venipuncture site by palpating the antecubital space. Use your index finger to trace the path of the vein and to judge its depth. The veins most often used are the medial or cephalic veins, which lie in the middle of the elbow (Fig. 2). Look at both arms, and use your critical thinking skills to find the vein that will give you the greatest chance of success for the venipuncture.
   PURPOSE: The index finger is most sensitive for palpating the vein. Do not use the thumb because it has a pulse of its own. Spend time to properly locate the best vein available; your patient will thank you.

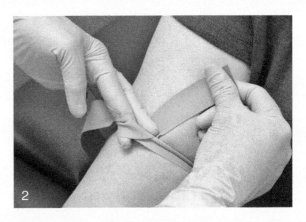

7. Remove the tourniquet, and cleanse the site with a 70% alcohol wipe (Fig. 3).
   PURPOSE: The tourniquet should only be tied for 60 seconds.

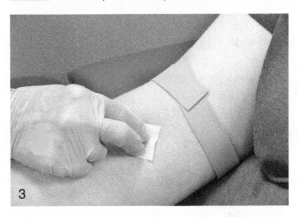

8. Assemble your equipment and supplies on the side of the patient's non-dominant arm. The choice of needle size depends on your inspection of the patient's veins. Attach the needle firmly to the vacuum tube holder. Keep the cover on the needle.
   PURPOSE: If the needle is loose, it may turn during the procedure, causing the bevel of the needle to turn away from its upward position.

9. Reapply the tourniquet when the alcohol is dry.
   PURPOSE: Puncturing an area that is still wet with alcohol stings and can cause hemolysis of the sample.

10. Hold the vacuum tube assembly in your dominant hand. Your thumb should be on top and your fingers underneath (Fig. 4). You may want to lay the first tube to be drawn in the needle holder, but do not push it onto the double-pointed needle. Remove the needle sheath.
    PURPOSE: Positioning the hand in this manner provides the best visibility of the needle entering the vein and accessibility to insert and withdraw tubes with the nondominant hand. Pushing the tube into the double-pointed needle before it is in the arm causes air to rush into the tube, destroying the vacuum.

Continued

PROCEDURE 32.1	**Perform a Venipuncture: Collect a Venous Blood Sample Using the Vacuum Tube Method**—*continued*

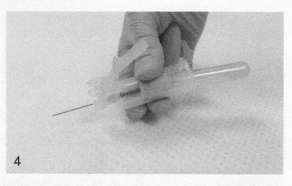

4

11. Grasp the patient's arm with the nondominant hand, and anchor the vein by gently stretching the skin downward below the collection site with the thumb of the nondominant hand.
    PURPOSE: Failure to anchor the vein may cause the vein to move away from the needle as it enters the arm.

12. With the bevel up and the needle aligned parallel to the vein, insert the needle at a 15- to 20-degree angle through the skin and into the vein with a quick but smooth motion (Fig. 5).
    PURPOSE: The sharpest point of the needle is inserted first. Inserting the needle quickly minimizes pain.

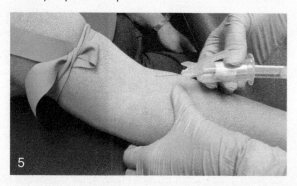

5

13. The dominant hand never lets go of the needle assembly once it is in the vein. Hold the assembly in place and steady through the venipuncture.
    PURPOSE: Holding the needle assembly steady will keep the needle from moving in the vein.

14. Place two fingers on the flanges of the needle holder, and use the thumb to push the tube onto the double-pointed needle (Fig. 6). Make sure you do not change the needle's position in the vein.
    PURPOSE: The thumb has the strength to push the needle swiftly through the stopper. Be careful and keep the position of the needle steady so it is not pushed farther into the site when the tube is pushed.

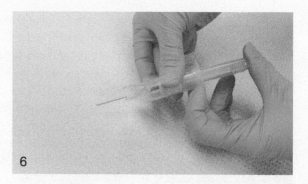

6

15. Allow the tube to fill to its maximum capacity. Remove the tube by placing the fingers at the end of the tube and pushing on the needle holder with the index finger (Fig. 7). Take care not to move the needle when removing the tube. Immediately after removing the tube from the needle holder, gently invert the tube to mix the additives and the blood.
    PURPOSE: Tubes must be full to ensure the proper anticoagulant-to-blood ratio. Moving the needle may result in the needle advancing farther into the vein or slipping out of the vein. Gentle inversion prevents blood from clotting. Do not vigorously mix or shake the tubes, because this may cause hemolysis.

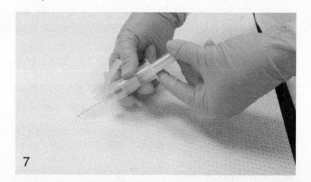

7

16. Insert the second tube into the needle holder, following the instructions in the previous steps. Continue filling tubes until the order on the requisition has been filled. Gently invert each tube after removing it from the needle holder. As the last tube begins filling, release the tourniquet. The tourniquet must be released before the needle is removed from the arm (Fig. 8).
    PURPOSE: The tourniquet should remain in place for no longer than 1 minute to prevent hemoconcentration.

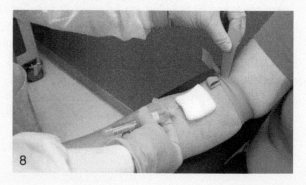

8

PROCEDURE 32.1	Perform a Venipuncture: Collect a Venous Blood Sample Using the Vacuum Tube Method—*continued*

17. Remove the last tube from the holder. Place gauze over the puncture site and quickly remove the needle, engaging the safety device (Fig. 9). Dispose of the entire needle/holder assembly into the sharps container.
PURPOSE: The gauze over the puncture site and activation of the safety needle ensure infection control.

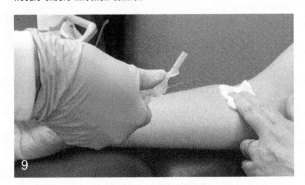

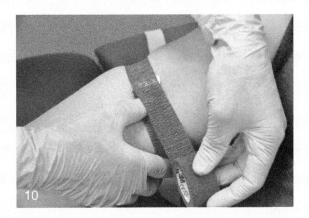

18. Apply pressure to the gauze, or instruct the patient to do so. The patient may elevate the arm but should not bend the elbow.
PURPOSE: Applying direct pressure and elevating the arm above the heart is the best method to stop bleeding.
19. While the patient is applying pressure to the site, label the tubes with the patient's name, the date, the time, and your initials, or affix the preprinted tube labels and print your initials on the label.
PURPOSE: Appropriate labeling will ensure proper specimen identification.
20. Check the venipuncture site. Make sure bleeding has stopped. Apply a hypoallergenic self-stick wrap, gauze and tape, or a bandage (Fig. 10).

21. Disinfect the work area. Dispose of blood-contaminated materials (e.g., gauze and gloves) in the biohazard waste container. Remove your protective eyewear and gloves. Wash hands or use hand sanitizer.
PURPOSE: It is important to ensure infection control.
22. Complete the laboratory requisition form, and route the specimen to the proper place. Record the procedure in the patient's record.
PURPOSE: A procedure is not considered done until it is recorded in the patient record.

Documentation Example
10/05/20XX 1:45 p.m.: Venous blood drawn from antecubital space of right arm. Lavender tube for CBC with differential, and red tube for Chemistry. Placed for pickup by Health Alliance Labs._____Maggie Brandt, CMA (AAMA)

PROCEDURE 32.2	Perform a Venipuncture: Collect a Venous Blood Sample Using the Syringe Method

Task: Collect a venous blood specimen using the syringe technique.

EQUIPMENT and SUPPLIES

- Patient's health record
- Provider's order or lab requisition
- Syringe with 21- or 22-gauge safety needle
- Vacuum tubes appropriate for tests ordered
- 70% isopropyl alcohol wipes
- Gauze
- Tourniquet
- Safety transfer device to transfer blood from syringe to vacuum tubes
- Hypoallergenic self-stick wrap, tape, or bandage
- Permanent marking pen or printed labels
- Fluid-impermeable lab coat, protective eyewear, and gloves
- Biohazard sharps container
- Biohazard waste container

PROCEDURAL STEPS

1. Check the provider's order or requisition form to determine the tests ordered. Gather the appropriate tubes and supplies. Put on a fluid-impermeable lab coat.
PURPOSE: Collect the specimen properly based on the tube requirements on the requisition. Donning a lab coat is part of ongoing infection control.
2. Greet the patient. Identify yourself. Verify the patient's identity with full name; ask the patient to spell the first and last names and to give his or her date of birth. Explain the procedure to be performed in a manner that the patient understands. Answer any questions the patient may have. Obtain permission for the venipuncture.
PURPOSE: It is important to identify the patient in two different ways to ensure that you have the correct patient. Explaining the procedure can make the patient feel more comfortable and reduces anxiety.

Continued

PROCEDURE 32.2	**Perform a Venipuncture: Collect a Venous Blood Sample Using the Syringe Method**—*continued*

3. Wash hands or use hand sanitizer. Put on gloves and protective eyewear.
   <u>PURPOSE</u>: It is important to ensure infection control.
4. Have the patient sit with the arm well supported in a slightly downward position. Ask the patient if he or she has a preference regarding which arm is used for the venipuncture.
   <u>PURPOSE</u>: The veins of the antecubital area are more easily located when the elbow is straight. Asking about a patient preference gives the patient a chance to participate in the procedure.
5. Apply the tourniquet around 3 to 4 inches above the elbow on the patient's preferred arm. The tourniquet should never be tied so tightly that it restricts blood flow in the artery (Fig. 1). Tourniquets should remain in place no longer than 60 seconds.
   <u>PURPOSE</u>: The tourniquet is used to make the veins more prominent.

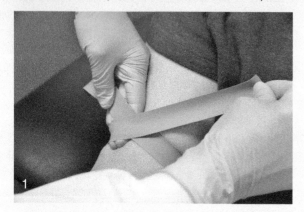

6. Select the venipuncture site by palpating the antecubital space. Use your index finger to trace the path of the vein and to judge its depth. The veins most often used are the medial or cephalic veins, which lie in the middle of the elbow (Fig. 2). Look at both arms, and use your critical thinking skills to find the vein that will give you the greatest chance of success for the venipuncture.
   <u>PURPOSE</u>: The index finger is most sensitive for palpating the vein. Do not use the thumb because it has a pulse of its own. Spend time to properly locate the best vein available; your patient will thank you.

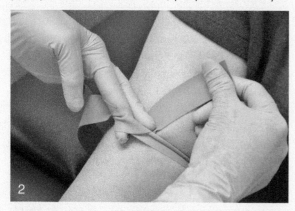

7. Remove the tourniquet, and cleanse the site with a 70% alcohol wipe (Fig. 3).
   <u>PURPOSE</u>: The tourniquet should only be tied for 60 seconds.

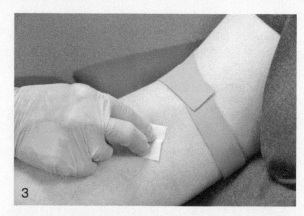

8. Assemble the equipment and supplies on the side of the patient's nondominant arm. Use your critical thinking skills to choose the proper syringe barrel size and needle size. This depends on the amount of blood required for the ordered tests and your inspection of the patient's veins. Attach the needle firmly to the syringe. Pull and depress the plunger several times to loosen it in the barrel while keeping the cover on the needle (Fig. 4). The plunger must be pushed in completely after you have loosened it in the barrel.
   <u>PURPOSE</u>: Using the smallest syringe possible minimizes the chance of hemolysis. Engaging the plunger ensures that you will not have to use as much force to pull the blood into the barrel, thereby minimizing the chance of hemolysis.

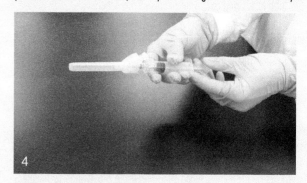

9. Reapply the tourniquet when the alcohol is dry.
   <u>PURPOSE</u>: Puncturing an area that is still wet with alcohol stings and can cause hemolysis of the sample.
10. Hold the syringe in your dominant hand. Your thumb should be on top and your fingers underneath, the same as when using the vacuum tube method. Remove the needle sheath.
    <u>PURPOSE</u>: Positioning the hand in this manner provides the best visibility of the needle entering the vein and accessibility to the syringe plunger.
11. Grasp the patient's arm with the nondominant hand, and anchor the vein by stretching the skin downward below the collection site with the thumb of the nondominant hand.
    <u>PURPOSE</u>: Failure to anchor the vein may cause the vein to move away from the needle when it is inserted, resulting in a missed vein.
12. With the bevel up and the needle aligned parallel to the vein, insert the needle at a 15- to 20-degree angle through the skin and into the vein with a quick but smooth motion (Fig. 5). Observe for a "flash" of blood in the hub of the syringe.

| PROCEDURE 32.2 | **Perform a Venipuncture: Collect a Venous Blood Sample Using the Syringe Method**—*continued* |

PURPOSE: The sharpest point of the needle is inserted first. The angle ensures that the needle does not penetrate through the vein. The appearance (flash) of blood in the hub ensures that the needle is in the vein.

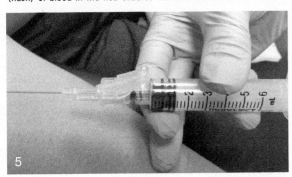

5

13. Slowly pull back the plunger of the syringe with the nondominant hand. Do not allow more than 1 mL of head space between the blood and the top of the plunger. Make sure you do not move the needle after entering the vein. Fill the barrel to the needed volume (Fig. 6).
PURPOSE: Pulling back the plunger slowly allows for a consistent vacuum and less chance of vein collapse.

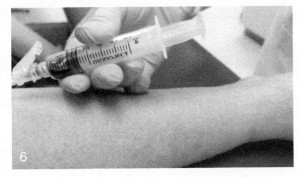

6

14. Release the tourniquet when the proper volume is reached. The tourniquet must be released before the needle is removed from the arm.
PURPOSE: Removal of the tourniquet releases pressure on the vein and helps prevent blood from getting into adjacent tissues, causing a hematoma.
15. Place sterile gauze over the puncture site at the time of needle withdrawal (Fig. 7). Then immediately activate the needle safety device using the syringe hand, and apply pressure to the site with the nondominant hand.
PURPOSE: The gauze over the puncture site and activation of the safety needle ensure infection control.

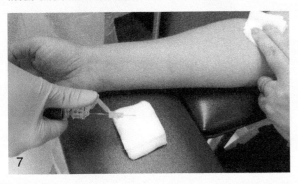

7

16. Instruct the patient to apply direct pressure on the puncture site with gauze. The patient may elevate the arm but should not bend the elbow.
PURPOSE: Applying direct pressure and elevating the arm above the heart is the best method to stop bleeding.
17. Remove the syringe safety needle, and transfer the blood immediately to the required tube or tubes using a safety transfer device. Do not push on the syringe plunger during transfer. Discard the entire unit in the sharps container when transfer is complete. Gently invert the tubes after the addition of blood. Label the tubes with the patient's name, the date, the time, and your initials, or affix the preprinted tube labels and print your initials on the label (Fig. 8).
PURPOSE: The safety transfer device protects against accidental needlesticks and allows the correct amount of blood to be transferred into the tube by vacuum. Pushing the plunger hemolyzes the blood and may alter the amount of blood intended in each tube. Blood begins to clot shortly after collection, so it must be transferred into the vacuum tube and mixed with anticoagulant immediately after collection. Gently inverting the tubes ensures anticoagulation. Labeling ensures proper patient identification.

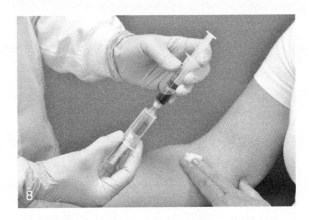

8

18. Check the venipuncture site. Make sure bleeding has stopped. Apply a hypoallergenic self-stick wrap, gauze and tape, or a bandage (Fig. 9).

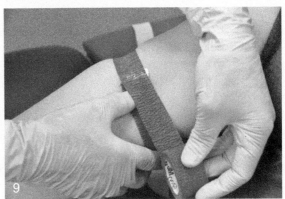

9

Continued

PROCEDURE 32.2	Perform a Venipuncture: Collect a Venous Blood Sample Using the Syringe Method—*continued*

19. Disinfect the work area. Dispose of blood-contaminated materials (e.g., gauze and gloves) in the biohazard waste container. Remove your eyewear and gloves. Wash hands or use hand sanitizer.
 <u>PURPOSE:</u> It is important to ensure infection control.

20. Complete the laboratory requisition form, and route the specimen to the proper place. Record the procedure in the patient's record.
 <u>PURPOSE:</u> A procedure is not considered complete until it is recorded in the patient's record.

PROCEDURE 32.3	Perform Venipuncture: Obtain a Venous Sample With a Safety Winged Butterfly Needle Assembly

Task: Obtain a venous sample accurately from a hand or arm vein using a butterfly needle and syringe.

EQUIPMENT and SUPPLIES

- Patient's health record
- Provider's order or lab requisition
- Safety winged (butterfly) needle set
- Syringe of appropriate volume for testing
- Vacuum tubes appropriate for tests ordered
- 70% isopropyl alcohol wipes
- Gauze
- Tourniquet
- Hypoallergenic self-stick wrap, tape, or bandage
- Permanent marking pen or printed labels
- Fluid-impermeable lab coat, protective eyewear, and gloves
- Biohazard waste container
- Biohazard sharps container

PROCEDURAL STEPS

1. Check the provider's order or requisition form to determine the tests ordered. Gather the appropriate tubes and supplies. Put on a fluid-impermeable lab coat.
 <u>PURPOSE:</u> Collect the specimen properly based on the tube requirements on the requisition. Donning a lab coat is part of ongoing infection control.
2. Greet the patient. Identify yourself. Verify the patient's identity with full name; ask the patient to spell the first and last names and to give his or her date of birth. Explain the procedure to be performed in a manner that the patient understands. Answer any questions the patient may have. Obtain permission for the venipuncture.
 <u>PURPOSE:</u> It is important to identify the patient in two different ways to ensure that you have the correct patient. Explaining the procedure can make the patient feel more comfortable and reduces anxiety.
3. Wash hands or use hand sanitizer. Put on gloves and protective eyewear.
 <u>PURPOSE:</u> It is important to ensure infection control.
4. *If drawing from the antecubital region:* Have the patient sit with the arm well supported in a slightly downward position. Ask the patient if he or she has a preference regarding which arm is used for the venipuncture.

<u>PURPOSE:</u> The veins of the antecubital area are more easily located when the elbow is straight. Asking about a patient preference gives the patient a chance to participate in the procedure.
 a. *If drawing from the back of the hand:* Have the patient place the venipuncture hand over the other, fisted hand with the fingers lower than the wrist.
 <u>PURPOSE:</u> These positions help blood fill the veins in the hand; this makes it easier for you to identify the veins and choose the draw site.
5. *If drawing from the antecubital region:* Apply the tourniquet 3 to 4 inches above the elbow on the patient's preferred arm. The tourniquet should never be tied so tightly that it restricts blood flow in the artery. Tourniquets should remain in place no longer than 60 seconds.
 <u>PURPOSE:</u> The tourniquet is used to make the veins more prominent.
 a. *If drawing from the back of the hand:* Apply the tourniquet above the wrist just proximal to the wrist bone (Fig. 1). Do not apply the tourniquet so tightly that blood flow in the arteries is impeded.
 <u>PURPOSE:</u> The tourniquet is used to make the veins more prominent.

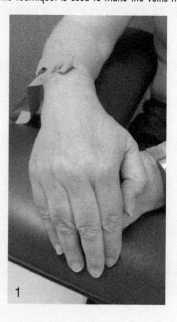

1

PROCEDURE 32.3	Perform Venipuncture: Obtain a Venous Sample With a Safety Winged Butterfly Needle Assembly—*continued*

6. *If drawing from the antecubital region:* Select the venipuncture site by palpating the antecubital space. Use your index finger to trace the path of the vein and to judge its depth. The veins most often used are the medial or cephalic veins, which lie in the middle of the elbow. Look at both arms, and use your critical thinking skills to find the vein that will give you the greatest chance of success for the venipuncture.

   PURPOSE: The index finger is most sensitive for palpating the vein. Do not use the thumb because it has a pulse of its own. Spend time to properly locate the best vein available; your patient will thank you.

   a. *If drawing from the back of the hand:* Select a vein on the back of the hand that is prominent, stable, and as straight as possible.

7. Remove the tourniquet, and cleanse the site with a 70% alcohol wipe.

   PURPOSE: The tourniquet should only be tied for 60 seconds.

8. Assemble your equipment and supplies on the side of the patient's non-dominant arm. Remove the butterfly device from the package, and stretch the tubing slightly. Take care not to activate the needle-retracting safety device accidentally.

   PURPOSE: It is important to keep the butterfly tubing from recoiling.

9. Attach the butterfly device firmly to the syringe (Fig. 2). If using a syringe, make sure to loosen the plunger a few times after the butterfly and syringe are attached.

   Note: The butterfly assembly can be attached to a needle holder *or* a syringe (see Fig. 2). Make sure the connection is firmly in place. When a vein on the back of the hand is used for the draw, a butterfly-syringe combination is almost always used.

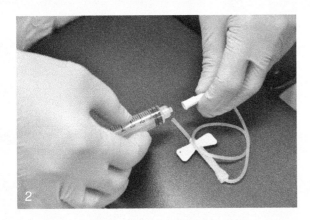

10. If using a needle assembly, lay the first tube in the vacuum tube holder and place the unit carefully where it will not roll away.

11. Reapply the tourniquet when the alcohol is dry.

    PURPOSE: Puncturing an area that is still wet with alcohol stings and can cause hemolysis of the sample.

12. Pinch the butterfly wings between your dominant hand thumb and index finger, or hold the base of the needle (Figs. 3 and 4). Remove the needle sheath.

PURPOSE: Positioning the hand in this manner provides the best visibility of the needle entering the vein and accessibility to insert and withdraw tubes with the nondominant hand.

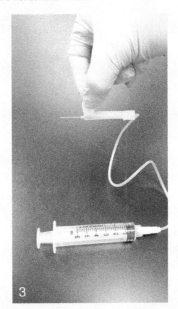

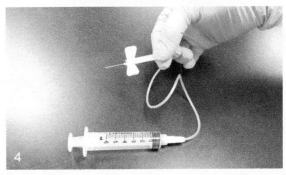

13. *If drawing from the antecubital region:* Grasp the patient's arm with the nondominant hand and anchor the vein by stretching the skin downward below the collection site with the thumb of the nondominant hand.

    PURPOSE: Failure to anchor the vein may cause the vein to move away from the needle when it is inserted, resulting in a missed vein.

    a. Using your thumb, pull the patient's skin taut over the knuckles.

    PURPOSE: Stretching the skin prevents the veins from rolling underneath.

14. With the bevel up and the needle aligned parallel to the vein, insert the needle at a 10- to15-degree angle through the skin and into the vein with a quick but smooth motion (Fig. 5).

    Note: According to CLSI, after insertion of the needle, the wings should be held in place to keep the needle from moving until the butterfly needle is removed. Make sure the safety device is not activated.

    PURPOSE: The sharpest point of the needle is inserted first. The angle ensures that the needle does not penetrate through the vein.

Continued

PROCEDURE 32.3	**Perform Venipuncture: Obtain a Venous Sample With a Safety Winged Butterfly Needle Assembly**—*continued*

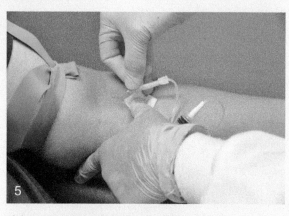

15. *If drawing with a needle holder assembly:* Push the blood collecting tube into the end of the holder. Note the position of the hands while drawing the blood.

    a. *If drawing with a syringe:* Make sure the vacuum you create is slow and steady and that no more than 1 mL of head space exists between the blood and the plunger. Slowly pull back the plunger of the syringe with the nondominant hand. Fill the barrel of the syringe to the needed volume (Fig. 6).

    PURPOSE: Drawing blood too forcefully into the syringe may collapse the vein or hemolyze the blood.

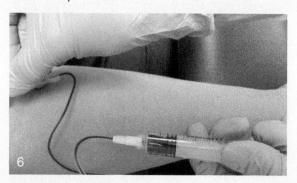

16. Release the tourniquet when the blood appears in the tubing or a "flash" of blood is seen in the hub of the syringe.
    PURPOSE: To prevent hemoconcentration, the tourniquet should remain in place no longer than 1 minute.

17. Always keep the tube and the holder in a downward position so that the tube fills from the bottom up.

18. Place a gauze over the puncture site and gently remove the needle, engaging the safety device. Dispose of the entire unit in the sharps container (Fig. 7).
    PURPOSE: The gauze over the puncture site and activation of the safety needle ensure infection control.

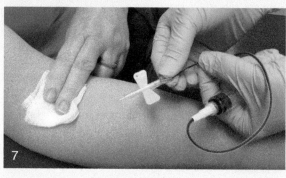

19. Complete the procedure as you would for an antecubital draw (see Procedure 32.1, steps 18 through 22).

PROCEDURE 32.4	**Perform a Capillary Puncture: Obtain a Blood Sample by Capillary Puncture**

Task: Collect a blood specimen suitable for testing using the capillary puncture technique.

EQUIPMENT and SUPPLIES

- Patient's health record
- Provider's order or lab requisition
- Sterile, disposable safety lancet
- 70% isopropyl alcohol wipes
- Gauze
- Hypoallergenic self-stick wrap, tape, or bandage
- Fluid-impermeable lab coat, protective eyewear, and gloves
- Appropriate collection containers (e.g., capillary tubes, Microtainer tubes)
- Permanent marking pen or printed labels
- Biohazard sharps container
- Biohazard waste container

PROCEDURAL STEPS

1. Check the provider's order or requisition form to determine the tests ordered. Gather the appropriate tubes and supplies. Put on a fluid-impermeable lab coat.

PROCEDURE 32.4   Perform a Capillary Puncture: Obtain a Blood Sample by Capillary Puncture—*continued*

PURPOSE: Collect the specimen properly based on the tube requirements on the requisition. Donning a lab coat is part of ongoing infection control.

2. Greet the patient. Identify yourself. Verify the patient's identity with full name; ask the patient to spell the first and last names and to give his or her date of birth. Explain the procedure to be performed in a manner that the patient understands. Answer any questions the patient may have. Obtain permission for the venipuncture.
   PURPOSE: It is important to identify the patient in two different ways to ensure that you have the correct patient. Explaining the procedure can make the patient feel more comfortable and reduces anxiety.

3. Wash hands or use hand sanitizer. Put on gloves and protective eyewear.
   PURPOSE: It is important to ensure infection control.

4. Select a puncture site, depending on the patient's age and the sample to be obtained (e.g., palmar side of the middle or ring finger of the nondominant hand for an adult or child; medial or lateral curved surface of the plantar surface of heel for an infant).
   PURPOSE: The nondominant hand may have fewer calluses. The palmar side of the finger is less sensitive, and the skin usually is not as thick. Use great caution when performing capillary puncture on infants (see Fig. 32.21A and B).

5. Gently rub the finger or have your patient wiggle the fingers and open and close the hand.
   PURPOSE: Movement promotes circulation. If the finger is very cold, you may immerse it in warm water or moisten it with warm towels.

6. Once the finger is warm, clean the site with a 70% isopropyl alcohol pad, and allow it to air dry (Fig. 1).
   PURPOSE: Puncturing skin that is wet with alcohol will sting and can hemolyze the specimen.

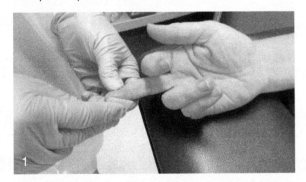

7. Hold onto the patient's finger above the puncture site with your nondominant hand.
   PURPOSE: Firmly holding the finger allows you to control the puncture and will not let the patient pull the hand away.

8. Hold the safety lancet firmly against the patient's finger, and press down on the safety trigger that activates the needle or blade to penetrate the skin. The sharp will then automatically retract into the plastic housing of the lancet. (Fig. 2).
   PURPOSE: Lancets are designed to puncture at specific depths that permit the free flow of blood.

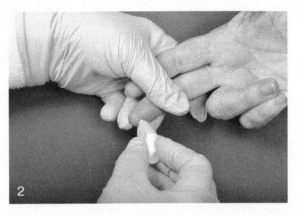

9. Dispose of the lancet in the sharps container. Wipe away the first drop of blood with gauze (Fig. 3).
   PURPOSE: The first drop of blood contains tissue fluid, which may alter test results. If there is any residual alcohol on the finger, it will hemolyze the blood.

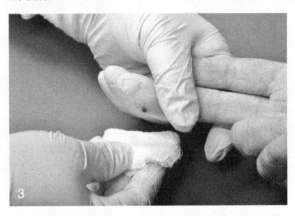

10. Apply gentle, intermittent pressure to cause the blood to flow freely (Fig. 4).
    PURPOSE: Forceful squeezing liberates fluid that dilutes the blood and causes inaccurate results. *Do not* milk the finger.

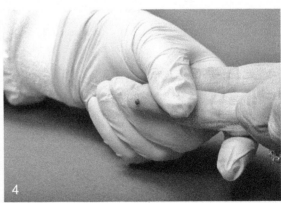

11. Collect the blood samples. Gently squeeze and release the finger two or three times to get a large drop of blood. Touch the capillary tube to the drop of blood. *Do not* scoop blood from the finger's surface. Fill the capillary

Continued

PROCEDURE 32.4   **Perform a Capillary Puncture: Obtain a Blood Sample by Capillary Puncture**—*continued*

tube to approximately three-fourths full or to the indicated line (Fig. 5). Then tip the tube with the presealed end down. When the blood flows down and touches the sealant, hold it for 30 seconds to allow it to seal automatically.

PURPOSE: The specimen should be free of air bubbles and then sealed in preparation for centrifuging.

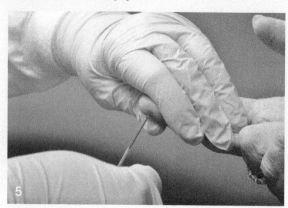

12. Wipe the patient's finger with gauze. Express another large drop of blood in the same way, and fill a Microtainer (Fig. 6). Do not touch the container to the finger. If more blood is needed, gently squeeze and release the finger to get another drop. Cap the Microtainer tube when the collection is complete.

PURPOSE: Touching the container to the finger irritates the puncture site and may cause infection. Touching the container also smears the blood in the fingerprint and does not allow the blood to form a good hanging drop.

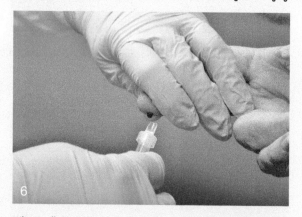

13. When collection is complete, apply pressure to the site with gauze (Fig. 7). The patient may be able to assist with this step.

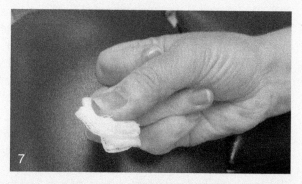

14. Select an appropriate means of labeling the containers. Sealed capillary tubes can be placed in a red-topped tube, which is then labeled. Microtainers can be placed in zipper-lock biohazard bags that are subsequently labeled. Follow your institution's procedures for labeling.

PURPOSE: Appropriate labeling will ensure proper patient identification.

15. Check the patient for bleeding and clean the site if traces of blood are visible. Apply a folded gauze square to the puncture site, and wrap with hypoallergenic self-stick wrap, tape, or a bandage (Fig. 8).

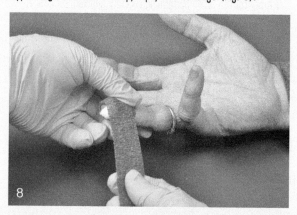

16. Disinfect the work area. Dispose of blood-contaminated materials (e.g., gauze and gloves) in the biohazard waste container. Remove your protective eyewear, and wash hands or use hand sanitizer.

PURPOSE: It is important to ensure infection control.

17. Complete the laboratory requisition form, and route the specimen to the proper location. Record the procedure in the patient's record.

PURPOSE: A procedure is not considered done until it is recorded in the patient's record.

ANALYSIS OF BLOOD

33

SCENARIO

Anita James, CMA (AAMA), has been working at the Walden-Martin Family Medical (WMFM) Clinic for 16 years. She loves her position as a medical assistant in a family medicine clinic. Every day is different. Each patient is unique. She has seen a number of children grow up over the years. Children who were toddlers when she started are now driving and thinking about college. The time has flown by.

Anita is working with Dr. Perez today, and they have a very busy schedule. A number of patients are in for follow-up visits, and a few new patients have appointments today, too.

While studying this chapter, think about the following questions:

- What is the anticoagulant of choice for hematology testing?
- What is the purpose of the following tests: microhematocrit test, hemoglobin test, erythrocyte sedimentation rate (ESR)?
- What is the purpose of performing a prothrombin time (PT) in coagulation testing?
- What tests are included in a complete blood count (CBC)? What are their reference ranges?
- When looking at hematology test results, can you differentiate between normal and abnormal test results?
- How would you describe the red blood cell (RBC) indices?
- Why would a provider order a white blood cell (WBC) count and differential?
- What is the medical assistant's role in blood transfusions?
- Why are the following test results important to a provider: blood glucose, hemoglobin A1c, cholesterol, liver enzymes, and thyroid hormones?
- What tests are part of a chemistry panel, and what are the reasons for performing each panel?

LEARNING OBJECTIVES

1. Name the main functions of blood.
2. Describe the appearance and function of erythrocytes, leukocytes, and platelets. Also, discuss plasma.
3. Explain the purpose of the microhematocrit test. Describe how to collect a microhematocrit specimen and perform a microhematocrit test.
4. Describe how to obtain a specimen for and perform a hemoglobin test.
5. Cite the reasons for performing an erythrocyte sedimentation rate (ESR) test, discuss the sources of error for ESR testing, and determine and record an erythrocyte sedimentation rate obtained by using a modified Westergren method.
6. Explain the purpose of a prothrombin time (PT) test, and describe how to obtain a specimen for and perform a CLIA-waived prothrombin time/international normalized ratio (PT/INR) test. Also, explain how you could reassure a patient of the accuracy of PT/INR test results.
7. Identify the tests included in a complete blood count (CBC) and their reference ranges and differentiate between normal and abnormal test results.
8. Explain the reasons for performing a white blood cell (WBC) count and differential and discuss the preparation of blood smears for the differential.
9. Differentiate between the ABO blood groupings and the Rh blood groupings. Also, discuss legal and ethical issues related to blood transfusions.
10. Do the following related to blood chemistry in the physician office laboratory:
    - Explain the reasons for testing blood glucose, hemoglobin A1c, cholesterol, liver enzymes, and thyroid hormones.
    - Assist a provider by performing a blood glucose test.
    - Determine a cholesterol level or lipid profile using a cholesterol chemistry analyzer.

albumin (al BYOO men) Most abundant plasma protein in human blood. It is important in regulating the water balance of blood.

anemia A deficiency of hemoglobin in the blood. Accompanied by a reduced number of red blood cells, pale skin, weakness, and shortness of breath among other symptoms.

antibody Protein produced in the blood or tissues in response to a specific antigen that destroys or weakens the antigen. Part of the immune system.

antigen A substance that stimulates the production of an antibody when introduced into the body. Antigens include toxins, bacteria, viruses, and other foreign substances.

artifact A substance, structure, or event that does not naturally occur in a situation. Examples include interference, or electrical "garbage" on an ECG, or crystals, lint, or contamination of a staining technique.

atypical lymphs In many viral infections stimulated or reactive lymphs are called *atypical lymphs*. They are commonly seen in infectious mononucleosis, or "mono."

autoimmune An immune response against a person's own tissues, cells, or cell parts.

centrifuge (SEN truh fyooj) A machine that rotates at high speed and separates substances of different densities by centrifugal force. Example: A tube of blood is separated into plasma/serum, white blood cells, platelets, and red blood cells.

cytoplasm The cell substance that fills the area between the nucleus and the cell membrane. Contains organelles of the cell.

density Describes how compact or concentrated something is.

dilution Reducing the concentration of a mixture or solution by adding a known volume of liquid.

enzyme A special protein that speeds up the chemical reaction in the body.

hematologist (hee mah TOL uh jist) A person trained in the nature, function, and diseases of the blood and blood-forming organs. Can be a physician, trained laboratory personnel, or researcher.

hemoglobin (HEE muh gloh bin) The oxygen-carrying pigment of red blood cells.

hormone A chemical substance produced in an endocrine gland and transported in the blood to a specific tissue, where it applies a specific effect.

immunoglobulins (im yuh noh GLOB yuh linz) A group of related proteins that function as antibodies. They are found in plasma and other body fluids.

intracellular pathogen A disease-causing organism that is within or inside a cell.

lateral flow immunoassay (im yuh noh AH say) A laboratory or clinical technique that uses the specific binding between an antigen and antibody to identify and quantify a substance in a sample. The sample in this technique moves in a sideways motion, usually on absorbent paper.

malignant A cell with uncontrolled growth that spreads rapidly, with the potential for serious harm.

metabolic Relating to or resulting from metabolism (the chemical process in which cells produce the substances and energy needed to sustain life).

microcuvette (MIE kroh koo vet) A small plastic or glass tube designed to hold samples for laboratory tests that detect light or color changes.

nucleus A structure in a cell that contains genetic material and controls the characteristics and growth of the cell.

pathologic Caused by or involving disease.

physiologic Consistent with the normal function of the body.

pipet (pie PET) A slender tube attached to or including a bulb, for transferring or measuring small amounts of a liquid, often used in a laboratory.

polycythemia (pohl ee sie THEE mee ah) A disorder characterized by an abnormal increase in the number of red blood cells in the blood.

reagent A substance used in a chemical reaction.

senescent (si NES ent) **cell** An old or aging cell that can no longer divide and reproduce.

The average body holds 10 to 12 pints of blood. The heart circulates the blood through the circulatory system more than 1000 times every day. More than 70,000 miles of passageways, most of which are narrower than a human hair, carry blood throughout the body. The blood is contained in a closed system of vessels; the largest is the aorta, and the smallest are the capillaries. The capillaries are only one cell layer thick, and their thin, permeable walls allow certain substances to move back and forth between blood vessels and surrounding tissue. The circulating blood contains more than 25 trillion cells, and every second the body replaces 8 million old red blood cells (RBCs) with 8 million new RBCs.

The circulating blood supplies the body's cells with nutrients and oxygen. The blood also distributes **enzymes**, **hormones**, and other chemicals needed for regulation of body activities. In addition, the blood functions to maintain body temperature, keep body fluids in balance, and maintain pH. Maintaining a constant internal environment is called *homeostasis*.

Blood tests are done routinely in the hematology, immunohematology (also referred to as the blood bank), chemistry, and immunology (also called *serology*) departments of the laboratory. The degree of blood testing performed by medical assistants depends on the level of service offered by the ambulatory care facility and the regulations established by the Clinical Laboratory Improvement Amendments (CLIA). As a medical assistant, you are qualified to perform CLIA-waived procedures described in the physician office laboratory (POL) sections of this chapter. More highly complex CLIA blood tests are performed at reference and hospital laboratories and are performed by medical laboratory personnel. This chapter explains more complex procedures to provide background information important to an understanding of the analysis of blood.

HEMATOLOGY

Whole blood is composed of visible formed elements suspended in *plasma* (a clear, yellow liquid). Plasma makes up approximately 55% of blood by volume. The remaining 45% consists of the following visible cellular elements; erythrocytes (RBCs), leukocytes (WBCs), and thrombocytes (platelets). The characteristics of blood and cellular components are reviewed in Chapter 24. A brief review of the components is presented in Table 33.1.

Plasma

Plasma is the highly complex liquid that transports the formed elements plus other substances, such as plasma proteins, throughout the body to every cell. Plasma proteins include **albumin**, the clotting proteins *prothrombin* and *fibrinogen*, and **immunoglobulins**. Plasma also transports nutrients (carbohydrates, fats, and amino acids), hormones, enzymes, mineral salts, gases, and waste products.

Plasma is composed of approximately 90% water, 9% protein, and 1% other chemical substances. The liquid portion of the blood in the body is plasma. In blood samples drawn for testing or other purposes, the body plasma must have an added anticoagulant to remain part of whole blood. The liquid that remains after blood has clotted is called *serum*.

HEMATOLOGY IN THE PHYSICIAN OFFICE LABORATORY (POL)

For many POL hematology tests, an adequate blood sample can be obtained from a capillary puncture of the finger. If a larger sample is required, blood can be obtained via venipuncture. For a complete blood count (CBC), venous blood is collected in a lavender-topped tube containing ethylenediaminetetraacetic acid (EDTA), an anticoagulant that prevents whole blood from clotting. EDTA is the anticoagulant of choice for hematology testing because it also acts as a preservative for the blood cells. It is very important to prevent blood from being hemolyzed during collection for hematology testing.

Hematocrit

The *hematocrit* (Hct) is a measurement of the percentage of packed RBCs in a volume of blood. A spun microhematocrit test is based on the principle of separating the cellular elements from plasma using a **centrifuge** (see Procedures 33.1 and 33.2, pp. 853–854). Drops of blood are collected from a capillary puncture into two capillary tubes that are placed in a specially designed microhematocrit centrifuge (Fig. 33.1). Capillary tubes can also be filled with EDTA-anticoagulated blood from a lavender-topped vacuum tube. As required by the

TABLE 33.1	Review of Blood Components			
COMPONENT	**FUNCTION**	**NORMAL VALUES**	**COMMENTS**
Plasma	To transport nutrients to cells and waste products away from cells	Approximately 55% of blood total volume	Plasma is the liquid portion of the blood inside the body.
Red blood cells (RBCs)	To carry oxygen to the cells and help carry some carbon dioxide away from cells	Approximately 4–6 million/mm³; may be slightly higher for men and slightly lower for women	About 120-day life span
Platelets	Help with the process of blood clotting	150,000–450,000/mm³	About 10-day life span
White Blood Cells (WBCs) – Granular			
Neutrophil	Engulfs and destroys foreign substances, particularly bacteria	Most abundant WBC in the blood, about 40%–60%	Also called *polymorphonuclear cells, PMNs, segs,* or *polys*
Eosinophil	Helps in the destruction of parasites and fungi	About 1%–4% of WBCs in the blood	Also called *eos*
Basophil	Helps in the destruction of allergens	About 0.5%–1% of WBCs in the blood	Also called *basos*
WBCs – Agranular			
Monocytes	Engulf and destroy foreign substances, particularly **senescent cells** and **malignant** cells	About 2%–8% of WBCs in the blood	Monocytes are found in the blood, but once they migrate into tissue, they are called *macrophages*; also called *monos*.
Lymphocyte B cells	Destroy foreign substances by producing **antibodies**	B and T cells combined are the second most abundant WBC in the blood, about 20%–40%	Looking under the microscope, you cannot see the difference between B- and T-cell lymphocytes. They look the same, but they function differently. Also called *lymphs*.
Lymphocyte T cells	Destroy foreign substances—particularly **intracellular pathogens**		

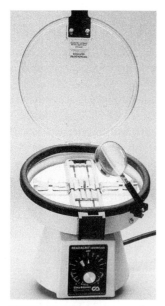

FIGURE 33.1 Microhematocrit centrifuge.

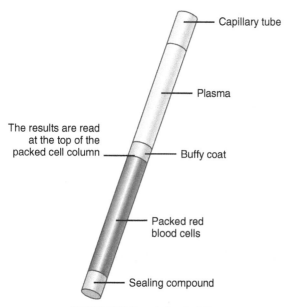

- Capillary tube
- Plasma

The results are read at the top of the packed cell column

- Buffy coat
- Packed red blood cells
- Sealing compound

FIGURE 33.2 Spun microhematocrit tube.

Occupational Safety and Health Administration (OSHA), capillary tubes must be safe. They are either made of plastic or plastic-coated glass to avoid sharps injuries. The most common type of microhematocrit tube is self-sealing at one end. A less used type is open-ended on both ends. If the tube is self-sealing, it must be tilted upright, causing the blood sample to flow down the tube and come into contact with the seal, and then held in place for 15 to 30 seconds. The open-ended tubes must be sealed with special clay before centrifugation.

After centrifugation, the packed RBCs are at the bottom of the tube against the sealant, the WBCs and platelets are in the center *buffy coat*, and plasma is on top (Fig. 33.2). The microhematocrit is determined by comparing the volume of RBCs to the total volume of the whole blood sample. The percentage is read by placing the tubes on a special microhematocrit reader. Some microhematocrit

TABLE 33.2 Hematocrit (Hct) Reference Values	
AGE/GENDER	Hct VALUE (%)
Neonate (newborn–<1 mo)	44–64
Infant (1 mo–1 yr)	37–41
Child (1–10 yr)	35–41
Male (>10 yr)	42–52
Female (>10 yr)	36–45

centrifuges have a built-in reading scale that reads the calibrated capillary tubes. Microhematocrit tests should be performed in duplicate and the average of the two results reported.

Normal hematocrit (Hct) values vary with gender and age (Table 33.2). They range from a low of 36% in women to a high of 52% in men. Low microhematocrit values can indicate **anemia** or the presence of bleeding. High values may be caused by dehydration or **polycythemia**. Values can be influenced by **physiologic**, **pathologic**, and even geographic factors and by collection techniques. Normal Hct ranges are affected by a person's geographic location. For example, people living at high altitudes have a higher percentage of RBCs, to compensate for the lower oxygen levels in the atmosphere.

The microhematocrit is a commonly performed test requested by providers either separately or as part of the CBC. Because it is a simple procedure that requires only a small amount of blood, it is an ideal screening test and often is part of a routine physical examination. Quality assurance includes care and maintenance of the microhematocrit instrument.

CRITICAL THINKING APPLICATION   33.1

One of Anita's patients today is Carl Bowden. Carl retired recently and has been enjoying his new, less hectic schedule. Carl is in good health, but he did mention at his physical today that he was feeling a little tired and lacked energy. Dr. Perez ordered a microhematocrit for Carl. The lab just sent the results to Carl's electronic health record.

Anita looks at the results and sees that his hematocrit is 38%. Is that value in the normal range for an adult male?

Hemoglobin

Hemoglobin (Hgb) determination is another way to measure the oxygen-carrying capacity of blood. The hemoglobin concentration can be part of the CBC or an individual test.

CLIA-waived methods include the STAT-Site M Hgb, Hemo-PointH2, and HemoCue, all portable, battery-operated hemoglobin analyzers that fit in the palm of the hand (Fig. 33.3 and Procedure 33.3 [p. 856]). The HemoCue uses plastic **microcuvettes** that contain **reagents** that *lyse* (break apart) the RBCs in the sample, releasing the hemoglobin. The hemoglobin reacts with the reagents and forms a color. The color is detected and measured in the instrument, producing a digital readout. Capillary, venous, or arterial blood can be used in the disposable microcuvette. The cuvettes have a long shelf life.

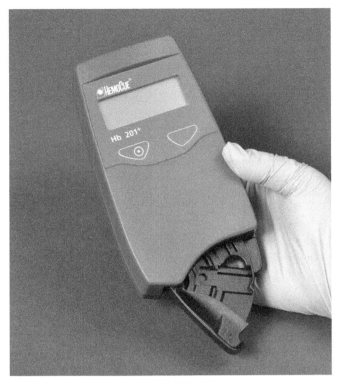

FIGURE 33.3 Handheld hemoglobin monitor.

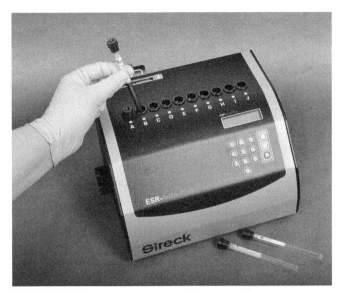

FIGURE 33.4 30-minute Streck ESR CLIA-waived test.

TABLE 33.3 Hemoglobin (Hgb) Reference Values

AGE/GENDER	Hgb LEVEL (g/dL)
Neonate (newborn–<1 mo)	17–23
Infant (1 mo–1 yr)	9–14
Child (1–10 yr)	10–15
Female (>10 yr)	12–16
Male (>10 yr)	14–18

TABLE 33.4 Erythrocyte Sedimentation Rate (ESR) Reference Values

	SEDIPLAST TEST (mm/hr)
Men	≤50 yr: 0–15 >50 yr: 0–20
Women	≤50 yr: 0–20 >50 yr: 0–30

Normal hemoglobin values vary throughout a lifetime (Table 33.3). Factors that affect the hemoglobin level include age, gender, diet, altitude, and existing disease states.

Hemoglobin and hematocrit tests are often performed together and are referred to as an *H&H*. A quick mental calculation should always be done before H&H results are reported: the hemoglobin value × 3 (± 3) should equal the hematocrit value. For example, if the hemoglobin is 15 g/dL, calculate the hematocrit as:

$$15\,g/dL \times 3 = 45 \pm 3 = 42 - 48$$

The hematocrit should be between 42% and 48%.

Erythrocyte Sedimentation Rate

The *erythrocyte sedimentation rate* (ESR) is a laboratory test that measures the rate at which red blood cells gradually separate from plasma and settle to the bottom of a specially calibrated tube in 1 hour. The test is not specific for any disease in particular but is used as a general indicator of inflammation. ESR and C-reactive protein (CRP) testing should correlate as indicators of inflammation. An increased ESR is seen in conditions such as:

- acute and chronic infections, including tuberculosis, hepatitis, and rheumatic fever
- rheumatoid arthritis, lupus erythematosus, and other **auto-immune** conditions
- some cancers, including multiple myeloma

Normal values vary slightly with age and gender (Table 33.4). An increased ESR is significant to the provider. It indicates the presence of inflammation in the body. A lower than normal ESR is not considered clinically significant. Several CLIA-waived methods of measuring the ESR are used, including the Sediplast procedure (see Procedure 33.4, p. 857). This closed system incorporates a pierceable stopper that ensures a leakproof seal when punctured by a **pipet**. An automatic self-zeroing cap and reservoir accurately bring the blood level to the zero mark and prevent overfilling. A prefilled vial of sodium citrate reagent is provided for **dilution** of blood before testing. A closed-tube Streck ESR method uses a Streck black-topped Vacutainer sample of blood that is directly placed in a Streck rack that provides results in 30 minutes (Fig. 33.4).

Many factors can affect the ESR. The tube must be filled with blood and must not have air bubbles. The tube must be allowed to sit in a vertical position, undisturbed, for the full designated time – careful timing is important. Tilting a tube even slightly may increase the sedimentation rate. Jarring or vibrations from nearby machinery will falsely increase the ESR.

Coagulation Testing

The medical assistant may be asked to perform a CLIA-waived test called a *prothrombin time* (PT; also called a *protime*). This test can be performed using a handheld, CLIA-waived instrument that uses whole blood from a fingerstick (Fig. 33.5). A PT is a method of measuring how long it takes blood to clot. Prothrombin is a protein in the liquid part of blood (*plasma*) that is converted to thrombin as part of the clotting process. Thrombin then causes fibrinogen to be converted to fibrin during the clotting process.

The PT is often used in combination with the partial thromboplastin time (PTT) to screen for hemophilia and other clotting disorders. The PT is also used to monitor patients taking anticoagulant drugs such as *warfarin* (Coumadin) and similar anticoagulants. Warfarin is given to prevent clots in deep veins of the legs and to treat a pulmonary embolism.

The CLIA-waived CoaguChek XS PT measures the time it takes a blood sample to form a fibrin clot. A precise amount of capillary sample blood is dispensed into the channels of a testing strip. The blood is mixed with a thromboplastin reagent. The blood is pumped back and forth in the channel, and a series of light-emitting diodes (LEDs) detect formation of a clot when blood movement in the channels stops (see Procedure 33.5, p. 859).

PT test results are reported as the number of seconds blood takes to clot when mixed with the thromboplastin reagent. The international normalized ratio (INR) was created by the World Health Organization (WHO) because PT test results can vary, depending on the thromboplastin reagent used. The INR is a conversion unit that considers the different sensitivities of reagents. It is widely accepted as the standard unit for reporting PT results rather than the actual clotting time. Normal PT values are 10 to 13 seconds, or an INR of 1 to 1.4. Patients who are taking warfarin to prevent the formation of blood clots or who have artificial heart valves should have an INR value of about 2 to 3. Their blood should take longer to clot than that of a normal healthy individual.

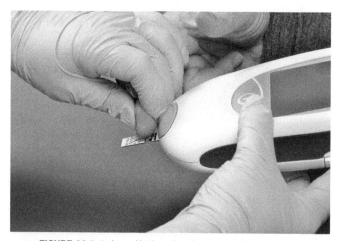

FIGURE 33.5 Applying a blood sample to the CoaguChek XS PT test monitor.

It is important that the medical assistant knows how to accurately document INR follow-up and related warfarin dosages on a patient flow sheet. The provider will balance repeated INR levels with the warfarin dosage so the INR is maintained at about 2 throughout the anticoagulant treatment (Fig. 33.6).

It is important to educate patients regarding their behaviors when a blood test such as the PT/INR is being monitored. Reassure these patients that follow-up testing is needed, accurate, and beneficial for their treatment. For example, if patients are taking the anticoagulant warfarin (Coumadin), they will need to follow up with the required lab work to monitor their PT/INR. Patients should understand how their vitamin K intake from food directly affects their lab results. Increased vitamin K can increase blood clotting time; this means that vitamin K is working against warfarin. Helping patients identify foods high in vitamin K is crucial to maintaining a proper PT/INR value. Many providers do not instruct patients to stop eating foods high in vitamin K, but rather stress the importance of eating the same amount of foods high in vitamin K consistently. Even though foods may change seasonally, keeping a consistent intake year-round will help their lab results to remain constant. Foods high in vitamin K include dark green leafy vegetables (e.g., kale, collards, spinach, and turnip greens), brussels sprouts, and broccoli.

CRITICAL THINKING APPLICATION   33.2

Anita just roomed Janine Butler. She has an appointment today, and Dr. Perez would like to check her PT/INR results. Janine is on warfarin, but her INR is still a bit low. Anita checks her chart, and the INR completed in the lab is 1.7. Is this an acceptable result for someone who is on medication to prolong clotting time? Is it too high, too low, or normal?

HEMATOLOGY IN THE REFERENCE LABORATORY

The most frequently ordered reference laboratory procedure for hematology is the CBC. This test requires a lavender-topped EDTA blood specimen. It gives a comprehensive look at the cellular components of blood and can provide a wealth of information about a patient's general health. It routinely includes the following:
- RBC count, hematocrit, hemoglobin, and RBC indices
- WBC count and differential
- Platelet count

Complete Blood Count (CBC) Laboratory Reports

It is important that medical assistants understand the hematology laboratory reports that arrive from reference and hospital laboratories. They should be able to distinguish between normal and abnormal results. Use the following references to complete the Critical Thinking Application exercise that follows:
- Hematology reference ranges (Table 33.5)
- The patient report form (Fig. 33.7), which is a sample lab report, also identifies the lab's reference ranges. Lab reports, both electronic and paper, must supply their own reference ranges, along with each patient's results.

Westhills Family Practice Center
Warfarin Anticoagulant Record

Patient's Name: _____   DOB: _____

Address: _____   SSN: _____

_____

Patient's Phone: _____

Dx for Anticoagulation: _____   ICDM Code: _____

Date Warfarin Started: _____   INR Goal: _____

Phone for Outside Lab: _____

Date	Warfarin Dose Pre-Test	PT	INR	Warfarin Dose Order	Next INR/PT	Signature

FIGURE 33.6 Warfarin flow sheet.

CRITICAL THINKING APPLICATION 33.3

Using the reference ranges in Table 33.5 and the lab report form in Fig. 33.7, decide if the following results are normal or abnormal.

1. Grace Sifuentes, age 4, has a hematocrit of 38%. Is that normal, high, or low?
2. Christian Washington, age 45, has a WBC count of 14,200/mm³. Is that normal, high, or low?
3. Brigitte Mulrooney, age 29, has a hematocrit of 32% and a hemoglobin of 10 g/dL. Are these results normal, high, or low?
4. Eleanor Jackson, age 81, has 23% bands in her white blood cell differential. Is that normal, high, or low?

Red Blood Cell Count

The RBC count is part of the CBC (see Table 33.5). It approximates the number of circulating RBCs in a person's blood. The function of an RBC is to transport oxygen to tissues. The RBC count often is decreased in patients with anemia. Increased RBC counts are found in people with dehydration, polycythemia, severe burns, and those living at high altitudes. Normal RBC values range from approximately 4 million to 6 million cells/mm³. RBC counts usually are higher in males than in females.

Red Blood Cell Indices

A variety of calculations can be performed using the information obtained from the CBC. The red cell *indices* provide information about RBC disorders. The indices are used to classify anemias and to select additional tests that may help determine the cause of anemia. Red cell indices are also helpful to monitor the treatment of anemia. Because indices may change in response to treatment, they can be used as an indicator of how well the patient is responding to a treatment. The indices are mathematical calculations using the three red blood cell tests: Hct, Hgb, and the RBC count.

- *Mean cell volume* (MCV): MCV = (Hct/RBC) × 10. The average size of the RBCs is the most important index for classifying anemias. Abnormally large RBCs are macrocytic and have a higher than normal MCV. Small RBCs are microcytic and have a lower than normal MCV. The normal reference range is 82 to 108 femtoliters (fL).
- *Mean cell hemoglobin* (MCH): MCH = (Hgb/RBC) × 10. The MCH is calculated to give the average weight of hemoglobin in the RBC. The reference range is 26 to 34 picograms (pg).
- *Mean cell ratio of Hgb and Hct* (MCHC): MCHC = (Hgb × 100)/RBC. The MCHC indicates the average weight of hemoglobin compared with the cell size. The reference range is 32 to 37 g/dL. A decreased MCHC shows *hypochromic* (pale, lacking color) RBCs in a stained blood smear. An increased MCHC is rare and should be flagged and brought to the attention of the provider.

TABLE 33.5   Reference Ranges for Complete Blood Count (CBC) Values[a]

TEST	NEONATES (NEWBORN–1 MO)	INFANTS (1 MO–1 YR)	CHILDREN (1–10 YR)	MALE (>10 YR)	FEMALE (>10 YR)
RBCs	4.8–7.1 million/mm³	3.8–5.5 million/mm³	4.5–4.8 million/mm³	4.5–6 million/mm³	4–5.5 million/mm³
Hematocrit (Hct)	44%–64%	30%–40%	35%–41%	42%–52%	36%–45%
Hemoglobin (Hgb)	17–23 g/dL	9–14 g/dL	11–16 g/dL	15–17 g/dL	12–16 g/dL
WBCs	9000–30,000/mm³	6000–16,000/mm³	5000–13,000/mm³	4000–11,000/mm³	
RBC Indices					
MCV	96–108 fL			82–99 fL	
MCH	32–34 pg			26–34 pg	
MCHC	31–33 g/dL			31–37 g/dL	
WBC Differential					
Neutrophils	≥45% by age 1 wk	32%	60% for children ≥2 yr	50%–65%	
Bands	—	—	—	0%–7%	
Eosinophils	—	—	0%–3%	1%–3%	
Basophils	—	—	1%–3%	0%–1%	
Monocytes	—	—	4%–9%	3%–9%	
Lymphocytes	≥41% by age 1 wk	61%	59% for children ≥2 yr	25%–40%	
Platelets	140,000–300,000/mm³	200,000–473,000/mm³	150,000–450,000/mm³	150,000–400,000/mm³	

fL, Femtoliter; *MCH*, mean corpuscular hemoglobin; *MCHC*, mean corpuscular hemoglobin concentration; *MCV*, mean corpuscular volume; *pg*, picograms; *RBC*, red blood cell; *WBC*, white blood cell.
[a]Lab reports, both electronic and paper, must supply their own reference ranges, along with each patient's results. This is because different methodologies may create different reference ranges and different units of measurement.

White Blood Cell Count

The WBC count gives an estimate of the total number of leukocytes in circulating blood. The count is performed to help the provider determine whether an infection is present or to aid in the diagnosis of leukemia. It also may be used to follow the course of a disease and indicate if the patient is responding to treatment.

The normal WBC count varies with age. It is higher in newborns and decreases throughout a lifetime. The average adult range is 4500 to 11,000 cells/mm³. Many factors can affect the WBC count.

An increase in the number of normal WBCs is a condition called *leukocytosis*. Increased WBC counts may normally be seen with pregnancy, stress, anesthesia, exercise, and exposure to temperature extremes, and also after treatment with corticosteroids. Pathologic causes of leukocytosis include many bacterial infections, leukemia, appendicitis, and pneumonia.

A decrease in the WBC count is called *leukopenia*. This condition may be caused by viral infection or by exposure to radiation and certain chemicals and drugs.

Differential Cell Count

The purpose of the differential, or *diff*, in the CBC is to analyze and count the types of WBCs found in a sample of blood. The differential can be manually performed using a stained blood smear and a microscope, or with an automated instrument. Automated cell counters

have the ability to analyze the WBCs and gather information about cell size, internal structures, and **density**.

Preparation of Blood Smears for the Differential. A *blood smear* enables the examiner to view the preserved cellular structures of blood. The *morphology* (form or shape) of WBCs, RBCs, and platelets can be studied. Their size, shape, and maturity can also be evaluated.

A blood smear is prepared by placing a drop of blood from a fingerstick or an EDTA tube (using a DIFF-SAFE blood dispenser) onto a clean glass slide (Fig. 33.8). The slide must be free of dust and grease. The best specimen for a blood smear is capillary blood that has no anticoagulant added. EDTA-anticoagulated blood can be used, provided the smear is made within 2 hours of specimen collection. Because timing is important, the medical assistant may be asked to prepare a smear during collection of the CBC specimen.

The wedge smear is used most frequently and would follow these steps:

1. Place a small drop of blood ½ inch from the frosted end (placed to the right) of a glass slide.
2. The end of a second glass spreader slide is placed in front (to the left) of the drop of blood at an angle of 30 to 35 degrees.
3. The spreader slide is brought back into the drop with a quick but smooth gliding motion until the blood spreads along the edge of the spreader slide.

	DATE & TIME RECEIVED		ACCESSION NUMBER
	10/ 20/ 20XX 20:45		
	LOCATION		DATE REPORTED
			10/ 21/20XX

PHYSICIAN		PATIENT INFORMATION		

TEST		RESULTS	REFERENCE RANGE	UNITS
HEMOGRAM	LO	2.9	4. 5-10. 5	CU.MM.
WHITE BLOOD COUNT	LO	2. 39	4.40-5.90	CU.MM.
RED BLOOD COUNT	LO	7.4	14.0-18.0	GM/100ML
HEMOGLOBIN	LO	22.3	40. 0-52.0 %	
MEAN CORPUSCULAR VOLUME		93	80-100	fL
MEAN CORPUSCULAR HGB		31.0	27. 0-32.0	PG
MEAN CORPUSCULAR HgB CONC		33.2	31.0-36.0	%
DIFFERENTIAL, WBC				
SEGMENTED NEUTROPHILS		57	38-80	%
LYMPHOCYTE		29	15-45	%
MONOCYTES		7	1-10	%
EOSINOPHILS		1	0-4	%
BAND NEUTROPHILS	HI	6	0-5	%
ANISOCYTOSIS	ABN	SLIGHT		
HYPOCHROMIA	ABN	SLIGHT		
PLATELET ESTIMATE	ABN	DECREASED		
PARTIAL THROMBOPLASTIN TIME				
PARTIAL THROMBOPLASTIN TIME		31.7	20.0-40.0	SECONDS
CONTROL PTT		30.4	20.0-40.0	SECONDS
PROTHROMBIN TIME				
PROTHROMBIN TIME		12.2	10.0-13.5	SECONDS
CONTROL PT		12.0	11.0-13.0	SECONDS
FINAL Report (Summary)				

FIGURE 33.7 Sample lab report with normal and abnormal patient results.

4. The spreader slide is then pushed to the left with a quick, steady motion, spreading the blood across the slide (Fig. 33.9).

A good wedge smear should cover ½ to ¾ of the slide. It should show a gradual transition from a thick to a thin end with a feathered edge (Fig. 33.10). It should have a smooth appearance with no ridges, holes, lines, streaks, or clumps. On microscopic examination, the cells should be evenly distributed.

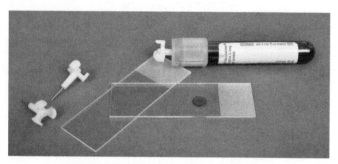

FIGURE 33.8 DIFF-SAFE device used to make a blood smear.

After the smear has been made, the patient's name is written on the frosted end of the slide with a pencil and the smear is allowed to air dry. The slide should be propped up to dry with the thick end down. Do not blow on the blood slide to dry it. The moisture in your breath can cause **artifacts** to form in the RBCs. Once dry, the slide is *fixed*, which preserves the cells and prevents changes in the cells. Many of the quick stains available on the market contain the fixative in the stain.

Staining Blood Smears.   Stains commonly used to make blood smears are described as *polychromatic*. They contain dyes that stain cell components different colors. These stains are attracted to different parts of the cell, which makes the cells and their structures easier to see and tell apart. The most commonly used differential blood stain is Wright's stain.

Identification of Normal Blood Cells

Useful information can be gathered from a microscopic evaluation of blood cells in a stained smear. The three features **hematologists** look for in blood cells are the cell size, the appearance of the **nucleus,**

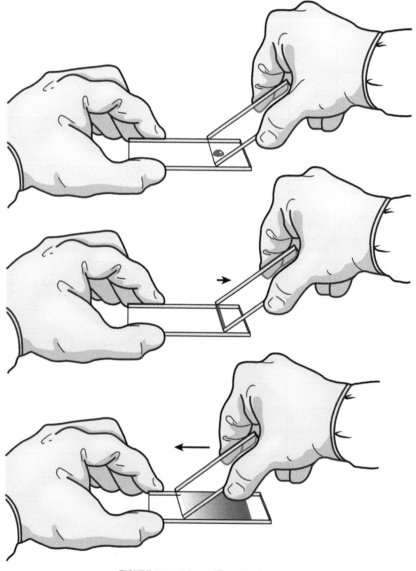

FIGURE 33.9 Making a differential wedge smear.

and the appearance of the **cytoplasm.** In Table 33.6 you will see a summary of the cells seen in a differential and a description of normal characteristics. To review additional information on blood cells, see Chapter 24.

Differential Examination

A specific area of a stained smear is examined under the microscope for a differential. The slide is examined near the feathered end of the smear, where cells are barely touching one another and are easiest to identify. Cells are examined with the oil immersion objective of the microscope. The differential involves counting and classifying 100 consecutive WBCs while moving in a winding pattern through the smear (see Fig. 33.10). A count of the cells observed is kept on a differential cell counter or a computer.

Normal values for a differential vary with age. As mentioned previously, laboratory reports must include the lab's own reference ranges, along with each patient's results.

Disease states may give differential results that are unlike a normal diff. The types of leukocytes, their maturity, and the appearance of the differential can be very useful for the provider in making a diagnosis. The differential exam typically is performed in a reference laboratory.

Red Blood Cell Morphology

After the differential cell count has been determined, the RBCs are observed and evaluated. Normally, stained RBCs are the same size and shape and are well filled with hemoglobin. Any variations from the normal state are reported. (Fig. 33.11 shows examples of abnormal cells.) The appearance of the RBCs should correlate with the RBC indices.

Size. Normal-sized RBCs are said to be *normocytic*. If the cells are larger than normal, they are *macrocytic;* if the cells are smaller than normal, they are *microcytic*. The condition in which different sizes of RBCs are present is known as *anisocytosis*.

Shape. Normal RBCs are round or slightly oval. Cells may be shaped like sickles, targets, crescents, or burs. *Poikilocytosis* is a significant variation in the shape of RBCs.

Content. An RBC with a normal amount of hemoglobin is said to be *normochromic*. Pale-staining cells are *hypochromic* and have less

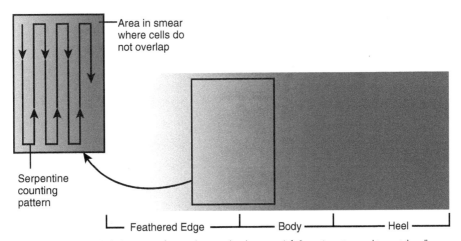

FIGURE 33.10 *Right,* Appearance of a properly prepared wedge smear. *Left,* Serpentine pattern used to count the cells.

TABLE 33.6	Cells in a Differential	
CELL NAME	**NORMAL CHARACTERISTICS**	**PHOTOGRAPH OF A NORMAL CELL**
Red blood cell	Most numerous cell on diff. A small, red, biconcave disk with no nuclei.	
Platelet	Smallest cell on diff. May be round or oval. Has no nucleus. A fragment of cytoplasm from a large bone marrow cell called a *megakaryocyte*. Note the platelets, indicated by the arrows.	

Continued

TABLE 33.6	Cells in a Differential—*continued*	
CELL NAME	NORMAL CHARACTERISTICS	PHOTOGRAPH OF A NORMAL CELL
Neutrophil — mature	Most numerous white blood cell (WBC) on diff. Nucleus has many lobes. Increased numbers seen with bacterial infections.	
Neutrophil — immature	Called a *band* or *stab cell*. Horseshoe-shaped nucleus. Increased numbers seen with some types of leukemia, and infections.	
Eosinophil	Has large, red-orange granules. Increased numbers seen with allergies, asthma, and certain parasitic infections.	
Basophil	Has large, dark blue/purple granules. Granules contain *histamine*, which is involved in the inflammatory response. Natural anticoagulant.	
Lymphocyte	Smallest WBC, but most numerous in the blood. Large, dark blue/purple nucleus. Increased numbers seen with viral and some bacterial infections. Viral infections may show **atypical lymphs**.	
Monocyte	Largest WBC in the blood. Increased numbers seen with viral and some bacterial infections	

CRITICAL THINKING APPLICATION   33.4

Anita checks Reuven Ahmad's CBC and differential results as she prepares information for Dr. Perez. Reuven's RBC count is 5.1 million/mm³. Is that a normal value for an adult male? In the notes from the differential, the laboratory technologist comments that Reuven's RBCs are normocytic and slightly hypochromic. Define normocytic and hypochromic in your own words. Be ready to share your definitions with the class.

hemoglobin than normal. Any inclusions within red cells should be reported.

Platelet Analysis

On a stained smear, the platelets are observed for any abnormalities. Platelets are small and irregularly shaped and may vary considerably in size. The normal platelet count is 150,000 to 450,000/mm³. An increase in platelets is called *thrombocytosis*, and a decrease is called *thrombocytopenia*. Excessive clumping of platelets is also reported in a platelet analysis.

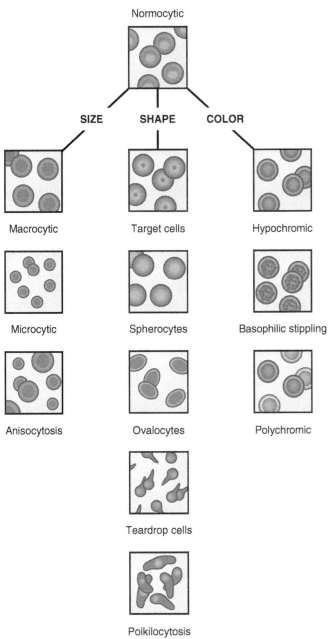

FIGURE 33.11 Abnormal red blood cells.

Normocytic

SIZE — SHAPE — COLOR

Macrocytic

Microcytic

Anisocytosis

Target cells

Spherocytes

Ovalocytes

Teardrop cells

Poikilocytosis

Hypochromic

Basophilic stippling

Polychromic

TABLE 33.7 Blood Compatibility

RBC ANTIGEN	PLASMA ANTIBODIES	COMPATIBLE WITH DONOR TYPES[a]
Type O (no antigens)	Anti-A and anti-B	O
Type A (type A antigen)	Anti-B	O and A
Type B (type B antigen)	Anti-A	O and B
Type AB (type AB antigen)	None	O, A, B, and AB

RBC, Red blood cell.
Patients with type AB blood are considered universal recipients.
[a]Patients with type O blood are considered universal donors.

major blood groups: A, B, O, and AB. Another major blood group is the Rh group. A person is either Rh positive (Rh+) or Rh negative (Rh−). Determinations of ABO and Rh blood groups are simple tests that can be performed easily. But because the consequences of performing the test incorrectly can be life-threatening, blood typing is not a CLIA-waived test. Table 33.7 presents blood transfusion compatibility types.

Blood Type Populations

This table gives you an idea of the blood type frequency in a few different populations in the United States.

TYPE	CAUCASIAN	AFRICAN-AMERICAN	HISPANIC	ASIAN
O+	37%	47%	53%	39%
O−	8%	4%	4%	1%
A+	33%	24%	29%	27%
A−	7%	2%	2%	0.5%
B+	9%	18%	9%	25%
B−	2%	1%	1%	0.4%
AB+	3%	4%	2%	7%
AB−	1%	0.3%	0.2%	0.1%

Data from the American Red Cross. *www.redcrossblood.org/learn-about-blood/blood-types.* Accessed September 9, 2018.

CRITICAL THINKING APPLICATION 33.5

Griffin Jones is in for a physical today, but she would also like to have her blood type tested. She and her husband are thinking of starting a family soon and would like to know her ABO/Rh type. She thinks she is A−. If Griffin is A−, what antigen or antigens are on her RBCs?

IMMUNOHEMATOLOGY

Formerly called the *blood bank*, the immunohematology department of the laboratory is responsible for blood typing. The major reason for performing immunohematology tests is to prevent problems caused by incompatible blood types during blood transfusions. Compatibility testing (also called *cross-matching*) is performed to prevent transfusion reactions in patients receiving blood from a donor. Identifying potential Rh incompatibility problems in expectant mothers is another procedure done in immunohematology. Rh incompatibility between an expectant mother and the unborn child may result in hemolytic disease of the newborn (HDN). (See Chapter 27 for more details on HDN.)

Blood Typing

The two major blood **antigen** systems are the ABO system and the Rh system (see Chapter 24 for details). The ABO system has four

Other Blood Types

In addition to the A and B antigens that characterize the ABO blood grouping, more than 600 antigens and more than 20 other blood antigen systems are known. Many are named after the person or family in which the blood antigen system was discovered. A medical assistant should be aware that other blood antigens exist. They may cause incompatibility issues in rare cases.

Beyond ABO and Rh Typing

There are many blood types beyond ABO and Rh. Here are a few blood antigens or antigen systems. Just so that you have seen the terms:

Diego – Found only among East Asians and Native Americans

MNS – Useful in maternity and paternity testing

Duffy – The malarial parasite requires the Duffy antigen to enter the red blood cells. Lack of the antigen confers resistance to malaria. Duffy-negative blood is found only in descendants of African populations.

Lewis – Antigens are soluble in blood rather than attached to the red blood cells. These are the only blood group antibodies that have never been implicated in hemolytic disease of the newborn.

Other blood group systems – Colton, M, Kell, Kidd, Landsteiner-Wiener, P, Yt or Cartwright, XG, Scianna, Dombrock, Chido/Rodgers, Kx, Gerbich, Cromer, Knops, Indian, Ok, Raph, and JMH.

Legal and Ethical Issues Related to Blood Transfusion

The Blood Safety Act was passed in 1991 to ensure that all donor blood is tested for human immunodeficiency virus (HIV) and other bloodborne pathogens. The impact of this law can be seen in the ambulatory care environment. The law requires providers to explain to each elective surgery patient the chances that he or she may need a blood transfusion. The discussion must include positive and negative aspects of *autologous transfusion* (i.e., transfusion with a person's own blood). The pros and cons of transfusions from family, friends, or other donors should also be discussed. The conversation must be documented in the patient's health record. Before the surgery, the patient must sign a form giving consent to any needed blood transfusions. The medical assistant should be aware that certain populations (e.g., Jehovah's Witnesses) do not believe in blood transfusions.

If the patient decides to use autologous transfusions, this may require the patient to donate blood several weeks before the procedure. Usually autologous transfusions are performed for stable patients undergoing major orthopedic, vascular, cardiac, or thoracic surgery. The medical assistant might need to help make arrangements for the blood donation. Another type of autologous transfusion can occur if the surgeon inserts an autologous drain in the surgical wound. The drain collects the blood from the surgical wound to prevent postoperative hematomas. The collected blood is then washed and reinfused into the patient.

BLOOD CHEMISTRY IN THE PHYSICIAN OFFICE LABORATORY

CLIA-waived chemistry tests using whole blood from capillary punctures have become popular in ambulatory practices. With the increase in diabetes and cardiovascular disease in the United States, patients with either (or both) of these **metabolic** diseases benefit from early diagnosis. Treatment is based on continued monitoring of glucose and hemoglobin A1c for diabetes and of cholesterol, lipid panels, and liver enzymes for cardiovascular diseases related to fatty deposit in the arteries.

Blood Glucose Testing

Glucose is used as a fuel by all body cells. Under normal circumstances, it is the only substance used to nourish brain cells. Maintenance of

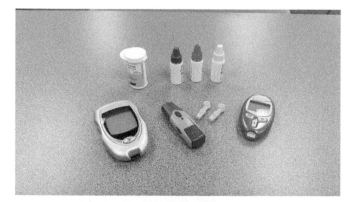

FIGURE 33.12 Glucometer and supplies.

blood glucose levels within a normal range is vital to homeostasis of the human body. Understanding the importance of glucose can help the medical assistant understand why glucose is the most frequently tested chemical analyte in the blood.

Elevated blood glucose levels are most often associated with diabetes mellitus. They also may indicate pancreatitis, endocrine disorders, or chronic renal failure. Diabetes mellitus is a disorder of carbohydrate metabolism that results in elevated blood and urine glucose levels. In diabetes mellitus, either the pancreas is unable to produce sufficient insulin to meet the body's needs, or insulin resistance develops at the cellular level (see Chapter 23).

For the initial screening of a patient for diabetes type 2, a fasting blood sample is usually taken in the morning, after a fast of 10 to 12 hours. The patient's fasting blood glucose (FBG) level should be less than 100 mg/dL. If it is higher than 105 mg/dL, the provider may request a blood *glucose tolerance test* (GTT). For this test, the fasting patient receives a sugary liquid to drink that contains 100 g of glucose. (The amount may be adjusted according to the patient's weight.) A blood sugar level of less than 140 mg/dL after 2 hours is normal. A reading of more than 200 mg/dL after 2 hours may indicate diabetes. A reading between 140 and 199 mg/dL indicates impaired glucose tolerance, or prediabetes.

Self-monitoring of blood glucose levels has become an important part of diabetes management. A very small amount of blood from a capillary puncture is drawn into a test strip in a glucose monitor. The test strip electronically calibrates the monitor and then tests the patient sample for blood glucose. These rapid-test glucose strips test the blood with the help of enzymes that convert glucose into a colored product that is measurable. The monitor detects and records the results and displays them on a small screen.

The medical assistant can screen a patient's blood glucose levels by using a glucometer cleared for home use by the US Food and Drug Administration (FDA) (see Procedure 33.6, p. 860). The blood glucose level is routinely monitored by patients with diabetes mellitus type 1 or type 2. Glucose levels may also be monitored by women with *gestational diabetes*, a condition seen during pregnancy in which the effect of insulin is partially blocked by hormones produced by the placenta (Fig. 33.12).

Hemoglobin A1c Testing

Hemoglobin A1c is also described as *glycosylated hemoglobin* (sugar-coated hemoglobin). Glycosylated hemoglobin is the result of glucose irreversibly binding to the hemoglobin molecules in the RBCs. It is also referred to as the A1c.

TABLE 33.8 Relationship Between Glycosylated Hemoglobin Levels and Blood Glucose Levels

GLYCOSYLATED HEMOGLOBIN A1c (%)	BLOOD GLUCOSE (mg/dL)
13.0	326
12.0	298
11.0	269
10.0	240
9.0	212
8.0	183
7.0	154
6.0	126
5.0	97
4.0	67

RBCs have a life span of approximately 120 days. Measuring the amount of glucose that has been irreversibly bound to hemoglobin provides an assessment of the average blood sugar during the 60 to 90 days before the test. The A1c test is performed every 3 months in patients with diabetes to monitor the person's average blood glucose level during those months. An A1c value higher than normal indicates that the average blood sugar has been elevated during the past 2 to 3 months. A normal A1c level for a person without diabetes ranges from 4% to 5.6%. For patients with diabetes, the goal is to maintain the glycosylated hemoglobin level below 7%. In Table 33.8 glycosylated hemoglobin A1c levels are associated with blood glucose levels. With higher levels, the risk of developing complications from diabetes increases.

Several methods can be used to measure the A1c level, and the medical assistant can perform A1c testing using several CLIA-waived devices. Patients also can perform A1c testing at home using FDA-approved instruments, such as the A1CNow SelfCheck (Bayer) and the in2it (II) Self-Test A1c System (Bio-Rad).

Cholesterol Testing

Cholesterol is a fatlike substance (lipid) present in cell membranes. It is needed to form bile acids, steroid hormones, the coverings of our nerves, and some of our brain tissue. Cholesterol travels in the blood as distinct particles containing both lipid and proteins. These particles are called *lipoproteins.* The cholesterol level in the blood is determined partly by inheritance and partly by acquired factors, such as diet, calorie and nutrient balance, and level of physical activity.

Patients often are confused by cholesterol testing. Cholesterol is often a catchall term for both the cholesterol a person eats and the cholesterol that is produced in the body. A high blood level of low-density lipoprotein, or LDL, cholesterol reflects an increased risk of heart disease. LDL cholesterol is often referred to as "bad" cholesterol. Lower levels of LDL cholesterol reflect a lower risk of heart disease.

When too much LDL cholesterol circulates in the blood, it can slowly build up in the walls of arteries that feed the heart and brain. Together with other substances, it can form *plaque,* a thick and sticky deposit that can clog arteries. This condition is known as *atherosclerosis.* If a clot (thrombus) forms at the site of plaque, blood flow can be blocked in the coronary arteries of the heart muscle, causing a heart attack. If a clot blocks blood flow to part of the brain, a stroke may result. LDL results are often interpreted as follows:

LDL >100 mg/dL = Optimal
LDL 100–129 = Near or above optimal
LDL 130–159 = Borderline high
LDL 160–189 = High
LDL 190+ = Very high

About one-third to one-fourth of blood cholesterol is carried by high-density lipoprotein (HDL). HDL cholesterol is known as the *good* cholesterol. High levels of HDL cholesterol seem to protect against heart attack. HDL can carry cholesterol away from the arteries and back to the liver. It is believed that cholesterol is removed from the lining of the arteries when high levels of HDL exist. Low levels of HDL cholesterol (i.e., lower than 40 mg/dL) may result in a greater risk of heart disease.

CRITICAL THINKING APPLICATION   33.6

One of Anita's favorite patients is in today, Sophie McCoy. She is 86 years young, still lives in her own home, and works in her garden every chance she gets. Sophie had a cholesterol screen at a local senior citizens health fair recently, and her results were as follows:

Total cholesterol 202 mg/dL, LDL 104 mg/dL, HDL 42 mg/dL

Given Sophie's age and general good health, are the cholesterol results concerning? Are they normal, high, or low?

Adults older than 20 years of age should have a cholesterol test at least once every 5 years. Total cholesterol and the combination of LDL and HDL typically are screened and monitored. All three tests are considered screening tests, and elevated results require additional testing. In general, total cholesterol levels under 200 mg/dL are considered normal. Results over 240 mg/dL are considered elevated and may place a person in the high-risk category for coronary heart disease. An HDL cholesterol level of 40 mg/dL or higher is considered acceptable for men, and values of 50 or higher are acceptable for women. HDL levels below 40 mg/dL for men and below 50 mg/dL for women place a person at risk of coronary heart disease.

Although total cholesterol and HDL cholesterol levels are not significantly affected by food consumption, most providers prefer that patients fast from food and liquids, with the exception of water, for 12 hours before cholesterol levels are checked. If the total cholesterol is elevated, the provider is likely to order a *lipid profile,* which is a series of tests that measures the total cholesterol, HDL and LDL cholesterol levels, and triglyceride levels. Triglycerides are fat in the blood related to caloric intake. Therefore, the patient must be instructed to fast from all food and alcoholic beverages 12 hours before the triglyceride test and/or lipid profiles. Consistently high triglyceride levels may lead to heart disease, especially in people with low levels of "good" HDL cholesterol and high levels of "bad" LDL cholesterol, and in people with diabetes type 2. Elevated levels of triglycerides are typically stored in belly fat and are associated with central obesity.

CLIA-waived cholesterol monitors can measure total cholesterol from a fingerstick specimen. The Cholestech LDX analyzer performs a lipid panel and provides a risk assessment using a capillary blood sample (see Procedure 33.7, p. 862). This system uses a cassette testing device capable of measuring glucose, total cholesterol (TC), HDL, LDL, very-low-density lipoprotein (VLDL), triglycerides, and the TC/HDL ratio. It uses a combination of testing methods to detect the color changes caused by each of the lipid panel analytes.

Thyroid Hormone Testing

The thyroid gland is located anterior to the trachea in the throat. It produces the hormones triiodothyronine (T_3) and thyroxine (T_4). These hormones are essential for life and regulate body metabolism, growth, and development. The thyroid gland is influenced by hormones produced by two other glands found in the brain, the pituitary gland and the hypothalamus. The pituitary gland produces thyroid-stimulating hormone (TSH), and the hypothalamus produces thyrotropin-releasing hormone (TRH). (Regulation of thyroid hormone production and thyroid disorders are discussed in Chapter 23.)

CLIA-waived rapid diagnostic tests are available to qualitatively measure TSH. These tests are available for point-of-care testing (POCT). Using whole blood from a fingerstick, CLIA-waived tests can screen patients for *hypothyroidism,* which is deficient activity of the thyroid gland. Hypothyroidism is indicated with elevated TSH levels. The tests use **lateral flow immunoassay** technology housed in a plastic cassette. One such commercially available test is the ThyroTest Whole Blood TSH Test.

REFERENCE LABORATORY CHEMISTRY PANELS AND SINGLE ANALYTE TESTING AND MONITORING

Automated blood chemistry analyzers are often used to perform blood chemistry testing in a reference laboratory. It is common for several analytes to be detected at once. A provider may order a chemistry panel, such as a renal or liver panel, to determine the levels of several related analytes (Fig. 33.13). Analytes commonly detected in the chemistry department are listed in Table 33.9. In general, serum from a clotted specimen is needed to perform these tests. Typical panels are shown in Table 33.10. As noted previously, laboratory reports, both electronic and paper, must provide their own reference ranges, along with each patient's results. Different methodologies may generate different reference ranges and may use different units of measurement.

CLOSING COMMENTS

Patient Coaching

As with all other procedures, the laboratory test is only as valid as the specimen and the procedure performed on that specimen. You, as the provider's agent, are responsible for that validity when you instruct the patient and when you perform the test. Be clear in your instructions. Give written materials to reinforce your instructions. Ask the patient if he or she has any questions and take the time and effort to answer the questions in a way that is clear and understandable to the patient. If the patient has additional questions that you cannot answer, have the provider talk to the patient directly.

Legal and Ethical Issues

A medical assistant who is responsible for POL testing must clearly understand the basic concepts of laboratory medicine. Therefore, you must stay current with the rapid technologic advances in laboratory medicine and help establish a protocol for testing that best suits your provider-employer.

You are responsible for properly collecting specimens and testing them accurately. Patient confidentiality is paramount when testing is performed, as is strictly conforming to all established quality control procedures.

Patient-Centered Care

The MA plays an important role in the laboratory and patient care. Often many different tests are needed to assess a patient's health. Many patients appreciate that they can have CLIA-waived tests done during a routine visit to their provider. With a simple fingerstick a patient can have tests such as a hemoglobin and hematocrit, protime, A1c, blood glucose, cholesterol, and ALT/AST completed in the POL. Saving patients time and the inconvenience of going to a different location are just a few benefits of having a CLIA-waived POL. Also, having test results available quickly and while patients are still in the clinic gives them the opportunity to ask questions and have them answered on the spot.

TABLE 33.9 Blood Chemistry Tests[a]				
TEST	**ABBREVIATION**	**NORMAL VALUES**	**DESCRIPTION**	**PURPOSE**
Alanine aminotransferase *Some CLIA-waived available*	ALT (SGPT)	<45 units/L	Enzyme found predominantly in the liver but also in the kidney	To detect liver disease
Albumin *Some CLIA-waived available*		3.5–5 g/dL	Protein	To assess kidney function
Alkaline phosphatase *Some CLIA-waived available*	ALP	20–70 units/L	Enzyme found in several tissues	To detect liver and bone disease

TABLE 33.9 Blood Chemistry Tests[a]—*continued*

TEST	ABBREVIATION	NORMAL VALUES	DESCRIPTION	PURPOSE
Aspartate aminotransferase *Some CLIA-waived available*	AST (SGOT)	<40 units/L	Enzyme found in several tissues	To detect tissue damage
Blood urea nitrogen *Some CLIA-waived available*	BUN	7–18 mg/dL *or* 2.5–6.4 mmol/L	Metabolic product of protein catabolism	To detect renal disease
Calcium *Some CLIA-waived available*	Ca	8.4–10.2 mg/dL *or* 2.1–2.6 mmol/L	Mineral	To assess parathyroid function and calcium metabolism
Chloride *Some CLIA-waived available*	Cl	98–106 mmol/L	Electrolyte	To determine acid-base and water balance
Cholesterol *Some CLIA-waived available*	CH, Chol	*Total:* <200 mg/dL *or* <5.18 mmol/L *LDL:* <130 mg/dL *or* <3.37 mmol/L *HDL:* >35 mg/dL *or* >0.91 mmol/L	Lipid	To screen for atherosclerosis related to heart disease
Creatine kinase *Some CLIA-waived available*	CK	Specific to testing method used	Enzyme found in several tissues	To assess source of muscle damage (myocardial infarct)
Creatinine *Some CLIA-waived available*	creat	0.2–0.8 mg/dL	Metabolic product of protein catabolism	To screen for renal function
Ferritin		20–50 ng/mL	Iron-carrying protein	To detect amount of iron stored in the body
Gamma glutamyl transferase *Some CLIA-waived available*	GGT	0–45 units/L	Enzyme found mainly in liver cells	To detect liver disease
Globulin	glob, Ig	Varies according to type	Protein	To detect abnormalities in protein synthesis and removal
Glucose fasting blood sugar *Some CLIA-waived available*	FBS	70–100 mg/dL *or* 3.9–6.1 mmol/L	Carbohydrate	To detect disorders of glucose metabolism (diabetes)
Glucose tolerance test	GTT	Varies with time	Carbohydrate	To detect disorders of glucose metabolism (diabetes)
Iron	Fe	35–140 mcg/dL	Mineral	To assist in diagnosis of anemia
Lactate dehydrogenase	LDH	<240 units/L	Enzyme found in several tissues	To assist in confirmation of myocardial or pulmonary infarct
pH *Some CLIA-waived available*	pH	7.35–7.45	Measurement of the acid-base (acidity and alkalinity)	To assess acidity or alkalinity of blood
Phosphorus *Some CLIA-waived available*	P	3–4.5 mg/dL *or* 0.97–1.45 mmol/L	Mineral	To assist in proper evaluation of calcium levels and to detect endocrine system disorders
Potassium *Some CLIA-waived available*	K	3.5–5.1 mmol/L	Mineral	To assist in diagnosis of acid-base and water balance
Sodium *Some CLIA-waived available*	Na	135–146 mmol/L	Mineral	To assist in diagnosis of acid-base and water balance

Continued

TABLE 33.9 Blood Chemistry Tests[a]—*continued*

TEST	ABBREVIATION	NORMAL VALUES	DESCRIPTION	PURPOSE
Total bilirubin *Some CLIA-waived available*	TB	0.2–1 mg/dL *or* 3.4–17.1 mmol/L	Metabolic product of hemoglobin catabolism	To evaluate liver function and to aid in diagnosis of anemia
Total iron-binding capacity	TIBC	245–400 mcg/dL		A measure of the potential to transport iron
Total protein *Some CLIA-waived available*	TP	6–8 g/dL; 60–80 g/L		To assess the state of hydration; to screen for diseases that alter protein balance
Troponin I and T		<0.4	Cardiac-specific protein found only with heart muscle damage	To aid in diagnosis of myocardial infarction
Thyroid-stimulating hormone (thyrotropin) *Some CLIA-waived available*	TSH	5–6 milliunits/L	Hormone produced by the pituitary	To assess thyroid and pituitary gland function
Thyroxine	T_4	5–12 mcg/dL *or* 64–155 mmol/L	Hormone produced by the thyroid gland	To assess thyroid function
Triglycerides *Some CLIA-waived available*	Trig	30–190 mg/dL *or* 0.34–2.15 mmol/L		To screen for atherosclerosis related to heart disease
Triiodothyronine	T_3	27%–47%	Hormone produced by the thyroid gland	To assess thyroid function
Uric acid *Some CLIA-waived available*	UA	*Male*: 3.4–7 mg/dL *or* 202–416 mcmol/L *Female*: 2.4–6 mg/dL *or* 143–357 mcmol/L	Metabolic product of protein catabolism	To evaluate renal failure, gout, and leukemia

[a]Lab reports, both electronic and paper, must supply their own reference ranges, along with each patient's results. This is because different methodologies may create different reference ranges and different units of measurement.

TABLE 33.10 Typical Chemistry Panels

PANEL	COMPONENT	PANEL	COMPONENT
Liver	Alkaline phosphatase (ALP) Gamma glutamyl transferase (GGT) Aspartate aminotransferase (AST) Alanine aminotransferase (ALT) Lactate dehydrogenase (LDH)	**Cardiac**	Creatine kinase (CK) Troponin I Troponin T
Anemia	Iron Total iron-binding capacity Ferritin Transferrin	**Electrolyte**	Sodium Potassium Chloride
Thyroid	Thyroid-stimulating hormone (TSH) Thyroxine (T_4) Triiodothyronine (T_3)	**Renal**	Creatinine Blood urea nitrogen (BUN) Uric acid Glucose

Physician's Medical Center
77332 E. Capital Drive
Anytown, USA 11123

Ronald J. Haldor, M.D.
Kaye M. Jones, M.D.
Nicholas P. Stepp, M.D.

PATIENT – PLEASE NOTE

If this box is checked, don't eat or drink anything, except water, for 14 hours before going to the lab.

PATIENT NAME_____
LAST   FIRST   M.I.
ADDRESS _____ DOB_____
CITY_____ STATE____ ZIP_____ SEX: M F
TELEPHONE # _____ SOCIAL SECURITY #____–__–____
ORDERING PHYSICIAN_____ DATE_____
BILLING: ☐ HMO ☐ MEDICARE ☐ MEDICAL ☐ OTHER #_____
GUARANTOR (If other than patient)_____
☐ PHONE RESULTS TO_____
☐ SEND ADDITIONAL COPIES OF REPORT TO_____
(Please attach copy of eligibilty card.)

Patient Diagnosis _____

☐ 906 ARTERIAL BLOOD GASES
ROOM AIR_____
RESP. ASSIST_____
☐ 105 BLOOD CELL PROFILE (Hgb + Hct)
☐ 862 BILIRUBIN (NEONATAL)
☐ 868 BILIRUBIN (TOTAL & DIRECT)
☐ 100 CBC (Complete Blood Count & Diff)
☐ 3000 ELECTROLYTES
☐   (NA, K, CO2, Cl)
☐   FANA
☐   GLUCOSE
☐ 915 GLUCOSE, PRE-NATAL DIABETIC SCR.
(1 Hour Post-Glucola)
☐   GLUCOSE TOLERANCE TEST
OF HOURS_____DOSE_____
☐ 3398 HEPATITIS PANEL
(B-Surf Ag/Ab, B-Core Ab, A-Ab)
☐ 988 LIPID PROFILE
(Chol, Trig, HDL, LDL, Cardiac Risk)
☐ 3380 LIVER PANEL
(Alk Phos, Bili, TP, Alb, GGT, SGOT
(AST) SGPT (ALT), & Consult)
☐ 3006 METABOLIC 7
(Na, K, CO2, Cl, Glu, Mg)

☐ 3035 PANEL 17
(Panel 13 + Na + K + Cl + CO2)
☐ 3020 METABOLIC 10
(Na, K, CO2, Cl, Glu, BUN, Creat)
☐ 3015 METABOLIC 11
(Met 10 & Phos)
☐ 3160 OBSTETRICAL PANEL 1
(CBC, UA, ABO/Rh, Antibody
Screen, Rubella, RPR)
☐ 3172 OBSTETRICAL PANEL 3
(CBC, ABO/Rh, Antibody Screen,
Rubella, RPR)
☐ 3445 OBSTETRICAL PANEL 7
(ABO/Rh, Antibody Screen,
Rubella, RPR)
☐ 3447 OBSTETRICAL PANEL 7A
(ABO/Rh, Antibody Screen,
Rubella, RPR, Hepatitis B Surt Ag)
☐ 3025 PANEL 13
(Glu, BUN, Creat, Uric Acid, Ca,
Tp, Alb, Bili, Chol, Alk, Phos,
SGOT (AST), LDH, Phos)
☐ 3030 PANEL 15
(Panel 13 + Na + K)

☐ 3010 METABOLIC 8
(Na, K, CO2, Cl, Glu, BUN)
☐ 3040 PANEL 20 - SMAC
(Panel 17 + SGPT (ALT) +
GGT + Osmolality)
☐ 3043 S-1 Panel (Panel 20 + Triglyceride)
☐ 500 PROTHROMBIN TIME (PT)
☐ 505 Partial Thromboplastin Time (PPT)
☐ 7500 RPR
☐ 7515 RUBELLA
☐ 2030 THYROID SCREEN
(T4, T3, Uptake, Adj T4)
☐ 704 URINALYSIS

BACTERIOLOGY

SPECIMEN SOURCE (REQUIRED)
COLLECTION DATE_____
☐ ____ ROUTINE CULTURE
☐ 8919 AFB CULTURE
☐ 8921 FUNGAL CULTURE

ADDITIONAL LABORATORY TESTS: _____

2804 (4/2019)

LABORATORY OUTPATIENT REQUEST

OFFICE USE ONLY
Telephone Order per_____
Order Received by_____

FIGURE 33.13 Panel request form.

Professional Behaviors

An ever-increasing number of CLIA-waived hematology and chemistry blood tests are relatively simple to perform and require minimal training. This allows the provider to share the results with the patient quickly, which may result in greater patient compliance with the prescribed treatment plan. Proper patient care demands attention to detail in all three areas of the testing process:

- *Preanalytic:* Proper care of the testing supplies and equipment, and proper patient identification and specimen collection

- *Analytic:* Running the tests according to the specific manufacturer's instructions; recording and analyzing the controls and the patient results
- *Postanalytic:* Proper disposal of biohazard supplies; routing of test results to the provider and patient

The medical assistant is involved in all three areas of testing. He or she is responsible for the organization and documentation of each performed test on the appropriate lab flow sheet and in the patient's health record.

SUMMARY OF SCENARIO

It has been another busy day for Anita at WMFM. She had a chance to see a variety of patients with a variety of concerns. It was a normal day at work! Anita enjoys the variety. She also enjoys the work she does with the laboratory. Anita prepares specimens for transport to the reference lab. She checks on results once they are posted in patients' electronic medical records. She knows that Dr. Perez and all the providers at WMFM rely on lab results as part of patient diagnosis and monitoring treatment.

Another good day at work. Now Anita is going to go home and try to get a little gardening done!

SUMMARY OF LEARNING OBJECTIVES

1. **Name the main functions of blood.**

   Blood contains RBCs to deliver oxygen to tissues through hemoglobin, WBCs to fight infections, and platelets to aid in coagulation and the formation of clots. The plasma carries needed nutrients to the cells throughout the body and removes waste products from the cells and carries them to the lungs and kidneys for elimination.

2. **Describe the appearance and function of erythrocytes, leukocytes, and platelets. Also, discuss plasma.**

   Erythrocytes are also called *red blood cells* because of their red color, which comes from hemoglobin. The biconcave disks lack a nucleus and are responsible for transporting oxygen and carbon dioxide to and from tissues.

   Leukocytes are also called *white blood cells.* Agranular leukocytes lack granules in the cytoplasm, and granular leukocytes have granules. All leukocytes function in fighting infection.

   A thrombocyte (platelet) is a fragment of a larger cell (megakaryocyte) found in the bone marrow. Thrombocytes play an important role in clot formation, both physically and chemically. Clot formation begins with the aggregation of thrombocytes, which release a substance that initiates the clotting cascade, resulting in a network of minute threads that trap plasma and blood cells. Plasma is approximately 90% water and is the carrier for the formed elements and other substances.

3. **Explain the purpose of the microhematocrit test. Describe how to collect a microhematocrit specimen and perform a microhematocrit test.**

   A microhematocrit (or hematocrit) test is performed to assess the volume of erythrocytes in relation to the total blood volume. The test is performed by centrifuging a small amount of whole blood in a capillary tube. Whole blood normally consists of slightly less than 50% RBCs. Hematocrit is reported as a percentage and is roughly three times the value of hemoglobin in the same specimen. See Procedure 33.2 for specimen collection and how to perform a microhematocrit test.

4. **Describe how to obtain a specimen for and perform a hemoglobin test.**
   Refer to Procedure 33.3.

5. **Cite the reasons for performing an erythrocyte sedimentation rate (ESR) test, discuss the sources of error for ESR testing, and determine and record an erythrocyte sedimentation rate obtained by using a modified Westergren method.**

   An ESR test is performed to assess inflammation and often is used to monitor rheumatoid arthritis. This test measures the rate at which RBCs fall in a calibrated tube in a 60-minute period.

   An ESR test result may be erroneous if a tube is not standing vertically in the rack; bubbles are present in the Sediplast or Streck ESR tube; dilutions are incorrect; vibrations or jarring occurs; the blood is at a temperature other than room temperature; and the blood has hemolyzed.

   Refer to Procedure 33.4 for the steps in determining the erythrocyte sedimentation rate using a modified Westergren method.

6. **Explain the purpose of a prothrombin time (PT) test, and describe how to obtain a specimen for and perform a CLIA-waived prothrombin time/international normalized ratio (PT/INR) test. Also, explain how you could reassure a patient of the accuracy of PT/INR test results.**

   The PT is a method of measuring how well the blood clots and is used in combination with the partial thromboplastin time (PTT) to screen for hemophilia and other hereditary clotting disorders. It is important to educate patients who take warfarin (Coumadin) about the need for follow-up laboratory monitoring of their protime/INR. Helping patients identify foods high in vitamin K is crucial to maintaining a balance between the warfarin dosage and the lab values.

   Refer to Procedure 33.5 for information on how you can reassure a patient of the accuracy of PT/INR test results.

7. **Identify the tests included in a complete blood count (CBC) and their reference ranges and differentiate between normal and abnormal test results.**

   In the hematology laboratory, blood cells are counted, WBCs are differentiated, and the oxygen-carrying capacity of blood is determined. Hematology testing provides an excellent overview of homeostasis. The CBC involves an erythrocyte count, leukocyte count, thrombocyte

SUMMARY OF LEARNING OBJECTIVES—*continued*

count, hemoglobin and hematocrit determination, differential examination of leukocytes, and calculation of red cell indices. Refer to the hematology diagnostic reference ranges in Table 33.5 and Fig. 33.7.

8. **Explain the reasons for performing a white blood cell (WBC) count and differential and discuss the preparation of blood smears for the differential.**

A differential WBC count is performed to assess the percentages of the five types of WBCs in the blood. In addition, the red cells and platelets are examined for distribution and abnormalities. A blood smear is prepared by placing a drop of blood from a fingerstick, or from an EDTA tube using a DIFF-SAFE blood dispenser, onto a clean glass slide that is free of dust and grease. A thin smear of whole blood is spread across the slide, and then stained, typically with Wright's stain, followed by microscopic examination.

9. **Differentiate between the ABO blood groupings and the Rh blood groupings. Also, discuss legal and ethical issues related to blood transfusions.**

Both the ABO blood type and the Rh type result from antigens on the surfaces of RBCs, and both groups are crucial when it comes to transfusion. There are four different ABO types (A, AB, B, and O). The body produces natural antibodies against the AB antigens that are not present in the blood cells. For example, if a person has type A antigens on the cells, there will be anti-B antibodies in the plasma. A type O blood type would have both anti-A antibodies and anti-B antibodies because they are both foreign to someone with type O blood. There are only two Rh types (positive and negative). Unlike the ABO group,

an Rh-negative blood type does not have natural antibodies against Rh-positive cells. The Rh-negative individual must first be exposed to Rh-positive cells via transfusion or childbirth, which initiates the formation of anti-Rh antibodies that attack and destroy Rh-positive cells.

10. **Do the following related to blood chemistry in the physician office laboratory:**
    - *Explain the reasons for testing blood glucose, hemoglobin A1c, cholesterol, liver enzymes, and thyroid hormones.*
    The blood glucose level is monitored routinely in patients with diabetes type 1 or type 2 and in women who have gestational diabetes during pregnancy. Hemoglobin A1c levels are measured to determine the average blood glucose level during the 2 to 3 months before the test; this test assists in the management of diabetes. Cholesterol testing generally refers to assessing levels of total cholesterol, HDL, and LDL; it is done to help determine a patient's susceptibility to coronary artery disease. Liver enzyme testing (ALT and AST) is performed in the POL primarily to monitor the side effects of certain therapeutic drugs, such as those used to treat elevated cholesterol and diabetes. Thyroid testing is performed in the POL to detect elevated TSH levels and to assist in the diagnosis of hypothyroidism. Refer to Table 33.10.
    - *Assist a provider by performing a blood glucose test.*
    Refer to Procedure 33.6 on p. 860.
    - *Determine a cholesterol level or lipid profile using a cholesterol chemistry analyzer.*
    Refer to Procedure 33.7 on p. 862.

PROCEDURE 33.1 Perform Preventive Maintenance for the Microhematocrit Centrifuge

Task: Perform daily, monthly, semiannual, and annual maintenance on a microhematocrit centrifuge.

EQUIPMENT and SUPPLIES

- Microhematocrit centrifuge
- Maintenance logbook
- Utility gloves
- Fluid-impermeable lab coat, eye protection, and gloves
- Disinfectant
- Biohazard waste container

PROCEDURAL STEPS

- *Note:* These are general recommendations. Always check the manufacturer's guidelines for specific instructions.
- *Personal protective equipment* (PPE): Wash hands or use hand sanitizer. Put on fluid-impermeable lab coat, eye protection, and gloves. In all maintenance procedures, gloves are worn under the utility gloves.
- Always unplug the power cord before cleaning or servicing the centrifuge.

Daily Maintenance
1. Clean the inside of the centrifuge and the gasket with a disinfectant recommended by the manufacturer. Plastic and nonmetal parts may be cleaned

with a fresh solution of 5% sodium hypochlorite (bleach) mixed to a 1:10 dilution with water (1 part bleach plus 9 parts water).
PURPOSE: To remove any dried blood or shattered glass. Do not use bleach on the gasket because it may harden the rubber.

Monthly Maintenance
1. Check the reading device. Misuse and zeroing of reading devices can result in considerable error. Always use a second, simple reading device as a cross-check. Use a ruler or a flat plastic card specially made for this purpose. To use these cards, lay the spun hematocrit tube on the card and align the red cells with a line on the card to obtain the reading.
PURPOSE: To ensure accuracy of quality control and patient results
2. Check the rotor for cracks or corrosion and check the interior for signs of white powder.
PURPOSE: Cracks, corrosion, or powder may indicate impending rotor failure; these findings require the immediate attention of a service technician.
3. Record all preventive maintenance in the laboratory logbook.
PURPOSE: Recording maintenance is necessary to maintain warranties and to comply with regulations established by CLIA and other regulatory agencies.

Continued

PROCEDURE 33.1   Perform Preventive Maintenance for the Microhematocrit Centrifuge—*continued*

Semiannual Maintenance

1. Check the gasket for cuts and breaks.
   PURPOSE: Cut gaskets allow tubes to leak and must be replaced.
2. Check the timer with a stopwatch to verify timer accuracy.
   PURPOSE: To ensure timer accuracy.
3. Perform a maximum cell pack to verify the time required for complete packing by reading a sample after centrifugation and then recentrifuging for 1 minute. The results should be the same. If they are not, perform preventive maintenance and/or call the service technician.
   PURPOSE: If the cells compact further during recentrifugation, the centrifuge is not rotating at the proper speed, and hematocrit results will be falsely elevated.
4. Record all preventive measures in the equipment maintenance log.
   PURPOSE: Recording maintenance is necessary to maintain warranties and to comply with regulations established by CLIA and other regulatory agencies.

Annual Maintenance (or Maintenance Performed as Needed)

1. The centrifuge functions and maintenance verification should be performed by qualified personnel. This includes checking the centrifuge mechanism, rotors, timer, speed, and electrical leads.
   PURPOSE: To ensure proper centrifuge function.
2. Record all professional service calls in the laboratory logbook.
   PURPOSE: Proper documentation is essential for all laboratory maintenance.

MICROHEMATOCRIT CENTRIFUGE MAINTENANCE LOG

DATE	SERVICE	INITIALS
10/7/20XX	Performed routine daily and monthly preventive maintenance	AJ

Comments:

PROCEDURE 33.2   Perform CLIA-Waived Hematology Testing: Perform a Microhematocrit Test

Task: Perform a microhematocrit test accurately.

EQUIPMENT and SUPPLIES

- Patient's health record
- Provider's order and/or lab requisition
- Microhematocrit lab log
- Fresh sample of blood collected in a tube containing ethylenediaminetetraacetic acid (EDTA) anticoagulant (or equipment for fingerstick specimen: lancet, alcohol wipe, gauze, bandage)
- Plastic-coated self-sealing capillary tubes, or plain capillary tubes (blue-tipped)
- Sealing clay (if capillary tubes are not self-sealing)
- Gauze
- Microhematocrit centrifuge
- Fluid-impermeable lab coat, protective eyewear, and gloves
- Biohazard waste container
- Biohazard sharps containers

PROCEDURAL STEPS

1. Wash hands or use hand sanitizer. Put on fluid-impermeable lab coat, protective eyewear, and gloves.
   PURPOSE: To ensure infection control.
2. Assemble the materials needed.
   a. *If the capillary tubes are self-sealing:* Fill two tubes by inserting the end opposite the sealed end into the well-mixed EDTA blood sample. *Note:* If the capillary tube and the EDTA tube are held almost parallel to the table, the capillary tubes fill easily by capillary action. When the self-sealing capillary tubes are two-thirds to three-fourths filled, tilt them upright, causing the blood sample to flow down the tube and meet the sealant. Continue to hold the tube vertical when the blood contacts the sealant for an additional 15 seconds.
   PURPOSE: Duplicates should always be done as a means of quality control.

   b. *Alternative:* Fill two plain (blue-tipped) capillary tubes two-thirds to three-fourths full of a well-mixed EDTA blood sample. Tip the blood tube slightly, touching the capillary tube into the blood using the side that is opposite the blue band. When enough blood has filled the capillary tube, tip the blue end of the tube down, causing the blood to flow toward the blue tip. Then readjust the tube horizontally while inserting the blue tip of the capillary tube into the clay sealant. Insert the tube as many times as needed to achieve a plug up to the blue band (see Fig. 1).
   PURPOSE: Duplicates should always be done as a means of quality control. Tubes are not filled completely to provide space for the sealing clay.

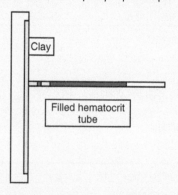

1

3. Wipe the outside of the tubes with clean gauze without touching the wet open end of the tube.
   PURPOSE: Wiping the outside of the capillary tube removes any blood. Touching the blood inside the capillary tube with absorbent material removes more plasma than blood cells and can alter the hematocrit.

PROCEDURE 33.2 Perform CLIA-Waived Hematology Testing: Perform a Microhematocrit Test—*continued*

4. Place the tubes opposite each other in the centrifuge with the sealed ends securely against the gasket (see Fig. 33.1).
   PURPOSE: The centrifuge must always be balanced to prevent damage. If the clay ends of the capillary tubes are not outermost against the gasket, the sample will spin out of the tubes, contaminating the centrifuge.
5. Note the numbers on the centrifuge slots and record the numbers on the log sheet, along with the patient's name
   PURPOSE: The sample must be identified throughout the entire procedure.
6. Secure the locking top, fasten the lid down, and lock it.
   PURPOSE: If the locking top is not firmly in place during the spinning cycle, the tubes will come out of their slots and break. The lid is always locked during centrifugation for safety purposes, to prevent the ejection of aerosols or broken glass.
7. Set the timer and adjust the speed as needed.
   PURPOSE: The prescribed time is 3 to 5 minutes at 11,000 to 12,000 rpm. Check the manufacturer's instructions for time and speed.
8. Allow the centrifuge to come to a complete stop. Unlock the outer locking top and then remove the inner lid.
   PURPOSE: Opening the centrifuge before it has stopped could result in harm to the user.
9. Remove the tubes immediately and read the results. If this is not possible, store the tubes in an upright position.
   PURPOSE: Tubes left in the centrifuge will show altered results because the red blood cell (RBC) layer will spread out horizontally
10. Determine the microhematocrit values using one of the following methods:
    a. Centrifuge with built-in reader using calibrated capillary tubes.
       (1) Position the tubes as directed by the manufacturer's instructions.
       (2) Read both tubes.
       (3) The average of the two results is reported.
       (4) The two values should not vary by more than 2%.
    b. Centrifuge without a built-in reader.
       (1) Carefully remove the tubes from the centrifuge.
       (2) Place a tube on the microhematocrit reader.
       (3) Align the clay-RBC junction with the zero line on the reader. Align the plasma meniscus with the 100% line. The value is read at

the junction of the red cell layer and the buffy coat. The buffy coat is not included in the reading (see Fig. 2).
(4) Read both tubes.
(5) The average of the two results is reported.
(6) The two values should not vary by more than 2%.

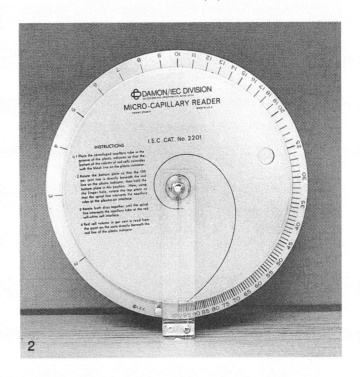

2

11. Dispose of the capillary tubes in a biohazard sharps container.
12. Disinfect the work area and properly dispose of all biohazard materials. Remove your gloves, eyewear, and lab coat. Wash hands or use hand sanitizer.
    PURPOSE: To ensure infection control.
13. Record the results in the Hematocrit Patient Log and document the results in the patient's medical record.
    PURPOSE: A procedure is not considered done until it is charted.

HEMATOCRIT—PATIENT LOG

Hematocrit expected values:	Adult Males = 42–52%
	Adult Females = 36–48%
	Infants = 32–38%
	Children = increase to adult

DATE	TECH	PATIENT I.D.	SLOT #	RESULT	CHARTED
10/7/20–	dc	# 12345	1 & 4	44% & 44%	✓

Documentation Example
10/07/20XX 11:25 a.m. Hct 44%._____Anita James, CMA (AAMA)

| PROCEDURE 33.3 | Perform CLIA-Waived Hematology Testing: Perform a Hemoglobin Test |

Task: Accurately determine the level of hemoglobin present in a blood sample using the HemoCue B-Hemoglobin System.

EQUIPMENT and SUPPLIES

- Patient's health record
- Provider's order and/or lab requisition
- Hemoglobin laboratory log
- HemoCue monitor
- HemoCue microcuvette
- Safety blood lancet
- Alcohol wipes
- Gauze
- Fluid-impermeable lab coat, protective eyewear, and gloves
- Biohazard waste container
- Biohazard sharps containers

PROCEDURAL STEPS

1. Perform an instrument quality control check by inserting the control cuvette into the instrument. Make sure the reading is within acceptable limits before proceeding.
   PURPOSE: Only instruments that record values within acceptable control limits can be used for patient testing. If the value is outside the control limits, refer to the troubleshooting guide for the instrument or contact the manufacturer.
2. Wash your hands or use hand sanitizer. Put on fluid-impermeable lab coat, protective eyewear, and gloves.
   PURPOSE: To ensure infection control.
3. Assemble all equipment and supplies needed.
4. Greet the patient. Identify yourself. Verify the patient's identity with the full name; ask the patient to spell the first and last name and to give his or her date of birth. Explain the procedure to be performed in a manner that is understood by the patient. Answer any questions the patient may have on the procedure. Obtain permission for the capillary puncture.
   PURPOSE: It is important to identify the patient in two different ways to ensure that you have the correct patient. Explaining the procedure can make the patient feel more comfortable and helps to reduce anxiety.
5. Examine the patient's fingers and choose the site to be used to obtain the blood sample.
   PURPOSE: The site must be free of trauma, calluses, and scarring.
6. Clean the site with an alcohol wipe or another recommended antiseptic preparation.
   PURPOSE: To ensure a properly cleaned puncture site; infection control.
7. Perform a capillary puncture and wipe away the first drop of blood.
   PURPOSE: This drop may contain tissue fluid or antiseptic that may hemolyze the blood.
8. Obtain a large drop of blood on the surface of the finger.
   PURPOSE: To ensure enough blood for an adequate sample.
9. Touch the microcuvette to the drop of blood. Do not touch the finger. The correct volume is drawn into the cuvette by capillary action. Wipe off any excess blood from the sides of the cuvette (see Figs. 1 and 2).

PURPOSE: Blood on the cuvette may alter the readings or contaminate the instrument.

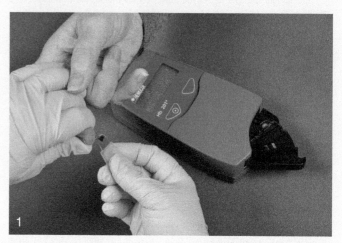

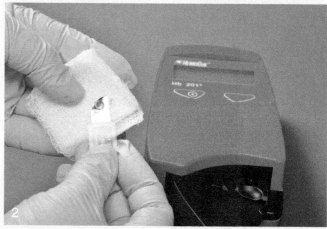

10. Place the cuvette in the cuvette holder of the HemoCue sample door and close the door of the instrument (see Fig. 3).
    PURPOSE: To begin the testing process.

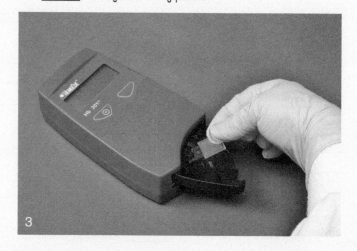

PROCEDURE 33.3 | Perform CLIA-Waived Hematology Testing: Perform a Hemoglobin Test—*continued*

11. Read the result and record it in the lab's hemoglobin log and the patient's health record.
PURPOSE: A procedure is not completed until the results are recorded.
12. Dispose of biohazard waste in the biohazard waste containers. Turn off the instrument. Properly disinfect the work area.

13. Remove your gloves and dispose of them in the biohazard waste container. Remove the lab coat and protective eyewear. Wash hands or use hand sanitizer.
PURPOSE: To ensure infection control.

HEMOCUE B HEMOGLOBIN SYSTEM PATIENT LOG

TEST: _____ KIT LOT # _____

Hemoglobin expected values= Adult Males = 13.0–18.0 g/dL
Adult Females = 12.0–16.0 g/dL
Infants = 10.0–14.0 g/dL
Children = increase to adult

DATE	TECH	PATIENT I.D.	RESULT	CHARTED
10/09/20–	DC	# 12345	15.5 g/dL	✓

Documentation Example
10/09/20 9:30 a.m. Hgb 15.5 g/dL._____Anita James, CMA (AAMA)

PROCEDURE 33.4 | Perform CLIA-Waived Hematology Testing: Determine the Erythrocyte Sedimentation Rate Using a Modified Westergren Method

Task: Fill a Westergren tube properly and observe and record an erythrocyte sedimentation rate (ESR) obtained by using a modified Westergren method.

EQUIPMENT and SUPPLIES

- Patient's health record
- Provider's order and/or lab requisition
- Erythrocyte sedimentation rate (ESR) laboratory log
- Ethylenediaminetetraacetic acid (EDTA) — anticoagulated blood specimen
- Safety tube decapper (if tubes do not have Hemogard plastic tops)
- Disposable transfer pipet
- Sediplast ESR system (prefilled Sediplast vial)
- Sediplast rack
- Timer
- Fluid-impermeable lab coat, eye protection, and gloves
- Biohazard waste container
- Biohazard sharps container

PROCEDURAL STEPS

1. Wash hands or use hand sanitizer. Put on a fluid-impermeable lab coat, eye protection, and gloves.
PURPOSE: To ensure infection control.
2. Assemble the materials needed.
3. Check the leveling bubble of the Sediplast rack.
PURPOSE: The rack must be horizontal on the table or bench to ensure that the tube is vertical.
4. Bring the blood sample to room temperature if it has been refrigerated and mix the sample well by gently inverting the tube 6 to 8 times, making sure the tube has no bubbles.
PURPOSE: Cells settle when a specimen stands, and blood must always be well mixed before sampling. Test results will be altered if refrigerated blood is not brought to room temperature.

Continued

PROCEDURE 33.4	Perform CLIA-Waived Hematology Testing: Determine the Erythrocyte Sedimentation Rate Using a Modified Westergren Method—*continued*

5. Remove the plastic Hemogard stopper on the blood sample by twisting and slowly pushing up on the stopper with your thumbs (or by using a tube decapper on rubber-stoppered blood tubes). Also remove the stopper on the prefilled Sediplast vial.
   PURPOSE: Using the Hemogard cover or removing the rubber cap with a protective device blocks blood splashes and helps prevent aerosolization of the specimen.

6. Fill the Sediplast vial with blood to the indicated line using a disposable transfer pipet (see Fig. 1). Replace the stopper on the prefilled vial and invert it several times to mix. Recap the blood collection tube with its stopper.
   PURPOSE: This dilutes the blood in accordance with the Westergren procedure.

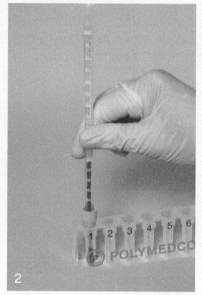

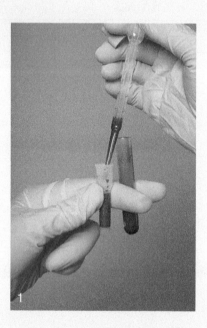

7. Insert a Sediplast pipet through the pierceable stopper on the prefilled vial and push down until the pipet touches the bottom of the vial. The pipet automatically draws the blood up and over the zero mark (see Fig. 2).

8. Insert the filled Sediplast pipet and its vial into the Sediplast rack, making sure the vial is vertical.
   PURPOSE: A pipet that is not vertical produces incorrect results.

9. Note the start time on the ESR log sheet and allow the vial to stand undisturbed for 60 minutes.
   PURPOSE: Jarring or moving the vial increases the sedimentation rate.

10. After 60 minutes, measure the distance the erythrocytes have fallen at the top of the tube. The scale reads in millimeters — each line is 1 mm.
    PURPOSE: Precise timing is important with this test method.

11. Properly dispose of all biohazard materials. Disinfect the work area. Dispose of the plastic Sediplast pipet and its vial into a biohazard sharps container. Remove your gloves, protective eyewear, and lab coat. Wash hands or use hand sanitizer.
    PURPOSE: To ensure infection control.

12. Record the findings in the lab's ESR log and the patient's health record. Remember: the Westergren ESR is reported in millimeters per hour (mm/hr).
    PURPOSE: A procedure is not considered complete until it is recorded.

ESR—SEDIPLAST—PATIENT LOG

ESR expected values: Adult Males < 50 years = 0–15 mm/hr
                       Adult Males > 50 years = 0–20 mm/hr
                       Adult Females < 50 years = 0–20 mm/hr
                       Adult Females > 50 years = 0–30 mm/hr

DATE	TECH	PATIENT I.D.	SLOT #	TIME	RESULT	CHARTED
10/09/20–	DC	# 12345	2	60 min	15 mm	✓

Documentation Example
10/09/20XX 9:30 a.m. ESR 15 mm in 60 minutes._____ Anita James, CMA (AAMA)

PROCEDURE 33.5   Perform a CLIA-Waived Protime/INR Test

Task: Perform a coagulation test to determine protime/INR using the CoaguChek XS instrument with built-in quality control.

EQUIPMENT and SUPPLIES

- Patient's health record or flow chart (see Fig. 33.6)
- Provider's order and/or lab requisition
- PT/INR lab log
- Gauze, alcohol wipes, bandage
- CoaguChek XS PT Test monitor (see Fig. 33.5)
- CoaguChek lancet
- CoaguChek test strip container and code chip
- Package insert or flow chart with directions
- Fluid-impermeable lab coat, protective eyewear, and gloves
- Biohazard waste container
- Biohazard sharps containers

PROCEDURAL STEPS

1. Wash hands or use hand sanitizer. Put on fluid-impermeable lab coat, protective eyewear, and gloves.
   PURPOSE: To ensure infection control.
2. Assemble the materials needed.
3. If you are using test strips from a new, unopened container, you must change the test strip code chip. The three-number code on the test strip container must match the three-number code on the code strip. To install the code strip, follow the instructions in the Code Chip section of the *User's Manual.*
   PURPOSE: To ensure that the instrument is calibrated correctly, to produce accurate, precise, and reliable results.
4. Place the meter on a flat surface so that it will not vibrate or move during testing.
   PURPOSE: The test results are based on the back-and-forth movement of the blood sample that stops when the clot has formed. Vibrations or other movements will result in an error message, and the test will have to be repeated.
5. Greet the patient. Identify yourself. Verify the patient's identity with full name; ask the patient to spell the first and last name and to give his or her date of birth. Explain the procedure to be performed in a manner that is understood by the patient. Answer any questions the patient may have on the procedure. Obtain permission for the capillary puncture.
   PURPOSE: It is important to identify the patient in two different ways to ensure that you have the correct patient. Explaining the procedure can make the patient feel more comfortable and helps to reduce anxiety.
6. Examine the patient's fingers and choose the site to obtain the blood sample.
   PURPOSE: Proper site choice will help ensure a good sample.
7. Prepare the site:
   (1) Warm the hand by placing it under the arm, using a hand warmer, and/or washing the hand in warm water.

   (2) Have the patient hold his or her arm down to the side so that the hand is below the waist.
   (3) Massage the palm of the hand toward the base of the finger and toward the tip until the fingertip has increased color.
   (4) If necessary, immediately after lancing, gently squeeze the finger from its base to encourage blood flow.
   PURPOSE: The hanging drop blood sample must be sufficient to travel down the three channels on the test strip. It must be free of contaminants, tissue fluids, and alcohol.
8. When you are ready to test, remove a test strip from the container and immediately close the container. Make sure it seals tightly. Do not open the container or touch the test strips with wet hands or wet gloves.
   PURPOSE: Exposure to moisture damages the test strips.
9. Insert the test strip as far as you can into the meter. This powers the meter ON (see Fig. 1).

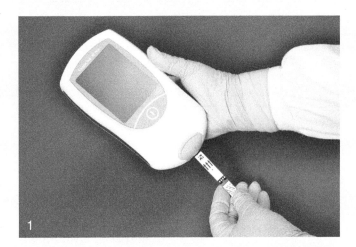

10. Disinfect the finger with an alcohol wipe and allow the finger to air dry. Perform the fingerstick.
    PURPOSE: To ensure infection control
11. Hold the finger with a blood drop very close to the target (the clear area of the test strip). Apply 1 drop of blood to the top or side of the target area and wait until you hear the beep. *You must apply a hanging drop of blood to the test strip within 15 seconds of the fingerstick. Do not add more blood. Do not touch or remove the test strip while the test is in progress.* The flashing blood drop symbol changes to an hourglass symbol when the meter detects a sufficient sample (see Fig. 33.5).
12. The result appears in approximately 1 minute. It may be displayed in three ways: as the international normalized ratio (INR); as the protime (PT) in seconds; or as %Quick (a unit used mainly in Europe). See the following chart.

Continued

PROCEDURE 33.5 | **Perform a CLIA-Waived Protime/INR Test**—*continued*

PROTIME EXPECTED VALUES FOR NORMAL AND THERAPEUTIC WHOLE BLOOD

	INR	PT (sec)
Normal	0.8–1.2	6.5–11.9[a]
Low anticoagulation therapy	1.5–2	Varies with method used
Moderate anticoagulation therapy	2–3	Varies with method used
High anticoagulation therapy	3–4	Varies with method used

[a]Laboratory reports and manufacturers must supply their own reference ranges for PT results along with each patient's results. This is because different methodologies may create different reference ranges and different units of measurement.

13. Record the result in the lab's PT/INR log and in the patient's warfarin therapy flow sheet and/or electronic health record. Any INR/PT results that do not fall into a normal range should be brought to the attention of the provider. Any INR/PT results that are considered critical in an institution should be relayed to the provider STAT so that medication changes are made a quickly as possible.
PURPOSE: The provider needs to know the result while the patient is still in the office, for proper follow-up with the patient.

WMFM CLINIC PROTIME PATIENT LOG

Protime expected values for both normal and therapeutic whole blood:

	INR	PT seconds (ISI = 1.0)
Normal	0.8–1.2	10.4–15.7 sec
Low anticoagulation	1.5–2.0	19.6–26.1 sec
Moderate anticoagulation	2.0–3.0	26.1–39.2 sec
High anticoagulation	3.0–4.0	39.2–52.2 sec

DATE	TECH	PATIENT I.D.	INR	PT SECONDS	CHARTED
10/09/20–	DC	# 12345	1.0	19.7	✓

14. Dispose of all sharps into the biohazard sharps container. Dispose of regulated medical waste into the biohazard waste container. Disinfect the test area and remove your PPE. Wash hands or use hand sanitizer.
PURPOSE: To ensure infection control.

Documentation Example
10/09/20XX 9:30 a.m. INR = 1.6 and PT = 19.7 seconds. Patient is on low anticoagulation therapy._____Anita James, CMA (AAMA)

PROCEDURE 33.6 | **Assist the Provider With Patient Care: Perform a Blood Glucose Test**

Task: Perform a blood test for blood glucose accurately.

EQUIPMENT and SUPPLIES

- Patient's record
- Glucometer glucose monitoring device[a]
- Blood glucose test strip[a]
- Lancet and autoloading finger-puncturing device
- Alcohol wipes
- Gauze
- Fluid-impermeable lab coat, protective eyewear, and gloves.
- Biohazard waste container
- Biohazard sharps container

[a]A variety of blood glucose monitors are available for testing blood sugar. Follow the specific instructions given by each individual manufacturer in the monitor/kit package insert.

PROCEDURAL STEPS

1. Check the provider's order and collect the necessary equipment and supplies. Perform quality control measures according to the manufacturer's guidelines and office policy.
2. Wash hands or use hand sanitizer. Put on fluid-impermeable lab coat, protective eyewear, and gloves.
PURPOSE: To ensure infection control.
3. Greet the patient. Identify yourself. Verify the patient's identity with full name; ask the patient to spell the first and last name and to give his or her date of birth. Explain the procedure to be performed in a manner that is understood by the patient. Answer any questions the patient may have on the procedure. Obtain permission for the capillary puncture.

PROCEDURE 33.6 | **Assist the Provider With Patient Care: Perform a Blood Glucose Test**—*continued*

<u>PURPOSE:</u> It is important to identify the patient in two different ways to ensure that you have the correct patient. Explaining the procedure can make the patient feel more comfortable and helps to reduce anxiety.

4. Ask the patient to wash his or her hands in warm, soapy water, then rinse them in warm water, and finally dry them completely.
<u>PURPOSE:</u> To clean the area that will be punctured; also, warming the fingers may increase peripheral blood flow.

5. Check the patient's middle and ring fingers and select the site for puncture (both forearm and fingertip testing can be done).
<u>PURPOSE:</u> To make sure the site of puncture is free of trauma.

6. Turn on the glucometer by pressing the ON button (see Fig. 1). Coding may or may not be necessary, depending on the monitor; follow the package insert directions for the specific glucose monitor you are using.

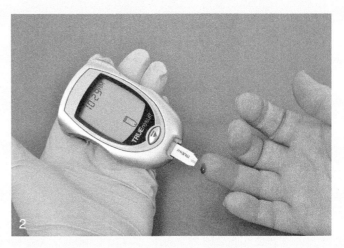

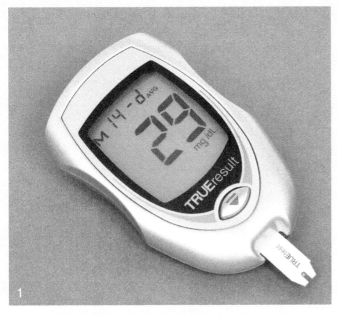

7. Check the expiration date on the test strip container. Take out a test strip and insert it into the glucometer.
<u>PURPOSE:</u> Tests strips should not be used if they have expired.

8. Cleanse the selected site on the patient's fingertip with an alcohol wipe and allow the finger to air dry.
<u>PURPOSE:</u> To ensure infection control.

9. Perform the capillary puncture and wipe away the first drop of blood.
<u>PURPOSE:</u> Tissue fluid may be present in the first drop of blood.

10. Apply a small blood sample to the end of the test strip (see Fig. 2).

11. Give the patient gauze to hold securely over the puncture site; apply a hypoallergenic bandage or wrap if needed.
<u>PURPOSE:</u> To aid in the stoppage of blood flow.

12. The glucometer automatically begins the measurement process, and results are obtained in a very short time frame.
<u>PURPOSE:</u> Automatic measurement makes for an easy-to-follow process.

13. The test result is shown in the display window.
<u>PURPOSE:</u> No calculations are involved obtaining a result.

14. The patient can set up testing reminders on most personal glucometers; a ketone alarm signal may also be available (depending on the monitor) when the blood glucose reading rises above a certain level.
<u>PURPOSE:</u> To ensure timely blood glucose monitoring.

15. Most glucometers store daily average test results and the date and time of each recording. Encourage patients to bring their personal glucometer to the clinic so the provider can review daily averages and previous test results.
<u>PURPOSE:</u> This helps the provider to monitor home results for the patient.

16. Most glucometers automatically turn off.
<u>PURPOSE:</u> To save battery life.

17. Discard all biohazard waste in biohazard waste containers.
<u>PURPOSE:</u> To ensure infection control.

18. Clean the glucometer according to the manufacturer's guidelines. Disinfect the work area. Remove your gloves and dispose of them properly. Remove protective eyewear and wash hands or use hand sanitizer.
<u>PURPOSE:</u> To ensure infection control.

19. Record the test results in the patient's health record.
<u>PURPOSE:</u> A procedure is not complete until the patient's results are recorded.

Documentation Example
08/16/20XX 1:00 p.m. Glucometer screening completed as ordered by Dr. Misha. NFBS 144. Pt took routine dose of 10 units Humalog insulin at noon. Pt had no questions._____Anita James, CMA (AAMA)

PROCEDURE 33.7	Perform a CLIA-Waived Chemistry Test: Determine the Cholesterol Level or Lipid Profile Using a Cholestech Analyzer

Task: Perform a Cholestech test for total cholesterol level and/or a lipid panel and accurately report the results.

EQUIPMENT and SUPPLIES

- Patient's health record
- Provider's order and/or lab requisition
- Cholestech analyzer
- Package insert or flow chart with directions
- Optics check cassette
- Test cassettes (provided by Cholestech)
- Levels 1 and 2 liquid controls
- Capillary tubes and plungers for fingerstick sample (provided by Cholestech)
- Mini-Pet pipet and pipet tips for venipuncture sample (provided by Cholestech)
- Lancet, gauze, alcohol wipes, bandage for capillary blood, or lithium heparin (green-topped) tube for venous blood
- Safety tube decapper (if tubes do not have a Hemogard plastic top)
- Fluid-impermeable lab coat, protective eyewear, and gloves
- Biohazard waste container
- Biohazard sharps containers

PROCEDURAL STEPS

1. Wash hands or use hand sanitizer. Put on a fluid-impermeable lab coat, protective eyewear, and gloves.
   <u>PURPOSE:</u> To ensure infection control.
2. Assemble the materials needed.
3. Perform quantitative quality control by performing a calibration check with the optics check cassette (see Fig. 1). Then test level 1 and level 2 liquid controls if using a new set of cassettes.
   <u>PURPOSE:</u> To ensure instrument is reading results accurately, precisely, and reliably.

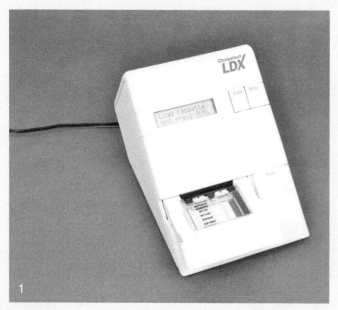

4. Allow refrigerated testing cassettes to come to room temperature (at least 10 minutes before opening).
   <u>PURPOSE:</u> Test is temperature and time sensitive when reading results.
5. Remove cassette from its pouch and place on flat surface without touching the black bar or magnetic strip.
   <u>PURPOSE:</u> The black bar is the testing area, and the magnetic strip must be read by the analyzer. Touching either may interfere with test results
6. Press RUN on the analyzer, allowing it to do a self-test; this will be followed by OK on the screen, then the test drawer will open. The drawer will stay open for 4 minutes while the specimen is prepared.
   <u>PURPOSE:</u> Ensures the instrument's electronics are working properly before patient testing.
7. Perform a fingerstick and collect the capillary blood to the black line of the Cholestech capillary tube with its plunger inserted into the red end of the tube. *Or* collect the fresh venous whole blood with the Cholestech Mini-Pet pipet.
   <u>PURPOSE:</u> Both collecting devices are provided by Cholestech to ensure that the exact volume of blood necessary is tested.
8. Place the whole blood sample into the well of the cassette. *Note:* The capillary specimen must be in the cassette within 5 minutes of collection (see Fig. 2).
   <u>PURPOSE:</u> Fingerstick blood will clot if not tested within 5 minutes.

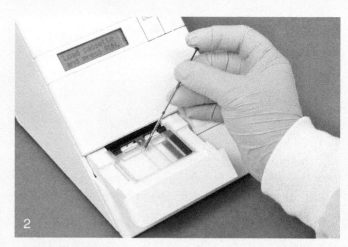

9. Immediately put the cassette into the drawer of the analyzer and press RUN. (*Note:* If the drawer has closed, press RUN again to open the drawer; load the specimen into the drawer and then press to close the drawer.)
   <u>PURPOSE:</u> This is a test with a color reaction that continues to change over time.
10. When the test is complete, the analyzer beeps. The screen displays and then prints out the results (see Fig. 3).
    <u>PURPOSE:</u> No calculations are required to obtain a patient result.

PROCEDURE 33.7	Perform a CLIA-Waived Chemistry Test: Determine the Cholesterol Level or Lipid Profile Using a Cholestech Analyzer—*continued*

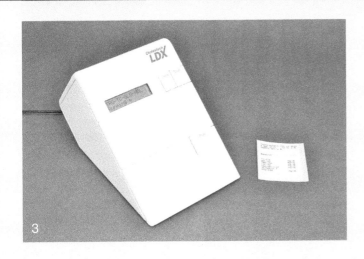

11. Record the findings in the laboratory log and in the patient's paper health record if they have not been transmitted electronically.
    <u>PURPOSE</u>: A procedure is not considered complete until it is recorded.
12. Any lipid profile or glucose results that do not fall into a normal range should be brought to the attention of the provider as quickly as possible.
    <u>PURPOSE</u>: The provider needs to know the results while the patient is still in the office, for proper follow-up with the patient.
13. Dispose of all sharps in the biohazard sharps container (i.e., lancet and capillary pipet with plunger). Place all regulated medical waste into the biohazard waste container (i.e., gauze, alcohol wipes, and cassettes). Disinfect test area, remove PPE, and dispose of gloves in biohazard waste container. Wash hands or use hand sanitizer.
    <u>PURPOSE</u>: To ensure infection control.

CHOLESTECH LDX PATIENT/CONTROL LOG

Cassette Lot #: _____   Expiration Date: _____   LDX Serial #: _____

DATE	TECH	PT ID	TC	HDL	LDL	TRG	TC/HDL	GLU	CHARTED
10/09/20–	DC	#12345	190	50	120	135	4.3	80	✓

Documentation Example

Attach printed readout, or record results in the electronic chart.

TEST	RESULTS	DESIRABLE RANGES[a]
Total cholesterol (TC)	190	<200 mg/dL
HDL cholesterol	50	>40 mg/dL
LDL cholesterol	120	<130 mg/dL
Triglycerides	135	<150 mg/dL
TC/HDL ratio	4.3	≤4.5
Other		
Glucose	80	Fasting: 60–110 mg/dL
		Nonfasting: <160 mg/dL

[a]Laboratory reports and manufacturers must supply their own reference ranges, along with each patient's results. This is because different methodologies may create different reference ranges and different units of measurement.

34

MICROBIOLOGY AND IMMUNOLOGY

SCENARIO

Laura Piper, a certified medical assistant (CMA) through the American Association of Medical Assistants (AAMA), has worked at Walden-Martin Family Medical (WMFM) Clinic for 6 years. She has seen many infectious diseases diagnosed over that time. Bacterial and viral infections are common, but Laura also knows that not all microorganisms are bad. Some diseases have been controlled using vaccines. Other infections can be treated with antibiotics. Not all infectious diseases can be treated with antibiotics, and improper use of antibiotics can lead to bacteria that are resistant to these very useful drugs. Laura knows that it is important to identify pathogens quickly so that proper treatment can begin. The identification of pathogens can involve various types of tests, many of which can be performed in the physician office laboratory (POL) where she works.

While studying this chapter, think about the following questions:

- What are the various bacterial shapes, oxygen requirements, and physical structures?
- What are the unusual characteristics of chlamydia, mycoplasma, and rickettsia?
- What are the characteristics of common viral diseases?
- What are the common methods for the collection, transport, and processing of microbiology and immunology specimens?
- What are three common CLIA-waived tests that use a rapid identification technique?
- What is the purpose of indirect immunology testing?
- What are three CLIA-waived immunology tests that could be done in the physician office laboratory?
- What is the importance of the Gram stain and acid-fast stains in microbiology?
- How does a reference laboratory assess a throat culture and a urine culture?

LEARNING OBJECTIVES

1. Describe the naming of microorganisms.
2. Describe various bacterial staining characteristics, shapes, oxygen requirements, and physical structures; also, explain the characteristics of common diseases caused by bacteria.
3. Describe the unusual characteristics of chlamydia, mycoplasma, and rickettsia organisms.
4. Do the following related to fungi, protozoa, and parasites:
   - Compare bacteria with fungi, protozoa, and parasites.
   - Identify the characteristics of common diseases caused by fungi, protozoa, and parasites.
   - Perform patient education on the collection of a stool specimen for ova and parasite testing.
5. Compare bacteria with viruses, and describe the characteristics of common viral diseases.
6. Cite the protocols for the collection, transport, and processing of specimens.
7. Explain how pinworm testing is done and when it is recommended.
8. Describe and perform CLIA-waived microbiology tests:
   - Describe three CLIA-waived microbiology tests that use a rapid identification technique.
   - Obtain a specimen, and perform the CLIA-waived rapid strep test.
9. Do the following related to CLIA-waived immunology testing:
   - Discuss the purpose of indirect immunology testing.
   - Describe three CLIA-waived immunology tests that could be done in the physician office laboratory.
   - Obtain a specimen, and perform a CLIA-waived mononucleosis test.
10. Detail the equipment needed in a microbiology reference laboratory, and discuss the identification of pathogens in the microbiology laboratory by describing various staining techniques.
11. Describe the reference laboratory assessment of a throat culture and a urine culture.
12. Explain the concepts used for culture and sensitivity testing.
13. Discuss patient education, in addition to legal and ethical issues, as it applies to laboratory testing.

VOCABULARY

acute phase The phase during which rapid multiplication of the pathogen takes place. Symptoms are very distinct. A strong response of the immune system takes place during this stage.

antibiotic A substance or medication that can destroy or inhibit the growth of bacteria.

antibody A protein substance produced in the blood or tissues in response to a specific antigen; antibodies destroy or weaken the antigen. Part of the immune system.

antigen A substance that stimulates the production of an antibody when introduced into the body. Antigens include toxins, bacteria, viruses, and other foreign substances.

antiseptic Substances that inhibit the growth of microorganisms on living tissue (e.g., alcohol and povidone-iodine [Betadine]); they are used to cleanse the skin, wounds, and so on.

arthropod Any animal that lacks a spine, such as insects, crustaceans, arachnids, and others.

asexual Describes reproduction that does not involve the fusion of male and female sex cells.

bacteria Microorganisms that are single-celled, lack a nucleus, reproduce asexually, or can form spores. Some can cause disease. The most abundant life form on earth.

binary fission Asexual reproduction in single-celled organisms during which one cell divides into two daughter cells.

binomial A name consisting of a generic and a specific term.

blood agar plate (BAP) A solid agar medium that contains nutrients and 5% washed sheep's blood. The blood is added as an extra nutrient source for bacteria.

bronchiolitis Occurs when the small airways of the lungs become inflamed because of a viral infection.

convalescent stage The phase during which the host recovers gradually and returns to baseline or normal health.

diluent (DIL yoo uh nt) A liquid substance that dilutes or lessens the strength of a solution or mixture.

disinfectants Chemical agents used on nonliving objects to destroy or inhibit the growth of harmful organisms.

eukaryote (yoo KAR ee oht) Any single-celled or multicellular organism that has genetic material contained in a distinct membrane-bound nucleus.

extraction A process by which a specific substance is separated from a group or solution.

fungus (plural, *fungi*) Any of a diverse group of single-celled organisms, including mushrooms, molds, mildew, smuts, rusts, and yeasts, and classified in the kingdom Fungi.

infectious agents Living and nonliving pathogens—such as bacteria, viruses, fungi, protozoa, parasites, helminths, and prions—that can cause disease. Also called infectious particles.

in vitro Latin term meaning "in glass" and commonly known as "in the laboratory."

macromolecules Molecules needed for metabolism: carbohydrates, lipids, proteins, amino acids, and nucleic acids.

microorganism Any living organism—such as bacterium, protozoan, fungi, parasite, or helminth—of microscopic size. Some definitions include viruses, which are not alive.

mold Growth of tiny fungi forming on a substance. Often looks downy or furry and is associated with dampness or decay.

molecule The simplest unit of a chemical compound that can exist, consisting of two or more atoms held together with chemical bonds.

nasal wash Also called a nasal aspirate. A syringe is used to gently squirt a small amount of sterile saline into the nose, and the resulting fluid is collected into a cup (for a wash). Or after the saline is squirted into the nose, gentle suction is applied (for the aspirate).

nomenclature (NOH muh n kley cher) A system of names or terms, used in science and art to categorize items.

normal flora A microorganism (usually a bacterium or yeast) that lives on or in the body. A normal microscopic resident of the body.

organelles Structures inside a cell that perform specific functions.

parasitic Pertaining to a parasite. (An organism that lives on or in another organism, known as the host. Benefits from the host; the host does not benefit from the parasite.)

pneumonia Inflammation of the lungs with congestion of the air sacs (alveoli). Can be caused by a bacterium or virus.

prokaryote (proh KAR ee ote) Any organism that is made up of at least one cell and has genetic material that is not enclosed in a nucleus. Bacteria are prokaryotes, primitive organisms.

protozoa (pro tuh ZOH ah) Single-celled organisms that are the most primitive form of animal life. Most are microscopic. Examples are amoebas, ciliates, flagellates, and sporozoans.

stains Reagents or dyes used to prepare specimens for microscopic examination.

subcultured Occurs when an organism (a bacterium) has been cultivated again on a new nutrient surface.

tissue culture The technique or process of keeping tissue alive and growing in a culture medium.

transport medium A medium used to keep an organism alive during transport to the laboratory.

wet mount A glass slide that holds a specimen suspended in a drop of liquid for microscopic examination.

yeast Any various single-celled fungi, which reproduce by budding and are able to ferment sugars.

Infectious diseases caused by **microorganisms** and **infectious agents** have gotten a lot of publicity in the news. We have all heard stories about **antibiotic**-resistant superbugs, food-borne illnesses, tick-borne diseases, and communicable infections. Listening to the news, it appears all microorganisms are harmful and can cause disease. In reality, less than 1% of known microorganisms

are *pathogens*. A pathogen is a disease-causing organism. Most microbes on and in our bodies are helpful and do not cause disease.

Most microorganisms are good. Without microorganisms, we could not survive. The **normal flora** in and on our bodies is needed for the following processes:

- Digesting food and making nutrients available to the body.
- Forming blood clots. Vitamin K is used in the clotting process and is made by **bacteria** in our intestines.
- Preventing pathogens from invading our skin, mucous membranes, and gastrointestinal and genitourinary tracts.

Saprophytes

Beneficial microorganisms that are responsible for breaking down organic matter are called *saprophytes*. They help break down plants and organic waste in farming, water purification, composting, and gardening.

Normal flora takes up space, requires nutrients, and excretes waste. When pathogens try to populate the skin or areas of the body that have normal flora, they must compete with the existing organisms. This makes it harder for pathogens to cause disease. Normal flora discourages pathogen populations.

When the body's normal flora is weakened (e.g., by antibiotic overuse or hormonal changes), certain *opportunistic organisms* that are normally present in low numbers can overgrow. An example is *Candida albicans*, which is a **yeast** that is normally found on mucous membranes in the body. When a patient is being treated with a broad-spectrum antibiotic for an infection, the antibiotics kill the pathogen, along with some of the normal flora. If enough normal flora is killed off, *Candida albicans* can increase in number and cause a secondary infection. For women who are taking antibiotics, a secondary vaginal yeast infection is possible after antibiotic use. *Candida albicans* is not normally a problem, but given the opportunity, it can cause disease.

As a medical assistant, you need to understand basic *microbiology* and the role of microorganisms in both health and disease. The main objective in medical microbiology is to identify the organisms responsible for illness so that the provider can properly treat the patient. Your responsibilities will also include preventing nosocomial infections, also known as healthcare-acquired infections (HAI), by observing infection control practices. Microbiology testing procedures may be performed in the physician office laboratory (POL) or in the microbiology department of a medical referral laboratory.

The study of *immunology*, or the immune system, is closely tied to microbiology. Invasive microorganisms stimulate an immune response, leading to the production of antibodies that come to our defense. Often a bacterial or viral infection is diagnosed by testing for the specific **antibody** that is produced to fight the infectious agent.

Chapter 4 discusses the chain of infection and how it can be broken by applying diligent infection control procedures, such as the following:

- Using frequent and proper hand hygiene
- Wearing appropriate personal protective equipment (PPE)
- Observing recommended precautions for infectious agent transmission
- Using appropriate **antiseptics** and **disinfectants**
- Performing sterilization procedures

This chapter covers the following topics:

- Major common infectious agents seen in a POL
- Quality control issues related to the collection and handling of microbiologic specimens

- Common CLIA-waived microbiology and immunology tests performed in the POL

The chapter concludes with an overview of the more complex microbiology procedures and tests performed in hospitals and reference laboratories.

CLASSIFICATION OF MICROORGANISMS

Although the medical assistant is not responsible for identifying microorganisms, a working knowledge of the terminology used in the naming microorganisms is essential.

Microorganisms are too small to be seen without magnification. Bacteria, **fungi**, and **protozoa** are all microorganisms that can be seen with a microscope. **Parasitic** worm infections are also identified in the microbiology laboratory because their eggs are visible under the microscope. Viruses are the smallest microbe and are visible only with a highly magnified electron microscope.

Naming Microorganisms

Scientists use the **binomial** system of **nomenclature** developed by Swedish botanist Carl Linnaeus to name all living organisms: animals, plants, fungi, protozoa, and bacteria. This binomial system assigns two names; the first name is the *genus* and the second name is the *species*. Both names are either *italicized* or underlined when written. The genus begins with a capital letter, the species with a lowercase letter. When microbiology laboratory results are reported, it is essential that both the genus and species names are recorded. Different species may cause different symptoms or require different antibiotic treatment. For example, *Streptococcus pyogenes* causes strep throat, whereas *Streptococcus viridans* is normal flora in the throat.

The genus name of the organism may be represented by a single letter, after the organism's full genus and species names have been written once in a report. For example, *Escherichia coli* is commonly referred to as *E. coli*.

CHARACTERISTICS OF BACTERIA

Bacteria are single-celled **prokaryote** organisms that reproduce by **binary fission**. This process of **asexual** reproduction results in a large number of bacteria being produced from a single cell. This is why bacterial infections can quickly overwhelm a person's immune system. Some bacteria reproduce in as little as 14 minutes, whereas others take days to divide. A single *E. coli* cell, which reproduces in about 30 minutes, produces 351,843,724,088,831 offspring in just 24 hours. This explains why a urinary tract infection (UTI) can appear so quickly and cause so much discomfort.

Learning about the different categories of bacteria is important for you as a medical assistant because it will increase your understanding of laboratory results and patient conditions. Bacteria are classified according to their staining characteristics, their shapes, and the environmental conditions in which they thrive. Both shape and staining characteristics are based on the structure of the bacterial cell wall.

Bacterial Staining Properties

Three types of cell wall structures are found among pathogenic bacteria: Gram-positive, Gram-negative, and acid-fast structures. These labels are based on reactions to specialized **stains** used to see bacteria under

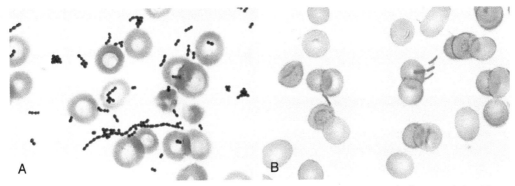

FIGURE 34.1 **(A)** Gram stain red blood cells (RBCs) and Gram-positive cocci. **(B)** RBCs with Gram-negative bacilli. (From De la Maza LM, Pezzlo MT, Baron EJ: *Color atlas of diagnostic microbiology*, St. Louis, 1997, Mosby.)

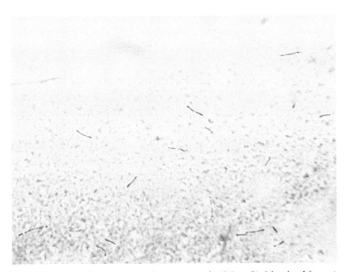

FIGURE 34.2 Acid-fast stain. (From De la Maza LM, Pezzlo MT, Baron EJ: *Color atlas of diagnostic microbiology*, St. Louis, 1997, Mosby.)

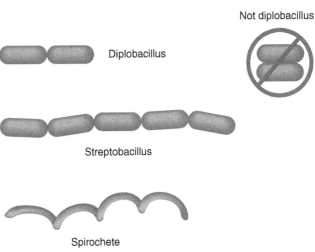

FIGURE 34.3 Typical bacterial arrangements.

a microscope. Bacterial cell walls are composed of *peptidoglycan* (PG), a **molecule** composed of carbohydrate and protein.

- *Gram-positive cells* contain a thick layer of PG, which looks deep blue/violet when stained with Gram stain (Fig. 34.1A).
- *Gram-negative cells* contain a thin layer of PG, which looks pinkish red when stained with Gram stain (Fig. 34.1B).
- *Acid-fast cells* contain a thin layer of PG surrounded by a thick layer of waxlike *lipids* (fats). Acid-fast bacteria do not stain well with a Gram stain, but they stain pink with the acid-fast stain (Fig. 34.2).

Bacterial Shapes

Pathogenic bacteria assume three different shapes:
- Round bacteria are called *cocci*.
- Rod-shaped bacteria are called *bacilli*.
- Spiral-shaped bacteria are called *spirilla*. Tightly coiled spirilla are called *spirochetes*.

Certain arrangements are also seen with different bacteria. For example, when bacteria are in a chain formation, the prefix *strepto-* is used. When bacteria are found in pairs, the prefix *diplo-* is used, and when they are found in grapelike clusters, the prefix *staphylo-* is used. Cocci

in packets of 4 are called *tetrads*, and in packets of 8 or 16 they are called *sarcinae* (Fig. 34.3).

Bacterial Oxygen Requirements

Bacteria are also classified according to oxygen requirements. Bacteria that require oxygen to live are called *aerobes*. Bacteria that die in the presence of oxygen are called *anaerobes*. Some bacteria are flexible regarding their oxygen needs; they can survive in the presence of oxygen but prefer to live without oxygen. These bacteria are called *facultative anaerobes*.

Oxygen Needs for Different Bacteria

Mycobacterium tuberculosis, which causes tuberculosis, thrives in white blood cells in the lungs; it is an aerobe. *Bacteroides fragilis* is a common Gram-negative bacillus found in the intestines; it is an anaerobe. *E. coli*, also an inhabitant of the intestines and the most common cause of urinary tract infections, can live in the presence of oxygen but prefers to live in the absence of oxygen; it is a facultative anaerobe.

Bacterial Physical Structures

Bacteria can be classified and identified according to additional physical structures. Some bacteria have long thin *flagella* (whiplike tails) that help them move. *Proteus vulgaris* is a Gram-negative bacillus with many flagella. It can move up the urethra and into the bladder and cause a UTI. Some bacteria produce a thick, jelly-like substance that surrounds the cell wall called a *capsule*. *Streptococcus pneumoniae* is nonpathogenic if it is not producing a capsule; however, when it produces a capsule it is the most common cause of pneumonia in older adults. The Pneumovax vaccine is given to older patients and to patients at high risk for respiratory complications (e.g., patients with asthma). Other bacteria form an intracellular structure called an *endospore*. An endospore allows the bacteria to remain viable when environmental conditions are poor. *Clostridium tetani* produces spores, and if spores enter a wound and grow, they cause the disease known as *tetanus*.

See Tables 34.1 to 34.3 for a list of some important infectious diseases caused by typical pathogenic bacilli, cocci, and spirilla.

CRITICAL THINKING APPLICATION   34.1

In your own words, write a brief description of the term *capsule*. What advantage does a bacterium have if a capsule surrounds it? Share your thoughts with the class.

UNUSUAL PATHOGENIC BACTERIA: *CHLAMYDIA, MYCOPLASMA*, AND *RICKETTSIA*

Typical pathogenic bacteria measure 1000 to 5000 nm in size. *Chlamydia*, *Mycoplasma*, and *Rickettsia* are tiny, unusual bacteria that fall between the size ranges of typical pathogenic bacteria and viruses (Table 34.4).

Chlamydiae are tiny bacteria that require host cells for growth. They once were considered viruses. *Chlamydia trachomatis* is the cause of a sexually transmitted infection (STI). Rickettsiae are tiny Gram-negative bacteria that are transmitted by blood-sucking insects. Rickettsia cannot multiply outside a living host cell. *Rickettsia rickettsii* causes Rocky Mountain spotted fever. Mycoplasmas are unusual in that they have no PG in the cell wall. Mycoplasmal pneumonia is also referred to as "walking pneumonia."

PATHOGENIC FUNGI

Mycology is the study of fungi and the diseases they cause (Table 34.5). Fungi are **eukaryotes** that are larger than bacteria and have a nucleus. Fungi include yeasts and **molds**. Fungi are present in the

TABLE 34.1   Common Diseases Caused by Bacilli

DISEASE STATE	CAUSATIVE AGENT	TRANSMISSION
Botulism	*Clostridium botulinum*	Improperly cooked canned foods
Clostridium difficile (C. diff) infection	*Clostridium difficile*	May be a healthcare-acquired infection (HAI), frequent antibiotic use increases likelihood; idiopathic
Diphtheria	*Corynebacterium diphtheriae*	Inhalation
Legionnaires disease	*Legionella pneumophilia*	Grows readily in air-conditioning systems (water)
Salmonella infection	*Salmonella* species	Food-borne illness
Tetanus (lockjaw)	*Clostridium tetani*	Open fractures, soil-contaminated wounds, open wounds, puncture wounds
Tuberculosis	*Mycobacterium tuberculosis*	Air-borne, inhalation
Urinary tract infection (UTI)	Various, most common include the following: • *Escherichia coli* • *Proteus* species • *Klebsiella* species • *Pseudomonas aeruginosa*	Bacteria-contaminated urethra, catheterization
Whooping cough	*Bordetella pertussis*	Respiratory secretions

TABLE 34.2   Common Diseases Caused by Cocci

DISEASE STATE	CAUSATIVE AGENT	TRANSMISSION
Gonorrhea	*Neisseria gonorrhoeae*	Sexually transmitted
Meningococcal meningitis	*Neisseria meningitidis*	Respiratory tract secretions
Methicillin-resistant *Staphylococcus aureus* (MRSA) infection	Methicillin-resistant *Staphylococcus aureus*	Healthcare-acquired infection (HIA), direct contact, fomites, carriers, poor hand washing technique
Pneumonia	*Streptococcus pneumoniae*	Direct contact, droplets
Staphylococcal food poisoning	*Staphylococcus aureus*	Poor hygiene, improper refrigeration of foods
Strep throat	*Streptococcus pyogenes*, also known as group A strep	Direct contact, droplets, fomites
Wound infections, abscesses, boils	*Staphylococcus aureus*	Direct contact, fomites, carriers, poor hand washing technique

TABLE 34.3   Common Diseases Caused by Spirilla

DISEASE STATE	CAUSATIVE AGENT	TRANSMISSION
Food-borne illness (most commonly seen in the United States)	*Campylobacter jejuni*	Contaminated and undercooked food, contaminated water and milk
Lyme disease	*Borrelia burgdorferi*	Tick bite
Pyloric ulcers	*Helicobacter pylori*	Unknown, possibly food/water-borne
Syphilis	*Treponema pallidum*	Sexually or congenitally

TABLE 34.4   Common Diseases Caused by Rickettsia, Mycoplasma, and Chlamydia

DISEASE STATE	CAUSATIVE AGENT	TRANSMISSION
Atypical or walking pneumonia	*Mycoplasma pneumoniae*	Respiratory secretions
Inclusion conjunctivitis or pneumonia	*Chlamydia trachomatis*	During the birth process
Nongonococcal urethritis or vaginitis	*Chlamydia trachomatis*	Sexually
Rocky Mountain spotted fever	*Rickettsia rickettsii*	Tick bite
Typhus (epidemic)	*Rickettsia prowazekii*	Body lice bite
Typhus (endemic)	*Rickettsia typhi*	Flea bite

soil, air, and water, but only a few species cause disease. They are transmitted by the following:

- Direct contact with infected persons
- Prolonged exposure to a moist environment
- Inhalation of contaminated dust or soil

Fungal infections may be superficial, affecting only the skin, hair, or nails. Some fungi can penetrate the tissues of the internal body structures and cause serious diseases of the mucous membranes, heart, and lungs. Fungal infections must be treated with specific antifungal medications.

A superficial fungal infection often is referred to as *tinea* (Latin for "ringworm"). The term *ringworm* arose because the infected area

is often circular. Chapter 17 discusses additional information about tinea infections. A diagnosis of fungal infections usually is based on culturing skin scrapings, microscopic observation of skin scrapings, or other sample sites. Usually, before microscopic observation, the samples are treated with *potassium hydroxide* (KOH) to dissolve away nonfungal material, making the fungal elements easier to observe.

CRITICAL THINKING APPLICATION   34.2

Fungi include two other types of organisms. Name these organisms. Share your answers with the class.

TABLE 34.5	Common Diseases Caused by Fungi	
DISEASE STATE	**CAUSATIVE AGENT**	**TRANSMISSION**
Candidiasis, vulvovaginal, monilial (vaginal yeast)	*Candida* species (yeast)	After antibiotic therapy; using hormonal birth control; diabetes-type I, II; gestational; AIDS
Cryptococcosis	*Cryptococcus neoformans*	Contact with poultry droppings
Fungal infections; athlete's foot, jock itch, ringworm	*Tinea* species and others	Direct contact with an infected person or animal, damp surfaces
Histoplasmosis	*Histoplasma capsulatum*	Inhaling dust contaminated with bird or bat droppings
Pneumocystis pneumonia	*Pneumocystis jiroveci* (formerly known as *Pneumocystis carinii*)	Contact with animals, most likely in immune-compromised patients, common in AIDS patients
Thrush (in the mouth)	*Candida* species (yeast)	Possibly during birth process, after antibiotic therapy, diabetes, or weakened immune system

TABLE 34.6	Common Diseases Caused by Protozoa and Parasites	
DISEASE STATE	**CAUSATIVE AGENT**	**TRANSMISSION**
Amoebic dysentery	*Entamoeba histolytica*	Fecal contamination of food or water
Giardiasis	*Giardia lamblia*	Contaminated water, opportunist in intestinal tract
Lice	*Pediculus humanus* (head and body lice), *Phthirus pubis* (pubic lice)	Direct contact, contaminated clothing, bedding, furniture, personal items (combs, hats, etc.)
Malaria	*Plasmodium* species	Bite of the *Anopheles* mosquito
Pinworm	*Enterobius vermicularis*	Fecal-oral contamination
Scabies	*Sarcoptes scabiei*	Direct contact, contaminated clothing, bedding
Tapeworm: beef or pork	*Taenia* species	Eating undercooked beef or pork
Tapeworm: fish	*Diphyllobothrium latum*	Eating undercooked fish
Toxoplasmosis	*Toxoplasma gondii*	Fecal contamination from cat litter, congenitally
Trichinosis	*Trichinella spiralis*	Eating undercooked pork or bear

PATHOGENIC PROTOZOA

Protozoa are single-celled parasitic organisms that contain a nucleus. They range in size from microscopic to *macroscopic* (visible to the naked eye) (Table 34.6). They are present in moist environments and in bodies of water, such as lakes and ponds. Protozoa are transmitted through contaminated feces, food, and drink. Some pathogenic protozoa inhabit the bloodstream, whereas others inhabit the intestines and genital tract. Diagnosis usually is based on the patient's signs and symptoms and on microscopic examination of stool or blood.

PATHOGENIC PARASITES

Parasitology includes the study of all parasitic organisms that live on or in the human body (see Table 34.6). In a parasitic relationship,

the host is harmed, and the parasite thrives. Parasites are transmitted by ingestion of contaminated food or water, direct penetration of the skin, or injection by an **arthropod**. A parasite cannot be identified accurately based on a single test or specimen. Most parasites are identified in feces, blood, urine, sputum, tissue fluids, or tissue biopsy samples.

PATHOGENIC HELMINTHS (WORMS)

Helminths are worms, a class of parasites. Helminths live on or in another living organism. They sustain themselves at the expense of the host organism. They can live in animals or humans. Worms are usually transmitted through the soil, by infected clothing or fingernails, through contact with infected persons, or by means of contaminated food/water. Helminths go through the same life cycle as other worms.

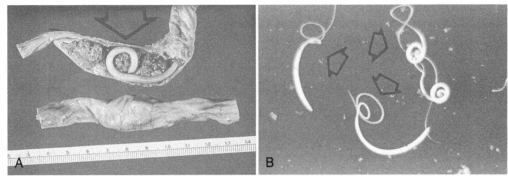

FIGURE 34.4 **(A)** Roundworms. **(B)** Whipworms. (From Stepp CA, Woods MA: *Laboratory procedures for medical office personnel,* Philadelphia, 1998, Saunders.)

The adult worm lays eggs (ova). The ova develop into larvae, which then grow into adult worms, and the cycle begins again. Diagnosis usually is based on microscopic examination of feces for ova and parasites and on patient signs and symptoms (Fig. 34.4).

Stool specimens are commonly examined for parasitic protozoa and helminths. The specimen is collected and placed into two vials, each with a preservative. From these preparations, a **wet mount** slide is made to observe moving organisms. A stained smear is made from a concentrated specimen. The smear is looked at under the microscope to observe *protozoal cysts* and helminth eggs. A protozoal cyst is a thick-walled protective membrane enclosing a cell, larva, or organism. The medical assistant should always consult the procedure manual provided by the referral laboratory when an ova and parasite stool examination (O&P) is ordered to make sure that proper collection and transport of the specimen takes place (see Procedure 34.1, p. 883).

PATHOGENIC VIRUSES

Many scientists do not consider viruses to be microorganisms because they are not alive. Viruses consist of a genetic core covered by a protein coat called a *capsid*. Some viruses have an additional spiked layer of protection over the capsid called an *envelope*. Viruses are not able to metabolize or reproduce unless they are inside a host cell. Viruses have their own enzymes but must use the host cell **organelles** and **macromolecules** to reproduce and metabolize. Because of the absolute need for a host cell, a virus can be considered an *obligate intracellular pathogen*. Viruses must be inside a host cell to reproduce and cause disease.

Recipe for a Virus

A viral genetic core is made up of either *ribonucleic acid* (RNA) or *deoxyribonucleic acid* (DNA). The RNA or DNA contains information about how and what the host cell needs to produce to form a new virus. The genetic material is like a recipe for a new viral particle.

A virus cannot be cultured on solid nutrient media, such as those used to culture bacteria and fungi. Viruses must be cultured in fertilized eggs or in a **tissue culture**, which is done by referral, research, or large hospital laboratories. It is a time-consuming and tedious process.

Usually, instead of culturing a specimen for a virus, the patient's blood sample is tested for a specific antibody produced to a specific virus. For example, in the diagnosis of HIV, patient serum is tested for the specific antibody produced in response to the HIV virus. This form of testing is referred to as *serology* or *immunology testing* (discussed later in the chapter). Table 34.7 lists common diseases caused by viruses.

CRITICAL THINKING APPLICATION   34.3
Looking at Table 34.7, pick four viral diseases that you are familiar with. Write down the disease, the virus that causes it, and two ways to prevent the infection. Be ready to share your answers with the class.

SPECIMEN COLLECTION AND TRANSPORT IN THE PHYSICIAN OFFICE LABORATORY

Specimen collection and handling are very important considerations in patient care because the results are only as good as the quality of the sample. Specimens for microbiology testing must be collected carefully so that contaminating microorganisms are not introduced into the specimen. This means not only using sterile collection and transport devices, but also taking steps to prevent contamination. Such steps include instructing a patient in the collection of a urine sample using the clean-catch midstream (CCMS) technique, as described in Chapter 31, as well as using antiseptics on the skin to avoid contamination of the site, described in Chapter 32.

Before collecting specimens for microbiologic testing, you should ask yourself two questions:

1. How can I prevent contamination of this sample?
2. How can I protect myself from pathogen exposure while I collect this sample?

To prevent sample contamination, do the following:
- Wash your hands properly, and then put on gloves.
- Cleanse the area to be sampled with an antiseptic.
- Open sterile containers only when necessary.
- Never touch a sterile swab or collection device to a nonsterile surface.

To protect yourself from pathogen exposure, do the following:
- Use frequent and proper handwashing methods.
- Wear gloves, a fluid-impermeable lab coat, and protective eyewear. It may be necessary to wear a surgical mask or a face shield in some cases (for droplet or airborne pathogens).

TABLE 34.7   Common Diseases Caused by Viruses

DISEASE STATE	CAUSATIVE AGENT	TRANSMISSION
Acquired immunodeficiency syndrome (AIDS)	Human immunodeficiency virus (HIV)	Sexual intercourse/contact, sharing needles, at-risk behavior
Common cold	Rhinovirus most common among many possible	Direct contact, inhaling droplets, fomites
Ebola	Ebola virus species (five identified)	Direct contact with infected blood or body fluids (bloodborne)
Infectious mononucleosis	Epstein-Barr virus	Direct contact and airborne
Influenza	Myxovirus, influenza A and B	Droplet and fomites
Measles	Paramyxovirus — measles virus	Direct contact, inhaling droplets
Molluscum contagiosum warts	Molluscipoxvirus	Direct contact with an infected person
Mumps	Paramyxovirus — mumps virus	Inhaling droplets, shared utensils with infected person
Polio	Poliovirus	Direct contact, via mouth
Rubella (German measles)	Rubella virus	Direct contact, inhaling droplets, congenitally
Warts (verruca)	Human papillomavirus (HPV)	Direct and indirect contact

- Always wear gloves when handling any patient specimen, even if you are not going to be testing the sample at that time.

Ideally, specimens should be collected during the **acute phase** of an illness and before antibiotics are prescribed. Many types of samples are collected:

- Sterile swabs can be used to collect samples from wounds and the upper respiratory tract.
- Serum or whole blood can be used to test for infectious organisms or antibodies.
- Urine samples are normally collected at a POL.
- Fecal samples can be collected by the patient at the POL or at home.

If patients are expected to collect a sample, it is crucial that they receive clear instructions on how to perform the procedure correctly and without contaminating the sample. The referral laboratory is responsible for providing a manual of written instructions to the POL. The POL is responsible for providing clear oral and written instructions to the patient. If the patient will be collecting the sample in private or at home, written instructions that are simple and straightforward should be supplied.

The transport of specimens to referral laboratories is also crucial. Different types of transport devices are available. Close attention must be given to their proper use. Microorganisms are living organisms, so they must be given conditions that ensure their survival. Care must also be taken so that any normal flora in the sample will not multiply and overgrow possible pathogens. The type and number of microorganisms in the sample should reflect the type and number of microorganisms at the site of collection and at the time of collection.

Specialized transport media are often included with specimen collection swabs or devices (Fig. 34.5). Collection devices typically consist of a plastic tube that encases a sterile Dacron swab and a sealed vial of **transport medium**. After the specimen has been collected on

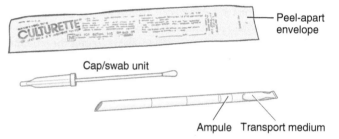

FIGURE 34.5 Collection and transport system for patient samples.

the swab, it is placed in the plastic tube with the transport medium. It is essential to follow the manufacturer's directions to prevent the swab and specimen from drying out. Transport system swabs also have a label that must be filled out completely, indicating the patient's full name, the date and time of collection, the collector's initials, and the source of the specimen (e.g., deep wound sample from left leg abscess).

CRITICAL THINKING APPLICATION   34.4

Each time Laura collects a wound swab that needs to be sent to the reference laboratory, she needs to put the swab in a transport medium. List three reasons why we use transport media when wound specimens cannot be tested immediately. Be ready to share your ideas with the class.

If possible, a specimen should be placed on culture media immediately after collection. If this is not possible, then the transport device must be sent to a referral laboratory or held in the POL until it can be cultured. For specimens that will be transported by a courier, make sure the specimen is safely packaged in a leak-proof container marked with warning labels (Fig. 34.6). The proper time and

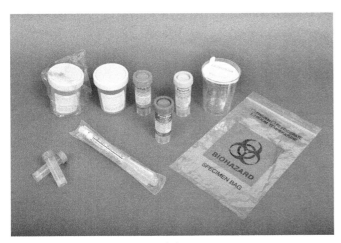

FIGURE 34.6 Microbiology specimen containers.

temperature of storage are vital. Most pathogenic organisms prefer body temperatures, approximately 37°C (98.6°F). They will remain viable for up to 72 hours if held at room temperature or refrigerator temperature (4°C [39.2°F]). Some organisms die if exposed to cold temperatures. Always check the referral laboratory's procedure manual for directions regarding sample time and temperature of storage. See Fig. 34.7 for some commonly used microbiology collection devices.

Devices used for both aerobic and anaerobic blood collection are shown in Fig. 34.7A, and Bactec blood culture bottles are pictured in Fig. 34.7B. Two other commonly used transportation devices are the Jembec plate for transporting *Neisseria gonorrhoeae* (Fig. 34.7C) and a viral-chlamydial transport medium (Fig. 34.7D).

See Table 34.8 for a description of the specimens, containers, patient preparation processes, and storage of specimens commonly collected or handled by medical assistants.

Collection of Pinworms

Enterobius vermicularis is commonly known as pinworm. This species of parasite primarily infects the colon of young children. Humans are infected by ingesting mature eggs through the following:

- Hand-to-mouth transfers
- Feces-contaminated fingers
- Feces-contaminated foods or liquids
- By inhaling eggs in air currents from infected areas

The eggs hatch in the small intestine, and the females migrate out of the anus, usually at night, to deposit the eggs. The eggs adhere to the skin and hair surrounding the anus, sleeping garments, and other clothing. Pinworms cause itching in the anal area, which may cause the eggs to come in contact with the hands and fingernails of the host.

In children, specimens are best collected late at night or early in the morning. Paraffin swabs impregnated with petroleum jelly or cellulose tape may be used to collect the eggs deposited by the adult worm during the night. The pinworm collection is then transferred to a clean glass microscope slide. The diagnosis is based on laboratory detection of the eggs on the pinworm-prepared slide. If the parent does not feel comfortable collecting the specimen, instruct the parent to bring the child to the office as soon as he or she wakes up in the morning. Instruct the parent not to change the child's clothing or diaper before coming into the office. When the child arrives, have

all the needed supplies ready to use, and perform the procedure immediately (Fig. 34.8).

CLIA-WAIVED MICROBIOLOGY TESTING

Often, growing a pathogen on a nutrient media plate is difficult, and it takes time to grow and isolate the pathogen. A rapid direct immunology test demonstrates the presence of the **antigen** in a specimen that is placed in a test kit containing its specific antibody. If the pathogen is present, it produces a colored reaction, indicating a positive result.

POLs with appropriate CLIA-waived certification can perform many rapid identification tests for a variety of infectious diseases. Rapid tests are designed to give the provider a positive test result quickly and efficiently, so that treatment can be started. If the test result is negative, the provider may need to order additional referral laboratory tests.

The first step in performing these tests is to review the package insert provided by the manufacturer. This gives the following valuable information about the test:

- Principle on which the test is based
- Reagents and equipment needed
- Proper specimen collection techniques
- Patient preparation requirements
- Test procedures
- Any precautions or warnings pertaining to the procedure

The insert also provides information about quality control, interpretation of results, limitations of the procedure, and references.

Rapid Strep Testing

Rapid strep testing is commonly performed in the POL and can be completed while the patient waits. The patient's throat is swabbed (see Procedure 34.2, p. 884). The test swab is placed in an **extraction** well, and the extract is tested for antigens found on the surface of *Streptococcus pyogenes* (also referred to as group A strep or GAS). The test kit uses a *lateral flow immunoassay*. This means that the specimen "flows" into the test area. If the strep A pathogen is present, it will have an antigen-antibody reaction with the group A strep antibodies in the testing area. The reaction of the strep A antigen and the strep A antibodies causes a color change that can be seen (see Procedure 34.3, p. 886).

Negative test results should be confirmed with a throat culture performed in the microbiology laboratory (explained later in the chapter). The rapid strep tests are highly specific, so if the test results are positive, there is confidence that *S. pyogenes* is present in the sample. If the test results are negative, the organism may not have been present in high enough numbers to be detected. Then a transport swab should be sent to the microbiology reference laboratory to be cultured.

CRITICAL THINKING APPLICATION   **34.5**

Frankie Burns, a 10-year-old, has a raw, sore throat, fever of 101°F, and just feels awful. Laura is going to collect a throat swab from Frankie for a rapid strep test. What bacteria cause strep throat? What is the scientific name of the bacteria? Which of the two names is the genus, and which of the two names is the species? Write down your answers, and share them with your classmates.

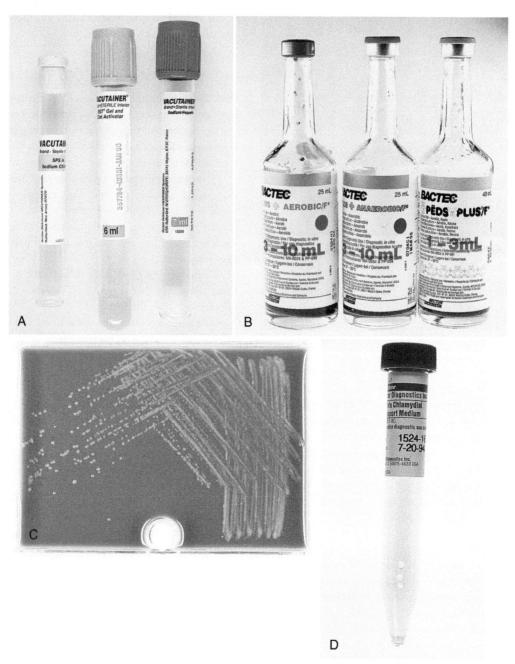

FIGURE 34.7 **(A)** Blood collection Vacutainer tubes, one for aerobic and one for anaerobic. **(B)** Bactec blood culture bottles. **(C)** Jembec plate. **(D)** Viral-chlamydial transport medium. (From De la Maza LM, Pezzlo MT, Baron EJ: *Color atlas of diagnostic microbiology*, St. Louis, 1997, Mosby.)

TABLE 34.8   Collection, Transport, and Processing of Specimens Commonly Collected in the Physician Office Laboratory[a]

SPECIMEN	CONTAINER	PATIENT PREPARATION	SPECIAL INSTRUCTIONS	STORAGE BEFORE PROCESSING
Throat	Transport swab (see Fig. 34.5)	Have patient sitting with head tilted back	Swab pharynx and tonsils, not mouth, tongue, or teeth	Transport and plate within 24 hr; room-temperature storage
Superficial wound	Aerobic transport swab (see Fig. 34.5)	Wipe area with sterile saline before collection	Rotate swab while gently swiping wound	Transport swab stored at room temperature

TABLE 34.8 Collection, Transport, and Processing of Specimens Commonly Collected in the Physician Office Laboratory[a]—*continued*

SPECIMEN	CONTAINER	PATIENT PREPARATION	SPECIAL INSTRUCTIONS	STORAGE BEFORE PROCESSING
Eye	Aerobic transport swab (see Fig. 34.5)	Pull lower lid down while gently collecting exudate along rim	Not applicable	Transport swab may be stored up to 24 hr at room temperature
Ova and parasite (O&P)	O&P transport containers (with formalin and PVA) (see Fig. 34.6)	See Procedure 34.1 for collection of a stool specimen for ova and parasites	Wait 7–10 days if patient has been taking Pepto-Bismol, Kaopectate, or milk of magnesia	Store at room temperature and deliver to laboratory within 24 hr
Stool	Clean, leak-proof containers (see Fig. 34.6)	Outpatients: At minimum, three specimens are collected every other day	Transport to laboratory within 24 hr if storing at 4°C (39.2°F)	Laboratory must plate within 72 hr if storing at 4°C (39.2°F)
Sputum	Sterile, screw-cap container (see Fig. 34.6)	Patient should rinse or gargle with mouthwash before collection	Have patient collect from deep cough; do not collect saliva	Store at 4°C (39.2°F); laboratory must plate within 24 hr
Urine	Vacutainer collection system or sterile, screw-cap container (see Fig. 34.6)	Instruct patient in clean-catch midstream collection	Hold at 4°C (39.2°F), and deliver to laboratory within 24 hr	Hold at 4°C (39.2°F), and plate within 24 hr
Skin scraping (fungal culture)	Clean, screw-top tube (see Fig. 34.6)	Wipe skin with alcohol wipe	Scrape skin at leading edge of lesion	Can be held indefinitely at room temperature but best to process within 72 hr of collection
Blood	Blood culture tube with SPS medium (see Fig. 34.7A) or Vacutainer blood culture medium (see Fig. 34.7B)	Disinfect venipuncture site with alcohol wipe and Betadine	Draw blood during febrile episodes	Deliver to laboratory within 2 hr; incubate at 37°C (98.6°F) on receipt in the laboratory
Gonorrhea culture	Jembec transport system (see Fig. 34.7C)	Wipe away exudate before obtaining culture specimen; obtain culture specimen with swab	Do not refrigerate	Transport to laboratory within 2 hr
Chlamydia culture	Specialized antibiotic *Chlamydia* transport medium (see Fig. 34.7D)	Urogenital swabs preferred; necessary to obtain epithelial cells, not exudate	Transport immediately on ice to laboratory	Store up to 24 hr at 4°C (39.2°F); inoculate cultures within 15 min of collection if swab is not on ice
Body fluids (e.g., peritoneal, synovial, pleural)	Sterile, screw-cap container or anaerobic transporter	Disinfect aspiration site with alcohol wipe and Betadine	Needle aspirations are preferable to swab collections	Transport immediately to laboratory
Rectal swab	Swab placed directly into enteric transport medium	Not applicable	Insert swab approximately 1 inch past anal sphincter	Store at 4°C (39.2°F), transport within 24 hr to laboratory, and plate within 72 hr
Deep wound or abscess	Anaerobic transport device	Wipe area with sterile saline or alcohol wipe before collection	Aspirate material, excise tissue, or insert swab deep into wound	Store at room temperature; transport to laboratory and plate within 4 hr

[a]Reference laboratories also have specific directions for collecting specimens based on their testing methods.
O&P, Ova and parasites; *PVA,* polyvinyl alcohol; *SPS,* Sodium polyanethole sulfonate.
Modified from Forbes BA, Sahm DF, Weissfeld AS: *Bailey and Scott's diagnostic microbiology,* ed 11, St. Louis, 2002, Mosby.

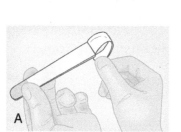
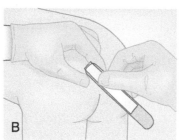
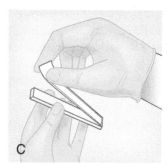

FIGURE 34.8 The three steps for collecting a pinworm specimen from a child. **(A)** Place cellulose tape over a tongue depressor with the sticky side out. **(B)** Press the tape firmly against the right and left anal folds. **(C)** Place the tape with adhesive side down onto the microscope slide.

Influenza A and B Testing

The *influenza* virus causes influenza, or "the flu." This is a highly contagious, acute viral infection of the respiratory tract. The infection is highly communicable through respiratory exposure, and outbreaks are typically seen in the fall and winter. Type A viruses usually are more common than type B viruses. Type A viruses typically are associated with epidemics, and type B viruses cause a milder infection. A rapid diagnosis of influenza can help with the decision to give antiviral medications. They should be given early in the infection cycle to be the most effective. CLIA-waived rapid lateral flow immunoassays detect both influenza A and influenza B antigens from **nasal washes** or nasopharyngeal swabs.

Respiratory Syncytial Virus Testing

Respiratory syncytial virus (RSV) is a major cause of upper and lower respiratory tract infections. It is the major cause of **bronchiolitis** and **pneumonia** in children and infants. Outbreaks typically occur yearly in the fall, winter, and spring and can be severe for very young children. The CLIA-waived rapid direct immunoassay for RSV uses a nasopharyngeal swab specimen or nasal washings to detect the virus. Because antiviral agents are available to treat RSV infection, rapid diagnosis can lead to the following:

- Shorter hospital stays
- Reduced need for antibiotic therapy to treat secondary bacterial infection
- Lower cost for hospital care

The tests are intended for children under age 5. Fig. 34.9 shows the proper placement of the swab when collecting a nasal specimen.

CLIA-WAIVED IMMUNOLOGIC TESTING

Immunology testing provides information about past or present infections with bacteria or viruses. It also detects certain types of cancers. Testing done in the immunology laboratory is designed to demonstrate the reaction between an antigen and its specific antibody. Antibodies are formed when the body encounters a foreign agent. In the acute stage of a disease, the antibody level is high. During the **convalescent stage**, the antibody level declines. Once the immune system recognizes an antigen, then antibodies are made. The antibody will remain in the blood at a low but detectable level for a lifetime. The amount of antibody can be measured with a specific test called a *titer*. The definition of a titer is the lowest concentration of a specific antibody that is still able to neutralize (or precipitate) an antigen.

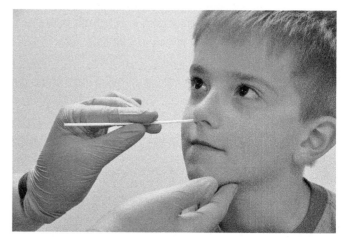

FIGURE 34.9 Note the proper angle of insertion for the swab when collecting a nasal specimen. The swab is inserted at least 1 inch along the base of the nostril on the side that has the most discharge. Once inside, the swab is rotated and rocked back and forth gently for 5 to 10 seconds to obtain a sufficient specimen for influenza and respiratory syncytial virus (RSV) testing.

Most serologic/immunologic testing performed in the ambulatory care center is done using individual test kits (e.g., rapid strep, influenza, infectious mononucleosis [mono], and HIV tests). The difference is the source of the specimen and what the test is looking for.

The direct immunologic tests in the previous section (strep test and influenza test) used a throat swab and nasal swab specimen. The test kits were detecting the antigen or pathogen causing the disease directly. In the indirect immunologic tests, the specimen is the patient's blood or serum. The blood or serum is tested to see whether the patient has produced the specific antibody to the pathogen in question. CLIA-waived immunology tests that may be performed by a medical assistant include infectious mononucleosis, *Helicobacter pylori*, Lyme disease, and human immunodeficiency virus (HIV) tests.

Infectious Mononucleosis Testing

Infectious mononucleosis, commonly called mono, is an acute infectious disease caused by the *Epstein-Barr* virus (EBV). EBV is one of the many herpes viruses. The viral infection is especially common in teenagers. It is found most frequently in people 10 to 25 years of age and is seen occasionally in adults over the age of 25. In the United States, about 95% of adults between ages 35 and 40 have already been infected.

In children, the infection may pass unrecognized or result in a mild illness lasting only a few days. It is marked by sore throat, fever, swollen tonsils, and enlarged lymph nodes in the neck. In young people, some of the most common complications include the abrupt onset of fatigue, headaches, very swollen tonsils, enlarged lymph glands, and loss of appetite often associated with nausea. There may be a short or prolonged period (days or weeks) after the initial illness when the fatigue continues. Occasionally, complications occur, including the development of a swollen spleen or liver, referred to as *hepatosplenomegaly*.

Testing for mononucleosis involves a complete blood count (CBC) and immunology tests. The CBC should reveal an increased number of lymphocytes that appear atypical on the blood smear. The infected lymphocytes undergo a cellular transformation, causing them to look like a monocyte (hence the name *mononucleosis*). Most patients exposed to EBV produce a nonspecific *heterophile antibody* in response to the virus. A heterophile antibody is an antibody that has an affinity for an antigen other than the specific antigen that stimulated its production.

The heterophile antibodies in the patient's blood react with the heterophile antigens supplied in the test kit, resulting in a positive color reaction in the testing area of the kit (see Procedure 34.4, p. 887).

CRITICAL THINKING APPLICATION   **34.6**

Allyson Anderson is 15 years old. She came into the clinic today with signs and symptoms of infectious mononucleosis. Laura is going to do a fingerstick on Allyson and do a mono test. What are the typical signs and symptoms of mono in a teenager? What is the mono test checking for in Allyson's blood?

Helicobacter pylori Testing

Helicobacter pylori is a spiral-shaped bacterium that can infect the stomach's mucous layer or lining. *H. pylori* causes more than 90% of *duodenal* (the first portion of the small intestine) ulcers and more than 80% of stomach ulcers (see Chapter 19). Several methods can be used to diagnose *H. pylori* infection. Serologic tests that measure specific *H. pylori* antibodies can determine whether a person has been infected. CLIA-waived rapid immunoassay tests use whole blood applied to a well in a test cartridge. The blood migrates from the well through the testing area of the cartridge. The presence of a line in the test area of the cartridge indicates the presence of antibodies to the pathogen *H. pylori*.

Lyme Disease Testing

Lyme disease is the most common insect-borne infectious disease in North America, and it is a significant public health concern. The spirochete bacterium *Borrelia burgdorferi* is the causative agent in Lyme disease.

The disease is contracted from an infected tick that bites a person. The bacteria are in the saliva of the tick. These ticks typically are found on deer, mice, dogs, horses, and birds. Infection occurs when the bacteria enter the tick bite. A characteristic bull's-eye rash, known as *erythema migrans* (EM), develops at the bite site in 60% to 80% of patients. Lyme disease progresses in three stages. If the person is not treated, the disease progresses. The spirochete bacterium invades the skin, joints, central nervous system (CNS), heart, and other locations. Arthritic or CNS syndromes often accompany late-stage disease and may be the only clinical symptoms that indicate the infection.

Lyme disease can be detected early with CLIA-waived antibody tests (e.g., Wampole PreVue *B. burgdorferi* test). This immunoassay tests for antibodies in whole blood. A sample of blood is applied to a test cartridge, a **diluent** is added, and the results are read in 20 minutes. The microbiology reference laboratory should verify any positive results.

HIV Testing

HIV attacks and destroys the *T-helper (CD4) lymphocytes*. The T-helper lymphocytes play a critical role in protecting the body against infection. They work with B lymphocytes to produce the specific antibodies that fight infections. As the HIV infection destroys more T-helper cells, the body becomes less able to fight off infections and more susceptible to opportunistic infections. If HIV is not treated with antiretroviral (ARV) medications, acquired immunodeficiency syndrome (AIDS) eventually develops. HIV infections become AIDS when life-threatening infections and cancers begin to appear (see Chapter 18 for more information on HIV and AIDS).

In 2013 the Centers for Disease Control and Prevention (CDC) and the World Health Organization (WHO) both advised preventive measures to control the disease. This requires early detection and early treatment of individuals infected with HIV. The sooner the virus is detected via immunology testing, the sooner treatment with ARV medications may begin.

Two types of CLIA-waived HIV test are readily available to detect the presence of HIV antibodies in blood and in oral specimens.

Patients at risk of HIV infection are now strongly encouraged to take a blood test available in POLs or outpatient clinics. Note that HIV is a bloodborne pathogen. Therefore, the medical assistant testing for HIV should strictly follow the Bloodborne Pathogens Standard established by the Occupational Safety and Health Administration (OSHA).

The patient may also choose to perform an oral self-test from a kit that is available at pharmacies (Fig. 34.10). The test kit includes a testing device that is rubbed once over the upper and lower gums. It then is inserted into the test vial, which is placed in a plastic stand. The test results are read in 20 minutes. The test includes an internal

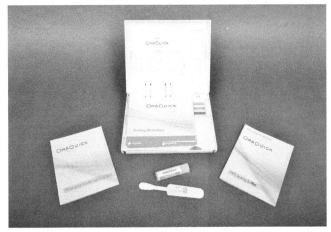

FIGURE 34.10 HIV home testing kit.

control band that verifies a specimen was added and that the test was run correctly.

MICROBIOLOGY REFERENCE LABORATORY: IDENTIFICATION OF PATHOGENS

After receiving the specimens collected in the POL described in the Specimen Collection and Transport in the Physician Office Laboratory section presented earlier in this chapter, the microbiology laboratory promptly prepares a smear of the specimen on a slide to be stained and then transfers the specimen contents onto culture plates (Fig. 34.11). The equipment and supplies in a microbiology laboratory vary with the size of the facility. Most laboratories have a refrigerator, an autoclave, a safety cabinet, a microscope, and an incubator.

Staining

Pathogenic microorganisms generally are colorless, and a microscope is needed to see them. Special stains (e.g., Gram stain and acid-fast stain) are used to differentiate bacteria based on cell membrane properties. As discussed previously, a Gram stain differentiates bacteria into two categories according to chemical makeup of the cell wall. The acid-fast stain differentiates bacteria into two categories based on the presence or absence of a waxy lipid in the cell wall.

Before staining can be done, the specimen must be applied to a labeled slide. The slide is then air dried and fixed. Either heat or methanol can be used to fix the sample to the slide. Fixing results in the material (sample) adhering to the slide. Both heat (e.g., from a Bunsen burner or an incinerator) and methanol cause protein in the sample to break down and stick to the slide. It is similar to how an egg would stick to a hot frying pan.

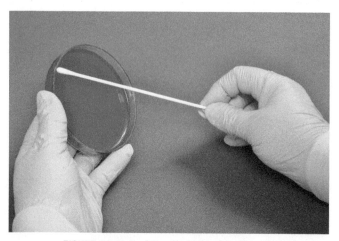

FIGURE 34.11 Inoculating a blood culture plate with a swab.

Gram Stain

The Gram stain, developed by Dr. Hans Christian Gram in the late 1800s, is still the most commonly used stain in microbiology. This procedure involves applying a sequence of reagents: a primary stain, *mordant* (which can fix or set a stain), *decolorizer* (which can wash out a stain), and counterstain (secondary stain) to the slide. The dyes are taken up differently according to the chemical composition of the bacterial cell walls. Bacteria react best in the Gram stain when they are less than 24 hours old. Gram-positive bacteria stain purple, and Gram-negative bacteria stain pink or red (see Fig. 34.1). It is useful for the medical assistant to understand the procedures and the microscopic results of a Gram stain. For example, when a Gram stain report is called in, the terms *GPCs* and *GNBs* mean "Gram-positive cocci" (deeply blue-stained circular cells) and "Gram-negative bacilli" (pink/red stained rod-shaped cells). See Tables 34.1 and 34.2 for the staining characteristics of various pathogenic bacilli and cocci.

CRITICAL THINKING APPLICATION   34.7
What are the four reagents used in the Gram stain? What color are Gram-positive organisms? What color are Gram-negative organisms? Share your answers with the class.

Acid-Fast Stain

The acid-fast stain is used in the identification protocol for *Mycobacterium* species. *M. tuberculosis* causes tuberculosis and can be isolated from sputum or tissue samples. A sputum sample is a respiratory sample from the lower respiratory tract and must be collected in a specific way to be useful. See Chapter 25 for more information about collecting a sputum sample. *M. avium* complex (MAC) is a common soil organism that enters through the respiratory tract and spreads throughout the body. MAC is one of the causes of death among patients with AIDS. An overview of the acid-fast stain is listed here:

- A red primary dye, *carbolfuchsin*, is applied first.
- Then the decolorizer, acid-alcohol, is applied.
- These are followed by a counterstain, *methylene blue*.

Acid-fast positive microbes stain fuchsia-red. Acid-fast negative microbes stain baby blue. Bacilli that are acid-fast positive often are referred to as *acid-fast bacillus* (AFB) (see Fig. 34.2).

Inoculating Equipment

Next, the specimen must be spread on specific culture media based on the source of the specimen. The inoculated culture media are placed in a body temperature incubator to grow overnight. Inoculating needles and loops (Fig. 34.12) are used to transfer samples to culture media or microbes to slides for staining. Needles and loops may be disposable and presterilized. They may also be made of wire and can be heat sterilized before and after each transfer (Fig. 34.13). An inoculating loop is shaped like a bubble wand, and a thin film of liquid adheres to the loop. The amount of fluid held by the loop can be calibrated. For example, a urine culture uses a loop that delivers a 1-mcL sample. The urine in the loop is spread across the culture medium and allowed to grow overnight. The next day, each bacterium becomes a visible *colony*, which is a discrete group of organisms.

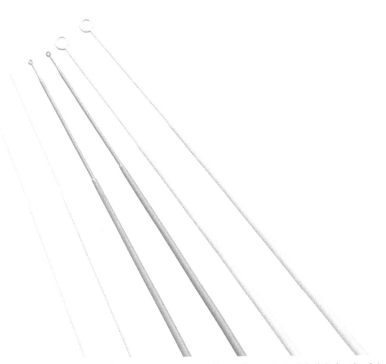

FIGURE 34.12 *(Left)* Inoculating needles. *(Right)* Inoculating loops. (Courtesy Simport Plastics, Beloeil, Quebec, Canada.)

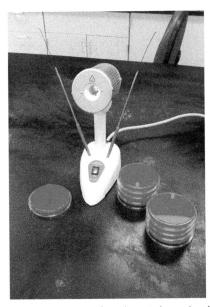

FIGURE 34.13 Incinerator for sterilizing wire loops and needles.

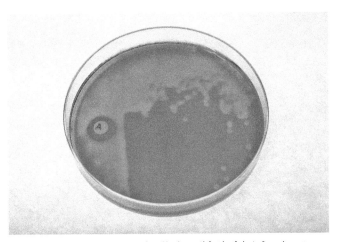

FIGURE 34.14 Positive strep test result on blood agar (*left side of plate*). Group A streptococcus (GAS) shows beta hemolysis (clearing) of the blood agar below the growing colonies. Notice there is no hemolysis, or clearing of the blood around the white bacitracin disk. That is because bacitracin can destroy GAS.

Colonies can then be counted and analyzed to determine the cause of a urinary tract infection.

Assessing a Culture

When the original (primary) culture has incubated at the appropriate temperature for 18 to 24 hours, it is examined for evidence of pathogens. Because normal flora is often present in samples in addition to pathogens, a trained eye is required to spot the organisms that might be causing an infection. Suspicious colonies are **subcultured** onto the appropriate medium to isolate them in *pure culture*. The definition of pure culture is growth of only one type of microorganism

in or on a culture medium. When an organism is in pure culture, staining and additional biochemical testing can be done to identify the organism. Throat and urine cultures may be performed in POLs that have been CLIA certified to perform moderately complex testing.

Throat Cultures

Streptococcus pyogenes, also known as *group A strep (GAS)* or *beta hemolytic streptococcus*, causes strep throat. If not diagnosed and treated promptly, this infection can cause severe complications, including scarlet fever, rheumatic fever, and glomerulonephritis. A throat swab is collected from the patient's throat. Then the swab is *streaked for isolation* on a **blood agar plate (BAP)**. An antibiotic disk is placed on the first quadrant of the streaked plate (Fig. 34.14) and incubated overnight at 37°C (98.6°F). The antibiotic disk contains *bacitracin*, which prevents the growth of *S. pyogenes*. Complete clearing of the agar around the colonies indicates *beta hemolysis*, which is caused by a toxin produced by *S. pyogenes*. The toxin breaks down the red blood cells in the agar, causing the agar to be a clear golden color around the colonies. The presence of beta hemolysis and a zone of no growth around the bacitracin disk indicate that the patient has strep throat. Additional testing may be needed to confirm the identity of the organism.

Streaking for Isolation

Streaking for isolation is also called a four-quadrant streak. To streak for isolation, an isolated colony of an organism growing on an agar plate is touched using a sterile inoculating loop. The organism is then methodically spread out onto solid nutrient media. The goal is to have colonies that are separate from other colonies. It is a procedure that is performed with most microbiology specimens. By distributing bacteria across the agar plate and isolating bacterial colonies, laboratory personnel can see characteristics of the bacteria that are useful in the identification process.

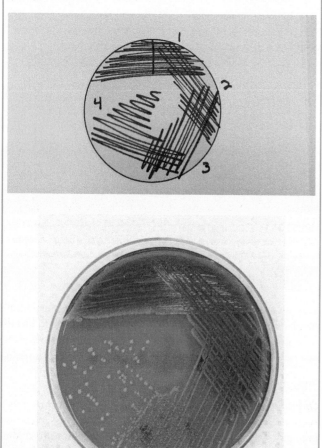

Urine Cultures

With urine cultures, the bacterial colonies that appear after incubation are counted. A calibrated inoculating loop is dipped into a well-mixed urine sample that was collected by the CCMS method or by catheterization. The urine from the loop is spread on solid culture media and incubated for 18 to 24 hours at 37°C (98.6°F). Each colony that grows on the plate represents 1000 colony-forming units (cfu) per milliliter. The final cfu results are interpreted as follows:

- Normal: <10,000 cfu/mL of urine; no urinary tract infection (UTI) is present
- Borderline: 10,000 to 100,000 cfu/mL of urine; a chronic or relapsing infection may be present, and the test should be repeated
- Positive: >100,000 cfu/mL of urine; a UTI is likely

The medical assistant needs to be aware of the terminology and values reported for urine cultures.

Microbiology Culture and Sensitivity Testing

Once a bacterial infection has been identified, an additional step is often required for successful treatment. To determine the appropriate antibiotic to destroy the pathogen, the provider will order a culture and sensitivity (C&S) test. *Culture* refers to growing the organisms, and *sensitivity* refers to the organism's susceptibility to antibiotics.

C&S test results provide vital information about which specific antibiotics work best against the particular infective pathogen. The healthcare provider must decide which medication to order based on initial test results and the patient's physical examination.

There are many methods of performing sensitivity testing. Some methods involve culture media and antibiotic disks. Other methods are fully automated and require a very small amount of the pure culture to be tested. No matter what method is used, sensitivity testing is reported to the provider in one of three categories for each antibiotic tested:

- **S** means that the pathogen is *susceptible*, or that the antibiotic is effective in destroying that particular organism.
- **R** means that the pathogen is *resistant*, or that the antibiotic is not effective in destroying that particular organism.
- **I** means *intermediate*, or that additional testing must be performed to determine the dosage of antibiotic necessary for successful treatment.

Some testing methods may give additional information regarding the dosage tested **in vitro**. This information may be helpful as the providers choose the appropriate antibiotic for treatment. The appropriate antibiotic agent meets the following criteria:

- Destroys the infectious agent with a reasonable level of the drug
- Is the least toxic to the patient
- Has the least impact on normal flora of the body
- Has the desired pharmacologic characteristics (preparation, route of delivery, effectiveness)
- If possible, is the most economical for the patient

CRITICAL THINKING APPLICATION   **34.8**

Laura is looking over the reference laboratory results from the day. Mrs. Liz Darcy was in for an office visit yesterday and collected a urine specimen for C&S. Her preliminary culture report came back as 82,000 cfu/mL, pure culture. The identification and susceptibility report is due to follow tomorrow.

- Does Mrs. Darcy have a urinary tract infection?
- Does Mrs. Darcy need any additional testing for this condition?
- In your own words, define *pure culture*.
- Describe C&S in your own words.

CLOSING COMMENTS

Patient Coaching

Microorganisms such as bacteria, viruses, fungi, and parasites are responsible for most human infectious diseases. Patient education plays an important role in helping the patient and family control the spread of infection. The teaching topics in the following list can help you educate a patient about infection control:

- An explanation of the patient's type of infection: bacterial, viral, fungal, or parasitic
- How infections spread
- Hand washing and sanitization, proper storage and cleaning of personal items, and disposal of contaminated supplies
- Risk factors for infection, such as poor nutritional habits or poor ventilation with airborne pathogens present
- The patient's role in specimen collection
- Patient preparation for laboratory tests, imaging tests, and other needed procedures

Explain to the patient that an infection can be transferred from person to person in many ways. Reinforce the importance of following directions for taking any medication. If patients do not follow the directions given to them by the provider and/or pharmacist, there is a real chance of the following:

- Developing complications
- Having a relapse of an infection
- Allowing an infection to spread to other areas or becoming systemic

Always listen to the patient. Be sure to answer all the patient's questions. Notify the provider of patient's concerns so that he or she can give further details or instructions before the patient leaves the facility.

Legal and Ethical Issues

Maintaining a laboratory in the office increases the physician's liability. By testing patients' specimens in the office, the physician assumes responsibility for the interpretation and accuracy of the results. As the person in the office who runs the tests and notes the results in the patient's record, you are responsible for maintaining optimum accuracy in testing results. A quality assurance (QA) program, including the running, interpreting, and recording of the internal controls supplied in each test kit, must be documented. Both microbiology and immunology tests allow the patient to benefit from the convenience of office testing. Strict confidentiality is essential. Never release information to anyone other than the patient or legal guardian.

Also note that certain infectious diseases must be reported to the CDC or local board of health. Each state legislature determines what diseases must be reported and how the data are to be reported. Additional data for nationally notifiable diseases is published weekly by the CDC in the *Morbidity and Mortality Weekly Report* (MMWR). For additional information on infectious disease reporting, please review the reporting procedure presented in Chapter 4 in the main text.

Patient-Centered Care

Hand hygiene should be foremost in your mind with each patient encounter. Making sure that you wash hands or use hand sanitizer as you enter and leave an exam room should be part of your routine. Sanitizing hands before and after gloving is also a must. But also remembering to sanitize hands when the patient is not in front of you is just as important. Anytime you handle specimens, containers, enter and leave a laboratory area, or put away laboratory supplies and equipment, you should also follow up with proper hand hygiene. The CDC states that the most effective means of stopping the transmission of disease is frequent and proper handwashing.

Professional Behaviors

Medicine is an ever-changing profession, and medical assistants need to remain current in all areas of their profession. The laboratory is no exception. Microbiology and immunology are areas of the laboratory where research, technical skills, and testing methods are changing rapidly. Making an effort to stay up to date with new ideas and concepts is critical to contributing to exceptional patient care.

SUMMARY OF SCENARIO

Laura has had another busy day at WMFM Clinic. Once again, she has seen infectious diseases in some of her patients today. Laura knows that most microorganisms are harmless, but knowing the signs and symptoms of common infectious diseases is important.

It is important to diagnose and treat most infectious diseases. Laura knows that proper specimen collection is essential. She is also aware that rapid CLIA-waived tests can identify pathogens and help treat patients in a timely manner.

Microbiology and immunology tests have become useful in the physician office laboratory. Meeting the needs of patients and quickly addressing their concerns are benefits of CLIA-waived testing. Laura feels comfortable collecting specimens, testing patient samples, and reporting the results for the provider to review. As a certified medical assistant, she knows that the work she does throughout the day is helping every one of her patients.

SUMMARY OF LEARNING OBJECTIVES

1. **Describe the naming of microorganisms.**

   The naming of all living organisms uses a binomial system consisting of two names; the first "family" name is the *genus,* and the second is the *species.* Both names are either italicized or underlined when written. The genus begins with a capital letter, the species with a lowercase letter. Often the name reveals some characteristic about the organism.

2. **Describe various bacterial staining characteristics, shapes, oxygen requirements, and physical structures; also, explain the characteristics of common diseases caused by bacteria.**

   Identification of bacteria begins with observation of their morphology. Cocci are spherical organisms, bacilli are rod-shaped organisms, and spirilla are spiral-shaped organisms. Staphylococci are cocci in clusters, streptococci and streptobacilli are organisms arranged in chains, and diplococci and diplobacilli are organisms arranged in pairs. Their staining characteristics are Gram positive (dark blue), Gram negative (pink), and acid-fast (pink). Organisms are classified by oxygen requirements as aerobic (needs oxygen to survive), anaerobic (lives without oxygen), or facultative (anaerobic but able to survive in the presence of oxygen). Tables 34.1 to 34.3 can help explain the characteristics of common diseases caused by bacteria.

3. **Describe the unusual characteristics of *Chlamydia, Mycoplasma,* and *Rickettsia* organisms.**

   Chlamydia and *Rickettsia* organisms are tiny bacteria; however, unlike most bacteria, they require a host cell for replication. *Rickettsia* organisms are transmitted by arthropods. *Mycoplasma* organisms are bacteria without cell walls (see Table 34.4).

4. **Do the following related to fungi, protozoa, and parasites:**
   - Compare bacteria with fungi, protozoa, and parasites.
     Bacteria are prokaryotic (containing no nucleus); fungi, protozoa, and parasites are eukaryotic. Bacteria, fungi, and protozoa must be observed microscopically; helminths, or worms, can be seen with the naked eye but their eggs may be microscopic in size.
   - Identify the characteristics of common diseases caused by fungi, protozoa, and parasites.
     Tables 34.5 and 34.6 present the characteristics of common diseases caused by fungi and protozoa.
   - Perform patient education on the collection of a stool specimen for ova and parasite testing.
     Stool is collected in special transport devices that contain preservatives and fixatives that aid microscopic examination of the specimen. Explicit instructions must be given to the patient to ensure proper collection (see Procedure 34.1, p. 883).

5. **Compare bacteria with viruses, and describe the characteristics of common viral diseases.**

   Viruses differ from bacteria in that they are not cells. Viruses have a core of nucleic acid surrounded by a protein coat. Unlike bacteria, viruses do not metabolize and cannot replicate on their own. They are called obligate intracellular parasites. Table 34.7 presents the characteristics of various viral diseases.

6. **Cite the protocols for the collection, transport, and processing of specimens.**

   Refer to Table 34.8.

7. **Explain how pinworm testing is done and when it is recommended.**

   Pinworm testing detects the eggs of the pinworm, *E. vermicularis.* The worm deposits eggs in the anal folds at night. The eggs can be retrieved by using a sticky collection device either late in the evening or in the morning before a bowel movement. The diagnosis is made if the eggs are found microscopically.

8. **Describe and perform CLIA-waived microbiology tests:**
   - Describe three CLIA-waived microbiology tests that use a rapid identification technique.
     Often, growing a pathogen on a culture plate is difficult, and it takes time to grow and isolate the pathogen. A rapid "direct" immunology test demonstrates the presence of the pathogen's antigen in a specimen that is placed in a test kit containing its specific antibody. If the pathogen is present, it produces a colored reaction, indicating a positive result. The *rapid strep test* detects *S. pyogenes* and is used in the diagnosis of strep throat. The *influenza A and B rapid test* detects surface antigens of the viruses that cause influenza. The *RSV rapid test* detects antigens from RSV, which causes pneumonia and bronchiolitis in young children.
   - Obtain a specimen, and perform the CLIA-waived rapid strep test. Refer to Procedures 34.2 and 34.3, pp. 884–886.

9. **Do the following related to CLIA-waived immunology testing:**
   - Discuss the purpose of indirect immunology testing.
     "Indirect" immunology testing detects antibodies in whole blood, serum, or plasma that react to the specific antigen in the test kit, producing a colored reaction. A positive reaction indicates that the antibodies have been produced and attack the pathogen in question (e.g., heterophile antibodies seen in mononucleosis).
   - Describe three CLIA-waived indirect immunology tests that could be done in the physician office laboratory.
     Mononucleosis testing detects the heterophile antibodies made in reaction to an infection of the Epstein-Barr virus. The *H. pylori test* detects antibodies to the bacterium that commonly causes stomach ulcers. Early detection of *Lyme disease* can be accomplished using a CLIA-waived test that detects the antibodies that attack the *B. burgdorferi* pathogen. Rapid HIV testing detects the HIV antibodies made in reaction to an HIV infection that could develop into AIDS.
   - Obtain a specimen, and perform the CLIA-waived microbiology strep test.
     Refer to Procedure 34.4, p. 887.

10. **Detail the equipment needed in a microbiology reference laboratory, and discuss the identification of pathogens in the microbiology laboratory by describing various staining techniques.**

    Microbiology viewing equipment includes slides, stains, and microscopes. Culturing equipment includes inoculating loops and needles, petri dishes with the appropriate growth media, and incubators. Sterilizing equipment includes incinerators and autoclaves. The Gram stain is the most commonly used stain in the microbiology laboratory. The acid-fast stain is used in the identification protocol for *Mycobacterium* species.

11. **Describe the reference laboratory assessment of a throat culture and a urine culture.**

The throat culture is observed on the blood agar plate for beta hemolysis and no growth around the bacitracin disk (Fig. 34.14). Urine growth is assessed after incubation to determine whether a urinary tract infection is present. Each colony that grows on the plate represents 1000 colony-forming units (cfu) per milliliter. The final cfu results are interpreted as normal (<10,000 cfu/mL, no UTI is present), borderline (10,000 to 100,000 cfu/mL, a chronic or relapsing infection may be present, and the test should be repeated), and positive (>100,000 cfu/mL, a UTI is likely).

12. **Explain the method used for culture and sensitivity testing.**

There are many methods of performing sensitivity testing. Some methods involve culture media and antibiotic disks. Other methods are fully automated and require a very small amount of the pure culture to be tested. No matter what method is used, sensitivity testing is reported to the provider in one of three categories for each antibiotic tested: susceptibility, resistance, or an intermediate reaction to the antimicrobial agent.

13. **Discuss patient education, in addition to legal and ethical issues, as it applies to laboratory testing.**

The medical assistant must be aware that patient confidentiality is of utmost importance; however, certain infections must be reported to the CDC and to the local board of health.

PROCEDURE 34.1	Instruct Patients in the Collection of Fecal Specimens to Be Tested for Ova and Parasites

Task: Instruct a patient in the proper collection of stool for an ova and parasite microscopic examination.

EQUIPMENT and SUPPLIES

- Patient's health record
- Provider's order or lab requisition
- Clean, dry container for stool collection
- Two parasitology collection vials*
- Plastic biohazard zipper-lock bag

*Please note that several types of preservatives are available. Check with the referral laboratory to make sure the patient is given the proper vials for collection. Preservatives include low-viscosity polyvinyl alcohol (LV-PVA), zinc sulfite polyvinyl alcohol (ZN-PVA), sodium acetate acetic acid formalin (SAF), and 10% neutral buffered formalin.

PROCEDURAL STEPS

1. Greet the patient. Identify yourself. Verify the patient's identity with full name, then ask the patient to spell the first and last names and to state his or her date of birth. Explain the procedure in a manner that the patient understands. Answer any general questions the patient may have about the collection procedures before you give detailed instructions.
   PURPOSE: It is important to identify the patient in two different ways to ensure that you have the correct patient. Explaining the procedure can make the patient feel more comfortable and reduces anxiety.

2. Instruct the patient not to take any antacids, laxatives, or stool softeners before collecting the specimen.
   PURPOSE: Laxatives increase fecal transit time and may result in a false-negative test result.

3. Instruct the patient to urinate before collecting the specimen.
   PURPOSE: This eliminates the possibility of the stool becoming contaminated with urine.

4. The patient then collects the specimen.
   - *Adults:* Instruct the patient to defecate into the container. Stool cannot be retrieved from the toilet bowl.
   - *Children:* Loosely drape the toilet rim with plastic wrap and lower the seat. The child should have a bowel movement into the toilet, onto the wrap. Remove the stool using a disposable plastic spoon.
   PURPOSE: The stool cannot be contaminated by or diluted with water.
   - *Infants:* Fasten a "diaper" made of plastic wrap over the child, using tape. Remove the plastic wrap immediately after a bowel movement and remove the stool using a plastic spoon. *Never leave the child unattended with the plastic wrap in place because of the risk of suffocation.*
   PURPOSE: Stool cannot be collected in a diaper.

5. Instruct the patient to add stool to the collection containers.
   - If the stool is formed, use the scoop on the lid of the containers to add a large, jelly bean–sized piece of stool to the liquid in the containers (Fig. 1).
   - If the stool is liquid, pour it into the containers.
   - In both of the previous cases, keep adding the specimen until the liquid preservative in the vial reaches the indicated level on the containers.
   PURPOSE: Proper instructions will give patients confidence in what they need to do to ensure a proper specimen.

Continued

PROCEDURE 34.1	**Instruct Patients in the Collection of Fecal Specimens to Be Tested for Ova and Parasites**—*continued*

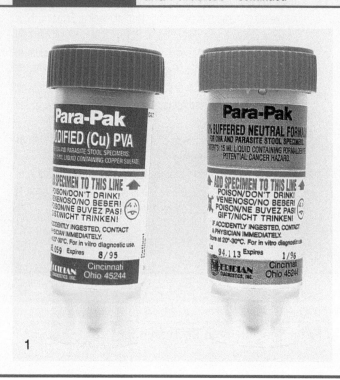

1

6. Instruct the patient to tighten the caps completely and wipe the outside of the vials with rubbing alcohol or to wash carefully with soap and water.
   PURPOSE: These actions ensure infection control.
7. The vials should be labeled, placed in a biohazard bag with a zippered closure, and transported to the laboratory immediately, if possible. *The vials should not be refrigerated.*
8. Instruct the patient to wash his or her hands after the specimen collection procedure.
   PURPOSE: It is important to ensure infection control.

Figure 1 Courtesy Meridian Bioscience, Cincinnati, Ohio.

PROCEDURE 34.2	**Collect a Specimen for a Throat Culture**

Task: Collect a throat culture, using sterile technique, for immediate testing or for transportation to the laboratory.

EQUIPMENT and SUPPLIES

- Patient's health record
- Provider's order
- Laboratory requisition
- Fluid-impermeable lab coat, face shield, and gloves
- 1 sterile swab if transporting to a reference lab for culture, and/or 1 sterile swab from the rapid strep test kit if testing patient in the POL.
- Sterile tongue depressor
- Transport medium
- Biohazard waste container

PROCEDURAL STEPS

1. Wash hands or use hand sanitizer. Put on a fluid-impermeable lab coat.
   PURPOSE: It is important to ensure infection control.
2. Gather the materials needed.
3. Greet the patient. Identify yourself. Verify the patient's identity with full name, then ask the patient to spell the first and last names and to state his or her date of birth. Explain the procedure in a manner that the patient understands. Answer any general questions the patient may have about the collection procedures before you give detailed instructions.
   PURPOSE: It is important to identify the patient in two different ways to ensure that you have the correct patient. Explaining the procedure can make the patient feel more comfortable and reduces anxiety.
4. Put on face shield and gloves. Position the patient so that the light shines into the mouth.
   PURPOSE: It is important to ensure infection control and to illuminate the area to be swabbed.
5. Remove the sterile swab from the sterile wrap with your dominant hand, and grasp the sterile tongue depressor with your nondominant hand.
   PURPOSE: These actions allow better control of the swabbing process.
6. Instruct the patient to open the mouth and say, "Ah." Depress the tongue with the depressor.
   PURPOSE: Saying "Ah" helps elevate the uvula and reduces the tendency to gag. The tongue is depressed so that you can see the back of the throat and prevent contamination of the sterile swab.

PROCEDURE 34.2 | Collect a Specimen for a Throat Culture—*continued*

7. Swab the back of the throat between the tonsillar pillars in a figure-8 pattern, especially any reddened, patchy areas of the throat, white pus pockets, purulent areas, and the tonsils; take care not to touch any other areas in the mouth (Fig. 1).
   PURPOSE: Pathogenic organisms are found in the back of the throat and on the tonsils.

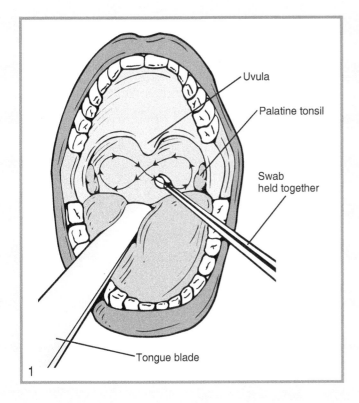

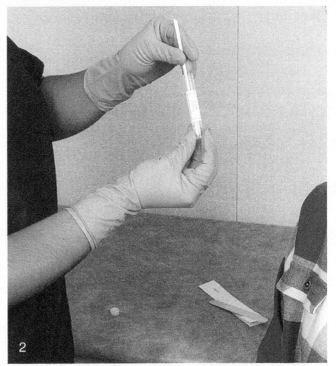

9. Dispose of contaminated supplies in the biohazard waste container.
   PURPOSE: Disposing of contaminated supplies prevents the spread of infection.
10. Disinfect the work area.
    PURPOSE: Disinfection will ensure infection control.
11. Remove your gloves, and discard them in the biohazard waste container. Remove the face shield.
12. Wash hands or use hand sanitizer.
    PURPOSE: Hand sanitization is an important step for infection control.
13. Document the procedure in the patient's health record.
    PURPOSE: Procedures are not complete until they are recorded.

   8/14/20 8:35 a.m. Throat specimen collected via swab from tonsillar area. Sent to University Laboratories for strep testing. _____
   _____Laura Piper, CMA (AAMA)

8. Place the swab in the transport medium, label it, and follow appropriate procedures to send it to the referral laboratory (Fig. 2). If rapid strep testing is requested, it may be done in the POL or sent to a reference laboratory.
   PURPOSE: A transport medium prevents the swab from drying out. Labeling immediately after collection prevents specimen misidentification.

PROCEDURE 34.3   **Perform a CLIA-Waived Microbiology Test: Perform a Rapid Strep Test**

Task: Perform a rapid strep screening test to assist in the diagnosis of strep throat.

EQUIPMENT and SUPPLIES

- Patient's health record
- Provider's order or lab requisition
- QuickVue In-Line Strep A test kit contents (Fig. 1):
  - Extraction solution bottles
  - Individually packaged test cassettes
  - Individually wrapped sterile rayon swabs provided in kit
  - Positive (+) control swab provided in kit
  - Visual flow chart outlining the steps of the test
- Rapid Strep Test Log Sheet
- Stopwatch or laboratory timer
- Fluid-impermeable lab coat, eye protection, and gloves
- Biohazard waste container
- Biohazard sharps container

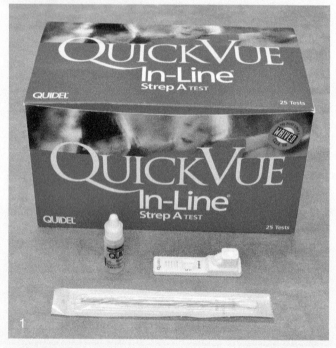

PROCEDURAL STEPS

1. Collect all necessary supplies and equipment. Bring all reagents to room temperature. Check the expiration date on the test kit package.
   PURPOSE: Follow manufacturer's directions for reagent temperature. Do not use any supplies that are outdated.
2. Put on fluid-impermeable lab coat.
   PURPOSE: Always wear proper PPE when doing laboratory testing.
3. Note: Before running the first patient test from a new test kit, a positive and negative control test must be run using the control swabs provided in the kit. Confirm that both controls reacted correctly, and record the control results on the log sheet.
   PURPOSE: Both control swabs must be checked before patients are tested. If the controls show the appropriate results, the test kit is reliable.

4. Greet the patient. Identify yourself. Verify the patient's identity with full name, then ask the patient to spell the first and last names and to state his or her date of birth. Explain the procedure in a manner that the patient understands. Answer any general questions the patient may have about the collection procedures before you give detailed instructions.
   PURPOSE: It is important to identify the patient in two different ways to ensure that you have the correct patient. Explaining the procedure can make the patient feel more comfortable and reduces anxiety.
5. Wash hands or use hand sanitizer.
   PURPOSE: Hand sanitization is an important step for infection control.
6. Put on gloves and face protection. Collect a throat specimen using the rayon swab provided in the test kit.
   PURPOSE: Always wear proper PPE when doing laboratory testing. The test kit provides a rayon swab to avoid the use of cotton swabs, which can kill bacteria, possibly causing a false-negative result.
7. Remove the test cassette from the foil pouch, and place it on a clean, dry, level surface. Using the notch at the back of the chamber as a guide, insert the patient's swab completely into the swab chamber (Fig. 2).

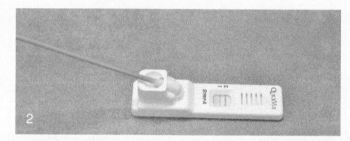

8. Place the extraction bottle between your thumb and forefinger, and squeeze once to break the glass ampule inside the extraction solution bottle. Vigorously shake the bottle five times to mix the solutions. The solution should turn green.
   PURPOSE: The color change is an indicator of extraction reagent integrity and that the extraction procedure was performed correctly.
9. Immediately remove the cap on the extraction solution bottle, hold the bottle vertically over the chamber, and quickly fill the chamber to the rim (approximately 8 drops).
   PURPOSE: The liquid extract reacts with the swab and then flows into the test cassette, passing through the test area (T) and then through the internal control area (C).
10. Remove your face shield. Wait 5 minutes to read the results, and record them in the lab log.
    - *Positive result:* A pink line shows in the T area, indicating the presence of *Streptococcus pyogenes* antigen; a blue line appears in the C area, indicating that the fluid activated the internal control.
    - *Negative result:* No pink line appears in the T test area; a blue line appears in the C control area, indicating that the internal control worked.
    - *Invalid result:* The blue control line does not appear next to the letter C at 5 minutes. The test result cannot be reported.

PROCEDURE 34.3 Perform a CLIA-Waived Microbiology Test: Perform a Rapid Strep Test—*continued*

11. Discard all the test materials in the appropriate biohazard waste container.
    PURPOSE: Items that come in contact with samples are considered potentially infectious.
12. Disinfect the work area; remove your gloves and fluid-impermeable lab coat. Wash hands or use hand sanitizer.
    PURPOSE: Hand sanitization is an important step for infection control.
13. Record the test results in the patient's health record.
    PURPOSE: A procedure is considered not complete until it is properly documented.

14. If the test results are negative, a second throat swab should be obtained and sent to the reference laboratory for a throat culture. Often two swabs are used simultaneously when the sample is initially collected from the throat to prevent the need to re-collect a specimen.
    PURPOSE: Negative rapid strep test results should be confirmed with a throat culture.

QUALITATIVE CONTROL/PATIENT LOG SHEET

TEST: _____ STREP A TEST _____
KIT NAME AND MANUFACTURER: QuickVue In-Line Strep A Test — Quidel
LOT # _____ 12345 _____   EXPIRATION DATE: _____ 11/22/20XX _____
STORAGE REQUIREMENTS: _ Room Temp _ TEST FLOW CHART __ yes __

DATE	SPECIMEN I.D. (CONTROL/PATIENT)	RESULT (+ OR −)	INTERNAL CONTROL PASSED (Y OR N)	CHARTED IN PATIENT RECORD	TECH INITIALS
7/11/20XX	POSITIVE CONTROL	+	Y		DC
7/11/20XX	NEGATIVE CONTROL	−	Y		DC
7/11/20XX	PT ID: 5432	+	Y	✓	DC

Documentation in the Medical Record

10/9/20– 9:30 a.m. Rapid Strep A Test performed with a positive result.
Second swab sent to lab for culture and sensitivity. _____
_____ Laura Piper, CMA (AAMA)

PROCEDURE 34.4 Perform a CLIA-Waived Immunology Test: Perform the QuickVue+ Infectious Mononucleosis Test

Task: Perform and interpret a rapid CLIA-waived test for infectious mononucleosis.

EQUIPMENT and SUPPLIES

- Patient's health record
- Provider's order or lab requisition
- CLIA-waived QuickVue+ test kit for infectious mononucleosis and blood collecting supplies (Fig. 1):
  - Package with test kit supplies
  - Color-coded bottles of positive and negative controls and the developer
  - Test cassette in foil-wrapped protective pouch

- Pipettes supplied in kit with black line indicating amount of capillary blood to collect
- Alcohol prep pad, gauze, and bandage
- Lancet
- Laboratory timer, stopwatch, or wristwatch with sweep second hand
- Fluid-impermeable lab coat, eye protection, and gloves
- Biohazard waste container

Continued

PROCEDURE 34.4	Perform a CLIA-Waived Immunology Test: Perform the QuickVue+ Infectious Mononucleosis Test—*continued*

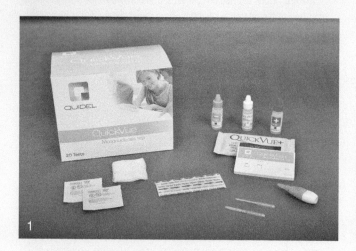

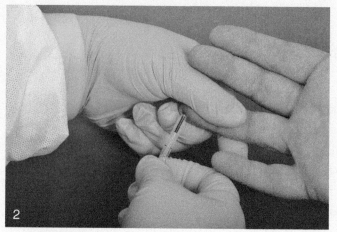

PROCEDURAL STEPS

1. Remove the test kit from the refrigerator, and allow the reagents to warm to room temperature. Check the expiration date of the kit.
   <u>PURPOSE:</u> Follow the manufacturer's directions for reagent use. Do not use outdated reagents or kits.

2. Put on the fluid-impermeable lab coat and protective eyewear.
   <u>PURPOSE:</u> Always wear proper PPE when doing laboratory testing.

3. Before running the first patient test from a new test kit, run the positive and negative liquid controls provided in the kit to see whether they react correctly. Record your control results on the log sheet.
   <u>PURPOSE:</u> Both control swabs must be checked before patients are tested. If the controls show the appropriate results, the test kit is reliable.

4. Greet the patient. Identify yourself. Verify the patient's identity with full name, then ask the patient to spell the first and last names and to state his or her date of birth. Explain the procedure in a manner that the patient understands. Answer any general questions the patient may have about the collection procedures before you give detailed instructions.
   <u>PURPOSE:</u> It is important to identify the patient in two different ways to ensure that you have the correct patient. Explaining the procedure can make the patient feel more comfortable and reduces anxiety.

5. Wash hands or use hand sanitizer. Put on gloves
   <u>PURPOSE:</u> It is important to ensure infection control.

6. Remove the test device from its protective pouch, and label it with the patient's identification.
   <u>PURPOSE:</u> Proper labeling ensures correct patient identification on the test cassette.

7. Disinfect the patient's finger with the alcohol swab. Allow it to air dry, and then perform a capillary puncture.
   <u>PURPOSE:</u> Disinfection will ensure infection control. If the alcohol is wet, the capillary puncture will sting and be uncomfortable for the patient.

8. Wipe away the first drop of blood, and then fill the disposable pipette provided in the kit to the calibration mark with capillary blood (see Chapter 32 for proper blood collection methods) (Fig. 2).
   <u>PURPOSE:</u> The plastic capillary tube measures the exact amount of sample, for accurate testing.

9. Dispense all the blood from the capillary tube into the "Add" well of the testing device. (Or, if you are using venous blood, transfer a large drop from the venous whole blood specimen using the longer capillary pipette provided in the kit.)
   <u>PURPOSE:</u> Proper specimen type and volume is required for accurate testing.

10. Hold the developer bottle vertically above the "Add" well, and allow 5 drops to fall freely.
    <u>PURPOSE:</u> Holding a dropper vertically ensures delivery of the same-size drop. If the dropper touches other materials, it becomes contaminated and the results will be inaccurate.

11. Read the results at 5 minutes. Note: The "Test Complete" box must be visibly colored by 10 minutes.
    - *Positive result:* A vertical line in any shade of blue forms a plus sign in the "Read Result" window, along with a blue "Test Complete" line. Even a faint blue plus sign should be reported as a positive.
    - *Negative result:* No vertical blue line appears, leaving a minus sign in the "Read Result" window, along with a blue "Test Complete" line.
    - *Invalid result:* After 10 minutes, no line is seen in the "Test Complete" window, or a blue color fills the "Read Result" window. If either of these is noted, the test must be repeated with a new testing device. If the problem continues, request technical support.
    <u>PURPOSE:</u> Always follow manufacturer's instructions for reading the test result.

12. Dispose of biohazard waste in the biohazard waste container. Disinfect the work area.
    <u>PURPOSE:</u> It is important to ensure infection control.

13. Remove your personal protective equipment. Dispose of gloves in the biohazard waste container. Wash hands or use hand sanitizer.
    <u>PURPOSE:</u> Hand sanitization is an important step for infection control.

14. Document control results in the appropriate laboratory log. Document patient results in the appropriate laboratory log and in the patient's health record.
    <u>PURPOSE:</u> A procedure is not considered complete until it is properly documented.

| PROCEDURE 34.4 | Perform a CLIA-Waived Immunology Test: Perform the QuickVue+ Infectious Mononucleosis Test—*continued* |

Quality Control Procedures

External positive and negative liquid controls are provided with each new kit. Each new operator of the test should perform liquid positive and negative external controls once to confirm that his or her testing technique is correct. Also, external controls should be tested and charted when a new kit is used.

The *internal* control occurs in the "Test Complete" window built into each reaction unit. Chart the control results on the control log with the operator's initials.

QUALITATIVE CONTROL/PATIENT LOG SHEET

TEST: _____MONONUCLEOSIS RAPID TEST_____
KIT NAME & MANUFACTURER: QUICK VUE+ Infectious Mononucleosis Test -QUIDEL
LOT # ___12345_____   EXPIRATION DATE: _____11/22/20XX_____
STORAGE REQUIREMENTS: _REFRIGERATOR___   TEST FLOW CHART ___yes_____

DATE	SPECIMEN I.D. (CONTROL/PATIENT)	RESULT (+ OR −)	INTERNAL CONTROL PASSED (Y OR N)	CHARTED IN PATIENT RECORD	TECH INITIALS
7/11/20XX	POSITIVE CONTROL	+	Y		DC
7/11/20XX	NEGATIVE CONTROL	−	Y		DC
7/11/20XX	PT ID: 5432	−	Y	✓	DC

Documentation in the Medical Record

10/9/20 9:30 a.m.: Mononucleosis rapid test performed with a negative result. Lavender-topped EDTA blood sample sent to lab for CBC and differential.
_____Laura Piper, CMA (AAMA)

35

SKILLS AND STRATEGIES

SCENARIO

Michelle, Krysia, and Zacarias (or "Zac" to his friends) met during their first semester of college. They have developed a great friendship over the past few months. They will be graduating from the medical assistant program in less than 6 weeks. Michelle just graduated from high school a year ago. Krysia entered the military just after her high school graduation. She spent 10 years in the Marines. Zac has been out of high school for several years and worked in a factory. He started as a line worker and gradually advanced to supervisory positions. Due to downsizing, his position was eliminated. He went back to school. These friends are looking forward to graduation and getting jobs as medical assistants.

As these three friends discuss finding a job, Michelle is hesitant about the job search experience. Her only work experience is 2 years as a waitress at a local restaurant. She has never created a resume or a cover letter. She only had a very informal interview with the restaurant owner before she was given the job. Krysia is concerned about her military career. The positions she held were not related to healthcare. She managed inventory and supervised others. She was also deployed to many hot spots around the world. Zac has a lot of experience in the factory setting, but he feels that that world is so different from healthcare. As they talk with each other, it is clear that each person has a unique situation, and they all must take a closer look at their past experiences as they prepare for their job search adventure.

While studying this chapter, think about the following questions:
- What personality traits are important to employers?
- What are the best job search methods?
- How do you develop a resume and cover letter?
- How do you complete a job application?
- How do you prepare for an interview?

LEARNING OBJECTIVES

1. Describe personality traits important to employers.
2. Discuss personality traits, technical skills, and transferable job skills.
3. Describe how to develop a career objective and identify your personal needs.
4. Explain job search methods.
5. Create a resume and cover letter.
6. Complete an online profile and job application.
7. Describe how to create a career portfolio.
8. Practice interview skills during a mock interview.
9. List legal and illegal interview questions.
10. Create a thank-you note for an interview.
11. Explain common human resource hiring requirements when starting a new job.

VOCABULARY

clarification Allows the listener to get additional information.
collaboration (kuh lab uh RAY shun) The act of working with another or other individuals.
counteroffer Return offer made by one who has rejected an offer or a job.
dignity The inherent worth or state of being worthy of respect.
interpersonal skills The ability to communicate and interact with others; sometimes referred to as "soft skills."
job boards Websites where employers post jobs; they can be used by job seekers to identify open positions.
mock Simulated; intended for imitation or practice.

reflecting Putting words to the patient's emotional reaction, which acknowledges the person's feelings.
reverse chronologic order The most recent item is on top and the oldest item is last.
paraphrasing Rewording a statement to check the meaning and interpretation; also shows you are listening to and understanding the speaker.
proofread To read and mark corrections.
skill set A person's abilities, skills, or expertise in an area.
summarizing Allowing the listener to recap and review what was said.

As you move toward graduation, you may be experiencing many emotions. You might be excited about finishing your medical assistant program. You might be scared of the future changes. The thought of finding a job might be overwhelming. These are common feelings of all graduates. The important step before graduation is to prepare for the next phase: getting a job.

Preparing for the job-seeking phase is very important. This chapter will help you:

- Understand the characteristics that employers want
- Identify your strengths, experiences, and skills
- Develop your career objectives

When you have done these things, you are ready to market yourself to potential employers. You will market yourself through your resume and interview experiences. Remember that an early job search, even before graduation, can be the key to landing a job soon after graduation.

UNDERSTANDING PERSONALITY TRAITS IMPORTANT TO EMPLOYERS

It is important to understand what employers are looking for in employees. Employers spend money and time training new employees. It is critical that they initially find the right employees. Many employers will agree that they can help refine technical skill proficiencies. It is more difficult to help grow or change personality traits. We will examine the five personality traits that are most important to employers. These include collaboration, interpersonal skills, professionalism, compassion, and a sincere interest in the job.

Collaboration and Interpersonal Skills

Collaboration and **interpersonal skills** are crucial to the efficiency of the healthcare environment. Employers look for people who can blend well with the current staff. New employees need to be flexible, dependable, supportive of peers, and remain calm under pressure. Employers want employees who will provide excellent customer service by having outstanding interpersonal skills, including the following:

- *Effective verbal communication*: Involves using clear, thoughtful, and easily understood language.
- *Professional nonverbal communication*: Relays more information to patients and peers than any words you could use. Eye contact, posture, voice, and gestures provide insights into a person's attitude. Being focused, calm, polite, and interested in the other person are traits of effective nonverbal communication.
- *Good listening skills*: Critical when working with peers and patients. For effective communication to occur, listening must occur. Appropriate questions can draw others into the conversation and show others you are listening and care. Communication techniques such as **reflecting**, **paraphrasing**, **summarizing**, and asking for **clarification** are also excellent ways of demonstrating active listening skills.
- *Good manners*: Are essential, along with a basic understanding of the diversity of your patient population.

Professionalism

A person's professionalism is being evaluated from the cover letter to the interview and beyond. Employers are looking for employees who project a professional image in all situations. Professionalism includes a person's appearance (i.e., dress and grooming habits) and behaviors. The behaviors include a person's flexibility, punctuality, honesty, attention to detail, time management skills, ability to following directions, and ability to prioritize.

Compassion

Compassion is another trait employers look for. *Compassion* means to have a deep awareness of another's suffering and the desire to lessen it. **Dignity** and respect are part of providing compassionate care to others. Many people go into healthcare to help others. They may like the technical skills involved with patient care. Providing dignity and respect during patient care is just as important. Compassion and respect help healthcare employees connect to patients and their families. Acts of kindness and thoughtfulness that lessen stress are welcomed by patients.

Dignity and Respect Example

Imagine being a patient in your 70s. You have a walker. You spent 4 months in a wheelchair recovering from a stroke. You are proud to be walking today, even if you are slow. You know that walking is important, so that you do not get stiff and then cannot walk.

The medical assistant calls you in for the visit. You slowly walk to her and then she takes you down the hall. She is far ahead of you as you slowly make your way. It appears the room is at the end of the long hall. You hear the medical assistant calling to a peer to get a wheelchair. She looks back at you and states, "We have a wheelchair for you to speed things up." How do you feel? Do you feel that she values you? Is she showing you respect?

If you reverse the roles, how could you, as a medical assistant, show that you respect and value the patient?

Genuine Interest

Employers also look for people genuinely interested in the job. This trait can be seen during the interview. Does the person ask thoughtful questions regarding the position and the facility? Genuine interest in the job extends beyond the hiring phase into day-to-day operations. Being interested in one's job is critical. Looking for ways to improve procedures and provide better patient care is an important behavior to demonstrate to the employer. This genuine interest is reflected in your attitude and performance in the workplace. It helps ease your transition into a new job and promotes your success.

CRITICAL THINKING APPLICATION   35.1

Think of the three friends in the Scenario. Michelle just graduated from high school and has 2 years of waitressing experience. Krysia has 10 years in the military, where she managed inventory, supervised others, and was deployed to many hot spots around the world. Zac has been working in a factory, advancing to supervisory positions. Now think about the personality traits that employers want. What personality traits might each friend possess? Explain your answer.

- Create your own list of the personality traits that employers want, and you possess.

ASSESSING YOUR STRENGTHS AND SKILLS

As you prepare to market yourself to potential employers, you need to examine your strengths and skills in three different areas. What personality traits do you possess? What technical skills are your strengths? What are the transferable job skills that you possess?

Personality Traits

In addition to the typical personality traits required by employers, the job posting may list extra traits, including personality traits. Which of these skills and strengths do you possess? Many people will tell potential employers what they think employers want to hear. They claim to be "a team player," to "communicate well," to be "dependable," and so on. Listing these phrases on your resume or during the interview is not enough to convince the potential employer that you truly have those characteristics. They like "supporting evidence"!

Early on in the preparation phase, make a list of the qualities that you believe you possess. For each quality provide one or two pieces of "evidence" to support your claims. Your "evidence" may be a past job review or practicum evaluation in which the author indicates your strengths and characteristics. These are excellent documents to include in your portfolio, which will be discussed later in the chapter. Using stories of situations in which you portrayed those characteristics is another way to illustrate your qualities. It is important to share these during the interview, if pertinent to the questions asked.

Technical Skills

Employers are also interested in your technical skills. Technical skills for medical assistants can be related to clinical procedures, such as phlebotomy, injections, electrocardiograms (ECGs), and obtaining vital signs. Technical skills can also be related to administrative procedures, including software proficiency, keyboard speed, reception duties, and coding procedures.

You may be able to provide supporting documentation of your technical skills through the use of practicum skill checklists or through a portfolio. Technical skills might also include skills that you developed outside the medical assistant program but that still relate to your chosen career. For instance, if you worked as a pharmacy technician at a local hospital, several of the technical skills you acquired may relate to a clinic position.

Transferable Job Skills

Transferable job skills are the last area to examine. A person develops these skills in one job or experience. The skills can be "transferred" to another job. This means the person will use these skills in other jobs. Many of these skills may sound familiar. They are also characteristics employers are looking for.

Potential Transferable Skills

- Customer service
- Compassion and empathy
- Strong communication and listening skills
- Computer skills
- Leadership skills
- Organizational skills
- Teamwork
- Time management and prioritizing skills
- Creativity
- Grace under pressure
- Problem-solving skills

Identifying transferable job skills can be difficult for many people. Job descriptions for past experiences can be very useful. To start, make a list of your past jobs, military experience, and volunteer opportunities. Make a list of potential transferable skills you developed and used for each experience. Some examples of transferable skills for different jobs and situations include:

- Wait staff jobs: Strong communication and listening skills, prioritizing, and customer service skills
- Factory jobs: Communication skills, teamwork, and problem solving
- Military experience: Strong communication skills, grace under pressure, and prioritizing
- Stay-at-home parent: Organization, prioritizing, budgeting, time management, and problem solving

This list of transferable job skills will be used as you create your resume and prepare for your interview.

CRITICAL THINKING APPLICATION   35.2

What might be some transferable skills that the three friends, Michelle, Krysia, and Zac, possess? Explain your answer.

- Using the list you have already started, add on the personality traits, technical skills, and transferable job skills that you possess. Also, indicate why you believe you have these skills (e.g., which job or experience helped you develop the skill).

DEVELOPING CAREER OBJECTIVES

Each medical assistant has a reason for entering the healthcare field. This basic desire should influence decisions concerning his or her career choices. Because medical assisting is such a versatile profession, a medical assistant has numerous options after graduation.

Medical assistant students should take some time to think about what they want from their careers. While the medical assistant is attending school and subsequently completing the practicum, ideas may surface about the area of healthcare or a specific facility in which she or he most wants to work.

When developing career objectives, the medical assistant should start by asking several questions:

- What areas and skills did I enjoy in practicum?
- Where do I want to be in 5 years?
- Where do I want to be in 10 years?
- What additional skills do I need to get where I want to go?

Write down the questions and answers and go into specific detail. Set realistic goals and develop a plan as to how and when they will be reached. Remember, career objectives are reached over time. It is important to know where you want to be, so you can start down the right path to reach your goals. Keep your list of goals available and visible so you can revisit it frequently.

CRITICAL THINKING APPLICATION   35.3

For the following four questions, write down your answers and explain them. These answers will help you as you start the job search process.

- What areas and skills did I enjoy in practicum?
- Where do I want to be in 5 years?
- Where do I want to be in 10 years?
- What additional skills do I need to get where I want to go?

IDENTIFYING PERSONAL NEEDS

The next step in the process is to identify personal needs. What do you need in a job? Do you need a specific wage to meet your living expenses? What benefits do you need? What hours do you need to work? Some people need to consider day care and school hours for their children. How far are you willing to travel for a job? Do you have a reliable mode of transportation? Evaluating your personal needs will help you find a job that matches your requirements.

CRITICAL THINKING APPLICATION 35.4

What are your personal needs? Make a list identifying your needs that must be considered when seeking a new position.

FINDING A JOB

Finding employment and staying employed in healthcare are typically not difficult. Usually healthcare employment needs remain high, even in a poor economy. However, graduation from a medical assisting program does not guarantee employment. Completion of the program gives the medical assistant the job skills needed to work. A good attitude and positive outlook are essential for success in the job search. The medical assistant should always be open to new and better opportunities.

Some job seekers assume that potential employers will not interact with students until they have passed a credential examination. However, searching for a job before graduation is a smart idea. Some employers do not require credentialing examinations. Others may hire a medical assistant before the exam is taken. They may have an agreement that the medical assistant obtain the credential within a specified period of time. Many employers are interested in hiring new graduates. They consider new graduates "teachable." This means they can train and "mold" them into the employee they require. Employers recognize that new graduates have more current knowledge and skills.

Certification Exams

- Certified Medical Assistant (CMA) through the American Association of Medical Assistants (AAMA)
- Registered Medical Assistant (RMA) through the American Medical Technologists (AMT)
- Certified Clinical Medical Assistant (CCMA) through the National Healthcare Association (NHA)
- National Certified Medical Assistant (NCMA) through the National Center for Competency Testing (NCCT)
- Clinical Medical Assistant Certification (CMAC) through the American Medical Certification Association (AMCA)

Two Best Job Search Methods

There are many ways to find employment. Networking and checking **job boards** are the best and most effective methods.

Networking

Networking is the exchange of information among others in your field. For medical assistant graduates or students searching for a

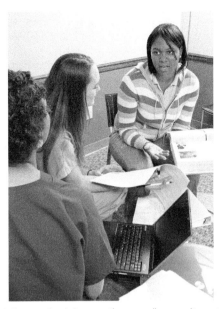

FIGURE 35.1 Stay in touch with classmates. They are excellent networking contacts and may be able to provide job leads.

job, networking involves meeting individuals in healthcare. It also involves sharing information on available opportunities. Through the medical assistant program, a student forms a network of friends and acquaintances (Fig. 35.1). Staying in contact with these people allows for networking opportunities. Email, LinkedIn, Facebook, Twitter, and other social networking advances make staying in touch very easy.

The practicum experience gives medical assistant students opportunities to network. During the practicum (externship), you will be working with many healthcare professionals. It is crucial that you look at the practicum as a continuous job interview. It is important to be professional, follow the guidelines, and strive to do your very best. It is not uncommon that, when staff members find a student who portrays the characteristics of a professional medical assistant, they are willing to help the student find a job.

Strategies Medical Assistants Can Use in Practicum to Assist With Job Seeking

During practicum, medical assistant students can:
- Inquire about potential job openings, either through their mentor, supervisor, or the facility's human resource department.
- Ask their mentors if they would be willing to provide a reference or a letter of recommendation.
- Show their gratitude by formally thanking their mentors for the opportunity. In most cases, the practicum agencies provide assistance to help train the medical assistant student. It is important to send a thank-you note to the mentor, the supervisor, and to the department.
- Provide the supervisor with a resume and cover letter.

Another networking technique is to join a medical assistant organization. The members who attend regular meetings often know about job leads in the area. Creating connections with currently employed medical assistants can be helpful in the job search process.

Job Boards

Job boards are websites where employers post job openings. There are two types of job boards:

- *Facility job boards*: Larger healthcare facilities post job openings on their websites. The employment website can use different tools that make the process easier for the job seeker and the employer. Some sites allow the job seeker to register for a specific type of job. The software will generate emails to job seekers when new jobs are posted. Some websites allow job seekers to complete online profiles or applications and upload a resume and cover letter. These tools are useful to both the job seeker and the facility.
- *Public job boards*: These job boards include jobs from a variety of employers. The job boards can be local, state, or national. Local job boards may be found through your school or your community's media (i.e., newspaper, television, radio) agencies. These websites target the local audience. They are usually cheaper for employers. Smaller healthcare organizations tend to advertise using these boards. The Department of Workforce Development in each state addresses unemployment. It provides a job board for job seekers. National job boards, such as Monster, Indeed, alliedhealthjobcafe.com, and glassdoor.com, provide job seekers the ability to search for openings across the country. Medical assistant jobs available in the federal government can be found at the website *http://www.usajobs.gov*.

Many positions for medical assistants use alternative job titles. Some agencies may use "technician" or "coordinator" for medical assistant jobs. It is important to research the local job titles that are used for medical assistants. If you do not know the local job title, try looking at the allied health positions. Look at a job posting. What are the educational requirements? Are the duties skills you have? Make a list of job titles related to medical assisting and search by those as you identify potential openings.

Additional Job Search Methods

Besides using networking and checking job boards, the medical assistant can find job postings by other, more traditional methods. The school's placement office resources, newspaper ads (online and print), and employment agencies also can have medical assistant job postings.

School Career Placement Offices

Students usually have lifetime access to their school placement offices. Students and graduates should take advantage of the opportunities offered. Many schools offer resume building, job search classes, and interviewing assistance. School placement offices may also work with local employers to advertise their openings online to graduates. The school has a vested interest in helping you find employment. The placement office should be the first resource for the student's job search.

Newspaper Ads

Smaller healthcare facilities usually use newspaper ads to find potential employees. Many newspaper companies post their ads online. This allows more job seekers to view those positions.

Employment Agencies

Employment agencies hire staff to fill in at healthcare facilities. The employment agency is paid by the facility to staff different positions. Some employment agencies hire and pay the medical assistant. The medical assistants work in a healthcare facility as employment agency employees. After a period of time, if the medical assistant proves to be a good employee, the healthcare facility then hires that person. This allows the employment agency to do the hiring, firing, and managing of employees until the employees "prove themselves" to the healthcare facility.

Being Organized in Your Job Search

As you submit your resume and cover letter for various positions, it is important that you stay organized and track the jobs you applied for. You should also keep the original electronic files of your customized documents.

Create a handwritten or an electronic log of the jobs you apply for. Include the job title, number, and facility name. When you submit your resume and cover letter, update the log with the date of those activities. As you are notified about an interview, add the interview information (e.g., date, time, location, interview team members) to your log. Continually update the status of each job in the log.

It is important for you to save the customized documents for each job position. If you are called for an interview, it is important to bring copies of your customized resume and cover letter. The easiest method is to create a job-seeking folder on your computer. For each job you apply for, create a subfolder in the job-seeking folder. Save your customized resume and cover letter in the subfolder. Save any other documents related to that job in that subfolder, including the job posting. If you get called for an interview, print the customized resume and cover letter for your interview portfolio and for the interviewer(s). You may also want to print the job posting as a reference during the interview.

One of the most important things to remember with job searching is that it takes time, stamina, and persistence to find a job. Do not expect to get a job with the first resume and cover letter you send or with the first interview you have. By keeping good records, you will not apply for the same job twice or overlook job opportunities because you thought you had applied for them already.

DEVELOPING A RESUME

The purpose of a resume is to "market" yourself. You want an employer interested in you. You want your resume to be included in those selected for an interview. A resume summarizes your qualifications, education, and experience. Medical assistants must determine what to include in the resume. The resume should be developed before the cover letter is written. Strengths for the posted job must be

identified and emphasized on all documents. These documents include the resume, cover letter, and application.

Resume Formats

There are three commonly used resume formats: chronologic, combination, and targeted resumes. The resume format used will depend on the medical assistant's situation.

A *chronologic resume* is the most popular format used. It is useful when people are seeking employment in the same field as their education or previous experience. The chronologic resume focuses on the person's employment history. Job duties for each position are bulleted out (Fig. 35.2). See Procedure 35.1 on p. 912 for the steps in creating a chronologic resume.

Michelle Marison

1234 Cedar Way, Mytown, OH 45458
Home phone: 715.555.1899
Cell phone: 715.555.1355
mmarison@elsevier.net

Education
Community College, Mytown, OH
Medical Assistant Diploma, 20XX
- GPA 3.6

Health Care Experience
Family Practice Associates, Mytown, OH
Medical Assistant Practicum, April 20XX to May 20XX (220 hours)
- Performed injections, electrocardiogram, wound care, phlebotomy, throat swabs, and waived tests.
- Obtained vital signs and measurements on children and adults.
- Utilized an electronic health record to document patients' histories, test results and treatments.
- Answered calls, checked-in patients, and updated patients' demographic and insurance information.

Mytown Hospital, Mytown, OH
Volunteer, January 20XX to May 20XX
- Provided hospital information to visitors.
- Maintained confidentiality of patients.
- Assisted with deliveries of mail and flowers to patients.
- Assisted nursing staff as needed.

Work Experience
Mytown Family Diner, Mytown, OH
Waitress, June 20XX to present
- Provide efficient, accurate, and timely service to customers.
- Prioritize duties to meet customer needs.
- Provide exceptional customer service.

Special Skills
Fluent in Spanish.
Keyboarding speed: 73 wpm
Proficient in word processing and spreadsheet software

Credentials
Certified Medical Assistant, American Association of Medical Assistants (expires May 20XX)
BLS for Healthcare Providers, American Heart Association (expires March 20XX)

FIGURE 35.2 Chronologic resume.

The *combination resume* is sometimes confused with a functional resume. A true functional resume showcases a person's **skill sets**. It does not include a work history. A combination resume is preferred over a functional resume. A combination resume:

- Lists a person's abilities and skill sets, as does the functional resume
- Includes the person's employment history, as does the chronologic resume (Fig. 35.3)

A combination resume may be used if a person is switching careers. Transferable skills related to the new position will be emphasized. It can also be used by applicants who have a gap in their work history. The focus is on the person's skills and ability, rather than the employment history.

The third type of resume is the *targeted resume*. This type of resume is customized to a unique job posting (Fig. 35.4). Targeted resumes:

- Detail key skills required for the position
- Indicate how the applicant has demonstrated those skills
- Take longer to create, but can be the most effective format

---

CRITICAL THINKING APPLICATION   35.7

The three friends have very different backgrounds. Michelle has the waitressing experience, Krysia was in the military, and Zac worked in a factory. What type of resume might each use? Explain your answers.

- What type of resume would work best for you with your experience and background?

Zacarias Garcia
523 River Way, Mytown OH 45459

Cell phone: 715.555.5472
ZacGarcia@elsevier.net

Education
Community College, Mytown, OH
Medical Assistant Diploma, 20XX
- Medical Assistant Practicum at Mytown Orthopedic and Massage Center, Mytown, OH
  o Obtained and charted history and vital signs in electronic health record.
  o Assisted providers with tests and treatments.

Credentials
Certified Medical Assistant, American Association of Medical Assistants, expires May 20XX.
BLS for Healthcare Providers, American Heart Association, expires March 20XX.

Skills and Achievement
Strong communication skills
- Supervised 60 employees in a factory setting for over 3 years.
- Initiated procedures to improve communication between employees and management.
- Promoted in union to assist with negotiations with upper management.
- Fluent in Spanish.

Excellent problem-solving skills
- Problem-solved factory issues that delayed shipments to customers.
- Initiated solutions to expedite shipments and increased the profit margin of the company.

Excel in Teamwork
- Assisted team on assembly line, helping fill in when others were absent.
- Promoted to Team Lead within 6 months of hire.
- Received "Outstanding Employee" award in 20XX, 20XX, and 20XX.

Work Experience
Mytown Doors, Mytown, OH
Supervisor, (March 20XX – January 20XX)
Team Lead – Door Assembly, (January 20XX – March 20XX)
Door Assembler, (August 20XX – January 20XX)

FIGURE 35.3 Combination resume.

Krysia Debski

111 Mall Drive • Mytown, OH 45457
Cell phone: 715.555.6956 • Email: KDebski@elsevier.net

Education
Community College, Mytown, OH
A.S. in Medical Assisting, 20XX
- Medical Assistant Practicum at Mytown Associates, Mytown, OH
  - o Obtained and charted patients' histories and vital signs in the electronic health record.
  - o Assisted providers with tests and treatments in a busy internal medicine practice.
  - o Performed injections, throat swabs, and phlebotomy.

Skills
ORGANIZATION SKILLS
- Organized supplies to expedited restocking procedures and decrease financial loss .
- Exceptional organizational and filing skills utilized to maintain purchase and delivery records from over 300 suppliers.
- Assisted with the install and training for inventory tracking software for warehouse.

TEAMWORK
- Refined teamwork skills with over ten years in the U.S. Marines.
- Taught teambuilding courses.
- Promoted teamwork among staff by incorporating incentives.

COMMUNICATION SKILLS
- Assertive when working with suppliers to meet deadlines.
- Utilized excellent listening skills to identify needs of various teams that impact the warehouse.
- Composed frequent emails and letters for supervisors.
- Fluent in Spanish and Polish

Credentials
Certified Medical Assistant, American Association of Medical Assistants, (expires May 20XX)

BLS for Healthcare Providers, American Heart Association (expires March 20XX)

Work Experience
United States Marines
Supply Administration and Operations Specialist (May 20XX – September 20XX)
Warehouse Clerk (August 20XX – May 20XX)

FIGURE 35.4 Targeted resume customized for a medical assistant posting. The medical assistant should possess strong organizational skills, experience with teamwork, and exceptional communication skills. The posting indicated it required a person with a Certified Medical Assistant (CMA) credential and a current Basic Life Support (BLS) certification.

Resume Content

Between the resume formats, there are similarities and differences in the information presented. The following discussion will describe the content found in the different sections of a resume. See Procedure 35.1 on p. 912 for the steps in creating a chronologic resume.

Header

The person's contact information is found in the header of the document. This includes the person's name, mailing address, professional email address, phone number, and personal websites (e.g., LinkedIn).

This information or a variation of the information should appear on each sheet if the resume is more than one page long.

Professional email addresses may include your first and last name or first initial and last name. Email addresses that include expressions such as "one_hot_chick" or "party_dude" are not professional and are not used on resumes. An old email format may indicate that you are not knowledgeable about the current technology. If you do not have a professional email address or have an old email address, free email sites are available (e.g., gmail.com). Like professional emails, personal websites should be professional and contain a professional image of you.

Education

The education section includes information on the schooling that the person has received after high school. The information should appear in **reverse chronologic order**. Information should include:

- *If a diploma was obtained:* List the school's name, city, and state, the degree, and the year it was obtained.
- *If no degree was obtained:* Summarize the coursework completed. List the school's name, city, and state, and the years of the coursework.
- *Practicum (externship) information:* Include the location, dates, and duties (optional; some will include this information in the Healthcare Experience section, discussed later in the chapter).
- *Academic recognition:* Include academic awards, scholarships, and overall GPA if greater than 3.0.

The location of the education section can differ based on the person's situation. For new graduates, the education section should appear toward the top of the resume. If the degree is not related to the position or the degree is older, the education section would come toward the end of the resume. Moving education to the end allows the person's achievements and work history to be emphasized.

Work Experience

This section can be titled several different ways. If a person is strictly including job information, then "Work Experience" or "Job Experience" can be used. Using the word "job" or "work" implies the person got paid for the position. If a person wants to include volunteer positions with job positions, then the section should be titled "Related Experience" or "Other Experience." "Related" means it relates to the position the person is applying for. If the section contains unrelated experience, then use "Other Experience." For those with military experience, it is recommended to add a special section to discuss the military experience.

If you have prior healthcare experience, you may want to separate your volunteer and job experiences into two sections. First, use "Healthcare Experiences." Include any healthcare jobs and volunteer positions you have had. Some students may opt to include their practicum in this section. Second, use a topic header, such as "Other Experience" or "Additional Experience." Include all of your non-healthcare jobs and volunteer positions. Do not repeat information you included in prior sections.

The information in this section should be presented in reverse chronologic order. All three resumes discussed require the following elements for each position:

- Name of the facility
- City and state of the facility
- Title of position or positions held at that facility
- Dates in that position (include start date [month and date] and end date [month and date]; for a current position, include the start date and use "to present")

For those in the workforce for 10 years or longer, employers want to see 10 years of employment information. For those working at the same facility for over 10 years, it is important to list changes and advancements in the position over the duration of employment. Any gaps in the employment history should be explained to the potential employer during the interview or discussed in the cover letter.

For the chronologic resume, the most relevant job duties need to be listed. For instance, if you worked as a housekeeper in a motel, making beds is not related to medical assisting. Providing customer service would be relevant.

The statements regarding the duties should be bulleted and begin with an active verb. For present positions, use active verbs in the present tense (e.g., administer, provide). For past positions, use active verbs in the past tense (e.g., administered, provided) (Fig. 35.5).

The position of the work experience section is dependent on the resume format. Chronologic resumes typically have work experience near the top, whereas combination and targeted resumes list it toward the end of the resume.

Summary and Skills

A "Summary" section appears at the top in the targeted resume. This section summarizes why the applicant is the best candidate for the job. It is helpful to use key words from the job posting when describing skills one possesses. This helps to make the connection of why the person is the best candidate for the job.

A "Skills" or "Skills and Achievements" section is found in combination resumes. It showcases specific transferable skills that relate to the new position. These transferable skills may have been obtained in the military, by a stay-at-home parent, or by a person switching careers.

A "Special Skills" section is found in a chronologic resume. Information that may appear in this section includes:

- Fluency in another language (e.g., fluent in Spanish)
- Keyboarding speed (e.g., keyboarding speed: 85 wpm)
- Computer skills and experiences (e.g., used electronic health records during practicum)

Certifications

Many employers may require specific certifications or credentials for a job position. It is important to include those that relate to the job position. When listing the information, include these items:

- Title of the certification or license
- Awarding agency
- Expiration date

An example for all resume formats would be: "BLS for Healthcare Providers, American Heart Association, expires 10/2022."

Appearance of the Resume

As you create your resume, keep in mind the eye appeal or interest the resume will create for the reader. It is recommended to bold-face only important information. A job title should be bold, whereas the facility should not be bold. Simple bullets help organize information and provide a neat appearance to the resume. Changing the font size in certain areas can emphasize more important elements and help keep content on one page.

Spacing is crucial to the appearance of a resume. A lot of spacing creates too much "white space." This can give the reader a negative impression of the resume. Too little spacing creates a busy, text-heavy

Administered	Copied	Performed
Advocated	Developed	Posted
Aided	Distributed	Prepared
Answered	Documented	Processed
Arranged	Established	Provided
Assigned	Filed	Purchased
Assisted	Guided	Reconciled
Balanced	Helped	Restocked
Calculated	Instructed	Reviewed
Cared	Listened	Scanned
Coded	Logged	Scheduled
Collected	Mailed	Sorted
Compiled	Maintained	Supported
Composed	Monitored	Taught
Computed	Operated	Trained
Contacted	Ordered	Wrote
Coordinated	Organized	

FIGURE 35.5 Action verbs in the past tense.

resume that is difficult to read. Make sure to use the same spacing between the sections. Use less spacing, but be consistent between subsections (e.g., different employment positions).

It is important to have resume paper available. Even if you submit your resume online, you should bring copies of your resume on resume paper to the interview. Use a light solid-colored resume paper (e.g., cream, light gray). The light colors will duplicate better than a pattern or dark-colored paper.

Before submitting your resume, have another person review it. Obtain the person's initial impression of the resume's appearance. Is there too much white space? Does the resume look too wordy? Does it look too plain? Does it look too busy? Then have the person read the content in the resume and provide you with feedback. Use the feedback to revise your resume.

Tips for creating a resume include:
- Do not add clipart or other pictures.
- Do not include personal information (e.g., married, children, and religious affiliation).
- Do not lie or exaggerate the truth.
- Do not add unrelated content, such as hobbies and interests.
- Do not include "References available upon request" or a similar statement, because it is understood references will be requested and required.
- Do not use personal pronouns, such as "I."
- Do not repeat content.
- Do not include any pay/salary information.
- Always keep the resume to one page, unless you have been in the workforce for multiple years. Then use an additional page, but your content must fill both pages.
- Be concise and clear.
- Use key terms found in the job posting or job description in your resume.
- Put important details first.
- Perform a grammar and spelling check on your resume.
- Limit abbreviations to only the abbreviations used in the job posting (e.g., BLS for basic life support, CPR for cardiopulmonary resuscitation).

CRITICAL THINKING APPLICATION   35.8

Zac, Michelle, and Krysia drafted their resumes. They read each other's and provided feedback. Who else might they give their resumes to for proofreading and feedback?
- Think of your circle of family and friends. List three people who might be great candidates to provide feedback on your resume.

DEVELOPING A COVER LETTER

A cover letter must always accompany the resume (Fig. 35.6). The cover letter is a critical tool that gains the reader's attention. The goal is to have the cover letter create enough interest that the reader wants to look at the resume. The cover letter gives the reader more information on the applicant's personality than the factual resume. Cover letters allow applicants to express themselves.

Strategies When Writing a Cover Letter

To create a professional cover letter, it is important to follow these strategies:
- *Match the appearance of the cover letter and resume*
  - Headers on both documents should be identical.
  - Font type and margins should be identical.
  - If using paper, use the same paper for both documents.
- *Address the inside address and the salutation (greeting) to a specific person*
  - Address the letter to the person who is hiring the new employee. This shows that you took time to find out the details.
  - Use the person's name and job title in the inside address.
  - Use a formal salutation (e.g., *Dear Mr. Jones:*).
  - Call the healthcare facility or use online resources, such as LinkedIn, to find out the information.
- *Start the body of your cover letter off with a bang!*
  - In the first paragraph: Show enthusiasm as you summarize why you believe you are the best candidate for the job. Also include the job title and the number for easy reference for the reader.
  - For example: "Having a strong customer service background and a degree in medical assisting, I am confident that I can fulfill your expectations for the family practice medical assistant position (#123)."
- *Sell yourself to the reader*
  - In the second paragraph: Provide a snapshot of your experiences.
  - Weave in the key "requirement" words from the job posting. Address the requirements first, followed by the lesser requirements or "would like" qualities. Some experts recommend using bold font for these key words.
  - You can bullet your qualifications and abilities but limit the bullets to four or five points.
  - Be concise, yet clear. Do not repeat the resume. You want the reader to move onto the resume for the details.
- *Reaffirm that you are an excellent match for the job*
  - In the final paragraph: Use such phrases as "I believe I have the qualities you require" or "I am confident I will meet your expectations."
  - If you include an action you will take (e.g., "I will call the week of…"), do not be overly aggressive in your tone.
  - Finish the paragraph by expressing your interest in and enthusiasm for an interview (e.g., "I am very excited about this opportunity and would enjoy meeting with you to explore how my qualifications could meet your needs.").
- *Be professional*
  - Express your thanks to the reader for his or her consideration.

Proofreading the Cover Letter

After writing the cover letter, review it for inaccuracies. Use the spell-check tool in your word processing software to help identify errors. Also **proofread** your letter. Make sure your spelling, punctuation, grammar, and sentence structure are correct. Common cover letter weaknesses include:

Michelle Marison

1234 Cedar Way, Mytown, OH 45458
Home phone: 715.555.1899
Cell phone: 715.555.1355
mmarison@elsevier.net

May 15, 20XX

Ms. Alex Brown
Medical Assistant Supervisor
Mytown Medical Clinic
555 Clover Drive
Mytown OH 45457

Dear Ms. Brown:

I was excited to see the posting on the Mytown Telegram job board for the medical assistant position (#1243) and would like to be considered for that position. I am graduating from Community College on May 30, 20XX and will be taking my AAMA CMA exam June 2, 20XX.

With two years of customer service experience and five months of being a hospital volunteer, I have learned the importance of prioritizing, teamwork, and communication. During my medical assistant practicum, I have utilized these skills along with my attention to detail and my medical assistant knowledge, as I assist providers with procedures and treatments. The knowledge and skills I am learning in practicum combined with the skills I have developed as a waitress and volunteer will help me provide the best care to my future patients.

I have heard excellent things about Mytown Medical Clinic and would love to be a part of the staff of such a caring agency. I am available for interviews whenever it is convenient for you. I am available either by phone or email.

Thank you so much for considering me for this position.

Sincerely,

Michelle Marison

Enclosure: 1

FIGURE 35.6 Basic cover letter.

- Starting a majority of sentences with "I"
- Introducing yourself in the first sentence (for instance, "*Hi, I am Sally Green.*")
- Spelling, grammar, punctuation, and sentence structure errors
- Missing parts of the letter (e.g., date, inside address)
- Not including the position title and posting number
- Too busy (overuse of font styles), too wordy, or too much white space
- Inappropriate spacing that leads to the body of the letter being too high or too low on the page. Remember, the body should be centered vertically on the page.
- Creating a generic letter that does not contain the key requirement words from the job posting. (Many larger employers use software to screen letters and resumes for key words. Those with key words are reviewed more closely. Those that lack the key words are discarded.)

Create an error-free cover letter. It must have a professional tone and appearance. Also, have a few people proofread your letter. Use their advice as you make your changes. Refer to Chapter 7 in the main text if you need assistance with composing a business letter.

Procedure 35.2 on p. 913 will help guide you in writing a professional cover letter.

COMPLETING ONLINE PROFILES AND JOB APPLICATIONS

Many healthcare agencies use the internet during the employment process. The online human resource software may require applicants to create a profile before applying for open positions. The online profile collects the information that previously was collected by paper applications.

Online profiles have many advantages over paper applications for both the employer and the applicant. An applicant completes the profile once and updates the information as needed. Typically, the agencies keep the profiles active for years. Employers can:

- Track the activities of applicants
- Easily read a person's information
- Advertise new postings to potential applicants whose profiles meet certain requirements

If a healthcare facility does not use online profiles, then the applicant will need to complete a job application (Fig. 35.7). Some organizations require the application to be submitted with the cover letter and resume. Others have applicants arriving for interviews complete the application. If you need to complete an application before an interview, come prepared with your information. Arrive at least 20 minutes before the interview so you can complete the application. See Procedure 35.3 on p. 913 for the steps in completing a job application.

Regardless of whether you need to complete a profile or an application, you will need to provide the same information. Even if you have the information on your resume, you still need to add it to the application or profile. Having the reference information in a word-processed document will save you time. If you are providing the information online, the copy and paste feature will speed up completion time. Table 35.1 contains the information you should include in the word-processed document.

When filling out the application or profile, answer the questions carefully. When addressing your current and past employment, keep these points in mind:

- When giving your availability date, make sure you know how long you have to give notice at your current position. Most employers have a 2-week notice policy. If you are hired, your new employer will understand that you need to give a 2-week notice.
- When giving the reason you left prior positions, make sure to write the reason using a positive tone. For instance, "Obtained a

---

APPLICATION FOR EMPLOYMENT

Date:_____

Name: (First, Middle Initial, Last)_____

Social Security No.:_____   Phone: _____

Address:_____

EDUCATION

	Name, City, State	Graduation Date	Degree Obtained
High School:			
College:			
Other:			

LICENSURE/CERTIFICATION/REGISTRATION

Type of Certification, License or Registration	Agency/State	Registration Name

List any special skills or qualifications which you possess and feel are relevant to health care and the position for which you are applying._____

_____

EMPLOYMENT HISTORY

May we contact and communicate with your present employer? ☐ Yes ☐ No

Employer:	Phone:
Address:	Supervisor:
Employed	Hourly Pay:
Position title and responsibilities:	
Reason for leaving:	

FIGURE 35.7 Application for employment.

TABLE 35.1   Information Required for Online Profiles and Applications

INFORMATION	DETAILS NEEDED
Education	Institution's name and address; dates and titles of coursework or diploma
Past and present jobs	Facility name and address; supervisors' names, titles, and contact information; job title, duties, start and end salary, start and end dates; and reason for leaving
Certifications and credentials	Certifying agency's name and address; certification/credential; expiration date (a copy of your certification and BLS card may be required by the employer)
References	Name, title, facility, address, phone number, and email address

Typical Items Found in Career Portfolios

Using a three-ring binder with plastic sheet protectors and divider tabs, include the following:

- Table of contents at the beginning with identified tabbed sections
- Cover letter and resume (a copy of what was sent to that facility)
- References
- Certifications (e.g., copy of BLS card, copy of credentials [e.g., CMA or RMA card])
- Education-related documents
  - Copies of letters of recommendation
  - Copies of transcripts, awards, and honors
  - A list of the courses successfully completed with a short description of each course (optional, but consider if you are moving to another location where your institution may not be known)
  - Copies of practicum evaluation forms and skill document form
  - Scholarships awarded
  - Copies/details of school-related activities (e.g., officer in student medical assistant group, athlete, volunteer activities)
- Prior employment documents
  - Copies of past employment evaluations
  - Copies of letters of recommendations
- Documentation showing the student balancing work and education (this can help exhibit a strong work ethic, organizational skills, and prioritizing skills)
- Examples of work or summaries of projects that can provide evidence of abilities and skills
- Criminal background documentation, blood titers, vaccination history, and current tuberculosis (TB) skin or blood tests results (optional)

position that would advance my skill set" or "Resigned to focus on my education" sounds more professional than "I hated the job."

If you have a unique situation (e.g., sick parent, new baby), ask the advice of your school's placement counselor if you are unsure what to say in these sections. Most employers require an explanation for time not employed.

As you complete the online profile or paper application, you will be required to read important legal statements and add your signature (or electronic signature). This is a legal document. It should be filled out accurately and completely.

CREATING A CAREER PORTFOLIO

Many job seekers claim to have the skill sets required by the potential employer. Very few actually show the employer evidence of those qualifications. A career portfolio is a fantastic tool to show that you have the skills required for the job.

The portfolio should be developed along with the cover letter and resume. Creating a different portfolio for each type of job applied for is a great strategy. A receptionist portfolio would look different from a phlebotomy portfolio. There will be similarities in the information for all portfolios, but different "evidence" of skills will be in each. The medical assistant should be prepared to leave the portfolio with the interviewer, so no originals should be included.

The documents placed in the career portfolio binder should be positive and helpful to you in your mission of getting a job. You may want to consider adding the following:

- *A transcript*: Some experts state that a B average GPA or better is considered appropriate to add to a resume for an entry level position. Thus, you may want to add your transcript to the portfolio if you have a B average GPA or higher. Some employers require a higher GPA, and in these situations, only include your transcript if you meet their GPA requirement.

- *Performance evaluations*: Include positive employment or school-related performance evaluations.
- *Projects*: Include projects that provide evidence of personal characteristics or specific skills mastered.

Be creative as you prepare your portfolio, keeping the appearance professional and neat.

Just before an interview, the medical assistant should customize the portfolio for that employer (see Procedure 35.4, p. 914). A copy of the cover letter and resume sent to the employer should be in the portfolio. A list of references should also be included. All three of these documents should be printed on the same type of resume paper. The medical assistant should do additional customization of the portfolio. The examples of work or the summary of projects should reflect the skills required and key words in the job posting.

JOB INTERVIEW

Interviewers can consist of one or two people or a panel of employees. The job seeker may interview with a human resource employee, the office manager, the provider, and/or potential peers. The job seeker may have a number of interviews before the actual decision is made.

For many people, the interview is a stressful part of the job search. Some individuals dread job interviews and become extremely nervous at the prospect of interviewing. Others are very comfortable and consider the interview to be as much for their own purposes as for the employer's. The more interviews people do, the more comfortable they become with each subsequent interview.

We will examine the four phases of an interview. These include preparation for the interview, the interview itself, the follow-up, and the negotiation.

Preparation for the Interview

When preparing for an interview, the job seeker needs to:
- Research the facility
- Practice answering potential questions
- Select interview attire
- Prepare for the day of the interview

We will discuss each of these in depth. The better prepared the job candidate is, the more comfortable he or she will be during the interview.

Research the Healthcare Facility

The job seeker should learn everything possible about the employer. The organization's website is an excellent source of information. A job seeker should research the following topics:
- Mission and value statements
- Size of the organization
- Size of the department with the open position
- Names and types of providers in the department

It is important to ask questions at the interview. Possible questions can relate to your research on the facility:
- "I see that there are two providers in this department. Would I be working with both of them?"
- "There are three locations for your clinic on your website; how will I interact with the other locations?"
- "Given the size of your organization, is there an opportunity to interact with the other departments?"

Questions that relate to your research show the interviewer you are truly interested in the position. They also show that you prepared for the interview.

Practice Answers to Questions

Organizations need to follow federal and state hiring laws. The agencies cannot discriminate. During the interview phase, most organizations use a preset list of questions. All candidates are asked the same questions. You will not know the exact questions that will be asked. It is important to practice answering some standard interview questions (Fig. 35.8). This practice will help you prepare for the interview and also appear more confident during the actual interview.

When practicing your answers to standard interview questions, start by writing down your answer. Review your answer. Does it answer the question? What perception might you be giving to the interviewers by your answer? Is it the perception you want to be giving? How might you strengthen your answer? Is it really short or does it ramble on? Be clear and concise. Expand on the topic, but do not get too wordy. Provide examples to support what you say. When you have refined your answers, practice your answers before the interview.

Decide on Your Interview Attire

Prior to the interview, it is important to select an interview outfit. Be conservative with wardrobe choices. For example:
- Females: Business suit; skirt or dress pants and blouse. Skirt or dress should be of modest length (i.e., at the knee or longer). Blouse should not be sheer or show cleavage.
- Males: Business suit; dress pants and shirt. Conservative tie.

Be sure clothing is clean, wrinkle free, and well fitting, and that shoes are clean and shined. For a medical assistant, scrubs may be acceptable for an interview. (It is appropriate to ask the person arranging the interview if scrubs can be worn.) Take care in washing and pressing your scrubs, and use a lint roller on them, before wearing them on an interview.

Pay particular attention to other aspects of appearance. Make sure your hair is clean and styled attractively, your teeth are clean, and your breath is fresh. Nails should be clean and well-groomed. Nails should not be excessively long or painted in highly visible colors. Do not wear perfumes or colognes. Do not wear excessive jewelry or makeup. Do not chew gum during the interview. Do not smoke in your interview attire. Remember the appearance guidelines that applied to the practicum. Some employers will react negatively to tattoos, piercings, extravagant hairstyles, unnatural hair colors, or other excessive wardrobe choices. Always dress appropriately and conservatively for an interview. Once hired, the new employee may be allowed to wear more diverse styles that comply with the employee handbook or procedures manual.

Prepare for the Interview Day

Do a test run before the day of the interview to identify the travel time. Always arrive 15 minutes early for the interview. Never take anyone along on a job interview, especially children. Expect to be a little nervous. Any interview can be a stressful situation. If necessary, practice stress-relieving strategies (e.g., deep breathing) that you can use before the interview. The better prepared a person is, the more successful the interview will be.

You should also prepare what you need to bring for the interview. These items include:
- An interview portfolio
- A copy of your cover letter and resume for each interviewer
- A notepad and pen to take notes
- A list of references on resume paper
- A list of questions for the interviewer

If you will be completing an application, bring the information discussed in the prior section regarding completing online profiles and applications.

During the Interview

During the interview it is important to be professional. Your professionalism may be tested if the interviewer asks illegal questions. We will discuss how to answer interview questions. We will also discuss professionalism during the different types of interviews.

Answering Interview Questions

It is important to give the interviewers a good impression of you. As discussed in a prior section, it is important to practice answering questions before the interview. This will help you to prepare and to feel more confident during the interview.

1. Tell me about yourself.	16. What do you know about this facility and our competitors?
2. Why do you want to work for this company?	17. What has been your most rewarding experience at work?
3. Why should I hire you?	18. What was your single most important accomplishment for the company on your last job?
4. How do you work under pressure?	19. What was the toughest problem you have ever solved and how did you do it?
5. How do you handle criticism?	20. How do you see yourself fitting in with our company?
6. What do you think your co-workers think about you?	21. What skills did you learn on your last job that can be used here?
7. Describe your last supervisor.	22. What immediate contribution could you make if you came to work for us today?
8. What would you like to change about yourself?	23. Do you prefer working with others or by yourself?
9. What is your best asset?	24. Can you take instructions or criticism without being upset?
10. What adjectives would you use to describe yourself?	25. What job in this company would you choose if you could?
11. How would you describe the perfect job?	26. What have you done that shows initiative and willingness to work?
12. Why did you leave your last job?	27. What will previous supervisors say about you?
13. Why did you choose this type of profession?	28. Why would you be successful in this job?
14. What are your strongest and weakest personal qualities?	29. Can you explain the gap in your employment history?
15. What personal characteristics are necessary for success in your chosen field?	30. Are you a member of any professional organizations?

FIGURE 35.8 Top 30 interview questions.

Tips for All Interviews

- For simple, straightforward questions, do not pause before you answer. Any pause would be hinting at insincerity.
- For complex questions, pause for a few seconds as you think about your answer. Write down some key words to help you focus and answer the question.
- Refrain from saying "um."
- Do not volunteer any negative information.
- Be honest and do not exaggerate experiences or lengths of employment.
- Never speak negatively about former employers.
- Write down the names of the interviewers to help you as you follow up after the interview.
- Avoid a "know-it-all" attitude, which indicates overconfidence and reluctance to take direction.
- Express a sincere interest in the employer and his or her projects, rather than in what the employer can do for the employee.
- Ask intelligent questions at the end of the interview if given the opportunity. Your first question should never be, "How much will I be paid?" Money, although important, cannot appear to be your primary concern.

Many times, the interview will start with a question such as, "Tell me about yourself." The temptation is to answer the question focusing on your personal life. For example, "I'm a recent graduate, and I am married and have two children." The answer to this question should not reflect information about personal issues. Answer instead with, "I am a recent graduate and completed a 6-week practicum in a family practice." Focus all answers on your career, your strengths and attributes, and what skills you have to bring to the healthcare setting. Be able to prove the skills you claim. You can provide examples either by relating professional situations you have handled well, or by using your interview portfolio. Before the interview ends, the medical assistant should ask when a decision will be made and if it would be acceptable to call to follow up (see Procedure 35.5, p. 915).

Illegal Interview Questions

The interviewer should not ask any illegal questions. Table 35.2 lists such topics and potential illegal questions. Employers may either intentionally or accidentally ask illegal questions. The way that the medical assistant answers the questions can influence the employer's hiring decision. Here are some points to consider:

- If the medical assistant is openly offended: Employers may negatively conclude that the applicant will be offended by abrasive comments from patients.
- If the illegal question is answered: Discrimination may occur in the hiring process. The employer may use the information to weed out the medical assistant as a candidate.

The best approach is to politely address the question. Either answer the question or redirect the interviewer back to the job requirements. For example, an interviewer asks if the candidate plans to put his or her children in day care. This may be a way of determining the age of the dependent children. It could also provide information on the likelihood of absenteeism because of the children's illnesses. The medical assistant could answer, "I will be able to meet the work schedule and the responsibilities that this job requires."

Some questions that might normally be considered illegal, such as, "What organizations are you a member of?" might be job related. The employer may be interested in knowing if the medical assistant is a member of various professional organizations, such as the AAMA or the AMT.

CRITICAL THINKING APPLICATION   35.9

Krysia is enjoying a good interview when the interviewer, a male supervisor, asks her if she is married. When Krysia replies that she is not, he asks if she has a steady boyfriend.

- What might the supervisor's motive be with this line of questioning?
- How should Krysia respond?
- Are these questions inappropriate or do they serve a purpose?

Phone Interview

Phone interviews are usually done by the supervisor or the human resource representative. A phone interview may be done to:

- Screen applicants and narrow the candidate pool
- Provide additional information (e.g., benefits, job description) and verify the applicant wants an interview
- Replace a face-to-face interview, especially if the candidate is from out of town

It is important to treat a phone interview as a regular interview. Make sure to thank the interviewer at the end of the call.

Tips for Phone Interviews

- Prepare for the interview just as you would for a face-to-face interview.
- Take the call in a quiet environment. Make sure no dogs or children are in the room. Be alone in the room.
- Pay attention to the caller. Do not use other electronic devices or use the bathroom during the call.
- Have a copy of your resume and cover letter.
- Have your list of questions.
- Have a glass of water available should you need it.

TABLE 35.2	Illegal Versus Legal Interview Questions	
TOPIC	**EXAMPLES OF ILLEGAL QUESTIONS**	**EXAMPLES OF LEGAL QUESTIONS**
Birthplace, ancestry, or national origin	When did you move to the United States?	Are you eligible to work in this state?
Marital status, children, or pregnancy	Who will look after your child when he or she is born?	Are you able to work an 8 a.m. to 5 p.m. schedule?
Physical disability, health or medical history	What medications are you on?	Can you perform the essential job functions of a medical assistant with or without reasonable accommodation?
Religion or religious days observed	Where do you attend church services?	Can you work on weekends?
Age, race, ethnicity, gender, or color	How old are you?	Are you 18 or older? (or whatever the minimum age is for the facility)
Criminal record	Have you ever been arrested?	Have you ever been convicted of a crime?

Face-to-Face Interview

When you meet the interviewers, greet each person and shake hands. A firm handshake is recommended. Ensure each person has a copy of your resume and cover letter before the interview begins.

During the actual interview, maintain good eye contact. Many supervisors refuse to hire people who seem uncomfortable looking them directly in the eyes. Never take control of the interview. Allow the supervisor or panel members to ask questions at their own pace. Do not fidget in the chair or display any nervous habits (e.g., tapping your pen) (see Procedure 35.5).

Video Interview

A third interview possibility is a video interview using technology such as Skype. As with a phone interview, a video interview works well when the candidate is from out of town. There is a certain amount of technology needed for a video interview. Your school's placement office may be able to help you with that. The organization may have contacts for you to arrange your end of the interview. The benefit of a video interview over a phone interview is that the interviewers can actually see the interviewee. This allows the interviewers to assess the body language and the verbal message being presented. You should dress as you would for a face-to-face interview. You should have the same materials ready to access during the interview process. As with the face-to-face interview, you need to refrain from nervous habits.

Follow-Up After the Interview

Follow-up is critical after an interview. Always send a thank-you note, letter, or email to the person who conducted the interview (see Procedure 35.6, p. 915). It can be challenging to figure out what to send to the interviewer.

- *Send an email if:* the decision is going to be made quickly. Send an email later the day of the interview.
- *Send a written thank-you note or a letter if:* the facility is more conservative and formal. Also, it can be sent if the decision is going to be made in a week or two. Send the thank-you note within 24 hours of the interview.

Many employers see the thank-you as an expression of gratitude and professionalism. Even if you don't see yourself in that position, it is still important to send a thank you. This may be their last perception of you, and it may help you in the future at that facility.

Typically, at the end of the interview, there will be a discussion of how quickly the decision will be made. Many agencies using online hiring software will indicate the status of the job on the posting. Candidates not selected for the position usually receive an email or letter.

After the initial interviews are completed with all the candidates, several things can occur. With some employers, the list of interviewed candidates will be narrowed. The top two or three may be asked to come back for a second interview with additional team members (e.g., providers, medical assistants). With other employers, the top candidate is selected and references are checked. These processes take time, and the deadline may be extended if vacations or out-of-office times occur.

If the interviewer indicates a decision would be made in 2 weeks, wait to hear from the facility. Give a few days after the deadline before you follow up. At that time you can call and ask the status of the job. Remember, following up prior to the deadline may not be in your best interest. The employer may perceive that you do not follow directions if you make extra phone calls. If you receive a job offer from another facility but are waiting for a decision on your favorite position, it is appropriate to contact the interviewer. Explain that you were offered another position and wondered about the status of this position. Many employers will let you know if you are in the running for the position.

Never place all your hope in one job. Make sure to continue to search and interview until an offer is made and accepted. In addition, always be on the lookout for the next job opportunity.

Negotiation

The negotiation stage of job acceptance can be as stressful as the actual interviews. The salary and benefits must be considered when determining whether to accept a position or not. When a job offer is made, there should also be a discussion of the other benefits. If the salary offered is a bit lower than expected, but the employee's share of the health insurance premium is less than expected, the salary offer becomes more attractive. Medical assistants should know the lowest salary/benefit combination they can afford. They should ask for a little more than that figure.

Bracket salary requests are often helpful in this. Instead of asking for $13 per hour, ask for a salary in the "mid to high twenties." Let the employer mention a figure or a range of salary first. Usually the person who mentions a salary range first has the disadvantage. For example, if the medical assistant requests $13 per hour, but the facility was willing to pay $16 per hour, the medical assistant probably will get $13.

Many organizations have a starting pay level for new medical assistants. If you hope to get a higher pay level, you may need to:

- Obtain a national medical assistant credential (e.g., CMA [AAMA] or RMA)
- Show an advanced skills level acquired from previous work experience in healthcare. Having a well-designed interview portfolio will allow you to show the interviewer all that you have accomplished.

Never say "no" to a job offer on the spot. Request at least 24 hours to consider the offer. Before accepting or rejecting a job offer, consider whether the position carries any authority, the benefits, the hours, the distance from home, and the potential for advancement. People accept jobs for reasons other than the salary; remember the value of experience.

CRITICAL THINKING APPLICATION   35.10

Michelle has been on several interviews and likes the prospect of working for three different physicians. If an offer is made at each office, how can Michelle decide which to accept? What will help Michelle make this decision?

IMPROVING YOUR OPPORTUNITIES

We will examine ways to improve your opportunities for finding a job.

Finding Job Postings

Some students and graduates may not find job postings. This can be stressful, but it is important not to give up. Those who are not

UNIT SIX JOB SEEKING

having success with the job search may want to re-evaluate their search methods. Consider these questions:

- *Am I looking for a very selective opportunity?* For instance, are you looking for a dermatology medical assistant position in a specific facility? Those positions may be very limited. Try to broaden your search to other possible opportunities.
- *Am I looking for the correct job title?* Remember, employers may use a wide range of titles for a medical assistant.
- *Am I looking at all agencies that potentially could hire a person with my skill sets?* Depending on your area, medical assistants can be in many agencies besides a medical clinic, including a nursing home, hospital, school, assisted-living facility, and insurance company.
- *Can I increase the geographical search area for employment opportunities?* Can I relocate to an area with greater employment opportunities?
- *Where can I network to increase my awareness of job openings?*
- *What job boards are being used by local employers?*

Increasing Interview Opportunities

For people who apply for jobs but never get calls for interviews, it is important to re-evaluate their information given to employers. Consider these questions:

- *Is your cover letter, resume, online profile, or application negatively affecting the job search?* It may be important to get another opinion on the content and presentation. Often the school career placement officer will provide improvement tips.
- *Do you have spelling and grammar errors in your information?* Some employers may perceive that details are not important to you, and so they may not be interested in hiring you.
- *Do your cover letter and resume need to be reformatted or revised?* Applicants need their letter and resume to stand out from the crowd. People get very creative in how they make this occur.
- *Are your cover letter and resume customized to the job posting?* Do your documents reflect the key words in the posting? Or do your documents look "generic"? With generic-looking documents, employers perceive that the person is not into details and wasn't interested enough to spend the time to customize the documents.
- *Are you following the directions in the job posting?* For instance, an employer may want a handwritten cover letter to be included. Sometimes the employer provides a mailing address and states that no calls or visits will be allowed. If applicants do not follow the directions, they may not be considered for the job.
- *Are you providing a professional image with your email address and on social media sites, such as Facebook?* Graduates struggling to find positions may want to review their social media sites. Consider tighter security settings to limit outside viewers. You may want to remove any questionable content and pictures.

Increasing Job Offers

If you are getting interviews but no job offers, re-evaluate your interview strategies. Again, the school's career placement office may have interview assistance. **Mock** interviews can help you refine your interview skills and behavior.

The following is a ranked list of reasons interviewers do not hire job candidates, as expressed by surveyed career consultants and reported on the website *http://careers.workoplis.com*:

- Not sufficiently differentiating themselves from others
- Failure to successfully transfer past experience to the current job opportunity
- Not showing enough interest and excitement
- Focusing too much on what they want and too little on what the interviewer is saying
- Feeling they can "wing" the interview without preparation
- Not being able to personally connect with the interviewer
- Appearing overqualified or underqualified for the job
- Not asking enough or the right questions
- Not researching a potential employer/interviewer
- Lacking humor, warmth, or personality during the interview process

It is always important to prepare for the interview, show enthusiasm for the position, and ask the right questions. Other factors that may have negatively affected the decision include:

- *Inappropriate interview attire and grooming*: The outfit was too tight, neckline was too low, pants dragged on the ground, or the shoes were too casual (e.g., flip-flops). The perfume or cologne was too strong. The hairstyle or color was too extreme.
- *Didn't fit in the environment*: Each facility has a corporate environment. The interviewer looks to see which candidate would fit best. If a person is too shy, too talkative, or too loud, he or she might not be the best fit. Or, a person may have worn too many piercings, or too many tattoos were visible.
- *Used poor grammar*: Some employers correlate good grammar with intelligence. Employers look for candidates who sound intelligent and who will positively represent their facility.

If you have heard or feel that your resume lacks skills needed for specific positions you want to obtain, you may want to improve your skill sets. This can occur through education and experience. Some people improve their job history and skill sets by obtaining temporary employment through temp agencies. Temporary jobs can provide experience and also help you refine your skills. Another way to better your skill sets through experience is by volunteering at a healthcare facility or free clinic. Depending on the volunteer position, it may help enhance your skill sets and also provide you with potential job leads. Volunteer activities should be added to the resume, because these valuable experiences often can be used in a healthcare setting. It does not matter that the position was not a paid job; experience counts, whether paid or not.

YOU GOT THE JOB!

Human Resource Requirements

When you obtain a job, you will be required to complete a number of documents (Table 35.3). You will be asked to bring in proof of identity and employment authorization (e.g., US passport, Social Security account number card, and driver's license). These documents are required for the employer's portion of the Form I-9. Form I-9 must be completed within the set time period to meet governmental regulations. Make sure to complete all the required forms in a timely manner. Meet the deadlines given to you by the human resource representative.

TABLE 35.3 Forms to Complete When Hired	
FORM	**DESCRIPTION**
Form I-9: Employment Eligibility Verification Form	Form I-9 is used to verify a person's identity and employment authorization. All US employers must ensure the form is completed by both the new hire and the employer. The form requires the new hire to provide the employer with documents that prove identity and employment authorization proof.
Form W-4: Employee's Withholding Allowance Certificate	New hires must provide their tax status (e.g., single) and how many allowances they are claiming. This information is used when the employer withholds money from their paycheck for income taxes.
Insurance benefit form	Most agencies have health and life insurance benefits that the new hire can participate in. Completion of paperwork is required as part of the enrollment activities.
Background check form	Many healthcare providers will pay for background checks on new hires. Some hiring may be contingent based on a clean background check. Some types of background checks include criminal, sexual offender registry, and caregiver.
Emergency contact form	The new employee gives the employer information on whom to contact in case of an emergency.
Handbook acknowledgement form	Some agencies have handbooks for each employee. They may require that the employee sign a form to acknowledge receiving the handbook.
Direct deposit form	Most healthcare agencies will pay the employees using the direct deposit method. Funds are transferred into the employee's bank account instead of the employee receiving a paper paycheck.
Agreement forms	The newly hired employee must sign agreement forms related to the Health Insurance Portability and Accountability Act (HIPAA) and computer security.

Getting Started

When you get your first job, it can be an exciting and scary time. You may feel excited for the new opportunities yet scared of the new responsibilities. With any job, it takes time to learn the position. Most healthcare agencies have *probationary periods* for new employees. This time frame can vary. The purpose of the probationary period is to see if the new employee is the right fit for the job. If the employee is not able to do the job or is not the right person for the job, the employer can terminate the employee during the probationary period.

It is important for the medical assistant to do well during the probationary period. The first weeks to months of the job are usually devoted to orientation. The new employee learns the processes and becomes efficient and confident in the role. To be successful it is important for the medical assistant to:

- Arrive 10 to 15 minutes prior to the start of the day. Limit absences, especially during the probationary period.
- Be groomed appropriately according to the facility's dress code.
- Be honest, trustworthy, and respectful in all interactions with peers, patients, and providers.
- Be willing to try new things and ask questions.
- Take feedback professionally and with a positive attitude.
- Be motivated to do a good job and be willing to keep learning.
- Be a team player and be willing to help others.
- Provide safe care to patients, always working within the medical assistant scope of practice.
- Be open to new ideas, concepts, and procedures.

- Attempt to resolve simple differences with peers before involving the supervisor.
- Work with the supervisor to improve oneself and the department.
- Finish all assigned tasks in a timely manner and look for additional duties if time is available.

Maintaining Your Job

For the medical assistant to continue with the facility, it is important to be a reliable employee. It is also important to improve one's weaknesses. The medical assistant will get regular feedback from supervisors through performance appraisals. The performance appraisals inform employees of their strengths and weaknesses on the job. These appraisals are done after the probationary period and annually thereafter. Types of performance appraisals include:

- *180-degree style*: Supervisors evaluate their employees based on their observations of job performance over a given time period.
- *360-degree style*: Supervisors gather input from your co-workers and others whom you interact with on a regular basis.

Do not expect to receive a perfect appraisal. Employees are seldom perfect in all aspects of their jobs. If the supervisor gives perfect scores to an employee, there is no room for growth or improvement. The areas for growth are usually discussed during a meeting with the supervisor. You may be asked where you want to grow or improve and your goals for the coming year. It is important to consider these topics prior to the meeting with the supervisor.

Professional development is also important in maintaining one's job. Medical assistants must keep updated and current in the healthcare industry. It is important to meet the continuing education units (CEUs) needed to maintain your certification or registration. Information on the requirements can be found on the credentialing agency's website.

Leaving a Job

Always offer at least 2 weeks' notice when resigning from a job. Prepare a written notice of resignation and take it to the supervisor in person. Do not just leave it on a desk or place it in the interoffice mail.

Resigning from a job just as an attempt to get a salary increase is a dangerous practice. Once the employer doubts the employee's loyalty, the future is not usually bright for the employee at that facility. Resign only after a final decision has been made. If the medical assistant is resigning to take another position, the current employer may be expected to make a **counteroffer**. However, be wary about accepting counteroffers. What led you to look for a new job in the first place? Has the situation been resolved? Ask yourself these questions before agreeing to stay with the current employer. Often employees who accept a counteroffer and stay at their original job find that few changes are made, and the employee ends up leaving the position in the long run.

CLOSING COMMENTS

As you finish your medical assistant program, embrace the challenge of finding a job. Spend time preparing for the search. Design a professional resume and cover letter that positively set you apart from the other graduates. Network and check job boards for job openings. Apply for any jobs that interest you. Keep organized in your search so you don't overlook opportunities. Work with employment resources at your school to increase your confidence in interviewing. Your

preparation and hard work will help you find your first medical assistant job!

Legal and Ethical Issues

Always be completely honest when completing a job application and offering information on a resume. Most facilities stipulate that if an individual is not truthful on these documents, his or her employment can be terminated when the deception is discovered. Employers are more interested in honesty and a forthright explanation than in minor problems that affect the job performance.

If a medical assistant has had some brush with the law that requires disclosure on the job application, the best policy is to be honest and to deal with the ramifications of telling the truth. Most businesses can verify whether a potential employee has any type of criminal record. A solid explanation of the facts, admission of a past mistake, and excellent current references often prompt an employer to have faith and make a positive decision about offering employment.

Professional Behaviors

The development of professional behaviors must begin before the start of a new job. Use your time in school to develop those behaviors that employers are looking for: collaboration and interpersonal skills, professionalism, and compassion. By developing these behaviors in school, your teachers and practicum mentors will be able to give a recommendation that stresses those skills. By being on time and prepared for class, you are showing that you will be on time and prepared for work. By being diligent and self-directed in the classroom, you demonstrate that you have a strong work ethic, which is an important characteristic to employers.

SUMMARY OF SCENARIO

Before graduation, Michelle was offered a job at Walden-Martin Family Medical (WMFM) Clinic. She took her instructor's advice and sent a thank-you note to those who interviewed her. When she was offered the job, the supervisor mentioned how thoughtful the note was. During the call, the supervisor summarized the benefits and the starting salary. She mentioned to Michelle that all medical assistants start at the same wage, but after they pass the CMA (AAMA) certification examination, they get a raise. Michelle took 2 days to consider the position and decided to accept the job offer. The wage was lower than what she was hoping for, but the benefits were much better.

Krysia interviewed for several medical assistant positions over the past few weeks. She found that employers respected her service to her country and valued the skills she learned in military service. She just received her third job offer within the last few days and has decided to accept the position at the

local Veterans Affairs (VA) clinic. It is a full-time position with great benefits. The higher wage will help offset the extra mileage that she will be driving to work. She is very excited to be working with other veterans.

Zac has struggled identifying what type of clinic he wants to work for. With his strong leadership skills, he hopes to find a position where he can advance to a supervisory position. He has interviewed for job positions at small and large clinics. He is finding that he is more interested in working with surgeons than with family practitioners. He likes the complexity involved with surgical patients. He is hoping to receive a job offer shortly after graduation. He has decided that if his "dream job" is not offered to him, he will pursue a position in family medicine or internal medicine. This will give him a solid foundation for his new career and then someday he can move into orthopedics or surgery.

SUMMARY OF LEARNING OBJECTIVES

1. **Describe personality traits important to employers.**

   With the cost of training new employees, employers must find the best person to hire. Many employers struggle with assisting new employees to evolve or change personality traits. Thus, employers seek people who already have collaboration and interpersonal skills, professionalism, compassion, and a sincere interest in the job. Collaboration and interpersonal skills allow the new employee to blend well with the current staff. Being flexible, dependable, supportive of peers, remaining calm under pressure, listening, and having good manners are just some of the characteristics of a person with great collaboration and interpersonal skills. Being professional includes proper dress and grooming habits, punctuality, honesty, attention to detail, and the abilities to follow directions, prioritize, and manage time efficiently. Providing compassionate and respectful care and supporting the patient's dignity are crucial to good patient care. Lastly, being genuinely interested in the position positively affects the person's attitude and performance in the job.

2. **Discuss personality traits, technical skills, and transferable job skills.**

   A medical assistant must identify the personality traits, technical skills, and transferable job skills that he or she possesses. Using a portfolio will help the interviewee showcase the qualities that he or she has. Technical skills consist of administrative and clinical skills the person has developed during his or her medical assistant program. Transferable job skills are skills that were used in an unrelated position but relate or transfer to the new position.

3. **Describe how to develop a career objective and identify your personal needs.**

   Medical assistants should take some time to think about what they want from their career and develop a career objective. Your personal needs (e.g., wage, benefits, hours, locations) help you determine what job might be right for you, so you can focus your job search.

4. **Explain job search methods.**

   The two best methods to identify jobs are through networking and using job boards. Networking involves the medical assistant exchanging information with other professionals and family members in hopes of obtaining possible job leads. Job boards are online sites that list positions posted by employers. They can be specific to the healthcare facilities or they can be managed by local media organizations. National job boards can be very helpful for those who want to relocate to another part of the country. Traditional job search methods include school career placement offices, newspaper ads, and employment agencies.

5. **Create a resume and cover letter.**

   The three commonly used resume formats are chronologic, combination, and targeted resumes. Procedures 35.1 and 35.2 describe the steps involved with preparing a resume and cover letter. As you create your resume, keep in mind the eye appeal or interest the resume will create in the reader. A cover letter should always accompany a resume, and much attention to detail is necessary.

6. **Complete an online profile and job application.**

   Many healthcare agencies use the internet during the employment process, and an online profile can have many advantages over paper applications. However, not every employer uses online profiles, and students also may have to fill out job applications. Procedure 35.3 describes the steps involved in completing a job application.

7. **Describe how to create a career portfolio.**

   Procedure 35.4 describes the steps involved in creating a career portfolio.

8. **Practice interview skills during a mock interview.**

   Refer to Procedure 35.5.

9. **List legal and illegal interview questions.**

   See Table 35.2 for examples of illegal and legal interview questions that address the following topics: birthplace, ancestry, or national origin; marital status, children or pregnancy; physical disability, health or medical history; religion or religious days observed; age, race, ethnicity, gender, or color; and criminal record.

10. **Create a thank-you note for an interview.**

    Writing a thank-you note for an interview is a way to make you stand out from the other people who have interviewed for the same position. It shows that you are a courteous and conscientious person and also gives you another opportunity to show why you are the right person for the job. Refer to Procedure 35.6.

11. **Explain common human resources hiring requirements when starting a new job.**

    When you obtain a job, you will be required to complete a number of documents, including Form I-9, Form W-4, insurance benefit form, background check form, emergency contact form, handbook acknowledgement form, direct deposit form, and agreement form. You will be asked to bring in proof of identity and employment authorization (e.g., US passport, Social Security account number card, and driver's license). These documents are required for the employer's portion of Form I-9.

PROCEDURE 35.1 Prepare a Chronologic Resume

Task: Write an effective resume for use as a tool in obtaining employment.

EQUIPMENT and SUPPLIES

- Computer with word processing software and a printer
- Current job posting
- Resume paper
- Paper and pen

PROCEDURAL STEPS

1. Apply critical thinking skills as you create a list of the personality traits (wanted by employers), technical skills, and transfer job skills that you possess. Also write down your career goal(s).
   PURPOSE: To determine the strongest aspects of your abilities so that they can be emphasized on the resume.

2. Using the current job posting, identify the required and recommended qualifications and credentials needed for the position.
   PURPOSE: Identifying what the employer requires and would like will help you tailor your resume to address these qualifications and credentials.

3. Using the computer with word processing software, create a professional-looking header for your document. Include your name, address, telephone number(s), and email address. Select an appropriate font style for your name and a smaller font size for your contact information.
   PURPOSE: To make sure potential employers have a means of contacting you. Using a font style that is bold and a larger size for your name will help your name stand out. Make sure to have your contact information in a smaller, nonbold style so it will not detract from your name.

4. Create a section header for "Education." For the learning institution(s) you attended, list the school's name, city and state, degree obtained, or coursework successfully completed, and the year. Include any additional educational information, such as grade point average (GPA), awards, and practicum information.
   PURPOSE: It is important to provide the school's name, city, and state, along with the degree. Some employers may need to verify the information.

5. Create a section header for "Healthcare Experience" and/or "Work Experience." Provide details about your work experience, including the facility's name, city and state, title of your position, start and end date (month and year), and job duties. The job duties must start with an active verb using the appropriate tense (e.g., a past job would have past tense verbs and a current job would include present tense verbs).

PURPOSE: The potential employer will need to know your employment history and all the details.

6. Create a section header for "Special Skills" and list your special language skills, computer proficiencies, and other unique skills you possess that relate to the position.
   PURPOSE: This section can be a "marketing" area where you emphasize unique skills you possess.

7. Create a section header for "Certifications and Credentials" and list the active credentials and certifications you have. Include the title of the certification, awarding agency, and the expiration date.
   Note: You may want to consider adding in the date you are taking a credential examination. Employers like to know the status of your credential examination.
   PURPOSE: Employers need to know if you have your medical assistant credential (CMA or RMA). They also might like to know if you have an active cardiopulmonary resuscitation (CPR) card.

8. All information on the resume needs to appear in reverse chronologic order (i.e., newest information is on top). Work experiences should include both the start and end month and year.
   PURPOSE: Employers need to know how long you worked at a specific place. If the position was seasonal or temporary, it is important to note that.

9. The resume needs to look professional and interesting. Use font styles (e.g., bold, underline, italic) to emphasize important words and phrases. Use professional-looking bullets to list job duties and other information. Use the key words from the posting throughout the resume.
   PURPOSE: The more professional and interesting a resume appears, the better the chance that it will be reviewed by the potential employer.

10. Proofread the resume. Correct any spelling, grammar, punctuation, or sentence structure errors you find. If time allows, have another person review the resume and use the feedback to revise your resume.
    PURPOSE: Resumes submitted with errors often are discarded without consideration.

11. Print the resume on resume paper and proofread one final time. Any errors should be corrected, and the document should be reprinted or emailed to the instructor.

PROCEDURE 35.2 | Create a Cover Letter

Task: Write an effective cover letter that will accompany the resume.

EQUIPMENT and SUPPLIES

- Computer with word processing software and a printer
- Current job posting
- Resume paper
- Pen

PROCEDURAL STEPS

1. Using the job posting, read through the job description. With a pen, circle the position requirements and the key phrases.
   PURPOSE: Your letter should contain the key phrases and position requirements that are found in the job posting.
2. Using the computer with word processing software, create a professional-looking header in the document's header that matches your resume header. Include your name, address, telephone number(s), and email address.
   PURPOSE: To ensure potential employers have a means of contacting you. You can enhance the professional appearance of your documents by having the same header on each document.
3. Type the date in the correct location using the correct format. Have one blank line between the date line and the last line of the letterhead.
   PURPOSE: All letters require a date for legal purposes. The correct format would be month date, year (e.g., May 14, 2023).
4. Type the inside address using the correct spelling, punctuation, and location for the information. Leave 1 to 9 blank lines between the date and the inside address, depending on the location of the body of the letter.
   PURPOSE: The body of the letter needs to be centered vertically from top to bottom of the document. More blank lines can be added to move the body to the correct location.
5. Starting on the second line below the inside address, type the salutation using the correct format. Use a colon after the person's name.
   PURPOSE: A proper greeting helps set the tone of the letter.

6. Type the message in the body of the letter using the proper location and format. There should be a blank line after the salutation and between each paragraph. The message should be clear, concise, and professional. Use proper grammar, punctuation, capitalization, and sentence structure.
   PURPOSE: Proper grammar usage helps convey the message more accurately and professionally.
7. The first paragraph should contain the title and number of the job posting. The middle paragraph(s) should summarize your strengths and include key phrases from the posting. The final paragraph should discuss your availability for an interview. The body should end with an expression of gratitude to the reader.
   PURPOSE: It is important to thank the reader for considering you for the position.
8. Type a proper closing, leaving one blank line between the last line of the body and the closing. Use the correct format and location.
   PURPOSE: The closing helps end the message with a proper tone.
9. Type the signature block using the correct format and location. There should be four blank lines between the closing and the signature block.
   PURPOSE: The four blank lines will provide you with space to sign your name.
10. Spell-check and proofread the document. Check for proper tone, grammar, punctuation, capitalization, and sentence structure. Check for proper spacing between the parts of the letter.
    PURPOSE: The spell-check tool will identify only certain errors; proofreading will help to identify incorrect word usage, improper tone, and errors in formatting. The tone of the letter should be professional, but not aggressive.
11. Make any final corrections. Print the document on resume paper and sign the letter, or email the document to your instructor or employer.
    PURPOSE: It is professional to use resume paper when submitting a resume and cover letter to an employer.

PROCEDURE 35.3 | Complete a Job Application

Task: Complete an accurate, detailed job application legibly so as to secure a job offer.

EQUIPMENT and SUPPLIES

- Pen
- Application form
- Information regarding your past education, job experiences, and the skill sets you have developed (e.g., computer skills, keyboarding speed)
- Contact information for former supervisors and references
- Current resume

PROCEDURAL STEPS

1. Read the entire job application before completing any part of the document.
   PURPOSE: Reading through the entire application helps prevent errors when filling out the document.
2. Refer to your information on past jobs, education experiences, and skill sets you have developed as you complete the application. Answers to the questions need to be accurate and honest.

Continued

PURPOSE: The application is a legal document, and the answers must be correct and true.

3. Use proper grammar, sentence structure, punctuation, spelling, and capitalization. Handwriting should be legible to the reader.
PURPOSE: Errors on the application or illegible sections may affect whether you are hired.

4. Do not leave any space blank. Answer each question on the document. If the question does not apply, write "not applicable."
PURPOSE: Leaving a space blank on the application may suggest that the candidate did not want to answer a certain question or accidentally overlooked it. By writing "not applicable" on such questions, the candidate demonstrates competence and attention to detail.

5. Do not write "See resume" anywhere on the document.
PURPOSE: Many supervisors view this practice as laziness. Always fill out the job application completely and do not leave blank spaces.

6. Include information on the application that exhibits dependability, punctuality, teamwork, attention to detail, a positive work ethic and initiative, the ability to adapt to change, a responsible attitude, and use of technology.
PURPOSE: These phrases send an important message to employers. It is important to use words they are looking for.

7. Sign the document and date it.
PURPOSE: Because this is a legal document, read the fine print before signing the document and dating it.

8. Proofread the document and make sure none of the information conflicts with the resume.
PURPOSE: Proofreading helps the candidate to catch any errors before submitting the application.

PROCEDURE 35.4   Create a Career Portfolio

Task: Create a custom portfolio that provides potential employers evidence of your skills and knowledge as a medical assistant.

EQUIPMENT and SUPPLIES

- Three-ring binder or folder
- Plastic sleeves for the three-ring binder
- Dividers with tabs for the three-ring binder
- Current resume and cover letter
- Documents providing evidence of your skills and knowledge (e.g., transcripts, job and practicum evaluation forms, practicum skill checklist, projects completed in school, letters of recommendation, copies of certifications [e.g., CPR card])

PROCEDURAL STEPS

1. Group documents in a logical manner, putting similar documents together. Identify the arrangement for the portfolio. An arrangement could include cover letter and resume, education section (e.g., transcript, practicum evaluation form and skills checklist, awards), prior job-related documents (e.g., evaluations), reference letters, and work products (e.g., projects you created in your medical assistant program).
PURPOSE: Organizing the documents in a logical manner will help the reader identify the important documents. The arrangement will also show the reader your ability to organize content.

2. Insert one document per plastic pocket. Place all documents in plastic pockets.
PURPOSE: The plastic pockets will keep the documents clean and neat.

3. Neatly write the topic area on the tab of the dividers. Insert the tabbed dividers in the binder or folder.
PURPOSE: This will help the reader find the content easier.

4. Place all documents in the binder or folder behind the correct divider. Place your cover letter and resume in the front of all the other documents.
PURPOSE: The reader can review the letter and resume as needed before looking at the other documents in the portfolio.

5. Create a table of contents to identify the tabbed areas.
PURPOSE: Organizing the documents in a logical manner will help the reader identify the important documents. The arrangement will also show the reader your ability to organize content.

6. After the portfolio is assembled, review the entire portfolio to ensure it looks professional and the documents provide positive support of your skill set and knowledge.
PURPOSE: Minimize the negative documents in your portfolio. They will not help you obtain a job as much as the positive, supporting documents.

PROCEDURE 35.5 Practice Interview Skills During a Mock Interview

Task: Project a professional appearance during a job medical assistant interview and to be able to express the reasons you are the best candidate for the medical assistant position.

EQUIPMENT and SUPPLIES

- Current job posting
- Resume
- Cover letter
- Interview portfolio (optional)
- Application (optional)
- Interviewer
- Mock interview questions

PROCEDURAL STEPS

1. Wear interview-appropriate attire and be groomed professionally.
   PURPOSE: Your appearance will influence the first impression made on this potential employer. Most medical facilities prefer conservative dress.
2. Portray a professional image by shaking hands firmly prior to the start of the interview. Ensure that each interviewer has a copy of your resume and cover letter. Refrain from nervous behaviors (e.g., saying "um," tapping a pen or your foot) during the interview.
   PURPOSE: Many employers feel a firm handshake is important. Each interviewer may need a copy of your documents to reference during the interview.
3. Answer introductory questions by providing only professional information. This may include information about your education, experience, and career goals.

PURPOSE: Many people are tempted to answer with personal information (e.g., if they are married, have children). Personal information should not be discussed during the interview.

4. Answer interview questions with open, honest, and positive responses. Completely answer questions, provide information or examples, and do not answer in single sentences or with limited responses.
   PURPOSE: The goal of the interview is for the employer to get to know you. Limited responses negatively affect this goal.
5. Use key words from the job posting when answering the interview questions.
   PURPOSE: This helps to prove the interviewee has exactly what the organization is looking for.
6. Ask the interviewer two to three appropriate questions about the facility or the position.
   PURPOSE: This demonstrates an interest in the organization and the position.
7. Express interest in the job and politely complete the interview by shaking hands and thanking the interviewer for the opportunity for the interview.
   PURPOSE: The employer wants to know that you are interested in the job. It is professional to thank the interviewer for the interview opportunity.

PROCEDURE 35.6 Create a Thank-You Note for an Interview

Task: Create a meaningful thank-you note to be sent after the interview process.

EQUIPMENT and SUPPLIES

- Computer with word processing software and a printer
- Job description
- Contact name from interview

PROCEDURAL STEPS

1. Using word processing software, compose a professional letter using the business letter format. Include all of the required elements in the letter. Use correct spacing between the elements.
   PURPOSE: Creating a letter that reflects a professional business letter shows the employer you pay attention to detail.
2. Emphasize the particulars of the interview in the body of the letter.
   PURPOSE: Providing highlights of the interview will assure the employer that you took the time to write an individual thank-you letter.

3. Include positive information you wish you had covered in the interview.
   PURPOSE: This allows you to present any missed skills or details in a professional manner.
4. Create a message that is concise and to the point.
   PURPOSE: Keep the letter short and concise. Employers look for employees who can summarize a message and communicate that message.
5. Proofread the letter and make any revisions as needed. Sign and send the thank-you note.
   PURPOSE: It is important to make sure your note is written correctly. You want to leave a positive perception with the employer.

GLOSSARY

Abscess Localized collections of pus, which may be under the skin or deep in the body, that cause tissue destruction.

Abstract Collecting important information from the health record.

Abuse An action that purposely harms another person.

Accessory muscles Muscles in the neck, abdomen, and back that assist in breathing.

Accommodation Adjustment of the eye that allows a person to see various sizes of objects at different distances.

Accounts payable Money owed by a company to other companies for services and goods; pertains to paying the facility's bills.

Acute phase The phase during which rapid multiplication of the pathogen takes place. Symptoms are very distinct. A strong response of the immune system takes place during this stage.

Addiction A disease that occurs when a person cannot stop or limit the use of a drug, even after negative consequences have been experienced.

Adherence (ad HEER ehns) The act of sticking to something.

Adhesions (ad HEE zhuns) Bands of scar tissue that can bind anatomic structures together.

Adjudicate (uh JOO di kayt) To settle or determine judicially.

Advance directives Written instructions about healthcare decisions in case a person is unable to make them.

Affect The external emotional expression.

Afferent (AF er uhnt) Pertaining to carrying toward a structure.

Age of majority The age at which the law recognizes a person to be an adult; it varies by state.

Albumin (al BYOO men) Most abundant plasma protein in human blood. It is important in regulating the water balance of blood.

Allopathic (al uh PATH ik) A system of medical practice that treats disease by the use of remedies, such as medications and surgery, to produce effects different from those caused by the disease under treatment; medical doctors (MDs) and osteopaths (DOs) practice allopathic medicine; also called *conventional medicine*.

Alphabetic filing Any system that arranges names or topics according to the sequence of the letters in the alphabet.

Alphanumeric Describes systems made up of combinations of letters and numbers.

Amblyopia (am blee OH pee ah) Dull or dim vision, with no apparent organic defect.

Amenorrhea (ey men uh REE uh) Lack of menstrual flow.

Amino (ah MEE noe) acids Released during the digestion of protein foods in the intestines; carried by the blood to cells, where they are used to make proteins. Used for growth, maintenance, and repair of cells; they also transport nutrients.

Amnesia (am NEE zhah) Memory loss.

Amygdala (ah MIG dah lah) A small mass of gray matter found in each temporal lobe of the cerebrum and involved with memories, emotions, and activating the fight-or-flight response; part of the limbic system.

Analgesic (an ahl JEE zik) A drug that reduces or eliminates pain.

Analyte (AN e lit) The substance or chemical being analyzed or detected in a specimen.

Anaphylaxis (an ah fah LAK sis) A rapidly progressing, life-threatening allergic reaction; characterized by hives, swelling of the mouth and airway, difficulty breathing, wheezing, and loss of consciousness.

Anaplastic (an uh PLAS tic) A rapidly dividing cancer cell that has little to no similarity to normal cells.

Anemia A deficiency of hemoglobin in the blood. Accompanied by a reduced number of red blood cells, pale skin, weakness, and shortness of breath among other symptoms.

Anencephaly (an en SEF uh lee) Congenital absence of part or all of the brain.

Anesthetic (an ehs THET ik) An agent that causes partial or complete loss of sensation.

Aneurysm (AN yeh rizm) An abnormal blood fill sac formed from a localized dilatation of the wall of a vein, artery, or heart.

Anhedonia (an hee DOE nee ah) The inability to feel or experience pleasure during a pleasurable activity.

Anovulation Failure of the ovaries to release an ovum at the time of ovulation.

Answering service A commercial service that answers telephone calls for its clients.

Anthropometric (an thruh PO me trik) The measurement of the size and proportions of the human body.

Antiarrhythmic (an tee ah RITH mik) A drug that prevents or alleviates heart arrhythmias.

Antibiotic (an ti bie OT ik) A drug that destroys or inhibits the growth of bacteria.

Antibody A protein substance produced in the blood or tissues in response to a specific antigen, which destroy or weaken the antigen; part of the immune system.

Anticoagulant (an tee koe AG yuh lunt) A substance (i.e., medication or chemical) that prevents clotting of blood.

Anticonvulsant (an tee kahl VUL sahnt) A drug used to prevent or treat seizures.

Antigen A substance that stimulates the production of an antibody when introduced into the body. Antigens include toxins, bacteria, viruses, and other foreign substances.

Antihistamine (an tee HIS tah meen) A drug that counteracts the effects of histamine.

Antihyperlipidemic (an tie hie per lip i DEE mik) A drug that lowers the lipid levels in the blood.

Antihypertensive A drug that reduces high blood pressure.

Anti-inflammatory (an TEE in FLAM ah tor ee) A medication that prevents or reduces inflammation.

Antimalarial (an TEE mah LAR ee ahl) A drug used to treat or prevent malaria.

Antioxidant (an tee OK si dahnt) Synthetic or natural substance found in food and supplements; may prevent or delay some types of cell damage.

Antipyretic (an tee pie RET ik)   A drug that is used to reduce a fever.

Antiseptic (an ti SEP tik)   Substances that inhibit the growth of microorganisms on living tissue (e.g., alcohol and povidone-iodine solution [Betadine]); they are used to cleanse the skin, wounds, and so on.

Aphasia (ah FAY zhah)   Partial or complete loss of the ability to articulate ideas or understand written or spoken language.

Apnea (AP nee ah)   Abnormal, periodic cessation of breathing.

Approximated (uh PROK si may ted)   Near, close together.

Arbitration (ahr bi TRAE shuhn)   The process in which conflicting parties in a dispute submit their differences to a court-appointed person (arbitrator), who submits a legally binding decision.

Arrhythmia (ah RITH mee ah)   An abnormal heart rate or rhythm.

Arterioles (ar TEER ee ohlz)   Small arteries.

Arteriosclerosis (ar teer ee oh sklah ROH sis)   Thickening, decreased elasticity, and calcification of arterial walls.

Arteriovenous   Pertains to the arteries and veins.

Arteriovenous fistula   An abnormal joining of an artery and vein.

Arthropod   Any animal that lacks a spine, such as insects, crustaceans, arachnids, and others.

Artifact   A substance, structure, or event that does not naturally occur in a situation. Examples include interference, or electrical "garbage," on an ECG, or crystals, lint, or contamination of a staining technique.

Artificial insemination   The injection of semen into the vagina or uterus using a catheter or syringe. Nonsexual.

Aseptically (ay SEP tick ah lee)   Free from living pathogenic organisms.

Asexual   Describes reproduction that does not involve the fusion of male and female sex cells.

Aspirate (AS pi rayt)   To withdraw fluid using suction. Example: a specimen that has been removed from the body using a needle and syringe.

Aspirating (AS puh rayt ing)   To draw off or remove by suction.

Assets   All property available for the payment of debts.

Atheroma (ath uh ROH mah)   A waxy lesion of cholesterol, fat, calcium, cells, and other substances that builds up on the inner wall of an artery.

ATP (adenosine triphosphate)   A high-energy molecule, found in every cell, that supplies large amounts of energy for various biochemical processes.

Attenuated (uh TEN yoo ayt ed)   Weakened or changed.

Atypical lymphs   In many viral infections stimulated or reactive lymphs are called atypical lymphs. They are commonly seen in infectious mononucleosis.

Audible (AW duh buh l)   Capable of being heard.

Audiologist (aw dee OL uh jist)   Allied healthcare professional who specializes in evaluation of hearing function, detection of hearing impairment, and determination of the anatomic site of impairment.

Audit   A process completed before claims submission in which claims are examined for accuracy and completeness.

Auditory cortex   The region of the cerebral cortex that receives auditory data.

Auscultated (AW skuh l teyt d)   Listened to with a stethoscope.

Authorized agent   A person who has written documentation that he or she can accept a shipment for another individual.

Autoimmune   An immune response against a person's own tissues, cells, or cell parts, as in autoimmune disease, leading to the deterioration of tissue.

Automatic call routing   A system that distributes incoming calls to a specific group or person based on customer need; for example, the customer presses 1 for appointments, 2 for billing questions, and so on.

Autonomy (aw TON uh mee)   The ability to function independently.

Axon (AK son)   A long extension of a nerve fiber that conducts the impulse away from the nerve cell body.

Backordered   An order placed for an item that is temporarily out of stock and will be sent at a later time.

Bacteria   Microorganisms that are single celled, lack a nucleus, reproduce asexually, or can form spores. Some can cause disease. The most abundant life form on earth.

Bartholin (BAR thoh lin) cyst   A fluid-filled cyst in one of the vestibular glands located on either side of the vaginal orifice.

Basal   Bottom layer.

Belligerent (buh LIG er ent)   Hostile and aggressive.

Beneficiary   A designated person who receives funds from an insurance policy.

Benign   A non-cancerous condition, not malignant, harmless.

Biconvex (bie KON veks)   Having two outward curving surfaces, on a lens.

Bilaterally (bie LAT er uhl ee)   Pertaining to, involving, or affecting two or both sides.

Bilingual (bie LING gwuhl)   Ability to communicate effectively in two languages.

Bilirubin (bil i ROO bin)   A reddish pigment that results from the breakdown of red blood cells in the liver.

Billable service   Assistance (i.e., service) that is provided by a healthcare provider and can be billed to the insurance company or patient.

Binary fission   Asexual reproduction in single-celled organisms during which one cell divides into two daughter cells.

Binocular (buh NOK yuh ler)   Involving, relating, or seeing with both eyes.

Binomial   A name consisting of a generic and a specific term.

Bioethicists (BYE oh eth i sists)   People who study the ethical effect of biomedical advances (e.g., drugs and genetic engineering).

Biomarkers   Detectable cellular indicators used as a marker for a substance or disease process.

Biopsy (BIE op see)   Process of viewing living tissue that has been removed for the purpose of diagnosis and/or treatment.

Bipolar   Having two poles or electrical charges.

Blood agar plate (BAP)   A solid agar medium that contains nutrients and 5% washed sheep's blood. The blood is added as an extra nutrient source for bacteria.

Blood culture   A microbiological procedure ordered when a provider suspects a bacterial infection is causing a fever of unknown origin (FUO). A blood sample is collected into a nutrient media and held at body temperature. If bacteria are in the blood sample, the culture media should encourage the growth of the infecting bacteria in the laboratory.

Bonded   A term describing employees for whom an employer has obtained a fidelity bond from an insurance company, which will cover losses from any dishonest acts (e.g., embezzlement, theft) committed by those employees.

Bookkeeping   The process of recording financial transactions.

Boot   The process of starting or restarting a computer when the operating system is loaded.

Bounding   Describes a pulse that feels full because of the increased power of cardiac contraction or as a result of increased blood volume.

Bradycardia (brad ee KAHR dee uh)   A slow heartbeat; a pulse below 60 beats per minute.

Bradypnea (brad IP nee ah)   Abnormally slow breathing.

Breach   Disclosure of protected health information, without a reason or permission, which compromises the security or privacy of the information.

Bronchiolitis   Occurs when the small airways of the lungs become inflamed because of a viral infection.

Bronchodilator   A drug that relaxes smooth muscle contractions in the bronchioles to improve lung ventilation.

Bruit (broot)   An abnormal sound or murmur heard on auscultation of an organ, vessel (e.g., carotid artery), or gland.

Business associate   A person or business that provides a service to a covered entity that involves access to PHI. Examples include legal, billing, and management services; accreditation agencies; consulting firms; and claims-processing organizations.

Buying cycle   Refers to how often an item is purchased and depends on how frequently the item is used and the storage space available for it.

Calcium   A naturally occurring element that is necessary for many body functions, including strong bones and teeth, proper blood clotting, nerve conduction, and muscle contractions.

Calculi (KAL kyuh lie)   Stones formed in the kidneys, gallbladder, and other parts of the body.

Calibrated (KAL uh bray ted)   Determined by or checked against those of a standard (as in readings).

Calibration (kal uh BRAY shun)   Determining the accuracy of an instrument by comparing its output with that of a known standard or another instrument known to be accurate.

Caliper   A pocket-sized tool used for measuring the height and width of the ECG waves and intervals.

Call forwarding   A telephone feature that allows calls made to one number to be forwarded to another specified number.

Caller ID   A feature that identifies and displays the telephone numbers of incoming calls made to a particular line.

Candidiasis (kan di DIE i sis)   An infection caused by a yeast, *Candida albicans*, that typically affects the vaginal mucosa and skin.

Cannula (KAN yuh la)   A rigid tube that surrounds a blunt trocar or a sharp, pointed trocar, which is inserted into the body; when the trocar is withdrawn, fluid may escape from the body through the cannula, depending on the insertion site.

Capitation (ka pi TAY shun)   A payment arrangement for healthcare providers. The provider is paid a set amount for each enrolled person assigned to him or her, per period of time, whether or not that person has received services.

Caption   A heading, title, or subtitle under which records are filed.

Cardiopulmonary resuscitation (ri sus i TAY shun) (CPR)   The application of manual chest compressions and ventilations (also called rescue breathing) to patients who are not breathing or do not have a pulse; also known as basic life support (BLS).

Cartilage (KAR tih lij)   Flexible connective tissue that covers the ends of many bones at the joint.

Cash on hand   The amount of money the healthcare facility has in the bank that can be withdrawn as cash.

Cataract (KAT ur ackt)   Progressive loss of transparency of the lens of the eye.

Catheter   A hollow, flexible tube that can be inserted into a vessel, organ, or cavity of the body to withdraw or instill fluid, monitor information, and visualize a vessel or cavity.

Caustic (KAW stik)   Capable of burning, corroding, or damaging tissue by chemical action.

Centrifuge (SEN truh fyooj)   A machine that rotates at high speed and separates substances of different densities by centrifugal force. Example: a tube of blood is separated into plasma/serum, white blood cells, platelets, and red blood cells.

Certified Registered Nurse Anesthetist (CRNA)   A nursing healthcare professional who is certified to administer anesthesia.

Cerumen (si ROO muhn)   A waxy secretion in the ear canal; commonly called *ear wax*.

Cessation (se SAY shuhn)   Bringing to an end.

Cheyne-Stokes respiration   Deep, rapid breathing followed by a period of apnea.

Chief complaint   A statement in the patient's own words that describes the reason for the visit.

Choroid plexus (KOR oid PLEK sus)   A network of capillaries found in the lateral ventricles and the third and fourth ventricles that secrete cerebrospinal fluid.

Chromosomes (KROE mah sohms)   Rod-shaped structures found in the cell's nucleus, which contain genetic information.

Chronic   Developing slowly and lasting for a long time, generally 3 or more months.

Chronic obstructive pulmonary disease (COPD)   A progressive, irreversible lung condition that results in diminished lung capacity.

Chronologic (kroon l OJ ick)   Arranged in the order of time.

Cicatrix (SIK uh triks)   Early scar tissue that appears pale, contracted, and firm.

Claim   An itemized statement of services and costs from a healthcare facility submitted to the health (insurance) plan for payment.

Claim scrubbers   Software that finds common billing errors before the claim is sent to the insurance company.

Claims clearinghouse   An organization that accepts the claim data from the provider, reformats the data to meet the specifications outlined by the insurance plan, and submits the claim.

Clarification (KLAR uh fa kay shuh n)   Allows the listener to get additional information.

Clitoris (KLIT uh ris)   Sensitive, erectile tissue.

Clot activators   Substances added to a venipuncture tube to enhance and speed up blood clotting.

Clubbing   Abnormal enlargement of the distal phalanges (fingers and toes) associated with cyanotic heart disease or advanced chronic pulmonary disease.

CMS-1500 Health Insurance Claim Form (CMS-1500)   The standard insurance claim form used for all government and most commercial insurance companies.

Coaching   Providing information in a supportive environment that allows people to grow, change, or improve their situation.

Code   A term used in healthcare settings to indicate an emergency situation and to summon the trained team to the scene.

Coding system   A system designed to use characters (i.e., numbers and letters) to represent something like a medical procedure or a disease.

Cohesive (koh HEE siv)   Sticking together tightly; exhibiting or producing cohesion.

Collaboration (kuh lab uh RAY shun)   The act of working with another or other individuals.

Collagen (KAH lah jen)   The most abundant structural protein found in skin and other connective tissues. It provides strength and cushioning to many parts of the body.

Colonoscopy (kohl uh NOS kuh pee)   A procedure in which a fiber-optic scope is used to examine the large intestine.

Colostomy (koh LOS tuh mee)   A surgical procedure in which the large intestine is brought though the abdominal wall, creating either a temporary or permanent opening (stoma) to allow stool to pass out of the body.

Colposcopy (kol PAW skoh pee)   Using a microscope with a light source, the vagina and cervix are visually examined to locate and evaluate abnormal cells. A biopsy of abnormal cells may be taken during this procedure.

Combining forms   The "subjects" of most terms. They consist of the word root with its respective combining vowel.

Common law   Unwritten laws that come from judicial decisions based on societal traditions and customs.

Communicable diseases (kuh MYOO ni kuh buh l)   Diseases spread from person to person either by direct contact or nondirect contact (i.e., insects).

Compartment syndrome   A serious condition that involves increased pressure, usually in the muscles; which leads to compromised blood flow and muscle and nerve damage.

Compassion   Having a deep awareness of the suffering of another and a wish to ease it.

Complementary and alternative medicine (CAM)   A group of diverse medical and healthcare systems, practices, and products that are not generally considered part of conventional medicine. Complementary medicine is used in combination with conventional medicine (allopathic or osteopathic); alternative medicine is used instead of conventional medicine.

Compliance (kuhm PLIE ahns)   The act of following through on a request or demand. Patient compliance sounds negative, thus patient adherence is now being used.

Compliant (kum PLIE unt)   Obeying, obliging, or yielding.

Computer network   A system that links personal computers and peripheral devices to share information and resources.

Computer on wheels (COW)   A wireless mobile workstation; also called a *workstation on wheels* (WOW).

Computerized provider/provider order entry (CPOE)   The process of entering medication orders or other provider instructions into the EHR.

Concise (kuhn SICE)   Using as few words as possible to express a message.

Concussion (kuhn KUSH uhn)   A traumatic brain injury caused by a blow to the head.

Cone biopsy   An extensive cervical biopsy during which a cone-shaped wedge of tissue is removed from the cervix and

examined under a microscope. Abnormal tissue, along with a small amount of normal tissue, is removed.

Conference call   A telephone call in which a caller can speak with several people at the same time.

Congruence (kuh n GROO uh ns)   Agreement; the state that occurs when the verbal expression of the message matches the sender's nonverbal body language.

Conscientious (kon shee EN shuhs)   Meticulous, careful.

Consensus (kun SEN sus)   General agreement.

Constrict   To contract or shrink.

Contamination (kun tam i NAY shun)   The process by which something becomes harmful or unusable through contact with something unclean.

Continuity of care   The smooth continuation of care from one provider to another. This allows the patient to receive the most benefit and no interruption or duplication of care.

Contraindicate (kon truh IN di keyt)   To suggest that it should not be used.

Control materials   Manufacturer-prepared samples that have a known quantity of a specific analyte. Used for quality control purposes. Testing results should fall within a manufacturer defined range of results. Also called *controls* or *quality controls.*

Convalescent stage   The phase during which the host recovers gradually and returns to baseline or normal health.

Copayment (copay)   A set dollar amount that the patient must pay for each office visit. There can be one copayment amount for a primary care provider, a different copayment amount (usually higher) to see a specialist or be seen in the emergency department.

Coping mechanisms   Behavioral and psychological strategies used to deal with or minimize stressful events.

Correlate (KAWR uh leyts)   To establish an orderly relationship or connection.

Corrosive (kuh ROH siv)   Causing or tending to cause the gradual destruction of a substance by chemical action.

Corticosteroids (kor ti koe STER oids)   A group of steroid hormones produced in the body or given as a medication. Some have metabolic functions, and others reduce tissue inflammation. Glucocorticoids and mineralocorticoids are two types.

Counterfeit (KOWN ter fit)   An imitation intended to be passed off fraudulently or deceptively as genuine; forgery.

Counteroffer   Return offer made by one who has rejected an offer or a job.

Covered entity (KUV er ed EN ti tee)   A healthcare facility, healthcare provider, pharmacy, health (insurance) plan, or claims clearinghouse that transmits protected health information electronically.

CPT Assistant   An online CPT coding journal, supported by the AMA, that addresses subjects such as appealing insurance denials, validating coding to auditors, training staff members, and answering day-to-day coding questions.

Crash cart   Emergency medications and equipment (e.g., oxygen, intravenous [IV] and airway supplies) stored in a cart and ready for an emergency.

Creatinine clearance rates   Result from a procedure used to evaluate the glomerular filtration rate of the kidneys.

Credential (kri DEN shus l)   Evidence of authority, status, rights, entitlement to privileges.

Crepitation (krep i TAY shun)   A dry, crackling sound or sensation.

Critical thinking   The constant practice of considering all aspects of a situation when deciding what to believe or what to do.

Cryopreservation (KRIE oh pri zur vae shun)   To preserve by freezing at low temperatures.

Cryosurgery   The technique of exposing tissue to extreme cold to produce a well-defined area of cell destruction.

Crystals   Solid substances with a regular shape that is due to the structure of molecules.

Culture media   A solid, liquid, or semi-solid medium designed to support the growth of microorganisms, especially bacteria and fungus.

Curettage (kyoo rhe TAHZH)   The act of scraping a body cavity with a surgical instrument, such as a curette.

Cystic fibrosis (CF)   A disorder that affects all the exocrine cells, but affects the respiratory system the most. Mucus is abnormally thick and blocks the alveoli, causing dyspnea.

Cytology (sie TOL oh jee)   The study of cells using microscopic methods.

Cytoplasm   The cell substance that fills the area between the nucleus and the cell membrane. It contains the organelles of the cell.

Damages   A monetary settlement the defendant pays the plaintiff in a civil case for loss or injury. Also, one of the 4 Ds of negligence, meaning the patient suffers a legally recognized injury.

Data server   Computer hardware and software that perform data analysis, storage, and archiving; also called a *database server.*

Debridement   The surgical removal of dead, damaged, or infected tissue to improve the function of healthy tissue.

Debris (duh BREE)   The remains of anything broken down or destroyed; ruins, rubble.

Decanting   Pouring a liquid gently so that it does not disturb the remaining sediment.

Declaratory judgment   A court judgment that defines the legal rights of the parties involved.

Decongestant   A drug that is used for nasal congestion.

Decryption (dee KRIP shun)   The computer process of changing encrypted text to readable or plain text after a user enters a secret key or password.

Decubitus ulcers (deh KYOO bi tus)   Sores or ulcers that develop over a bony prominence as the result of ischemia from prolonged pressure; also called *bed sores* or *pressure sores.*

De-escalating   Reducing the level or intensity; bringing down a person's anger or elevated emotions.

Defecation (DEF i kay shun)   The act of voiding waste from the bowels through the anus; the act of having a bowel movement.

Defendant (dih FEN dant)   An individual or business against whom a lawsuit is filed.

Defense (di FENS)   A strategy used by the defendant to avoid liability in a lawsuit.

Defense mechanisms   Unconscious mental processes that protect people from anxiety, loss, conflict, or shame.

Degenerative (dih JEN er uh tiv)   An illness resulting from the deterioration of tissues and organs.

Delegate   To appoint a person as a representative.

Delusion (de LOO zhun)   Unshakable belief in something untrue; may be accompanied by hallucinations and/or paranoia.

Demeanor (dih MEE ner)   Behavior toward others; outward manner.

Dementia (dih MEN shah)   A mental disorder in which the individual experiences a progressive loss of memory, personality alterations, confusion, loss of touch with reality, and stupor (seeming unawareness of, and disconnection with, one's surroundings).

Demographic (dem uh GRAF ik)   Statistical data of a population. In healthcare this includes the patient's name, address, date of birth, employment, and other details.

Density   Describes how compact or concentrated something is.

Deoxygenated   Oxygen deficient; oxygen was removed.

Dependent adults   People between the ages of 18 and 64 who have a mental or physical impairment that prevents them from doing normal activities or from protecting themselves.

Depersonalization   Alternative perception of the self; a person's own reality is lost. People feel they are not in control of their own actions or speech.

Deposition (dep ah ZISH uhn)   A sworn testimony made before a court-appointed officer; it is used in the discovery process and may be used in the trial.

Depreciate   To diminish in value (such as the value of an item) over a period of time; a concept used for tax purposes.

Derealization   Loss of sensation of the reality of one's surroundings.

Dermatome (DUR mah tome)   Skin surface areas supplied by a single afferent spinal nerve.

Detrimental (de truh MEN tl)   Harmful.

Dextrocardia (dek stro KAHR dee ah)   The heart is located on the right side of the chest and the apex is pointing to the right.

Diabetic retinopathy (die ah BET ik reh tin OP ah thee)   Diabetes mellitus damages the blood vessels in the retina leading to loss of vision and eventual blindness.

Diagnosis (die ag NOH sis)   Determining the cause of a condition, illness, disease, injury, or congenital defect.

Diagnostic statement   Information about a patient's diagnosis or diagnoses that has been taken from the medical documentation.

Diaphragm (DIE uh fram)   A broad, dome-shaped muscle used for breathing. It separates the thoracic and abdominopelvic cavities.

Dictation (dik TEY shuh n)   To say something aloud for another person to write down.

Differentiate (dif uh REN shee eyt)   To distinguish one thing from another. To make a distinction between items.

Differentiated (dif uh REN shee ayt)   Describes how malignant tissue looks like the normal tissue it came from; poorly differentiated means it does not look like the normal tissue, and well differentiated means it looks like the normal tissue.

Diffuse   To spread, scatter, disperse, or move.

Dignity (DIG ni tee)   The inherent worth or state of being worthy of respect.

Dilation (die LAY shuhn)   The opening or widening of the circumference of a body orifice with a dilating instrument.

Diluent (die LU ent)   A liquid substance that dilutes or lessens the strength of a solution or mixture.

Dilution   Reducing the concentration of a mixture or solution by adding a known volume of liquid.

Direct filing system   A filing system in which materials can be located without consulting another source of reference.

Discipline   A branch of knowledge, learning, or instruction; for instance medicine, nursing, social work, and physical therapy.

Discrepancy   A lack of similarity between what is stated and what is found; for instance, the computer inventory count is different than the physical count.

Discretionary income   Money in a bank account that is not assigned to pay for any office expenses.

Discrimination (dis krim eh NAE shuhn)   Unfair treatment of another person based on the person's age, gender (sex), ethnicity, sexual orientation, disability, marital status, or other selective factors.

Disinfect   To destroy or render pathogenic organisms inactive; does not include spores, tuberculosis bacilli, and certain viruses.

Disinfectant (dis in FEK tuh nt)   Any chemical agent used on nonliving objects to destroy or inhibit the growth of harmful organisms; not effective against bacterial spores.

Disparaging (di SPAR a jing)   Slighting; having a negative or degrading tone.

Disruption   An unexpected event that throws a plan into disorder; an interruption that prevents a system or process from continuing as usual or as expected.

Dissect   To cut or separate tissue with a cutting instrument or scissors.

Diuretic   A drug that increases the amount of urine produced.

Diurnal (die UR nl) variation   Fluctuations that occur during each day.

Diversity   The differences and similarities in identity, perspective, and points of view among people.

Docking station   Also known as a *universal port replicator*; this hardware device allows laptops to connect with other devices, making it into a desktop computer.

Dosage   May also be referred to as *dose*; the quantity of medication to be administered at one time.

Down syndrome   A genetic disorder in which abnormal cell division results in an extra chromosome 21.

Downtime   The interval of time where something, such as hardware or software, is not functioning.

Drive   A computer device that reads data from and may write data to a storage medium.

Dumb terminal   A personal computer that does not contain a hard drive and allows the user only limited functions, including access to software, the network, or the internet.

Dynamic (die NAM ik) equilibrium   Relating to balance when moving at an angle or rotating.

Dysmenorrhea (dis men uh REE uh)   Painful menstrual flow, cramps.

Dyspareunia (dis ph ROO nee ah)   Painful or difficult intercourse.

Dysphagia   Difficulty swallowing.

Dyspnea (DISP nee uh)   Difficult or painful breathing.

Ecchymosis (ek i MOH sis)   Discoloration of the skin caused by the escape of blood into the tissues from ruptured blood vessels; typically caused by bruising.

Echocardiography (ECHO) (eck oh KAR dee AH gruh fee)   The use of ultrasonic waves directed through the heart to study the structure and motion of the heart. The visual record produced is called an *echocardiogram*.

Ectopic pregnancy (eck TAH pick)   A pregnancy in which the fertilized egg implants outside of the uterus (e.g., fallopian tubes).

Efferent (EF er uhnt)   Pertaining to carrying away from a structure.

Egress (EE gress)   Leaving a place; exit route.

Elastin (ih LAS tin)   A highly elastic protein in connective tissue that allows tissues to resume their shape after stretching or contracting. It is found abundantly in the dermis of the skin.

Electrocardiogram (ECG, EKG)   A record or recording of electrical impulses of the heart produced by an electrocardiograph.

Electrodes   Adhesive patches that conduct electricity from the body to the machine wires (e.g., ECG and transcutaneous electrical nerve stimulation [TENS] unit).

Electrolyte   An inorganic compound, usually a salt. A major factor in controlling fluid balance within the body.

Electronic health record (EHR)   An electronic record conforms to nationally recognized standards and contains health-related information about a specific patient. It can be created, managed, and consulted by authorized clinicians and staff from more than one healthcare organization.

Electronic transaction   The electronic exchange of information between two agencies to accomplish financial or administrative healthcare activities.

Eligibility (el i ji BILL i tee)   Meeting the stipulated requirements to participate in the healthcare plan.

Emancipated minor (i MANS i pa ted MIE nohr)   A minor who has been granted emancipation by the court; the minor can assume the rights and responsibilities of adulthood.

Embezzlement (em BEZ uh l ment)   The misuse of funds for personal gain.

Embolus (EM boh lus)   An air bubble, blood clot, or foreign body that travels through the bloodstream and blocks a blood vessel.

Embryo (EM bree oh)   A developing organism from the moment of conception through the eighth week of development.

Emergency   An unexpected, life-threatening situation that requires immediate action.

Empathy (EM pah thee)   The ability to understand another's perspective, experiences, or motivations.

Emphysema (em fuh ZEE muh)   Thinning and eventual destruction of the alveoli; usually accompanies chronic bronchitis.

Emulsifies (ee MUL sih fyez)   When a substance suspends tiny droplets of one liquid into a second liquid. By creating an emulsion, you can mix two liquids that usually do not mix well, such as oil and water.

EMV chip technology   Global technology that includes imbedded microchips that store and protect cardholder data; also called *chip and PIN* and *chip and signature*.

Encoder   Software that will apply diagnostic or procedure codes to medical conditions or procedures.

Encounter form   A document used to capture the services/procedures and diagnoses for a patient visit. The fees for the services/procedures are usually included on the encounter form.

Endocrine   A glandular secretion that is released into the blood or lymph directly (does not go through a duct).

Endoscopy (en DOS kuh pee)   An examination using a scope with a camera attached to the long, thin tube that can be inserted into the body.

Endoscope   A scope with a camera attached to a long, thin tube that can be inserted into the body.

Endotracheal (EN doe TRAY kee al) (ET) tube   A catheter that is inserted into the trachea through the mouth; provides a patent airway.

Enriched   Nutrients are added back into a food, after they were loss during food processing.

Enunciation (ih nuhn see EY shuh n)   The use of articulate, clear sounds when speaking.

Enzymes (EN zimes)   Special proteins that speed up a chemical reaction in the body.

Epidemiological (ep i dee mee o LOJ i kuh l)   The branch of medicine dealing with the incidence, distribution, and control of disease in a population. It also involves the prevalence of disease in large populations, in addition to detection of the source and cause of epidemics of infectious disease.

Epiglottis (ep i GLOT is)   Lid-like structure over the glottis that prevents food and liquids from entering the trachea when swallowing occurs.

Epiphyseal plate (eh pi FIZ ee uhl)   A thin layer of cartilage located at the ends of a long bone where new bone forms.

Epithelial cells (ep i THEE lee al)   Form cellular sheets that cover surfaces, both inside and outside the body. Epithelial cells are closely packed, take on different shapes, and strongly stick to each other.

Eponym (EP uh nim)   In medical terms, a medical diagnosis or procedure named for the person who discovered it.

E-prescribing   The use of electronic software to communicate with pharmacies and send prescribing information. It takes the place of writing a prescription by hand and giving it to a patient; most new or refill prescriptions can be submitted electronically, cutting down on fraud and errors.

Equilibrium (ee kwuh LIB ree uh m)   A state of rest or balance due to the equal action of opposing forces.

Ergonomics (ur guh NOM iks)   An applied science concerned with designing and arranging things needed to do your job, in an efficient and safe way.

Erythema (er ee THEE mah)   Redness.

Erythropoietin (eh rith roh POY eh tin)   A hormone that is produced by the kidney cells and travels to the bone marrow to stimulate red blood cell formation.

Essential hypertension   Elevated blood pressure of unknown cause that develops for no apparent reason; sometimes called *primary hypertension.*

Established patient   A patient who has been treated previously by the healthcare provider within the past 3 years.

Esterase   Any enzyme that breaks down esters (a type of organic molecule) into alcohols and acids.

Ethernet (EE thuhr net)   A communication system for connecting several computers so information can be shared.

Ethics (ETH iks)   Rules of conduct that differentiate between acceptable and unacceptable behavior.

Ethics committee   A group composed of members from a variety of disciplines that analyzes ethical issues.

Etiology (ee tee OL uh jee)   The study of the causes or origin of diseases.

Eukaryote (yoo KAR ee oht)   Any single-celled or multicellular organism that has genetic material contained in a distinct membrane-bound nucleus.

Euphoria (yoo FOR ee ah)   An exaggerated sense of physical and mental well-being.

Evacuated   To create a vacuum in a tube, flask, or reaction vessel.

Evert (ih VURT)   To turn the eyelid inside out; this typically is done by the provider to inspect the area for foreign bodies.

Evidence-based practice   Healthcare practice that incorporates the most current and valid research results, thus providing the best patient care.

Evoked potential test   A nerve response test that uses electrodes, which are placed on the scalp to measure brain reaction to a stimulus.

Exclusivity (ik SKLOO siv i tee)   The sole right to market an approved medication granted by the FDA; may occur with the patent.

Excoriated (ik SKOHR ee ay ted)   To strip off or remove the skin from an area.

Excoriation (ik skawr ee EY shun n)   Inflammation and irritation of the skin.

Executor   An individual assigned to make financial decisions about the estate of a deceased patient.

Exocrine   A glandular secretion released through a duct.

Expediency (ik SPEE dee uh n see)   A means of achieving a particular end, as in a situation requiring urgency or caution.

Expert witnesses   People who are educated and knowledgeable in the area of concern; they testify in court and provide an expert opinion on the topic of concern.

Expiration   Exhaling; movement of waste gases from the alveoli into the atmosphere.

Explanation of benefits (EOB)   A document sent by the insurance company to the provider and the patient explaining the allowed charge amount, the amount reimbursed for services, and the patient's financial responsibilities.

Expletive (EK sple tiv)   An oath or swear word.

Explicit (ik SPLIS it)   Fully and clearly expressed or demonstrated; leaving nothing merely implied.

Exploitation (EKS ploi TAY shuhn)   The act of using another person for one's own advantage.

Extension   The process of stretching out; increasing the angle of a joint.

Extraction   A process by which a specific substance is separated from a group or solution.

Exudates (EKS yoo dayts)   Fluids with high concentrations of protein and cellular debris that have escaped from the blood vessels and have been deposited in tissues or on tissue surfaces.

Fact witnesses   People who observed the situation and testify in court about the facts of the case.

Familial (fuh MIL yuh l)   Occurring in or affecting members of a family more than would be expected by chance.

Fascia (FASH ee ah)   A tough fibrous covering of the muscles.

Fatigue (fuh TEEG)   Extreme tiredness.

Fatty acids   Result when fats are broken down; used by the body for energy and tissue development.

Febrile (FEB ruh l)   Pertaining to an elevated body temperature.

Federal Reserve Bank   The central bank of the United States. The Federal Reserve system consists of a seven-member Board of Governors with headquarters in Washington, D.C., and 12 Federal Reserve banks in major cities throughout the country.

Fee schedule   A list of fixed fees for services.

Filamentous (fil ah MEN tuhs)   Composed of or containing filaments or strands of a substance.

File   A collection of data or program records stored as a unit with a specific name.

Filtrate   Fluid and substances that are filtered out of the blood in the Bowman capsule.

Fire doors   Doors made of fire-resistant materials; they close manually or automatically during a fire to prevent it from spreading.

Fissure (fish EHR)   A groove that divides an organ into lobes or parts.

Flexion   The process of decreasing the angle of a joint.

Fluctuate (FLUHK choo ayt)   To shift back and forth.

Follicle-stimulating hormone (FSH)   A glycoprotein hormone secreted by the anterior pituitary gland. It stimulates the growth of ovum (eggs) in the ovary and induces the formation of sperm in the testis.

Follow-up appointment   An appointment type used when a patient needs to see the provider after a condition should have been resolved or to monitor an ongoing condition, such as hypertension. Also known as a *recheck appointment*.

Fontanel / Fontanelle (fon tah NEL)   A soft membranous gap between the incompletely formed cranial bones of an infant; also called a *soft spot*.

Foramen magnum   A large opening in the base of the skull. It forms a passageway for the spinal cord.

Forensic (fuh REN sik)   Scientific tests or techniques used regarding the detection of crime.

Form   Physical characteristics of a medication (e.g., tablet, suspension).

Fornix (FORE niks)   A recess in the upper part of the vagina caused by protrusion of the cervix into the vaginal wall.

Fortified   Nutrients are added to a food; these nutrients were never originally in the food.

Fungus   Any of a diverse group of single-celled organisms, including mushrooms, molds, mildew, smuts, rusts, and yeasts and classified in the kingdom Fungi.

Gait   The manner or style of walking.

Gamete (GAM eet)   A mature sexual reproductive cell; spermatozoa or ovum.

Gatekeeper   The primary care provider, who is in charge of a patient's treatment. Additional treatment, such as referrals to a specialist, must be approved by the gatekeeper.

Germicides (JUR muh sahyds)   Agents that destroy pathogenic organisms.

Germline cells   Sperm and egg cells.

G-force   A force acting on an object because of gravity. Example: A centrifuge spins and exerts g-force.

Girth   The measurement around something; when referring to mail, it is the measurement around the middle of the package that is being shipped.

Glasgow coma scale   A scale used to measure the level of consciousness and severity of a head injury; ability to open eyes, verbal response, and motor response are evaluated and the score is determined based on the findings.

Glaucoma (glou KOE mah)   Increase in the fluid pressure in the eye; can lead to blindness if not treated.

Global services   For purposes of CPT coding, medical services and procedures performed for the patient before, during, and after a surgical procedure, that are included with the assigned CPT code.

Glomerulonephritis (gloh mer yuh loh neh FRIE tis)   Kidney disease affecting the capillaries of the nephron (glomeruli); characterized by albuminuria, edema, and hypertension.

Glucagon (GLOO kah gon)   A hormone produced by the alpha cells in the pancreas; works on the liver to release glycogen and thereby prevent dangerously low blood glucose levels.

Glucose   A simple sugar that is absorbed by the intestines and found in the blood. Used by cells for energy and the extra is stored in the liver as glycogen.

Glycolysis (glie KOL uh sis)   The chemical breakdown of carbohydrates (glucose) by enzymes, with the release of energy.

Gonads (GOH nad)   Organs that produce sex cells in both males and females.

Gonioscopy (goh nee AH skuh pee)   Used to diagnose glaucoma and to inspect ocular movement.

Graduated cylinder   A narrow, tube-shaped container marked with horizontal lines to represent units of measurement. Used to precisely measure the volume of liquids.

Graft   Tissue taken from one area in the body and inserted into another area or person.

Gray matter   Nerve tissue that lacks the insulation that causes a white appearance to other nerves; thus, gray matter looks gray.

Gross   The amount earned before any tax deductions or adjustments.

Guarantor   The person legally responsible for the entire bill. This is usually the patient, but in the case of a minor it would be a parent or legal guardian.

Gyri (JIE rie)   Folds or convolutions on the surface of the cerebral hemisphere, which increase the gray matter surface area.

Gyrus (JIE rus) is the singular form.

Hackers   Unauthorized users who attempt to break into computer networks.

Hallucination (hah LOO si nae shun)   A sensory experience (e.g., a smell, sound, sight, touch, or taste) involving something that is not present.

Harassment (hah RAS ment)   The continued, unwanted, and annoying actions done to another person.

Hardware   Physical equipment of the computer system required for communication and data processing functions.

Headset   A set of headphones with a microphone attached, used especially in telephone communication.

Health insurance exchange   An online marketplace where you can compare and buy individual health insurance plans. State health insurance exchanges were established as part of the Affordable Care Act.

Hematologist (hee mah TOL uh jist)   A person trained in the nature, function, and diseases of the blood and blood-forming organs. Can be a physician, trained laboratory personnel, or researcher.

Hematoma (hee mah TOH mah)   An abnormal buildup of blood in an organ or tissue of the body, caused by a leak or cut in a blood vessel.

Hematopoiesis (hee mah toh poh EE sis)   The formation of the blood cells and platelets.

Hemoconcentration (hee muh kon sun TRAY shun)   A condition in which the concentration of blood cells is increased in proportion to the plasma.

Hemoglobin (HEE muh gloh bin)   The oxygen-carrying pigment of red blood cells.

Hemolysis (hee MOL i sis)   The breakdown of red blood cells with the release of hemoglobin.

Hemolytic uremic syndrome   Kidney disorder that can occur after a digestive infection with E. coli, shigella, or salmonella; red blood cells are destroyed and block the kidneys' filtering system causing acute kidney failure.

Hemolyzed (HEE muh liezd)   A blood sample in which the red blood cells have ruptured.

Hemophilia (hee moh FEE lee ah)   A group of inherited blood disorders characterized by a deficiency of one of the factors necessary for the coagulation of blood.

Hemostasis (hee muh STAY sis)   The stoppage of bleeding.

Hereditary (huh RED i ter ee)   Passed from parents to offspring through the genes.

Hertz (hurts)   The unit of measurement used in hearing examinations; a wave frequency equal to one cycle per second.

Hierarchy (HIE er ar kee)   Things arranged in order and rank.

Hippocampus (Hip oh KAM pus)   A ridge in the floor of the lateral ventricle; composed of gray matter. Involved with the limbic system and with creating and filing new memories.

Histology (hi STOL oh jee)   The study of tissues.

History of present illness (HPI)   Describes the signs and symptoms from the time of onset.

Holistic (hoh LIS tik)   A form of healing that considers the whole person (i.e., body, mind, spirit, and emotions) in individual treatment plans.

Homeostasis (hoh mee oh STAY sis)   The internal environment of the body that is compatible with life. A steady state that is created by all the body systems working together to provide a consistent and unvarying internal environment.

Hormone   A chemical substance produced in an endocrine gland and transported in the blood to a specific tissue, where it applies a specific effect.

Hospice (HOS pis)   A concept of care that involves health professionals and volunteers who provide medical, psychological, and spiritual support to terminally ill patients and their loved ones.

Human resources file (HR file)   Contains all documents related to an individual's employment.

Hydrocephalus (HIE droe sef ah luhs)   An abnormal accumulation of cerebrospinal fluid that causes enlargement of the skull and compression of the brain.

Hydronephrosis (hie droh nuh FROH sis)   A backup of urine that causes dilation of the ureters and calyces; can increase pressure on the nephron units.

Hyperlipidemia (hie per lip i DEE mee ah)   An elevated level of lipids in the blood.

Hyperplasia (hahy per PLEY zhee uh)   Enlargement due to an abnormal multiplication of cells.

Hyperpnea (hie PURP nee ah)   Excessively deep breathing.

Hyperventilation (hie pur ven ti LAY shun)   Abnormally increased breathing.

Hypoalbuminemia (hie poh al byoo mi NEE mee ah)   A decreased level of albumin (protein) in the blood.

Hypotension   Blood pressure that is below normal (systolic pressure below 90 mm Hg and diastolic pressure below 50 mm Hg).

Hysterectomy   Surgical removal of the uterus and cervix. The ovaries and fallopian tubes may also be removed.

Idiopathic (id ee uh PATH ik)   Of unknown cause.

Immunoglobulins (im yuh noh GLOB yuh linz)   A group of related proteins that functions as antibodies. Are found in plasma and other body fluids.

Immunosuppressant   A drug used to suppress the immune system.

Impending   A term used in the diagnosis of a condition that can be imminently threatening. For example, a patient showing signs of prediabetes may in the near future develop diabetes; therefore, in this case, diabetes is an impending condition.

Impervious (im PUR vee uhs)   Not permitting penetration.

In vitro   Latin term meaning "in glass" and commonly known as "in the laboratory."

Inanimate   Not animate; lifeless.

Incentive   Things that incite or spur to action; rewards or reasons for performing a task.

Incidence (IN si duh ns)   How often something happens or occurs.

Incompetence (in KOM pi tahns)   The state of being incompetent or lacking the ability to manage personal affairs due to mental deficiency; an appointed guardian or conservator manages the person's affairs.

Incompetent valves   Valves do not close completely and blood leaks backward into the prior chamber; also called "leaky valves."

Inconspicuous (in kuh n SPIK yoo uh s)   Not noticeable or prominent.

Incurred   To come into or acquire.

Indicator (IN di kay ter)   An important point or group of statistical values that, when evaluated, indicates the quality of care provided in a healthcare facility.

Indigent (IN di juh nt)   Poor, needy, impoverished.

Infarction (in FARK shuhn)   Tissue death.

Infection   Invasion of body tissues by microorganisms, which then multiply and damage tissues.

Infectious agents   Living and nonliving pathogens—such as bacteria, viruses, fungi, protozoa, parasite, helminths, and prions—that can cause disease. Also called infectious particles.

Inflammation (in fluh MAY shuhn)   A pathology characterized by redness, swelling, pain, tenderness, heat, and disturbed function of an area of the body. Especially a reaction of tissues to injury.

Ingested   Taken, as food, into the body.

Inhalant (in HAY lunt)   Any substance that can be breathed into the lungs.

Inhalation (in huh LEY shuh n)   The act of breathing in.

Initiative (i NISH eh tive)   The ability to determine what needs to be done and take action on your own.

Injunction (in JUNGK shuhn)   A court order by which an individual or institution is required to perform or restrain from performing a certain act.

INR   INR stands for International Normalized Ratio and is also called a prothrombin time (PT). It is used to test the effectiveness of blood thinning medication.

Insidious (in DID ee uh s)   Proceeding in a gradual, subtle way, but with harmful effects.

Inspiration   Inhaling; movement of O_2 from the atmosphere into the alveoli.

Insufficiency   Also called regurgitation or incompetence; the valve does not close completely, and blood leaks backward across the valve into the prior chamber.

Insulin (IN suh lin)   A hormone produced by the beta cells in the pancreas; moves glucose into the cells so it can be used for energy.

Intact (in TAKT)   Complete or whole. Not altered; unbroken.

Intangible (in TAN juh buhl)   Something of value that cannot be touched physically.

Integral (IN ti gruhl)   Essential; being an indispensable part of a whole.

Integrity (in TEG ri tee)   Adhering to ethical standards or right conduct standards.

Intercellular   Located between cells.

Intercom   A two-way communication system with a microphone and loudspeaker at each station; often a feature of business telephones.

Intercostal muscles (in tur KOS tul)   Muscles located between the ribs that help with quiet respiration.

Interest   Money the bank pays the account holder, on the amount in his or her account, for using the money in the account.

Interface   An interconnection between systems.

Interferon (in ter FEER on)   A protein formed when a cell is exposed to a virus; the protein blocks viral action on the cell and protects against viral invasion.

Intermittent   Occurring in intervals.

Intermittent pulse   A pulse in which beats occasionally are skipped.

Interoperability (in ter OP er uh bi li tee)   The ability to work with other systems.

Interpersonal skills   The ability to communicate and interact with others; sometimes referred to as "soft skills."

Interrogatory (IN tah rog ah TOOR ee)   Written or oral questions that must be answered under oath.

Interstitial (in ter STISH ul)   Between the cells.

Interstitial cells   Testosterone-secreting cells of testes that are found in the spaces between the seminiferous tubules.

Interval   Space of time between events.

Intracellular pathogens   A disease causing organism that is within or inside of a cell.

Intranet (IN trah net)   A private computer network that can only be accessed by authorized people (e.g., employees of the facility, that owns the network).

Intraosseous (in tra OS ee us)   Within bone; route for delivery of fluids and medications through a needle inserted into the marrow of certain bones (e.g., humerus, tibia, and femur).

Intravenous (IV)   Through a vein; fluids and medications can be given through a vein.

Intrinsic factor   Secreted by the parietal cells of the stomach; necessary for the absorption of vitamin B_{12} to prevent pernicious anemia.

Inventory   A detailed list of equipment and supplies owned and stored; the process of counting the supplies in stock.

Invoices   Billing statements that list the amount owed for goods or services purchased.

Ion (AHY ons)   An electrically charged atom, or the smallest component of an element.

Jargon (JAHR guhn)   The vocabulary of a particular profession as opposed to common, everyday terms.

Jaundice   A yellow discoloration of the skin and mucous membranes caused by deposits of bile.

Job boards   Websites where employers post jobs, that can be used by job seekers to identify open positions.

Judicious (joo DISH uhs)   Using good judgment; being discreet, sensible.

Labia majora (LAY bee ah muh JOR ah)   The larger external folds of skin surrounding the opening of the vagina.

Labia minora (LAY bee ah min NOR uh)   The smaller inner folds of skin surrounding the opening of the vagina.

Lacrimation (lak ri MAY shun)   The secretion or discharge of tears.

Laparoscopy (lap ar AW scoh pee)   A procedure used to visually examine the abdomen.

Larynx (LAR inks)   The voice box.

Lateral flow immunoassay (im yuh noh AH say)   A laboratory or clinical technique that uses the specific binding between an antigen and antibody to identify and quantify a substance in a sample. The sample in this technique moves in a sideways motion, usually on an absorbent paper.

Learning style   The way an individual perceives and processes information to learn new material.

Lethargy (LETH er jee)   The state of being drowsy and dull, listless and unenergetic.

Leukoderma   Lack of skin pigmentation, especially in patches.

Liability (LIE ah bil i tee)   The state of being liable or responsible for something.

Liable   Legally responsible or obligated.

Libido   Sexual drive or instinct.

Licensure (LIE sen shur)   A mandatory process established by state law that ensures a person has met the legal standards for practicing an occupation in that state.

Ligaments (LIH gah ments)   Supportive connective tissue that connects bones at a joint.

Limbic system   Consists of several structures including the amygdala, hippocampus, and hypothalamus; plays an important role with behavior, memories, and emotions.

Litigious (LI ti jehs)   Prone to lawsuits.

Local   Affecting the area where applied.

Locum tenens **(LOE kuhm TEE nenz)**   Latin for "to substitute for"; physicians or advance practice professionals who temporarily contracted to provide healthcare services when a facility has a vacancy, vacation, or a leave of absence.

Loop electrosurgical excision procedure (LEEP)   After an anesthetic has been injected into the cervix, a high-frequency electrical current running through a wire is used to remove abnormal tissue from both the cervix and the endocervical canal.

Lumen   The cavity, channel, or open space within a tube or tubular organ.

Lumpectomy (luhm PEK tuh mee)   Removal of the breast tumor and a small amount of the surrounding tissue.

Luteinizing hormone (LH)   A hormone produced by the anterior pituitary gland. LH stimulates ovulation and the development of the corpus luteum in females and the production of testosterone in males.

Lymph (limf)   A clear, yellowish fluid containing white blood cells in a liquid similar to plasma. The fluid comes from the tissues of the body and is moved through the lymphatic vessels and the bloodstream.

Lymphedema (lin fuh DEE mah)   A condition in which extra lymph fluid builds up in tissues and causes swelling. It may occur in an arm or leg if lymph vessels are blocked, damaged, or removed by surgery.

Lymphocyte (LIM fuh site)   A type of white blood cell that has a large, round nucleus that is surrounded by a thin layer of agranular cytoplasm.

Lymphostasis (lim foh STAY sis)   Obstruction or interruption of normal lymph flow.

Macromolecules   Molecules needed for metabolism: carbohydrates, lipids, proteins, amino acids, and nucleic acids.

Macrophages (MACK roh fay jehs)   Large white blood cells that live in the tissues. They engulf foreign particles, microorganisms, and cell debris.

Malaise (ma LAYZ)   A condition of general bodily weakness or discomfort, often marking the onset of a disease.

Malignant   A cell with uncontrolled growth that spreads rapidly, with the potential for serious harm.

Malpractice (mal PRAK tis)   A type of negligence in which a licensed professional fails to provide the standard of care, causing harm to a person.

Malware (MAL wair)   Malicious software designed to damage or disrupt a system (e.g., a virus).

Mania (MAY nee ah)   Abnormally elated mental state; the person may have feelings of euphoria, lack of inhibitions, sleeplessness, talkativeness, risk-taking behaviors, and irritability.

Manipulation   Movement or exercise of a body part by means of an externally applied force.

Mastectomy (ma STEK tuh mee)   Removal of the entire breast.

Matrix (MAY triks)   The environment where something is created or takes shape. A base on which to build.

Mature minor   A person under the age of adulthood who demonstrates the maturity to make a personal healthcare decision and can give informed consent for treatment.

Meatus   A body opening or passage, especially the external opening of a structure.

Media (ME de ah)   Types of communication (e.g., social media sites); with computers, the term refers to data storage devices.

Mediastinum (mee dee AH sti nuhm)   The space in the thoracic cavity that lies between the lungs, containing the heart, trachea, and esophagus.

Mediation (MEE dee ae shuhn)   The process of facilitating conflicting parties to make an agreement, settlement, or compromise.

Medical necessity   Services or supplies (CPT and HCPCS codes) that are used to treat the patient's diagnosis (ICD codes) meet the accepted standard of medical practice.

Medically necessary   Accepted healthcare services that are appropriate for the evaluation and treatment of a disease, condition, illness or injury and are consistent with the applicable standard of care.

Medulla oblongata (muh DUHL uh ob lawng GAH tuh)   The lowest part of the brain, continuous with the top of the spinal cord.

Melanocytes (meh LAN oh sites)   Cells of the stratum germinativum that produce a brownish pigment called melanin. Melanin gives us our skin color.

Ménière's (mayn YAIRZ) disease   Chronic disease of the inner ear causing recurrent episodes of vertigo, progressive sensorineural hearing loss, and tinnitus.

Meninges (meh NIN jeez)   A protective covering around the brain and spinal cord.

Meningocele (meh NING goh seel)   The protrusion of the meninges through an opening in the spinal column or skull.

Menometrorrhagia (men oh meh troh RAH zsa)   Excessive menstrual flow and uterine bleeding other than that caused by menstruation.

Menorrhagia (men or RAH zsa)   Abnormally heavy menstrual flow or prolonged menstrual periods.

Mentor   A steady employee whom a new staff member can approach with questions and concerns.

Metabolic   relating to or resulting from metabolism (the chemical process where cells produce the substances and energy needed to sustain life).

Metabolism (me TAB oh lizm)   The chemical process that occurs within a living organism in order to maintain life.

Metabolites (meh TAB uh lites)   By-products of drug metabolism.

Microbiome (mie kroh BIE ohm)   The total collection of microorganisms, and their genetic material, present on or in the human body or a specific site in the human body.

Microcephaly (mie kroh SEF ul ee)   Abnormally small head associated with incomplete brain development.

Microcuvette (MIE kroh koo vet)   A small plastic or glass tube designed to hold samples for laboratory tests that detect light or color changes.

Microorganism   Any living organism—such as bacterium, protozoan, fungi, parasite, or helminth—of microscopic size. Some definitions include viruses, which are not alive.

Minor   One who has not reached adulthood; usually age 18 or 21, depending on the jurisdiction.

Miotic (my OT ik)   Any substance or medication that causes constriction of the pupil.

Mitosis (mie TOH sis)   A cell division process by which two daughter cells are formed from one parent cell; each daughter has a complete copy of parent's chromosomes.

Mnemonic (ni MON ik)   A learning device (e.g., an image, a rhyme, or a figure of speech) that a person uses to help him or her remember information.

Mock   Simulated; intended for imitation or practice.

Modalities (moe DAL i tees)   A therapeutic treatment for a disorder.

Modem (MOE duhm)   Peripheral computer hardware that connects to the router to provide internet access to the network or computer.

Mold   Growth of tiny fungi forming on a substance. Often looks downy or furry and is associated with dampness or decay.

Molecule   The simplest unit of a chemical compound that can exist, consisting of two or more atoms held together with chemical bonds.

Monocytes (MON uh site)   Agranulocyte that engulfs foreign particles, microorganisms, and cell debris.

Monotone (MON uh tohn)   A succession of syllables, words, or sentences spoken in an unvaried key or pitch.

Morale (muh RAL)   Emotional or mental condition with respect to cheerfulness or confidence.

Morals (MORE ahls)   Internal principles that distinguish between right and wrong.

Morbidity (more BID i tee)   The rate of a disease in a population.

Mortality (more TAL i tee)   The relative frequency of deaths in a specific population.

Mucous membrane   A mucus-producing membrane that lines tracts and structures of the body (e.g., GI tract, respiratory tract); also called *mucosa*.

Multiple-line telephone system   A business telephone system that allows for more than one telephone line.

Murmur   An abnormal sound heard during auscultation of the heart that may or may not have a pathologic origin; it is associated with valve disease or a congenital heart defect.

Myelin sheath (MIE uh lin sheeth)   A protective insulation that covers the axons and help with the transmission of nerve impulses.

Myocardium (mie oh KAR dee um)   The middle layer and the thickest layer of the heart; composed of cardiac muscles.

Myoglobin   Type of hemoglobin found in the muscle.

Myxedema (mick suh DEE mah)   Advanced hypothyroidism in adulthood.

Nasal wash   Also called a nasal aspirate. A syringe is used to gently squirt a small amount of sterile saline into the nose, and the resulting fluid is collected into a cup (for a wash). Or after the saline is squirted into the nose, gentle suction is applied (for the aspirate).

Nasopharyngeal (nae zoe fah RIN jee ahl) airway (NPA)   A soft flexible tube that is inserted in the nose and provides a patent airway; also known as a *nasal trumpet*.

National Provider Identifier (NPI)   An identifier assigned by the Centers for Medicare and Medicaid Services (CMS) that classifies the healthcare provider by license and medical specialties.

Necrosis (neh KROH sis)   Tissue death.

Negative feedback   An output or response that affects the input of a system.

Neglect   Failure to provide proper attention or care to another person.

Negligence (NEG li juhns)   Failure to act as a reasonably prudent person would under similar circumstances; such conduct falls below the standards of behavior established by law for the protection of others against unreasonable risk of harm.

Negotiable (ni GOH shee uh buhl) instrument   A document guaranteeing payment of a specific amount of money to the payer named on the document.

Nephrectomy   Surgical removal of a kidney.

Nephrotoxic   Damaging or destructive to the kidneys.

Net   The amount someone is paid after taxes and other deductions have been subtracted.

Neuralgia (noo RAL jah)   Sharp, spasm-like pain in a nerve or along the course of one or more nerves.

Neuropathy (nu ROP a thee)   A nervous system disorder of the peripheral nerves that causes discomfort, numbness, and weakness, especially in the extremities.

Neurotransmitter   A chemical that helps a nerve cell communicate with another nerve cell or muscle.

Nocturia (nok TOOR ee uh)   Frequent urination at night.

Nodules (NOJ ool)   Small lumps, lesions, or swellings that are felt when the skin is palpated.

Nomenclature (NOH muh n kley cher)   A system of names or terms, used in science and art to categorize items.

Nondecodable terms   Words used in healthcare whose definitions must be memorized without the benefit of word parts.

Noninvasive procedures   Procedures that do not penetrate human tissue.

Nonorganic (nahn or GAN ik)   Not having an organic or physiologic cause; a disorder that does not have a cause that can be found in the body.

Nonverbal communication   A type of communication that occurs through body language and expressive behaviors rather than with verbal or written words.

Normal flora   Microorganisms (mostly bacteria and yeast) that live on or in the body. Normal microscopic residents of the body.

No-show   Failure of a patient to keep an appointment without advance notice.

Nosocomial (nos uh KOH mee uh l)   Also known as Healthcare-Acquired Infections (HAI).

Nosocomial (nos uh KOH mee ul) infections   Infections acquired in a healthcare setting.

Notice of Privacy Practices (NPP)   A written document describing the healthcare facility's privacy practices. The patient must be provided with the NPP and sign an acknowledgment of receipt.

Nucleus   A specialized organelle of a cell that is encased in a membrane and directs growth, metabolism, and reproduction of the cell.

Numeric filing   The filing of records, correspondence, or cards by number.

Objective information   Data obtained through physical examination, laboratory and diagnostic testing, and by measurable information.

Obliteration (uh blit uh REY shun)   To remove or destroy all traces of; do away with; destroy completely.

Obturator (OB tuh rayt oar)   A metal rod with a smooth, rounded tip that is placed in hollow instruments to reduce injury to body tissues during insertion.

Occlude   To close, shut, or stop up.

Occult   Hidden or unseen.

Oncologist   A specially trained doctor who diagnoses and treats cancer.

Online insurance web portal   An online service provided by various insurance companies for providers to look up a patient's insurance benefits, eligibility, claims status, and explanation of benefits.

Oocyte (OO eh site)   An immature ovum (egg).

Oophorectomy (oo for ECK tuh mee)   Surgical removal of the ovaries.

Opaque (oh PAYK)   Not transparent; cloudy or murky.

Operating system   System software; it acts as the computer's software administrator by managing, integrating, and controlling application software and hardware. Windows is an example.

Organelles   Structures inside of a cell that perform specific functions.

Orientation   Awareness of one's environment, with reference to people, place, and time.

Orifice (ORE ih fis)   The vaginal opening.

Orthopnea (or THOP nee ah)   Condition of difficult breathing unless in an upright position.

Orthostatic (postural) hypotension   A temporary fall in blood pressure that occurs when a person rapidly changes from a recumbent position to a standing position.

Ossicles (OS i kahls)   The three small bones of the middle ear (malleus, incus, and stapes) that transmit sound vibrations from the eardrum to the inner ear.

Osteoblasts (OS tee oh blasts)   Bone-forming cells.

Osteoclasts (OS tee oh clasts)   Bone cells that break down bone.

Osteoporosis (os tee oh puh ROH sis)   Abnormal thinning of the bone structure causing bones to become brittle and weak.

Otitis externa   Inflammation or infection of the external auditory canal; commonly called *swimmer's ear.*

Otosclerosis (oh tuh skli ROH sis)   The ossicles of the middle ear (malleolus, incus, and stapes) become fused and act as a single unit instead of individual bones.

Ototoxic (oh tuh TOK sik)   A medicine or substance capable of damaging cranial nerve VIII or the organs of hearing and balance.

Out guides   Sturdy cardboard or plastic file-sized cards used to replace a folder temporarily removed from the filing space.

Output device   Computer hardware that displays the processed data from the computer (e.g., monitors and printers).

Overlearn   To learn or memorize beyond the point of proficiency or immediate recall.

Ovulation (OV yuh ley shun)   The release of the ovum from the ovarian follicle.

Packing slip   A document that accompanies purchased merchandise and shows what is in the box or package.

Palpation (PAL pey shuh n)   The use of touch during the physical examination to assess the size, consistency, and location of certain body parts.

Parameters (puh RAM it ers)   Rules that control how something should be done; guidelines or boundaries.

Paranasal sinuses (pair uh NAY zul SIE nus suhs)   Hollow, air-filled cavities in the skull and facial bones. They lighten the weight of the skull and increase the tone, or resonance, of speech.

Paraphrasing   Rewording a statement to check the meaning and interpretation; also shows you are listening and understanding the speaker.

Parasitic   Pertaining to a parasite (an organism that lives on or in another organism, known as the host). Benefits from the host; the host does not benefit from the parasite.

Parenteral (pa REN ter uh l)   Taken into the body by any route other than the digestive tract (e.g., subcutaneous, intravenous, or intramuscular administration).

Participating provider   A physician or other healthcare provider who enters into a contract with a specific insurance company or program and by doing so agrees to abide by certain rules and regulations set forth by that particular third-party payer.

Patency (PAT en see)   Open condition of a body cavity or canal.

Patent (PAT nt)   A grant from the government that gives a creator (or manufacturer) of an invention the sole right to produce, use, and sell the product for a set period of time.

Patent (PAY tent)   Open.

Pathogen   A disease-causing organism.

Pathogenic   Capable of producing disease.

Pathologic   Caused by or involving disease.

Pathologist (pah THOL uh jist)   A physician specially trained in the nature and cause of disease.

Pathology   Study of disease.

Patient abandonment   A form of medical malpractice, also called *negligent termination*; the provider ends the provider-patient relationship without reasonable or adequate notification.

Patient account   A running balance of all financial transactions for a specific patient.

Patient navigator   A person who identifies patients' needs and barriers; then assists by coordinating care and identifying community and healthcare resources to meet the needs. May also be called *care coordinator.*

Patient portal   A secure online website that gives patients 24-hour access to personal health information using a username and password.

Pegboard system   A manual bookkeeping system that uses a day sheet to record all financial transactions for the date of service and maintains patient account balances by using physical ledger cards.

Perceiving (per SEEV ing)   How an individual looks at information and sees it as real.

Percutaneous   Puncture through the skin.

Performance measurement   The regular collection of data to assess whether the correct processes are being performed and desired results are being achieved.

Perineal (pair ih NEE uhl)   Pertaining to the area between the vaginal opening and the rectum (perineum).

Perineum (pair ih NEE um)   The area between the opening of the vagina and the anus.

Peripheral (puh RIF er uhl)   Refers to an area outside of or away from an organ or structure.

Peripheral neuropathy (puh RIF er uh l noo ROP uh thee)   A problem with the function of the nerves outside the spinal cord; symptoms include weakness, burning pain, and loss of reflexes; a frequent complication of diabetes mellitus.

Peristalsis (payr i STAHL sis)   Wave-like movement from alternating contraction and relaxation of a tubular structure (e.g., intestine), which propels the content forward.

Peritoneum (per i tuh NEE um)   A serous membrane lining of the abdominal cavity, which folds inward to enclose the viscera (internal organs).

Peritubular capillaries (PER i too bu lar)   Blood capillaries surrounding the proximal and distal convoluted tubules in the kidneys.

Permeability (PUR mee ah bil i tee)   A quality or characteristic of a material that allows another substance to pass through it.

Permeable (PUR mee uh buhl)   Allowing for penetration.

Personal ethics   An individual's code of conduct.

Petechiae (pi TEEK kee uh)   Very small, round hemorrhage in the skin or mucous membrane.

Peyer patches (PEYH urh PACH ehs)   Small masses of lymphatic tissue found mostly in the ileum of the small intestine. They are an important part of the immune system, because they monitor intestinal bacteria populations and prevent the growth of pathogenic bacteria in the intestines.

Pharyngitis   Inflammation or infection of the pharynx, usually causing the symptoms of a sore throat.

Phenylalanine   An essential amino acid found in milk, eggs, and other foods.

Phenylketonuria (PKU)   A deficiency in the enzyme phenylalanine hydroxylase, which is responsible for converting phenylalanine into tyrosine.

Photophobia (foh toh FOH bee ah)   Extreme sensitivity to light.

Photosensitivity (FOE toe sen si TIV i tee)   Increase in the reactivity of the skin to sunlight or ultraviolet radiation.

Physiologic   Consistent with the normal function of the body.

Pineal gland   A small organ in the brain that secretes melatonin, a hormone that regulates the sleep/awake cycle.

Pipet (pie PET)   A slender tube attached to or including a bulb, for transferring or measuring small amounts of a liquid, often used in a laboratory.

Pitch   The depth of a tone or sound; a distinctive quality of sound.

Pitting edema   Excessive fluid in the intercellular spaces in the tissue; when external pressure (e.g., socks, finger pressure) is relieved, a depression is seen in the tissue.

Plaintiff (PLAIN tif)   An individual or party who brings a lawsuit to court.

Plaque   Sticky substance made of mucus, food particles, and bacteria that builds up on the exposed part of the tooth.

Plasma (PLAZ muh)   The liquid portion of a whole blood sample that has not clotted due to an anticoagulant. Liquid portion of blood that contains clotting factors. Liquid portion of the blood found in the body.

Plume   Vapor, smoke, and particle debris produced by laser procedures.

Pneumonia   Inflammation of the lungs with congestion of the air sacs (alveoli). Can be caused by a bacterium or virus.

Pocket face mask   A device used to deliver a rescue breath.

Point-of-care   Something designed to be used at or near where the patient is seen; point-of-care tools and apps are resources for the provider to use when working directly with the patient.

Poised (poizd)   Having a composed and self-assured manner.

Policy   A written agreement between two parties, in which one party (the insurance company) agrees to pay another party (the patient) if certain specified circumstances occur.

Polycythemia (pol ee sie THEE mee ah)   A disorder characterized by an abnormal increase in the number of red blood cells in the blood.

Pores   Tiny openings in the surface of the skin that allow gases, liquids, or microscopic particles to pass.

Portrait orientation   The most common layout for a printed page; the height of the paper is greater than its width.

Postherpetic neuralgia (noo RAL juh)   Nerve pain that occurs after a shingles outbreak and may become chronic.

Practice management software   A type of software that allows the user to enter demographic information, schedule appointments, maintain lists of insurance payers, perform billing tasks, and generate reports.

Preauthorization   A process required by some insurance carriers in which the provider obtains permission to perform certain procedures or services.

Precedence (PRES i dehns)   Followed first.

Precedent (PRES i dent)   A prior court decision that serves as a model for similar legal cases in the future.

Precertification   The process of determining if a procedure or service is covered by the insurance plan and what the reimbursement is for that procedure or service.

Precipitate (pri SIP i tate)   Solid particles that settle out of a liquid.

Preeclampsia (pree ih KLAMP see ah)   A form of toxemia during pregnancy, characterized by high blood pressure, fluid retention, and protein in the urine. May progress to eclampsia.

Preexisting condition   A health problem that was present before new health insurance coverage started.

Prefixes   Word parts that appear at the beginning of some terms.

Premium   The amount paid or to be paid by the policyholder for coverage under the contract, usually in periodic installments.

Privacy filters   Devices attached to the monitor that allow visualization of the screen contents only if the user is directly in front of the screen; also called *monitor filters* or *privacy screens*.

Privileged communication   Communication that cannot be disclosed without authorization of the person involved; includes provider-patient and lawyer-client communications.

Processing (prah CES ing)   How an individual internalizes new information and makes it his or her own.

Product   The number obtained by multiplying two or more numbers together.

Productive cough   A cough that produces phlegm or mucus.

Proficiency (pruh FISH uh n see)   Skilled as a result of training or practice.

Prognosis (prog NOH sis)   The likely outcome of a disease, including the chance of recovery.

Progress notes   Documentation in the paper health record that can be used to track the patient's condition and progress.

Prokaryote (proh KAR ee ote)   Any organism that is made up of at least one cell and has genetic material that is not enclosed in a nucleus. Bacteria are prokaryotes, primitive organisms.

Proofread   To read and mark corrections.

Protected health information (PHI)   Individually identifiable health information stored or transmitted by covered entities or business associates. Includes verbal, paper, or electronic information.

Protozoa (pro tuh ZOH ah)   Single-celled organisms that are the most primitive form of animal life. Most are microscopic. Examples are amoebas, ciliates, flagellates, and sporozoans.

Provider network   An approved list of physicians, hospitals, and other providers.

Provider Web portal   A secure online website that gives contracted providers a single point of access to insurance companies. This allows the provider to determine patient eligibility and deductible status, submit preauthorizations/precertifications, and check the status of claims.

Provider   An individual or company that provides medical care and services to a patient or the public.

Provisional diagnosis (dahy uh g NOH sis)   A temporary diagnosis made before all test results have been received.

Pruritus (proo RYE tuss)   Itching.

Psoriasis (sah RIE ah sis)   A usually chronic, recurrent skin disease marked with bright red patches covered with silvery scales.

Psychiatrists   Medical doctors who have been specially trained to diagnose and treat patients with mental, emotional, and behavioral conditions.

Psychotherapy (sie KOE ther ah pee)   The treatment of behavioral health disorders through the use of psychological techniques, which encourage communication of conflicts and insights into the person's problems. The goals of this treatment include symptoms relief, changes in behavior leading to improved social and vocational function, and personality growth.

Psychotherapy notes   Patient-provider details from private, group or family therapy, including what the patient stated and the provider's analysis of the statements and situation.

Puberty (PYOO bur tee)   The stage of life in which males and females become functionally capable of sexual reproduction.

Pulmonary hypertension   High blood pressure that affects the pulmonary system (pulmonary arteries and the right side of the heart).

Pulse deficit   A condition in which the radial pulse is less than the apical pulse; it may indicate a peripheral vascular abnormality.

Pulse pressure   The difference between the systolic and diastolic blood pressures (30 to 50 mm Hg is considered normal).

Purchase order number   A unique number assigned by the ordering facility that allows the facility to track or reference the order.

Pure culture   The growth of only one microorganism in a culture, or on a nutrient surface.

Purulent (PYOOR yoo lent)   Pus like.

Pyemia (pahy EE mee uh)   The presence of pus-forming organisms in the blood.

Pyrexia (pahy REK see uh)   A febrile condition or fever.

Qualified Medicare Beneficiaries (QMBs)   Low-income Medicare patients who qualify for Medicaid for their secondary insurance.

Quality control   A process to ensure the reliability of test results, often using manufactured samples with known values.

Quantitative   Describes a test result that is expressed as a number, usually with units of measure attached to numeric values.

Rales [rayls]   An abnormal lung sound heard on auscultation, characterized by discontinuous bubbling noises.

Rapport (ra PORE)   A relationship of harmony and accord between the patient and the healthcare professional.

Reagent (re-AY-jent)   A substance for use in a chemical reaction.

Rebound pain   Pain felt when the pressure on the abdomen is released.

Receptors   Structures or sites on or in a cell that bind with substances such as hormones, antigens, or drugs.

Recommended dietary allowance (RDA)   Average daily level of food intake needed to meet the nutrient requirements of most healthy people.

Reconciliation (rek uh n sill ee EY shuh n)   To bring into agreement.

Reconciling   Comparing a document with another document to ensure that they are consistent.

Reconstituted (ree KON sti toot ed)   A dried substance (powder) that has been restored to a fluid form, so it can be injected.

Recovery position   A position on the person's side that helps to keep the airway open and clear.

Referral   An order from a primary care provider for the patient to see a specialist or to get certain medical services.

Referral laboratory   A laboratory that performs testing for another laboratory. Testing varies from high-volume routine testing to low-volume unique or unusual testing. Also called reference,

diagnostic, or commercial testing laboratories. Often privately owned.

Reflecting   Putting words to the patient's emotional reaction, which acknowledges the person's feelings.

Reflection (ree FLEK shun)   The process of thinking about new information so as to create new ways of learning.

Reflexes   Movements or processes caused by a reflex response; reflex is an automatic response that doesn't require thought.

Registered dietitian (die eh TISH an)   A credentialed healthcare professional who is trained in nutrition and is able to apply the information to the dietary needs of healthy and ill patients.

Regular diet   The food and drink a person typically consumes when there are no dietary limitations.

Reimbursement (ree im BURS ment)   To make repayment for an expense or a loss incurred.

Relapse   The recurrence of the symptoms of a disease after apparent recovery.

Release of information   A form completed by the patient that authorizes the medical office to release medical records to the insurance company for health insurance reimbursement.

Reliable (ree LIE ah bul)   Dependable, able to be trusted.

Remission   The partial or complete disappearance of the clinical and subjective characteristics of a chronic or malignant disease.

Renal ischemia   A blood flow deficiency to the kidney(s).

Renal threshold   The blood level of a substance, above which the kidneys fail to reabsorb it, so the substance will appear in the urine.

Replication   The production of exact copies of a complex molecule, such as DNA.

***Res ipsa loquitur* (RASE ipsah low kwah tuhr)**   Latin term meaning "the thing speaks for itself." A legal concept under which the plaintiff's burden to prove malpractice is minimal, since the jury can clearly understand the details of the injury. For example, a surgical instrument was left in the body during surgery.

***Res judicata* (RASE JOO di kah tah)**   Latin for "a thing decided." Once a case has been decided by the court, it cannot be litigated again.

Resection   Surgical removal of all or part of an organ.

Resident   A physician who has graduated from medical school and is finishing specialized clinical training.

Residual urine   Urine that remains in the bladder after micturition or urination.

Resource-based relative value system (RBRVS)   A system used to determine how much providers should be paid for services provided. It is used by Medicare and many other health insurance companies.

Respect   Showing consideration or appreciation for another person.

Respiratory arrest   Stoppage of breathing.

***Respondeat superior* (re SPON dee at soo PIR ee ahr)**   Latin for "let the master answer"; a legal doctrine by which the employer/provider is legally responsible for the wrongful actions or lack of actions of employees if done within the scope of employment.

Restock   The process of replacing the supplies that were used.

Retaliation (ree tal ee A shuhn)   Getting back at others for something they did to you.

Retention   A term referring to actions taken by management to keep good employees.

Retention schedule A method or plan for retaining or keeping health records and for their movement from active to inactive to closed.

Retractions (re TRAK shuns) The sucking in of tissues between the intercostal spaces and neck due to respiratory distress; classic sign of severe asthma.

Retribution (reh trih BYOU shuhn) Punishment inflicted on someone as vengeance for a wrong or criminal act; the act of taking revenge.

Revenue (REV eh noo) Money collected for providing a product or service.

Reverse chronologic order The most recent item is on top and the oldest item is last.

Review of systems A list of questions related to each organ system, designed to uncover potential disease processes.

Rhonchi (RON kye) An abnormal rumbling sound heard on auscultation, caused by airways blocked by secretions or muscle contractions.

Route The means by which a drug enters the body.

Rugae (ROO gah) Folds in the wall of the organ; when organ (e.g., stomach, bladder, uterus) fills or needs to expand, the rugae unfold.

Salary A fixed compensation periodically paid to a person for regular work.

Salpingo-oophorectomy (sal ping goh oh of or EK toh mee) Surgical removal of the fallopian tube and ovary.

Sanitize The process of cleaning equipment and instruments with detergent and water in order to remove debris and reduce the number of microorganisms.

Sclera (SKLEER uh) The white part of the eye that forms the orbit.

Scope of practice Range of responsibilities and practice guidelines that determine the boundaries within which a healthcare worker practices.

Scored tablet A tablet with a groove on the surface, used for splitting it in half.

Screen A system for examining and separating into different groups; in the healthcare facility, it means determining the severity of illness that patients experience and prioritizing appointments based on that severity.

Screening A system for examining and separating into different groups; in the healthcare facility, it means determining the severity of illness that patients experience, and prioritizing appointments based on that severity.

Seborrhea (seb uh REE ah) An excessive discharge of sebum from the sebaceous glands, forming greasy scales or crusty areas on the body.

Secondary storage devices Media (e.g., jump drive, flash drive, hard drive) capable of permanently storing data until they are replaced or deleted by the user.

Security risk analysis Identification of potential threats of computer network breaches, for which action plans for corrective actions are instituted.

Sediment An insoluble material that settles to the bottom of a liquid specimen and to the bottom of centrifuged sample.

Senescent (si NES ent) cell An old or aging cell that can no longer divide and reproduce.

Sensorineural (sen suh ree NOOR uhl) Involving the sensory nerves, especially as they affect hearing.

Sentinel node biopsy Removal of a limited number of lymph nodes to determine if the cancer has spread to the lymph nodes.

Septicemia (sep tih SEE mee ah) A systemic infection involving pathologic microbes in the blood as a result of an infection that has spread from elsewhere in the body.

Sequela (si KWEL uh) (singular), Sequelae (plural) An abnormal condition resulting from a previous disease.

Serous (SEER uhs) A thin, watery serum-like drainage.

Serum (SEER um) The liquid portion of a clotted blood specimen. It no longer contains active clotting agents.

Shaken baby syndrome Condition resulting from internal head injuries that occur when a baby or young child is violently shook.

Sharps Medical term for devices with sharp points or edges that can puncture or cut skin. Examples include needles, scalpels, or broken glass.

Sickle cell anemia An inherited anemia characterized by crescent-shaped red blood cells (RBCs). This causes RBCS to block capillaries, reducing the oxygen supply to the cells.

Side effects Unpleasant effects of a drug in addition to the desired or therapeutic effect.

Signs Objective findings determined by a clinician, such as a fever, hypertension, or rash.

Sinus arrhythmia An irregular heartbeat that originates in the sinoatrial node (pacemaker).

Skill set A person's abilities, skills, or expertise in an area.

Small claims court A special court established to handle small claims or debts without the services of lawyers.

Software A set of electronic instructions to operate and perform different computer tasks.

Solvent A liquid that is able to dissolve other substances.

Solvent (SOL vuhnt) Able to pay all debts.

Somatic cells (soe MAT ik) Nonreproductive cells; they do not include sperm and egg cells.

Speakerphone A telephone with a loudspeaker and a microphone; it can be used without having to pick up and hold the handset.

Special report Additional medical documentation required to confirm the need for the use of unlisted, unusual, or newly adopted medical procedures code.

Specificity (spes i FIS i tee) The quality or state of being specific.

Speed dialing A telephone function in which a selected stored number can be dialed by pressing only one key.

Spermatozoa (spur mat ah ZOH ah) (singular, spermatozoon) Mature male reproductive cells.

Sphincter (SFINGK ter) A circular muscle that either constricts and closes the opening or relaxes and allows substances to pass through the opening.

Spina bifida (SPY nah BIF id dah) A condition in which the spinal column has an abnormal opening that allows protrusion of the meninges and/or the spinal column.

Spore A thick-walled, dormant form of bacteria that is very resistant to disinfection measures.

Stains Reagents or dyes used to prepare specimens for microscopic examination.

Standard of care The level and type of care an ordinary, prudent healthcare professional with the same training and experience in a similar practice would have provided under a similar situation.

Standard operating procedures (SOP)   A set of step-by-step instructions to help employees carry out routine operations efficiently, with high quality, and uniformity of performance.

Standard Precautions   A set of infection control practices used to prevent the transmission of diseases that can be acquired by contact with blood, body fluids, nonintact skin, and mucous membranes.

STAT   The medical abbreviation for the Latin term *statum,* meaning immediately; at this moment.

Static (STAT ik) equilibrium   Relating to balance when moving in a straight line.

Stem cells   Undifferentiated cells that can become specialized cells in the body.

Stenosis (sten OH sis)   Occurs when the heart valve flaps are stiff or fused together, thus narrowing the valve.

Sterile (STER il)   Free of all microorganisms, pathogenic and nonpathogenic.

Sterilize   The process of removing all microorganisms.

Stertorous (STUR ter uhs)   Heavy, as related to snoring.

Stoma (STOH mah)   A temporary or permanent surgically created opening used for drainage (i.e., urine, stool).

Strata   Naturally or artificially formed layers of material, usually multiple layers.

Stretch receptor   A sensory nerve ending that responds to a stretch stimulus.

Stylus (STI luhs)   A metal probe that is inserted into or passed through a catheter, needle, or tube used for clearing purposes or to facilitate passage into a body orifice.

Stylus (STI luhs)   A pen-shaped device with a variety of tips that is used on touchscreens to write, draw, or input commands.

Subcultured   Occurs when an organism (a bacterium) has been cultivated again on a new nutrient surface.

Subjective information   Data or information obtained from the patient, including the patient's feelings, perceptions, and concerns; obtained through interview or questions.

Subpoena (suh PEE nuh)   A court order requiring a person to appear in court at a specific time to testify in a legal case.

Subpoena duces tecum **(suh PEE nuh DOO seez TEE kuhm)**   A legal document commanding a person to bring a piece of evidence (such as the plaintiff's health record) to court.

Subsequent (SUHB si kwuhnt)   Occurring later or after.

Suction (SUHK shun)   The production of a partial vacuum by the removal of air in order to force fluid into a vacant space.

Suffixes   Word parts that appear at the end of some terms.

Sulci (SUL sie)   Grooves or depressions on the surface of the brain between the gyri. **Sulcus (SUL kus)** is the singular form.

Summarizing   Allowing the listener to recap and review what was said.

Supernatant   The clear liquid above the sediment in a centrifuged urine specimen.

Suppurative (SUHP yuh ray tiv)   Characterized by the formation and/or discharge of pus.

Surfactant (sur FACK tunt)   A mixture of protein and fats that lines the alveoli and prevents the tissues from sticking together and collapsing during exhalation.

Surrogate (SUR ah git)   A person who acts on behalf of another person or takes the place of another person. Examples include a surrogate mother or a healthcare agent.

Symmetry (SIM ih tree)   Similarity in size, form, and arrangement of parts on opposite sides of the body.

Symptoms   Subjective complaints reported by the patient, such as pain or nausea.

Synapse (SIN aps)   A point of communication between two cells.

Syncope (SING kuh pee)   Fainting; a brief lapse in consciousness.

Synthesis (SIN theh sis)   Formation of a chemical compound from simpler compounds or elements.

Syringe (suh RINJ)   A device with a slender barrel and needle used to withdraw blood from a vein or artery.

Systemic   Affecting the entire body.

Tachycardia (tak i KAHR dee uh)   A rapid but regular heart rate; one that exceeds 100 beats per minute.

Tachypnea (tack ip NEE ah)   Rapid, shallow breathing.

Tactful   The quality of having a sense of what to do or say to maintain good relations with others or to prevent offense.

Target cells   A cell selectively affected by a specific agent, such as a drug, hormone, or virus.

Target tissue   The destination, or intended tissue in the nervous impulse (e.g., a muscle).

Telehealth   Refers to remote clinical services and nonclinical services, such as provider training, meetings, and continuing education.

Telemedicine (TEL i med i sin)   The use of telecommunication technology to provide healthcare services to patients at a distance; it is usually used in rural communities.

Template (TEM plit)   A document or file that has a preset format; used as a starting point when composing something and saves from recreating it each time it is used.

Tendons   (TEN duns) Connective tissue that attaches muscles to bone.

Termination letters   Documents sent to patients explaining that the provider is ending the physician-patient relationship and the patients need to see other providers.

Testis (TES tis) (plural, testes)   The male gonad, also called a **testicle (TESS tick kul)**.

Testosterone (tess TOSS tur rohn)   Male sex hormone produced by the interstitial cells in the testes.

Thalamus (THAL uh muh s)   The middle part of the brain through which sensory impulses pass to reach the cerebral cortex.

Therapeutic range   Is reached when the blood concentration of a medication is high enough for the therapeutic effect to occur.

Third-party administrator (TPA)   An organization that processes claims and provides administrative services for another organization. Often used by self-funded plans.

Thoracentesis (thor ah sen TEE sis)   Aspiration of a fluid from the pleural cavity.

Thready   Describes a pulse that is thin and feeble.

Thrombus (THRAHM bus)   A blood clot that blocks the flow of blood.

Tickler file   A chronologic file used as a reminder that something must be dealt with on a certain date.

Tinea (TIN ee uh)   Any fungal skin disease that results in scaling, itching, and inflammation; examples include ringworm and athlete's foot.

Tinnitus (TIN it uh s)   A noise sensation of ringing heard in one or both ears.

Tissue culture   The technique or process of keeping tissue alive and growing in a culture medium.

Tonometer (toh NOM i ter)   An instrument used to measure intraocular pressure.

Tort   A civil wrongdoing that causes harm to a person or property; excludes breach of contract.

Tortfeasor (TORTE fee zahr)   The individual or entity who committed the tort, either intentionally or as a result of negligence.

Toxicity   The harmful and deadly effect of a medication that can develop due to the buildup of medication or by-products in the body.

Toxicology (tok si KOL oh jee)   The study and science dealing with the effects, antidotes, and detection of poisons or drugs.

Toxins   Substances created by microorganisms, plants, or animals and poisonous to humans.

Tract   A system of tissues (e.g., neuronal axons) and/or organs (e.g., intestines) that function together.

Transcription (tran SKRIP shuh n)   To make a written copy of dictated material.

Transient (TRAN zee uhnt)   Not lasting, enduring or permanent; transitory.

Transillumination (trans i LOO muh ney shun)   Inspection of a cavity or organ by passing light through its walls.

Transitional epithelium   A type of cell found in the lining of hollow organs. It has the ability to stretch with the contraction and distention of the organ.

Transmission   The passage or spread disease.

Transport medium   A medium used to keep an organism alive during transport to the laboratory.

Trauma (TRAW muh)   A physical injury or wound caused by external force or violence.

Triage (tree AHZH)   The process of sorting patients to determine medical need and the priority of care.

Triaging flow map   A written flow map to make triage decisions; based on answers to questions, the person moves through the map until a triage decision is made.

Tripod position   The standing position when using crutches; crutch tips are 4 to 6 inches to the side and front of each foot.

Trustee   The coordinator of financial resources assigned by the court during a bankruptcy case.

Turgor (TUR ger)   Referring to normal skin tension; the resistance of the skin to being grasped between the fingers and released. Turgor decreases with dehydration and increases with edema.

Unipolar   Having one pole or electrical charge.

Unit dose packaging   A packaging method for drugs; holds a specified quantity of medication in a single-use container (e.g., syringe, blister pack).

Unsecured debt   Debt that is not guaranteed by something of value; credit card debt is the most common type of unsecured debt.

Urgent   An acute situation that requires immediate attention but is not life-threatening.

Urostomy (yoo ROS te mee)   A surgically created opening on the abdominal wall used to drain urine.

Urticaria (ur ti KAYR ee ah)   Hives.

Utilization management   A decision-making process used by managed care organizations to manage healthcare costs. It involves case-by-case assessments of the appropriateness of care.

Vascular (VAS kyuh ler)   Having vessels that conduct or circulate liquids (blood).

Vascular access   A surgical procedure that creates a vein to remove and return blood during the hemodialysis procedure.

Vasoconstriction (vas oh kuhn STRIK shuhn)   Contraction of muscles, causing the narrowing of the inside tube of the vessel.

Vectors   Animals or insects (e.g., ticks, rodents, mosquitos) that transmit a pathogen.

Vendors   Companies that sell supplies, equipment, or services to other companies or individuals.

Venule (VEN yuhl)   A very small vein.

Verification of eligibility   The process of confirming health insurance coverage for the patient.

Vertebrae (VUR teh bray)   A series of small, irregular-shaped bones that form the spine. Each vertebra has several projections, joint surfaces, areas for muscle attachment, and a hole where the spinal cord passes.

Vertigo (VER ti goe)   Dizziness; an abnormal sensation of movement when there is none.

Vested   Granted or endowed with a particular authority, right, or property; to have a special interest in.

Viability (vie a BIL ih tee)   The ability to live.

Vigilance (VIJ uh lahns)   Keen watchfulness to detect danger.

Viscosity (vi SKOS I tee)   Resistance to flow; the thicker the liquid, the higher the viscosity.

Voice mail   An electronic system that allows messages from telephone callers to be recorded and stored.

Waiting period   The length of time a patient waits for disability insurance to pay after the date of injury.

Water deprivation test   A test to measure the amount and concentration of urine produced when water is withheld from a patient for a period of time.

Wet mount   A glass slide that holds a specimen suspended in a drop of liquid for microscopic examination.

Wheezing (WHEE zeeng)   Whistling sound made during breathing.

Whistleblower   A person (usually an employee) who reports a violation of the law within the organization. The person reports the information to the public or to a person in authority.

Workplace emergencies   Unforeseen situations that threaten employees and visitors; can disrupt services provided.

Yeast   Any various single-celled fungi, which reproduce by budding and are able to ferment sugars.

Zone   A region or geographic area used for shipping.

ABBREVIATIONS

%TBSA percent of total burn surface area

°C Celsius

(D)HHS Department of Health and Human Services

°F Fahrenheit

s̄ without

3D three-dimensional

A

A&Ox3 alert and oriented to person, place, and time

A/P accounts payable

A/R accounts receivable

A1c glycated hemoglobin

a͞a of each (used in prescriptions)

AAA abdominal aortic aneurysm

AAFP American Academy of Family Physicians

AAMA American Association of Medical Assistants

AAMT American Association for Medical Transcriptions

AAP American Academy of Pediatrics

AAT alpha-1 antitrypsin

ABG arterial blood gas

ABHES Accrediting Bureau of Health Education Schools

ac before meals

ACA The Affordable Care Act

ACE inhibitor angiotensin converting enzyme inhibitor

Ach acetylcholine

ACL anterior cruciate ligament

ACTH adrenocorticotropic hormone

AD Alzheimer's disease

ad lib as desired

ADA Americans with Disabilities Act

ADA American Diabetes Association

ADAAA Americans with Disabilities Act Amendment Act

ADF scanner automatic document feeder

ADH antidiuretic hormone

ADHD attention deficit hyperactivity disorder

ADLs activities of daily living

ADR alternative dispute resolution

AED automated external defibrillator

AFB acid-fast bacilli

AFP alpha-fetoprotein

AgNO₃ silver nitrate

AHA American Heart Association

AHRQ Agency for Healthcare Research and Quality

AIDS acquired immunodeficiency syndrome

AK astigmatic keratotomy

ALL acute lymphocytic leukemia

ALP alkaline phosphatase

ALS amyotrophic lateral sclerosis

ALT alanine aminotransferase

AM, a.m. morning

AMA American Medical Association

AML acute myeloid leukemia

AML acute myelogenous leukemia

AMT American Medical Technologists

ANA antinuclear antibody test

ANLL acute myeloid leukemia

ANS autonomic nervous system

Anti-CCP anti-cyclin citrullinated peptide

AP Anteroposterior

APAP acetaminophen

APRN advanced practice registered nurse

aq water

ARB angiotensin II receptor blocker

ART assistive reproductive technology

ARV antiretroviral

ASA aspirin

ASA The Anesthesia Society of America

ASCP American Society of Clinical Pathologists

ASD atrial septal defect

ASD autism spectrum disorder

AST aspartate aminotransferase

ATP adenosine triphosphate

AUD alcohol use disorder

AV atrioventricular

aV augmented voltage

B

BAP blood agar plate

BBB blood-brain barrier

BBPS bloodborne pathogen standard

BCG bacille Calmette-Guérin

BD Blu-Ray disc

beta-hCG beta human chorionic gonadotropin

bid twice a day

BLS basic life support

BMI body mass index

BMR basal metabolic rate

BOO bladder outlet obstruction

BP blood pressure

BPD bronchopulmonary dysplasia

BPH benign prostatic hyperplasia

BSE breast self-examination

BTL bottle

BUN blood urea nitrogen

BX box

C

c̄ with

C Celsius

c centi

C&S culture and sensitivity

Ca calcium

CAAHEP Commission on Accreditation of Allied Health Education Programs

CABG coronary artery bypass graft

CAD   coronary artery disease
CAM   complementary and alternative medicine
cap   capsule
CAP   College of American Pathologists
CAPTA   Child Abuse Prevention and Treatment Act
CARD   check, assign, reverse, define
CAT   computerized axial tomography
CBC   complete blood count
CBT   cognitive behavioral therapist
CC   chief complaint
cc   cubic centimeter
CCB   calcium channel blocker
CCK   cholecystokinin
CCMA   certified clinical medical assistant
CCMS   clean-catch midstream urine
CD   collecting duct
CD   compact disc
CD   conduct disorder
CDC   Centers for Disease Control and Prevention
CEJA   Council of Ethical and Judicial Affairs
CEU   continuing education unit
CF   cystic fibrosis
cfu   colony-forming units
CHAMPVA   Civilian Health and Medical Program of the Department of Veterans Affairs
CHD   coronary heart disease
CHF   congestive heart failure
CHIP   Children's Health Insurance Program
Chol   cholesterol
CIS   clinically isolated syndrome
CK   creatine kinase
CKD   chronic kidney disease
CK-MB   creatine kinase-MB
Cl   chloride
CLIA   Clinical Laboratory Improvement Amendments
CLL   chronic lymphocytic leukemia
CLS   clinical laboratory scientist
CLSI   Clinical and Laboratory Standards Institute
CLT   clinical laboratory technician/technologist
cm   centimeter
CMA   certified medical assistant
CML   chronic myeloid leukemia
CMLA   certified medical laboratory assistant
CMP   comprehensive metabolic profile
CMPs   civil monetary penalties
CMS   Centers for Medicare and Medicaid Services
CNM   certified nurse midwife
CNS   central nervous system
CNS   clinical nurse specialist
CO₂   carbon dioxide
COPD   chronic obstructive pulmonary disease
COW   computer on wheels
CoW   certificate of waiver
CPAP   continuous positive airway pressure
CPK   creatinine phosphokinase
CPOE   computerized provider/physician order entry
CPR   cardiopulmonary resuscitation

CPT   current procedural terminology
CPT   certified phlebotomy technician
CPU   central processing unit
Creat   creatinine
CRNA   certified registered nurse anesthetist
CRP   C-reactive protein
CS   case
CSF   cerebrospinal fluid
CSMT   color, sensation, motion, and temperature
CT   computed tomography
CTA   computerized tomography angiography
CVA   cerebrovascular accident
CVS   cyclic vomiting syndrome
CVS   chorionic villus sampling
CWP   coal workers' pneumoconiosis
CXR   chest x-ray
D
d   day
DAP test   draw-a-person test
DASH   Dietary Approaches to Stop Hypertension
DBS   deep brain stimulation
DBT   dialectical behavioral therapy
DC   Doctor of Chiropractic
DCT   distal (convoluted) tubule
DDL   digital data loggers
DEA   Drug Enforcement Agency
DEA   Drug Enforcement Administration
DHE   dihydroergotamine
DI   diabetes insipidus
DJD   degenerative joint disease
DKA   diabetic ketoacidosis
DM   diabetes mellitus
DMARDs   disease-modifying antirheumatic drugs
DNA   deoxyribonucleic acid
DNR   do not resuscitate
DO   Doctor of Osteopathy
DOB   date of birth
DRE   digital rectal exam
DSL modem   digital subscriber line modem
DSM   Diagnostic and Statistical Manual of Mental Disorders
DTP   diphtheria-tetanus-pertussis
DUB   dysfunctional uterine bleeding
DV   daily value
DVD   digital versatile/video disc
DVT   deep vein thrombosis
E
E/M   evaluation and management
EA   each
EAP   employee assistance program
EBV   Epstein-Barr virus
ECG   electrocardiogram
ECHO   echocardiography
ED   emergency department
ED   erectile dysfunction
EDTA   ethylenediaminetetraacetic acid
EEG   electroencephalography
EFT   electronic funds transfers

EGD   esophagogastroduodenoscopy

EHR   electronic health record

EIA   enzyme immunoassay

EIN   employer identification number

EKG   electrocardiogram

ELISA   enzyme-linked immunosorbent assay

EM   erythema migrans (sometimes called erythema chronicum migrans)

EMDR   eye movement desensitization and reprocessing

EMG   electromyography

EMG   emergency

EMG   electromyography

EMR   electronic medical record

EMS   emergency medical services

EMTs   emergency medical technicians

ENT   ear, nose, throat

EOB   explanation of benefits

EOM   extraocular movement

EP   established patient

EPA   Environmental Protection Agency

EPDS   Edinburgh Postnatal Depression Scale

ePHI   electronic protected health information

EPO   exclusive provider organization

EPS   electrophysiology study

EPSDT   early and periodic screening, diagnosis, and treatment

ER   endoplasmic reticulum

ERCP   endoscopic retrograde cholangiopancreatography

ERV   expiratory reserve volume

ESR   erythrocyte sedimentation rate

ESRD   end-stage renal disease

ESU   electrosurgical unit

ESWL   extracorporeal shock wave lithotripsy

ET   endotracheal

F

F   Fahrenheit

FAERS   FDA adverse event reporting system

FBG   fasting blood glucose

FBS   fasting blood sugar

FDA   Food and Drug Administration

Fe   iron

FECA   Federal Employees Compensation Act

FEV₁   forced expiratory volume in 1 second

FH   family history

FIT   fecal Immunochemical test

fl oz   fluid ounce

FOB   fecal occult blood

FOBT   fecal occult blood test

FRC   functional residual capacity

FSH   follicle-stimulating hormone

FTC   Federal Trade Commission

FUO   fever of unknown origin

FVC   forced vital capacity

G

g   gram

G   gauge

GAD   generalized anxiety disorder

GAS   general adaptation syndrome

GAS   group A streptococcus

GB   gigabyte

GER   gastroesophageal reflux

GERD   gastroesophageal reflux disease

gFOBT   guaiac fecal occult blood test

GGT   gamma glutamyl transferase

GH   growth hormone

GHRL   ghrelin

GI   gastrointestinal

GI   glycemic index

GINA   Genetic Information Nondiscrimination Act

GMOs   genetically modified organisms

GNB   Gram negative bacilli

GN-RH   gonadotropin-releasing hormone

GPC   Gram positive cocci

GPOs   group purchasing organizations

gr   grain

GTT   glucose tolerance test

gtt(s)   drop(s)

H

H&H   hemoglobin and hematocrit

H&P   history and physical

h, hr   hour

H⁺   hydrogen

HAV   hepatitis A virus

HAV   hepatitis A virus

HbA1C or A1C   glycosylated hemoglobin

HBV   hepatitis B virus

hCG   human chorionic gonadotropin

HCPCS   Healthcare Common Procedure Coding System

HCS   hazard communication standard

HCT   hematocrit

HCV   hepatitis C virus

HD   hoarding disorder

HD   Huntington's disease

HDD   hard disk drive

HDL   high-density lipoprotein

HDN   hemolytic disease of the newborn

HDV   hepatitis D virus

HEV   hepatitis E virus

Hgb   hemoglobin

HHR   hybrid health record

HHS   Department of Health and Human Services

HIDA scan   hepatobiliary iminodiacetic acid scan

HIE   health information exchange

HIPAA   Health Insurance Portability and Accountability Act

HITECH   Health Information Technology for Economic and Clinical Health Act

HIV   human immunodeficiency virus

HMIS   hazardous materials information system

HMO   health maintenance organization

HPI   health plan identifier

HPI   history of present illness

HPV   human papilloma virus

HRT   hormone replacement therapy

HSV   herpes simplex virus

HSV-1   herpes simplex virus-1

HZV   herpes zoster vaccine

I

I&D   incision and drainage
IAPS   International Academy of Phlebotomy Sciences
IBD   inflammatory bowel disease
IBS   irritable bowel syndrome
IC   inspiratory capacity
IC   interstitial cystitis
ICD   implantable cardioverter defibrillator
ICD   International Classification of Disease
ICD-10-CM   *International Classification of Diseases, 10th revision, Clinical Modification*
ICP   intracranial pressure
ICS   intercostal space
ID   identification
ID   intradermal
IDS   integrated delivery system
IE   infective endocarditis
IFA   immunofluorescence assay
iFOBT   immunochemical fecal occult blood test
Ig   Immunoglobulin
IM   intramuscular
INR   international normalized ratio
IOL   intraocular lens
IPA   independent practice associations
IPAA   ileal pouch-anal anastomosis
IPT   interpersonal psychotherapy
IQ   intelligent quotient
IRV   inspiratory reserve volume
ISCLT   International Society of Clinical Laboratory Technology
ISP   internet service provider
IT   information technology
ITP   idiopathic thrombocytopenic purpura
IUD   intrauterine device
IUFD   intrauterine fetal death
IUI   intrauterine insemination
IV   intravenous
IVIg   intravenous immunoglobulin
IVP   intravenous pyelogram

J

JA   juvenile arthritis
JIA   juvenile idiopathic arthritis

K

K   potassium
k   kilo
KB   kilobyte
kg   kilogram
KOH   potassium hydroxide
KS   Kaposi sarcoma

L

L   liter
LA   left arm
LAGB   laparoscopic adjustable gastric band
LAN   local area network
LASIK   laser-assisted in-situ keratomileusis
lb   pound
LCD monitor   liquid crystal display monitor
LCL   lateral collateral ligament

LCSW   licensed clinical social worker
LDH   lactate dehydrogenase
LDL   low-density lipoprotein
LED   light-emitting diodes
LEEP   loop electrosurgical excision procedure
LES   lower esophageal sphincter
LH   luteinizing hormone
LICSW   license independent clinical social worker
LL   left leg
LLQ   left lower quadrant
LP   lumbar puncture
LPN   licensed practical nurse
LSW   licensed social worker
LUQ   left upper quadrant

M

m   meter
m   milli
MA   medical assistant
MAC   Mycobacterium avium complex
MB   megabyte
mc   micro
mcg   microgram
MCH   mean cell hemoglobin
MCHC   mean cell ratio of hemoglobin and hematocrit
MCL   medial collateral ligament
MCO   managed care organization
MCV   mean cell volume
MD   doctor of medicine
MD   muscular dystrophy
MDI   metered-dose inhaler
med   medicine
mg   milligram
MGUS   monoclonal gammopathy of undetermined significance
mHealth   mobile health
MI   myocardial infarction
min   minute
mL   milliliter
mL   milliliter
MLA   medical laboratory assistant
MLT   medical laboratory technician
mm   millimeter
MMPI   Minnesota Multiphasic Personality Inventory
MMR   measles-mumps-rubella
MOM   milk of magnesia
Mono   infectious mononucleosis
MPM   medical practice management
MRA   magnetic resonance angiography
MRI   magnetic resonance imaging
MS   musculoskeletal system
MS   multiple sclerosis
MSAFP   maternal serum alpha-fetoprotein (test)
MT   medical technologist
MT-sDNA   multi-targeted stool DNA (test)
MUGA   multiple-gated acquisition
MVD   coronary microvascular disease
MVV   maximum voluntary ventilation
MY   myopia

N

Na   sodium

NAFLD   nonalcoholic fatty liver disease

NAS   nasal

NCA   National Certification Agency

NCA   National Certification Agency for Medical Laboratory Personnel

NCCI   National Corrective Coding Initiative

NCCT   National Center for Competency Testing

NCMA   National Certified Medical Assistant

NCQA   National Committee for Quality Assurance

NCV   nerve conduction velocity

NCVIA   The National Childhood Vaccine Injury Act

NDC   National Drug Code

NH$_3$ ammonia

NHA   National Healthcareer Association

NHI   National Institutes of Health

NIDA   National Institute on Drug Abuse

NIH   National Institutes of Health

NK   natural killer

NKA   no known allergies

NKDA   no known drug allergies

nm   nanometer

NMJ   neuromuscular junction

noc, noct   night

NOTA   National Organ Transplant Act

NP   new patient

NP   nurse practitioner

NPA   National Phlebotomy Association

NPI   national provider identifier

NPO   nothing by mouth

NPP   notice of privacy practices

NS   normal saline

NSAID   nonsteroidal anti-inflammatory drug

NTM   nontuberculous mycobacteria

NUCC   National Uniform Claim Committee

O

O&P   ova and parasite

O$_2$ oxygen

OA   osteoarthritis

OAE   otoacoustic emission

OB/GYN   obstetrics and gynecology

OCD   obsessive-compulsive disorder

OCP   oral contraceptive pills

OCR   Office for Civil Rights

OCR   optical character recognition

ODD   oppositional defiant disorder

OGTT   oral glucose tolerance test

OMT   osteopathic manipulative therapy

ONC   The Office of the National Coordinator for Health Information Technology

OPIM   other potentially infectious materials

OPTN   Organ Procurement and Transplant Network

ORIF   open reduction and internal fixation

OSA   obstructive sleep apnea

OSH Act   Occupational Safety and Health Act

OSHA   Occupational Safety and Health Administration

OT   oxytocin

OTC   over-the-counter (drugs)

OUI   operating under the influence

OWI   operating while intoxicated

oz   ounce

P

p̄   after

P   phosphorus

PA   physician assistant

PA   posteroanterior

PA-C   physician assistant-certified

PACs   premature atrial contractions

PAD   peripheral artery disease

PAP   Papanicolaou

PAR   participating provider

PBGs   physician buying groups

PBS   painful bladder syndrome

PBS   prune belly syndrome

pc   after meals

PC   personal computer

PCL   posterior cruciate ligament

PCMH   patient-centered medical home

PCP   primary care provider

PCT   proximal (convoluted) tubule

PCV13   13-valent pneumococcal conjugate vaccine

PD   Parkinson's disease

PDA   patent ductus arteriosus

PDD   pervasive developmental disorder

PDR   proliferative diabetic retinopathy

PDR   Physician Desk Reference

PDT   photodynamic therapy

PE   pulmonary embolism

PEP   post-exposure prophylaxis

PET   positron emission tomography

PFO   patent foramen ovale

PG   peptidoglycan

PH   pulmonary hypertension

PH   past history

PHI   protected health information

PHQ-2   Patient Health Questionnaire-2

PHQ-9   Patient Health Questionnaire-9

PHR   personal health record

PID   pelvic inflammatory disease

PIN   personal identification number

PKD   polycystic kidney disease

PKG   package

PKU   phenylketonuria

PLMD   periodic limb movement disorder

PM, p.m.   afternoon

PMDD   premenstrual dysphoric disorder

PMH   past medical history

PMN   polymorphonucleocyte

PMS   practice management software

PMS   premenstrual syndrome

PNL   percutaneous nephrolithotripsy

PNS   peripheral nervous system

PO   purchase order

po   oral (route)

po, PO   by mouth

POCT   point-of-care testing

POL   physician office laboratory

POLST   Physician Orders for Life-Sustaining Treatment

POR   problem-oriented record

POS   place of service

POS   point-of-sale

POTS   postural orthostatic tachycardia syndrome

PPD   purified protein derivative (tuberculin skin test)

PPD   prepaid

PPD   purified protein derivative

PPD   postpartum depression

PPE   personal protective equipment

PPI   proton pump inhibitor

PPM(P)   provider-performed microscopy (procedures)

PPMS   primary progressive multiple sclerosis

PPO   preferred provider organizations

PPP   2-hour postprandial urine specimen

PPSA   Physician Payments Sunshine Act

PPSV23 or PPSV   23-valent pneumococcal polysaccharide vaccine

PRL   prolactin

prn   as needed

PSA   prostate-specific antigen

PSDA   Patient Self-Determination Act

PSI   pounds per square inch

PST   plasma separator tubes

PT   prothrombin time

pt   pint

PT   protime

Pt, pt   patient

PTH   parathyroid hormone

PTSD   post-traumatic stress disorder

PTT   partial thromboplastin time

PTT   activated partial thromboplastin time

PTT   partial thromboplastin time

PUVA   psoralen plus ultraviolet A

PVCs   premature ventricular contractions

PYMT   payment

Q

q2h   every 2 hours

q3h   every 3 hours

q4h   every 4 hours

q6h   every 6 hours

q8h   every 8 hours

QA   quality assurance

qam   every morning

QC   quality control

QFT   QuantiFERON-TB

QFT-GIT   QuantiFERON-TB Gold In-Tube

qh   every hour

qid   four times a day

QMBs   qualified Medicare beneficiaries

qs   quantity sufficient

qt   quart

QTY   quantity

R

RA   remittance advice

RA   right arm

RA   rheumatoid arthritis

RAAS   renin-angiotensin aldosterone system

RAIU   radioactive iodine uptake

RAM   random access memory

RBC   red blood cell

RBRVS   resource-based relative value system

RCC   renal cell carcinoma

RDS   respiratory distress syndrome

REM   rapid eye movement

RF   rheumatoid factor

RICE   rest, ice, compression, and elevation

RL   right leg

RLQ   right lower quadrant

RLS   restless leg syndrome

RLS/WED   restless legs syndrome/Willis-Ekborn disease

RMA   registered medical assistant

RMT   registered medical technician

RN   registered Nurse

RNA   ribonucleic acid

ROM   range of motion

ROM   read-only memory

ROS   review of systems

RPM   remote patient monitoring

RPM   revolutions per minute

RRMS   relapsing-remitting multiple sclerosis

RSV   respiratory syncytial virus

RUQ   Right upper quadrant

RV   residual volume

RVG   relative value guide

RW   read/write

Rx   take

S

SA node   sinoatrial node

SA   sinoatrial

SAFER   Safety Assurance Factors for EHR Resilience

SAMHSA   Substance Abuse and Mental Health Services Administration

SBS   shaken baby syndrome

SDS   safety data sheet

SH   social history

SI   Système International

SIBO   small intestinal bacterial overgrowth

SIDS   sudden infant death syndrome

Sig   give the following directions

SL   semilunar

SL   sublingual

SLADH   syndrome of inappropriate antidiuretic hormone

SLE   systemic lupus erythematosus

SNRI   serotonin and norepinephrine reuptake inhibitor

SOB   shortness of breath

sol, soln   solution

SOP   standard operating procedure

SOR   source-oriented record

SPECT   single-photon emission computerized tomography

SPMS   secondary progressive multiple sclerosis
SpO$_2$ pulse oximetry
SR   systems review
SS   symptom severity (score)
SSD   solid-state disk or drive
SSN   Social Security number
SSRI   selective serotonin reuptake inhibitors
SST   serum separator tubes
STAT   immediately
STI   sexually transmitted infection
subcut   subcutaneous
T
T$_3$ triiodothyronine
T$_4$ thyroxine
tab(s)   tablet(s)
TAT   thematic apperception test
TB   terabyte
TB   tuberculosis
TB   total bilirubin
TBI   traumatic brain injury
Tbs, tbsp   tablespoon
TC   total cholesterol
Td   tetanus and diphtheria
Tdap   tetanus-diphtheria-pertussis (vaccine)
TEE   transesophageal echocardiogram
TENS   transcutaneous electrical nerve stimulation
TFT   thyroid function test
TIA   transient ischemic attack
TIBC   total iron-binding capacity
tid   three times a day
TILA   Truth in Lending Act
TIM   topical immunomodulators
tinct   tincture
TLC   total lung capacity
TM   tympanic membrane
TNF   tumor-necrosis factor
TNM   tumor, number of lymph nodes, metastasized
TOF   tetralogy of Fallot
TP   total protein
TPA   third-party administrator
TPR   temperature, pulse, respirations
TRH   thyrotropin-releasing hormone
Trig   triglyceride
TSE   testicular self-exam
TSE   testicular self-examination
TSH   thyroid-stimulating hormone
tsp   teaspoon
T-Spot   T-SPOT *TB* (test)

TST   tuberculin skin test
TTE   transthoracic echocardiogram
TTM   transtelephonic monitor
TURP   transurethral resection of the prostate
TV   tidal volume
U
UA   urinalysis or uric acid
UAGA   Uniform Anatomical Gift Act
UCD or UCHD   usual childhood diseases
UCR   usual, customary, and reasonable
UDDA   Uniform Determination of Death Act
UES   upper esophageal sphincter
UGI   upper gastrointestinal
ung   ointment
UNHS   universal newborn hearing screening test
UPJ   ureteropelvic junction
US   ultrasound
USAN   U.S. adopted name (council)
USB   universal serial bus
USDA   U.S. Department of Agriculture
USMLE   U.S. Medical Licensing Examination
USP-NP   U.S. Pharmacopeia and the National Formulary
USPS   U.S. Postal Service
UTI   urinary tract infection
UV   ultraviolet
V
VA   visual acuity
VAERS   vaccine adverse event reporting system
VC   vital capacity
V-fib   ventricular fibrillation
VICP   Vaccine Injury Compensation Program
VIS   vaccine information statement
VLDL   very low-density lipids
VO   verbal order
VQ scan   lung ventilation/perfusion scan
VS   vital signs
VSD   ventricular septal defect
V-tach   ventricular tachycardia
VUR   vesicoureteral reflux
W
WAIS   Wechsler Adult Intelligent Scale
WAN   wide area network
WBC   white blood cell
WHO   World Health Organization
WOW   workstation on wheels
WPI   widespread pain index (score)
X
x   times

INDEX

Page numbers followed by "*f*" indicate figures, "*t*" indicate tables, and "*b*" indicate boxes.

948 INDEX

Harvey, William, 14t
hCG. see Human chorionic gonadotropin
HDL. see High-density lipoprotein
Head, examination of, 157–158
Headaches, 538–539
Health belief model, 174, 174t, 174b
Health information
   exchanges, 42
   management professional, 17t–18t
   meaningful use and, 36, 36b
   technologic terms in, 35–36
Health Information Technology for
   Economic and Clinical Health
   (HITECH) Act, 36
Health Insurance Portability and
   Accountability Act (HIPAA), 35, 137
Health maintenance and wellness
   additional screenings, 184–186
   one-time screenings, 183–184
   patient coaching and, 181–186
   regular screening, 183, 183b, 184t
   self-exams, 181–183
Health records, 29–54
   accurate, importance of, 31
   contents of, 31–35
   corrections and alterations to, 44, 46f
   electronic. see Electronic health records
   filing equipment, 45–47
   filing methods, 49–50
   filing supplies, 47–48
      divider guides, 47
      file folders, 47–48
      labels, 48
      out guides, 47, 47f
   health information exchanges and, 42
   indexing rules, 48–49, 48t
   information, releasing of, 40–42, 41f
   legal and ethical issues in, 51
   medical assistant's role in, 35
   objective information, 34–35
   organization of, 42
      problem-oriented, 42, 43f
      source-oriented, 42
   ownership of, 35, 35b
   paper
      documenting, 44
      management system for, 45–48
   patient-centered care and, 51–52
   retention and destruction of, 40
   stickers for, 32
   subjective information, 31–34
      chief complaint, 34
      family history, 32, 33f
      past health history, 32, 33f
      personal demographics, 31
      social history, 33, 33f
   types of, 30–31, 31b
Health-related correspondence, 50
Healthcare facility. see also Medical office
   types of, 16–21
Healthcare rules, when writing numbers,
   344
Healthcare team, 21–22, 21f
   medical assistant and, 1–28
Hearing, aging and, 737, 737b
Hearing loss, 410, 411f
Heart
   anatomy of, 599–601, 601f–602f, 601b
   chambers of, 266, 266f, 599, 601f
   conduction system of, 267–268, 267f,
      268b, 606–607, 607b
   disease, 266
   disorders of, 609–617
      congestive heart failure, 611–612,
         612f
      legal and ethical issues in, 623
      patient coaching on, 623
      risk factors for, 614t
   structure, 266–267, 266f
   valves of, 599–601
   wall, 267
Heart block, 278
Heart-healthy diet, 208, 208t
Heart valve diseases, 613, 613f
Heartbeat, 601

Heat applications, for orthopedic
   conditions, 511f, 512, 512t,
   522b–523b
Hegar uterine dilators, 225t
Height measurement, 120–121, 121f,
   121b–122b, 133f–134f, 133b–134b
Helicobacter pylori bacterium, 473
Helicobacter pylori testing, 877
Helminths, 77t
   pathogenic, 870–871, 871f
Hematemesis, 471
Hematocrit, 835–836, 836f, 836t, 836b
Hematologist, 834, 842–843
Hematology, 746, 835, 835t
Hematoma, 803
   during venipuncture, 814, 814t
Hematopoiesis, 491
Hematuria, 660, 777
Hemochromatosis, 478
Hemoconcentration, 803
Hemodialysis, 660–661, 661f
Hemogard, 805
Hemoglobin, 473, 834, 836–837, 837f,
   837t
   test, 856f–857f, 856b–857b
Hemoglobin A1c testing, 846–847, 847t
Hemoglobin glycosylated test (HbA1C or
   A1C), 74t–75t
Hemoglobinuria, 777, 778f
Hemolysis, 803
   venipuncture, 815t
Hemolytic anemia, 616t
Hemolytic disease of the newborn (HDN),
   694f, 695
Hemolytic uremic syndrome, 466
Hemolyzed, definition of, 744, 756
Hemophilia, 616–617, 678
Hemoptysis, 631t
Hemorrhagic stroke, 303
Hemorrhoids, 474
Hemostasis, 238, 246–247, 609
Hemostat forceps, 220, 220f
Henle loop, 655
Hepatic portal circulation, 602
Hepatitis, 477, 477b
Hepatitis A virus (HAV), 458t, 474, 477t
   vaccine for, 718t–719t
Hepatitis B virus (HBV), 458t, 477t
   vaccination, 94, 94f, 718t–719t
Hepatitis C virus (HCV), 458t, 477t
Hepatitis D virus (HDV), 458t, 477t
Hepatitis E virus (HEV), 458t, 477t
Hepatobiliary (HIDA) scan, 480t–481t
Herbal supplements, 335, 337t–338t
Hereditary, definition of, 30, 84
Hernia, 474–475
   hiatal, 472, 472f
Herniated disk, 500, 500f
Heroin, 567t–569t
Herpes simplex virus type 1 (HSV-1), 437
Hertz, 403, 416–417
Hiatal hernia, 472, 472f
High-complexity tests and laboratories, 747
High-density lipoprotein (HDL), 197–198
High-fiber diet, 208–209
High ligation and vein stripping, for
   varicose veins, 615
Hilum, 653
Hinged needle shields, 365, 365f
HIPAA. see Health Insurance Portability
   and Accountability Act
Hippocampus, 529–530
Hippocrates, 12
Hippocratic Oath, 12, 13f
Hirschsprung's disease, 476
Hirsutism, 586f
Histology, 65–66, 744
Histoplasmosis, fungi and, 870t
History of present illness, 136
HIV. see Human immunodeficiency virus
Ho, David, 14t
Hoarding disorder, 559, 559b
Holistic, definition of, 2, 136
Holter monitor, 281, 281b, 285b–287b
Home health agencies, 20–21

Homeostasis, 59, 66–67, 106, 448–449,
   529, 531, 576, 580, 745, 770, 834
Honesty, 5
Hordeolum, 408
Horizontal recumbent position, 154, 166f,
   166b
Horizontal shelf files, 46
Hormonal contraceptives, 687–689, 688t
Hormonal patch, 688t
Hormone, 834
Hospice, definition of, 2
Hospice care, 20–21
Hospital system, 20
Hospitalists, 16
Hospitals, types of, 16–20
Household system, 345, 345b, 346t
Housekeeping controls, 92–93, 93f,
   93b–94b
HPV. see Human papillomavirus
Human chorionic gonadotropin (hCG),
   680, 786
Human immunodeficiency virus (HIV),
   455–456, 459t
   nutritional needs and, 210
   testing, 184, 877–878, 877f, 878b
Human papillomavirus (HPV)
   cervical cancer and, 681
   vaccines for, 718t–719t
Humoral immunity, 87, 87b, 452
Hunter, John, 14t
Huntington's disease, 537–538
Hyaline casts, 780, 780f
Hydrocele, 668, 669f
Hydrocephalus, 529, 543b
Hydrocephaly, 704, 713
Hydrocortisone, 579
Hydrogenated, 198t
Hydronephrosis, 653, 664f, 666
Hypercapnia, 631t
Hyperextension, 494f, 494t–495t
Hyperlipidemia, 653
Hyperopia (farsightedness), 406
Hyperparathyroidism, 579, 584, 584b
Hyperplasia, 430, 436
Hyperpnea, 106, 114, 631t
Hypersensitivity reactions, 453, 453b, 454t
Hypertension, 613–614, 614t, 660
   signs and symptoms of, 116b
   stages of, 115t
Hyperthyroidism, 583, 583t
Hyperventilation, 106, 114, 304
Hypoalbuminemia, 653
Hypocalcemia, 580t
Hypochlorhydria, 473
Hypodermic needles, 364–365, 364f
Hypodermic puncture, 247f–248f
Hypodermic syringes, 365, 365f–366f
Hypoglycemic, 580t, 587–588, 588b
Hypoparathyroidism, 579, 584–585
Hypospadias, 668
Hypotension, 106, 116
Hypothalamus, 577
Hypothyroidism, 583, 584, 584b, 848
Hypovolemia, 614
Hypovolemic shock, 306, 615
Hypoxemia, 631t
Hysterectomy, 678

Iatrogenic crystals, 782
Idiopathic, definition of, 106
Idiopathic thrombocytopenic purpura,
   617
Ileoanal anastomosis, 475, 475f
Ileostomy, 475
Ileum, 468
Illustrator, medical, 17t–18t
Immersion oil, 761
Immune disorders, 78
Immune system
   anatomy of, 67t, 449–450, 450f
   levels of defense, 450–453, 451f
Immunity
   acquired, 454, 454f, 454b
   nonspecific, 451, 451b, 452f
   specific, 451–453, 453f

Immunizations, pediatric, 716–719, 717f,
   718t–719t, 719b–720b, 725b–726b,
   726f
Immunodeficiency, 78
Immunoglobulin, 834–835
Immunologist, 14t–15t
Immunology, 449, 864–883, 881b. see also
   Microbiology
Immunology testing, CLIA-waived,
   876–878
Immunosuppressants, 491
Impacted cerumen, 413
Impacted fractures, 498f, 498t–499t
Impaired hearing, patients with, 179
Impaired vision, patients with, 179, 179f
Impervious, definition of, 84, 92, 216
Impetigo, 433b, 435, 435f
Implantable cardioverter defibrillator (ICD),
   279, 280f
   medical assistant in, 621–622, 622f
Implantable device rhythms, 279
Implantable loop recorder, 281–282
Implants, 688t
In vitro, definition of, 744, 747, 865
In vitro fertilization (IVF), 14t
Inactive poliovirus (IPV), 718t–719t
Inanimate, definition of, 84, 86
Incidence, definition of, 30, 73
Incision, 247f–248f
Incompetent valves, definition of, 598
Incomplete proteins, 197
Inconspicuous, definition of, 136
Incubation period, 76, 88
Incubator, 762, 762f, 763t
Indexing rules, 48–49
Indicator, definition of, 2, 20
Indirect filing system, 49
Indirect transmission, 86
Individual diversity, respect for, 4–5
Induration, 374
Infants, therapeutic approaches for, 706b
Infarction, 599, 612
Infection control, 83–100
   aseptic techniques, 95–98
      disinfection, 97–98, 98b
      hand hygiene, 95–97, 97b, 102f–103f,
         102b–103b
      sanitization, 97, 103b–104b, 104f
      sterilization, 98, 98b
   chain of infection, 84–87, 85f, 85b–87b
   disease, 84
   inflammatory response, 87–88, 88f, 88b
   in laboratories, 752–754
   legal and ethical issues, 99, 99b
   Occupational Safety and Health
      Administration Standards, for the
      healthcare setting, 89–95
      Bloodborne Pathogens Standard,
         89–90, 89f–90f
      compliance guidelines, 90–95, 91f
   patient coaching, 98
   professional behaviors, 99b
   role of the medical assistant in asepsis, 98
   types of infection, 88–89
      acute, 88
      chronic, 88
      latent, 88
      opportunistic, 89
Infections
   definition of, 216
   of eye, 408
   pathogens, 76, 76b, 77t
Infectious agents, definition of, 865
Infectious arthritis, 502t
Infectious diseases, 448–463
   diagnostic procedures in, 461–462, 461t
   medical assistant's role in examinations,
      460–463, 461f
Infectious mononucleosis, 460, 460f
   testing, 876–877, 877b, 887b–889b,
      888f
   viral causes of, 872t
Inferior vena cava, 267
Inflammation, 448–451, 497
   of respiratory system, 632f